Varcarolis's
Canadian Psychiatric Mental Health Nursing

A Clinical Approach

SECOND EDITION

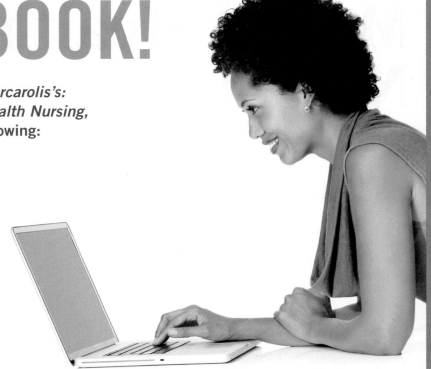

Varcarolis's
Canadian Psychiatric Mental Health Nursing
A Clinical Approach

SECOND EDITION

Cheryl L. Pollard, RPN, RN, BScN, MN, PhD (Nursing)
Associate Dean & Associate Professor
Faculty of Nursing
MacEwan University
Edmonton, Alberta

Sonya L. Jakubec, RN, BHScN, MN, PhD (Nursing)
Associate Professor
Faculty of Health & Community Studies, School of
    Nursing and Midwifery
Mount Royal University
Calgary, Alberta

American Editor
Margaret (Peggy) Jordan Halter, PhD, APRN
Clinical Nurse Specialist
Cleveland Clinic Akron General
Akron, Ohio;
Adjunct Faculty
Ohio State University
Columbus, Ohio

ELSEVIER

ELSEVIER

VARCAROLIS'S CANADIAN PSYCHIATRIC MENTAL HEALTH NURSING:
A Clinical Approach, SECOND EDITION

Copyright © 2019 Elsevier Canada, a division of Reed Elsevier Canada, Ltd.

This adaptation of *Varcarolis' Foundations of Psychiatric Mental Health Nursing: A Clinical Approach,* Eighth Edition, by Margaret Jordan Halter, is published by arrangement with Elsevier Inc.

ISBN 978-0-3233-8967-9 (soft cover)

Copyright © 2018, Elsevier Inc. All Rights Reserved.
Previous editions copyrighted 2014, 2010, 2006, 2002, 1998, 1994, 1990.

Notices

Knowledge and best practice in this field are constantly changing. As new research and experience broaden our understanding, changes in research methods, professional practices, or medical treatment may become necessary.

Practitioners and researchers must always rely on their own experience and knowledge in evaluating and using any information, methods, compounds, or experiments described herein. In using such information or methods, they should be mindful of their own safety and the safety of others, including parties for whom they have a professional responsibility.

With respect to any drug or pharmaceutical products identified, readers are advised to check the most current information provided (i) on procedures featured or (ii) by the manufacturer of each product to be administered, to verify the recommended dose or formula, the method and duration of administration, and contraindications. It is the responsibility of practitioners, relying on their own experience and knowledge of their patients, to make diagnoses, to determine dosages and the best treatment for each individual patient, and to take all appropriate safety precautions.

To the fullest extent of the law, neither the Publisher nor the authors, contributors, or editors, assumes any liability for any injury and/or damage to persons or property as a matter of products liability, negligence or otherwise, or from any use or operation of any methods, products, instructions, or ideas contained in the material herein.

The Publisher

Library and Archives Canada Cataloguing in Publication

Varcarolis's Canadian psychiatric mental health nursing : a clinical approach / [edited by] Margaret (Peggy) Jordan Halter, PhD, APRN (Clinical Nurse Specialist, Cleveland Clinic Akron General, Akron, Ohio; Adjunct Faculty, Ohio State University, Columbus, Ohio); Canadian editors, Cheryl L. Pollard, RPN, RN, BScN, MN, PhD (Nursing) (Associate Dean & Associate Professor, Faculty of Nursing, MacEwan University, Edmonton, Alberta), Sonya L. Jakubec, RN, BHScN, MN, PhD (Nursing) (Associate Professor, Faculty of Health & Community Studies, School of Nursing and Midwifery, Mount Royal University, Calgary, Alberta). – Second Canadian edition.

Includes bibliographical references and index.
ISBN 978-1-77172-140-0 (softcover)

1. Psychiatric nursing–Canada–Textbooks.   2. Mental health–Canada–Textbooks.   3. Textbooks.
I. Halter, Margaret J. (Margaret Jordan), editor   II. Pollard, Cheryl L., editor   III. Jakubec, Sonya L., editor

RC440.V37 2018   616.89'0231   C2017-904751-5

Elsevier Canada
420 Main Street East, Suite 636, Milton, ON, Canada L9T 5G3
Phone: 416-644-7053

Printed in Canada
2 3 4 5 6   23 22 21 20 19

Ebook ISBN: 978-177172-143-1

Vice President, Medical and Canadian Education: Madelene J. Hyde
Content Strategist (Acquisitions): Roberta A. Spinosa-Millman
Content Development Specialist: Sandy Matos
Publishing Services Manager: Julie Eddy
Senior Project Manager: Marquita Parker
Copy Editor: Susan Broadhurst
Proofreader: Leslie Saffrey
Cover Designer: Brett J. Miller, BJM Graphic Design and Communications
Cover Image: nature photos/Shutterstock.com
Book Designer: Paula Catalano
Printing and Binding: Transcontinental

Working together to grow libraries in developing countries

www.elsevier.com • www.bookaid.org

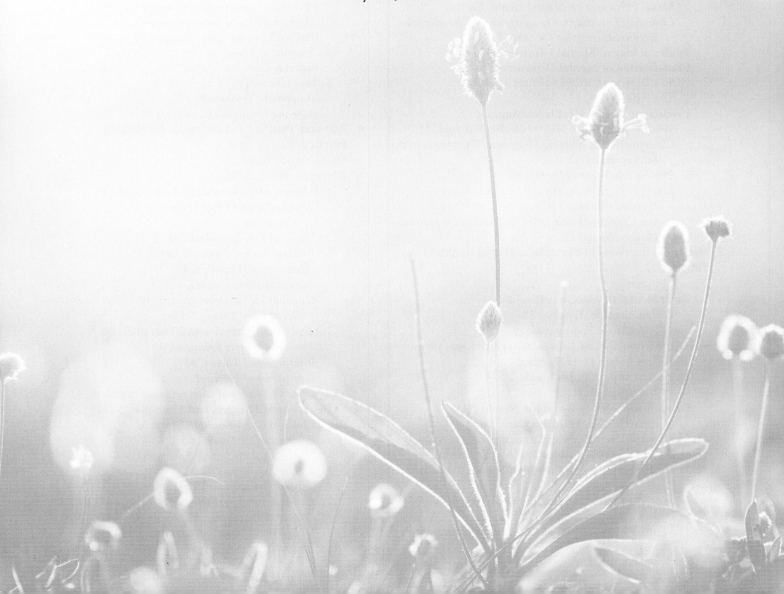

Walk gently in the lives of others, as not all wounds are visible.
This text is dedicated to those individuals who have courageously shared their
lived experience of mental illness with me. It has been through this sharing that
caring moments were created and transformational understanding happened.
—Cheryl L. Pollard

For those holding this text, the faculty looking to enliven teaching and practice,
and the students who already know mental health and practice in novel ways; for you
to inspire us in our shared responsibility for more compassionate and expanded
experiences of mental wellbeing in our daily lives; in our natural helping environments
as well as our families, communities, workplaces, institutions and politics. This text
is also dedicated to those who have taught me about the power and possibilities of
listening, recovery, and inclusion—in particular to Fran, Elizabeth, Cecile and Don:
I am privileged to have worked alongside you all.
—Sonya L. Jakubec

CONTENTS

Acknowledgements, xvi
Contributors, xvii
Contributors to US Eighth Edition, xviii
Reviewers, xix
To the Instructor, xx
To the Student, xxii

UNIT 1 Foundations in Theory

1 Mental Health and Mental Illness, 2
Sonya L. Jakubec
  Mental Health and Mental Illness, 3
    *Two Conceptualizations of Mental Health and
      Mental Illness, 3*
    Contributing Factors, 5
    Perceptions of Mental Health and Mental Illness, 7
    Human Genome Project, 7
    Social Influences on Mental Health Care, 8
    *Changing Directions, Changing Lives: The Mental
      Health Strategy for Canada, 8*
  Epidemiology of Mental Disorders, 9
  Classification of Mental Disorders, 10
    The Diagnostic and Statistical Manual, 10
    The ICD-10-CA, 11
  Psychiatric Mental Health Nursing, 11
    What Is Psychiatric Mental Health Nursing?, 11
    *Classification of Nursing Diagnoses, Outcomes, and
      Interventions, 12*
    Evidence-Informed Practice, 12
    *Levels of Psychiatric Mental Health Clinical
      Nursing Practice, 12*
    *Future Challenges and Roles for Psychiatric Mental
      Health Nurses, 12*

**2 Historical Overview of Psychiatric Mental Health
Nursing, 17**
Sonya L. Jakubec
  Early Mental Illness Care, 17
    Early Canadian Asylums, 18
  Early Psychiatric Treatments, 19
  The Introduction of Nurses to Asylum Care, 19
  Shifts in Control Over Nursing, 20
    Eastern and Atlantic Canada, 20
    Western Canada, 21
  **Deinstitutionalization and the Nursing Role in
    Psychiatric Mental Health Care, 21**
  University-Based Nursing Curriculum, 21
  **National Organizations for Psychiatric Mental
    Health Nursing and Canadian Nurses Association
    Certification, 22**
  **Advanced-Practice Nursing in Psychiatric Mental
    Health Care, 22**
  The Future of Psychiatric Mental Health Nursing, 23

**3 Overview of Psychiatric Mental Health Nursing Care
Within Various Settings, 26**
Cheryl L. Pollard
  Funding Psychiatric Mental Health Care, 27
  The Continuum of Mental Health Care, 28
    Evolving Venues of Practice, 28
  Psychiatric Mental Health Care Settings, 28
    Community Mental Health Centres, 29
    Crisis Intervention Team, 31
    Disaster Response Teams, 32
    Partial Hospitalization Programs, 32
    Inpatient Psychiatric Mental Health Programs, 32
    Assertive Community Treatment, 34
    Ensuring Safety, 34
  Roles and Responsibilities, 36
    Community Psychiatric Mental Health Nursing, 36
    Biopsychosocial Assessment, 36
    Treatment Goals and Interventions, 37
    Interprofessional Team Member, 37
    Biopsychosocial Care Manager, 37
    Treatment Team, 38
    Nursing Care, 39
  Future Issues, 41
    Barriers to Treatment, 41
    Meeting Changing Demands, 42

**4 Relevant Theories and Therapies for Nursing
Practice, 45**
Margaret Jordan Halter
Adapted by Cheryl L. Pollard
  Psychoanalytic Theories and Therapies, 46
    *Sigmund Freud's Psychoanalytic
      Theory, 46*
    Classical Psychoanalysis, 48
    Psychodynamic Therapy, 48
  Developmental Theories, 48
    Cognitive Development, 48
    Stages of Moral Development, 49
    Ethics of Care Theory, 50
  Interpersonal Theories and Therapies, 50
    Theory of Object Relations, 50
    Interpersonal Theory, 51
    Interpersonal Psychotherapy, 51
    Peplau's Theory of Interpersonal Relations, 51
  Behavioural Theories and Therapies, 52
    Classical Conditioning Theory, 53
    Behaviourism Theory, 53
    Operant Conditioning Theory, 53
    Behavioural Therapy, 53
  Cognitive Theories and Therapies, 55
    Rational Emotive Behaviour Therapy (REBT), 55
    Cognitive Behavioural Therapy (CBT), 55
    Dialectic Behavioural Therapy (DBT), 56

Humanistic Theories, 58
  Abraham Maslow's Humanistic Psychology Theory, 58
Biological Theories and Therapies, 60
  The Advent of Psychopharmacology, 60
  The Biological Model, 60
Additional Therapies, 60
  Milieu Therapy, 60

5 Understanding Responses to Stress, 65
Margaret Jordan Halter
Adapted by Sonya L. Jakubec
Responses to and Effects of Stress, 66
  Early Stress Response Theories, 66
  Neurotransmitter Stress Responses, 66
  Immune Stress Responses, 67
Mediators of the Stress Response, 68
  Stressors, 68
  Perception, 69
  Personality, 69
  Social Support, 69
  Culture, 69
  Spirituality and Religious Beliefs, 69
Nursing Management of Stress Responses, 70
  Measuring Stress, 70
  Assessing Coping Styles, 71
  Managing Stress through Relaxation Techniques, 71

UNIT 2 Foundations for Practice

6 The Nursing Process and Standards of Care for Psychiatric Mental Health Nursing, 80
Elizabeth M. Varcarolis
Adapted by Sonya L. Jakubec
Assessment, 82
  Age Considerations, 83
  Language Barriers, 84
  Psychiatric Mental Health Nursing Assessment, 84
Nursing Diagnosis, 89
Outcomes Identification, 90
Planning, 90
Implementation, 91
  Basic-Level Interventions, 92
  Advanced-Practice Interventions, 92
Evaluation, 92
Documentation, 92

7 Ethical Responsibilities and Legal Obligations for Psychiatric Mental Health Nursing Practice, 96
Cheryl L. Pollard
Ethical Concepts, 97
Mental Health Legislation, 100
Establishing Best Practice, 102
  Standards of Practice, 102
  Standards of Care, 103
  Policies and Procedures, 103
  Traditional Practice Knowledge, 103

Guidelines for Ensuring Adherence to Standards of Care, 103
Patients' Rights Under the Law, 104
  Authorization of Treatment, 104
  Autonomy, 104
  Beneficence and Nonmaleficence, 105
  Rights Regarding Confidentiality, 106
Civil Obligations and Responsibilities, 109
  Tort Law, 109

8 Cultural Considerations for Psychiatric Mental Health Nursing, 115
Gwen Campbell McArthur, Sonya L. Jakubec
Understanding the Landscape of Culture in Mental Health, 116
  Culture, Race, Ethnicity, and the Social Determinants of Health, 116
  Cultural Views and Contexts Affecting Mental Health Care, 116
  Culture, Mental Health, and Mental Illness, 119
The Cultural Landscape of Canada, 120
  Indigenous and Multicultural Contexts, 120
Mental Health Concerns of Indigenous Peoples, 121
  Intergenerational Trauma, 121
  Hopelessness and Suicide, 122
  Family Violence and Separation and Community Violence, 122
  Substance Use, 122
  Need for Culturally Relevant and Appropriate Services, 122
Mental Health Concerns of Immigrants, 123
Mental Health Concerns of Refugees, 124
Barriers and Facilitators to Mental Health Care in a Multicultural Context, 125
  Stigma and Discrimination, 125
  Communication Barriers, 125
  Misdiagnosis, 126
  Ethnic Variation in Pharmacodynamics, 127
Cultural Competence in Psychiatric Mental Health Nursing, 127
Culturally Competent Care, 127
  Cultural Awareness, 128
  Cultural Knowledge, 128
  Cultural Encounters, 128
  Cultural Skill, 128
  Cultural Desire, 130

UNIT 3 Biopsychosocial Nursing Techniques

9 Therapeutic Relationships, 135
Elizabeth M. Varcarolis
Adapted by Cheryl L. Pollard
Concepts of the Nurse–Patient Relationship, 136
  Goals and Functions, 137
  Social Versus Therapeutic, 137
  Relationship Boundaries, 139
Values, Beliefs, and Self-Awareness, 140

Peplau's Model of the Nurse–Patient Relationship, 142
  Preorientation Phase, 143
  Orientation Phase, 143
  Working Phase, 146
  Termination Phase, 146
What Hinders and What Helps the Nurse–Patient
  Relationship, 147
Factors That Encourage and Promote Patients'
  Growth, 147
  Genuineness, 148
  Empathy, 148
  Positive Regard, 148

10 Communication and the Clinical Interview, 152
Elizabeth M. Varcarolis
Adapted by Sonya L. Jakubec
The Communication Process, 153
Factors That Affect Communication, 153
  Personal Factors, 153
  Environmental Factors, 154
  Relationship Factors, 154
Verbal and Nonverbal Communication, 155
  Verbal Communication, 155
  Nonverbal Communication, 155
  Interaction of Verbal and Nonverbal
    Communication, 156
Communication Skills for Nurses, 157
  Therapeutic Communication Strategies, 157
  Cultural Considerations, 163
  Assertive Communication, 164
  Evaluation of Communication Skills, 164
The Clinical Interview, 164
  Preparing for the Interview, 164
  Introductions, 165
  Initiating the Interview, 165
  Tactics to Avoid, 165
  Helpful Guidelines, 166
  Attending Behaviours: The Foundation of
    Interviewing, 166
  Clinical Supervision, 167
  Process Recordings, 167

11 Psychotropic Drugs, 171
Adapted by Martin Davies, Paul M. Kerr
Structure and Function of the Brain, 172
  Functions and Activities of the Brain, 172
  Cellular Composition of the Brain, 175
  Organization of the Brain, 177
  Visualizing the Brain, 179
  Disturbances of Mental Function, 183
Use of Psychotropic Drugs, 184
  Drugs Used to Treat Anxiety and Insomnia, 185
  Drug Treatment for Depression, 186
  Drug Treatment for Bipolar Disorders, 190
  Drugs Used To Treat Psychosis, 192
  Drug Treatment for Attention-Deficit/
    Hyperactivity Disorder, 194
  Drug Treatment for Alzheimer's Disease, 195
  Natural Health Products, 195

UNIT 4 Psychobiological Disorders

12 Anxiety and Related Disorders, 200
Margaret Jordan Halter
Adapted by Cheryl L. Pollard
Anxiety, 202
Levels of Anxiety, 202
  Mild Anxiety, 202
  Moderate Anxiety, 202
  Severe Anxiety, 202
  Panic, 203
Defences Against Anxiety, 203
Clinical Picture, 204
Anxiety Disorders, 204
  Panic Disorder, 204
  Phobias, 206
  Generalized Anxiety Disorder, 207
  Substance-Induced Anxiety Disorder, 209
  Anxiety Due to Nonpsychiatric Medical
    Conditions, 209
Epidemiology, 209
Comorbidity, 209
Somatic Symptom and Related Disorders, 209
Clinical Picture, 210
  Somatic Symptom Disorder, 210
  Illness Anxiety Disorder, 210
  Conversion Disorder, 210
Epidemiology, 211
Comorbidity, 211
Obsessive-Compulsive Disorders, 211
Epidemiology, 212
Comorbidity, 212
Trauma- and Stressor-Related Disorders, 214
Acute Stress Disorder, 214
Post-Traumatic Stress Disorder, 214
Dissociative Disorders, 214
Clinical Picture, 215
  Depersonalization/Derealization Disorder, 215
  Dissociative Amnesia, 215
  Dissociative Identity Disorder, 216
Epidemiology, 216
Comorbidity, 216
Etiology of Anxiety-Related Disorders, 216
Biological Factors, 216
  Genetic, 216
  Neurobiological, 216
Psychological Factors, 216
  Psychodynamic Theories, 216
  Behavioural Theory, 217
  Cognitive Theory, 217
  Learning Theory, 217
Environmental Factors, 217
Sociocultural Factors, 217
  Culture-Bound Syndromes, 218
Application of the Nursing Process, 218
Assessment, 218
  General Assessment, 218

Rating Scales, 218
Psychosocial Factors, 221
Self-Assessment, 221
Diagnosis, 222
Outcomes Identification, 222
Planning, 224
Implementation, 225
Determining Levels of Distress, 225
Psychosocial Interventions, 226
Counselling, 227
Health Teaching and Health Promotion, 227
Milieu Therapy, 229
Promotion of Self-Care Activities, 229
Pharmacological Interventions, 232
Integrative Therapy, 233
Advanced Interventions, 233
Evaluation, 234

13 Depressive Disorders, 244
Margaret Jordan Halter, Mallie Kozy
Adapted by Cheryl L. Pollard
Clinical Picture, 245
Disruptive Mood Dysregulation Disorder, 245
Persistent Depressive Disorder, 246
Premenstrual Dysphoric Disorder, 247
Substance/Medication-Induced Depressive Disorder, 247
Depressive Disorder Due to Another Medical Condition, 247
Epidemiology, 248
Children and Adolescents, 248
Older Adults, 248
Comorbidity, 249
Etiology, 249
Biological Factors, 249
Psychological Factors, 251
Application of the Nursing Process, 251
Assessment, 251
General Assessment, 251
Assessment of Suicide Potential, 251
Key Assessment Findings, 253
Areas to Assess, 253
Age Considerations, 254
Self-Assessment, 254
Diagnosis, 256
Outcomes Identification, 256
The Recovery Model, 256
Planning, 256
Implementation, 257
Counselling and Communication Techniques, 257
Health Teaching and Health Promotion, 257
Promotion of Self-Care Activities, 258
Milieu Management: Teamwork and Safety, 258
Pharmacological Interventions, 258
Biological Interventions, 266
Electroconvulsive Therapy, 266
Transcranial Magnetic Stimulation, 267
Nerve Stimulation, 267

Advanced-Practice Interventions, 269
Future of Treatment, 269
Evaluation, 269

14 Bipolar Disorders, 275
Margaret Jordan Halter
Adapted by Cheryl L. Pollard
Clinical Picture, 277
Bipolar I Disorder, 277
Bipolar II Disorder, 277
Cyclothymic Disorder, 278
Other Bipolar Disorders, 278
Epidemiology, 278
Children and Adolescents, 278
Cyclothymic Disorder, 279
Comorbidity, 279
Bipolar I Disorder, 279
Bipolar II Disorder, 279
Cyclothymic Disorder, 279
Etiology, 279
Biological Factors, 279
Environmental Factors, 280
Psychological Factors, 280
Application of the Nursing Process, 281
Assessment, 281
General Assessment, 281
Self-Assessment, 283
Nursing Diagnosis, 284
Outcomes Identification, 284
Acute Phase, 284
Continuation Phase, 284
Maintenance Phase, 285
Planning, 285
Acute Phase, 285
Continuation Phase, 285
Maintenance Phase, 286
Implementation, 286
Acute Phase, 286
Pharmacological Interventions, 286
Mood Stabilization, 286
Electroconvulsive Therapy, 290
Milieu Management, 290
Support Groups, 292
Health Teaching and Health Promotion, 292
Psychotherapy, 292
Advanced-Practice Interventions, 293
Evaluation, 293

15 Schizophrenia Spectrum and Other Psychotic Disorders, 300
Edward A. Herzog
Adapted by Sonya L. Jakubec
Clinical Picture, 302
Epidemiology, 302
Comorbidity, 303
Etiology, 303
Biological Factors, 304
Psychological, Social, and Environmental Factors, 304

Course of the Disorder, 305
Prognosis, 306
Phases of Schizophrenia, 306
Application of the Nursing Process, 307
Assessment, 307
During the Prepsychotic Phase, 307
General Assessment, 307
Self-Assessment, 312
Diagnosis, 314
Outcomes Identification, 314
Phase I—Acute, 314
Phase II—Stabilization, 314
Phase III—Maintenance, 314
Planning, 314
Phase I—Acute, 315
Phase II—Stabilization and Phase III—Maintenance, 315
Implementation, 315
Phase I—Acute, 316
Phase II—Stabilization and Phase III—Maintenance, 317
Milieu Management, 317
Counselling and Communication Techniques, 317
Health Teaching and Health Promotion, 319
Pharmacological Interventions, 321
Specific Interventions for Paranoia, Catatonia, and Disorganization, 325
Advanced-Practice Interventions, 328
Evaluation, 330

16 Eating and Feeding Disorders, 338
Carissa R. Enright
Adapted by Sonya L. Jakubec
Clinical Picture, 338
Avoidant/Restrictive Food Intake Disorder, 339
Pica, 340
Rumination Disorder, 340
Epidemiology, 340
Comorbidity, 341
Etiology, 342
Biological Factors, 342
Psychological Factors, 342
Environmental Factors, 343
Anorexia Nervosa, 343
Application of the Nursing Process, 343
Assessment, 343
General Assessment, 345
Self-Assessment, 345
Diagnosis, 345
Outcomes Identification, 345
Planning, 345
Implementation, 346
Acute Care, 346
Psychosocial Interventions, 346
Pharmacological Interventions, 346
Health Teaching and Health Promotion, 346
Milieu Management, 347
Advanced-Practice Interventions, 347

Evaluation, 348
Bulimia Nervosa, 348
Application of the Nursing Process, 349
Assessment, 349
General Assessment, 349
Self-Assessment, 349
Diagnosis, 350
Outcomes Identification, 350
Planning, 350
Implementation, 351
Acute Care, 351
Milieu Management, 351
Pharmacological Interventions, 351
Counselling, 351
Health Teaching and Health Promotion, 351
Advanced-Practice Interventions, 351
Evaluation, 352
Binge Eating Disorder, 352

17 Neurocognitive Disorders, 362
Jane Stein-Parbury
Adapted by Cheryl L. Pollard
Delirium, 363
Clinical Picture, 363
Epidemiology, 365
Comorbidity and Etiology, 365
Application of the Nursing Process, 365
Assessment, 365
General Assessment, 365
Self-Assessment, 367
Diagnosis, 367
Outcomes Identification, 368
Planning, 368
Implementation, 369
Evaluation, 370
Mild and Major Neurocognitive Disorders, 370
Clinical Picture, 370
Progression of Alzheimer's Disease, 371
Epidemiology, 373
Etiology, 373
Biological Factors, 373
Environmental Factors, 374
Application of the Nursing Process, 374
Assessment, 374
General Assessment, 374
Diagnostic Tests, 374
Self-Assessment, 375
Diagnosis, 375
Outcomes Identification, 376
Planning, 376
Implementation, 378
Counselling and Communication Techniques, 378
Health Teaching and Health Promotion, 378
Pharmacological Interventions, 381
Integrative Therapy, 384
Evaluation, 384

18 Psychoactive Substance Use and Treatment, 390
Rick Csiernik
   **Distinguishing Between an Addiction and a
      Compulsive Behaviour,** 391
   The Process of Addiction Development, 392
      No Contact, 392
      Experimentation, 393
      Integrated Use, 393
      Excessive Use, 393
      Addiction, 394
   Epidemiology, 394
   Comorbidity, 394
      Psychiatric Comorbidity, 394
      Medical Comorbidity, 395
   Etiology, 396
      Biological Factors, 396
      Psychological Factors, 397
      Sociocultural Factors, 397
   Application of the Nursing Process, 398
   Assessment, 398
      *Assessment of Substance Use and
         Substance-Induced Disorders, 398*
      *Assessment of Acute Intoxication and Active and
         Historical Substance Use, 398*
      Signs of Intoxication and Withdrawal, 400
   Helping Patients Change, 411
      Self-Assessment and Self-Awareness, 411
      Psychological Changes, 411
      The Transtheoretical Model of Change, 411
      Motivational Interviewing, 413
      *Communication Techniques for Assessment and
         Interventions, 413*
   Diagnosis, 415
   Outcomes Identification, 415
      Withdrawal, 416
      Initial and Active Substance Abuse Treatment, 416
      Health Maintenance, 416
   Planning, 416
   Implementation, 416
   Substance Abuse Interventions, 416
      Pharmacological Interventions, 416
      *Implementation at Primary, Secondary, and
         Tertiary Levels of Prevention, 418*
   Evaluation, 427

19 Personality Disorders, 432
Christine A. Tackett, Margaret Jordan Halter, Claudia A. Cihlar
Adapted by Cheryl L. Pollard
   Clinical Picture, 433
   Epidemiology, 434
   Comorbidity, 434
   Etiology, 434
      Biological Factors, 434
      Psychological Factors, 435
      System Factors, 435
   Cluster a Personality Disorders, 435
      Paranoid Personality Disorder, 435
      Schizoid Personality Disorder, 436

      Schizotypal Personality Disorder, 437
   Cluster B Personality Disorders, 438
      Borderline Personality Disorder, 438
      Antisocial Personality Disorder, 441
      Histrionic Personality Disorder, 442
      Narcissistic Personality Disorder, 443
   Cluster C Personality Disorders, 443
      Avoidant Personality Disorder, 443
      Dependent Personality Disorder, 444
      Obsessive-Compulsive Personality Disorder, 445
   Application of the Nursing Process, 445
   Assessment, 445
      Assessment Tools, 445
      Patient History, 446
      Self-Assessment, 446
   Diagnosis, 446
   Outcomes Identification, 447
   Planning, 447
   Implementation, 448
      Safety and Teamwork, 450
      Pharmacological Interventions, 450
      Case Management, 451
      Advanced-Practice Interventions, 452
   Evaluation, 453

20 Sleep–Wake Disorders, 457
Margaret Jordan Halter, Margaret Trussler
Adapted by Sonya L. Jakubec
   Sleep, 458
   Consequences of Sleep Loss, 458
   Normal Sleep Cycle, 459
   Regulation of Sleep, 460
   Functions of Sleep, 461
   Sleep Requirements, 461
   Sleep Patterns, 461
   Sleep–Wake Disorders, 462
   Clinical Picture, 462
      Insomnia Disorders, 462
      Hypersomnia Disorders, 463
      Confusional Arousal Disorders, 463
      Kleine–Levin Syndrome, 464
      *Sleep–Wake Disorders Related to
         Breathing, 464*
      Circadian Rhythm Sleep Disorder, 464
      *Restless Legs Syndrome (Willis-Ekbom
         Disease), 464*
   Epidemiology, 465
   Comorbidity, 465
      Sleep–Wake Disorders and Mental Illness, 465
      Sleep and General Health, 466
   Application of the Nursing Process, 466
   Assessment, 466
      General Assessment, 466
      Sleep Studies, 468
      Self-Assessment, 469
   Diagnosis, 469
   Outcomes Identification, 469
   Planning, 469

Implementation, 469
    Counselling, 469
    Health Teaching and Health Promotion, 470
    Pharmacological Interventions, 470
    Cognitive Behavioural Therapy for Insomnia, 470
    Advanced-Practice Interventions, 472
Evaluation, 472

UNIT 5 Trauma Interventions

21 Crisis and Disaster, 477
Sonya L. Jakubec
    The Development of Crisis Theory, 478
        Types of Crisis, 479
        Phases of Crisis, 480
    Application of the Nursing Process, 480
    Assessment, 480
        General Assessment, 480
        Self-Assessment, 482
    Diagnosis, 483
    Outcomes Identification, 484
    Planning, 485
    Implementation, 485
        Counselling, 485
    Evaluation, 487

22 Suicide and Nonsuicidal Self-Injury, 495
Sonya L. Jakubec
    Epidemiology, 496
        Racial and Ethnic Statistics, 496
        Risk Factors, 497
    Etiology, 498
        Biological Factors, 498
        Psychosocial Factors, 500
        Cultural Factors, 500
        Societal Factors, 500
    Application of the Nursing Process, 501
    Assessment, 502
        Verbal and Nonverbal Clues, 502
        Lethality of Suicide Plan, 503
        Assessment Tools, 503
        Self-Assessment, 503
    Implementation, 503
        Primary Intervention, 504
        Secondary Intervention, 505
        Tertiary Intervention, 505
        Milieu Management, 505
        Counselling, 505
        Health Teaching and Health Promotion, 506
        Case Management, 506
        Pharmacological Interventions, 506
        Postvention for Survivors of Suicide, 506
    Evaluation, 507
    Nonsuicidal Self-Injury, 507
    Epidemiology, 507
    Comorbidity, 508
    Risk Factors, 508
        Biological Factors, 508
        Environmental Factors, 508

    Clinical Picture, 508
    Assessment, 508
        Self-Assessment, 508
    Diagnosis, 508
    Outcomes Criteria, 508
    Planning, 508
    Interventions, 509
    Evaluation, 509

23 Anger, Aggression, and Violence, 512
Melodie B. Hull
    Clinical Picture, 512
    Epidemiology, 514
    Comorbidity, 514
    Etiology, 514
        Biological Factors, 514
        Psychological Factors, 515
        Sociological Factors, 516
    Application of the Nursing Process, 517
    Assessment, 517
        General Assessment, 517
        Self-Assessment, 517
    Diagnosis, 517
    Outcomes Identification, 517
    Planning, 517
    Implementation, 517
        Psychosocial Interventions, 518
        Pharmacological Interventions, 520
        Health Teaching and Health Promotion, 520
        Case Management, 521
        Milieu Management, 521
        Caring for Patients in General Hospital
          Settings, 524
        Caring for Patients in Inpatient Psychiatric
          Settings, 525
        Caring for Patients With Cognitive Deficits in
          Long-Term Residential Care Settings, 525
    Evaluation, 526

24 Interpersonal Violence: Child, Older Adult, and Intimate Partner Abuse, 530
Margaret Jordan Halter, Judi Sateren
Adapted by Sonya L. Jakubec
    Clinical Picture, 531
        Violence, 532
        Cycle of Violence, 535
    Epidemiology, 535
        Child Abuse, 535
        Intimate Partner Violence, 535
        Older Adult Abuse, 536
    Comorbidity, 537
    Etiology, 537
        The Ecological Model of Violence, 537
        Environmental Factors, 537
    Application of the Nursing Process:
    **   Interpersonal Violence, 539**
    Assessment, 539
        General Assessment, 539
        Self-Assessment, 544
        Level of Anxiety and Coping Responses, 544

Family Coping Patterns, 544
Support Systems, 545
Suicide Potential, 545
Homicide Potential, 545
Drug and Alcohol Use, 545
Diagnosis, 546
Outcomes Identification, 546
Planning, 546
Implementation, 547
Reporting Abuse, 547
Counselling, 548
Case Management, 548
Milieu Management, 548
Promotion of Self-Care Activities, 549
Health Teaching and Health Promotion, 549
Prevention of Abuse, 550
Advanced-Practice Interventions, 550
Evaluation, 552

25 **Sexual Assault,** 560
Jodie Flynn
Adapted by Sonya L. Jakubec
Epidemiology, 561
Profile of Sexual Perpetrators, 562
Clinical Picture, 562
Relationships Between Victims and
Perpetrators, 562
Psychological Effects of Sexual Assault, 562
Rape-Trauma Syndrome, 562
Application of the Nursing Process, 564
A Trauma-Informed Approach, 564
Assessment, 564
General Assessment, 565
Self-Assessment, 566
Diagnosis, 567
Dissociative Disorders, 568
Outcomes Identification, 568
Planning, 568
Implementation, 569
Counselling, 569
Promotion of Self-Care Activities, 570
Follow-Up Care, 570
Advanced-Practice Interventions, 570
Evaluation, 571

UNIT 6 Interventions for Distinct Populations

26 **Sexuality and Gender,** 577
Erin Ziegler
Sexuality, 577
Gender, 578
Gender Dysphoria, 579
Clinical Picture, 579
Epidemiology, 579
Nursing Care for Gender Dysphoria, 579
Advanced Interventions, 579
Pharmacological, 579
Surgical, 580
Application of the Nursing Process, 580

Assessment, 580
Self-Assessment, 580
General Assessment, 581
Diagnosis, 581
Outcomes Identification, 581
Planning, 582
Implementation, 582
Mental Health Issues in the LGBTQ
Population, 582
Clinical Picture, 582
Depression, 583
Self-Harm and Suicide, 584
Substance Abuse, 584
Evaluation, 584

27 **Disorders of Children and Adolescents,** 587
Cheryl L. Pollard
Epidemiology, 588
Comorbidity, 589
Risk Factors, 589
Etiology, 590
Biological Factors, 590
Environmental Factors, 591
Child and Adolescent Psychiatric Mental Health
Nursing, 591
Assessing Development and Functioning, 591
General Interventions, 594
Neurodevelopmental Disorders, 598
Intellectual Disabilities, 599
Communication Disorders, 599
Autism Spectrum Disorder, 599
Attention-Deficit/Hyperactivity Disorder, 599
Specific Learning Disorder (SLD), 600
Motor Disorders, 600
Application of the Nursing Process, 601
Assessment, 601
Diagnosis, 601
Outcomes Identification, 601
Implementation, 601
Disruptive, Impulse Control, and Conduct
Disorders, 603
Oppositional Defiant Disorder, 603
Conduct Disorder, 603
Bullying, 604
Application of the Nursing Process, 604
Assessment, 604
Diagnosis, 604
Outcomes Identification, 604
Implementation, 604
Anxiety Disorders, 606
Separation Anxiety Disorder, 606
Generalized Anxiety Disorder (GAD), 607
Application of the Nursing Process, 607
Assessment, 607
Diagnosis, 608
Outcomes Identification, 608
Implementation, 608
Other Disorders of Children and
Adolescents, 608

Depressive Disorders and Bipolar and Related
Disorders, 608
Post-Traumatic Stress Disorder (PTSD), 609
Feeding and Eating Disorders, 609

28 Psychosocial Needs of the Older Adult, 614
Leslie A. Briscoe
Adapted by Cheryl L. Pollard
Developmental Theories of Aging, 615
Mental Health Issues Related to Aging, 616
Late-Life Mental Illness, 616
Trauma, 618
Caregiver Burden, 618
Access to Care, 618
Ageism, 619
Ageism and Public Policy, 619
Ageism and Drug Testing, 620
Distinguishing Between Psychiatric and Physical
Symptoms, 620
Pain, 620
Nursing Care of Older Adults, 624
Assessment Strategies, 624
Intervention Strategies, 626
Care Settings, 629

29 Living With Recurrent and Persistent Mental Illness, 633
Edward A. Herzog
Adapted by Sonya L. Jakubec
Serious Mental Illness Across the Lifespan, 634
Older Adults, 634
Younger Adults, 634
Development of Serious Mental Illness, 635
Rehabilitation Versus Recovery: Two Models
of Care, 635
Issues Confronting Those With Serious Mental
Illness, 635
Establishing a Meaningful Life, 635
Comorbid Conditions, 636
Social Problems, 636
Economic Challenges, 637
Treatment Issues, 637
Resources for People With Serious Mental
Illness, 639
Comprehensive Community Treatment, 639
Substance Abuse Treatment, 639
Evidence-Informed Treatment Approaches, 640
Assertive Community Treatment, 640
Cognitive Behavioural Therapy, 640
Cognitive Enhancement Therapy, 640
Family Support and Partnerships, 640
Social Skills Training, 640
Supportive Psychotherapy, 640
*Vocational Rehabilitation and Related
Services, 641*
Other Potentially Beneficial Services or Treatment
Approaches, 641
Consumer-Run Programs, 641
Wellness and Recovery Action Plans, 641
Exercise, 641

Nursing Care of Patients With Serious Mental
Illness, 641
Assessment Strategies, 641
Intervention Strategies, 642
Evaluation, 643
Current Issues, 643
Involuntary Treatment, 643
Criminal Offences and Incarceration, 643

**30 Psychological Needs of Patients With Medical
Conditions,** 647
Cheryl L. Pollard
Psychological Factors Affecting Medical
Conditions, 647
Psychological Responses to Serious Medical
Conditions, 649
Depression, 649
Anxiety, 649
Substance Use, 650
Grief and Loss, 650
Denial, 650
Fear of Dependency, 651
Human Rights Abuses of Stigmatized Persons With
Medical Conditions, 651
Application of the Nursing Process, 651
Assessment, 651
Psychosocial Assessment, 651
Self-Assessment, 652
Diagnosis, 653
Outcomes Identification, 653
Planning, 653
Implementation, 653
Health Teaching and Health Promotion, 653
Coping Skills, 653
Advanced-Practice Interventions, 654
Evaluation, 654

31 Care for the Dying and for Those Who Grieve, 657
Sonya L. Jakubec
Hospice Palliative Care, 658
Nursing Care at the End of Life, 659
Hospice Palliative Care Nursing, 659
The Art, Presence, and Caring of Nursing, 659
Assessment for Spiritual Issues, 659
*Awareness and Sensitivity of Cultural
Contexts, 660*
Palliative Symptom Management, 660
The Importance of Effective Communication, 661
Self-Care, 664
Nursing Care for Those Who Grieve, 664
Grief Reactions, Bereavement, and Mourning, 665
Types of Grief, 665
Theories, 666
Helping People Cope With Loss, 668
Current Topics and Future Directions, 668
Medically Assisted Death Legislation, 668
*Palliative Care for Patients With
Dementia, 669*
Areas for Future Discovery, 670

32 Forensic Psychiatric Nursing, 674

Adapted by Sonya L. Jakubec

    Forensic Nursing, 676

        Education, 676

        Roles and Functions, 676

        The Forensic Mental Health System in Canada, 678

    Forensic Psychiatric Nursing, 678

        Roles and Functions, 678

UNIT 7 Advanced Intervention Modalities

33 Therapeutic Groups, 684

Donna Rolin, Sandra Snelson Yaklin

Adapted by Cheryl L. Pollard

    Therapeutic Factors Common to All Groups, 685

    Planning a Group, 685

    Phases of Group Development, 685

    Group Member Roles, 686

    Group Leadership, 686

        Responsibilities, 686

        Styles of Leadership, 687

        Clinical Supervision, 687

        Group Observation, 688

    Nurse as Group Leader, 688

        Ethical Issues in Group Therapy, 688

        Basic Groups, 689

        Advanced-Practice Nurse or Nurse Therapist, 691

        Dealing With Challenging Member Behaviours, 691

    Expected Outcomes, 693

34 Family Interventions, 696

Laura G. Leahy, Laura Cox Dzurec

Adapted by Sonya L. Jakubec

    Family, 697

        Family Functions, 698

        Families and Mental Illness, 698

    Canadian Models of Family Nursing Care and Assessment, 698

        McGill Model of Nursing, 698

        Calgary Family Assessment Model (CFAM) and Calgary Family Intervention Model (CFIM), 698

    Family Therapy, 699

        Issues Associated With Family Therapies, 699

        Family Life Cycle, 700

        Working With the Family, 700

    Family Therapy Theory, 702

        The Family as a System, 703

    Application of the Nursing Process, 704

    Assessment, 704

        Sociocultural Context, 704

        Intergenerational Issues, 705

        Self-Awareness, 707

    Diagnosis, 708

    Outcomes Identification, 708

    Planning, 708

    Implementation, 708

        Counselling and Communication Techniques, 708

        Family Therapy, 709

        Case Management, 710

        Pharmacological Interventions, 710

    Evaluation, 711

35 Integrative and Complementary Therapies, 714

Cheryl L. Pollard, Karen Scott Barss

    Integrative Health Care in Canada, 715

        Research, 716

    Patients and Integrative Care, 716

        Safety, 716

        Efficacy, 717

    Integrative Nursing Care, 717

    Classification of Integrative Therapies, 717

        Whole Medical Systems, 717

        Mind–Body–Spirit Approaches, 719

        Biologically Based Therapies, 721

        Manipulative Practices, 724

        Energy Therapies, 725

Appendix A: Standards of Practice, Code of Ethics, Beliefs, and Values, 729

Appendix B: NANDA-International Nursing Diagnoses 2018–2020, 733

Glossary, 737

Index, 748

ACKNOWLEDGEMENTS

First, we would like to acknowledge the text from which this text has been adapted. To work from the years of work and expertise of Elizabeth Varcarolis and Margaret Halter and their contributors is to stand on the shoulders of giants. Our first edition of this adaptation was developed by a remarkable team. The second edition would not be possible without the foundation of that strong adaptation which was carefully crafted and edited over many years with outstanding contributors. This second edition was especially important, with its publication coinciding with beginning implementation of recommendations building on the Truth and Reconciliation Commission (TRC) and Canada's adoption of the UN Declaration of the Rights of Indigenous Peoples. It is too early to report on how these changes will manifest in mental health policy and practice in order to address many years of legislated wrongs, trauma and inequities. In recognition of these forthcoming changes, however, we would like to recognize our use of the terms *Indigenous Peoples* and *Indigenous health* which are emphasized throughout this text to acknowledge the inherent rights and political views of the diverse groups of people with historical and cultural ties to Canada. This is distinct from the term *Aboriginal*, which is a broad term that does not account for the various original peoples (First Nations, Métis, or Inuit) in our country. Throughout the text, it is important for readers to critically reflect on the terms used to reference the diverse Indigenous populations in Canada. In this textbook, we use the term *First Nations, Métis, and Inuit peoples* to replace the term *Aboriginal* unless otherwise specified (for instance in original source reference material). Mental health nursing practice depends on an informed reading and ability to value the rights of Indigenous Peoples to act and claim their identity according to their original names as a form of resistance to the legislated terms that have created inequity and harm over many years. The context and considerations surrounding these terms are discussed in greater depths in Chapter 8, and approaches to culturally safe practice and trauma-informed care are elaborated in Chapters 9 and 22.

Additional changes include, reorganizing and updating clinical chapters. These changes were based on the most recent evidence available, including Canadian research and statistics, current pharmacological practices, as well as content in a number of contemporary mental health concerns (including substance abuse and treatment, harm reduction, as well as gender and sexuality diversity) which provide a current perspective of mental health and mental health practice in Canada.

Our heartfelt appreciation also goes out to the talented group of writers who contributed to both the first edition and the updates and changes to this second Canadian edition. Your contributions figuratively bind us together in this text, which is a collective source of current knowledge for Canadian practice. Special thanks go to those authors who significantly revised and adapted chapter content, in particular Gwen Campbell McArthur who, from her experiences as a person of Métis ancestry and a long-time community mental health practitioner, activist, advisor and researcher, carefully updated the Indigenous mental health section in Chapter 8. Meegiwch (thank you) for sharing your wisdom, Gwen. We would also like to recognize the work of Richard Csiernik who brought his finesse and expertise as a contributor, author and editor of his own books, alongside his in-depth understanding of assessment and treatment of substance use disorders to Chapter 18. Rick, you make it seem easy. Martin Davies and Paul Martin Kerr must be recognized for their extensive pharmacology expertise that has come together for the expanded exploration of pharmacological treatment in Chapter 11. Chapter 23 has benefited from the careful work on anger, aggression and violence by Melodie B. Hull. We are very proud to congratulate Melodie on her being the recipient of the 2017 Nursing Excellence Award for Lifetime Achievement by the Association of Registered Psychiatric Nurses of British Columbia. This award is given in recognition of her professional and academic achievements, dynamic and innovative approach to patient care and her long career in psychiatric nursing. Finally, Erin Ziegler has skillfully contributed to the significant revision of Chapter 26, on sexuality and gender that adds this most current thinking and practice to our text and the discourse. We have indeed sought the expertise of a talented pool of contributors. Their knowledge and passion has had a powerful influence on this edition. It has truly been a joy working with each of you. Thanks for the countless hours you spent researching, writing, and rewriting!

A huge debt of gratitude goes to the many educators and clinicians who reviewed the manuscript and offered valuable suggestions, ideas, opinions, and criticisms. All comments were appreciated; they helped refine and strengthen the individual chapters. In particular, we would like to thank Dr. Lisa Bourque Bearskin at Thompson Rivers University for her thoughtful suggestions that have been part of our framing of Indigenous mental concepts and terminology for this edition.

Throughout this project, a number of people at Elsevier provided superb, and patient, support and encouragement. Sincere thanks go to the Elsevier team: our Content Strategist, Roberta A. Spinosa-Millman, who held the project and us all together with the perfect combination of strong vision, diplomacy and good humour; Sandy Matos, our patient, organized, respectful, and always encouraging Content Development Specialist; and finally to the Copy Editing and Production team, who have made our work shine.

A shared thank-you goes out to each other as Canadian co-editors, we could ask for no more respectful, clear and focused companions on this journey. Finally, we must express our deep gratitude to the first edition Canadian Editorial team that included our colleague Mary Hasse and her visionary work with ongoing support of this textbook while retired, in addition to Susan Ray, who is so deeply missed. Susan has left us all a strong legacy of her work that lives on in this text and elsewhere. Good works have a way of enduring.

CONTRIBUTORS

Karen Scott Barss, RPN, BHSc, MA
Faculty
Nursing Division
Saskatchewan Institute of Applied Science &
    Technology (SIAST)
Saskatoon, Saskatchewan
Adjunct Undergraduate Professor
College of Nursing
University of Regina
Regina, Saskatchewan

**Gwen Campbell McArthur, RPN RN
    BSCN- MH Spec. MN**
Clinical Psychiatric Mental Health Nurse
    Specialist
Kamloops, British Columbia

Richard Csiernik, BSc, MSW, PhD
Professor
Social Work
King's University College
London, Ontario

Martin Davies, BSc, PhD
Undergraduate Program Coordinator
Faculty of Medicine and Dentistry,
    Pharmacology
University of Alberta
Edmonton, Alberta

**Melodie B. Hull, RPN, BA, MSc, MEd,
    PID, TESOL**
Faculty
Nursing
College of the Rockies
Cranbrook, British Columbia
Open Learning Faculty—Nursing & Health
Thompson Rivers University
Kamloops, British Columbia

Dr. Paul Martin Kerr, PhD, BSc
Associate Professor
Department of Nursing Science
Faculty of Nursing
MacEwan University
Edmonton, Alberta

Erin Ziegler, BScN, MN, PHC-NP
Instructor
Daphne Cockwell School of Nursing
Ryerson University
Toronto, Ontario

CONTRIBUTORS TO US EIGHTH EDITION

Leslie A. Briscoe, MSN, RN, PMHCNP
Psychiatric Nurse Practitioner
Louis Stokes Cleveland VA Medical Center
Geriatric Psychiatry: Outpatient and
  Consultation/Liaison Service
Cleveland, Ohio
Nursing Editorial Advisory Panel
Wolters Kluwer Publishing
Clinical Drug Information / Nursing
  division
Hudson, Ohio

Claudia A. Cihlar, PMHCNS-BC, PhD
Coordinator of Behavioral Health Services
Center for Psychiatry
Akron General Medical Center
Akron, Ohio

**Laura Cox Dzurec, FAAN, ANEF,
  PMHCNS-BC, PhD**
Dean
School of Nursing
Widener University
Chester, Pennsylvania

Carissa Enright, MSN, RN, PMHNP BC
Associate Clinical Professor
Texas Woman's University
Dallas, Texas

**Jodie A. Flynn, MSN, RN, SANE-A,
  SANE-P, D-ABMDI**
Instructor
Capital University
Columbus, Ohio

Edward A. Herzog, APRN-CNS
Senior Lecturer, College of Nursing
Kent State University
Kent, Ohio

Mallie Kozy, PMHCNS-BC, PhD
Professor
School of Nursing
University of Portland
Portland, Oregon

**Laura G. Leahy, DrNP, APN, PMH-CNS/
  FNP, BC**
Family Psychiatric Advanced Practice Nurse
APN Solutions, LLC
Sewell, New Jersey

**Donna Rolin, PhD, APRN, PMHCNS-BC,
  PMHNP-BC**
Assistant Professor
Director of Family Psychiatric Mental
  Health Nurse Practitioner Graduate
  Program
University of Texas at Austin, School of
  Nursing
Austin, Texas

Judi Sateren, RN, MS
Associate Professor Emerita
St. Olaf College
Northfield, Minnesota

**Jane Stein-Parbury, RN, BSN, MEd, PhD,
  FRCNA**
Adjunct Professor
University of Technology Sydney
Sydney, Australia

Christine Tackett, MSN RN
Associate Professor
Herzing University
Akron, Ohio

Margaret Trussler, MSN, MS, ANP-BC
Instructor
Graduate School of Nursing
University of Massachusetts Medical School
Worcester, Massachusetts

Elizabeth M. Varcarolis, RN, MA
Professor Emeritus
Formerly Deputy Chairperson and
  Psychiatric Nursing Coordinator
  Department of Nursing
Borough of Manhattan Community College,
  Associate Fellow
Albert Ellis Institute for Rational Emotional
  Behavioral Therapy (REBT)
Former Major, Army Nurse Corps Reserve
New York, New York

**Sandy Snelson Yaklin, MSN, APRN,
  PMHNP-BC, CNE, CHPN**
Bluebonnet Trails Community Service
Round Rock, Texas

Pamela Adams, RN, BN, MScN, PhD, JD
Professor
School of Health Sciences
Humber College Institute of Technology
    and Advanced Learning
Toronto, Ontario

**Michelle Bayard, RN, BN, M.Ed.
    (candidate)**
Teacher
Nursing
Vanier College
Montreal, Quebec

Melissa Brereton, RN, BN, MN
Nurse Clinician
PICU
Montreal Children's Hospital
Montreal, Quebec

**Sharon Chin, BSc(Hons.), MHScN,
    CPMHN(C)**
Professor
Nursing, Collaborative BScN Program
Canadore College/Nipissing University
North Bay, Ontario

Patricia Anne Hart, BSN, MN
Faculty
Saskatchewan Collaborative Bachelor of
    Science in Nursing
Saskatchewan Polytechnic
Saskatoon, Saskatchewan

Carmen Hust, RN, MScN, PhD (c)
Professor
Nursing
Algonquin College
Ottawa, Ontario

**Kristen Jones-Bonofiglio, BScN,
    MPH(N), PhD**
Assistant Professor
School of Nursing, Faculty of Health and
    Behavioural Sciences
Lakehead University
Thunder Bay, Ontario

Tania Killian, BScN, BEd, MEd, CCN
Professor
Health Sciences, Department of Nursing
Seneca College
Toronto, Ontario

Annette M. Lane, RN PhD
Associate Professor
Faculty of Health Disciplines, Centre for
    Nursing and Health Sciences
Athabasca University
Athabasca, Alberta

**Robert J. Meadus, BN, BVocED, MSc(N),
    PhD, CPMHN (C)**
Associate Professor
School of Nursing
Memorial University
St. John's, Newfoundland

Lynn C. Musto, PhD(c), MSN, BSN
Assistant Professor
School of Nursing
Trinity Western University
Langley, British Columbia

Bhavik Bhavan Patel, RN, BScN
Professor
Practical Nursing
Loyalist College
Belleville, Ontario

**J. Craig Phillips, PhD, LLM, RN, ARNP,
    ACRN, FAAN**
Associate Professor
Faculty of Health Sciences, School of
    Nursing
University of Ottawa
Ottawa, Ontario

Diana Snell, MN, RN
Instructor
Faculty of Nursing
University of Calgary
Calgary, Alberta

**Mary Jean Thompson, RN, BN, MHS,
    MPC**
Nursing Instructor
Nursing Faculty, Division of Science and
    Health
Medicine Hat College
Medicine Hat, Alberta

Stephen VanSlyke, RN, BN, MN
Senior Teaching Associate
Faculty of Nursing
University of New Brunswick
Fredericton, New Brunswick

TO THE INSTRUCTOR

The role of the health care provider continues to become more challenging as competing funding priorities, lack of trained personnel, and the dictates of municipal, provincial and territorial, and federal governments compromise our health care system. We nurses and our patients are from widely diverse historical, cultural, religious, and socioeconomic contexts, bringing together a wide spectrum of knowledge, beliefs, and practices. An in-depth consideration and understanding of these contextual and social experiences are paramount in the administration of responsive and evidence-informed nursing care and are emphasized throughout this text.

We have made a concentrated effort to align diagnostic terms, where appropriate, with the *Diagnostic and Statistical Manual of Mental Disorders, fifth edition*. However, note that we have decided to use the term *dementia* when referring to progressive degenerative neurocognitive disorders. Although the term *dementia* was dropped from the *DSM-5*, many current practitioners still frequently use it. Therefore, an editorial decision was made to include and use the term to ensure that readers using this text as a basis for clinical practice would be able to understand what is meant when *dementia* is used by more experienced health care providers.

We are living in an age of fast-paced research in neurobiology, genetics, and psychopharmacology that strives to find the most effective evidence-informed approaches for patients and their families. Legal issues and ethical dilemmas faced by the health care system are magnified accordingly. Given these myriad challenges, knowing how best to teach our students and serve our patients can seem overwhelming. Well researched, with contributions from knowledgeable and experienced nurse educators and interdisciplinary clinical experts with pan-Canadian perspectives, our goal is to bring to you the most current and comprehensive trends and evidence-informed practices in psychiatric mental health nursing.

CONTENT NEW TO THIS EDITION

The following topics are at the forefront of nursing practice and, as such, are considered in detail in this second edition:

- Neurotransmitter and immune stress responses, stress-inducing events and stress-reducing techniques, self-assessment of the nurse's stress level, and mindfulness (Chapter 5)
- Emphasis on Indigenous and refugee mental health concerns, approaches and related trauma-informed practices (Chapter 8)
- Evidence-informed practices and an emphasis on health promotion, resiliency, and recovery in the disorders chapters (Unit 4)
- Issues involving opioid withdrawal, harm reduction and an emphasis on motivational interviewing in substance use disorders (Chapter 18)
- Disaster preparedness in light of climate change and other disasters of our times (Chapter 21)

- Attention to the language and distinctions of assessment and treatment with suicide and nonsuicidal self-injury (Chapter 22)
- Exploration of legislative changes in medically assisted death (MAID) and issues for psychiatric mental health nursing (Chapter 31)
- The important mental health issues concerning gender and sexual diversity, in particular issues surrounding stigma and discrimination for people from the LGBTQ community (Chapter 26)
- Special attention to lifespan mental health assessment, treatment and promotion and prevention (Chapters 27 and 28)
- Emphasis throughout the text on recovery versus rehabilitation, victimization, social isolation and loneliness, unemployment and poverty, involuntary treatment, incarceration, wellness and recovery action plans, mental health first aid, interventions to promote adherence to treatment, and more
- A recognition of the increased prevalence and implications of sleep disturbances and sleep–wake disorders with a focus on their relationship to psychiatric illness and the nurse's role in assessment and management (Chapter 20)

Refer to the *To the Student* section of this introduction for examples of thoroughly updated familiar features with a fresh perspective, including How a Nurse Helped Me boxes, Research Highlight boxes, Integrative Therapy boxes, Patient and Family Teaching boxes, Drug Treatment boxes, Considering Culture boxes, Key Points to Remember, Assessment Guidelines, and Vignettes, among others.

ORGANIZATION OF THE TEXT

Chapters are grouped in units to emphasize the clinical perspective and facilitate location of information. All clinical chapters are organized in a clear, logical, and consistent format with the nursing process as the strong, visible framework. The basic outline for clinical chapters is as follows:

- Clinical Picture: Identifies disorders that fall under the umbrella of the general chapter name. Presents an overview of the disorder(s) and includes *DSM-5* criteria as appropriate.
- Epidemiology: Helps the student to understand the pattern of the problem and characteristics of those who would most likely be affected. This section provides information related to prevalence, lifetime incidence, age of onset, and gender differences.
- Co-Morbidity: Describes the most commonly associated co-morbid conditions. Knowing that co-morbid disorders are often part of the clinical picture of specific disorders helps students and clinicians understand how to better assess and treat their patients.
- Etiology: Provides current views of causation along with formerly held theories. It is based on the biopsychosocial triad and includes biological, psychological, and environmental factors.

- Assessment:
  - General Assessment: Appropriate assessment for a specific disorder, including assessment tools and rating scales. Rating scales, for instance—used to gauge suicide risk, assess anxiety, or assess substance use problems—help to highlight important areas in the assessment. Because the ratings provided by patients are subjective in nature, experienced clinicians use these tools as a guide when planning care, in addition to their knowledge of their patients.
  - Self-Assessment: Discusses topics relevant to the nurse's self-reflection required to enhance self-growth and provide the best possible and most appropriate care to the patient.
  - Assessment Guidelines: Provides a summary of specific areas to assess by disorder.

  Diagnosis: NANDA International–approved nursing diagnoses are used in all relevant nursing process sections, and *DSM-5* (2013) taxonomy and criteria are used throughout.
- Outcomes Identification: *NIC* classifications for interventions and *NOC* classifications for outcomes are introduced in Chapter 1 and used throughout the text when appropriate.
- Planning
- Implementation: Interventions follow Canadian Standards of Psychiatric-Mental Health Nursing (2014) set by the Canadian Federation of Mental Health Nurses under the umbrella of the Canadian Nurses Association (CNA). These standards are incorporated throughout the chapters and are listed for easy reference in Appendix A, "Psychiatric Mental Health Nursing Standards of Practice, Code of Ethics, Beliefs, and Values."
- Evaluation

TEACHING AND LEARNING RESOURCES

For Instructors

Instructor Resources on Evolve, available at http://evolve.elsevier.com/Canada/Varcarolis/psychiatric/, provide a wealth of material to help you make your psychiatric nursing instruction a success. In addition to all of the Student Resources, the following are provided for Faculty:

- **TEACH** includes an expansive introduction with course preparation guidelines and teaching tips, Objectives and Key Terms from each chapter, Thoughts About Teaching the Topic, teaching strategies, and collaborative/learning activities.

- **PowerPoint Presentations** are organized by chapter, with approximately 525 slides for in-class lectures. These are detailed and include customizable text and image lecture slides to enhance learning in the classroom or in Web-based course modules. If you share them with students, they can use the Notes feature to help them with your lectures.
- **Audience Response Questions for i>clicker and other systems** are provided with two to five multiple-answer questions per chapter to stimulate class discussion and assess student understanding of key concepts.
- The **Test Bank** has more than 1000 test items, complete with correct answers, rationales, the cognitive level of each question, the corresponding step of the nursing process, appropriate NCLEX Client Needs labels, and text page reference(s).

For Students

Student Resources on Evolve, available at http://evolve.elsevier.com/Canada/Varcarolis/psychiatric/, provide a wealth of valuable learning resources.

The Evolve Resources page near the front of the book gives login instructions and a description of each resource.

- The **Answer Key to Critical Thinking** questions provides possible outcomes for the Critical Thinking questions at the end of each chapter.
- The **Answer Key to Chapter Review** questions provides answers and rationales for the Chapter Review questions at the end of each chapter.
- **Case Studies and Nursing Care Plans** provide detailed case studies and care plans for specific psychiatric disorders to supplement those found in the textbook.
- The **Glossary** highlights psychiatric mental health nursing terms with definitions.
- **Review Questions** provided for each chapter will help students prepare for course examinations and for the nursing licensure examination.
- **Pre-Tests and Post-Tests** provide interactive self-assessments for each chapter of the textbook, including instant scoring and feedback at the click of a button.

We are grateful to educators who send suggestions and provide feedback, and hope this second edition helps students learn and appreciate the scope of psychiatric mental health nursing practice.

Cheryl L. Pollard
Sonya L. Jakubec

Psychiatric mental health nursing challenges us to understand the complexities of human behaviour. In the chapters that follow, you will learn about people with psychiatric mental health disorders and how to provide them with quality nursing care and promote their mental health. As you read, keep in mind these special features.

READING AND REVIEW TOOLS

1 Key Terms and Concepts and **2 Objectives** introduce the chapter topics and provide a concise overview of the material discussed.

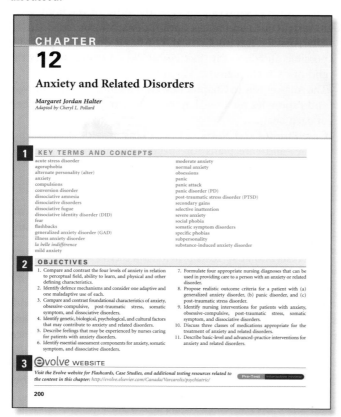

Key Points to Remember listed at the end of each chapter reinforce essential information.

Critical Thinking activities at the end of each chapter are scenario-based critical thinking problems to provide practice in

applying what you have learned. **Answer Keys** can be found on the Evolve website.

Multiple-choice **Chapter Review** questions at the end of each chapter help you review the chapter material and study for exams. **Answers** with **rationales** are located on the Evolve website.

ADDITIONAL LEARNING RESOURCES

Your **3** Evolve Resources at http://evolve.elsevier.com/Canada/Varcarolis/psychiatric/ offer more helpful study aids, such as additional Case Studies and Nursing Care Plans.

CHAPTER FEATURES

4 How a Nurse Helped Me boxes are patient accounts and narratives that introduce select chapters and invite exploration into the lived experiences of patients and families.

5 Considering Culture boxes reinforce the importance of providing culturally competent care.

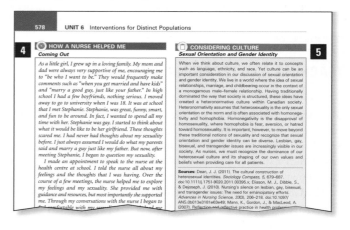

6 Vignettes describe the unique circumstances surrounding individual patients with psychiatric disorders.

7 Assessment Guidelines at the end of each Assessment section in most clinical chapters provide summary points for patient assessment.

8 Research Highlight boxes demonstrate how current research findings affect psychiatric mental health nursing practice and standards of care.

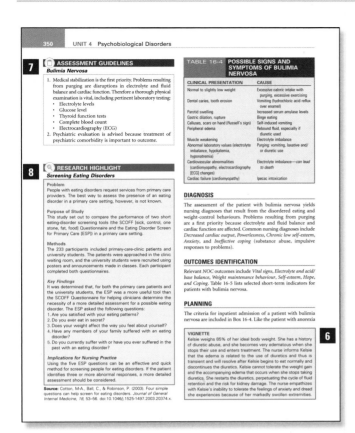

10 Guidelines for Communication boxes provide tips for communicating therapeutically with patients and their families.

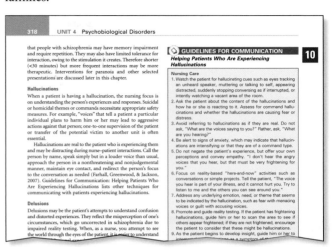

11 Patient and Family Teaching boxes underscore the nurse's role in helping patients and families understand psychiatric disorders, treatments, complications, and medication adverse effects, among other important issues.

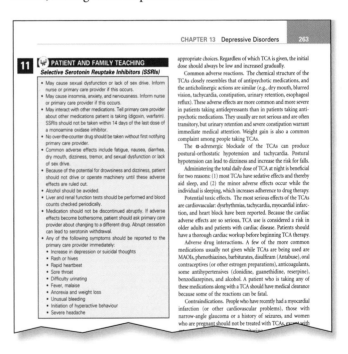

9 Self-Assessment sections discuss topics relevant to a nurse's process of self-reflection needed to enhance self-growth and provide the best possible and most appropriate care to the patient.

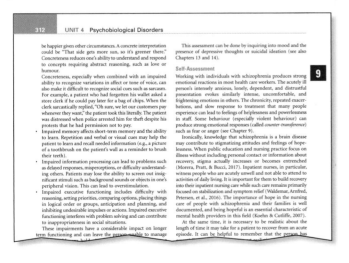

12 Drug Treatment boxes present the latest information on medications used to treat psychiatric disorders.

13 Integrative Therapy boxes discuss significant nursing considerations for complementary and alternative therapies and examine relevant study findings.

15 Case Studies and Nursing Care Plans present individualized histories of patients with specific psychiatric disorders following the steps of the nursing process. Interventions with rationales and evaluation statements are presented for each patient goal.

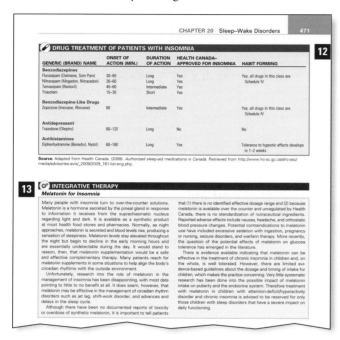

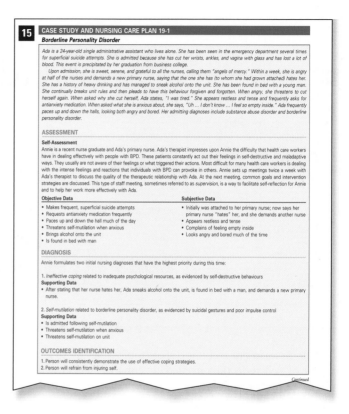

14 DSM-5 boxes identifies the criteria of disorders identified and described in the *Diagnostic and Statistical Manual of Mental Disorders, fifth edition*.

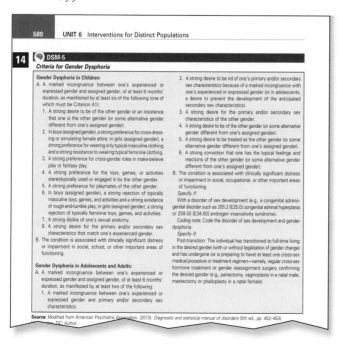

Foundations in Theory

1. Mental Health and Mental Illness

2. Historical Overview of Psychiatric Mental Health Nursing

3. Overview of Psychiatric Mental Health Nursing Care Within Various Settings

4. Relevant Theories and Therapies for Nursing Practice

5. Understanding Responses to Stress

1

Mental Health and Mental Illness

Sonya L. Jakubec

KEY TERMS AND CONCEPTS

clinical epidemiology
comorbid condition
Diagnostic and Statistical Manual of Mental Disorders, fifth edition (*DSM-5*)
electronic health care
epidemiology
evidence-informed practice

incidence
mental health
mental illness
Nursing Interventions Classification (NIC)
Nursing Outcomes Classification (NOC)
prevalence
resilience

OBJECTIVES

1. Describe the two conceptualizations of mental health and mental illness.
2. Explore the role of resilience in the prevention of and recovery from mental illness, and consider your own resilience in response to stress.
3. Identify how culture influences our view of mental illnesses and behaviours associated with them.
4. Define and identify attributes of positive mental health.
5. Discuss the nature/nurture origins of psychiatric disorders.
6. Summarize the social determinants of health in Canada.
7. Explain how findings of epidemiological studies can be used to identify areas for medical and nursing interventions.
8. Identify how the *DSM-5* can influence a clinician to consider a broad range of information before making a diagnosis.
9. Describe the specialty of psychiatric mental health nursing.
10. Compare and contrast a *DSM-5* medical diagnosis with a NANDA nursing diagnosis.

⊖volve WEBSITE

Visit the Evolve website for Flashcards, Case Studies, and additional testing resources related to the content in this chapter: http://evolve.elsevier.com/Canada/Varcarolis/psychiatric/

Pre-Test | interactive review

Because they are frequently mentioned in our daily conversations and in the media, it is likely you routinely hear about people's mood, thinking, emotions, and behaviours. Terms like *depression, anxiety, psychosis, dementia, addiction, crisis*, and *stress* are used in many different ways. But what does this mean for people who are experiencing problems in their mental health and well-being? How are you to understand and work knowledgeably in this changing and rapidly evolving area of nursing? Certainly, people living with mental illnesses and their families and caregivers experience a range of physical symptoms that result both from the illness itself—and as a consequence of treatment, the social determinants of health—and from the stigma and discrimination that contribute further to distress (Gaebel, Rössler, & Sartorius, 2017). Your understanding of the theories of mental health and illness is an important place to begin to establish psychiatric mental health nursing practice that can treat, support, and empower people who suffer unnecessarily from mistreatment, misunderstanding, and social exclusion (Ungar, Knaak, & Szeto, 2016).

HOW A NURSE HELPED ME

When a Nurse Becomes a Patient

I am a registered nurse working in the area of mental health. I always prided myself on my ability to give caring and compassionate care to all of my patients. Little did I know that one day I would be the patient. I was diagnosed with bipolar disorder when I was 34 years old. For many years, I struggled with devastating depressions and periods of acute mania. I felt stupid, shameful, and embarrassed about my behaviour during these times. Whenever I needed hospitalization, I begged the ambulance driver to take me to any hospital but the one I worked in. On one occasion, that did not happen, and I was admitted to the unit where I worked as a nurse. I thought I could have died of the deep shame I felt. Judy, the nurse assigned to me, seemed scared and embarrassed to come and speak with me, so I felt uncomfortable when I spoke with her. On about the fourth day of that admission, Brenda, another nurse I knew, was assigned to my care. Brenda started out by telling me that she would be my nurse for the shift and that she would make herself available to me for a one-on-one later in the day. When she came to speak with me, she said, "Let's talk about the elephant in the room, and then we can move into talking about how I can support you in getting well." We talked about my embarrassment and shame. I felt so relieved that she was willing to address my feelings about my mental illness. Over the next several weeks, we had many one-on-one sessions, and I was able to share my story with Brenda. Brenda helped me see that there was hope for my future and that I could learn to live well despite my diagnosis. I would love to say that I got well and stayed well, but actually, I have continued to struggle with my health. I can tell you that Brenda's acknowledgement of my feelings helped me deal with the stigma I felt about my illness. I no longer feel ashamed of having a mental illness.

MENTAL HEALTH AND MENTAL ILLNESS

The World Health Organization (WHO, 2014a) maintains that a person cannot be considered healthy without taking into account mental and physical health. The WHO defines mental health as "a state of well-being in which each individual is able to realize his or her own potential, cope with the normal stresses of life, work productively and fruitfully, and make a contribution to the community" (WHO, 2016a). Our quality of life and our ability to enjoy life are enhanced by positive mental health and a sense of well-being (Mental Health Commission of Canada, 2017). Good mental health is associated with better physical health outcomes, improved educational attainment, increased economic participation, and rich social relationships (Canadian Institute for Health Information, 2009). Mental health is described

as more than merely the absence of mental disorders or disabilities (WHO, 2016a). The Public Health Agency of Canada (2014) offers the following definition of mental health: "the capacity of each and all of us to feel, think, and act in ways that enhance our ability to enjoy life and deal with the challenges we face. It is a positive sense of emotional and spiritual well-being that respects the importance of culture, equity, social justice, interconnections and personal dignity." Some of the attributes of positive mental health are presented in Figure 1-1.

Societal and psychiatric definitions of *mental health* are continually evolving. Defining concepts are shaped by the prevailing culture and social values, and reflect changes in cultural norms, society's expectations, dominant medical discourse, as well as corporate and political climates. In the past, the term *mental illness* was applied to behaviours considered "strange" or "different"—behaviours that occurred infrequently and deviated from an established norm. Such criteria are inadequate because they suggest that mental health requires conformity. But there is a further problem in viewing people whose behaviour is unusual as mentally ill. Such a definition would mean that nonconformists and independent thinkers like Socrates, Mahatma Gandhi, and Canada's suffragettes such as Nellie McClung and Emily Murphy would be considered mentally ill. And although the determination of Steven Jobs, the dedication of Terry Fox, and the artistic abilities of Leonard Cohen are uncommon, virtually none of us would consider their much-admired behaviours to be signs of mental illness.

Alterations in cognition, mood, or behaviour that are coupled with significant distress and impaired functioning characterize mental illness (Public Health Agency of Canada, 2015a). *Mental illness* refers to all mental disorders with definable diagnoses. Cognition may be impaired, as in Alzheimer's disease; mood may be affected, as in major depression; behaviour may change, as in schizophrenia; or a combination of the three types of symptoms may be apparent.

Two Conceptualizations of Mental Health and Mental Illness

Published in 1988, *Mental Health for Canadians: Striking a Balance*, commonly called the Epp Report, highlighted the importance of issues related to mental health and mental illness in Canada. It proposed seven guiding principles for the development of public policies to support mental health. Despite the forward thinking of this report, it was not until 2009 that Canada developed a mental health strategy framework (Mental Health Commission of Canada, 2009), with a framework for action established in 2017 (Mental Health Commission of Canada, 2017).

The Epp Report (Epp, 1988) proposed two continua to depict the relationship between mental health and mental disorder. The Mental Disorder Continuum assigns one endpoint as maximal mental disorder and the opposite endpoint as absence of mental disorder, allowing for a range of impairment and distress. For instance, a person with a severe clinical depression would be at the endpoint of maximal mental disorder, but as the depression subsided, he or she would move along the continuum toward absence of mental disorder. The Mental Health Continuum

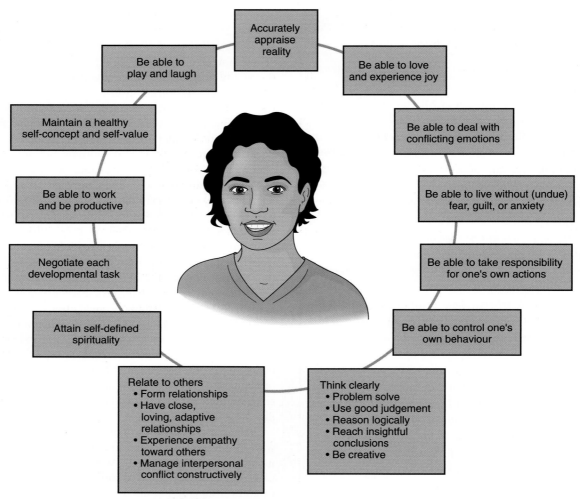

FIGURE 1-1 Some attributes of mental health.

assigns one pole as optimal mental health and the opposite pole as minimal mental health. On this scale, a person with optimal mental health would demonstrate good coping skills and resilience when faced with stressors, and a person with minimal mental health may decompensate and not be able to cope with stressors.

Considering the interaction between the continua suggested by Epp (see Figure 1-2) is interesting and could provide a basis for many research studies. For example, how can nurses increase health-related hardiness in people with schizophrenia?

This depiction of mental health and mental illness allows for four possible outcomes: (1) maximal mental disorder and optimal mental health; (2) optimal mental health and absence of mental disorder; (3) absence of mental disorder and minimal mental health; and (4) minimal mental health and maximal mental disorder. We will look at each outcome:

1. A person may have a severe mental disorder *and* optimal mental health. How could this be possible? Think of the person with a diagnosis of chronic schizophrenia who is stable on her medications, maintains contact with health care providers, has a social network, possibly works or volunteers, and follows a healthy diet and exercises. This person still has a mental disorder, yet she meets the criteria for optimal mental health.

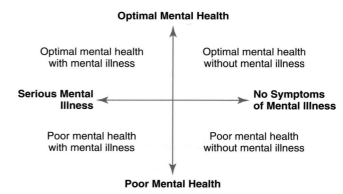

FIGURE 1-2 Continua from the Epp Report. Source: Public Health Agency of Canada. (1988). *Mental health for Canadians: Striking a balance.* Reproduced with permission from the Minister of Health, 2013.

2. This quadrant is the one in which we would all like to be. Imagine a world with no mental illness and good mental health.

3. It is possible for a person to have poor coping skills and no resilience when faced with stressors and yet not have a mental disorder.

4. This quadrant is the one in which we would not like to be, yet many patients find themselves here. A person with borderline personality disorder would most likely be placed in this quadrant.

It is important to note that it is possible to be anywhere along the continua, not just at one end.

Contributing Factors

Many factors can affect the severity and progression of a mental illness, as well as the mental health of a person who does not have a mental illness (Figure 1-3). If possible, these influences need to be evaluated and factored into an individual's plan of care. In fact, the *Diagnostic and Statistical Manual of Mental Disorders, fifth edition (DSM-5)*, classifies around 350 mental disorders with evidence that suggests the symptoms and causes of a number of them are influenced by cultural and ethnic factors. The *DSM-5* is discussed in further detail later in this chapter.

Resilience

Researchers, clinicians, and patients are all interested in actively facilitating mental health and reducing mental illness. A characteristic of mental health increasingly being promoted as essential to the recovery process is **resilience**. Canadian researcher Michael Ungar (2015) understands *resilience* as a process and outcome of complex, cultural systems, rather than as an individual capacity to overcome adversity. In this way, when exposed to adversity, one's resilience depends on the navigation and negotiation of resources that can support well-being. Ungar's (2015) research emphasizes that resilience depends far more on the quality of the social and physical ecologies surrounding people than on individual personality traits, cognitions, or talents. Closely associated with the process of *adapting*, resilience helps people face tragedies, loss, trauma, and severe stress. We can see evidence of resilience in the wake of disasters such as the fire in Fort McMurray, Alberta, in 2016 and the civil war in Syria resulting in mass casualties and refugees. Being resilient does not mean being unaffected by stressors; rather, it means that instead of falling victim to negative emotions, resilient people recognize such feelings and negotiate complex personal and societal systems in order to deal with their responses and the responses of others.

Alongside social and environmental understanding of resilience, accessing and developing resilience in turn assists people to recover from painful experiences and difficult events. It is characterized by optimism and a sense of mastery and competence. Research demonstrates that early experiences in mastering difficult or stressful situations enhance the prefrontal cortex's ability to

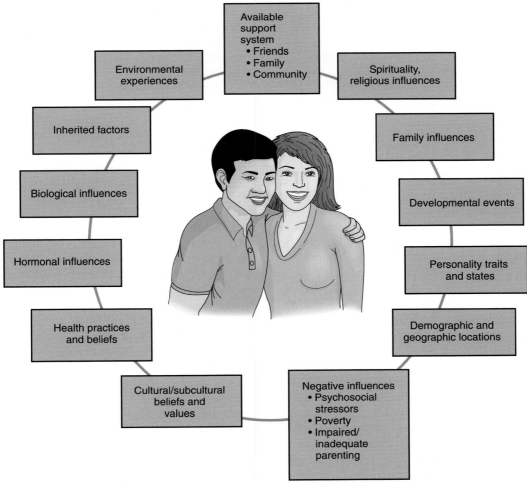

FIGURE 1-3 Influences that can have an impact on an individual's mental health.

cope with such situations later (Siegel, 2015). You can get an idea of how good you are at regulating your emotions by taking the assessment in Box 1-1.

Mental health recovery. According to the Mental Health Commission of Canada (2015), recovery rests on several key concerns: respect for individual contexts and wishes, hope for a better future, dignity and self-determination, collaboration and reflection, and a focus on strengths and personal responsibility. Recovery practices insist that all people are respected for the experience, expertise, and strengths they contribute. Recovery approaches challenge traditional notions of professional power and expertise by helping to break down the conventional notions of expertise that privileges professional expertise over lived experience (of patients and families).

VIGNETTE

Elizabeth Anderson lives with schizophrenia. Involvement in a recovery support group has changed her view of her illness, herself, her marriage, and her potential. She has taken the lead role in her own recovery and supports others to do the same through her writing, speaking, and community work. This leadership and her book *Being Mentally Healthy (in spite of a mental illness)* highlight a recipe for recovery and for being mentally healthy while living with a mental illness. According to Elizabeth, the recipe requires six ingredients: "timely intervention; the right medications; supportive people (especially loved ones); a reason to be well; a reason to hope; something important to do, or a higher purpose or calling." Elizabeth describes her life with mental illness in terms of resiliency—and with hope for the future and any number of possibilities, stating: "Yes, I'm doing well and I've got a mental illness."

Learn more about Elizabeth's story here: http://beingmentally-healthy.com/bio/

Culture

There is no standard measure for mental health, in part because it is culturally defined and is based on interpretations of effective functioning according to societal norms (WHO, 2016a). One approach to differentiating mental health from mental illness is to consider what a particular culture regards as acceptable or unacceptable behaviour. In this view, mentally ill people are those who violate social norms and thus threaten (or make anxious) those observing them. For example, traditional Japanese may consider suicide to be an act of honour, and Middle Eastern "suicide bombers" are considered by some to be holy warriors or martyrs. Contrast these viewpoints with those in the West, where people who attempt or complete suicides are nearly always considered mentally ill.

Throughout history, people have interpreted health or sickness according to current views. A striking example of how cultural change influences the interpretation of mental illness is an old definition of *hysteria*. According to *Webster's Dictionary* (Porter, 1913), hysteria was "a nervous affection, occurring almost exclusively in women, in which the emotional and reflex excitability is exaggerated, and the will power correspondingly

---

BOX 1-1   ASSESSING YOUR RESILIENCE

The following questions are intended to provide you with an opportunity to reflect on and perhaps discover your own resilience.

1. What about my life gives me the most meaning?
2. What do others depend on you for?
3. What do you do that others value?
4. What is your philosophy, beliefs about life that guide your day to day choices?
5. What do you hope for?
6. How do you respond in difficult times?
7. How have you gotten through difficult times?
8. How do I handle disappointments in life?
9. What is my general outlook in life (optimist, pessimist)?
10. In what ways can you depend on yourself?
11. What has changed in your life?
12. What has stayed the same in your life?

As you reflect on your answers those related to your inner strength, competence, optimism, flexibility, and the ability to cope effectively when faced with adversity are all positively linked to increased levels of resilience.

---

diminished, so that the patient loses control over the emotions, becomes the victim of imaginary sensations, and often falls into paroxysm or fits." Treatment for this condition often involved sexual outlets for afflicted women, whose condition was thought to be the result of sexual deprivation. According to some authors, this diagnosis fell into disuse as women gained rights, the family atmosphere became less restrictive, and societal tolerance of sexual practices increased.

Cultures differ not only in their views regarding mental illness but also in the types of behaviour categorized as mental illness. Culture-bound syndromes seem to occur in specific sociocultural contexts, identify local idioms of distress, and are easily recognized by people in those cultures (Scull, 2014; Stern, Freudenreich, Smith, et al., 2017). For example, one syndrome recognized in parts of Southeast Asia is *running amok*, in which a person (usually a male) runs around engaging in furious, almost indiscriminate violent behaviour. *Pibloktoq*, an uncontrollable desire to tear off one's clothing and expose oneself to severe winter weather, is a recognized psychological disorder in parts of Greenland, Alaska, and the Arctic regions of Canada. In Canada, *anorexia nervosa* (see Chapter 16) is recognized as a psychobiological disorder that entails voluntary starvation. The disorder is well known in Europe, North America, and Australia but unheard of in many other parts of the world.

What is to be made of the fact that certain disorders occur in some cultures but are absent in others? One interpretation is that the conditions necessary for causing a particular disorder occur in some places but are absent in others. Another interpretation is that people learn certain kinds of abnormal behaviour by imitation. However, the fact that some disorders may be culturally determined does not prove that all mental illnesses are so determined. Evidence suggests that schizophrenia (see Chapter 15) and bipolar disorders (see Chapter 14) are found throughout the world. The symptom patterns of schizophrenia have been observed among indigenous Greenlanders and West African villagers as well as in Western culture.

Perceptions of Mental Health and Mental Illness

Mental Illness Versus Physical Illness

People commonly make a distinction between mental illnesses and physical illnesses. It is an odd distinction, considering that *mental* refers to the brain, the most complex and sophisticated part of the body, the organ responsible for the higher thought processes that set us apart from other creatures. Surely the workings of the brain—the synaptic connections, the areas of functioning, the spinal innervations and connections—are *physical*. One problem with this distinction is that it implies that psychiatric disorders are "all in the head" and, therefore, under personal control and indistinguishable from a choice to indulge in bad behaviour. Although some physical disorders, such as a broken arm from skiing or lung cancer from smoking, are blamed on the victim, the majority of physical illnesses are considered to be beyond personal responsibility.

Perhaps the origin of this distinction between mental and physical illness lies in the religious and philosophical tradition of explaining the unexplainable by assigning a mystical or spiritual origin to cognitive processes and emotional activities. Despite many advances in understanding, mental illnesses continue to be viewed differently from illnesses that originate in other parts of the body.

Consider that people with epilepsy were once thought to be possessed by demons, under the attack of gods, or cursed; they were subjected to horrible "cures" and treatments. Today, most people would say that epilepsy is a disorder of the brain and not under one's personal control because epilepsy appears on brain scans as areas of overactivity and excitability. But there are no specific biological tests to diagnose most psychiatric disorders—for example, no blood test to diagnose obsessive-compulsive disorder (OCD). However, researchers are convinced that the root of most mental disorders lies in intercellular abnormalities, and they can now see clear signs of altered brain function in several mental disorders, including schizophrenia, OCD, stress disorders, and depression. Further details about these signs are discussed in Chapter 5 and throughout Unit 3.

Nature Versus Nurture

For students learning about mental illness, one of its most intriguing aspects is its origins. Although for centuries people believed that extremely unusual behaviours were due to demonic forces, in the late 1800s the mental health pendulum swung briefly to a biological focus with the "germ theory of diseases" (Nolan, 1993). Germ theory explained mental illness in the same way other illnesses were being described—that is, they were caused by a specific agent in the environment (Morgan, McKenzie, & Fearon, 2008). This perspective led to the segregation and isolation of people who were thought to be "mad," in the same way that those with infections were isolated in order to prevent the infection of others. This theory was abandoned rather quickly since clinicians and researchers could not identify single causative factors for mental illnesses; there was no "mania germ" that

could be viewed under a microscope and subsequently treated. Nonetheless, the practices of isolation persisted.

Although biological treatments for mental illness continued to be explored and ultimately dismissed as ineffective, over the next half century, psychological theories dominated and focused on the science of the mind and behaviour. These theories explained the origin of mental illness as faulty psychological processes that could be corrected by increasing personal insight and understanding. For example, a patient experiencing depression and apathy might be assisted to explore feelings left over from childhood, when his attempts at independence were harshly discouraged by overly protective parents.

This psychological focus was challenged in 1952, when the medication chlorpromazine (Largactil) was found to have a calming effect on agitated, out-of-control patients. Imagine what this discovery must have been like for clinicians who had resorted to every biological treatment imaginable, including wet wraps, insulin shock therapy, and psychosurgery (in which holes were drilled in the head of a patient and probes inserted in the brain), in a futile attempt to change behaviour. Many began to believe that if psychiatric problems respond to medications that alter intercellular components, then the illness must be a disruption of intercellular components to begin with. At this point, the pendulum made steady and sure progress toward a biological explanation of psychiatric problems and disorders.

Currently, the diathesis–stress model—in which diathesis represents biological predisposition and stress represents environmental stress or trauma—is the most accepted explanation for mental illness. This nature-plus-nurture argument asserts that most psychiatric disorders result from a combination of genetic vulnerability and negative environmental stressors. While one person may develop major depressive disorder (MDD) largely as the result of an inherited and biological vulnerability that alters brain chemistry, another person with little vulnerability may develop depression from changes in brain chemistry caused by the insults of a stressful environment. MDD is discussed in Chapter 13.

Human Genome Project

The Human Genome Project was a 13-year project (1990–2003) that was completed on the fiftieth anniversary of the discovery of the DNA double helix. The project has strengthened some biological and genetic explanations for psychiatric conditions (Cowan, Kopnisky, & Hyman, 2002). The goals of the project were to:

- Identify the approximately 20 000 to 25 000 genes in human DNA
- Determine the sequences of the three billion chemical base pairs that make up human DNA
- Store this information in databases
- Improve tools for data analysis
- Address the ethical, legal, and social issues that may arise from the project

Although researchers have begun to identify some genetic links to mental illness and gene-environment interactions (as you will see in the chapters on clinical disorders), it will be some time before we understand the exact nature of genetic influences on mental illness (Uher, 2014). What we do know is that most psychiatric disorders are the result of multiple mutated or defective genes, each of which in combination may contribute to the disorder.

Social Influences on Mental Health Care

Self-Help Movement

In January 1918, the Canadian Mental Health Association (CMHA) was formed by Dr. Clarence M. Hincks and Clifford W. Beers to promote mental health. The CMHA is one of the oldest and most respected voluntary health organizations in Canada (CMHA, 2016). In the latter part of the twentieth century, the CMHA and other organizations and individuals expended tremendous energy on putting the notion of equality—treating people fairly and extinguishing stigmatizing labels—into widespread practice in Canada. In regard to mental illness, decades of institutionalization had created political and social concerns that gave rise to a mental health movement similar to the rights movements for women, people with disabilities, and the LGBTQ (lesbian, gay, bisexual, transgender, and queer) communities. Groups of people with mental illnesses—or mental health patients—began to advocate for their rights and the rights of others with mental illness and to fight stigma, discrimination, and forced treatment. Practitioners and activists who are concerned with these service user, human rights, and critical approaches are establishing alternative ways of understanding and addressing the conditions and contexts that organize contemporary psychiatry in Canada and elsewhere (Burstow, 2015; Burstow, LeFrançois, & Diamond, 2014; Menzies, Reaume, & LeFrançois, 2013).

Decade of the Brain

In 1990, the United States Congress designated the last decade of the past century the "Decade of the Brain." This American initiative stimulated a worldwide growth of scientific research (Abi-Rached, 2008). Among the advances and progress made during the Decade of the Brain were the following:

- Understanding of the genetic basis of embryonic and fetal neural development
- Mapping of genes involved in neurological illness, including mutations associated with Parkinson's disease, Alzheimer's disease, and epilepsy
- Discovery that the brain uses a relatively small number of neurotransmitters but has a vast assortment of neurotransmitter receptors
- Uncovering of the role of cytokines (proteins involved in the immune response) in such brain disorders as depression
- Refinement of neuroimaging techniques, such as positron emission tomography (PET) scans, magnetic resonance imaging (MRI), magnetoencephalography, and event-related electroencephalography (EEG), which have improved our understanding of normal brain functioning as well as areas of difference in pathological states
- Bringing together of computer modelling and laboratory research, which resulted in the new discipline of computational neuroscience.

While the Decade of the Brain ended in 2000, the so-called neuro-age of expanded scientific exploration of the brain continues to influence society in numerous ways, including biomedical, clinical, political, marketing, and business.

Mental Health for Canadians: Striking a Balance

Mental Health for Canadians: Striking a Balance (Epp, 1988) was one of the first government-generated reports that acknowledged the challenges of the mentally ill population. The purpose of the report was to assist Canadians engaged in developing and reviewing mental health–related policies and programs. Three challenges in mental health were identified: (1) reducing inequities, (2) increasing prevention, and (3) enhancing coping. These challenges continue. For example, the Mental Health Commission of Canada (2012) identified similar challenges, which are reflected in its six strategic directions: (1) promoting mental health across the lifespan; (2) fostering recovery and well-being for people, while upholding their rights; (3) providing timely access to treatment and supports; (4) reducing disparities; (5) recognizing the distinct circumstances, rights, and cultures in addressing mental health needs of individuals and communities; and (6) ensuring effective leadership and collaboration across sectors, agencies, and communities.

Changing Directions, Changing Lives: The Mental Health Strategy for Canada

In November 2009, the Mental Health Commission of Canada released a report titled *Toward Recovery & Well-Being: A Framework for a Mental Health Strategy for Canada*. Until this time, Canada did not have a national plan for the development of a mental health strategy. Seven interconnected goals were identified to define what it would take to have a system oriented toward both enabling the recovery of people living with mental health problems and illnesses and fostering the mental health and well-being of everyone living in Canada (p. 19). This framework was the first phase in the development of a comprehensive Canadian mental health strategy, instrumental in both health reform and social change (Rosen, Goldbloom, & McGeorge, 2010). It put forward the vision and broad goals for the strategy in 2012 and a later action plan in 2017.

The aim of the strategy and action plan is to improve mental health and well-being for all Canadians. The large collaborative teams who have developed the strategy and plan strongly believe that we can create a mental health system that will meet the needs of people of all ages living with mental health problems and illnesses, and their families. Implementation of this strategy will help to ensure that people who experience mental health problems and illnesses, especially those with the most severe and complex ones, are treated with respect and dignity and enjoy the same rights as all Canadians. Six key strategic directions (see Box 1-2) were outlined in the report. Students are encouraged to access the full report to get an understanding of how health care providers, patients, families, and communities can work together to implement the strategies throughout Canada.

The 2017–2022 action plan for this strategy goes on to focus on four key pillars: leadership and funding, promotion and prevention, access and services, and data and research.

BOX 1-2 STRATEGIC DIRECTIONS IDENTIFIED IN CHANGING DIRECTIONS, CHANGING LIVES: THE MENTAL HEALTH STRATEGY FOR CANADA

Strategic Direction 1: Promotion and Prevention
Promote mental health across the lifespan in homes, schools, and workplaces, and prevent mental illness and suicide wherever possible. Reducing the impact of mental health problems and illnesses and improving the mental health of the population require promotion and prevention efforts in everyday settings where the potential impact is greatest.

Strategic Direction 2: Recovery and Rights
Foster recovery and well-being for people of all ages living with mental health problems and illnesses, and uphold their rights. The key to recovery is helping people to find the right combination of services, treatments, and supports, and eliminating discrimination by removing barriers to full participation in work, education, and community life.

Strategic Direction 3: Access to Services
Provide access to the right combination of services, treatments, and supports, when and where people need them. A full range of services, treatments, and supports includes primary health care, community-based and specialized mental health services, peer support, and supported housing, education, and employment.

Strategic Direction 4: Disparities and Diversity
Reduce disparities in risk factors and access to mental health services, and strengthen the response to the needs of diverse communities and Northerners. Mental health should be taken into account when acting to improve overall living conditions and addressing the specific needs of groups such as new Canadians and people in northern and remote communities.

Strategic Direction 5: First Nations, Inuit, and Métis
Work with First Nations, Inuit, and Métis to address their mental health needs, acknowledging their distinct circumstances, rights, and cultures. By calling for access to a full continuum of culturally safe mental health services, the *Mental Health Strategy for Canada* can contribute to truth, reconciliation, and healing from intergenerational trauma.

Strategic Direction 6: Leadership and Collaboration
Mobilize leadership, improve knowledge, and foster collaboration at all levels. Change will not be possible without a whole-of-government approach to mental health policy, without fostering the leadership roles of people living with mental health problems and illnesses, and their families, and without building strong infrastructure to support data collection, research, and human resource development.

Source: Mental Health Commission of Canada. (2012). *Changing directions, changing lives: The mental health strategy for Canada.* Retrieved from http://strategy.mentalhealthcommission.ca/pdf/strategy-images-en.pdf.

EPIDEMIOLOGY OF MENTAL DISORDERS

Epidemiology, as it applies to psychiatric mental health, is the quantitative study of the distribution of mental disorders in human populations. Once the distribution of mental disorders has been determined quantitatively, epidemiologists can identify high-risk groups and high-risk factors associated with illness onset, duration, and recurrence. The further study of risk factors for mental illness may then lead to important clues about the causes of various mental disorders.

Two different but related words used in epidemiology are *incidence* and *prevalence*. Incidence refers to the *number of new cases* of mental disorders in a healthy population within a given period of time—for example, the number of Vancouver adolescents who were diagnosed with major depressive disorder between 2008 and 2018. Prevalence describes the *total number of cases*, new and existing, in a given population during a specific period of time, regardless of when the subjects became ill—for example, the number of adolescents who screen positive for major depressive disorder in Toronto schools between 2008 and 2018. Each level of investigation supplies information that can be used to improve clinical practice and plan public-health policies.

Report From the Canadian Chronic Disease Surveillance System: Mental Illness In Canada, a report from the Public Health Agency of Canada published in 2015, describes the major mental illnesses and reports their incidence and prevalence over a 14-year period. The report identified individuals as having used health services for a mental illness if they met the criteria for diagnosed illness meeting the International Classification of Diseases (ICD) from a hospital or other physician visit. Select highlights from the report include the following:

- "Approximately five million Canadians (or about one in seven people) use health services for a mental illness annually."
- "Women are more likely than men to use health services for a mental illness, especially those between the ages of 25 to 39 years. A combination of genetic, biological, behavioural and sociocultural factors may explain this difference."
- "Almost one in four people aged 80 and over use health services for a mental illness, a trend likely driven by the inclusion of dementias in the International Classification of Diseases under mental disorders."
- "The largest relative increase [of the use of health services for mental illness] occurred among young adolescents (aged 10 to 14)."
- "Boys (under 15 years of age) are more likely to use health services for a mental illness than girls; likely driven by certain disturbance of conduct disorders and attention deficit disorder which are known to occur more frequently among boys."

Many individuals have more than one mental disorder at a time; this state is known as a comorbid condition.

Some disorders may have a high incidence but a low prevalence, and vice versa. A disease with a short duration, such as the common cold, tends to have a high incidence (many new cases in a given year) and a low prevalence (not many people suffering from a cold at any given time). Conversely, a chronic disease such as diabetes will have a low incidence because a year (or whatever time increment is used) after diagnosis, the person will be dropped from the list of new cases. Lifetime risk data, or the risk that one will develop a disease in the course of his or her lifetime, will be higher than both incidence and prevalence. Table 1-1 shows the prevalence of some psychiatric disorders in Canada.

Clinical epidemiology is a broad field that addresses what happens after people with illnesses are seen by clinical care providers. Using traditional epidemiological methods, studies are conducted in groups usually defined by the illness or symptoms or by diagnostic procedures or treatments given to address the illness or symptoms. Clinical epidemiology includes the following:

- Studies of the natural history of an illness
- Studies of diagnostic screening tests
- Observational and experimental studies of interventions used to treat people with the illness or symptoms

Results of epidemiological studies are now routinely included in the *Diagnostic and Statistical Manual of Mental Disorders* (discussed below) to describe the frequency of mental disorders. Analysis of such studies can reveal the frequency with which psychological symptoms appear together with physical illness. For example, epidemiological studies demonstrate that depression is a significant risk factor for death in people with cardiovascular disease and for premature death in people with breast cancer.

CLASSIFICATION OF MENTAL DISORDERS

The Diagnostic and Statistical Manual

The first *Diagnostic and Statistical Manual of Mental Disorders (DSM)* was published by the American Psychiatric Association in 1952. Its purpose was to provide clinicians, educators, and researchers with a common framework to understand and communicate about mental disorders. With a common understanding about mental disorders, researchers and clinicians could work together in their attempts to improve care for people with mental illness.

Today, its fifth edition, the *DSM-5*, serves as the official guide for diagnosing psychiatric disorders. Listing more than 350 diagnoses, this authoritative manual was influenced by psychiatrists, psychologists, licensed clinical social workers, licensed counsellors, licensed marriage and family therapists, and advanced-practice psychiatric mental health nurses. Consistent with the purposes of previous editions, the *DSM-5* also serves as a tool for collecting epidemiological statistics about the diagnosis of psychiatric disorders.

A common misconception is that a classification of mental disorders classifies *people*, when actually the *DSM-5* classifies *disorders* people have. For this reason, the *DSM-5* and this textbook avoid the use of expressions such as "a schizophrenic" or "an

TABLE 1-1	MENTAL HEALTH PROFILE: PREVALENCE OF MENTAL ILLNESS AND INDICATORS (OVER 12 MONTHS)	
DISORDER	**PREVALENCE OVER 12 MONTHS (%)**	**COMMENTS**
Any mental illnesses (including substance use disorder)	10.1%	33.1% (lifetime prevalence)
Schizophrenia or psychosis	1.3%	Population aged 15 and over who reported that they have ever been diagnosed by a health professional with schizophrenia or psychosis.
Substance use disorder (alcohol or drug)	4.4%	21.6% lifetime prevalence
All mood disorders	7.8% (males 6%; females 9.6%)*	Leading cause of disability in Canada and established economies worldwide
Major depressive episode	4.7%	11.3% lifetime prevalence
Bipolar disorder	1.5%	2.6% lifetime prevalence
Generalized anxiety disorder	2.6%	8.7% lifetime prevalence. Can begin across life cycle; risk is highest between childhood and middle age
Panic disorder	0.7%	Typically develops in adolescence or early adulthood
Obsessive-compulsive disorder (OCD)	1.8%	Symptoms begin in childhood or adolescence
Post-traumatic stress disorder (PTSD)	1.7%	Current diagnosed condition
Eating disorders	0.4%	Current diagnosed condition
Attention deficit disorder	2.6%	Current diagnosed condition
Other		
Suicidal behaviour (not classified as a mental disorder but has significant impact on mental well-being, and people with mental illness are at higher risk for suicide)	11.5 per 100,000	Over 4000 suicides reported in Canada in 2013. Rates vary by population. The largest population of suicides in Canada are from men and women 45-59. The suicide rate for Inuit peoples living in Northern Canada is between 60 and 75 per 100,000 people, significantly higher than the general population.
Suicidal thoughts	3.3%	11.9% (lifetime)

Source: Statistics Canada. (2013). Mental health profile, Canadian Community Health Survey—Mental Health (CCHS), by age group and sex, Canada and provinces. Retrieved from http://www5.statcan.gc.ca/cansim/a26?id=1051101&retrLang=eng&lang=eng.
*Statistics Canada. (2017). Latest indicator tables: Mental health and well-being. Retrieved from http://www.statcan.gc.ca/tables-tableaux/sum-som/l01/ind01/l3_2966_2443-eng.htm?hili_health87.

alcoholic." Viewing the person as a person first and not an illness requires more accurate terms such as "an individual with schizophrenia" or "my patient has major depression."

The *DSM-5* Organizational Structure

The *DSM-5* (American Psychiatric Association, 2013) organizes diagnoses for psychiatric disorders on a developmental hierarchy, meaning that disorders that are usually seen in infancy, childhood, and adolescence are listed in the first chapter and neurodevelopmental disorders and disorders that occur later in life, such as the neurocognitive disorders, are further down the list. Also, within each chapter, specific disorders are listed based on the typical age of onset, from youngest to oldest. Diagnostic groups that are related to one another have been closely situated (for example, schizophrenia spectrum disorders are next to bipolar-related disorders, and feeding and eating disorders are next to elimination disorders).

- Neurodevelopmental disorder
- Schizophrenia spectrum disorder
- Bipolar and related disorders
- Depressive disorders
- Anxiety disorders
- Obsessive-compulsive disorders
- Trauma and stressor disorders
- Dissociative disorders
- Somatic symptom disorders
- Feeding and eating disorders
- Elimination disorders
- Sleep–wake disorders
- Sexual dysfunctions
- Gender dysphoria
- Disruptive, impulse control, and conduct disorders
- Substance and addictive disorders
- Neurocognitive disorders
- Personality disorders
- Paraphilias
- Other disorders

When making a diagnosis based on the *DSM-5*, clinicians and researchers need to consider presenting symptoms and how these symptoms are affecting the patient's life. Assessing the impact that the mental disorder is having on a person's day-to-day functioning requires the Disability Assessment Schedule 2.0, a tool developed by the WHO (see http://www.who.int/classifications/icf/whodasii/en/).

The *ICD-10-CA*

The *International Classification of Diseases (ICD)* (WHO, 2014b, 2016b) sets the global health information standard for mortality and morbidity statistics. Clinicians and researchers use this classification system to define diseases, study disease patterns, monitor outcomes, and subsequently allocate resources based on the prevalence of disease. The *ICD* is used globally and has been translated into 43 languages. An eleventh revision is expected in 2018.

The Canadian Institute for Health Information developed an enhanced version of the *ICD-10*, referred to as the *ICD-10-CA*. The *ICD-10-CA* goes beyond defining and classifying diseases to describe conditions and situations that are not diseases, including, for example, risk factors to health and psychosocial circumstances. Also, the *ICD-10-CA* better represents the social determinants of health than the *ICD-10* did. It has 23 categories of diseases, including diseases of the circulatory system, diseases of the nervous system, mental and behavioural disorders, certain conditions originating in the perinatal period, and factors influencing health status and contact with health services (Canadian Institute for Health Information, 2017). A complete listing of all *ICD-10-CA* chapters can be found at https://www.cihi.ca/en/submit-data-and-view-standards/codes-and-classifications/icd-10-ca.

PSYCHIATRIC MENTAL HEALTH NURSING

In all clinical settings, nurses work with people who are going through crises, including physical, psychological, mental, and spiritual distress. You will encounter patients who are experiencing feelings of hopelessness, helplessness, anxiety, anger, low self-esteem, or confusion. You will meet people who are withdrawn, suspicious, elated, depressed, hostile, manipulative, suicidal, intoxicated, or withdrawing from a substance. Many of you have already come across people who are going through difficult times in their lives. You may have handled these situations skillfully, but at other times, you may have wished you had additional skills and knowledge. Basic psychosocial nursing concepts will become central to your practice of nursing and increase your competency as a practitioner in all clinical settings. Whatever setting you choose to work in, you will have the opportunity to improve the lives of people who are experiencing mental illness as an additional challenge to their health.

Your experience in the mental health nursing rotation can help you gain insight into yourself and greatly increase your insight into the experiences of others. This part of your nursing education can also give you guidelines for and the opportunity to learn new skills for dealing with a variety of challenging behaviours. The following sections of this chapter present a brief overview of the work of professional psychiatric nurses, their scope of practice, and the challenges and evolving roles in the future health care environment.

What Is Psychiatric Mental Health Nursing?

Psychiatric mental health nurses enrich the health and well-being of Canadians (Canadian Federation of Mental Health Nurses, 2017). They work with people throughout the lifespan and assist healthy people who are in crisis or who are experiencing life problems, as well as those with long-term mental illness. Their patients may include people with concurrent disorders (i.e., a mental disorder and a coexisting substance disorder), homeless people and families, people in jail, individuals who have survived abusive situations, and people in crisis. Psychiatric mental health nurses work with individuals, couples, families, and groups in every nursing setting: in hospitals, in patients' homes, in halfway houses, in shelters, in clinics, in storefronts, on the street—virtually everywhere.

Uniquely, Canada has two bodies that provide standards of practice for mental health nursing. In the four western provinces and Yukon, registered psychiatric nurses follow the standards of practice issued by the Registered Psychiatric Nurses of Canada (RPNC). Registered nurses working in the specialty area of psychiatric mental health nursing follow the standards of practice issued by the Canadian Federation of Mental Health Nurses (CFMHN), an associate group of the Canadian Nurses Association (CNA).

Classification of Nursing Diagnoses, Outcomes, and Interventions

To provide the most appropriate and scientifically sound care, the psychiatric mental health nurse uses standardized classification systems developed by professional nursing groups. The *Nursing Diagnoses: Definitions and Classification 2012–2014* of the North American Nursing Diagnosis Association International (NANDA-I) (Herdman & Kamitsuru, 2014) provides 235 standardized diagnoses, more than 40% of which are related to psychosocial and psychiatric nursing care. These diagnoses provide a common language to aid in the selection of nursing interventions and ultimately lead to positive outcome achievement.

DSM-5– and NANDA-I–Approved Nursing Diagnoses

A nursing diagnosis is "a clinical judgment about individual, family, or community responses to actual or potential health problems and life processes" (Herdman & Kamitsuru, 2014, p. 25). A well-defined nursing diagnosis provides the framework for setting priorities and identifying appropriate nursing interventions for dealing with the patient's reaction to the disorder. Those reactions might include confusion, low self-esteem, impaired ability to function in job or family situations, and so on, differing from the diagnoses that are made based on the criteria contained within the *DSM-5* that are used to label the patient's disorder.

Appendix B lists NANDA-I–approved nursing diagnoses, and the individual clinical chapters offer suggestions for potential nursing diagnoses for the behaviours and phenomena often encountered in association with specific disorders.

Nursing Outcomes Classification (NOC)

The *Nursing Outcomes Classification (NOC)* provides "a comprehensive list of standardized outcomes, definitions, and measures to describe client outcomes influenced by nursing practice" (Moorhead, Johnson, Maas, et al., 2013). Outcomes are organized into seven domains: functional health, physiological health, psychosocial health, health knowledge and behaviour, perceived health, family health, and community health. The psychosocial health domain, which this text is most concerned with, includes four classes: psychological well-being, psychosocial adaptation, self-control, and social interaction.

Nursing Interventions Classification (NIC)

The *Nursing Interventions Classification (NIC)* is another tool used to standardize, define, and measure nursing care. Bulechek and colleagues (2013) define a nursing intervention as "any treatment, based upon clinical judgment and knowledge, that a nurse performs to enhance patient/client outcomes", including direct and indirect care through a series of nursing activities.

There are seven domains: basic physiological, complex physiological, behavioural, safety, family, health system, and community. Two domains relate specifically to psychiatric nursing: behavioural, including communication, coping, and education; and safety, covering crisis and risk management.

Evidence-Informed Practice

The nursing diagnosis classification systems mentioned have been researched extensively by nurses across a variety of treatment settings. They form a foundation for the novice or experienced nurse to participate in evidence-informed practice—that is, care based on the collection, interpretation, and integration of valid, important, and applicable patient-reported, clinician-observed, and research-derived evidence (Jakubec & Astle, 2017). In the chapters that follow, you will see examples of the application of these classifications to specific patients in vignettes and case studies, along with brief descriptions of other relevant research in the Research Highlight boxes, and evidence-informed practice description.

Levels of Psychiatric Mental Health Clinical Nursing Practice

Registered nurses in Canada may choose to work in psychiatric mental health nursing settings without additional certifications. However, many will choose to write the CNA's psychiatric/mental health nursing certification exam for the specialty. Registered psychiatric nurses (in the western provinces and Yukon) write national registration examinations.

Registered nurses and registered psychiatric nurses can further their education at a baccalaureate level or at the graduate level (master's, doctorate) and can become qualified to practise psychiatric mental health nursing at two levels—basic and advanced—depending on their educational preparation. Table 1-2 describes basic and advanced psychiatric nursing interventions.

Future Challenges and Roles for Psychiatric Mental Health Nurses

There has been a great demand for psychiatric mental health nurses, and indications suggest this need will increase in the future. Four significant trends that will affect the future of psychiatric mental health nursing in Canada are the aging population, increasing cultural diversity, expanding technology, and an increased awareness of the impact of health determinants on mental illness.

Aging Population

As the population of older adults grows, the prevalence of Alzheimer's disease and other dementias requiring the support of skilled and knowledgeable nurses will increase. Healthier older adults will need more services at home, in retirement communities, or in assisted-living facilities. For more information on the needs of older adults, refer to Chapters 17, 25, and 28.

Increasing Cultural Diversity

Cultural diversity is steadily increasing in Canada. Recent immigrants represent about 16% of Canada's population (Citizenship and Immigration Canada, 2012). These new Canadians add to and

TABLE 1-2	BASIC-LEVEL AND ADVANCED-PRACTICE PSYCHIATRIC MENTAL HEALTH NURSING INTERVENTIONS	
BASIC-LEVEL INTERVENTION	**DESCRIPTION**	
Coordination of care	Coordinates implementation of the nursing care plan and documents coordination of care	
Health teaching and health maintenance	Provides individualized anticipatory guidance to prevent or reduce mental illness or enhance mental health (e.g., community screenings, parenting classes, stress management)	
Milieu therapy	Provides, structures, and maintains a safe and therapeutic environment in collaboration with patients, families, and other health care clinicians	
Pharmacological, biological, and integrative therapies	Applies current knowledge to assessing patients' responses to medication, provides medication teaching, and communicates observations to other members of the health care team	
ADVANCED-PRACTICE INTERVENTION	**DESCRIPTION**	
All of the above plus:		
Medication prescription and treatment	Prescribes psychotropic medications, with appropriate use of diagnostic tests; has hospital admitting privileges	
Psychotherapy	Provides individual, couple, group, or family therapy using evidence-informed therapeutic frameworks	
Consultation	Shares clinical expertise with nurses or those in other disciplines to enhance their treatment of patients or address systems issues	

Source: Adapted from American Psychiatric Nurses Association, International Society of Psychiatric-Mental Health Nurses, & American Nurses Association. (2014). *Psychiatric-mental health nursing: Scope and standards of practice.* Silver Spring, MD: NurseBooks.org.

form an important part of our social, cultural, and economic institutions. Potential immigrants to Canada are required to undergo health screening; those who do not meet the requirements for health are denied entry to the country. It is important for nurses to know how immigrants may be affected by a mental illness. In the report *Mental Health and Well-Being of Recent Immigrants in Canada* (Citizenship and Immigration Canada, 2012), cases of depression and alcohol dependence were examined and compared between immigrant and Canadian-born populations. The rate of depression in the Canadian-born population was 2.5%, compared to 6.2% for immigrants. Immigrants, however, had lower rates of alcohol dependence: 0.5% compared to 2.5% for the Canadian-born population. The gap between the two groups increased for more recent immigrants than for those who had arrived earlier to Canada. Rates of depression and alcohol dependence for immigrants living in Canada for 10 to 14 years were on par with those of the Canadian-born population. Going forward, psychiatric mental health nurses will need to increase their cultural competence—that is, their sensitivity to different cultural views regarding health, illness, and response to treatment (see Chapter 8 for more on this topic).

Expanding Technology

Genetic mapping from the Human Genome Project has resulted in a steady stream of research discoveries concerning genetic markers implicated in a variety of psychiatric illnesses. This information could be helpful in identifying at-risk individuals and in targeting medications specific to certain genetic variants and profiles. However, the legal and ethical implications of responsibly using this technology are staggering and generate questions such as:
• Would you want to know you were at risk for a psychiatric illness like bipolar disorder?

• Who should have access to this information—your primary care provider, your future spouse, a lawyer in a child-custody battle?
• Who will regulate genetic testing centres to protect privacy and prevent twenty-first-century problems like identity theft and fraud?

Despite these concerns, discoveries and technology provide great promise in the diagnosis and treatment of psychiatric disorders, and nurses will be central as informed educators and caregivers.

Scientific advances through research and technology are certain to shape psychiatric mental health nursing practice. Magnetic resonance imaging (MRI) research, in addition to comparing healthy people to people diagnosed with mental illness, is now focusing on the development of preclinical profiles of children and adolescents. The hope of this type of research is to be able to identify people at risk for developing mental illness, thereby allowing earlier interventions to try to decrease impairment.

Electronic health care services provided from a distance are gaining wide acceptance. In the early days of the Internet, patients were cautioned against the questionable wisdom of seeking advice through an unregulated medium. However, the Internet has transformed the way we approach our health care needs. It is used liberally by young and old alike, with particularly strong associations found in mobile phone platform-based mental health alerts and tools (Whitton, Proudfoot, Clarke, et al., 2015). Internet-delivered mental health care has empowered people to advocate for themselves and explore health problems and options related to treatment.

Telepsychiatry, also known as telemedicine, has evolved over the past 20 years in an attempt to reach the population in rural and remote districts (25% of the Canadian population). Through the use of telepsychiatry, the mental health needs of these populations can be met with timely professional assessments and prescribed interventions (Lauckner & Whitten, 2016). In this practice, real-time consultations typically occur in health care facilities using a secured telecommunications connection to enable a psychiatric assessment or consultation.

Twelve Key Social Determinants of Health

Psychiatric mental health nurses use the social determinants of health to facilitate their practice. An ever-increasing body of evidence that addresses what Canadians need to be healthy suggests that spending more on the treatment of illness and disease will not actually improve a person's health (Public Health Agency of Canada, 2011). Rather, it is suggested that factors such as income, social status, and education directly affect the health of individuals and populations (Compton & Shim, 2015). Psychiatric mental health nurses will be required to address patient needs related to disease prevention and health promotion, which are identified through the assessment of the social determinants of health. Twelve key social determinants of health have

been identified. Each stands alone but is at the same time closely linked to the other determinants of health. The 12 determinants are as follows:

1. Income and social status
2. Social support networks
3. Education
4. Employment/working conditions
5. Social environments
6. Physical environments
7. Personal health practices and coping skills
8. Healthy child development
9. Biology and genetic endowment
10. Health services
11. Gender
12. Culture

For a brief explanation of each health determinant, see "Key Determinants" (Public Health Agency of Canada, 2011) at http://www.phac-aspc.gc.ca/ph-sp/determinants/index-eng .php#determinants.

▋ KEY POINTS TO REMEMBER

- Resilience is a process and outcome that supports people to navigate stressors and accompanying negative emotions and to negotiate resources in order to deal with the stressor and reactions. This process can be promoted and improved to strengthen supportive environments at individual and broader community and societal levels.
- Mental health and mental illness exist along two distinct but intersecting continua.
- Culture influences behaviour, and symptoms may reflect a person's cultural patterns or beliefs. Symptoms, therefore, must be understood in terms of a person's cultural background.
- The study of epidemiology can help identify high-risk groups and behaviours, which can lead to a better understanding of

the causes of some disorders. Incidence rates provide us with the number of new cases in a given period of time. Prevalence rates help us to identify the proportion of a population experiencing a specific mental disorder at a given time.
- Comorbid conditions are those disorders that occur at the same time as another condition. For example, a person with schizophrenia may also have comorbid diabetes, depression, and hypertension.
- Psychiatric mental health nurses work with a broad population of patients in diverse settings to promote optimal mental health.
- Due to social, cultural, scientific, and political factors, the future holds many challenges and possibilities for the psychiatric mental health nurse.

▋ CRITICAL THINKING

1. Amir, a 19-year-old first-year university student with a grade point average of 3.4, is brought to the emergency department after a suicide attempt. He has been extremely depressed since the death of his girlfriend 5 months previously, when the car he was driving crashed. His parents are devastated. They believe taking one's own life prevents a person from going to heaven. Amir has epilepsy and has had more seizures since the auto accident. He says he should be punished for his carelessness and does not care what happens to him. Over the past month, he has not been to school or shown up for his part-time job tutoring children in reading.
   a. What might be a possible NANDA-I nursing diagnosis for Amir? Before you plan your care, what are some other factors you would like to assess regarding aspects of Amir's

   overall health and other influences that can affect his mental health?
   b. Do you think that an antidepressant could help Amir through the grieving process? Why or why not? What additional care do you think Amir needs?
   c. Formulate at least two potential nursing interventions for Amir.
   d. Would the religious beliefs of Amir's parents factor into your plan of care? If so, how?
2. In a small study group, share experiences you have had with others from unfamiliar cultural, ethnic, religious, or racial backgrounds, and identify two positive learning experiences from these encounters.
3. Consider what it would be like working with a group of healthy women preparing for parenthood versus working with a group

of depressed women in a mental health clinic. What do you feel are the advantages and disadvantages of working with each group?

4. Would you feel comfortable referring a family member to a mental health clinician? What factors make you feel that way?

5. How do basic-level and advanced-practice psychiatric mental health nurses work together to provide the highest quality of care?

6. Would you consider joining a professional group or advocacy group that promotes mental health? Why or why not?

CHAPTER REVIEW

1. Resilience, the capacity to rebound from stressors via adaptive coping, is associated with positive mental health. Your friend has just been laid off from his job. Which of the following responses on your part would most likely contribute to his enhanced resilience?
   a. Using your connections to set up an interview with your employer
   b. Connecting him with a friend of the family who owns his own business
   c. Supporting him in arranging, preparing for, and completing multiple interviews
   d. Helping him to understand that the layoff resulted from troubles in the economy and is not his fault

2. Which of the following situations best supports the diathesis–stress model of mental illness development?
   a. The rate of suicide increases during times of national disaster and despair.
   b. A woman feels mildly anxious when asked to speak to a large group of people.
   c. A man with no prior mental health problems experiences sadness after his divorce.
   d. A man develops schizophrenia, but his identical twin remains free of mental illness.

3. Of the following statements about mental illness, identify all correct ones:
   a. About 20% of Canadians experience a mental disorder during their lifetime.
   b. Mental disorders and diagnoses occur very consistently across cultures.

   c. Most serious mental illnesses are psychological rather than biological in nature.
   d. The Mental Health Commission of Canada's report *Changing Directions, Changing Lives* outlines the mental health strategy for Canada.

4. Jane is a 32-year-old mother of four. She is active with her family and in her community despite having a diagnosis of severe anxiety. Refer to the mental health–mental illness continuum shown in Figure 1-2 and consider where you would place Jane.
   a. Optimal mental health with mental illness
   b. Optimal mental health without mental illness
   c. Poor mental health with mental illness
   d. Poor mental health without mental illness

5. Which of the following actions represent the primary focus of psychiatric nursing for a basic-level registered nurse? Select all that apply.
   a. Determining a patient's diagnosis according to the *DSM-5*
   b. Ordering diagnostic tests such as EEGs or MRI scans
   c. Identifying how a patient is coping with a symptom such as hallucinations
   d. Guiding a patient to learn and use a variety of stress-management techniques
   e. Helping a patient without personal transportation find a way to his or her treatment appointments
   f. Collecting petition signatures seeking the removal of stigmatizing images on television

Post-Test | interactive review

⊖volve WEBSITE

Visit the Evolve website for Chapter Review Answers and Rationales, Critical Thinking Answer Guidelines, and additional resources related to the content in this chapter: http://evolve.elsevier.com/Canada/Varcarolis/psychiatric/

REFERENCES

Abi-Rached, J. M. (2008). The implications of the new brain sciences: The "Decade of the Brain" is over but its effects are now becoming visible as neuropolitics and neuroethics, and in the emergence of neuroeconomies. *EMBO Reports, 9*(12), 1158–1162. doi:10.1038/embor.2008.211.

American Psychiatric Association (2013). *Diagnostic and statistical manual of mental disorders* (5th ed.). Arlington, VA: American Psychiatric Publishing.

Bulechek, G. M., Butcher, H. K., Dochterman, J. M., et al. (Eds.), (2013). *Nursing Interventions Classification (NIC)* (6th ed.). St. Louis, MO: Mosby.

Burstow, B. (2015). *Psychiatry and the business of madness: An ethical and epistemological accounting.* New York: Palgrave Macmillan.

Burstow, B., LeFrançois, B. A., & Diamond, S. (2014). *Psychiatry disrupted: Theorizing resistance and crafting the (r)evolution.* Montreal: McGill-Queen's University Press.

Canadian Federation of Mental Health Nurses. (2017). *Professional practices.* Retrieved from http://cfmhn.ca/professionalPractices.

Canadian Institute for Health Information. (2009). *Improving the health of Canadians: Exploring positive mental health.* Retrieved from https://www.cihi.ca/en/improving_health_canadians_en.pdf.

Canadian Institute for Health Information. (2017). *International statistical classification of diseases and related health problems, 10th revision, Canada.* Retrieved from https://www.cihi.ca/en/submit-data-and-view-standards/codes-and-classifications/icd-10-ca.

Canadian Mental Health Association (CMHA). (2016). *History of CMHA.* Retrieved from http://www.cmha.ca/about-cmha/history-of-cmha/#.WO3Pj_nyt0w.

Citizenship and Immigration Canada. (2012). *Mental health and well-being of recent immigrants in Canada: Evidence from the Longitudinal Survey of Immigrants to Canada.* Retrieved from http://www.cic.gc.ca/english/pdf/research-stats/mental-health.pdf.

Compton, M. T., & Shim, R. S. (2015). *The social determinants of mental health* (1st ed.). Arlington, VA: American Psychiatric Association Publishing.

Cowan, W. M., Kopnisky, K. L., & Hyman, S. E. (2002). The human genome project and its impact on psychiatry. *Annual Review of Neuroscience, 25*(1), 1–50. doi:10.1146/annurev.neuro.25.112701.142853.

Epp, J. (1988). *Mental Health for Canadians: Striking a Balance.* Ottawa: Minister of National Health and Welfare.

Gaebel, W., Rössler, W., & Sartorius, N. (2017). *The stigma of mental illness: End of the story?* Cham, Switzerland: Springer.

Herdman, T. H., & Kamitsuru, S. (Eds.), (2014). *NANDA International nursing diagnoses: Definitions and classification, 2014–2017.* Oxford, UK: Wiley-Blackwell.

Jakubec, S. L., & Astle, B. J. (2017). *Research literacy for health and community practice.* Toronto: Canadian Scholars' Press.

Lauckner, C., & Whitten, P. (2016). The state and sustainability of telepsychiatry programs. *The Journal of Behavioral Health Services & Research, 43*(2), 305–318. doi:10.1007/s11414-015-9461-z.

Mental Health Commission of Canada. (2009). *Toward recovery & well-being: A framework for a mental health strategy for Canada.* Retrieved from http://www.mentalhealthcommission.ca/SiteCollectionDocuments/boarddocs/15507_MHCC_EN_final.pdf.

Mental Health Commission of Canada. (2012). *Changing directions, changing lives: The mental health strategy for Canada.* Retrieved from strategy.mentalhealthcommission.ca/pdf/strategy-images-en.pdf.

Mental Health Commission of Canada (2015). Recovery guidelines. Ottawa, ON: Author. Retrieved from http://www.mentalhealthcommission.ca/sites/default/files/2016-07/MHCC_Recovery_Guidelines_2016_ENG.PDF.

Mental Health Commission of Canada. (2017). *Advancing the mental health strategy for Canada: A framework for action 2017–2022.* Retrieved from http://www.mentalhealthcommission.ca/sites/default/files/2016-08/advancing_the_mental_health_strategy_for_canada_a_framework_for_action.pdf.

Menzies, R. J., Reaume, G., & LeFrançois, B. A. (2013). *Mad matters: A critical reader in Canadian mad studies.* Toronto: Canadian Scholars' Press.

Moorhead, S., Johnson, M., Maas, M. L., et al. (Eds.), (2013). *Nursing outcomes classification (NOC)* (5th ed.). St. Louis, MO: Mosby.

Morgan, C., McKenzie, K., & Fearon, P. (2008). *Society and psychosis.* Cambridge, UK: Cambridge University Press.

Nolan, P. (1993). *A history of mental health nursing.* New York: Chapman and Hall.

Porter, N. (Ed.), (1913). *Webster's revised unabridged dictionary.* Boston: Merriam.

Public Health Agency of Canada. (2011). *Determinants of health: What makes Canadians healthy or unhealthy.* Ottawa: Author. Retrieved from http://www.phac-aspc.gc.ca/ph-sp/determinants/index-eng.php#determinants.

Public Health Agency of Canada. (2014). *Mental health promotion.* Retrieved from http://www.phac-aspc.gc.ca/mh-sm/mhp-psm/index-eng.php.

Public Health Agency of Canada. (2015a). *Chronic diseases: Mental illness.* Retrieved from http://www.phac-aspc.gc.ca/cd-mc/mi-mm/index-eng.php.

Public Health Agency of Canada. (2015b). *Report from the Canadian Chronic Disease Surveillance System: Mental illness in Canada, 2015.* Retrieved from https://www.canada.ca/content/dam/canada/health-canada/migration/healthy-canadians/publications/diseases-conditions-maladies-affections/mental-illness-2015-maladies-mentales/alt/mental-illness-2015-maladies-mentales-eng.pdf.

Rosen, A., Goldbloom, D., & McGeorge, P. (2010). Mental health commissions: Making the critical difference to the development and reform of mental health services. *Current Opinion in Psychiatry, 23*(6), 593.

Scull, A. (2014). *Cultural sociology of mental illness: An A-to-Z guide.* Thousand Oaks, CA: SAGE Reference.

Siegel, D. J. (2015). Interpersonal neurobiology as a lens into the development of wellbeing and resilience. *Children Australia, 40*(2), 160–164. doi:10.1017/cha.2015.7.

Stern, T. A., Freudenreich, O., Smith, F. A., et al. (2017). *Handbook of general hospital psychiatry* (7th ed.). Philadelphia: Elsevier.

Uher, R. (2014). Gene–environment interactions in common mental disorders: An update and strategy for a genome-wide search. *Social Psychiatry and Psychiatric Epidemiology, 49*(1), 3–14. doi:10.1007/s00127-013-0801-0.

Ungar, M. (2015). Social ecological complexity and resilience processes. *The Behavioral and Brain Sciences, 38*, e124. doi:10.1017/S0140525X14001721.

Ungar, T., Knaak, S., & Szeto, A. C. (2016). Theoretical and practical considerations for combating mental illness stigma in health care. *Community Mental Health Journal, 52*(3), 262–271. doi:10.1007/s10597-015-9910-4.

Whitton, A. E., Proudfoot, J., Clarke, J., et al. (2015). Breaking open the black box: Isolating the most potent features of a web and mobile phone-based intervention for depression, anxiety, and stress. *JMIR Mental Health, 2*(1), e3. doi:10.2196/mental.3573.

World Health Organization (WHO). (2014a). *Mental health: A state of well-being.* Retrieved from http://www.who.int/features/factfiles/mental_health/en/.

World Health Organization (WHO) (2014b). *ICD 10: International Statistical Classification of Diseases and Related Health Problems (10th rev.): Instruction Manual* (2nd ed., Vol. 1). Geneva, Switzerland: Author. Retrieved from https://www.cdc.gov/nchs/data/dvs/2e_volume1_2014.pdf.

World Health Organization (WHO). (2016a). *Mental health: Strengthening our response (Fact sheet no. 220).* Retrieved from http://www.who.int/mediacentre/factsheets/fs220/en/.

World Health Organization (WHO). (2016b). *ICD 10: 2016 version.* Retrieved from http://apps.who.int/classifications/icd10/browse/2016/en.

Historical Overview of Psychiatric Mental Health Nursing

Sonya L. Jakubec

KEY TERMS AND CONCEPTS

advanced-practice nursing (APN)
asylums
Canadian Federation of Mental Health Nurses
custodial care
deinstitutionalization
Dorothea Dix

moral treatment
Philippe Pinel
Registered Psychiatric Nurses of Canada
Weir Report
William Tuke

OBJECTIVES

1. Identify the sociopolitical, economic, cultural, and religious factors that influenced the development of psychiatric mental health nursing.
2. Summarize the influence of psychiatric treatment trends on the role of the nurse.
3. Identify the factors that led to the separate designations of registered nurse and registered psychiatric nurse.
4. Analyze the factors that have enhanced and delayed the professionalization of psychiatric mental health nursing.
5. Consider the future potentials and challenges for psychiatric mental health nursing in Canada.

℮volve WEBSITE

Visit the Evolve website for Flashcards, Case Studies, and additional testing resources related to the content in this chapter: http://evolve.elsevier.com/Canada/Varcarolis/psychiatric/

Pre-Test   interactive review

Exploring the history of nursing in Canada, and specifically of psychiatric mental health nursing, can enrich our understanding of the factors that have shaped the profession in the past and that will shape it in the future. Throughout history, the evolution of the role of nursing has been affected by sociopolitical, economic, cultural, medical, and religious trends in Canada and around the world. Although there has been much historical analysis of psychiatric mental health nursing in England, Holland, and the United States, Canadian nursing historians have only recently focused on the mental health field (see, for example, Boschma, 2012; Hicks, 2011; Smith & Khanlou, 2013). For many reasons, it is a convoluted history, unique to Canada and separate from that of generalist registered nursing. Understanding this history provides us with insights into the past challenges and accomplishments

of psychiatric mental health nursing and prepares us for the continuing development of the role and further advanced-practice nursing.

EARLY MENTAL ILLNESS CARE

Trends in approaches to the treatment of mental illness have significantly contributed to the emergence and evolution of the role of psychiatric nursing. These trends stem largely from societal values, politics, culture, and economics.

Asylums, designed to be retreats from society, were built with the hope that, with early intervention and several months of rest, people with mental illness could be cured (Weir, 1932). Eighth-century Middle Eastern Islamic societies such as those in Baghdad and Cairo established the first asylums (Youssef, Youssef, & Dening, 1996). Even that early, these treatment centres, guided by Islamic beliefs, provided a compassionate and peaceful environment in which to care for people with mental illnesses. In medieval Western Europe, however, strong religious influences inspired the belief that mental illness indicated demonic possession or sin. Unfortunately, mentally ill people without protective support systems were commonly subjected to torture or isolation from the community (Cellard & Thifault, 2006). By the fifteenth century, several asylums had been built across Europe, but attitudes had not evolved much. Patients in these settings were often chained or caged, and cruelty or neglect was not uncommon (Digby, 1983). This type of treatment reflected the societal view that people with mental illness were bestial or less human in nature and, therefore, required discipline and were immune to human discomforts such as hunger or cold (Digby, 1983).

In the late 1700s, Philippe Pinel, a French physician, along with other humanitarians, began to advocate for more humane treatment of people with mental illness by literally removing the chains of the patients, talking to them, and providing a calmer, soothing environment. Pinel and another reformer from England, William Tuke, described this use of social and psychological approaches to treatment as "moral treatment" (Digby, 1983). Critics such as French philosopher Michel Foucault argued that the asylum movement was little more than a shift from physical restraint to psychological and social control of people considered undesirable by societal norms (Foucault, 1971). Regardless, this revolutionary way of treating people with mental illness swept across Europe and influenced the design of early asylums in North America.

In Canada, the country's size, location, and history have played a significant part in how people with mental illness are treated. Indigenous peoples in Canada had a variety of approaches to caring for people with mental illness. Most were holistic—treating mind, body, and soul—and included sweat lodges, animistic charms, potlatch, and Sundance (Kirkmayer, Brass, & Tait, 2000). In the sixteenth century, colonial settlers from France and, later, England brought with them their own approaches to mental illness care. As in their European homelands, much of the responsibility of caring for people with mental illness fell on the family and the asylums established in the communities (Cellard & Thifault, 2006). Some Canadian religious orders, such as the Grey Nuns, were early providers of care for people with mental illness (Hardill, 2006). Those who could not be cared for in the community, however, often ended up in jails, where they received minimal shelter at best and abuse at worst (Moran, 1998). By the 1800s, migration to Canada increased, as did its urbanization. This relocation of families to cities or isolated settlements changed support systems and families' ability to care for people with mental illness (Cellard & Thifault, 2006). In Europe, the move to asylum care was well under way, and the Canadian colonies began to explore similar options.

Early Canadian Asylums

Beauport, the first asylum in what would soon become Canada, was opened in Quebec in 1845 (Sussman, 1998). Soon, more asylums were established in Upper and Lower Canada, the

Maritime colonies, and Canada's West. Despite the creation of asylums, early historical records demonstrate that most families of people with a mental illness maintained the care of those individuals themselves (Cellard & Thifault, 2006), so the asylums predominantly housed patients who were poor and had no family support. Many asylums were built in countrylike settings on large parcels of land that could provide opportunity for occupational therapies such as farming. Toward the end of the nineteenth century, asylum care became more acceptable, and, with family support systems becoming diluted due to urbanization and relocation, the inpatient population grew exponentially (Cellard & Thifault, 2006). Although the moral treatment era had moved psychiatric treatment toward more humane treatment, the lack of success in treating mental illnesses combined with increased admissions to asylums led to overcrowding and less than humane conditions in many asylums. In most settings, a large population of people received only minimal custodial care—assistance with performing the basic daily necessities of life, such as dressing, eating, using a toilet, walking, and so on.

This situation caught the attention of many social reformers who, in the late nineteenth and early twentieth centuries, lobbied governments to create more humane environments of care for people with mental illness. Among them was Dorothea Dix, a retired schoolteacher from New England who became the superintendent of nurses during the American Civil War. Dix was educated in the asylum reform movements in England while she was there recuperating from tuberculosis. In 1841, during an encounter at a Boston jail, Dix was shocked to witness the degrading treatment of a woman with mental illness who was imprisoned there. Passionate about social reform, Dix began advocating for the improved treatment and public care of people with mental illness. She met with many politicians and even the Pope to push her agenda forward. Ultimately, she was influential

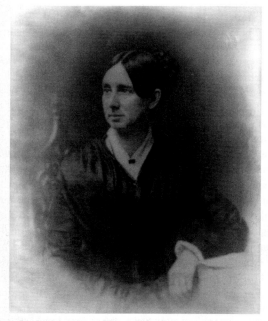

Dorothea Dix, advocate, 1802–1887. Source: Library of Congress Prints and Photographs Division. Washington, DC, 20540, USA.

in lobbying for the first public mental hospital in the United States and for reform in British and Canadian institutions.

EARLY PSYCHIATRIC TREATMENTS

By the end of the nineteenth century, the new field of psychiatry was being challenged to provide a medical cure for mental illness. Since there were few medications available other than heavily alcohol-based sedatives, doctors used many experimental treatments—for example, leeching (using bloodsucking worms), spinning (tying the patient to a chair and spinning it for hours), hydrotherapy (forced baths), and insulin shock treatment (injections of large doses of insulin to produce daily comas over several weeks). In the mid-twentieth century, treatment choices expanded to include electroconvulsive therapy (see Chapter 13) and lobotomies, through which nerve fibres in the frontal lobe were severed. As treatments became more invasive, the need for patient monitoring beyond custodial care led many medical superintendents to recruit nurses to work in their institutions.

THE INTRODUCTION OF NURSES TO ASYLUM CARE

In Canada, prior to the late 1800s, there were no nurses working in psychiatric settings; instead, asylums used predominantly male attendants to provide custodial care for patients. Changes in treatment approaches and the increased medicalization of psychiatry prompted a need for more specially trained providers, especially for female patients (Connor, 1996). In 1888, Rockwood Asylum in Kingston, Ontario, became the first psychiatric institution in Canada to open a training program for nurses (Kerrigan, 2011). The 2-year program was overseen by the asylum's medical director and included one lecture a week combined with work experience training. The curriculum, taught by physicians, included courses in physiology, anatomy, nursing care of the sick, and nursing care of the insane (Legislature of the Province of Ontario, 1889). Consistent with societal beliefs of the time about women's innate caring capacity, the training was offered only to females. This exclusion of males from the program hindered the recognition of the importance of nursing knowledge and skills and lowered the status of male attendants at the time (Yonge, Boschma, & Mychajlunow, 2005). Both of these factors would greatly affect the future development of psychiatric mental health nursing in Canada.

Asylum-based training schools opened across Canada, and the training curriculum, similar to that of the hospital-based programs of generalist nurses, varied among institutions. Medical superintendents controlled the content and delivery of the programs, and hospital administrators valued highly the inexpensive labour provided by the female workforce, so much so that their cross-training in other medical settings was discouraged so as to maintain staffing supplies (Tipliski, 2004). The asylum-based programs were founded heavily on a medical model of training nurses to be obedient, orderly, and focused on the discipline of the inpatients (Cowles, 1916). Nursing duties at the beginning of the twentieth century often included extensive cleaning, serving meals, counting cutlery after meals, and assisting

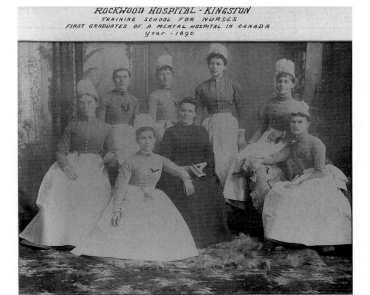

First graduating class of Rockwood Asylum Nursing School, Kingston, Ontario, 1890. Source: Providence Care Archives, http://providencecarearchives.files.wordpress.com/2011/03/image2011-03-24-102507-1.jpg.

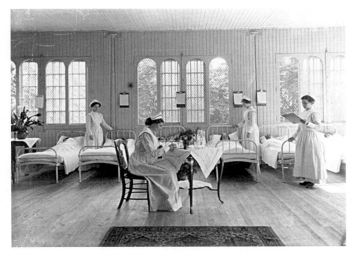

Nurses at Toronto Hospital for the Insane in 1910. Source: RG 10-276-2-0-8. Ministry of Health. Queen Street Mental Health Centre miscellaneous historical materials. Queen Street Mental Health Centre miscellaneous photographs. Female infirmary at the Hospital for the Insane, Toronto, ca. 1910. Archives of Ontario, I0018987.

patients with hygiene activities, as well as administering treatments such as the long baths referred to as "hydrotherapy," sedation with alcohol, and postoperative care (Forchuk & Tweedell, 2001). Nurses also played a key role in the care of patients in the infirmary. The custodial environment of asylums did not promote a sense of professional knowledge for nurses and limited their ability to question the treatment approaches being offered at the time (Leishman, 2005). Societal trends for women in the workforce reinforced nurses' lack of power in controlling their education programs and work environments (Anthony & Landeen, 2009).

SHIFTS IN CONTROL OVER NURSING

In the early part of the twentieth century, nurses' lack of control over their own profession began to shift with changes to nursing education models and blossoming political advocacy by nursing groups across Canada, particularly with the formation of the Canadian National Association of Trained Nurses in 1908. This early group expanded, and by 1926 each province had an affiliate group and the organization was renamed the Canadian Nurses Association (CNA). The CNA provided a united voice for nurses and increased advocacy for control over nursing by nurses (Canadian Nurses Association, 2011a). At this time, nursing training programs still varied by institution, but many had long hours of hospital ward service taking precedence over instructional hours for students. The CNA's mandate included the profession-alization of nursing, so it began to advocate for standardization of nursing education (Tipliski, 2004). This was a politically loaded issue for several reasons: physicians wanted control over nursing education, patriarchal society structures devalued nursing knowledge, nursing skills were seen as natural women's work, and hospitals relied on the economical service hours of nursing students (Anthony & Landeen, 2009). Some vocal physicians expressed concerns that giving nurses too much education may lead to their disobedience and boredom (Kirkwood, 2005).

In 1927, the Canadian Medical Association and the Canadian Nurses Association performed a joint study on the state of nursing education in Canada. The result, known as the "Weir Report," was released in 1932 and concluded that drastic changes were needed in nursing education programs, including standardization of curriculum, work hours, and instructor training, and that care of people with mental illnesses needed to be integrated into all generalist programs (Fleming, 1932). The uptake of the recommendations varied across Canada and even within regions. Since psychiatric hospitals and asylums had a harder time recruiting nurses, the idea of giving up their workforce so that students could complete an affiliation in general hospital settings was considered very costly. The medical superintendent psychiatrists were protective of their asylum-based training programs, which they felt developed specialized skills compared to general nursing skills (Tipliski, 2004). They argued that a 3- to 6-month affiliation in psychiatry was too short to learn the skills required in their institutions.

At the time, provincial legislation in the form of nursing acts was coming into existence and further formalizing the title and licensure of the registered nurse. There were provincial differences in government-legislated power over licensure and nursing education as well as variable interest in psychiatric training by provincial nursing associations (Tipliski, 2004). This, combined with the political influence of some medical superintendents from provincial psychiatric hospitals, led registered nursing associations in Manitoba, Saskatchewan, Alberta, and British Columbia to be less inclusive of the psychiatric hospital–trained nurse than the associations in Eastern Canada were, which in turn led to the exclusion of registered nurse licensure for graduates of asylum programs. This division of perspectives eventually resulted in a split between Western and Eastern Canada in training programs and the creation in the western provinces of the specialty-focused psychiatric nursing training programs and the registered psychiatric nurse designation.

 RESEARCH HIGHLIGHT

An Analysis of Canadian Psychiatric Mental Health Nursing History and Possibilities

Problem
Given the need for increased accessibility to mental health care and treatment, there is a need to understand the circumstances of nurses with regards to occupational stress and barriers to advanced education in mental health nursing.

Purpose of Study
This study sought to compile a more complete analysis of what current Canadian mental health nursing looks like, considering important issues facing nurses regarding history, gender, education, and quality of work life.

Methods
An integrative review and historical analysis of existing literature was undertaken using a critical and gendered sociological lens.

Key Findings
Fourteen articles were selected, which provided a partial reflection of contemporary Canadian psychiatric mental health nursing. Findings included the identification of an association between gender and professional status, inconsistencies in psychiatric nursing education, and the limitations for Canadian nurse practitioners to advance the role of the psychiatric mental health nurse practitioner at this time.

Implications for Nursing Practice
The authors recommend facilitating advanced education in mental health so that people within primary care settings can benefit from the knowledge and expertise of nurses with additional mental health education. Additional educational opportunities for psychiatric nurses who wish to become advanced nurse practitioners and to prescribe psychiatric treatments or medications are encouraged. Partnerships are recommended for provincial and national nursing bodies to foster national standards and regulation for psychiatric mental health nursing education and bridging programs.

Source: Smith, M., & Khanlou, N. (2013). An analysis of Canadian psychiatric mental health nursing through the junctures of history, gender, nursing education, and quality of work life in Ontario, Manitoba, Alberta, and Saskatchewan. *ISRN Nursing.* Retrieved from http://pubmedcentralcanada.ca/pmcc/articles/PMC3655684/.

Eastern and Atlantic Canada

From the outset, the Registered Nurses' Association of Ontario (RNAO) accepted the asylum-based programs for licensing of prospective nurses who were affiliated with a general hospital (Tipliski, 2004). It also represented nurses working in asylum settings, providing them with advocacy and nursing leadership (Tipliski, 2004). With the support of nurse leaders like Nettie Fiddler and the publication of the Weir Report, more generalist hospital programs began adding a psychiatry rotation to the curriculum. Also influential in the addition of a psychiatry rotation was the RNAO addressing the nursing shortage in psychiatric settings and the care concerns of mentally ill patients at the organization's 1945 annual meeting (Tipliski, 2004). At this point, many psychiatric hospitals had large numbers of patients, inadequate staffing, and minimal enrollment of new students (Tipliski, 2004). The advocacy of nurse leaders, combined with the post–World War II mental hygiene movement, led to the addition of psychiatric nursing theory for all registered nurse education programs (Tipliski, 2004). Some asylum programs added training in general medical settings; however, by the 1950s, all of the psychiatric hospital training programs in Eastern Canada had closed. Nurses in psychiatric mental health were trained as generalist registered nurses with affiliations in psychiatry and the chance to specialize after graduation.

Western Canada

In the western provinces, where the population was much smaller and asylums were located in rural settings, recruiting an adequate labour force was a major concern. In the early 1900s, British Columbia, Alberta, Saskatchewan, and Manitoba attempted different approaches to training nurses for psychiatric settings. Selkirk, Manitoba, opened the first asylum training school in Western Canada in 1920, followed closely by Brandon, Manitoba, in 1921 (Hicks, 2011). Manitoba implemented several combination programs between general hospitals and psychiatric hospitals, but similar attempts at other institutions in the western provinces failed due to lack of investment from administrators and nurse leadership groups and difficulty enticing nurses to remain in the psychiatric settings after their graduation (Hicks, 2011; Tipliski, 2004).

In the 1930s, Saskatchewan's two provincial psychiatric hospitals began a training program for their attendants. Unlike in the rest of Canada, this training was offered to both male and female attendants and, upon completion, gave graduates the title "nursing attendant" (Tipliski, 2004). However, the specialized training did not bestow upon graduates any professional title or licensure, so several attendants lobbied for the creation of the designation "psychiatric nurse." The movement for the designation of psychiatric nurse was supported by medical superintendents, unions, and politicians at the time, so despite opposition by provincial nursing leaders, the *Registered Psychiatric Nurses Act* was enacted in Saskatchewan in 1948 (Tipliski, 2004). This step toward professionalization of the role of the nurse in psychiatric hospitals was soon adopted by other western provinces. At the same time, the Saskatchewan Registered Nurses' Association's leader, Kathryn Ellis, was also trying to address the nursing shortage in mental hospitals by convincing provincial hospitals to become more involved in training, but she was unable to negotiate satisfactory psychiatric or general hospital affiliations (Hicks, 2011; Tipliski, 2004).

Much of the professionalization movement was facilitated by the Canadian Council of Psychiatric Nurses (CCPN), an interprovincial organization of psychiatric nurses focused on increasing the standards and recognition of psychiatric nurse training (Hicks, 2011). The CCPN, along with the efforts of provincial psychiatrists, was successful in advocating for the registered psychiatric nurse specialty designation across the western provinces; subsequently, British Columbia passed its psychiatric nurses act in 1951, Alberta followed in 1955, and Manitoba followed in 1960. To date, the separate designation has remained, although the CCPN evolved first into Registered Psychiatric Nurses of Canada and now is Registered Psychiatric Nurse Regulators of Canada (RPNRC). The organization has more than 5 600 practising members (Registered Psychiatric Nurse Regulators of Canada, 2017a), resulting in both registered nurses and registered psychiatric nurses working in psychiatric mental health settings in the four western provinces and Yukon.

DEINSTITUTIONALIZATION AND THE NURSING ROLE IN PSYCHIATRIC MENTAL HEALTH CARE

Psychiatric nursing continued to take place predominantly in hospital settings until the 1960s, when deinstitutionalization—the shift from caring for people with mental illness in institutions to caring for them in communities—began, significantly changing the role of the nurse. (See Chapter 3 for further discussion of deinstitutionalization.) The "pioneer" community mental health nurses set up many programs and frameworks for the delivery of psychiatric mental health care in the community (Boschma, 2012). The wide range of community-based mental health services that eventually developed (e.g., crisis management, consultation-liaison, primary care psychiatry) created new settings and skill requirements for psychiatric mental health nurses. The ability to assess and monitor clients and their environment changed nursing approaches toward mental health care. Assessment, autonomy, collaboration, crisis management, and resource finding became key skills for community-based nurses.

UNIVERSITY-BASED NURSING CURRICULUM

In 1919, the University of British Columbia (UBC) launched the first university-based program in nursing. The program was a "sandwich model," with 3 years of hospital-based nursing sandwiched between the first and final years of university studies (Anthony & Landeen, 2009). At the time, the idea of a university program for nursing was considered so risky that UBC refused to fund or administer the middle years of the program. A leader in nursing education at the time, E. Kathleen Russell at the University of Toronto, supported by the Rockefeller Foundation, set up one of the first university-based training programs in public health nursing, leadership, and education. This revolutionary postdiploma certification program for registered nurses was attended internationally. Later, in 1928, Russell coordinated the first solely university-based nursing program at the University of Toronto; in 1942, it began granting bachelor of science degrees in nursing (BScN) (University of Toronto, 2011). These university programs initiated a critical change in nursing education: for the first time, education for nurses was separated from and prioritized over their service in the hospitals (Anthony & Landeen, 2009). Despite this revolution in nursing education, nursing programs remained under the control of medical faculties until 1962, when the University of Montreal set up the first independent nursing faculty (Anthony & Landeen, 2009).

Many other Canadian universities began to offer diploma programs in specialty areas such as public health. In the 1950s, the University of Saskatchewan became the first to offer a 1-year post–registered nurse training diploma in advanced psychiatric nursing (University of Saskatchewan, 2011). The inception of university education for nurses led to the growth and formalization of nursing knowledge. The University of Western Ontario launched Canada's first graduate program in nursing in 1959, and the first PhD program in nursing began at the University of Alberta in 1991. The growth of graduate programs gave rise to increased research and theory in psychiatric nursing practice. The influence of nurse theorists such as American Hildegard Peplau, the first published nursing theorist since Florence Nightingale, contributed to the expansion of specialized nursing knowledge and related skills in the psychiatric mental health field. Much of Peplau's work focused on the role of the nurse in therapeutic relationships and anxiety management. The growth of academic study in nursing, in turn, influenced nursing in the practice setting: the Hamilton Psychiatric Hospital became the first health care institution in Canada to employ a clinical nurse specialist and to require theory-based nursing practice (Forchuk & Tweedell, 2001).

Currently, entry-to-practice mental health and addiction competencies for undergraduate nursing education in Canada have been established by the Canadian Association of Schools of Nursing and Canadian Federation of Mental Health Nurses (CASN & CFMHN, 2015). The CFMHN (2016) recommends that the curricula of all undergraduate nursing programs in Canada include entry-to-practice mental health and addiction competencies in both theoretical knowledge and clinical practice. The CFMHN recommends delivering mental health and addiction core competencies through a designated (stand-alone) theory course and a dedicated clinical experience. Regardless of pedagogical method, the obligatory outcome for undergraduate nurses is a strong knowledge base in mental health and addiction as outlined in the CFMHN practice standards (CFMHN, 2016). This body of core competency work and the nursing mandate to meet goals of key focus areas of the national mental health strategy (Mental Health Commission of Canada, 2017) are enhanced by growing nursing research. Nursing research in mental health continues to expand through the works of nurse researchers such as Bernie Pauly, Cheryl Forchuk, David Holmes, Kristin Cleverley, Cheryl L. Pollard, Nicole Letourneau, and Kimberley Ryan-Nicholls.

In Western Canada, over the past 25 years, the shift to the role of the registered psychiatric nurse and the increased range of practice settings (i.e., away from inpatient facilities and into primary care and community-based clinics) have also brought about changes in educational programs. Registered psychiatric nursing programs have adjusted to ensure diversification of skills and knowledge base related to consumer-oriented primary health care and health promotion activities (Ryan-Nicholls, 2004). Registered psychiatric nurse training continued to be diploma-based across the western provinces until 1995, when Brandon University began its baccalaureate program in psychiatric mental health nursing. Registered Psychiatric Nurses of Canada (RPNC) issued a position statement in 2012 advocating for baccalaureate degree entry to practice for registered psychiatric nurses due to the increasingly complex needs and roles of the registered psychiatric nurse (RPNC, 2012). The RPNC earlier issued a position statement on the need for graduate programs for registered psychiatric nurses that could help foster the professional development, research, and clinical training of baccalaureate registered psychiatric nursing students (RPNC, 2008). The first graduate program in psychiatric nursing for registered psychiatric nurses began at Brandon University in January 2011.

NATIONAL ORGANIZATIONS FOR PSYCHIATRIC MENTAL HEALTH NURSING AND CANADIAN NURSES ASSOCIATION CERTIFICATION

The division of Eastern and Western Canada in psychiatric nursing training and designation resulted in separate organizational groups. Although having multiple organizations has led to some duplication and fragmentation of a voice for nurses in psychiatric settings, the groups have also worked collaboratively toward common goals. Since 1995, the CNA has offered registered nurses certification in psychiatric mental health nursing (CNA, 2011b). Under the umbrella of the CNA and with consumer input, the Canadian Federation of Mental Health Nurses, an organization of registered nurses across Canada who specialize in psychiatric mental health nursing, established the standards of practice for psychiatric mental health nursing, now in a fourth edition (see http://cfmhn.ca/professionalPractices). The 2014 Standards for Psychiatric Mental Health Nursing build on the Canadian Nurses Association Code of Ethics (CNA, 2008a). Despite the separations in licensure and professional bodies, in workplaces in Western Canada, registered nurses and registered psychiatric nurses work closely together in mental health settings and have much opportunity for collaboration and advocacy for the people they serve.

ADVANCED-PRACTICE NURSING IN PSYCHIATRIC MENTAL HEALTH CARE

Advanced-practice nursing (APN) includes the roles of nurse practitioner and clinical nurse specialist (CNA, 2008b). Each province has its own regulations guiding the licensing and scope of practice for APN. The clinical nurse specialist (CNS) role has been well established in psychiatry since 1972, when Hamilton Psychiatric Hospital employed Pat Barry, a nurse with a graduate degree, to educate staff and increase theoretical-based nursing practice (Forchuk & Tweedell, 2001). CNSs can provide psychotherapy and have worked as consultants, educators, and clinicians in inpatient and outpatient psychiatry throughout Canada. Nurse practitioners, on the other hand, work as consultants or collaborative team members and can diagnose, prescribe and manage medications, and provide psychotherapy. While the role of psychiatric nurse practitioner has been well established in the United States, where specialized graduate programs and advanced certification exams are offered, the role has remained virtually nonexistent in Canada, likely because the nurse practitioner role itself is relatively new to Canada compared to the United States, where it has been well established and regulated since the 1970s.

There has been a recent attempt in Canada to standardize the requirements for advanced-practice nursing nationally through the use of exam certification. Currently, nurse practitioner certification falls under particular areas of specialization that are unique to certain provinces and include adult, family, primary care, pediatric, or neonatal. All of these certifications are focused more on physical health than on mental health knowledge. Further, differences in licensure for nurse practitioners exist among provinces due to hospital legislation and funding methodology for health care billing. Because of the strong need for psychiatric care throughout Canada and the lack of providers available, especially in rural areas, the role of the advanced-practice nurse in psychiatric mental health is expected to expand in the near future.

THE FUTURE OF PSYCHIATRIC MENTAL HEALTH NURSING

As its history has shown, the role of the nurse in psychiatric mental health care will continue to evolve and be influenced by societal trends. The change in structure of health care delivery toward a primary health model and an integrative mental health care approach has led to new roles for nurses in psychiatric mental health, including shared-care roles in primary care and consultation-liaison psychiatry within the general hospital setting.

The Association of Registered Nurses of Newfoundland and Labrador (2008) took some key steps in articulating the range of competencies and role development required for community mental health nursing in its 2008 policy paper *Advancing the Role of the Psychiatric–Mental Health Nurse in the Community*. These competencies and role development are in line with the CNA 2020 vision statement, which has called for an increased role for nurses working in integrative mental health care roles and primary care (Villeneuve & MacDonald, 2006). Career pathways for nurse practitioners who specifically work in mental health are lacking at this time in Canada. Based on the success of this and other advanced-practice psychiatric mental health nursing roles in the United States, it is hoped that these models will develop in Canada in the near future (Smith & Khanlou, 2013). The changes in public perception of mental illness and efforts toward addressing stigma are placing a new emphasis on mental health promotion and illness prevention in schools and workplace settings (Mental Health Commission of Canada, 2017). Evidence-informed approaches to treatment—for example, concurrent treatment for people with mental illnesses and addictions, harm reduction, and dialectical behavioural therapy for people with borderline personality disorder—have led to the creation of related nursing roles, education, and research.

▌ KEY POINTS TO REMEMBER

- Early asylum care for people with mental illness predominantly focused on containment and sometimes on punishment.
- Philippe Pinel and William Tuke were eighteenth-century reformers who introduced the moral treatment era of psychiatry, which attempted to focus on providing peaceful, nurturing environments for people with mental illness. Their theories influenced the rural, farmlike settings of early Canadian asylums.
- Nursing within asylums began in the late nineteenth century as a result of the increased medicalization of psychiatry.
- Psychiatric mental health nursing development in Canada was heavily influenced by societal values toward gender and toward mental illness, by politics, and by psychiatric care approaches.
- Early nursing roles in psychiatry were largely custodial until the introduction of new treatments such as electroconvulsive therapy, insulin shock therapy, and lobotomies.
- The division between western provinces and eastern provinces in the creation of the registered psychiatric nurse designation was largely related to differences in nursing leadership power, advocacy, and labour supply issues.

- The development of university-based programs in nursing in the 1920s was a key step in the professionalization of nursing and in the transition of nursing education from medical dominance to nursing-led knowledge development.
- Psychiatric mental health nursing led the way in reinforcing theory-based nursing practice with the use of clinical nurse specialists.
- Registered nurses work within psychiatric mental health settings across Canada.
- Registered psychiatric nurses work in psychiatric mental health settings in Manitoba, Saskatchewan, Alberta, British Columbia, and Yukon.
- The deinstitutionalization of patients in favour of community-based treatment led to the development of new nursing roles in psychiatric mental health care, including community mental health, crisis management, consultation-liaison, and primary care psychiatry.
- Advanced-practice nursing roles have had varied implementation in Canada. The clinical nurse specialist role has been well established, whereas the nurse practitioner role has had limited development.

▌ CRITICAL THINKING

1. Consider the first students at Rockwood Asylum in 1888. What factors might have influenced their decision to enter into asylum nursing (a new program and role)?
2. How have educational programs for nurses evolved with the professionalization of nursing in Canada?

3. What are the potential implications of having two different designations and educational programs for nurses in psychiatric mental health nursing in four Canadian provinces?

CHAPTER REVIEW

1. Asylum care of people with mental illness in Canada began in which year?
   a. 1620
   b. 1932
   c. 1845
   d. 1798

2. The Weir Report was considered influential in which of the following areas?
   a. Asylum reform
   b. Nursing education curriculum reform
   c. Deinstitutionalization
   d. The establishment of the registered psychiatric nurse designation

3. Psychiatric mental health nursing in the community setting was influenced by which of the following factors?
   a. The Weir Report
   b. Deinstitutionalization
   c. The registered psychiatric nurse designation
   d. The increased medicalization of psychiatry

evolve WEBSITE

Post-Test   interactive review

Visit the Evolve website for Chapter Review Answers and Rationales, Critical Thinking Answer Guidelines, and additional resources related to the content in this chapter: http://evolve.elsevier.com/Canada/Varcarolis/psychiatric/

REFERENCES

Anthony, S. E., & Landeen, J. (2009). Evolution of Canadian nursing curricula: A critical retrospective analysis of power and caring. *International Journal of Nursing Education Scholarship*, 69, 1–14. doi:10.2202/1548-923X.1766.

Association of Registered Nurses of Newfoundland and Labrador (2008). *Advancing the role of the psychiatric–mental health nurse in the community (Policy paper)*. St. John's: Author.

Boschma, G. (2012). Community mental health nursing in Alberta, Canada: An oral history. *Nursing History Review*, 20(1), 103–135. doi:10.1891/1062-8061.20.103.

Canadian Association of Schools of Nursing & Canadian Federation of Mental Health Nurses (2015). *Entry-to-practice mental health and addiction competencies for undergraduate nursing education*. Ottawa, ON: Author. Retrieved from http://www.casn.ca/wp-content/uploads/2015/11/Mental-health-Competencies_EN_FINAL-3-Oct-26-2015.pdf.

Canadian Federation of Mental Health Nurses (2016). *CFMHN's 3rd position statement 2016: Mental health and addiction curriculum in undergraduate nursing education in Canada*. Toronto, ON: Author. Retrieved from http://www.cfmhn.ca/positionpapers.

Canadian Nurses Association (2008a). *Code of ethics for registered nurses*. Ottawa: Author.

Canadian Nurses Association (2008b). *Advanced nursing practice: A national framework*. Ottawa: Author.

Canadian Nurses Association. (2011a). *History*. Retrieved from http://www.nurseone.ca/Default.aspx?portlet=StaticHtmlViewerPortlet&stmd=False&plang=1&ptdi=582.

Canadian Nurses Association. (2011b). *CNA certification*. Retrieved from http://www.nurseone.ca/Default.aspx?portlet=StaticHtmlViewerPortlet&plang=1&ptdi=153.

Cellard, A., & Thifault, M. C. (2006). The uses of asylums: Resistance, asylum propaganda and institutionalization strategies in turn of the century Quebec. In J. Moran (Ed.), *Mental illness and Canadian society: A historical perspective* (pp. 97–116). Montreal: McGill-Queen's University Press.

Connor, P. (1996). "Neither courage nor perseverance enough": Attendants at the Asylum for the Insane, Kingston 1877–1905. *Ontario History*, 88(4), 251–272.

Cowles, E. (1916). Training schools for nurses and the first school in McLean Hospital. In H. Hurd (Ed.), *The institutional care of the insane in the United States and Canada* (pp. 289–300). New York: Arno Press.

Digby, A. (1983). Changes in the asylum: The case of York, 1777–1815. *Economic History Review*, 36, 218–239. doi:10.1111/j.1468-0289.1983.tb01230.x.

Fleming, G. (1932). Survey on nursing education. *Canadian Medical Association Journal*, 26(4), 471–474.

Forchuk, C., & Kohr, R. (2009). Prescriptive authority for nurses: The Canadian perspective. *Perspectives in Psychiatric Care*, 45(1), 3–8. doi:10.1111/j.1744-6163.2009.00194.x.

Forchuk, C., & Tweedell, D. (2001). Celebrating our past. *Journal of Psychosocial and Mental Health Services*, 39(10), 16–24.

Foucault, M. (1971). *Madness and civilization: A history of insanity in the age of reason*. New York: Routledge.

Hardill, K. (2006). From the Grey Nuns to the streets: A critical history of outreach nursing in Canada. *Public Health Nursing*, 24(1), 91–97.

Hicks, B. (2011). Gender, politics, and regionalism: Factors in the evolution of registered psychiatric nursing in Manitoba, 1920–1960. *Nursing History Review*, 19, 103–126. doi:10.1891/1062-8061.19.103.

Kerrigan, M. (2011). *Providence Care family connection to Rockwood Nursing [Blog post]*. Retrieved from http://providencecarearchives.wordpress.com/2011/03/25/providence-care-family-connection-to-rockwood-nursing/.

Kirkmayer, L. J., Brass, G. M., & Tait, C. L. (2000). The mental health of Aboriginal peoples: Transformations of identity and community. *The Canadian Journal of Psychiatry*, 45(7), 607–616.

Kirkwood, L. (2005). Enough but not too much: Nursing education in English language Canada. In C. Bates, D. Dodd, & N. Rousseau (Eds.), *On all frontiers: Four centuries of Canadian nursing* (pp. 183–196). Ottawa: University of Ottawa Press.

Legislature of the Province of Ontario (1889). *Sessional papers: Volume xxi—Part 1*. Toronto: Queen's Printer.

Leishman, J. (2005). Back to the future: Making a case for including the history of mental health nursing in nurse education programmes. *The International Journal of Psychiatric Nursing Research*, 10(3), 1157–1164.

Mental Health Commission of Canada. (2017). *Focus areas*. Retrieved from http://www.mentalhealthcommission.ca/English/focus-areas.

Moran, J. (1998). The ethics of farming-out: Ideology, the state, and the asylum in nineteenth-century Quebec. *Canadian Bulletin of Medical History*, 15, 297–316.

Registered Psychiatric Nurse Regulators of Canada. (2017a). *About us*. Retrieved from http://www.rpnc.ca/about-us.

Registered Psychiatric Nurse Regulators of Canada. (2017b). *Registered psychiatric nurse entry level competencies*. Retrieved from http://www.rpnc.ca/sites/default/files/resources/pdfs/RPNRC-ENGLISH%20 Compdoc%20%28Nov6-14%29.pdf.

Registered Psychiatric Nurses of Canada. (2008). *Position statement on master's preparation in psychiatric nursing*. Retrieved from http://www.rpnc.ca/sites/default/files/resources/pdfs/Masters_Preparation_PositionStatement_June2008.pdf.

Registered Psychiatric Nurses of Canada. (2012). *Position statement on baccalaureate preparation as entry to practice in psychiatric nursing*. Retrieved from http://www.rpnc.ca/sites/default/files/resources/pdfs/BACCAL_Prep_PositionStatement_2012.pdf.

Ryan-Nicholls, K. D. (2004). Impact of health reform on registered psychiatric nursing practice. *Journal of Psychiatric and Mental Health Nursing, 11,* 644–653. doi:10.1111/j.1365-2850.2004.00761.x.

Smith, M., & Khanlou, N. (2013). An analysis of Canadian psychiatric mental health nursing through the junctures of history, gender, nursing education, and quality of work life in Ontario, Manitoba, Alberta, and Saskatchewan. *ISRN Nursing*. Retrieved from http://pubmedcentralcanada.ca/pmcc/articles/PMC3655684/.

Sussman, S. (1998). The first asylums in Canada: A response to neglectful community care and current trends. *Canadian Journal of Psychiatry, 43*(3), 260–264.

Tipliski, V. M. (2004). Parting at the crossroads: The emergence of education for psychiatric nursing in three Canadian provinces, 1909–1955. *Canadian Bulletin of Medical History, 21*(2), 253–279.

University of Saskatchewan. (2011). *History of the College of Nursing*. Retrieved from http://www.usask.ca/nursing/college/history.php.

University of Toronto. (2011). *Historic contributions*. Retrieved from http://bloomberg.nursing.utoronto.ca/about/history-of-the-faculty.

Villeneuve, M., & MacDonald, J. (2006). *Toward 2020: Visions for nursing*. Ottawa: Canadian Nurses Association.

Weir, G. M. (1932). *Survey of nursing education in Canada*. Toronto: University of Toronto Press.

Yonge, O., Boschma, G., & Mychajlunow, L. (2005). Gender and professional identity in psychiatric nursing practice in Alberta, Canada, 1930–1975. *Nursing Inquiry, 12,* 243–255. doi:10.1111/j.1440-1800.2005.00287.x.

Youssef, H. A., Youssef, F. A., & Dening, T. R. (1996). Evidence for the existence of schizophrenia in medieval Islamic society. *History of Psychiatry, 7,* 55–62.

Overview of Psychiatric Mental Health Nursing Care Within Various Settings

Cheryl L. Pollard

KEY TERMS AND CONCEPTS

admission criteria

assertive community treatment (ACT)

barriers to treatment

biopsychosocial model

case management

clinical pathway

continuum of psychiatric mental health treatment

decompensation

elopement

interdisciplinary

multidisciplinary

recovery

OBJECTIVES

1. Identify key features of the Canadian health care system and funding structure.
2. Discuss the continuum of psychiatric treatment.
3. Describe primary, secondary, and tertiary treatment outcomes and interventions by setting.
4. Explain the evolution of the community mental health movement.
5. List the criteria for admission to inpatient care
6. Explain the role and responsibilities of the nurse as care manager.
7. Discuss the process for preparing patients to return to the community for ongoing care.
8. Describe the role of the community psychiatric mental health nurse in disaster preparedness.
9. Discuss barriers to mental health treatment.
10. Examine influences on the future of community psychiatric mental health nursing.

๑volve WEBSITE

Visit the Evolve website for Flashcards, Case Studies, and additional testing resources related to the content in this chapter: http://evolve.elsevier.com/Canada/Varcarolis/psychiatric/

Pre-Test   interactive review

Mental illness is a significant problem faced by Canadians (at least 33% of Canadians will experience a mood disorder, anxiety disorder, or substance-related disorder in their lifetime), and hospitalization continues to be a treatment option for some individuals with mental disorders and emotional crises (Public Health Agency of Canada, 2015, p. 5). About 1 in 7 people use health services for mental illness annually (Public Health Agency of Canada, 2015, p. 2). The prevalence of mental illness has increased 43.8% among youth 10 to 14 years old between 1993 and 2010 (Public Health Agency of Canada, 2015, p. 8). Although most psychiatric treatment today takes place in the community, or in general hospital psychiatric units, there continue to be specialized provincial psychiatric organizations that serve individuals with very complex needs, including those individuals referred by the court system (forensic psychiatric services).

HOW A NURSE HELPED ME

When Hope Fades

I'm Amanda, just 23 years old, but I reached a dark place where my life seemed intolerably painful and without hope. I felt weighted down by problems in my home community in Nunavut. At the same time, I felt the incredible pressure of my community, my family, and my own dream to complete a medical degree at McGill University Faculty of Medicine so that I could contribute to the healing of my people.

It was so strange and lonely at university. I felt isolated and without supports. I started to have trouble finding enough energy to keep up with the relentless pace of my studies. I couldn't concentrate, couldn't sleep, and couldn't be bothered eating, so I lost weight. I was anxious and afraid. In order to cope with my anxiety, I started to drink alone in my residence. I wanted to give up and felt I had no option other than suicide. I ate a whole bottle of Tylenol and drank it down with a bottle of gin.

When I was admitted to an acute care psychiatric facility, I felt so ashamed, so hopeless, and so angry. I just wanted to scream, but instead I was polite and withdrawn because that is proper behaviour for an Inuk. Luckily, a nurse, Andrea, reached out and helped me change my life. How? I think mostly by listening respectfully—that's important where I come from. When I whispered, "You can't understand my life," she said, "I know, but maybe I can help you understand your life better."

Andrea listened, but she also taught me about the symptoms of and treatment for depression. Andrea and I made a plan to keep me safe while I explored some options to make my life seem livable again. She was very clear that she had a responsibility to keep me safe while in hospital and explained the suicide precautions needed. I felt safe. Andrea helped me identify my health priorities (like getting back to healthy eating and sleeping), and she also helped me identify some community supports. I didn't know there was an Inuk medical resident at McGill. It was a huge relief to talk with him about university. Andrea also helped me talk with my family when they came all the way from home to visit me. Gradually, I began to see hope for life again. Andrea helped me by listening and respecting me. I will always be grateful for her care.

FUNDING PSYCHIATRIC MENTAL HEALTH CARE

The Canadian mental health care system has many areas of strength—for example, most citizens have access to mental health services—but it also has gaps, such as equitable access to specialized care at the primary, secondary, and tertiary levels. Canada has a predominately publicly financed and administered health care system whereby all eligible residents have reasonable access to medically necessary hospital and physician services (referred to as "insured services") (Health Canada, 2015). Federal government and provincial and territorial government roles and responsibilities for health care are set out, primarily, in the *Medicare Act* (1966) and the *Canada Health Act* (1984). Provincial and territorial governments are responsible for health care within their jurisdictions. The federal government is responsible for transferring health care funds to the provincial and territorial governments and for ensuring that insured health care services are publicly funded and administered by the provinces and territories according to five basic principles: public administration, comprehensiveness, universality, portability, and accessibility. The federal government continues to maintain health care responsibility for select populations (First Nations communities, armed forces, Royal Canadian Mounted Police, individuals in federal penitentiaries, and refugees) and select functions (such as health promotion, disease surveillance, and drug regulation). For instance, the federal government operates Operational Stress Injury Social Support (OSISS) programs across Canada for military members, veterans, and their families to help them cope with the psychological effects of stress and trauma associated with warfare. (For more information on OSISS programs, visit https://www.cfmws.com/en/AboutUs/DCSM/OSISS/Pages/Operational-Stress-Injury-Social-Support-(OSISS).aspx.) The mental health strategy for Canada includes a First Nations, Inuit, and Métis advisory committee to promote mental health and wellness in Indigenous individuals and communities in Canada (Mental Health Commission of Canada, 2012). Responsibility for health care services is further devolved from the provincial and territorial governments to regional organizations—for instance, regional health boards, regional health authorities, and hospitals—the type of which depend on the province or territory. This distribution of roles and responsibilities within the Canadian health care system has resulted in services gaps within the continuum of mental health care.

Although differences exist among the various provinces or territories, mental health and addiction services generally include primary, secondary, and tertiary services that are provided in inpatient and outpatient psychiatric hospital settings and in community-based settings. These services may include crisis response and emergency services, temporary and long-term housing, psychoeducational or support groups, and vocational or educational services. Services are generally delivered by a number of professionals—for example, registered nurses, registered psychiatric nurses, licensed/registered practical nurses, psychiatrists, psychologists, counsellors, occupational therapists, recreation therapists, and social workers. Not all of these services, however, are publicly funded. Canadians pay directly or indirectly for all health care: 70% through taxation, 12% through private or employment insurance plans, 15% out of pocket, and another 3% through other means (Canadian Institute for Health Information, 2016). Individuals with mental health problems often have financial challenges as a result of the signs and symptoms of their illness, which makes the private or employment health insurance plans difficult or impossible to access and out-of-pocket expenses—including medication costs, counselling, appropriate housing, re-entry to employment or education support, and dental care—burdensome.

THE CONTINUUM OF MENTAL HEALTH CARE

Health care services can generally be divided into three different levels: primary, secondary, and tertiary. Primary-level activities are delivered to healthy populations and include providing information and teaching coping skills to reduce stress, with the goal of avoiding mental illness (e.g., a nurse may teach parenting skills in a well-baby clinic). These services are generally provided in a community or outpatient setting. Secondary-level services involve the early detection and treatment of psychiatric symptoms, with the goal of minimizing impairment (e.g., a nurse may conduct screening for depression at a work site). These services are also generally provided in a community or outpatient setting. Tertiary-level services involve the treatment of psychiatric symptoms and address residual impairments in psychiatric patients in an effort to promote the highest level of community functioning. These are very specialized services that may be delivered in a clinic or a hospital (e.g., a nurse may provide long-term treatment in a clinic, or the person may be admitted to a specialized inpatient unit). In the past, tertiary care models focused on providing inpatient services.

Evolving Venues of Practice

Many psychiatric mental health nurses originally practised within tertiary care settings, but practice locations have evolved because of financial, technological, health care, regulatory, cultural, and population changes. Nurses are now providing primary mental health care at therapeutic day care centres, schools, partial hospitalization programs, and shelters. In addition to these more traditional environments for care, psychiatric mental health nurses are entering forensic settings and drug and alcohol treatment centres. Box 3-1 presents examples of practice sites for the psychiatric mental health nurse.

Mobile mental health units have been developed in some service areas. In a growing number of communities, mental health programs are collaborating with other health or community services to provide integrated approaches to treatment. A prime example of this is the growth of concurrent disorder programming (programs that address the diagnosis of a mental illness and substance use disorder) at both mental health and chemical dependency clinics.

Technology has also contributed to changes in venues for providing community care. Telephone crisis counselling, telephone outreach, and the Internet are being used to enhance access to mental health services, particularly in remote areas of the provinces. Although face-to-face interaction is still preferred, technology has the potential to improve support, confidence, and health status among mental health care consumers (Hollis, Morriss, Martin, et al., 2015).

Over the course of a mental illness, patients may receive care from a range of psychiatric services. Figure 3-1 illustrates the continuum of psychiatric mental health treatment. A patient's movement along the continuum is fluid, from higher to lower levels of intensity of care, and changes are not necessarily made

---

BOX 3-1   POSSIBLE COMMUNITY MENTAL HEALTH PRACTICE SITES

Primary Prevention
Adult and youth recreational centres
Churches, temples, synagogues, mosques
Day care centres
Ethnic cultural centres
Public health clinics
Schools

Secondary Prevention
Assisted-living facilities
Chemical dependency programs
Community outreach treatment programs
Correctional community facilities
Crisis centres
Early intervention psychosis programs
General inpatient units
Hospices and acquired immunodeficiency syndrome (AIDS) programs
Industry/work sites
Nursing homes
Partial hospitalization programs
Primary care networks
Shelters (homeless, women subjected to domestic violence, adolescents)
Youth residential treatment centres

Tertiary Prevention
Psychosocial rehabilitation programs
Specialized community mental health centres
Specialized inpatient units

---

step by step. Upon discharge from acute hospital care or a 24-hour supervised crisis unit, many patients need intensive services to maintain their initial gains or to "step down" in care. Failure to follow up in outpatient treatment increases the likelihood of rehospitalization and other adverse outcomes (Henzen, Moeglin, Giannakopoulos, et al., 2016). It is also notable that patients may pass through the continuum of treatment in the reverse direction; that is, if symptoms do not improve, a lower-intensity service may refer the patient to a higher level of care in an attempt to prevent decompensation (deterioration of mental health) and hospitalization.

PSYCHIATRIC MENTAL HEALTH CARE SETTINGS

The following sections describe various psychiatric settings, and each section offers examples of basic-level nursing interventions:
- Counselling—assessment interviews; crisis intervention; problem solving in individual, group, or family sessions
- Promotion of self-care activities—fostering grooming, guidance in use of public transportation, instruction in budgeting (in home settings, the nurse may directly assist as necessary)
- Psychobiological interventions—medication administration, instruction in relaxation techniques, promotion of sound eating and sleep habits

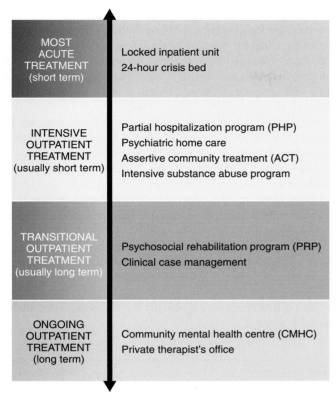

MOST ACUTE TREATMENT (short term)	Locked inpatient unit 24-hour crisis bed
INTENSIVE OUTPATIENT TREATMENT (usually short term)	Partial hospitalization program (PHP) Psychiatric home care Assertive community treatment (ACT) Intensive substance abuse program
TRANSITIONAL OUTPATIENT TREATMENT (usually long term)	Psychosocial rehabilitation program (PRP) Clinical case management
ONGOING OUTPATIENT TREATMENT (long term)	Community mental health centre (CMHC) Private therapist's office

FIGURE 3-1 The continuum of psychiatric mental health treatment.

- Health teaching—medication use, illness characteristics, coping skills, relapse prevention
- Case management—liaising with family, significant others, and other health care or community resource personnel of care regarding referrals, assistance with paperwork applications, connection to resources, and overall navigation of the health care system to coordinate an effective plan

Community Mental Health Centres

Since the 1950s. the trend of deinstitutionalization has occurred internationally (Hudson, 2016). In Canada, several factors contributed to this shift, including financial pressures on the provincially funded psychiatric hospitals, changing societal values, and new mental health treatment philosophies (LaJeunesse, 2002). Many hospitals were indeed grossly overcrowded, patients' rights were often disregarded, and seclusion and restraint were overused. Due to the largely custodial nature of inpatient treatment, patients were left with little incentive for growth or participation in their own care; this phenomenon became known as *institutionalization*. Grassroots efforts, increased advocacy, and legal initiatives on behalf of people with mental illness and their right to humane care resulted in the provincial health care systems looking for alternative treatment settings (LaJeunesse, 2002).

Policymakers came to believe that community care would be more humane and less expensive than hospital-based care, and the introduction of psychotropic drugs, beginning with chlorpromazine (Largactil), made community living a more realistic option for many people. Organizations like the Canadian Mental Health Association (CMHA) established housing and support services for people living with mental illness in the community. From 1960 to 1980, all Canadian provinces implemented some type of deinstitutionalization of psychiatric services, although the timing and degree of bed closures varied greatly across regions (Sealy & Whitehead, 2004). For example, between 1965 and 1981, Canada saw a 70.6% decrease in psychiatry beds across the nation, but during that time Saskatchewan had an 81.6% decrease and Prince Edward Island had only a 34.5% decrease (Sealy & Whitehead, 2004). A second pattern associated with deinstitutionalization was the change in duration of stay and admission rates to psychiatric inpatient beds. Days of care in inpatient units gradually shortened from the 1970s to the 1990s, with a drastic drop between 1994 and 1999 (Sealy & Whitehead, 2004).

Government promises to expand funding for community services were not kept, mental health funding continued to decline, and patients outnumbered resources. Many patients with serious mental illness resisted treatment with available providers, so providers began to use up scarce resources for the less mentally disabled but more committed population. While deinstitutionalization, in principle, was largely considered to have been a step toward improved care for people with mental illness, the lack of funding and available community supports negated many of the benefits. In reality, many people with mental illness were discharged to inadequate supports, a situation that led to increased homelessness and criminalization (McCauley, Montgomery, Mossey, et al, 2015).

Through the 1990s, advocacy by the CMHA and others continued. Increasing awareness resulted in increasing pressure on government to redesign the mental health system in Canada and to ensure adequate community supports. The 2006 Senate report led by Michael Kirby and Wilbert Keon, *Out of the Shadows at Last*, was an optimistic step toward transforming the delivery system of mental health care. However, until 2012 Canada remained the only G7 country without a national mental health strategy. At that time, the Mental Health Commission of Canada (2012) issued *Changing Directions, Changing Lives: The Mental Health Strategy for Canada*, which was a call to action in an effort to unite people's efforts to improve mental health. Unfortunately, Canada continues to have lower rates of spending on mental health than most other G7 countries focused on an underlying recovery principle for mental health care (Lurie & Mulvale, 2015).

Recovery is a critical aspect to improving the well-being and mental health of all Canadians. It is described as the ability of the individual to work, live, and participate in the community. It is a journey that provides patients with hope, empowerment, and confidence to take an active role in determining their own treatment paths. Ideally, recovery would be facilitated by interconnected community agencies that work in harmony to assist consumers of mental health care as they navigate an often confusing system. Realistically, funding has always been an issue in treating people with mental illness, and current economic realities have not improved the situation. Registered nurses and registered psychiatric nurses may be the answer to transforming an illness-driven and dependency-oriented system into a one that emphasizes recovery and empowerment. Nurses are adept at understanding the system and coordinating care as well as taking a health-oriented approach.

Over the past 50 years—with advances in psychopharmacology and psychosocial treatments—psychiatric care in the community has become more sophisticated, with a continuum of care that provides more options for people with mental illness. The role of the psychiatric mental health nurse has grown to include service provision in a variety of community settings. Nurses may also provide care to individuals as they leave the criminal justice system and re-enter the community. The range of community services available varies but generally includes emergency services and services for adults and children such as medication administration, treatment for concurrent disorders, individual therapy, group therapy, family therapy, psychoeducational services, and education to other professionals. A clinic may also be aligned with a psychosocial rehabilitation program that offers a structured day program, vocational services, and residential services. Some community mental health centres have an associated intensive case-management service to assist patients in finding housing or obtaining funding.

Community mental health centres often provide services using an interprofessional team model. The psychiatric mental health nurse will work with a number of patients. Patients are either self-referred or referred by inpatient units or primary care providers for long-term or short-term follow-up. Patients may attend the clinic for years or be discharged when they improve and reach desired goals. Each clinic varies in design of service delivery; the nurse sees the majority of patients in the clinic but often will see patients in other settings such as primary care offices or their homes.

Walking into a person's home creates a different set of dynamics from that commonly seen in a clinical setting. Boundaries become important. The nurse may find it best to begin a visit informally by chatting about the patient's family events or by accepting refreshments offered. This interaction can be a strain for the nurse who has difficulty maintaining boundaries between the professional relationship and a personal one. However, there is great significance to the therapeutic use of self (i.e., the personality, insights, perceptions, and judgements of the nurse as part of the therapeutic process) in such circumstances, to establish a level of comfort for the patient and family.

The vignette illustrates a typical day for a nurse in a community mental health centre.

VIGNETTE

Nita Desai is a nurse at a community mental health centre. She is on the adult team and carries a caseload of 80 patients diagnosed with chronic mental illness.

0830–0900: Upon arriving at the clinic, Nita receives a voicemail message from Ms. DiTomasso, who is crying and says she is out of medication. Nita consults with the psychiatrist and calls Ms. DiTomasso to arrange for an emergency appointment later that day.

0900–0930: Nita's first patient is Mr. Enright, a 35-year-old man diagnosed with schizophrenia, who has been in treatment at the clinic for 10 years. During their 30-minute counselling session, Nita assesses Mr. Enright for any exacerbation of psychotic symptoms (he has a history of grandiose delusions) and any changes in eating and sleep habits or social functioning in the psychosocial rehabilitation program that he attends 5 days a week. Today, he presents as stable. Nita gives Mr. Enright his decanoate injection and schedules a return appointment for a month from now, reminding him of his psychiatrist appointment the following week.

1000–1100: Nita's second patient of the day is Susan, a 28-year-old mother with postpartum depression. Nita sees Susan weekly to assess her response to the antidepressant medication prescribed by her family physician and to work on anxiety coping strategies. She also spends time assessing Susan's attachment to her 6-month-old baby and provides education on any parenting questions that Susan may have. They discuss the idea of Susan attending a support group for postpartum depression as an adjunct to individual treatment. Susan is agreeable to the idea now that she is feeling less anxious and has more energy. Nita calls the group facilitator and arranges for Susan's intake for the following week.

1100–1200: Nita writes progress and medication notes; responds to telephone calls from patients and other agencies, such as home care and public-health nursing agencies; and prepares for the team conference.

1200–1400: All adult-team staff members attend the weekly intake meeting, at which new admissions are discussed and individual treatment plans are written with team input. Nita presents a patient intake, reading from the standardized interview form. She also gives nursing input about treatment for the other five newly admitted patients. The new patient she presented is assigned to her, and she plans to call him later in the afternoon to set up a first appointment.

1400–1500: Nita co-leads a concurrent disorders therapy group with the addictions specialist, who is a social worker. The group is made up of seven patients who have concurrent diagnoses of substance abuse and a major psychiatric illness. The leaders take a psychoeducational approach, and today's planned topic is teaching about the physical effects of alcohol on the body. Nita focuses on risks associated with the interaction between alcohol and medications and answers the members' questions. Because this is an ongoing group, members take a more active role, and discussion may vary according to members' needs instead of following planned topics. After the session, the co-leaders discuss the group dynamics and write progress notes.

1530–1600: Nita meets with Ms. DiTomasso, who arrives at the clinic tearful and agitated. Ms. DiTomasso says that she missed her appointment this month because her son died suddenly. Nita uses crisis intervention skills to assess Ms. DiTomasso's status (e.g., any risks for her safety related to her history of suicidal ideation). After helping Ms. DiTomasso clarify a plan to increase support from her family, Nita notes that insomnia is a new problem. She takes Ms. DiTomasso to the psychiatrist covering "emergency prescription time" and explains the change in the patient's status. The psychiatrist refills Ms. DiTomasso's usual antidepressant and adds a medication to aid sleep. Nita makes an appointment for the patient to return to see her in 1 week instead of the usual 1 month and also schedules her to meet with her assigned psychiatrist that same day.

1600–1630: Nita completes all notes, makes necessary telephone calls to staff working with her patients in the psychosocial rehabilitation program, and phones her new patient to schedule an appointment.

Crisis Intervention Team

When psychiatric mental health care moved to a community setting, the need to address some of the acute mental health care concerns of individuals living in the community increased. Initially, the necessary response was left to local police departments, which often felt unprepared to deal effectively with mental health concerns. Crisis intervention teams were set up in many communities across Canada to address this issue and are now considered an essential part of comprehensive community mental health services (Fahim, Semovski, & Younger, 2016). Various service-delivery models for crisis intervention teams are being used, but some commonalities among them exist, such as the use of an interprofessional team, mobile units, and collaborative partnerships with police (Forchuk, Jensen, Martin, et al., 2010). Often the crisis intervention team is an interprofessional team made up of nurses, social workers, and psychologists. Psychiatrists often are used as consultants for the team. Crisis teams operate out of community clinics, emergency departments, or stand-alone offices.

Partnership with local police authorities has been found to be an extremely effective way to meet the needs of individuals in acute psychiatric crisis and has led to decreased criminalization and improved access to services for people with severe chronic mental illness (Fahim, Semovski, & Younger, 2016). When required, the interprofessional team may act as consultants to the police. Some crisis intervention models in Canada even include specially trained police members on the interprofessional team. Crisis services offer 24/7 phone support and in-person mental health assessments in homes, public places, and emergency departments (Fahim, Semovski, & Younger, 2016).

VIGNETTE

Ben Thien is a nurse working on the mobile crisis team in a large urban setting; the following describes a typical evening shift.

1500–1530: Ben comes onto his shift and meets with the evening team to get a report from the day shift and plan for the evening shift. The team is told by day-shift staffers of any outstanding calls that have not been assessed and any updates regarding patients that are being case-managed by the team currently. The team decides that Ben and Officer George will go out at 1700 hours to try to see a man whom a neighbour has called about today but who had not been at home when the day team went out earlier.

1530–1630: Ben answers the phone and receives a call from a woman who is feeling very sad and hopeless. Ben conducts a mental status exam over the phone and assesses the woman for risk. The woman appears to be suffering from depression but is not currently suicidal, so Ben offers her support and some psychoeducation about depression and its treatment. He gives her a phone number for the mental health clinic in her area, and she agrees to follow up. Ben asks for permission to fax a copy of his assessment to her family physician to ensure continuity of care, and the patient agrees. Ben completes his documentation and then faxes the report to the family physician.

1630–1830: Ben and his partner, Officer George, leave the office to follow up on the call from the day shift. They drive to the person's house in an unmarked police car. They both go to the door and ring the doorbell. A young man in his early 20s answers, and Ben explains who they are and that they would like to talk to him about how he has been feeling lately. The man agrees to speak to them. Officer George and Ben enter the house and assess it for any safety risks such as environmental issues, uncontrolled dogs, or other people present. Ben and George sit down at the kitchen table with the patient and begin the interview. The patient reports recent difficulties with his sleep and mood. He denies any history of mental illness or physical illness. He tells of his ability to control the weather and his fear that perhaps people in the government are out to get him. He denies any risk for harm or self-harm, and he agrees that this is a recent change for him but does not feel the need to seek medical treatment. He does not demonstrate any impulsive behaviour during the interview, but Ben notices that many of the kitchen appliances are wrapped in tin foil. The patient vaguely refers to this as "antiradar devices." At the completion of the interview, Ben concludes that although the patient seems to be showing signs of psychosis, he is not currently demonstrating risk and does not meet criteria under the mental health act for involuntary admission. Ben decides to try to engage the patient further and arranges a follow-up meeting for 2 days later. Prior to leaving, Ben ensures that the patient has adequate food supplies in his fridge and does some basic wellness teaching about sleep hygiene for the patient. Ben and George return to the office and document the visit.

1830–2030: George receives a call from a fellow police officer requesting an assessment of a person in the community who was reported for disturbing the peace at a bus shelter. Ben and George leave to drive to the scene. On the way to the scene, Ben takes a crisis call over the cellphone from a young man looking for resources for panic attacks. Upon arrival at the scene, Ben and George meet briefly with the police officers on-site, who bring them up to date on the situation. According to witnesses, the woman has been pacing at the bus stop for the past 6 hours, occasionally stepping into traffic. George and Ben go into the bus shelter and begin talking to the woman, who is dressed in shorts despite the cold weather, is pacing back and forth muttering to herself, and refuses to go to the hospital, stating, "I've had enough of all you FBI agents." Ben conducts the mental status and risk assessment and then, conferring with George, decides that this woman does meet the criteria of the mental health act for an involuntary assessment because she appears to have a mental illness, is at risk for self-harm (walking into traffic, continued exposure to the cold weather) and further deterioration, and refuses to go to the hospital voluntarily. George and Ben explain that they need to take her to the hospital for an assessment. George puts her safely in the back of the police car, and Ben documents his assessment en route to the hospital. At the hospital, Ben informs the triage nurse of his assessment and arranges a secure room for the patient. Ben ensures that the patient is given food and fluids by the emergency staff and then discusses his assessment with the psychiatry resident on call. Ben and George then return to the office.

2030–2230: Ben continues to answer the phone and provide support, referrals, and assessments to callers. He arranges a home visit for the following day for a woman who is concerned about her father-in-law and his recent changes in behaviour.

2230–2300: Ben gets an update from the three other teams working the evening shift and then prepares his report for the night shift.

Nurses who work on crisis teams collaborate with other interprofessional members to assess patients in crisis; provide early intervention; provide crisis intervention counselling and support; offer short-term case management, including referrals to other resources; and advocate on behalf of families and patients.

The vignette describes a typical day of a nurse working on a crisis team.

Disaster Response Teams

Nurses who work in community mental health are often part of the intersectoral disaster response planning committee for the community in which they work. Following a disaster, the immediate goal is to ensure that those affected have shelter, food, and first aid as necessary. Then the community mental health nurse provides crisis management for victims and volunteers who are assisting in the relief efforts. After the crisis passes, the community psychiatric mental health nurse must find those individuals whose care was disrupted and help them to link back into the system. The nurse administers "psychological first aid" by assisting victims to meet basic needs, listening to individuals who need to share their stories, directing individuals to agencies that can help, and providing compassion and appropriate hope. Mental health nurses take on a leadership role in disaster situations to enhance the biopsychosocial outcomes for people living in a disaster-affected community (Ranse, Hutton, Wilson, et al, 2015). Chapter 21 offers a more detailed discussion of crisis and disaster.

Partial Hospitalization Programs

Partial hospitalization programs (PHPs) offer intensive, short-term treatment similar to inpatient care, except that the patient is able to return home each day. Criteria for referral to a PHP include serious symptoms that otherwise could lead to hospitalization or step-down from acute inpatient treatment, along with the presence of a responsible relative or caregiver who can assure the patient's safety (Joyce, Nordhagen, Ogrodniczuk, et al, 2015). Referrals come from inpatient or outpatient providers. Patients receive 5 to 6 hours of treatment daily, usually 5 days a week, although some programs operate on weekends. The average length of stay is approximately 2 to 3 weeks, depending on the program, and the interprofessional team consists of a psychiatrist, registered nurse or registered psychiatric nurse, social worker, occupational therapist, and recreational therapist.

The following vignette illustrates a typical day for a psychiatric mental health nurse in a PHP.

Inpatient Psychiatric Mental Health Programs

Inpatient psychiatric care has undergone significant change over the past half-century. Consequences of deinstitutionalization have included a reduction in long-stay psychiatric beds (as these are concentrated in the provincial psychiatric hospitals), decreased lengths of hospital stay, increased use of crisis services, and an increase in the number of individuals with mental illness who are homeless or in the penitentiary system. Fewer psychiatric in-patient beds means that acuity within psychiatric facilities has been increasing, wait times for admission are increasing, and admission is commonly reserved for those people who are acutely suicidal, actively homicidal, or extremely disabled and

in need of short-term acute care (Allison, Bastiampillai, & Goldney, 2014).

Entry to Inpatient Care

Although some patients are admitted directly based on a psychiatrist or primary care provider referral, most people receiving

---

VIGNETTE

Michael Sanders is a nurse in a partial hospitalization program (PHP) that is part of a general hospital's outpatient psychiatry department. Michael is the nurse member of the interprofessional team, and today his schedule is as follows:

0830–0900: Michael arrives at the PHP and meets with the team to review the patients expected to arrive in the program today. He prepares to meet with the patients who are scheduled for medication review with the psychiatrist. He also prepares the teaching outline for his daily psychoeducational groups.

0900–1230: Michael meets with a group of 10 patients and teaches them goal setting, medication management, and relapse prevention. Throughout the sessions, Michael assesses each patient's mental status and any concerns that have arisen.

1300–1400: Michael conducts an intake interview with a newly admitted patient. Ms. Brown is a 50-year-old woman with a history of major depression who was hospitalized for 2 weeks after a drug overdose following an argument with her boyfriend. Michael completes the standardized interview form, paying extra attention to risk factors for suicide. When asked about substance abuse, Ms. Brown admits that she has been drinking heavily for the past 2 years, including the night she took the drug overdose. When the interview is completed, the patient is referred to the psychiatrist for a diagnostic evaluation.

1400–1500: Michael meets with four patients scheduled to see the psychiatrist. He reviews the cases with the psychiatrist and ensures that the patients understand any changes in their medication regimens.

1500–1530: Michael has a discharge meeting with Mr. Callaghan, a 48-year-old man with a diagnosis of schizophrenia. He was referred to the PHP by his clinic therapist to prevent hospitalization due to increasing paranoia and agitation. After 2 weeks in the PHP, he has restabilized and recognizes that he must adhere to his antipsychotic medication regimen. Michael finalizes Mr. Callaghan's medication teaching and confirms his aftercare appointments with his previous therapist and psychiatrist.

1530–1600: To ensure Ms. Brown's safety, Michael meets with her again before she goes home, assessing her suicide risk potential. Michael also shares the preliminary individual treatment plan and begins a discussion of resources for alcohol treatment, including Alcoholics Anonymous.

1600–1700: Michael meets with the team for daily rounds. He presents Ms. Brown, and the team develops an individual treatment plan for her. In this treatment plan, the team notes discharge planning needs for referrals to a community mental health centre and an alcohol treatment program. As a critical member of the treatment team, Michael reviews the remaining cases and makes needed adjustments to their treatment plans. He completes his notes and discharge summary. He also makes case-management telephone calls to arrange for community referrals, communicate with families, and report to any mental health referral programs to review how often the client has used the services.

inpatient acute psychiatric care are assessed in the emergency department (ED) first and then are admitted through the ED if they meet the established admission criteria. The average ED wait time for a patient in need of hospitalization is increasing—in some areas, the wait can be days. Nurses who work on psychiatric units should recognize that patients admitted from the ED may need additional patience and attention. They may have been deprived of medication, treatments, sleep, or proper food.

People with psychiatric symptoms are often isolated and ignored from the outset of their hospitalization. However, an increasing number of Canadian EDs are using nurses who have experience working with people with mental illness in the ED to assist with triage and care of patients with mental health problems.

In the ED, the patient is generally evaluated by an emergency department physician and a social worker, who will determine if the patient meets the criteria to justify admission. The **admission criteria** begin with the premise that the person is suffering from a mental illness and include evidence of one or more of the following:

- High risk of harming self
- High risk of harming others
- Inability to care for basic needs, which will likely cause substantial mental or physical deterioration or serious physical impairments

Patients who meet the admission criteria are then given the option of being admitted on a voluntary basis, which means that they agree with the need for treatment and hospitalization. The vast majority of patient admissions to psychiatric inpatient units are voluntary. If patients do not wish to be hospitalized but mental health care providers feel that admission is necessary, the patients can be admitted against their wishes—commonly known as an "involuntary admission." Involuntarily admitted patients, sometimes referred to as certified patients, still have rights: right to receive information on their rights in a timely manner, right to retain counsel, and right to an independent

review of their committal (O'Reilly, Chaimowitz, Brunet, et al., 2010); Chapter 7 offers a more detailed discussion of this issue. If the admission is contested, a mental health review board (or panel or tribunal, depending on the province or territory) reviews the committal decision on behalf of the patient. Chapter 7 discusses legal requirements for admissions, commitment, and discharge procedures in more detail.

 RESEARCH HIGHLIGHT

"To Everything There Is a Season": Mental Health–Related Hospitalizations by Youth and Adults

Problem

The use of inpatient hospital and acute care services by children and adolescents has become a growing issue in Canada due to increases in hospital admissions and emergency department visits. Despite increasing rates of mental health–related hospitalizations among children and adolescents, little is known about the nondemographic or disease-related factors that influence the likelihood of young people being admitted to hospital for mental health problems.

Purpose of Study

The primary purpose of this study was to address this limitation in the literature by measuring seasonal variations in mental health–related hospitalizations by youth over a 9-year period using administrative health data from New Brunswick.

Methods

Hospital admission records from January 2004 to March 2014 were obtained from the provincial Discharge Abstract Database. Seasonal trends in mental health–related hospitalizations were analyzed

Key Findings

- The majority of mental health–related admissions to hospital were by adults 20 years of age and older; however, the odds of children and adolescents (ages 3 to 19 years) being admitted to hospital were 19% higher in 2014 compared to 2004.
- Youth ages 11 to 15 and 16 to 19 years had significantly greater admissions to hospital in the first quarter (January, February, March) in contrast to the third quarter (July, August, September). Hospital admissions for children and adolescents ages 3 to 19 years with neurosis and mood disorders had the greatest seasonal variation, whereas there were no identifiable seasonal differences in admissions attributed to substance use, behavioural disorders (i.e., eating disorders), personal disorders, or psychosis.

Implications for Nursing Practice

The results of this study indicate that mental health–related hospital admissions by children and adolescents are generally higher during the academic calendar. There are opportunities in schools for nurses to prevent and detect emerging mental health problems among youth.

Source: Ronis, S. T., Slaunwhite, A., Peters, P., et al. (2017). "To everything there is a season": Mental health–related hospitalizations by youth and adults. *Journal of Adolescent Health, 60*(2 Supp. 1), S23. doi:10.1016/j.jadohealth.2016.10.064.

VIGNETTE

Shane is a 22-year-old male who was brought to the emergency department by police after expressing thoughts of suicide. He reports having had difficulty sleeping and eating for the past several days and a weight loss of 5 pounds. He is restless and demanding. When approached, he becomes very irritable and threatening to the nurses and physicians, stating that he wants to leave and does not understand why he needs to be here. He states that he was tricked by his mother and brother, who are trying to have him admitted only so they can take his money. He is exhibiting poor judgement, insight, and impulse control. He has been nonadherent with his antipsychotic medication, risperidone, which he stopped taking 3 weeks ago because of adverse effects.

Shane did not want to be admitted, and despite several attempts by the nursing staff, he continued to refuse hospitalization. The decision was made to involuntarily admit him to the locked psychiatric inpatient unit. On arrival to the inpatient unit, Shane was informed of his rights and the fact that he was involuntarily committed to the unit.

Preparation for Discharge to the Community

Discharge planning begins upon admission and is continually modified as required by the patient's condition until the time of discharge. The reduction of overt symptoms and the development of an adequate outpatient plan signal that discharge is imminent. As members of the health care team, nurses assist patients and their families to prepare for independent or assisted living in the community.

The treatment plans are influenced by the clinical pathway (when available), which is a guideline that outlines the clinical standards—the usual care provided for a patient undergoing a certain procedure or for a patient who has a certain illness. Since each patient is unique, each person's care will be customized to meet his or her needs while keeping these guidelines in mind. The use of a clinical pathway is intended to improve patient care. The patient is expected to begin to progress toward a resolution of acute symptoms, assume personal responsibility, improve interpersonal functioning, and participate in discharge planning. Patients with prolonged mental illness benefit most from a seamless transition to community services. Such a transition is facilitated through collaboration with community mental health services and through the intensive case-management programs available there. Readiness for community re-entry should include preparation by members of the patient's support system for their role in enhancing the patient's mental health. Poverty, stigma, unemployment, and lack of appropriate housing are identified as major barriers to recovery of mental health. The nurse needs to consider these gaps when planning discharge for patients from acute care settings, as the gaps can delay discharge and increase the likelihood of readmission.

VIGNETTE

Tazmine meets with Shane and his mother on the day of discharge to review the aftercare arrangements. Tazmine reviews the goals that were established by the treatment team and Shane's own goal for hospitalization. She reviews the accomplishments Shane made during his hospitalization; reinforces the importance of medication adherence; reviews each prescription, highlighting how and when the medication must be taken; and tells Shane when and where his aftercare appointment is. Tazmine answers Shane's and his mother's questions.

Assertive Community Treatment

Assertive community treatment (ACT) is an intensive type of case management developed in response to the community-living needs of people with serious, persistent psychiatric symptoms (Linz & Sturm, 2016). Patients with severe symptoms are referred to ACT teams by inpatient or outpatient providers because of a pattern of repeated hospitalizations, along with an inability to participate in traditional treatment.

ACT teams work intensively with patients in their homes or in agencies, hospitals, or clinics—whatever settings patients find themselves in. Creative problem solving and interventions are hallmarks of the care provided by mobile teams. The ACT concept takes into account that people need support and resources after 1700 hours; teams are on call 24 hours a day. ACT teams are interprofessional and typically composed of psychiatric mental health nurses, social workers, psychologists, advanced-practice registered nurses, and psychiatrists. One of these professionals (often the nurse) serves as the case manager and may have a caseload of up to 10 patients who require visits three to five times per week. Length of treatment may extend to years, until the patient is ready to accept transfer to a less intensive site for care.

The vignette illustrates a typical day for a psychiatric mental health nurse on an ACT team.

Ensuring Safety

Safety is one of the most important aspects of care in any setting. Protecting the patient is essential, but equally important is the safety of the staff and other patients. Nurses maintain safety primarily through collaborative teamwork, good patient assessment, respectful attention to patient concerns, and recognition and de-escalation of potentially dangerous situations.

Safety needs are identified and individualized interventions begin on admission. In community, a through risk assessment is completed. In addition to this assessment in inpatient settings, staff should check all personal property and clothing to prevent any potentially harmful items from being taken onto the unit (e.g., medication, alcohol, sharp objects). Some people are at greater risk for suicide than others, and nurses must be skillful in evaluating this risk through questions and observations. Understanding the types of precautions used in each setting is one of the most important tasks a new staff member or nursing student can learn.

Accreditation Canada (2016) publishes required patient safety practices for Canadian hospitals (also see Brickell, Nicholls, Procyshyn, et al., 2009, for developing work on patient safety guidelines specific to mental health care in Canada). Box 3-2 lists important safety goals for care in mental health settings.

Due to the increased acuity of patients receiving care on an inpatient unit, further precautions are taken. The nurse supervises the unit for overall safety. One of the most important interventions is tracking patients' whereabouts and activities. These checks are done periodically or continuously, depending on patients' risk for a health crisis or self-harm. Visitors are another potential safety hazard. Although visitors can contribute to patients' healing through socialization, acceptance, and familiarity, visits may be overwhelming or distressing. Also, visitors may unwittingly or purposefully provide patients with unsafe items such as sharp objects, glass, or drugs; bags and packages brought onto the unit should be inspected by unit staff. Sometimes unsafe items take the form of comfort foods from home or a favourite restaurant, and these should be monitored because they may be incompatible with prescribed diets or medications.

When the patient's illness is affecting insight and judgement, intimate relationships between patients are discouraged or expressly prohibited. There are risks for sexually transmitted infections, pregnancy, and emotional distress at a time when patients are vulnerable and may lack the capacity for consent.

VIGNETTE

Maria Restrepo is a nurse who works on an assertive community treatment (ACT) team at a large, inner-city university medical centre. She had 5 years of inpatient experience before joining the ACT team, and she works with two social workers, two psychiatrists, and a mental health worker.

0800–0930: Maria starts the day at the clinic site with team rounds. Because she was on call over the weekend, she updates the team on three emergency department visits: two patients were able to return home after she met with them and the emergency department physician; one patient was admitted to the hospital because he made threats to his caregiver.

0930–1030: Maria's first patient is Mr. Zaman, a 35-year-old man with a diagnosis of bipolar disorder and alcohol dependence. He lives with his mother and has a history of five hospitalizations with nonadherence to outpatient clinic treatment. Except during his manic episodes, he isolates himself at home or visits a friend in the neighbourhood, at whose house he drinks excessively. Today he is due for his biweekly haloperidol decanoate (Haldol Decanoate) injection (a long-acting antipsychotic medication). Maria goes first to his house and learns that he is not at home. She speaks with his mother about his recent behaviour and an upcoming medical clinic appointment. Then she goes to the friend's house and finds Mr. Zaman playing cards and drinking a beer. He and his friend are courteous to her, and Mr. Zaman cooperates in receiving his injection. He listens as Maria repeats teaching about the risks of alcohol consumption. She encourages his attendance at an Alcoholics Anonymous meeting. He reports that he did go to one meeting yesterday. Maria praises him and encourages him and his friend to go again that night.

1100–1300: The next patient is Ms. Abbott, a 53-year-old single woman with a diagnosis of schizoaffective disorder and hypertension. She lives alone in a building for older adults and has no contact with family. Ms. Abbott was referred by her clinic team because she experienced three hospitalizations for psychotic decompensation over a period of a year despite receiving monthly decanoate injections. The ACT team is now the payee for her disability cheque. Today, Maria is taking Ms. Abbott out to pay her bills and to see her primary care physician for a checkup. Ms. Abbott greets Maria warmly at the door, wearing excessive makeup and inappropriate summer clothing. With gentle encouragement, she agrees to wear warmer clothes. She is reluctant to show Maria her medication box and briefly gets irritable when Maria points out that she has not taken her morning medications. As they stop by the apartment office to pay the rent, Maria talks with the manager briefly. This apartment manager is the team's only contact person and calls the team whenever any of the other residents report that Ms. Abbott is exhibiting unusual behaviour. Over the next hour and a half, Maria and Ms. Abbott drive to various stores and to Ms. Abbott's medical appointment.

1400–1630: The last patient visit of the day is with Mr. Hahn, a 60-year-old widowed man diagnosed with schizophrenia and cocaine dependence. Mr. Hahn was referred by the emergency department last year after repeated visits due to psychosis and intoxication. Initially he was homeless, but he now lives in a recovery house shelter and has been clean of illegal substances for 6 months. He receives a monthly decanoate injection and is socially isolated in the house. Now that he receives disability support payments, he is seeking an affordable apartment. Maria has made appointments at two apartment buildings. After greeting him, Maria notes that he is wearing the same clothes he had on 2 days earlier and his hair is uncombed. She suggests that he shower and change his clothes before they go out, and he agrees.

At the end of the day, Maria jots down information she will use to write her progress notes in patients' charts the next day when she returns to the clinic.

BOX 3-2 **PATIENT SAFETY GOALS IN MENTAL HEALTH CARE SETTINGS**

- Improve the accuracy of patient identification:
  - Use at least two ways, such as the patient's name and date of birth, to identify patients.
- Improve the effectiveness of communication among caregivers:
  - Read back verbal orders.
  - Create a list of abbreviations and symbols that are not to be used.
  - Promptly report critical tests and critical results.
- Improve the safety of using medications:
  - Create a list of look-alike and sound-alike medications.
- Reduce the risk of health care–associated infections:
  - Follow hand-cleaning guidelines from the World Health Organization.
- Record and report death or injury from infection.
- Accurately and completely reconcile medications across the continuum of care:
  - Compare current and newly ordered medications for compatibility.
  - Give a list of medications to the next provider and regular caregiver.
  - Provide a medication list to both the patient and the family.
- Encourage patients' active involvement in their own care:
  - Encourage patients and families to report safety concerns.
- Identify safety risks inherent in the patient population:
  - Identify individuals at risk for suicide.

Source: Adapted from Accreditation Canada. (2012). *Qmentum program standards*. Ottawa: Author

---

Aggression and violence are also risks when a patient's illness affects perception, thinking, insight, judgement, and behaviour. This risk also increases if patients have reduced outlets for frustration. Aggression in the mental health workplace is an important concern (Stevenson, Jack, O'Mara, et al., 2015). Psychiatric staff should have specialized training to minimize hostility while maintaining an atmosphere that promotes healthy and appropriate expression of anger and other feelings. Many psychiatric units are locked since some patients are hospitalized involuntarily, and elopement (absence from the unit without leave) must be prevented in a way that avoids an atmosphere of imprisonment, which can increase the risk for agitation and aggression.

One of the most important safety aspects of a psychiatric service area is the design of patient care areas. These areas are usually less institutional-looking than other hospital areas. Closets

TABLE 3-1	CHARACTERISTICS, TREATMENT OUTCOMES, AND INTERVENTIONS BY SETTING	
INPATIENT SETTING	**COMMUNITY MENTAL HEALTH SETTING**	
Characteristics		
Unit locked by staff	Home locked by patient	
24-hour supervision	Intermittent supervision	
Boundaries determined by staff	Boundaries negotiated with patient	
Milieu with food, housekeeping, security services	Patient-controlled environment with self-care, safety risks	
Treatment Outcomes		
Stabilization of symptoms and return to community	Stable or improved level of functioning in community	
Interventions		
Develop short-term therapeutic relationship	Establish long-term therapeutic relationship	
Develop comprehensive plan of care, with attention to sociocultural needs of patient	Develop comprehensive plan of care for patient and support system, with attention to sociocultural needs	
Enforce boundaries by seclusion or restraint as needed	Negotiate boundaries with patient	
Administer medication	Encourage adherence to medication regimen	
Monitor nutrition and self-care, with assistance as needed	Teach and support adequate nutrition and self-care and provide referrals as needed	
Provide health assessment and intervention as needed	Assist patient in self-assessment and self-management and provide referrals to meet health needs in community as needed	
Offer structured socialization activities	Use creative strategies to refer patient to positive social activities	
Plan for discharge to housing with family or significant other and plan for follow-up treatment	Communicate regularly with family or support system to assess and improve patient's level of functioning	

should be equipped with "break-bars" designed to hold a minimal amount of weight; windows, with shatterproof glass, are locked; beds are often platforms rather than mechanical hospital beds, which can be dangerous because of their crushing potential; and showers should have non–weight-bearing shower heads.

Differences in characteristics, treatment outcomes, and interventions between inpatient and community settings are outlined in Table 3-1. Note that all of these interventions fall within the practice domain of the basic-level registered nurse or registered psychiatric nurse.

ROLES AND RESPONSIBILITIES

As noted in Chapter 1, psychiatric mental health nurses are educated at a variety of levels, including diploma, baccalaureate, master's, and doctoral. Perhaps the most significant distinction among the multiple levels of preparation is the extent to which the nurse acts autonomously and provides consultation to other providers, both inside and outside the particular agency. The health professions acts of individual provinces and territories grant nurses authority to practise, and the standards of practice—developed for registered nurses by the Canadian Federation of Psychiatric Mental Health Nurses (2014) and for registered psychiatric nurses by the Registered Psychiatric Nurses of Canada (2010)—guide nurses in their practice (see Chapter 7). Table 3-2 describes the roles of psychiatric mental health nurses according to level of education.

Community Psychiatric Mental Health Nursing

Psychiatric mental health nursing in the community setting requires strong problem-solving and clinical skills, cultural

sensitivity, flexibility, solid knowledge of community resources, and comfort with functioning more autonomously than acute care nurses do. Patients need assistance with problems related to individual psychiatric symptoms, family and support systems, and basic living needs, such as housing and financial support. Community treatment hinges on enhancing patients' strengths in the same environment in which they maintain their daily life, which makes individually tailored psychiatric care imperative. Treatment in the community permits patients and those involved in their support to learn new ways of coping with symptoms or situational difficulties. The result can be one of empowerment and self-management for patients and their support systems.

Biopsychosocial Assessment

Assessment of the needs and capacities of patients living in the community requires expansion of the general psychiatric mental health nursing assessment (see Chapter 6). To be able to plan and implement effective treatment, the community psychiatric mental health nurse must also develop a comprehensive understanding of the patient's ability to cope with the demands of living in the community. The biopsychosocial model is a system that can guide the nursing assessment and interventions in a holistic manner, viewing clients comprehensively, including their biology, social environment and skills, and psychological characteristics. Box 3-3 identifies the elements of a biopsychosocial assessment.

Key elements of this assessment are strongly related to the probability that the patient will experience successful outcomes in the community. Problems in any of the following areas require immediate attention because they can seriously impair the success of other treatment goals:

TABLE 3-2	COMMUNITY PSYCHIATRIC MENTAL HEALTH NURSING ROLES RELEVANT TO EDUCATIONAL PREPARATION	
ROLE	**ADVANCED PRACTICE (MN, PHD)**	**BASIC PRACTICE (DIPLOMA, BSCN)**
Practice	Nurse practitioner or clinical nurse specialist; manage consumer care and prescribe or recommend interventions independently	Provide nursing care for consumer and assist with medication management as prescribed, under direct supervision
Consultation	Act as consultant to staff about plan of care, to consumer and family about options for care; collaborate with community agencies about service coordination and planning processes	Consult with staff about care planning and work with nurse practitioner or physician to promote health and mental health care; consult with consumer and family about options for care; collaborate with community agencies about service coordination and planning processes; collaborate with staff from other agencies
Administration	Assume administrative or contract consultant role within mental health agencies or mental health authority	Take leadership role within mental health treatment team
Research and education	Take on role as educator or researcher within agency or mental health authority	Participate in research at agency or mental health authority; serve as preceptor to undergraduate nursing students

- Housing adequacy and stability: A patient who faces daily fears of homelessness will not be able to focus on the treatment.
- Income and source of income: A patient must have a basic income—whether from an entitlement, a relative, or other sources—to obtain necessary medication and meet daily needs for food and clothing.
- Family and support system: The presence of a family member, friend, or neighbour supports the patient's recovery and gives the nurse a contact person (with the patient's consent).
- Substance abuse history and current use: Often hidden or minimized during hospitalization, substance abuse can be a destructive force, undermining medication effectiveness and interfering with relationships, safety, community acceptance, and procurement of housing.
- Physical well-being: Factors that increase health risks and decrease lifespan for individuals with mental illnesses include decreased physical activity, smoking, adverse effects of medications, and absence of routine health exams.

Individual cultural characteristics are also very important to assess. For example, working with a patient who speaks a different language from the nurse requires the nurse to consider the implications of language and cultural background. In such a case, the use of a translator or cultural consultant from the agency or from the family is essential (see Chapter 8).

Treatment Goals and Interventions

In the community setting, treatment goals and interventions are negotiated rather than imposed on the patient. To meet a broad range of patient needs, community psychiatric mental health nurses must approach interventions with flexibility and resourcefulness. Not unexpectedly, patient outcomes with regard to mental status and functional level have been found to be more positive and achieved with greater cost effectiveness when the community psychiatric mental health nurse integrates case management into the professional role (Chan, Mackenzie, & Jacobs, 2000). The complexity of navigating the mental health and social service funding systems is often overwhelming to patients. The 1980s brought increased emphasis on case management as a core nursing function in treating the patient with serious mental illness.

In the private domain as well, case management, or care management, found a niche. The intent was to charge case managers with designing individually tailored treatment services for patients and tracking outcomes of care. The new case management included assessing patient needs, developing a plan for service, linking the patient with necessary services, monitoring the effectiveness of services, and advocating for the patient as needed. Newer models, particularly team concepts, have since been developed and will be discussed later in this chapter.

Interprofessional Team Member

Interprofessional psychiatric nursing practice is one of the core mental health disciplines that work to the patient's benefit. In interprofessional team meetings, the individual and discipline-specific expertise of each member is recognized. Generally, the composition of the team reflects the availability of fiscal and professional resources in the area. The community psychiatric team may include psychiatrists, nurses, social workers, psychologists, addictions specialists, recreational therapists, occupational therapists, and mental health workers.

The nurse is able to integrate a strong nursing identity into the team perspective. At the basic- or advanced-practice level, the community psychiatric mental health nurse holds a critical position to link the biopsychosocial and spiritual components relevant to mental health care. The nurse also communicates a discipline-specific expertise in a manner that the patient, significant others, and other members of the health care team can understand. In particular, the management and administration of psychotropic medications have become significant tasks the community nurse is expected to perform.

Biopsychosocial Care Manager

The role of the community psychiatric mental health nurse includes coordinating mental health, physical health, spiritual health, social service, educational service, and vocational realms of care for the mental health patient. The reality of community practice in the new millennium is that few patients seeking treatment have uncomplicated symptoms of a single mental illness. The severity of illness has increased, and it is often

BOX 3-3 POTENTIAL MEMBERS OF PSYCHIATRIC MENTAL HEALTH TREATMENT TEAMS

Registered psychiatric nurses: Licensed professionals trained with an extensive focus on the knowledge and skills required for psychiatric mental health nursing (see the Registered Psychiatric Nurse Regulators of Canada website: http://www.rpnc.ca/pages/home.php).

Registered nurses: Registered nurses working in psychiatric mental health care do not necessarily have specific certification, but many have some specialty experience. Registered nurses in Canada can complete a specialty certificate in psychiatric mental health nursing (see the Canadian Nurses Association certification program: http://www.nurseone.ca/Default.aspx?portlet=StaticHtmlViewerPortlet&plang=1&ptdi=153). Among the responsibilities of a registered nurse are diagnosing and treating responses to psychiatric disorders, coordinating care, counselling, giving medication and evaluating responses, and providing education.

Licensed practical nurses or registered practical nurses: Provincial or territorial licensing or registration bodies regulate these professionals by determining entry-to-practice requirements and establishing and promoting standards for registration, practice, and professional conduct. These nurses are involved with the care of psychiatric patients by providing care within their scope of practice as determined by their provincial or territorial governing body.

Psychiatric mental health advanced-practice nurses: Psychiatric mental health advanced-practice nurses work as nurse therapists, clinical nurse specialists, or education specialists by virtue of advanced training (e.g., master's or doctorate prepared) or recognized advanced level of experience. These nurses may be involved in conducting therapy, case management, consulting, education, or research.

Social workers: Basic-level social workers help the patient prepare a support system that will promote mental health upon discharge from the hospital. They may help patients develop contacts with day treatment centres, employers, sources of financial aid, and landlords. Social workers can also undergo training in individual, family, and group therapies and function as primary care providers.

Counsellors: Counsellors prepared in disciplines such as psychology, rehabilitation counselling, nursing or psychiatric nursing, and addiction counselling may augment the treatment plan by co-leading groups, providing basic supportive counselling, or assisting in psychoeducational and recreational activities. Private counselling services in the community are not covered by medicare.

Psychologists: In keeping with their doctoral degree preparation, psychologists conduct psychological testing, provide consultation for the team, and offer direct services such as specialized individual, family, or marital therapies. Psychologists' services in the community are not covered by medicare.

Occupational, recreational, art, music, and dance therapists: Based on their specialist preparation, these therapists assist patients in gaining skills that help them cope more effectively, gain or retain employment, use leisure time to the benefit of their mental health, and express themselves in healthy ways.

Psychiatrists: Depending on their specialty of preparation, psychiatrists may provide in-depth psychotherapy or medication therapy or head a team of mental health providers functioning as a community-based service. Psychiatrists may be employed by the hospital or may hold practice privileges in the facility. Because psychiatry is a medical specialty, treatment and care by psychiatrists—with the exception of psychoanalysis—is covered by medicare. Because they have the legal power to prescribe and to write orders, psychiatrists often function as the leaders of the teams managing the care of patients individually assigned to them.

Medical physicians: Medical physicians provide medical diagnoses and treatments on a consultation basis. Medical physicians will also provide referrals to psychiatrists, mental health nurses, psychologists, and social workers when needed. Occasionally, a physician trained as an addiction specialist may play a more direct role on a unit that offers treatment for addictive disease.

Health care aides: Health care aides function under the direction and supervision of nurses. They provide assistance to patients in meeting basic needs and also help the community to remain supportive, safe, and healthy.

Community mental health workers: Community mental health workers are registered nurses or registered psychiatric nurses, social workers, or other trained professionals who offer case management and care in the community at various levels of intensity. Community mental health workers are sometimes involved in hospital-treatment-team and patient-discharge planning.

Pharmacists: In view of the intricacies of prescribing, coordinating, and administering combinations of psychotropic and other medications, the consulting pharmacist can offer a valuable safeguard. Physicians and nurses collaborate with the pharmacist regarding new medications, which are being introduced at a steady rate.

Spiritual carers: Spiritual advisors can play an important role in addressing the spiritual, and sometimes cultural, aspects of patients' lives and support spirituality as a coping resource.

---

accompanied by substance abuse, poverty, and stress. Repeated studies show that people with mental illnesses also have a higher risk for medical disorders than the general population (Robson & Gray, 2007).

The community psychiatric mental health nurse bridges the gap between the psychiatric and physical needs of the patient, meeting not only with the mental health treatment team but also with the patient's primary care team and serving as the liaison between the two. According to Griswold and colleagues (2010), integrating a primary care navigator to assist patients with primary care needs results in greater success with follow-up and attendance at appointments.

Treatment Team

Psychiatric nursing practice is one of the core mental health disciplines that work with a patient to improve well-being. The health care team may include psychiatrists, nurses, social workers, psychologists, addictions specialists, recreational therapists, occupational therapists, and mental health workers. Generally, the composition of the team reflects the availability of fiscal and professional resources in the area.

In team meetings, the individual and discipline-specific expertise of each member is recognized (see Box 3-3). The person with the mental illness is also an important member of the team.

It is the nurse's responsibility to ensure that a space is created for this person's voice within the team. Input from the patient and family (if available and desirable) is critical in formulating treatment goals. To take part in decision making, though, a patient must be knowledgeable about the illness and treatment options. Research demonstrates that people with mental illness want more than watered-down and simplistic information. (Imagine a pamphlet titled *You and Your Mental Illness*.) To fully participate in the treatment plan, patients need current, evidence-informed information about their illness and treatment options (Hamlett, Carr, & Hillbrand, 2016). Incorporating the patient's feedback in developing the treatment plan goals increases the likelihood of the success of established care outcomes.

Members of each discipline are responsible for gathering data and participating in the planning of care. Patients may find meeting with so many people and answering similar questions from each of them extremely stressful or threatening; team members, therefore, must consider appropriate timing. The urgency of the need for data should be weighed against the patient's ability to tolerate assessment. Assessments—in particular, suicide assessments—made by the nurse often provide the basis for initial care. In many inpatient settings, the psychiatrist must evaluate the patient and provide orders within a limited time frame.

There are three regulated nursing professions in Canada: licensed practical nurse (LPN) or registered practical nurse (RPN), licensed registered nurse (RN), and licensed registered psychiatric nurse (RPN). The nurse has a leadership role in the team meetings. This nursing leadership reflects the holistic nature of nursing, as well as the fact that nursing is the discipline that is represented on the unit at all times. Nurses are in a unique position to advocate on behalf of the patient and to contribute valuable information such as continuous assessment findings, the patient's adjustment to the unit, and any health concerns, psychoeducational needs, and patient self-care deficits.

Multidisciplinary teams use their team members' individual levels of expertise to develop individual care plans. A care plan is developed by each discipline. For example, nursing develops a nursing care plan, and physiotherapy develops its own care plan. Although these plans of care may be housed in the same patient chart, they are discipline specific, and each discipline is responsible for obtaining their own goals. In contrast, an interdisciplinary team develops one care plan. All of the health care professionals will work toward the same goals for the patient. For example, the goal may be for the patient to improve his or her self-concept; then nursing provides nursing interventions that lead to this outcome, and occupational therapy provides interventions that also lead to this outcome. With an interdisciplinary treatment plan, the overlap of professional scope of practice is recognized and shared goals are established. The team composes the plan of care, which is often based on the appropriate clinical pathway, revising the plan along the way if the patient's progress differs from that expected. A reduction in overt symptoms and the development of an adequate outpatient plan signal that discharge is near.

Within an interdisciplinary treatment team, the nurse may take on several roles. The role of the psychiatric mental health

> **VIGNETTE**
>
> Joelle is assigned as Shane's primary nurse, and Tazmine as his evening-shift nurse. Joelle met with the treatment team to plan Shane's care during his hospitalization. The physician's diagnosis was major depression with psychotic features. The major problems the team identified, based on reports of the past 2 days and nursing assessments, were safety, paranoia, nonadherence to medication regimens, and hypertension. Joelle identified that the nursing diagnoses were risk for self-directed violence, disturbed thought processes, noncompliance, and deficient knowledge. Along with the treatment team, Joelle identified the therapy and psychoeducation groups that Shane should participate in and recommended that suicide-precaution monitoring be maintained, owing to Shane's inability to promise that he would not harm himself on the unit or that he would tell one of the staff members if his thoughts about committing suicide changed.

nurse includes coordinating mental health, physical health, spiritual health, social service, educational service, and vocational realms of care for the mental health patient. The reality of practice in the new millennium is that few patients seeking treatment have uncomplicated symptoms of a single mental illness. The severity of illness has increased, and it is often accompanied by substance abuse, poverty, and stress. Repeated studies show that people with mental illnesses also have a higher rate of mental-physical disorder comorbidity than the general population (Kavalidou, Smith, & O'Connor, 2016).

The psychiatric mental health nurse bridges the gap between the psychiatric and physical needs of the patient, meeting not only with the mental health treatment team but also with the patient's primary care team and serving as the liaison between the two. Case management includes the care coordination activities the nurse does with or for the patient and includes referrals, assistance with paperwork applications, connection to resources, and overall navigation of the health care system. The complexity of navigating the mental health and social service funding systems is often overwhelming to patients. The 1980s brought increased emphasis on case management as a core nursing function in treating the patient with serious mental illness. According to Mohamed (2016), integrating a nurse case manager to assist patients with primary care needs results in greater success with follow-up and attendance at appointments. Many case managers assess patient needs, design individually tailored treatment services for patients, link the patient with necessary services, monitor the effectiveness of services, and advocate for the patient as needed.

Nursing Care
Establishing a Therapeutic Relationship
Being admitted to a psychiatric mental health care service is anxiety provoking for anyone, but anxiety can be severe for patients admitted to an inpatient psychiatric unit. Especially for the first-time patient, admission often summons preconceptions about psychiatric hospitals and the negative stigma associated with them. Patients may experience shame, and families may be reluctant to be forthcoming with pertinent information. Psychiatric mental health nurses can be most effective when they are

sensitive to both the patient and the family during the admission process. In this initial encounter with the patient, nurses must try to provide reassurance and hope.

Mental and Physical Health Assessment

Upon admission, the nurse will assess the patient with the goals of gathering information that will enable the treatment team to develop a suitable plan of care, ensuring that safety concerns are identified and addressed, identifying the learning needs of the patient so the nurse can prioritize the information needs, and initiating a therapeutic relationship between the nurse and the patient. Chapter 6 presents a more detailed discussion of how to perform an admission assessment, as well as a mental status examination.

The nurse is in an excellent position to assess not only mental health but also physical health. Rates of metabolic syndrome, diabetes, and heart disease are all higher for individuals with mental health problems. Nurses can play a key role in assessing for these problems and initiating patient teaching and supports for prevention and management (Kavalidou, Smith, & O'Connor, 2016).

Individuals with mental health problems may experience barriers to health care and healthy living practices necessary to maintain their health (Socias, Shoveller, Bean, et al, 2016). Often, when patients with pre-existing or comorbid conditions seek treatment in the ED for a physical medical condition, health care providers will downplay or attribute the patient's physical complaints to the psychiatric condition. Patients also report reluctance to seek out health care providers, owing to the stigma they encounter when they reveal they are being treated for a comorbid psychiatric illness. This reluctance to seek treatment not only adversely affects the patient's quality of life but also contributes to a decreased life expectancy.

Milieu Management

A well-managed milieu offers patients a sense of security and comfort. Structured aspects of the milieu include activities, program and unit rules, reality orientation practices, and the environment. In addition to the structured components of the milieu, Peplau (1989) described other less tangible factors, such as the interactions that occur among patients and staff, patients and patients, patients and visitors, and so forth. This interactivity is quite different from the environment of medical inpatient units, where patients generally remain in their rooms, often with closed doors, and rarely interact with other patients or the milieu. On psychiatric units, patients are in constant contact with their peers and staff. These interactions help patients engage and can increase their sense of social competence and worth.

The therapeutic milieu can serve as a real-life training ground for learning about the self and practising communication and coping skills in preparation for a return to the community. Even events that seemingly distract from the program of therapies can be turned into valuable learning opportunities for the members of the milieu. Nurses can support the milieu and intervene when necessary. They usually develop an uncanny ability to assess the mood of the unit (e.g., calm, anxious, disengaged, or tense) and predict environmental risk. Nurses observe the dynamics of interactions, reinforce adaptive social skills, and redirect patients during negative interactions. Reports from shift to shift provide information on the emotional climate and level of tension on the unit.

Structured Group Activities

In most mental health programs, experienced psychiatric mental health nurses conduct specific, structured activities involving the therapeutic community, special groups, or families. Examples of these activities include morning goal-setting meetings and evening goal-review meetings. Community meetings may be held daily or at other scheduled times of the week. At these meetings, new patients are greeted, and departing patients are given farewells; ideas for unit activities are discussed; community problems or successes are considered; and other business of the therapeutic community is conducted.

Nurses also offer psychoeducational groups for patients and families on topics such as stress management, coping skills, grieving, medication management, healthy-living practices, and communication skills. Group therapy is a specialized therapy led by a mental health practitioner with advanced training. This therapy addresses communication and sharing, helps patients explore life problems and decrease their isolation and anxiety, and engages patients in the recovery process. Chapter 33 presents a more detailed discussion of therapeutic groups led by nurses.

VIGNETTE

During the evening shift, Tazmine observes that Shane is restless and pacing in the hallway. Tazmine recalls that when he was admitted, Shane was asked if he had been aggressive in the past. He stated that he had periods of being angry when he felt people were not listening to him or were telling him what to do. Tazmine also recalls that Shane said that he has never struck or hit anyone before and that he usually handles anger by taking a walk around the neighbourhood or going to his room.

Tazmine asks Shane how things are going. He tells her he is upset because he told the doctor he wanted to be discharged, and the doctor said he was not ready yet. Tazmine affirms that this must be frustrating. She suggests that Shane practise some of the relaxation techniques he learned in the coping group today to manage his feelings of anger. Tazmine also asks Shane if he would like the medication that has been ordered to manage his feelings of agitation when necessary. Shane agrees to take 2 mg lorazepam orally and to relax in his room until he feels in better control of his anger. Tazmine goes to see Shane after 30 minutes. She provides positive feedback about his ability to successfully handle his aggressive feelings.

Documentation

Documentation of patient progress is the responsibility of the entire mental health care team. Although communication among team members and coordination of services are the primary goals when choosing a system for charting, practitioners in the inpatient setting must also consider professional standards, legal issues, and accreditation by regulatory agencies. Information must also be in a format that is retrievable for quality-assurance monitoring, utilization management, peer review, and research. Chapter 7 gives an overview of documentation options.

Medication Administration

The safe administration of medications and the monitoring of their effects is a responsibility for psychiatric mental health nurses, who are expected to have detailed knowledge of psychoactive medications and the interactions and psychological adverse effects of other medications. The nurse reports regarding the patient's adherence to the medication regimen, the presence or absence of adverse effects, and changes in the patient's behaviours exert great influence on the physician's medication decisions. For example, feedback about excessive sedation or increased agitation may lead to a decrease or increase in the dosage of an antipsychotic medication.

Nurses often have numerous decisions to make about medications that are prescribed to be administered prn (as needed). These decisions must be based on a combination of factors: the patient's wishes, the team's plan, attempts to use alternative methods of coping, and the nurse's judgements regarding timing and the patient's behaviour. Documentation for administering each prn medication must include the rationale for its use and its effects.

Medication adherence. One of the nurse's goals during hospitalization is to assist the patient to learn the importance of medication adherence during and after hospitalization. Taking medication regularly is a common challenge for psychiatric patients, often because of irritating adverse effects, lack of understanding about the medications, and lack of sufficient patient consultation in treatment decisions. Educating patients on how to recognize, report, and manage potential adverse effects can help empower patients and increase treatment success. This approach encourages the patient to seek out the nurse when it is time for medications to be administered and fosters responsibility and involvement in the treatment process.

Pain management. Just like others in the general population, psychiatric patients often suffer from medical problems that result in pain (e.g., neck, back, or spine problems; arthritis; migraine headaches). People with psychiatric conditions are often viewed as being unable to accurately assess their own sensations or are labelled "drug seeking," a situation that results in untreated or undertreated pain. Nurses can advocate for patients by stressing that relieving pain is a humanitarian consideration and that a patient in pain is less able to participate in formal activities on the unit and will have greater difficulty focusing on education. Psychological pain, which may manifest as anxiety, is equally distressing and can also decrease the ability of the individual to participate in activities of daily living and community life. Adequate assessment and treatment of pain within the psychiatric population may have a positive impact on the course of mental disorders.

Crisis Management

Medical crises may occur in any setting; however, they are more common on inpatient units. Nurses anticipate, prevent, and manage emergencies and crises on the unit. These crises may be of a medical or behavioural nature.

Medical crises. Mental health units must be able to assess and stabilize the condition of a patient who experiences a medical crisis. Mental health or addictive disease units that manage detoxification (withdrawal from alcohol or other drugs) must anticipate several common medical crises associated with that process. Mental health units, therefore, store crash carts containing the emergency medications used to treat shock and cardiorespiratory arrest. Nurses must maintain their cardiopulmonary resuscitation skills and be able to use basic emergency equipment. To be effective and practise at a high level of competency, nurses are advised to attend in-service sessions and workshops designed to teach and maintain skills. Nurses must also be able to alert medical support systems quickly and mobilize transportation to the appropriate medical facility.

Behavioural crises. Behavioural crises can lead to patient violence toward self or others and are usually, but not always, observed to escalate through fairly predictable stages. Crisis prevention and management techniques are practised by staff in most mental health facilities (see the Registered Nurses' Association of Ontario's *Best Practice Guideline for Crisis Intervention*, http://rnao.ca/bpg/guidelines/crisis-intervention). Many psychiatric hospitals have special teams made up of nurses, psychiatric aides, and other professionals who respond to psychiatric emergencies. Each member of the team takes part in the team effort to defuse a crisis in its early stages. If preventive measures fail, each member of the team participates in a rapid, organized movement designed to immobilize, medicate, or seclude a patient. The nurse is most often this team's leader, not only organizing the plan but also timing the intervention and managing the concurrent use of prn medications. The nurse can initiate such an intervention in the absence of a physician but must secure a physician's order for restraint or seclusion within a specified time. The nurse also advocates for patients in crisis by ensuring that their legal rights are preserved, no matter how difficult it may be to manage their behaviour. Refer to Chapters 7 and 24 for further discussions about and protocols for the use of restraints and seclusion.

Crises are upsetting and threatening to uninvolved patients and staff as well. A designated staff member usually addresses the uninvolved patient concerns and feelings. This person removes other patients from the area of the crisis and helps them express their fears. Patients may be concerned for their own safety or the welfare of the patient involved in the crisis. They may fear that they, too, might experience such a loss of control. The noninvolved staff members, staff members of the code team, and the patient in crisis all benefit from debriefing after these difficult situations.

FUTURE ISSUES

Barriers to Treatment

Despite the current availability and variety of community psychiatric treatments in Canada, many patients in need of services still do not receive them because of various barriers to treatment—factors that impede access to psychiatric care—including stigma, geographical challenges, financial limitations, policy issues, and system shortcomings. The *Canadian Community*

Health Survey: Mental Health, estimated that 2.8 million Canadians over age 15 have experienced mental health or substance abuse problems in the previous year. Thirty-three percent of these individuals identified having their needs partially unmet or not met at all (Sunderland & Findlay, 2013).

Although the stigma of mental illness has lessened over the past 40 years—in part because mental illnesses are now recognized as biologically based and also because many well-known people have admitted to having received psychiatric treatment—many people still are afraid to disclose a psychiatric diagnosis. Instead, they seek medical care for vague somatic complaints from primary care providers, who too often fail to diagnose anxiety or depressive disorders.

In addition to stigma, as mentioned, geographical, financial, and systems factors can impede access to psychiatric care. Mental health services are scarce in some rural areas, and due to funding shortfalls, mental health treatment programs often have wait lists. The 2006 Senate report *Out of the Shadows at Last* (Kirby & Keon, 2006) identified national system and policy problems, including fragmented care for children and adults with serious mental illness, high unemployment and disability among those with serious mental illness, undertreatment of older adults, and lack of national priorities for mental health and suicide prevention. Provincial and other insurance plans do not reimburse for community mental health care at the same level that they cover other health care.

Meeting Changing Demands

It is increasingly recognized that people with mental illness are receiving care in all areas of the health care system. With high rates of mental-physical comorbidities, nurses in all areas need to have a strong foundation of mental health nursing assessment and basic treatment skills. Disaster nursing will also become an increasing area of focus within mental health. There is increasing recognition of the mental-physical needs survivors of trauma and disaster. Certainly, many of these changing demands will occur within a context of a complex and adaptive health care system. As a result, nurses will need to become increasingly comfortable with ambiguity, have a willingness to be flexible, and become confident in their leadership skills.

KEY POINTS TO REMEMBER

- The basic-level community psychiatric mental health nurse practises in many sites.
- Inpatient psychiatric care is guaranteed for all Canadians, with costs and delivery responsibilities shared by regional, provincial or territorial, and federal governments.
- The continuum of psychiatric treatment includes numerous community treatment alternatives with varying degrees of intensity of care.
- Inpatient care has increasingly become more acute and short term.
- As part of the health care team, the psychiatric mental health nurse functions as a leader.
- Psychiatric mental health nurses require strong skills in management, communication, and collaboration.
- Discharge planning begins on the day of admission and requires input from the treatment team and the community mental health care provider.

- The nurse advocates for the patient and ensures that the patient's rights are protected.
- Monitoring the environment and providing for safety are important components of good care.
- Basic-level psychiatric mental health nursing interventions include admission, provision of a safe environment, psychiatric and physical assessments, milieu management, documentation, medication administration, and preparation for discharge to the community.
- Documentation is an important form of communication to promote consistency in patient care and to justify the patient's stay in the hospital.
- Barriers to mental health care still exist, but the psychiatric mental health nurse may be able to diminish them.

CRITICAL THINKING

1. Imagine that you were asked for your opinion in regard to your patient's ability to make everyday decisions for himself. What sort of things would you consider as you weighed out safety versus autonomy and personal rights? How would you incorporate your knowledge of protective empowering?
2. If nurses function as equal members of the multidisciplinary mental health team, what differentiates the nurse from the other members of the team?

3. Identify gaps in community care that might affect patient discharge planning.
4. How might the community be affected when patients with serious mental illness live in group homes?

CHAPTER REVIEW

1. A friend recognizes that his depression has returned and tells you he is suicidal and concerned he will harm himself. He is afraid that if he seeks help he will be involuntarily admitted to a psychiatric hospital, an idea that terrifies him. Which of the following responses best meets his immediate care needs?
   a. Provide emotional support and encourage him to contact his family.
   b. Express your concern for his safety, normalize psychiatric treatment as equal to treatment of any physical condition, and offer to accompany and support him through assessment at a nearby emergency department.
   c. Contact the police or a provincial/territorial magistrate to initiate involuntary assessment.
   d. Assist him to obtain an outpatient counselling appointment at an area community mental health centre, and call him frequently to ensure that he is safe until this appointment occurs.

2. You are about to interview a newly admitted patient on your inpatient mental health unit. This is his first experience with psychiatric treatment. Which of the following interventions would be appropriate for this patient? Select all that apply.
   a. Discuss outpatient care options for after discharge.
   b. Anticipate and address possible increased anxiety and shame.
   c. Ensure that the individual understands his rights as a patient on your unit.
   d. Assess the patient for physical health needs that may have been overlooked.
   e. Carefully check all clothing and possessions for potentially dangerous items.

3. Which of the following nursing actions are appropriate in maintaining a safe therapeutic inpatient milieu? Select all that apply.
   a. Interact frequently with both individuals and groups on the unit.
   b. Ensure that none of the unit fixtures can be used for suicide by hanging.
   c. Initiate and support group interactions via therapeutic groups and activities.
   d. Stock the unit with standard hospital beds and other sturdy hospital furnishings.
   e. Provide and encourage opportunities to practise social and other life skills.
   f. Collaborate with housekeeping to provide a safe, pleasant environment.

4. A patient becomes agitated and hostile, threatening to smash a chair into the nurses' station door. Which of the following responses would be most appropriate for the student nurse to make?

   a. Maintain a safe distance, and attempt to de-escalate the patient verbally.
   b. When the response team arrives, assist in physically restraining the patient.
   c. Assist in promptly moving other patients to a safe distance or separate location.
   d. Meet with the patient immediately after the crisis to help him process what happened.

5. A student is considering a career in mental health nursing. Which of the following statements accurately reflects the role and expectations of mental health nurses in acute care settings?
   a. The primary role of the nurse is to monitor the patients from the nurses' station.
   b. Psychiatric patients rarely need medical care, so nurses do not need medical nursing skills.
   c. The close relationships developed with patients can lead to later romantic relationships.
   d. Mental health nursing requires a high degree of interpersonal comfort and therapeutic skill.

6. You are a community mental health nurse meeting with a patient who has just been discharged from the hospital, where he had received psychiatric care for the first time. Which of the following activities would you expect to undertake in your role as the nurse on the treatment team caring for this patient?
   a. Take medications to the patient's home each day and administer them.
   b. Solve day-to-day problems for the patient to minimize his exposure to stress.
   c. Refer the patient to counsellors or other providers when he indicates a need to talk with someone.
   d. Take a ride on the local bus system with the patient to help him learn routes and schedules.

7. Mrs. Chan, a patient at the community mental health centre, tends to stop taking her medications at intervals, usually leading to decompensation. Which of the following interventions would most likely improve her adherence to her medications?
   a. Help Mrs. Chan understand her illness and allow her to share in decisions about her care.
   b. Advise Mrs. Chan that if she stops her medications, her doctor will hospitalize her.
   c. Arrange for Mrs. Chan to receive daily home care so her use of medications is monitored.
   d. Discourage Mrs. Chan from focusing on adverse effects and other excuses for stopping her pills.

ⒺVOLVE WEBSITE

Post-Test | interactive review

Visit the Evolve website for Chapter Review Answers and Rationales, Critical Thinking Answer Guidelines, and additional resources related to the content in this chapter: http://evolve.elsevier.com/Canada/Varcarolis/psychiatric/

REFERENCES

Accreditation Canada (2016). *Required organizational practices: Handbook 2017*. Ottawa, ON: Author. Retrieved from https://accreditation.ca/sites/default/files/rop-handbook-2017.pdf.

Allison, S., Bastiampillai, T., & Goldney, R. (2014). Acute versus sub-acute care beds: Should Australia invest in community beds at the expense of hospital beds? *The Australian and New Zealand Journal of Psychiatry, 48*(10), 952–956. doi:10.1177/0004867414538106.

Brickell, T., Nicholls, T., Procyshyn, R., et al. (2009). *Patient safety in mental health*. Edmonton: Canadian Patient Safety Institute and Ontario Hospital Association. Retrieved from http://www.patientsafetyinstitute.ca/en/toolsResources/Research/commissionedResearch/mentalHealthAndPatientSafety/Documents/Mental%20Health%20Paper.pdf.

Canadian Federation of Psychiatric Mental Health Nurses (2014). *Canadian standards of psychiatric–mental health nursing* (4th ed.). Toronto: Author.

Canadian Institute for Health Information. (2016). *National health expenditure trends, 1975 to 2016*. Retrieved from https://www.cihi.ca/sites/default/files/document/nhex-trends-narrative-report_2016_en.pdf.

Chan, S., Mackenzie, A., & Jacobs, P. (2000). Cost-effectiveness analysis of case management versus routine community care organization for patients with chronic schizophrenia. *Archives of Psychiatric Nursing, 14*(2), 98–104. doi: 10.1016/S0883-9417(00)80025-4.

Fahim, C., Semovski, V., & Younger, J. (2016). The Hamilton mobile crisis rapid response team: A first-responder mental health service. *Psychiatric Services, 67*(8), 929. doi:10.1176/appi.ps670802.

Forchuk, C., Jensen, E., Martin, M., et al. (2010). Psychiatric crisis services in three communities [Special issue]. *Canadian Journal of Community Mental Health, 29*(5), 73–86.

Griswold, K., Pastore, P., Homish, G., et al. (2010). Access to primary care: Are mental health peers effective in helping patients after a psychiatric emergency? *Primary Psychiatry, 17*(6), 42–45. Received from http://primarypsychiatry.com/.

Hamlett, N. M., Carr, E. R., & Hillbrand, M. (2016). Positive behavioral support planning in the inpatient treatment of severe disruptive behaviors: A description of service features. *Psychological Services, 13*(2), 178–182. doi:10.1037/ser0000070.

Health Canada (2015). *Canada Health Act annual report 2014–2015*. Ottawa: Author. Retrieved from http://www.hc-sc.gc.ca/hcs-sss/alt_formats/pdf/pubs/cha-ics/2015-cha-lcs-ar-ra-eng.pdf.

Henzen, A., Moeglin, C., Giannakopoulos, P., et al. (2016). Determinants of dropout in a community based mental health crisis centre. *BioMed Central Psychiatry, 16*(111), 1–7. doi:10.1186/s12888-016-0819-4.

Hollis, C., Morriss, R., Martin, J., et al. (2015). Technological innovations in mental healthcare: Harnessing the digital revolution. *The British Journal of Psychiatry, 206*(4), 263–265. doi:10.1192/bjp.bp.113.142612.

Hudson, C. G. (2016). A model of deinstitutionalization of psychiatric care across 161 nations: 2001–2014. *International Journal of Mental Health, 45*(2), 135–153. doi:10.1080/00207411.2016.1167489.

Joyce, A., Nordhagen, A., Ogrodniczuk, J. S., et al. (2015). Partial hospitalization treatment of the alexithymic patient: A case study. *Journal of Clinical Psychology, 71*(2), 167–177. doi:10.1002/jclp.22152.

Kavalidou, K., Smith, D. J., & O'Connor, R. C. (2016). The role of physical and mental health multimorbidity in suicidal ideation. *Journal of Affective Disorders, 19*(209), 80–85. doi:10.1016/j.jad.2016.11.026.

Kirby, M. L., & Keon, W. L. (2006). *Out of the shadows at last: Transforming mental health, mental illness and addiction services in Canada*. Ottawa: Standing Senate Committee on Social Affairs, Science and Technology.

Retrieved from http://www.mentalhealthcommission.ca/sites/default/files/out_of_the_shadows_at_last_-_full_0_0.pdf.

LaJeunesse, R. A. (2002). *Political asylums*. Edmonton: Muttart Foundation.

Linz, S., & Sturm, B. (2016). Facilitating social integration for people with severe mental illness served by assertive community treatment. *Archives of Psychiatric Nursing, 30*(6), 692–699. doi: 10.1016/j.apnu.2016.05.006

Lurie, S., & Mulvale, G. (2015). Special issue: Mobilizing Canada's mental health strategy: Introduction. *Canadian Journal of Community Mental Health, 34*(4), 1–3. Retrieved from http://www.cjcmh.com/journal/cjcmh.

McCauley, K., Montgomery, P., Mossey, S., et al. (2015). Canadian community mental health workers' perceived priorities for supportive housing services in northern and rural contexts. *Health and Social Care in the Community, 23*(6), 632–641. doi:10.1111/hsc.12187.

Mental Health Commission of Canada (2012). *Changing directions, changing lives: The mental health strategy for Canada*. Calgary: Author.

Mohamed, S. (2016). Comparison of intensive case management for psychotic and nonpsychotic patients. *Psychological Services, 13*(1), 10–19. doi:10.1037/ser0000041.

O'Reilly, R., Chaimowitz, G., Brunet, A., et al. (2010). Principles underlying mental health legislation [Position paper]. *Canadian Journal of Psychiatry, 55*(10), 1–5. Retrieved from http://publications.cpa-apc.org/media.php?mid=1037.

Peplau, H. E. (1989). Interpersonal constructs for nursing practice. In A. W. O'Toole & S. R. Welt (Eds.), *Interpersonal theory in nursing practice: Selected works of Hildegard E. Peplau* (pp. 42–55). New York: Putnam.

Public Health Agency of Canada (2015). *Report from the Canadian chronic disease surveillance system: Mental illness in Canada* (Cat. no. HP35-56/2015E-PDF). Ottawa: Public Health Agency of Canada. Retrieved from http://healthycanadians.gc.ca/publications/diseases-conditions-maladies-affections/mental-illness-2015-maladies-mentales/index-eng.php#s3a.

Ranse, J., Hutton, A., Wilson, R., et al. (2015). Leadership opportunities for mental health nurses in the field of disaster preparation, response, and recovery. *Issues in Mental Health Nursing, 36*(5), 391–394. doi:10.3109/01612840.2015.1017062.

Registered Psychiatric Nurses of Canada (2010). *Standards of practice and code of ethics*. Edmonton: Registered Psychiatric Nurses of Canada.

Robson, D., & Gray, R. (2007). Serious mental illness and physical health problems: A discussion paper. *International Journal of Nursing Studies, 44*(3) 457–466. doi: 10.1016/j.ijnurstu.2006.07.013.

Sealy, P., & Whitehead, P. C. (2004). Forty years of deinstitutionalization of psychiatric services in Canada: An empirical assessment. *Canadian Journal of Psychiatry, 49*(4), 249–257.

Socias, M. E., Shoveller, J., Bean, C., et al. (2016). Universal coverage without universal access: Institutional barriers to health care among women sex workers in Vancouver, Canada. *Public Library of Science One, 11*(5), 1–15. doi:10.1371/journal.pone.0155828.

Stevenson, K., Jack, S. M., O'Mara, L., et al. (2015). Registered nurses' experiences of patient violence on acute care psychiatric inpatient units: An interpretive descriptive study. *BioMedical Central Nursing, 14*(1), 1–13. doi:10.1186/s12912-015-0079-5.

Sunderland, A., & Findlay, L. (2013). Perceived need for mental health care in Canada: Results from the 2012 Canadian Community Health Survey—Mental Health. *Health Reports, 24*(9), 3–9. Retrieved from http://www.statcan.gc.ca/pub/82-003-x/2013009/article/11863-eng.pdf.

Relevant Theories and Therapies for Nursing Practice

Margaret Jordan Halter
Adapted by Cheryl L. Pollard

KEY TERMS AND CONCEPTS

automatic thoughts
behavioural therapy
biofeedback
classical conditioning
cognitive distortions
cognitive behavioural therapy (CBT)
conditioning
conscious
counter-transference
defence mechanisms
dialectic behavioural therapy (DBT)
ego
extinction
id

interpersonal psychotherapy
intrapsychic conflict
milieu therapy
negative reinforcement
operant conditioning
positive reinforcement
preconscious
psychodynamic therapy
punishment
reinforcement
superego
Tidal Model
transference
unconscious

OBJECTIVES

1. Evaluate the premises behind the various therapeutic models discussed in this chapter.
2. Describe the evolution of therapies for psychiatric disorders.
3. Identify ways each theorist has contributed to the nurse's ability to assess a patient's behaviours.
4. Drawing on clinical experience, provide the following:
   a. An example of how a patient's irrational beliefs influenced behaviour

   b. An example of counter-transference in your relationship with a patient
   c. An example of the use of behaviour modification with a patient
5. Identify Peplau's framework for the nurse–patient relationship.
6. Choose the therapeutic model that would be most useful for a particular patient or patient problem.

⊖volve WEBSITE

Visit the Evolve website for Flashcards, Case Studies, and additional testing resources related to the content in this chapter: http://evolve.elsevier.com/Canada/Varcarolis/psychiatric/

Pre-Test interactive review

Every professional discipline, from math, science, medicine, nursing, psychology, sociology, philosophy to religious studies, bases its work and beliefs on theories. Most of these theories can best be described as explanations, hypotheses, or hunches, rather than as testable facts. For example, psychological theories provide us with plausible explanations for various behaviours. Philosophical theories provide us with ways to understand problems. And nursing theories provide us with ways to look at and link the person, health, environment, and nursing.

45

Our patients challenge us to understand experiences that are complex and always unique. A broad base of knowledge about personality development, human needs, the determinants of mental health, contributing factors to mental illness, and the importance of relationships guide our nursing practice. The Canadian Federation of Mental Health Nurses (2014) emphasizes that nurses should build an evidence-informed practice built on evidence-based models and theories. This chapter provides you with a very brief overview of some of the most influential psychological and nursing theories relevant to mental health nursing. It also provides an overview of the treatment, or therapy, these theories inspired and the contributions they have made to our practice of psychiatric mental health nursing.

PSYCHOANALYTIC THEORIES AND THERAPIES

Sigmund Freud's Psychoanalytic Theory

Sigmund Freud (1856–1939), an Austrian neurologist, revolutionized thinking about mental health disorders with his groundbreaking theory of personality structure, levels of awareness, anxiety, the role of defence mechanisms, and the stages of psychosexual development. Freud came to believe that the vast majority of mental health disorders were caused by unresolved issues that originated in childhood. He arrived at this conclusion through his experiences treating people with hysteria—individuals who were experiencing physical symptoms despite the absence of an apparent physiological cause.

As part of his treatment, Freud initially used hypnosis, but this therapy had mixed therapeutic results. He then changed his approach to talk therapy, known as the *cathartic method.* Today, we about catharsis as a way of "getting things off our chests." This talk therapy evolved to include "free association," which requires full and honest disclosure of thoughts and feelings as they come to mind. Freud (1961, 1969) concluded that talking about difficult emotional issues had the potential to heal the wounds causing mental illness. Viewing the success of these therapeutic approaches led Freud to construct his psychoanalytic theory.

Levels of Awareness

As Freud's psychoanalytic theory developed, he came to believe that there were three levels of psychological awareness. He offered a topographical theory of how the mind functions, using the image of an iceberg to describe three levels of awareness (Figure 4-1).

Conscious. Freud described the conscious part of the mind as the tip of the iceberg. It contains all of the material a person is aware of at any one time, including perceptions, memories, thoughts, fantasies, and feelings.

Preconscious. Just below the surface of awareness is the preconscious, which contains material that can be retrieved rather easily through conscious effort.

Unconscious. The unconscious includes all repressed memories, passions, and unacceptable urges lying deep below the surface. Freud believed that the memories and emotions associated with trauma are often "placed" in the unconscious because the individual finds it too painful to deal with them. The

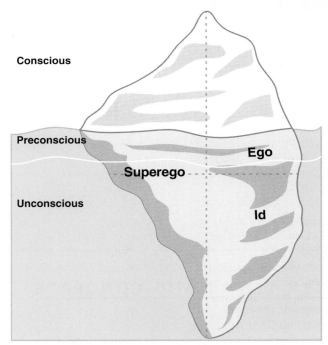

FIGURE 4-1 The mind as an iceberg.

unconscious exerts a powerful yet unseen effect on the conscious thoughts and feelings of the individual. The individual is usually unable to retrieve unconscious material without the assistance of a trained therapist; however, with this assistance, unconscious material can be brought into conscious awareness.

Personality Structure

Freud (1960) delineated three major and distinct but interactive components of the personality: the id, the ego, and the superego.

Id. At birth our personalities are all id. The id is the source of all drives, instincts, reflexes, needs, and wishes that motivate us. The id cannot tolerate frustration and seeks to discharge tension and return to a more comfortable state. The id lacks the ability to problem-solve; it is not logical and operates according to the pleasure principle. A hungry, screaming infant is the perfect example of id.

Ego. The ego develops because the needs, wishes, and demands of the id cannot be satisfactorily met through primary processes and reflex action. The ego emerges in the fourth or fifth month of life. It is the problem solver and reality tester. It is able to differentiate subjective experiences, memory images, and objective reality and attempts to negotiate a solution with the outside world. The ego follows the reality principle, which says to the id, "You have to delay gratification for right now," and then sets a course of action. For example, a hungry man feels tension arising from the id. His ego allows him not only to think about his hunger but also to plan where he can eat and to seek that destination. This process is known as *reality testing* because the individual is factoring in reality to implement a plan to decrease tension.

Superego. The superego, the last component of the personality to develop, represents the moral aspects of personality. The superego consists of the conscience (all the "should nots" internalized from parents) and the ego ideal (all the "shoulds" internalized from parents). The superego represents the ideal rather than the real; it seeks perfection, as opposed to seeking pleasure or engaging reason.

In a mature and well-adjusted individual, the three components of the personality—the id, the ego, and the superego—work together as a team under the administrative leadership of the ego. If the id is too powerful, the person will lack control over impulses; if the superego is too powerful, the person may be self-critical and suffer from feelings of inferiority.

Defence Mechanisms and Anxiety

Freud (1969) believed that anxiety is an inevitable part of living. The environment in which we live presents dangers, insecurities, threats, and satisfactions. It can produce pain and increase tension or produce pleasure and decrease tension. The ego develops defences, or defence mechanisms, to ward off anxiety by preventing conscious awareness of threatening feelings.

Defence mechanisms share two common features: (1) they all deny, falsify, or distort reality to make it less threatening; and (2) they (except suppression) operate on an unconscious level, and we are not aware of their operation. Although we cannot survive without defence mechanisms, it is possible for our defence mechanisms to distort reality to such a degree that we experience difficulty with healthy adjustment and personal growth. Chapter 12 offers further discussions of defence mechanisms.

Psychosexual Stages of Development

Psychoanalytic theorists believe that human development proceeds through five stages from infancy to adulthood. From this perspective, experiences that occur during the first 5 years of life determine an individual's lifetime adjustment patterns. In fact, many think that personality is formed by the time a child enters school and that subsequent growth consists of elaborating on this basic structure. The five psychosexual stages of development, proposed by Freud, are presented in Table 4-1.

TABLE 4-1 FREUD'S PSYCHOSEXUAL STAGES OF DEVELOPMENT

STAGE (AGE)	SOURCE OF SATISFACTION	PRIMARY CONFLICT	TASKS	DESIRED OUTCOMES	OTHER POSSIBLE PERSONALITY TRAITS
Oral (0–1 year)	Mouth (sucking, biting, chewing)	Weaning	Mastery of gratification of oral needs; beginning of ego development (4–5 months)	Development of trust in the environment, with the realization that needs can be met	Fixation at the oral stage is associated with passivity, gullibility, and dependence; the use of sarcasm; and the development of orally focused habits (e.g., smoking, nail-biting)
Anal (1–3 years)	Anal region (expulsion and retention of feces)	Toilet training	Beginning of development of a sense of control over instinctual drives; ability to delay immediate gratification to gain a future goal	Control over impulses	Fixation at the anal stage is associated with anal retentiveness (stinginess, rigid thought patterns, obsessive-compulsive disorder) or anal-expulsive character (messiness, destructiveness, cruelty)
Phallic (oedipal) (3–6 years)	Genitals (masturbation)	Oedipus and Electra	Sexual identity with parent of same sex; beginning of superego development	Identification with parent of same sex	Lack of successful resolution may result in difficulties with sexual identity and difficulties with authority figures
Latency (6–12 years)	—	—	Growth of ego functions (social, intellectual, mechanical) and the ability to care about and relate to others outside the home (peers of the same sex)	The development of skills needed to cope with the environment	Fixations can result in difficulty identifying with others and in developing social skills, leading to a sense of inadequacy and inferiority
Genital (12 years and beyond)	Genitals (sexual intercourse)	—	Development of satisfying sexual and emotional relationships with members of the opposite sex; emancipation from parents—planning of life goals and development of a strong sense of personal identity	The ability to be creative and find pleasure in love and work	Inability to negotiate this stage could result in difficulties in becoming emotionally and financially independent, lack of strong personal identity and future goals, and inability to form satisfying intimate relationships

Source: Adapted from Gleitman, H. (1981). *Psychology*. New York: W. W. Norton.

Classical Psychoanalysis

Classical psychoanalysis, as developed by Sigmund Freud, is seldom used today. Freud's premise that all mental illness is caused by early intrapsychic conflict—a mental struggle, often unconscious, between the id, ego, and superego—is no longer widely thought to be valid, and such therapy requires a lengthy period of treatment, making it prohibitively expensive for most. However, there are two concepts from classic psychoanalysis that used to guide contemporary mental health nursing practice: transference and counter-transference (Freud, 1969).

Transference develops when the patient experiences feelings toward the nurse or therapist that were originally held toward significant others in his or her life. When transference occurs, these feelings become available for exploration with the patient. Such exploration helps the patient to better understand certain feelings and behaviours. Counter-transference is the health care worker's unconscious personal response to the patient. For instance, if the patient reminds you of someone you do not like, you may unconsciously react as if the patient were that individual. Counter-transference underscores the importance of maintaining self-awareness and seeking supervisory guidance as therapeutic relationships progress. Chapter 9 talks more about counter-transference and the nurse–patient relationship.

Psychodynamic Therapy

Psychodynamic therapy uses many of the theoretical underpinnings of psychoanalytic models such as unconscious conflicts, relational attachments, personality development, and the use of defence mechanisms. As a result, therapy is approached from a standpoint that unconscious dynamics exist within normal human consciousness and that it is possible in therapy to engage many aspects of the human psyche in ways that are useful, creative, and healing. Techniques used include active listening, reflection, support of ego strength, empathetic communication, and identification of past patterns (Ramezani, Rockers, Wanlass, et al., 2016). Psychodynamic therapy tends to last longer than other common therapeutic modalities and may extend 20 or more sessions.

Clinicians who use this approach when working with patients with psychosis, severe depression, borderline personality disorders, and severe character disorders require advanced training, and work in collaboration with a practitioner who specializes in a biomedical approach. Supportive therapies, which are within the scope of practice of the basic-level psychiatric nurse, are useful for these patients. A variety of supportive therapies are described in chapters concerning specific disorders (see Chapters 12 to 22). Techniques common to the approaches discussed above and supportive therapies include identification of the presenting problem, identification of goals and values, open-ended questions, and psychoeducation. Many health care practitioners socialized in the biomedical model have difficulty adjusting to a nonauthoritarian approach when learning to use various psychotherapeutic modalities (Ramezani, Rockers, Wanlass et al., 2016).

Implications of Psychoanalytic Theory for Nursing Practice

Psychoanalytic theory has relevance to nursing practice at many junctures. It offers a comprehensive explanation of complex human processes and suggests that the formation of a patient's personality is influenced by many diverse sources rooted in past events. Freud's theory of the unconscious is particularly valuable as an explanation for understanding the complexity of human behaviour. By considering conscious and unconscious influences, a nurse can begin to think about meanings that might be behind certain behaviours. Psychoanalysts emphasize the importance of individual talk sessions characterized by attentive listening, with a focus on underlying themes as an important tool of healing in psychiatric care.

DEVELOPMENTAL THEORIES

Cognitive Development

Jean Piaget (1896–1980) was a Swiss psychologist and researcher. While working at a boys' school run by Alfred Binet, developer of the Binet Intelligence Test, Piaget helped to score these tests. He became fascinated by the fact that young children consistently gave wrong answers on intelligence tests, wrong answers that revealed a discernible pattern of cognitive processing that was different from that of older children and adults. He concluded that cognitive development was a dynamic progression from primitive awareness and simple reflexes to complex thought and responses. Our mental representations of the world, or schemata, depend on the cognitive stage we have reached.

- *Sensorimotor stage (birth to 2 years).* Begins with basic reflexes and culminates with purposeful movement, spatial abilities, and hand-eye coordination. Physical interaction with the environment provides the child with a basic understanding of the world. By about 9 months, object permanence is achieved, and the child can conceptualize objects that are no longer visible. This explains the delight of the game of peek-a-boo as an emerging skill, as the child begins to anticipate the face hidden behind the hands.
- *Preoperational stage (2 to 7 years).* *Operations* is a term used to describe thinking about objects. Children are not yet able to think abstractly or generalize qualities in the absence of specific objects, but rather think in a concrete fashion. Egocentric thinking is demonstrated through a tendency to expect others to view the world as they do. They are also unable to conserve mass, volume, or number. An example of this is thinking that a tall, thin glass holds more liquid than a short, wide glass.
- *Concrete operational stage (7 to 11 years).* Logical thought appears and abstract problem solving is possible. The child is able to see a situation from another's point of view and can take into account a variety of solutions to a problem. Conservation is possible. For example, two small cups of liquid are seen as being equal to a tall glass. The child is able to classify based on discrete characteristics, order objects in a pattern, and understand the concept of reversibility.
- *Formal operational stage (11 years to adulthood).* Conceptual reasoning commences at approximately the same time as does

puberty. At this stage, the child's basic abilities to think abstractly and problem-solve mirror those of an adult.

Theory of Psychosocial Development

Erik Erikson (1902–1994), an American psychoanalyst, was a follower of Freud. However, Erikson (1963) believed that Freudian theory was restrictive and negative in its approach. He also stressed that more than the limited mother–child–father triangle influences an individual's development. According to Erikson, personality is not set in stone at age 5 but continues to develop throughout the lifespan and is influenced by culture and society.

Erikson described development as occurring in eight predetermined and consecutive life stages (psychosocial crises), each of which consists of two possible outcomes (e.g., industry versus inferiority). The successful or unsuccessful completion of each stage affects the individual's progression to the next (Table 4-2).

For example, Erikson's crisis of industry versus inferiority occurs from the ages of 7 to 12. During this stage, the child's task is to gain a sense of personal abilities and competence and to expand relationships beyond the immediate family to include peers. The attainment of this task (industry) brings with it the virtue of confidence. The child who fails to navigate this stage successfully is unable to gain a mastery of age-appropriate tasks, cannot make a connection with peers, and will feel like a failure (inferiority).

Stages of Moral Development

Lawrence Kohlberg (1927–1987) was an American psychologist whose work reflected and expanded on Piaget's by applying his theory to moral development, which coincided with cognitive development (Crain, 1985). While visiting Israel, Kohlberg became convinced that children living in a kibbutz had advanced moral

TABLE 4-2	ERIKSON'S EIGHT STAGES OF DEVELOPMENT			
APPROXIMATE AGE	**DEVELOPMENTAL TASK**	**PSYCHOSOCIAL CRISIS**	**SUCCESSFUL RESOLUTION OF CRISIS**	**UNSUCCESSFUL RESOLUTION OF CRISIS**
Infancy (0–1½ years)	Forming attachment to mother, which lays foundation for later trust in others	Trust vs. mistrust	Sound basis for relating to other people; trust in people; faith and hope about environment and future, "I'm confident that my son will arrange for me to stay with his family until I'm able to live on my own again."	General difficulties relating to people effectively, suspicion, trust–fear conflict, fear of future, "I can't trust anyone; no one has ever been there when I needed them."
Early childhood (1½–3 years)	Gaining some basic control of self and environment (e.g., toilet training, exploration)	Autonomy vs. shame and doubt	Sense of self-control and adequacy, will power, "I'm sure that with the proper diet and exercise program, I can achieve my target weight."	Independence–fear conflict, severe feelings of self-doubt, "I could never lose the weight they want me to, so why even try?"
Late childhood (3–6 years)	Becoming purposeful and directive	Initiative vs. guilt	Ability to initiate one's own activities, sense of purpose, "I like to help Mom by setting the table for dinner."	Aggression–fear conflict, sense of inadequacy or guilt, "I know it's wrong, but I wanted the candy, so I took it."
School age (6–12 years)	Developing social, physical, and school skills	Industry vs. inferiority	Competence, ability to work, "I'm getting really good at swimming since I've been taking lessons."	Sense of inferiority, difficulty learning and working, "I can't read as well as the others in my class; I'm just dumb."
Adolescence (12–20 years)	Making transition from childhood to adulthood, developing sense of identity	Identity vs. role confusion	Sense of personal identity, fidelity, "I'm homosexual, and I'm okay with that."	Confusion about who one is, submersion of identity in relationships or group memberships, "I belong to the gang because without them, I'm nothing."
Early adulthood (20–35 years)	Establishing intimate bonds of love and friendship	Intimacy vs. isolation	Ability to love deeply and commit oneself, "My husband has been my best friend for 25 years."	Emotional isolation, egocentricity, "It's nearly impossible to find a man who is worth marrying."
Middle adulthood (35–65 years)	Fulfilling life goals that involve family, career, and society; developing concerns that embrace future generations	Generativity vs. self-absorption	Ability to give and to care for others, "I've arranged for a 6-month leave of absence to stay with my mother now that her illness is terminal."	Self-absorption, inability to grow as a person, "I've lived with this scar on my face for 3 years; it's worse than having cancer."
Later years (65 years to death)	Looking back over one's life and accepting its meaning	Integrity vs. despair	Sense of integrity and fulfillment, willingness to face death, wisdom, "I've led a happy, productive life, and I'm ready to die."	Dissatisfaction with life, denial of or despair over prospect of death, "I'm not ready to die; the doctors are wrong. You'll see they are wrong."

Sources: Altrocchi, J. (1980). *Abnormal psychology* (p. 196). New York: Harcourt Brace Jovanovich; and Erikson, E. H. (1963). *Childhood and society*. New York: W. W. Norton.

development, and he believed that the atmosphere of trust, respect, and self-governance nurtured this development. In the United States, he created schools or "just communities" that were grounded on these concepts. Based on interviews with youths, Kohlberg developed a theory of how people progressively develop a sense of morality (Kohlberg & Turiel, 1971).

His theory provides a framework for understanding the progression from black-and-white thinking about right and wrong to a complex, variable, and context-dependent decision-making process regarding the rightness or wrongness of action.

Preconventional level
Stage 1: Obedience and punishment. The hallmarks of this stage are a focus on rules and on listening to authority. People at this stage believe that obedience is the method to avoid punishment.

Stage 2: Individualism and exchange. Individuals become aware that not everyone thinks the way that they do, and that different people see rules differently. If they or others decide to break the rules, they are risking punishment.

Conventional level
Stage 3: Good interpersonal relationships. Children begin to view rightness or wrongness as related to motivations, personality, or the goodness or badness of the person. Generally speaking, people should get along and have similar values.

Stage 4: Maintaining the social order. A "rules are rules" mindset returns. However, the reasoning behind it is not simply to avoid punishment; it is because the person has begun to adopt a broader view of society. Listening to authority maintains the social order; bureaucracies and big government agencies often seem to operate with this tenet.

Postconventional level
Stage 5: Social contract and individual rights. People in stage 5 still believe that the social order is important, but the social order must be *good*. For example, if the social order is corrupt, then rules should be changed and it is a duty to protect the rights of others.

Stage 6: Universal ethical principles. Actions should create justice for everyone involved. We are obliged to break unjust laws.

Ethics of Care Theory
Carol Gilligan (born 1936) is an American psychologist, ethicist, and feminist who inspired the normative ethics of care theory. She worked with Kohlberg as he developed his theory of moral development and later criticized his work for being based on a sample of boys and men. In addition, she believed that he used a scoring method that favoured males' methods of reasoning, resulting in lower moral development scores for girls as compared with boys. Based on Gilligan's critique, Kohlberg later revised his scoring methods, which resulted in greater similarity between girls' and boys' scores.

Gilligan (1982) suggests that a morality of care should replace Kohlberg's "justice view" of morality, which maintains that we should do what is right no matter the personal cost or the cost to those we love. Gilligan's care view emphasizes the importance of forming relationships, banding together, and putting the needs of those for whom we care above the needs of strangers. Gilligan

asserts that a female approach to ethics has always been in existence but has been trivialized. Like Kohlberg, Gilligan asserts that moral development progresses through three major divisions: preconventional, conventional, and postconventional. These transitions are not dictated by cognitive ability but rather come about through personal development and changes in a sense of self.

Implications of Developmental Theories for Nursing Practice
Nurses continue to use developmental theories as an important part of patient assessment. For example, analysis of behaviour patterns using Erikson's framework can identify age-appropriate or arrested development of normal interpersonal skills. A developmental framework helps the nurse to know what types of interventions are most likely to be effective. For example, preschool and kindergarten-aged children in Piaget's preoperational stage of development respond best if they actively participate in imitative, imaginative, and dramatic play and ask questions in order to learn how to do things. When this model is used with older patients, they may respond well to a life review strategy that focuses on the integrity of their life as a tapestry of experience. In the therapeutic encounter, individual responsibility and the capacity for improving one's functioning are addressed. Treatment approaches and interventions can be tailored to the patient's developmental level.

INTERPERSONAL THEORIES AND THERAPIES
Theory of Object Relations
The theory of object relations was developed by interpersonal theorists who emphasize past relationships in influencing a person's sense of self as well as the nature and quality of relationships in the present. The term *object* refers to another person, particularly a significant person.

Margaret Mahler (1895–1985) was a Hungarian-born child psychologist who worked with emotionally disturbed children. She developed a framework for studying how an infant transitions from complete self-absorption, with an inability to separate from its mother, to a physically and psychologically differentiated toddler. Mahler and colleagues (1975) believed that psychological problems were largely the result of a disruption of this separation.

During the first 3 years of life, the significant other (e.g., the mother) provides a secure base of support that promotes enough confidence for the child to separate. This is achieved by a balance of holding (emotionally and physically) a child enough for the child to feel safe while encouraging independence and natural exploration.

Problems may arise in this process. If a toddler leaves his or her mother on the park bench and wanders off to the sandbox, the child should be encouraged with smiles and reassurance, "Go on honey. It's safe to go away a little." Then the mother needs to be reliably present when the toddler returns, thereby rewarding his or her efforts. Mahler notes that raising healthy children does not require that parents never make mistakes and that "good-enough parenting" will promote successful separation-individuation.

Interpersonal Theory

Harry Stack Sullivan (1892–1949), an American-born psychiatrist, initially approached patients using a Freudian framework, but he became frustrated by dealing with what he considered unseen and private mental processes within the individual. He turned his attention to interpersonal processes that could be observed in a social framework. Sullivan (1953) defined *personality* as behaviour that can be observed within interpersonal relationships.

According to Sullivan, the purpose of all behaviour is to get needs met through interpersonal interactions and to decrease or avoid anxiety. He defined *anxiety* as any painful feeling or emotion that arises from social insecurity or that prevents biological needs from being satisfied (Sullivan, 1953). Sullivan coined the term *security operations* to describe measures the individual uses to reduce anxiety and enhance security. For example, a person might imagine him- or herself to be right, muster up anger to fuel this righteousness, and try to act to reduce anxiety. Collectively, the security operations an individual uses to defend against anxiety and ensure self-esteem make up the self-system.

There are many parallels between Sullivan's notion of security operations and Freud's concept of defence mechanisms. Both are unconscious processes, and both are ways we reduce anxiety. However, Freud's defence mechanism of repression is an intrapsychic activity, whereas Sullivan's security operations are interpersonal relationship activities that can be observed.

Interpersonal Psychotherapy

Interpersonal psychotherapy is an effective short-term therapy that originated with Adolph Meyer and Harry Stack Sullivan. The assumption is that psychiatric disorders are influenced by interpersonal interactions and the social context. The goal of interpersonal psychotherapy is to reduce or eliminate psychiatric symptoms (particularly depression and anxiety) by improving interpersonal functioning and underlying relational dynamics. Interpersonal psychotherapy has been successful in the treatment of perfectionism, which increases a person's vulnerability for depression, suicidal symptoms, eating disorders, and anxiety (Hewitt, Mikail, Flett, et al., 2015). Treatment is predicated on the notion that disturbances in important interpersonal relationships (or a deficit in one's capacity to form those relationships) can play a role in initiating or maintaining symptoms. In interpersonal psychotherapy, the therapist identifies the nature of the problem to be resolved and then selects strategies consistent with that problem area.

Peplau's Theory of Interpersonal Relations

Hildegard Peplau (1909–1999) (Figure 4-2), influenced by the work of Sullivan and learning theory, developed the first systematic theoretical framework for psychiatric nursing in her groundbreaking book *Interpersonal Relations in Nursing*. Peplau was the first nurse to identify psychiatric mental health nursing both as an essential element of general nursing and as a specialty area that embraces specific governing principles. In shifting the focus from what nurses do *to* patients to what nurses do *with* patients, Peplau (1989) engineered a major paradigm shift from a model

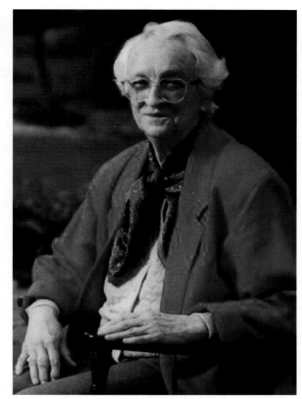

FIGURE 4-2 Hildegard Peplau. Source: Courtesy Anne Peplau.

focused on medical treatments to an interpersonal relational model of nursing practice. She viewed nursing as an educative instrument designed to help individuals and communities use their capacities to live more productively (Peplau, 1987). She believed that illness offered a unique opportunity for experiential learning, personal growth, and improved coping strategies and that psychiatric nurses play a unique role in facilitating this growth through the nurse–patient relationship (Peplau, 1982a, 1982b).

Peplau identified stages of the nurse–patient relationship (see Chapter 9) and also taught the technique of *process recording* to help her students hone their communication and relationship skills (see Table 10-4). The skills of the psychiatric nurse include observation, interpretation, and intervention. The nurse observes and listens to the patient, developing impressions about the meaning of the patient's situation. By employing this process, the nurse is able to view the patient as a unique individual. The nurse's inferences are then validated with the patient for accuracy. Peplau believed it was essential for nurses to observe the behaviour not only of the patient but also of themselves and so proposed an approach in which nurses are both participants and observers in therapeutic conversations. This self-awareness on the part of the nurse is essential in keeping the focus on the patient, as well as in keeping the social and personal needs of the nurse out of the nurse–patient conversation.

Perhaps Peplau's most universal contribution to the everyday practice of psychiatric mental health nursing is her application of Sullivan's theory of anxiety to nursing practice. She described the effects of different levels of anxiety (mild, moderate, severe, and

TABLE 4-3	SELECTED NURSING THEORISTS, THEIR MAJOR CONTRIBUTIONS, AND THEIR IMPACT ON PSYCHIATRIC MENTAL HEALTH NURSING	
NURSING THEORIST	**FOCUS OF THEORY**	**CONTRIBUTION TO PSYCHIATRIC MENTAL HEALTH NURSING**
Patricia Benner	"Caring" as foundation for nursing	Benner encourages nurses to provide caring and comforting interventions. She emphasizes the importance of the nurse–patient relationship and the importance of teaching and coaching the patient and bearing witness to suffering as the patient deals with illness.
Dorothea Orem	Goal of self-care as integral to the practice of nursing	Orem emphasizes the role of the nurse in promoting self-care activities of the patient; this has relevance to the seriously and persistently mentally ill patient.
Sister Callista Roy	Continual need for people to adapt physically, psychologically, and socially	Roy emphasizes the role of nursing in assisting patients to adapt so they can cope more effectively with changes.
Betty Neuman	Impact of internal and external stressors on the equilibrium of the system	Neuman emphasizes the role of nursing in assisting patients to discover and use stress-reducing strategies.
Joyce Travelbee	Meaning in the nurse–patient relationship and the importance of communication	Travelbee emphasizes the role of nursing in affirming the suffering of the patient and in being able to alleviate that suffering through communication skills used appropriately throughout the stages of the nurse–patient relationship.

Sources: Benner, P., & Wrubel, J. (1989). *The primacy of caring: Stress and coping in health and illness.* Menlo Park, CA: Addison-Wesley; Leddy, S., & Pepper, J. M. (1993). *Conceptual bases of professional nursing* (3rd ed., pp. 174–175). Philadelphia: Lippincott; Neuman, B., & Young, R. (1972). A model for teaching total-person approach to patient problems. *Nursing Research, 21*(3), 264–269; Orem, D. E. (1995). *Nursing: Concepts of practice* (5th ed.). New York: McGraw-Hill; Roy, C., & Andrews, H. A. (1991). *The Roy adaptation model: The definitive statement.* Norwalk, CT: Appleton & Lange; and Travelbee, J. (1961). *Intervention in psychiatric nursing.* Philadelphia: F. A. Davis.

panic) on perception and learning. She promoted interventions to lower anxiety, with the aim of improving patients' abilities to think and function at more satisfactory levels. More on the application of Peplau's theory of anxiety and interventions is presented in Chapter 12. Table 4-3 lists selected nursing theorists and summarizes their major contributions and the impact of these contributions on psychiatric mental health nursing.

Building on the work of Peplau (1952), who emphasized the importance of understanding people's relationships with their illnesses and their health, the Tidal Model focuses on the interpersonal relationships as the context for recovery. It relies heavily on metaphors that are used to empower people and uses each person's experience and wisdom to effect change. The Tidal Model emerged from the nursing practice. Through the use of this model, Dr. Barker and Poppy Buchanan-Barker (2005) suggest that mental well-being depends on individual experience or self, perceptions, thoughts, and actions. It is a recovery approach that can be used to inform person-centred collaborative care as listening to the person's "story" and experiences so that we can begin to understand and work out with the individual what might be done to help. The assumptions upon which this model is built are that people need to be encouraged to tell their story; in their own words, the account of their experiences must be listened to and respected, and it is through this sharing that assessments and collaborative care planning can occur. Each interaction is seen as an opportunity to repair, or damage still further, the person's vulnerable sense of self. When this model is used, assessment includes three primary questions: Why is this person experiencing this particular difficulty right now, how does the person see his or her problem, and what does the person think will work for or be counter-productive for him or her in the present circumstances? Nurses who use this model believe

that the therapeutic relationship is crucial to the delivery of truly collaborative care and that mental pain is eased if a person feels listened to, understood, and reassured.

Implications of Interpersonal Theories for Nursing Practice

Sullivan's theory is the foundation for Hildegard Peplau's nursing theory of interpersonal relationships, which we examine later in this chapter. Believing that therapy should educate patients and assist them in gaining personal insight, Sullivan introduced the term *participant observer*, which underscores that professional helpers cannot be isolated from the therapeutic situation if they are to be effective. Sullivan would insist that the nurse interact with the patient as an authentic human being. Mutuality, respect for the patient, unconditional acceptance, and empathy, which are considered essential aspects of modern therapeutic relationships, were important aspects of Sullivan's theory of interpersonal therapy. Sullivan also demonstrated that a psychotherapeutic environment, characterized by an accepting atmosphere that provided numerous opportunities for practising interpersonal skills and developing relationships, is an invaluable treatment tool. Group psychotherapy, family therapy, and educational and skill training programs, as well as unstructured periods, can be incorporated into the design of a psychotherapeutic environment to facilitate healthy interactions. This method is used today in virtually all residential and day hospital settings.

BEHAVIOURAL THEORIES AND THERAPIES

Behaviourists have no concern with inner conflicts and argue that personality simply consists of learned behaviours. Consequently, if behaviour changes, so does the personality. Therefore, contrary to what psychoanalyst theorists believe, a person's destiny was *not* carved in stone at a very early age.

The development of behavioural models began in the nineteenth century as a result of Ivan Pavlov's laboratory work with dogs. It continued into the twentieth century with John B. Watson's application of these models to shape behaviour and with B. F. Skinner's research on rat behaviour. These behavioural theorists developed systematic learning principles that could be applied to humans. Behavioural models emphasize the ways in which observable behavioural responses are learned and can be modified in a particular environment. Pavlov's, Watson's, and Skinner's models focus on the belief that behaviour can be influenced through a process referred to as *conditioning*. Conditioning involves pairing behaviour with a condition that reinforces or diminishes the behaviour's occurrence.

Classical Conditioning Theory

Ivan Pavlov (1849–1936) was a Russian physiologist. He won a Nobel Prize for his outstanding contributions to the physiology of digestion, which he studied through his well-known experiments with dogs. In incidental observation of the dogs, Pavlov noticed that the dogs were able to anticipate when food would be forthcoming and would begin to salivate even before actually tasting the meat. Pavlov labelled this process *psychic secretion*. He hypothesized that the psychic component was a learned association between two events: the presence of the experimental apparatus and the serving of meat.

Pavlov formalized his observations of behaviours in dogs in a theory of classical conditioning. Pavlov (1928) found that when a neutral stimulus (a bell) was repeatedly paired with another stimulus (food that triggered salivation), eventually the sound of the bell alone could elicit salivation in the dogs. An example of this response in humans is an individual who became very ill as a child after eating spoiled coleslaw at a picnic and later in life feels nauseated whenever he smells coleslaw. It is important to recognize that classical conditioned responses are involuntary—not under conscious personal control—and are not spontaneous choices.

Behaviourism Theory

John B. Watson (1878–1958) was an American psychologist who rejected the unconscious motivation of psychoanalysis as being too subjective. He developed the school of thought referred to as behaviourism, which he believed was more objective or measurable. Watson contended that personality traits and responses—adaptive and maladaptive—were socially learned through classical conditioning (Watson, 1919). In a famous (but terrible) experiment, Watson stood behind Little Albert, a 9-month-old who liked animals, and made a loud noise with a hammer every time the infant reached for a white rat. After this experiment, Little Albert became terrified at the sight of white fur or hair, even in the absence of a loud noise. Watson concluded that behaviour could be moulded by controlling the environment and that anyone could be trained to be anything, from a beggar to a merchant.

Operant Conditioning Theory

B. F. Skinner (1904–1990) represented the second wave of behavioural theorists. Skinner (1987) researched operant conditioning, in which voluntary behaviours are learned through consequences and behavioural responses are elicited through reinforcement, which causes a behaviour to occur more frequently. A consequence can be a positive reinforcement, such as receiving a reward (getting high marks after studying hard all semester), or a negative reinforcement, such as the removal of an objectionable or aversive stimulus (walking freely through a park once the vicious dog is picked up by animal services).

Other techniques can cause behaviours to occur less frequently. One technique is an unpleasant consequence, or punishment. Driving too fast may result in a speeding ticket, which—in mature and healthy individuals—decreases the chances that speeding will recur. Absence of reinforcement, or extinction, also decreases behaviour by withholding a reward that has become habitual. If a person tells a joke and no one laughs, for example, the person is less apt to tell jokes because his joke-telling behaviour is not being reinforced. Teachers employ this strategy in the classroom when they ignore acting-out behaviour that had previously been rewarded by more attention. Figure 4-3 illustrates the differences between classical conditioning (in which an involuntary reaction is caused by a stimulus) and operant conditioning (in which voluntary behaviour is learned through reinforcement).

Behavioural Therapy

Behavioural therapy is based on the assumption that changes in maladaptive behaviour can occur without insight into the underlying cause. This approach works best when it is directed at specific problems and the goals are well defined. Behavioural therapy is effective in treating people with phobias, alcoholism, schizophrenia, and many other conditions. Five types of behavioural therapy are discussed here: modelling, operant conditioning, systematic desensitization, aversion therapy, and biofeedback.

Modelling

In modelling, the therapist provides a role model for specific identified behaviours, and the patient learns through imitation. The therapist may do the modelling, provide another person to model the behaviours, or present a video for the purpose. Bandura, Blahard, and Ritter (1969) were able to help people lessen their phobias about nonpoisonous snakes by having them first view close-ups of filmed encounters between people and snakes that had successful outcomes and then view live encounters between people and snakes that also had successful outcomes. In a similar fashion, some behavioural therapists use role-playing in the

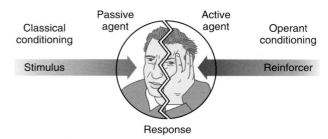

FIGURE 4-3 Classical versus operant conditioning. Source: From Carson, V. B. (2000). *Mental health nursing: The nurse–patient journey* (2nd ed., p. 121). Philadelphia: Saunders.

consulting room. For example, a student who does not know how to ask a professor for an extension on a term paper would watch the therapist portray a potentially effective way of making the request. The clinician would then help the student to practise the new skill in a similar role-playing situation.

Operant Conditioning

Operant conditioning is the basis for behaviour modification and uses positive reinforcement to increase desired behaviours. For example, when desired goals are achieved or behaviours are performed, patients might be rewarded with tokens. These tokens can be exchanged for food, small luxuries, or privileges. This reward system is known as a token economy.

Operant conditioning has been useful in improving the verbal behaviours of mute, autistic, and developmentally disabled children. In patients with severe and persistent mental illness, behaviour modification has helped increase levels of self-care, social behaviour, group participation, and more.

We all use positive reinforcement in our everyday lives. A familiar case in point occurs when a mother takes her preschooler along to the grocery store, and the child starts acting out, demanding candy, nagging, crying, and yelling. Here are examples of three ways the child's behaviour can be reinforced:

Action	Result
1. The mother gives the child the candy.	The child continues to use this behaviour. This is positive reinforcement of negative behaviour.
2. The mother scolds the child.	Acting out may continue, because the child gets what he really wants—attention. This positively rewards negative behaviour.
3. The mother ignores the acting out but gives attention to the child when he is behaving appropriately.	The child gets a positive reward for appropriate behaviour.

Systematic Desensitization

Systematic desensitization is another form of behaviour modification therapy that involves the development of behavioural tasks customized to the patient's specific fears; these tasks are presented to the patient while using learned relaxation techniques. The process involves four steps:

1. The patient's fear is broken down into its components by exploring the particular stimulus cues to which the patient reacts. For example, certain situations may precipitate a phobic reaction, whereas others do not. Crowds at parties may be problematic, whereas similar numbers of people in other settings do not cause the same distress.
2. The patient is incrementally exposed to the fear. For example, a patient who has a fear of flying is introduced to short periods of visual presentations of flying—first with still pictures, then with videos, and finally in a busy airport. The situations are confronted while the patient is in a relaxed state. Gradually,

over a period of time, exposure is increased until anxiety about or fear of the object or situation has ceased.
3. The patient is instructed in how to design a hierarchy of fears. For fear of flying, a patient might develop a set of statements representing the stages of a flight, order the statements from the most fearful to the least fearful, and use relaxation techniques to reach a state of relaxation as he or she progresses through the list.
4. The patient practises these techniques every day.

Aversion Therapy

Today, aversion therapy (which is akin to punishment) is used widely to treat behaviours such as alcoholism, sexual deviation, shoplifting, violent and aggressive behaviour, and self-mutilation. Aversion therapy is sometimes the treatment of choice when other less drastic measures have failed to produce the desired effects. The following are three paradigms for using aversive techniques:

1. Pairing of a maladaptive behaviour with a noxious stimulus (e.g., pairing the sight and smell of alcohol with electric shock), so that anxiety or fear becomes associated with the once-pleasurable stimulus
2. Punishment (e.g., punishment applied after the patient has had an alcoholic drink)
3. Avoidance training (e.g., patient avoids punishment by pushing a glass of alcohol away within a certain time limit)

Simple examples of extinguishing undesirable behaviour through aversion therapy include painting foul-tasting substances on the fingernails of nail biters or the thumbs of thumb suckers. Other examples of aversive stimuli are chemicals that induce nausea and vomiting, noxious odours, unpleasant verbal stimuli (e.g., descriptions of disturbing scenes), costs or fines in a token economy, and denial of positive reinforcement (e.g., isolation).

Before initiating any aversive protocol, the therapist, treatment team, or society *must* answer the following questions:

- Is this therapy in the best interest of the patient?
- Does its use violate the patient's rights?
- Is it in the best interest of society?

If aversion therapy is chosen as the most appropriate treatment, those administering it must provide ongoing supervision, support, and evaluation.

Biofeedback

Biofeedback is a form of behavioural therapy that uses sensitive instrumentation to acquire information about body functions such as muscle activity, brain waves, skin temperature, heart rate, and blood pressure. Biofeedback is successfully used today, especially for controlling the body's physiological response to stress and anxiety. This form of therapy is discussed in detail in Chapter 5.

Implications of Behavioural Theories for Nursing Practice

Behavioural models provide a concrete method for modifying or replacing behaviours. Behaviour management and modification programs based on his principles have proven to be successful in altering targeted behaviours. Programmed learning and token economies—in which tokens, or symbolic objects (e.g., check marks), can be exchanged for valued items, services, or privileges (e.g., food, passes out of the building, phone calls)—represent extensions of thoughts on learning. Behavioural methods are particularly effective with children, adolescents, and individuals with many forms of chronic mental illness.

COGNITIVE THEORIES AND THERAPIES

While behaviourists focused on increasing, decreasing, or eliminating measurable behaviours, little attention was paid to the thoughts, or cognitions, that were involved in these behaviours. Rather than thinking of people as passive recipients of environmental conditioning, cognitive theorists proposed that there is a dynamic interplay between individuals and the environment. These theorists believe that thoughts come before feelings and actions and that thoughts about the world and our place in it are based on our own unique perspectives, which may or may not be based on reality. Two of the most influential theorists and their therapies are presented here.

Rational Emotive Behaviour Therapy (REBT)

Rational emotive behaviour therapy (REBT) was developed by Albert Ellis (1913–2007) in 1955. The aim of REBT is to eradicate core irrational beliefs by helping people recognize thoughts that are not accurate, sensible, or useful. These thoughts tend to take the form of *shoulds* (e.g., "I should always be polite."), *oughts* (e.g., "I ought to consistently win my tennis games."), and *musts* (e.g., "I must be thin."). Ellis described negative thinking as a simple A-B-C process. *A* stands for the activating event, *B* stands for beliefs about the event, and *C* stands for the emotional consequence as a result of the event.

A   →   B   →   C
Activating Event   Beliefs   Emotional Consequence

Perception influences all thoughts, which in turn influence our behaviours. For example, imagine you have just received an invitation to a birthday party (activating event). You think, *I hate parties. Now I have to hang out with people who don't like me instead of watching my favourite television shows. They probably just invited me to get a gift* (beliefs). You will probably be miserable (emotional consequence) if you go. On the other hand, you may think, *I love parties!* (activating event). *This will be a great chance to meet new people, and it will be fun to shop for the perfect gift* (beliefs). You could have a delightful time (emotional consequence).

Although Ellis (Figure 4-4) admitted that the role of past experiences is instrumental in our current beliefs, the focus of REBT is on present attitudes, painful feelings, and dysfunctional behaviours. If our beliefs are negative and self-deprecating, we are more susceptible to depression and anxiety. Ellis noted that while we cannot change the past, we can change the way we are now. He was pragmatic in his approach to mental illness and colourful in his therapeutic advice: "It's too [darn] bad you panic, but you don't die from it! Get them over the panic about panic, you may find the panic disappears" (Ellis, 2000).

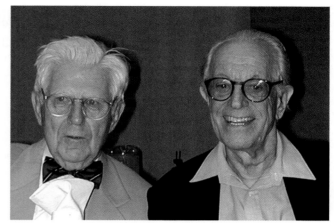

FIGURE 4-4 Aaron Beck *(left)* and Albert Ellis *(right)*. Source: Fenichel, 2000.

Cognitive Behavioural Therapy (CBT)

Aaron T. Beck (Figure 4-4), another follower of Sigmund Freud, was originally trained in psychoanalysis but is regarded as a neo-Freudian. When he attempted to study depression from a psychoanalytic perspective, he became convinced that people with depression generally had stereotypical patterns of negative and self-critical thinking that seemed to distort their ability to think and process information. **Cognitive behavioural therapy (CBT)** is based on both cognitive psychology and behavioural theory. It is a commonly used, effective, and well-researched therapeutic tool.

Beck's method (Beck, Rush, Shaw, et al., 1979), the basis for CBT, is an active, directive, time-limited, structured approach used to treat a variety of psychiatric disorders (e.g., depression, anxiety, phobias, pain problems). It is based on the underlying theoretical principle that how people feel and behave is largely determined by the way they think about the world and their place in it (Beck, 1967). Their cognitions (verbal or pictorial events in their stream of consciousness) are based on attitudes or assumptions developed from previous experiences. These cognitions may be fairly accurate, or they may be distorted. According to Beck, we all have schemata or unique assumptions about ourselves, others, and the world around us. For example, a person who has the schema "The only person I can trust is myself" will have expectations that everyone else has questionable motives, will lie, and will eventually hurt them. Other negative schemata include incompetence, abandonment, evilness, and vulnerability. We are typically not aware of such cognitive biases, but recognizing them as beliefs and attitudes based on distortions and misconceptions will help make apparent the dysfunctional schemata underlying our thinking.

Rapid, unthinking responses based on schemata are known as **automatic thoughts**. These responses are particularly intense and frequent in psychiatric disorders such as depression and anxiety. Often, automatic thoughts, or **cognitive distortions**, are irrational and lead to false assumptions and misinterpretations. For example, if a person interprets all experiences in terms of whether he or she is competent and adequate, thinking may be

TABLE 4-4   COMMON COGNITIVE DISTORTIONS

DISTORTION	DEFINITION	EXAMPLE
All-or-nothing thinking	Thinking in black and white, reducing complex outcomes into absolutes	Although Marcia earned the second highest score in the provincial figure-skating competition, she consistently referred to herself as "a loser."
Overgeneralization	Using a bad outcome (or a few bad outcomes) as evidence that nothing will ever go right again	Marty had a minor traffic accident. She refuses to drive and says, "I shouldn't be allowed on the road." When asked why, she answers, "I'm a horrible driver; I could have killed someone!"
Labelling	Generalizing a characteristic or event so that it becomes definitive and results in an overly harsh label for self or others	"Because I failed the advanced statistics exam, I am a failure. I should give up. I may as well quit my nursing program."
Mental filter	Focusing on a negative detail or bad event and allowing it to taint everything else	René's boss evaluated his work as exemplary and gave him a few suggestions for improvement. He obsessed about the suggestions and ignored the rest.
Disqualifying the positive	Maintaining a negative view by rejecting information that supports a positive view as being irrelevant, inaccurate, or accidental	"I've just been offered the job I've always wanted. No one else must have applied."
Jumping to conclusions	Making a negative interpretation despite the fact that there is little or no supporting evidence	"My fiancé, Ryan, didn't call me for 3 hours, which just proves he doesn't love me anymore."
a. Mind-reading	Inferring negative thoughts, responses, and motives of others	"The grocery store clerk was grouchy and barely made eye contact, so I must have done something wrong."
b. Fortune-telling error	Anticipating that things will turn out badly as an established fact	"I'll ask her out, but I know she won't have a good time."
Magnification or minimization	Exaggerating the importance of something (such as a personal failure or the success of others) or reducing the importance of something (such as a personal success or the failure of others)	"I'm alone on a Saturday night because no one likes me. When other people are alone, it's because they want to be."
a. Catastrophizing	Magnifying to the extreme so that the very worst is assumed to be a probable outcome.	"If I don't make a good impression on the boss at the company picnic, she will fire me."
Emotional reasoning	Drawing a conclusion based on an emotional state	"I'm nervous about the exam. I must not be prepared. If I were, I wouldn't be afraid."
Should and *must* statements	Assuming rigid self-directives that presume an unrealistic amount of control over external events	"My patient is worse today. I should give better care so she will get better."
Personalization	Assuming responsibility for an external event or situation that was likely outside personal control.	"I'm sorry your party wasn't more fun. It's probably because I was there."

Source: Adapted from Burns, D. D. (1989). *The feeling good handbook*. New York: William Morrow.

dominated by the cognitive distortion "Unless I do everything perfectly, I'm a failure." Consequently, the person reacts to situations in terms of adequacy, even when these situations are unrelated to whether he or she is personally competent. Table 4-4 describes common cognitive distortions.

The therapeutic techniques of the cognitive therapist are designed to identify, reality-test, and correct distorted conceptualizations and the dysfunctional beliefs underlying them. Patients are taught to challenge their own negative thinking and substitute it with positive, rational thoughts. They are taught to recognize when thinking is based on distortions and misconceptions. Homework assignments play an important role in CBT. A particularly effective technique is the use of a four-column format to record the precipitating event or situation, the resulting automatic thought, the proceeding feelings and behaviours, and, finally, a challenge to the negative thoughts based on rational evidence and thinking. The following is an example of the type of analysis done by a patient receiving CBT.

A 24-year-old nurse recently discharged from the hospital for severe depression presented this record (Beck, Rush, Shaw, et al., 1979):

Event	Feeling	Cognitions	Other Possible Interpretations
While at a party, Jim asked me, "How are you feeling?" shortly after I was discharged from the hospital.	Anxious	Jim thinks I am a basket case. I must look really bad for him to be concerned.	He really cares about me. He noticed that I look better than before I went into the hospital and wants to know if I feel better too.

Box 4-1 presents an example of CBT, and Table 4-5 compares and contrasts psychodynamic, interpersonal, cognitive behavioural, and behavioural therapies.

Dialectic Behavioural Therapy (DBT)

Dr. Marsha Linehan (1993) developed **dialectic behavioural therapy** (DBT), a specific type of cognitive behavioural

BOX 4-1 EXAMPLE OF COGNITIVE-BEHAVIOURAL THERAPY

The patient was an attractive woman in her early 20s. Her depression of 18 months' duration was precipitated by her boyfriend's leaving her. She had numerous automatic thoughts that she was ugly and undesirable. These automatic thoughts were handled in the following manner:

Therapist: Other than your subjective opinion, what evidence do you have that you are ugly?

Patient: Well, my sister always said I was ugly.

Therapist: Was she always right in these matters?

Patient: No. Actually, she had her own reasons for telling me this. But the real reason I know I'm ugly is that men don't ask me out. If I weren't ugly, I'd be dating now.

Therapist: That is a possible reason why you're not dating. But there's an alternative explanation. You told me that you work in an office by yourself all day and spend your nights alone at home. It doesn't seem like you're giving yourself opportunities to meet men.

Patient: I can see what you're saying, but still, if I weren't ugly, men would ask me out.

Therapist: I suggest we run an experiment: that is, for you to become more socially active, stop turning down invitations to parties and social events, and see what happens.

After the patient became more active and had more opportunities to meet men, she started to date. At this point, she no longer believed she was ugly.

Therapy then focused on her basic assumption that one's worth is determined by one's appearance. She readily agreed this didn't make sense. She also saw the falseness of the assumption that one must be beautiful to attract men or be loved. This discussion led to her basic assumption that she could not be happy without love (or attention from men). The latter part of treatment focused on helping her to change this belief.

Therapist: On what do you base this belief that you can't be happy without a man?

Patient: I was really depressed for a year and a half when I didn't have a man in my life.

Therapist: Is there another reason why you were depressed?

Patient: As we discussed, I was looking at everything in a distorted way. But I still don't know if I could be happy if no one was interested in me.

Therapist: I don't know either. Is there a way we could find out?

Patient: Well, as an experiment, I could not go out on dates for a while and see how I feel.

Therapist: I think that's a good idea. Although it has its flaws, the experimental method is still the best way currently available to discover the facts. You're fortunate in being able to run this type of experiment. Now, for the first time in your adult life, you aren't attached to a man. If you find you can be happy without a man, this will greatly strengthen you and also make your future relationships all the better.

In this case, the patient was able to stick to a "cold turkey" regimen. After a brief period of dysphoria, she was delighted to find that her well-being was not dependent on another person.

There were similarities between these two interventions. In both, the distorted conclusion or assumption was delineated, and the patient was asked for evidence to support it. An experiment to gather data was also suggested in both instances. However, to achieve the results, a contrasting version of the same experimental situation was required.

Source: Beck, A. T., Rush, A. J., Shaw, B. F., et al. (1979). *Cognitive therapy of depression.* New York: Guilford Press.

TABLE 4-5 COMPARISON OF PSYCHODYNAMIC, INTERPERSONAL, COGNITIVE BEHAVIOURAL, AND BEHAVIOURAL THERAPIES

	PSYCHODYNAMIC THERAPY	INTERPERSONAL THERAPY	COGNITIVE BEHAVIOURAL THERAPY	BEHAVIOURAL THERAPY
Treatment focus	Unresolved past relationships and core conflicts	Current interpersonal relationships and social supports	Thoughts and cognitions	Learned maladaptive behaviour
Therapist role	Significant other transference object	Problem solver	Active, directive, challenging	Active, directive teacher
Primary disorders treated	Anxiety, depression, personality disorders	Depression	Depression, anxiety/panic, eating disorders	Post-traumatic stress disorder, obsessive-compulsive disorder, panic disorder
Length of therapy	20+ sessions	Short term (12–20 sessions)	Short term (5–20 sessions)	Varies; typically fewer than 10 sessions
Technique	Therapeutic alliance, free association, understanding transference, challenging defence mechanisms	Facilitate new patterns of communication and expectations for relationships	Evaluating thoughts and behaviours, modifying dysfunctional thoughts and behaviours	Relaxation, thought stopping, self-reassurance, seeking social support

Source: Dewan, M. J., Steenbarger, B. N., & Greenberg, R. P. (2008). Brief psychotherapies. In R. E. Hales, S. C. Yudofsky, & G. O. Gabbard (Eds.), *Textbook of psychiatry* (5th ed., pp. 1155–1170). Washington, DC: American Psychiatric Publishing.

psychotherapy. This model was developed for use with individuals with intractable behavioural disorders involving emotional dysregulation. DBT suggests that these individuals' arousal levels increase more quickly than that of others, obtain a higher level of emotional stimulation, and take significantly more time to return to baseline arousal levels after the emotional situation. More recently, DBT has been found to be an effective treatment modality for other mental health symptoms, such as depression, suicidal ideation, hopelessness, anger, substance dependence, and dissociation (Lenz, Del Conte, Hollenbaugh, et al, 2016). DBT focuses on teaching people methods to help them deal with swings in emotions, seeing the world in black and white, and seemingly jumping from one crisis to another. There are three primary characteristics of DBT. First, it is support oriented. Individuals are helped to identify their strengths. Second, it helps people to identify thoughts and beliefs that make life harder, such as "I am a failure," and to learn different ways of thinking. Third, this model requires constant attention to the therapeutic relationship. This model is used in individual and group settings. Individual sessions generally focus on decreasing and dealing with responses from previous trauma. Group sessions often focus on learning skills related to interpersonal effectiveness, distress tolerance, reality acceptance skills, emotional regulation, and mindfulness.

Implications of Cognitive Theories for Nursing Practice

Recognizing the interplay between events, negative thinking, and negative responses can be beneficial from both a patient care standpoint and a personal one. Workbooks are available to aid in the process of identifying cognitive distortions. Personal benefits from this cognitive approach could help the nurse to understand his or her own response to a variety of difficult situations. One example might be the anxiety that some students feel regarding the psychiatric nursing clinical rotation. Students may overgeneralize ("All psychiatric patients are dangerous.") or personalize ("My patient doesn't seem to be better; I'm probably not doing him any good.") the situation. The key to effectively using the CBT approach in clinical situations is to challenge the negative thoughts not based on facts and then replace them with more realistic appraisals. Many cognitive therapy approaches use brief therapy modalities (see Box 4-2).

HUMANISTIC THEORIES

In the 1950s, humanistic theories arose as a protest against both the behavioural and the psychoanalytic schools, which were thought to be pessimistic, deterministic, and dehumanizing. Humanistic theories focus on human potential and free will to choose life patterns that are supportive of personal growth. Humanistic frameworks emphasize a person's capacity for self-actualization. This approach focuses on understanding the patient's perspective as she or he subjectively experiences it. There are a number of humanistic theorists. We explore Abraham Maslow and his theory of self-actualization.

Abraham Maslow's Humanistic Psychology Theory

Abraham Maslow (1908–1970), considered the father of humanistic psychology, introduced the concept of a "self-actualized personality" associated with high productivity and enjoyment of life (Maslow, 1963, 1968). He criticized psychology for focusing too intently on humanity's frailties and not enough on its strengths. Maslow contended that the focus of psychology must go beyond experiences of hate, pain, misery, guilt, and conflict to include love, compassion, happiness, exhilaration, and well-being.

Hierarchy of Needs

Maslow conceptualized human motivation as a hierarchy of dynamic processes or needs that are critical for the development

---

> **BOX 4-2 CHARACTERISTICS OF BRIEF THERAPIES**
>
> At the start of treatment, the patient and therapist agree on what the focus will be and concentrate their work on that focus. Sessions are held weekly, and the total number of sessions to be held is determined at the outset of therapy. There is a rapid, back-and-forth pattern between patient and therapist, with both participating actively. The therapist intervenes constantly to keep the therapy on track, either by redirecting the patient's attention or by interpreting deviations from the focus to the patient.
>
> Brief therapies share the following common elements:
> - Assessment tends to be rapid and early.
> - Clear expectations are established for time-limited therapy with improvement demonstrated within a small number of sessions.
> - Goals are concrete and focus on improving the patient's worst symptoms, improving coping skills, and helping the patient to understand what is going on in his or her life.
> - Interpretations are directed toward present life circumstances and patient behaviour rather than toward the historical significance of feelings.
> - There is a general understanding that psychotherapy does not cure, but that it can help troubled individuals learn to recognize that problems exist and can promote self-awareness as they deal with life's inevitable stressors.

of all humans. Central to his theory is the assumption that humans are active rather than passive participants in life, striving for self-actualization. Maslow (1968) focused on human need fulfillment, which he categorized into six incremental stages, beginning with physiological survival needs and ending with self-transcendent needs (Figure 4-5). The hierarchy of needs is conceptualized as a pyramid, with the strongest, most fundamental needs placed on the lower levels. The more distinctly human needs occupy the top sections of the pyramid. When lower-level needs are met, higher needs are able to emerge.

- *Physiological needs.* The most basic needs are the physiological drives—food, oxygen, water, sleep, sex, and a constant body temperature. If all needs were deprived, this level would take priority over the rest.
- *Safety needs.* Once physiological needs are met, safety needs emerge. They include security; protection; freedom from fear, anxiety, and chaos; and the need for law, order, and limits. Adults in a stable society usually feel safe, but they may feel threatened by debt, job insecurity, or lack of insurance. It is during times of crisis, such as war, disasters, assaults, and social breakdown, that safety needs really take precedence. Children, who are more vulnerable and dependent, respond far more readily and intensely to safety threats.
- *Belongingness and love needs.* People have a need for intimate relationships, love, affection, and belonging and will seek to overcome feelings of aloneness and alienation. Maslow stresses the importance of having a family and a home and of being part of an identifiable group.
- *Esteem needs.* People need to have a high self-regard and have it reflected to them from others. If self-esteem needs are met,

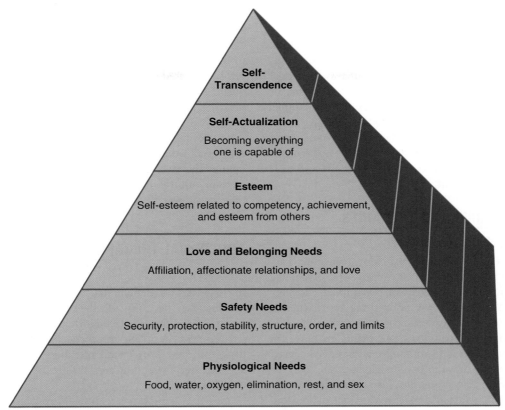

FIGURE 4-5 Maslow's hierarchy of needs. Source: Adapted from Maslow, A. H. (1972). *The farther reaches of human nature.* New York: Viking.

we feel confident, valued, and valuable. When self-esteem is compromised, we feel inferior, worthless, and helpless.

- *Self-actualization.* We are preset to strive to be everything we are capable of becoming. Maslow said, "What a man *can* be, he *must* be." What we are capable of becoming is highly individual—an artist must paint, a writer must write, and a healer must heal. The drive to satisfy this need is felt as a sort of restlessness, a sense that something is missing. It is up to each person to choose a path that will bring about inner peace and fulfillment.

Although his early work included only five levels of needs, Maslow (1970) later took into account two additional factors: (1) cognitive needs (the desire to know and understand) and (2) the aesthetic needs. He describes the acquisition of knowledge (our first priority) and the need to understand (our second priority) as being hard-wired and essential; he identified the aesthetic need for beauty and symmetry as universal. How else, after all, do we explain the impulse to straighten a crooked picture?

Maslow based his theory on the results of clinical investigations of people who represented self-actualized individuals, who moved in the direction of achieving and reaching their highest potentials. Among those Maslow chose to investigate were historical figures such as Henry David Thoreau, Walt Whitman, and Ludwig von Beethoven, as well as others like Albert Einstein and Albert Schweitzer, who were living at the time they were studied. This investigation led Maslow (1963, 1970) to identify some basic personality characteristics that distinguish self-actualizing people from those who might be called "ordinary" (Box 4-3).

BOX 4-3   SOME CHARACTERISTICS OF SELF-ACTUALIZED PERSONS (SAs)

- Accurate perception of reality; not defensive in their perceptions of the world
- Acceptance of themselves, others, and nature
- Spontaneity, simplicity, and naturalness (SAs do not live programmed lives)
- Problem-centred rather than self-centred orientation (possibly the most important characteristic); SAs have a sense of a mission to which they dedicate their lives
- Enjoyment of privacy and detachment; pleasure in being alone; ability to reflect on events
- Freshness of appreciation; not taking life for granted
- Mystical or peak experiences (a moment of intense ecstasy, similar to a religious or mystical experience, during which the self is transcended)*
- Active social interest
- An unhostile sense of humour
- Democratic character structure; displaying little racial, religious, or social prejudice
- Creativity, especially in managing their lives
- Resistance to conformity (enculturation); autonomy, independence, and self-sufficiency

*More recently, Mihaly Csikszentmihalyi developed the term *flow experience* to describe times when people become so totally involved in what they are doing that they lose all sense of time and awareness of self.
Source: Adapted from Maslow, A. H. (1970). *Motivation and personality.* New York: Harper & Row.

Implications of Motivation Theory for Nursing Practice

The value of Maslow's model in nursing practice is twofold. First, an emphasis on human potential and the patient's strengths is key to successful nurse–patient relationships. Second, the model helps establish what is most important in the sequencing of nursing actions in the nurse–patient relationship. For example, to collect any but the most essential information when a patient is struggling with drug withdrawal is inappropriate. Following Maslow's model as a way of prioritizing actions, the nurse meets the patient's physiological need for stable vital signs and pain relief before further assessment.

BIOLOGICAL THEORIES AND THERAPIES

The Advent of Psychopharmacology

In 1950, a French drug firm synthesized chlorpromazine (Largactil)—a powerful antipsychotic medication—and psychiatry experienced a revolution. The advent of psychopharmacology presented a direct challenge to psychodynamic approaches to mental illness. The dramatic experience of observing patients freed from the bondage of psychosis and mania by powerful drugs such as chlorpromazine and lithium left witnesses convinced of the critical role of the brain in psychiatric illness.

Since the discovery of chlorpromazine, many other medications have proven effective in controlling psychosis, mania, depression, and anxiety. These medications greatly reduce the need for hospitalization and dramatically improve the lives of people with serious psychiatric difficulties. Today, we know that psychoactive medications exert differential effects on different neurotransmitters and help restore brain function, allowing patients with mental illness to continue living productive lives with greater satisfaction and far less emotional pain.

The Biological Model

A biological model of mental illness focuses on neurological, chemical, biological, and genetic issues and seeks to understand how the body and brain interact to create emotions, memories, and perceptual experiences. This perspective views abnormal behaviour as part of a disease process or a defect and seeks to stop or alter it. The biological model locates the illness or disease in the body—usually in the limbic system of the brain and the synapse receptor sites of the central nervous system—and targets the site of the illness using physical interventions such as medications, diet, or surgery.

The recognition that psychiatric illnesses are as physical in origin as diabetes and coronary heart disease serves to decrease the stigma surrounding them. Just as people with diabetes or heart disease cannot be held responsible for their illness, patients with schizophrenia or bipolar affective disorder are not to blame for theirs. It often happens that one of the most helpful things we can tell those whose lives are affected by psychiatric illness is that they are not responsible or to blame.

Implications of the Biological Model for Nursing Practice

Historically, psychiatric mental health nurses always have attended to the physical needs of psychiatric patients. Nurses administer medications; monitor sleep, activity, nutrition, hydration, elimination, and other functions; and prepare patients for somatic therapies, such as electroconvulsive therapy. They have continued to do so with the advancement of the biological model, which has not altered the basic nursing strategies: focusing on the qualities of a therapeutic relationship, understanding the patient's perspective, and communicating in a way that facilitates the patient's recovery.

One of the risks in adopting a biological model to the exclusion of all other theoretical perspectives is that such a theory ignores the myriad other influences, including social, environmental, cultural, economic, spiritual, and educational factors, that play a role in the development and treatment of mental illness.

ADDITIONAL THERAPIES

Milieu Therapy

In 1948, Bruno Bettelheim coined the term milieu therapy to describe his use of the total environment to treat disturbed children. Bettelheim created a comfortable, secure environment (or milieu) in which psychotic children were helped to form a new world. Staff members were trained to provide 24-hour support and understanding for each child on an individual basis.

Milieu is sometimes a difficult concept to grasp. It is an all-inclusive term that recognizes the people, setting, structure, and emotional climate all as important to healing. Milieu therapy uses naturally occurring events in the environment as rich learning opportunities for patients. There are certain basic characteristics of milieu therapy, regardless of whether the setting involves treatment of psychotic children, patients in a psychiatric hospital, drug abusers in a residential treatment centre, or psychiatric patients in a day hospital. Milieu therapy, or a therapeutic community, has as its focus a living, learning, or working environment. Such therapy may be based on any number of therapeutic modalities, from structured behavioural therapy to spontaneous, humanistic-oriented approaches.

Implications of Milieu Therapy for Nursing Practice

Milieu therapy is a basic intervention in nursing practice. Although most commonly associated with inpatient treatment (Veale, Gilbert, Wheatley et al, 2015), other examples of milieu therapy include providing a safe environment for the suicidal patient or for a patient with a cognitive disorder (e.g., Alzheimer's disease), referring abused women to safe houses, and advocating for children suspected of being abused in their home environments.

You will be introduced to other therapeutic approaches later in the book. Crisis intervention (see Chapter 21) is an approach you will find useful, not only in psychiatric mental health nursing but also in other nursing specialties. Group therapy (see Chapter 33) and family interventions (see Chapter 34), which are appropriate for the basic-level practitioner, will also be discussed.

Table 4-6 lists additional theorists whose contributions influence psychiatric mental health nursing.

TABLE 4-6	ADDITIONAL THEORISTS WHOSE CONTRIBUTIONS INFLUENCE PSYCHIATRIC MENTAL HEALTH NURSING		
THEORIST	**SCHOOL OF THOUGHT**	**MAJOR CONTRIBUTIONS**	**RELEVANCE TO PSYCHIATRIC MENTAL HEALTH NURSING**
Carl Rogers	Humanism	Developed a person-centred model of psychotherapy; emphasized the concepts of: • Congruence—authenticity of the therapist in dealings with the patient • Unconditional acceptance and positive regard—climate in the therapeutic relationship that facilitates change • Empathic understanding—therapist's ability to apprehend the feelings and experiences of the patient as if these things were happening to the therapist	Encourages nurses to view each patient as unique; emphasizes attitudes of unconditional positive regard, empathic understanding, and genuineness that are essential to the nurse–patient relationship *Example:* The nurse asks the patient, "What can I do to help you regain control over your anxiety?"
Jean Piaget	Cognitive development	Identified stages of cognitive development, including sensorimotor (0–2 years), preoperational (2–7 years), concrete operational (7–11 years), and formal operational (11 years–adulthood); these stages describe how cognitive development proceeds from reflex activity to application of logical solutions to all types of problems	Provides a broad base for cognitive interventions, especially with patients with negative self-views *Example:* The nurse shows an 8-year-old all the equipment needed to start an intravenous when discussing the fact that he will need one prior to surgery.
Lawrence Kohlberg	Moral development	Posited a six-stage theory of moral development	Provides nurses with a framework for evaluating moral decisions *Example:* In stage 5, the nurse views laws as social contracts that promote "the greatest good for the greatest number of people." The nurse would advocate access to universal health care.
Albert Ellis	Existentialism	Developed approach of rational emotive behavioural therapy that is active and cognitively oriented; confrontation used to force patients to assume responsibility for behaviour; patients are encouraged to accept themselves as they are and are taught to take risks and try out new behaviours	Encourages nurses to focus on here-and-now issues and to help the patient live fully in the present and look forward to the future. *Example:* The nurse encourages the patient to vacation with her family even though she will be in a wheelchair until her leg fracture heals.
Albert Bandura	Social learning theory	Responsible for concepts of modelling and self-efficacy—that is, a person's belief or expectation that he or she has the capacity to effect a desired outcome through his or her own efforts	Includes cognitive functioning with environmental factors, which provides nurses with a comprehensive view of how people learn. *Example:* The nurse helps the teenage patient identify three negative outcomes of tobacco use.
Viktor Frankl	Existentialism	Developed "logotherapy," a future-oriented therapy offered to help people find their sense of self-respect and focused on their need to find meaning and value in living as their most important life task	Focuses the nurse beyond mere behaviours to understanding the meaning of these behaviours to the patient's sense of life meaning *Example:* The nurse listens attentively as the patient describes what life has been like since her daughter died.

Sources: Bandura, A. (1977). *Social learning theory.* Englewood Cliffs, NJ: Prentice-Hall; Bernard, M. E., & Wolfe, J. L. (Eds.). (1993). *The RET resource book for practitioners.* New York: Institute for Rational-Emotive Therapy; Ellis, A. (1989). *Inside rational emotive therapy.* San Diego: Academic Press; Frankl, V. (1969). *The will to meaning.* Cleveland: New American Library; Kohlberg, L. (1986). A current statement on some theoretical issues. In S. Modgil & C. Modgil (Eds.), *Lawrence Kohlberg.* Philadelphia: Palmer; and Rogers, C. R. (1961). *On becoming a person.* Boston: Houghton Mifflin.

RESEARCH HIGHLIGHT

Engaging Street-Involved Youth in Dialectical Behaviour Therapy: A Secondary Analysis

Problem

The issue of mental health problems in street-involved youth is complex. It is not known how best to provide services that are accessible and acceptable to this population.

Purpose of Study

One of the foundational requirements to provide effective mental health care is client engagement. However, the degree to which youth would engage in dialectical behavioural therapy (DBT) is relatively unknown.

Methods

A secondary analysis was conducted from the data gathered during a previous study that investigated the effectiveness of implementing a version of DBT, adapted for adolescents, to alleviate mental health challenges and strengthen their resiliency.

Key Findings

When a 12-week DBT intervention was offered, 13% of participants who expressed an intention to start the DBT intervention did not, 32% of the participants missed four or more sessions, and 55% completed the intervention. The street-involved youth who did engage and complete the intervention had statistically more years of education and were more likely to have seen a psychiatrist within the last month. In addition, those who engaged had higher levels of depression and suicidal ideation than those who did not engage. There was no significant difference in substance use between the groups.

Implications for Nursing Practice

When developing therapeutic relationships with clients, it is important to offer services in a safe and accessible environment. In addition, alternative engagement strategies need to be developed for street-involved youth with limited years of education.

Source: Lynk, M., McCay, E., Carter, C., et al. (2015). Engaging street-involved youth in dialectical behaviour therapy: A secondary analysis. *Journal of the Canadian Academy of Child & Adolescent Psychiatry, 24*(2) 116–122. Retrieved from http://www.cacap-acpea.org/en/cacap/Journal_p828.html.

KEY POINTS TO REMEMBER

- Sigmund Freud advanced the first theory of personality development.
- Freud articulated levels of awareness (unconscious, preconscious, conscious) and demonstrated the influence of our unconscious behaviour on everyday life, as evidenced by the use of defence mechanisms.
- Freud identified three psychological processes of personality (id, ego, superego) and described how they operate and develop.
- Freud articulated one of the first modern developmental theories of personality, based on five psychosexual stages.
- Various psychoanalytic therapies have been used over the years. Currently, a short-term, time-limited version of psychotherapy is common.
- Erik Erikson expanded on Freud's developmental stages to include middle age through old age. Erikson called his stages *psychosocial stages* and emphasized the social aspect of personality development.

- Harry Stack Sullivan proposed the interpersonal theory of personality development, which focuses on interpersonal processes that can be observed in a social framework.
- Hildegard Peplau, a nursing theorist, developed an interpersonal theoretical framework that has become the foundation of psychiatric mental health nursing practice.
- Abraham Maslow, the founder of humanistic psychology, offered the theory of self-actualization and human motivation that is basic to all nursing education today.
- Cognitive behavioural therapy is the most commonly used, accepted, and empirically validated psychotherapeutic approach.
- A biological model of mental illness and treatment dominates care for psychiatric disorders.
- Milieu therapy is a philosophy of care in which all parts of the environment are considered to be therapeutic opportunities for growth and healing. The milieu includes the people (patients and staff), setting, structure, and emotional climate.

CRITICAL THINKING

1. Consider the theorists and theories discussed in this chapter. The following questions address how they may affect your nursing practice.

   a. How do Freud's concepts of the conscious, preconscious, and unconscious affect your understanding of patients' behaviours?

   b. Do you believe that Erikson's psychosocial stages represent a sound basis for identifying disruptions in stages of development in your patients? Support your position with a clinical example.

   c. What are the implications of Sullivan's focus on the importance of interpersonal relationships for your interactions with patients?

   d. Peplau believed that nurses must exercise self-awareness within the nurse–patient relationship. Describe situations in your student experience in which this self-awareness played a vital role in your relationships with patients.

   e. Identify someone you believe to be self-actualized. What characteristics does this person have that support your assessment?

f. How do or will you make use of Maslow's hierarchy of needs in your nursing practice?

g. What do you think about the behaviourist point of view that a change in behaviour results in a change in thinking? Can you give an example of this in your own life?

2. Which of the therapies described in this chapter do you think are or will be the most helpful to you in your nursing practice? Explain your choice.

CHAPTER REVIEW

1. The nurse is working with a patient who lacks the ability to problem-solve and seeks ways to self-satisfy without regard for others. Which system of the patient's personality is most pronounced?
   a. Id
   b. Ego
   c. Conscience (superego)
   d. Ego ideal (superego)

2. Which behaviour, seen in a 30-year-old patient, would alert the nurse to the fact that the patient is not in his appropriate developmental stage according to Erikson?
   a. States he is happily married
   b. Frequently asks to call his brother "just to check in"
   c. Looks forward to visits from a co-worker
   d. Says, "I'm still trying to find myself."

3. A patient has difficulty sitting still and listening to others during group therapy. The therapist plans to use operant conditioning as a form of behavioural modification to assist the patient. Which action would the nurse expect to see in group therapy?
   a. The therapist will act as a role model for the patient by sitting still and listening.

   b. The patient will receive a token from the therapist for each session in which she sits still and listens.
   c. The patient will be required to sit in solitude for 30 minutes after each session in which she does not sit still or listen.
   d. The therapist will ask that the patient to sit still and listen for only 2 minutes at a time to begin with and will increase the time incrementally until the patient can sit and listen for 10 minutes at a time.

4. The nurse is planning care for a patient with anxiety who will be admitted to the unit shortly. Which nursing action is most important?
   a. Consider ways to assist the patient to feel valued during his stay on the unit.
   b. Choose a roommate for the patient so that a friendship can develop.
   c. Identify a room where the patient will have comfortable surroundings, and order a balanced meal plan.
   d. Plan methods of decreasing stimuli that could cause heightened anxiety in the patient.

⊖volve WEBSITE

Post-Test   interactive review

Visit the Evolve website for Chapter Review Answers and Rationales, Critical Thinking Answer Guidelines, and additional resources related to the content in this chapter http://evolve.elsevier.com/Canada/Varcarolis/psychiatric/

REFERENCES

Bandura, A., Blahard, E. B., & Ritter, B. (1969). Relative efficacy of desensitization and modeling approaches for inducing behavioural, affective, and attitudinal changes. *Journal of Personality and Social Psychology, 13*, 173–199. doi:10.1037/h0028276.

Barker, P., & Buchanan-Barker, P. (2005). *The tidal model: A guide for mental health professionals.* New York: Brunner-Routledge.

Beck, A. T. (1967). *Depression: Clinical, experimental and theoretical aspects.* New York: Harper & Row.

Beck, A. T., Rush, A. J., Shaw, B. F., et al. (1979). *Cognitive therapy of depression.* New York: Guilford.

Canadian Federation of Mental Health Nurses (2014). *Canadian standards for psychiatric-mental health nursing* (4th ed.). Toronto: Author.

Crain, W. C. (1985). *Theories of development.* New York: Prentice-Hall.

Ellis, A. (2000). *On therapy: A dialogue with Aaron T. Beck and Albert Ellis,* Symposium conducted at the American Psychological Association's 108th Convention. Washington, DC.

Erikson, E. H. (1963). *Childhood and society.* New York: W. W. Norton.

Freud, S. (1960). *The ego and the id.* J. Strachey, Trans. New York: W. W. Norton.

Freud, S. (1961). *The interpretation of dreams.* J. Strachey, Ed. & Trans. New York: Scientific Editions.

Freud, S. (1969). *An outline of psychoanalysis.* J. Strachey, Trans. New York: W. W. Norton.

Gilligan, C. (1982). *In a different voice.* Boston: Harvard University Press.

Hewitt, P. L., Mikail, S. F., Flett, G. L., et al. (2015). Psychodynamic/interpersonal group psychotherapy for perfectionism: Evaluating the effectiveness of a short-term treatment. *Psychotherapy, 52*(2), 205–217. doi:10.1037/pst0000016.

Kohlberg, L., & Turiel, E. (1971). Moral development and moral education. In G. S. Lesser (Ed.), *Psychology and educational practice* (pp. 410–465). Glenview, IL: Scott, Foresman, & Company.

Lenz, A. S., Del Conte, G., Hollenbaugh, K. M., et al. (2016). Emotional regulation and interpersonal effectiveness as mechanisms sof change for treatment outcomes within a DBT program for adolescents. *Counseling Outcome Research, 7*(2), 73–85. doi:10.1177/2150137816642439.

Linehan, M. M. (1993). *Cognitive behavioral treatment of borderline personality disorder.* New York: Guilford Press.

Mahler, M. S., Pine, F., & Bergman, A. (1975). *The psychological birth of the human infant*. New York: Basic Books.

Maslow, A. H. (1963). Self-actualizing people. In G. B. Levitas (Ed.), *The world of psychology* (Vol. 2). New York: Braziller.

Maslow, A. H. (1968). *Toward a psychology of being*. Princeton, NJ: Van Nostrands.

Maslow, A. H. (1970). *Motivation and personality* (2nd ed.). New York: Harper & Row.

Pavlov, I. (1928). W. H. Grant (Ed.), *Lectures on conditioned reflexes*. New York: International Publishers.

Peplau, H. E. (1952). *Interpersonal relations in nursing: A conceptual frame of reference for psychodynamic nursing*. New York: Putnam.

Peplau, H. E. (1982a). Therapeutic concepts. In S. A. Smoyak & S. Rouslin (Eds.), *A collection of classics in psychiatric nursing literature* (pp. 91–108). Thorofare, NJ: Slack.

Peplau, H. E. (1982b). Interpersonal techniques: The crux of psychiatric nursing. In S. A. Smoyak & S. Rouslin (Eds.), *A collection of classics in psychiatric nursing literature* (pp. 276–281). Thorofare, NJ: Slack.

Peplau, H. E. (1987). Interpersonal constructs for nursing practice. *Nursing Education Today, 7*, 201–208. doi:10.1016/0260-6917(87)90002-5.

Peplau, H. E. (1989). Future directions in psychiatric nursing from the perspective of history. *Journal of Psychosocial Nursing, 27*(2), 18–28.

Ramezani, A., Rockers, D., Wanlass, R. L., et al. (2016). Teaching behavioural medicine professionals and trainees an elaborated version of the Y-model: Implications for the integration of cognitive-behavioral therapy (CBT), psychodynamic therapy, and motivational interviewing. *Journal of Psychotherapy Integration, 26*(4), 207–424. doi:10.1037/int0000048.

Skinner, B. F. (1987). Whatever happened to psychology as the science of behavior? *American Psychologist, 42*, 780–786. doi:10.1037/0003-066X.42.8.780.

Sullivan, H. S. (1953). *The interpersonal theory of psychiatry*. New York: W. W. Norton.

Veale, D., Gilbert, P., Wheatley, J., et al. (2015). A new therapeutic community: Development of a compassion-focussed and contextual behavioural environment. *Clinical Psychology and Psychotherapy, 22*(4), 285–303. doi:10.1002/cpp.1897.

Watson, J. B. (1919). *Psychology from the standpoint of a behaviourist*. Philadelphia: Lippincott.

Understanding Responses to Stress

Margaret Jordan Halter
Adapted by Sonya L. Jakubec

KEY TERMS AND CONCEPTS

Benson's relaxation technique
cognitive reframing
coping styles
distress
eustress
fight-or-flight response
general adaptation syndrome (GAS)
guided imagery

journaling
meditation
mindfulness
physical stressors
progressive muscle relaxation (PMR)
psychological stressors
psychoneuroimmunology
stressors

OBJECTIVES

1. Recognize the short- and long-term physiological consequences of stress.
2. Compare and contrast Cannon's fight-or-flight response, Selye's general adaptation syndrome, and the psychoneuroimmunological models of stress.
3. Describe how responses to stress are mediated through perception, personality, social support, culture, and spirituality.
4. Assess stress level using the Recent Life Changes Questionnaire.
5. Identify and describe holistic approaches to stress management.
6. Teach a classmate or patient a behavioural technique to help lower stress and anxiety.
7. Explain how cognitive techniques can help increase a person's tolerance for stressful events.

⊖volve WEBSITE

Visit the Evolve website for Flashcards, Case Studies, and additional testing resources related to the content in this chapter: http://evolve.elsevier.com/Canada/Varcarolis/psychiatric/

Pre-Test   interactive review

Before turning our attention to the clinical disorders presented in the chapters that follow, we explore the subject of stress as a foundation to understanding the context and experiences of distress. Stress and our responses to it are central to psychiatric disorders and the provision of mental health care. The interplay among stress, the development of psychiatric disorders, and the exacerbation (worsening) of psychiatric symptoms has been widely researched. The old adage "What doesn't kill you will make you stronger" does not hold true with the development of mental illness; early exposure to stressful events actually sensitizes people to stress in later life. In other words, we know that people who are exposed to high levels of stress as children—especially during stress-sensitive developmental periods—have a greater incidence of all mental illnesses as adults (Paquola, Bennett, Hatton, et al., 2017). However, we do not know if severe stress causes a vulnerability to mental illness or if vulnerability to mental illness influences the likelihood of adverse stress responses. It is most important to recognize that severe stress is unhealthy and can weaken biological resistance to psychiatric pathology in any individual; however, stress is especially harmful for those who have a genetic predisposition to these disorders (Anisman, 2015).

While an understanding of the connection between stress and mental illness is essential in the psychiatric setting, it is also important when developing a plan of care for any patient, in any setting, with any diagnosis. Imagine having an appendectomy and being served with an eviction notice on the same day. How well could you cope with either situation, let alone both simultaneously? The nurse's role is to intervene to reduce stress by promoting a healing environment, facilitating successful coping, and developing future coping strategies. In this chapter, we explore how we are equipped to respond to stress, what can go wrong with the stress response, and how to care for our patients and even ourselves during times of stress.

RESPONSES TO AND EFFECTS OF STRESS

Early Stress Response Theories

The earliest research into the stress response (Figure 5-1) began as a result of observations that stressors brought about physical disorders or made existing conditions worse. Stressors are psychological or physical stimuli that are incompatible with current functioning and require adaptation. Walter Cannon (1871–1945) methodically investigated the sympathetic nervous system as a pathway of the response to stress, known more commonly as fight (aggression) or flight (withdrawal). The well-known fight-or-flight response is the body's way of preparing for a situation perceived as a threat to survival. This response results in increased blood pressure, heart rate, and cardiac output.

While groundbreaking, Cannon's theory has been criticized for being simplistic since not all animals or people respond by fighting or fleeing. In the face of danger, some animals (e.g., a deer) become still or freeze to avoid being noticed or to observe the environment in a state of heightened awareness. Also, Cannon's theory was developed primarily based on the responses of animals and men. Men and women, however, have different neural responses to stress. While men experience altered prefrontal blood flow and increased salivary cortisol in response to stress, women experience increased limbic (emotional) activity and, less significantly, altered salivary cortisol (Bangasser, 2013; Jones & Monfils, 2016).

Hans Selye (1907–1982), another pioneer in stress research, introduced the concept of stress into both the scientific and the popular literature. Selye (1974) expanded Cannon's 1956 theory of stress in his formulation of the general adaptation syndrome (GAS). The GAS occurs in three stages:

1. The *alarm* (or *acute stress*) stage is the initial, brief, and adaptive response (fight or flight) to the stressor. During the alarm stage, three principal *stress mediators* are involved:
   - The brain's cortex and hypothalamus signal the adrenal glands to release the catecholamine adrenaline. This release, in turn, increases sympathetic system activity (e.g., increased heart rate, respirations, and blood pressure) to enhance strength and speed. Pupils dilate for a broad view of the environment, and blood is shunted away from the digestive tract (resulting in dry mouth) and kidneys to more essential organs.

   - The hypothalamus also sends messages to the adrenal cortex. The adrenal cortex produces corticosteroids to help increase muscle endurance and stamina, whereas other nonessential functions (e.g., digestion) are decreased. Unfortunately, the corticosteroids also inhibit functions such as reproduction, growth, and immunity (Sadock & Sadock, 2017).
   - Endorphins that reduce sensitivity to pain and injury are released. The alarm stage is extremely intense, and no organism can sustain this level of reactivity and excitement for long. If the organism survives, the resistance stage follows.

2. The *resistance* stage could also be called the *adaptation stage*, because it is during this time that sustained and optimal resistance to the stressor occurs. Usually, stressors are successfully overcome; however, when they are not, the organism may experience the final stage: exhaustion.

3. The *exhaustion* stage occurs when attempts to resist the stressor prove futile. At this point, resources are depleted, and the stress may become chronic, producing a wide array of psychological and physiological responses and even death.

The body responds the same physiologically regardless of whether the stress is real or only perceived as a threat and whether the threat is physical, psychological, or social. In addition, the body cannot differentiate between the energy generated by positive and negative stimuli. Lazarus (2012) described these reactions as distress and eustress:

- Distress is a negative, draining energy that results in anxiety, depression, confusion, helplessness, hopelessness, and fatigue. Distress may be caused by such stressors as a death in the family, financial overload, or school or work demands.
- Eustress is a positive, beneficial energy that motivates and results in feelings of happiness, hopefulness, and purposeful movement. Eustress may be the result of a much-needed vacation, being called in for an interview, the birth of a baby, or buying a new car. Eustress could lead to a depletion of physiological resources if sustained, but, fortunately or unfortunately, one does not typically become chronically happy and motivated.

Selye's GAS remains a popular theory, but it has been expanded and reinterpreted since the 1950s (Contrada & Baum, 2011). Some researchers question the notion of "nonspecific responses" and believe that different types of stressors bring about different patterns of responses. Furthermore, the GAS is most accurate in the description of how males respond when threatened. Females do not typically respond to stress by fighting or fleeing but rather by tending and befriending, a survival strategy that emphasizes the protection of young and a reliance on the social network for support (Bangasser, 2013; Underwood, 2012).

Increased understanding of the exhaustion stage of the GAS has revealed that illness results from not only the depletion of reserves but also the stress mediators themselves. This finding is discussed in "Immune Stress Responses". Table 5-1 describes some reactions to acute and prolonged (chronic) stress.

Neurotransmitter Stress Responses

Serotonin is a brain catecholamine that plays an important role in mood, sleep, sexuality, appetite, and metabolism. It is one of

THE STRESS RESPONSE

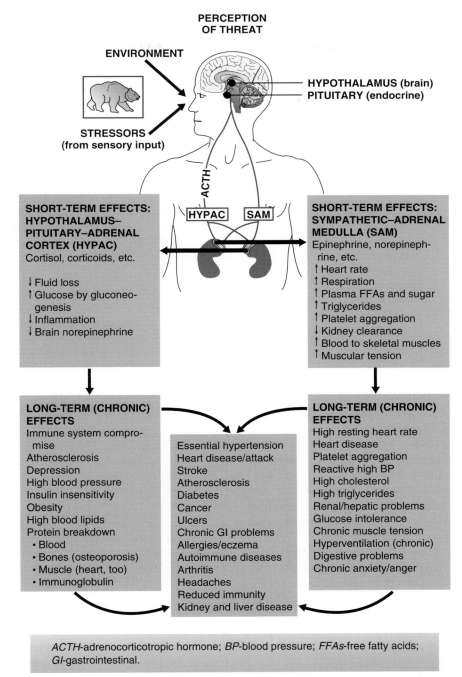

FIGURE 5-1 The stress response. Source: From Brigham, D. D. (1994). *Imagery for getting well: Clinical applications of behavioural medicine.* New York: W. W. Norton.

the main neurotransmitters implicated in depression, and many medications used to treat depression do so by increasing the availability of serotonin (see Chapter 11). During times of stress, serotonin synthesis becomes more active. This stress-activated turnover of serotonin is at least partially mediated by the corticosteroids, and researchers believe this activation may dysregulate (impair) serotonin receptor sites and the brain's ability to use serotonin (Sadock & Sadock, 2017). The influence of stressful life events on the development of depression is well documented, but researchers still do not fully understand the relationship. This neurotransmitter stress response research sheds some new light on the process.

Immune Stress Responses

Cannon and Selye focused on the physical and mental responses of the nervous and endocrine systems to acute and chronic stress.

TABLE 5-1	SOME REACTIONS TO ACUTE AND PROLONGED (CHRONIC) STRESS
ACUTE STRESS CAN CAUSE	**PROLONGED (CHRONIC) STRESS CAN CAUSE**
Uneasiness and concern	Anxiety and panic attacks
Sadness	Depression or melancholia
Loss of appetite	Anorexia or overeating
Suppression of the immune system	Lowered resistance to infections, leading to an increase in opportunistic viral and bacterial infections
Increased metabolism and use of body fats	Insulin-resistant diabetes
	Hypertension
Infertility	Amenorrhea or loss of sex drive
	Impotence, anovulation
Increased energy mobilization and use	Increased fatigue and irritability
	Decreased memory and learning
Increased cardiovascular tone	Increased risk for cardiac events (e.g., heart attack, angina, and sudden heart-related death)
	Increased risk for blood clots and stroke
Increased cardiopulmonary tone	Increased respiratory problems

Later work revealed that there is also an interaction between the nervous system and the immune system during the alarm phase of the GAS. In one classic study, rats were given a mixture of saccharine and a drug that reduces the immune system (Ader & Cohen, 1975). Afterward, when given only the saccharine, the rats continued to have decreased immune responses, which indicated that stress itself negatively affects the body's ability to produce a protective structure.

Studies in psychoneuroimmunology (the study of the relationship between the mind, the nervous system, and the immune system) continue to provide evidence that stress, through the hypothalamic–pituitary–adrenal and sympathetic–adrenal medullary axes, can induce changes in the immune system. This model helps explain what many researchers and clinicians have believed and witnessed for centuries: there are links among stress (biopsychosocial), the immune system, and disease—a clear mind–body connection that may alter health outcomes. Stress may result in malfunctions in the immune system that are implicated in autoimmune disorders, immunodeficiency, and hypersensitivities.

Stress influences the immune system in several complex ways. As discussed earlier, corticosteroids are released in response to stress and inhibit the immune system, which increases susceptibility to illness (Sadock & Sadock, 2017). Conversely, stress can enhance the immune system and prepare the body to respond to injury. Cytokines, which are proteins and glycoproteins used for communication between cells, are normally released by immune cells when a pathogen is detected; they serve to activate and recruit other immune cells. During times of stress, these cytokines are released, and immunity is profoundly activated. But the activation is limited since the cytokines stimulate further release of corticosteroids, which inhibit the immune system.

RESEARCH HIGHLIGHT
Urban Tree Canopy and Stress Recovery

Problem
While it is well established that viewing nature can help individuals to recover from illness or stressful experiences, the actual "dosage" or relationship of tree cover density and stress recovery is not known.

Purpose of Study
To determine the optimal urban tree canopy to aid in stress reduction.

Methods
An experiment was completed with 160 participants who engaged in a standard Trier Social Stress Test to induce stress. These participants were then randomly assigned to watch 1 of 10 three-dimensional videos of street scenes with varying degrees of tree cover density (from 2% to 62%). At three different points in the experiment participants completed a Visual Analogue Scale.

Key Findings
Analysis revealed a positive, linear association between the density of urban street trees and self-reported stress recovery. In short, an increase in tree density yields greater self-reported stress reduction. Compared with watching a 6-minute video with 2% tree cover density, watching a 6-minute video with 62% tree cover density resulted in a 60% increase in stress recovery. This relationship held after controlling for gender, age, and baseline stress levels. Participants' written narratives revealed a similar but even stronger association.

Implications for Nursing Practice
These results can help nurses in encouraging nature immersion for patients recovering from stress-related disorders and in general mental health promotion. Nurses can also advocate for a greater investment in urban tree planting and community parks and landscape design based on these significant findings.

Source: Jiang, B., Li, D., Larsen, L., et al. (2016). A dose-response curve describing the relationship between urban tree cover density and self-reported stress recovery. *Environment and Behavior, 48*(4), 607–629. doi:10.1177/0013916514552321.

The immune response and the resulting cytokine activity in the brain raise questions about their connection with psychological and cognitive states such as depression (Lovallo, 2015). Some cancers are treated with a type of cytokine molecules known as interleukins. These chemotherapy drugs tend to cause or increase depression. Furthermore, elevated cytokines and immune activation are often seen during episodes of severe depression.

MEDIATORS OF THE STRESS RESPONSE

Stressors

A variety of dissimilar situations (e.g., emotional arousal, fatigue, fear, loss, humiliation, loss of blood, extreme happiness, unexpected success) all are capable of producing stress and triggering the stress response (Lovallo, 2015; Selye, 1993). No individual factor can be singled out as the cause of the stress response; however, stressors can be divided into two categories: physical and psychological. **Physical stressors** include changes to environmental conditions (e.g., environmental trauma or disaster, excessive cold or heat), as well as physical conditions (e.g., injury, illness, hunger, pain). **Psychological stressors** include cognitive- or emotion-based changes, such as divorce, loss of a job, unmanageable debt, the death of a loved one, retirement, and fear of violence, as well as changes we might consider positive, such as marriage, the arrival of a new baby, or unexpected success.

Perception

Researchers have looked at the degree to which various life events upset a specific individual and have found that the perception of a stressor determines the person's emotional and psychological reactions to it (Rahe, Veach, Tolles, et al., 2000). When individuals perceive that stress will affect their health, this is associated with both poor health and poor mental health. Further, individuals who have this belief that stress affects their health, and who also report large amounts of stress, have an increased risk for premature death (Keller, Litzelman, Wisk, et al., 2012). Responses to stress and anxiety are affected by factors such as age, gender, culture, life experience, and lifestyle, all of which may work to either lessen or increase the degree of emotional or physical influence and the sequel of stress. For example, a man in his 40s who has a new baby, has just purchased a home, and is laid off with six months' severance pay may feel the stress of the job loss more intensely than a man in his 60s who is financially secure and is asked to take an early retirement.

Personality

As mentioned above, part of our response to stressors is based on our own individual perceptions, which are coloured by a variety of factors, including genetic structure and vulnerability, childhood experiences, coping strategies, and personal outlook on life and the world. All of these factors combine to form a unique personality with specific strengths and vulnerabilities.

Social Support

Social support is a mediating factor with significant implications for nurses and other health care providers (Underwood, 2012). Strong social support from significant others can enhance mental and physical health and act as a significant buffer against distress. A shared identity—whether with a family, social network, or colleagues—helps people overcome stressors more adaptively (Newman & Roberts, 2013). Numerous studies have found a strong correlation between lower mortality rates and intact support systems (Koenig, King, & Carson, 2012).

Self-Help Groups

The proliferation of self-help groups attests to the need for social supports, and the explosive growth of a great variety of support groups reflects their effectiveness for many people. Many of the support groups currently available are for people going through similar stressful life events, such as those experiencing grief and loss from death, suicide, divorce, or job loss and those seeking support through cancer survivorship, to note but a few.

Low- and High-Quality Support

It is important to differentiate between social support relationships of low quality and those of high quality. Low-quality support relationships (e.g., living in an abusive home situation or with a controlling and demeaning person) often negatively affect a person's coping effectiveness in a crisis. On the other hand, high-quality relationships have been linked to less loneliness, more supportive behaviour, and greater life satisfaction (Newman & Roberts, 2013). High-quality emotional support is a critical factor in enhancing a person's sense of control and in rebuilding feelings of self-esteem and competency after a stressful event. Supportive, high-quality relationships are relatively free from conflict and negative interactions and are close, confiding, and reciprocal (Newman & Roberts, 2013).

Culture

Each culture not only emphasizes certain problems more than others but also interprets emotional problems differently from other cultures, even when similar concepts are used to describe a problem. For example, the idiom (or common expression) of distress, "thinking too much," was explored in a qualitative research synthesis. Exploring numerous studies, researchers found that the expression was used across multiple cultural groups to describe ruminating thoughts, worry, reliving trauma, and a host of other characteristics (Kaiser, Haroz, Kohrt, et al., 2015). Although Western European and North American cultures subscribe to a psychophysiological view of stress and somatic distress, it must be said that this view does not dominate in other cultures. The overwhelming majority of Asian, African, and Central American cultural groups experience and describe distress in somatic terms. For more information about cultural implications for psychiatric mental health nursing, refer to Chapter 8.

Spirituality and Religious Beliefs

Linked in part to aspects of culture and social support, studies have demonstrated that spiritual practices can enhance the immune system and sense of well-being (Koenig, King, & Carson, 2012). Some scholars propose that spiritual well-being helps people to deal with health issues, primarily because spiritual beliefs help people to cope with issues of living. Thus, people with spiritual beliefs have established coping mechanisms they use in normal life and can use when faced with illness. Research also shows that religion and spirituality can be damaging to mental health through negative religious coping, community and relationship conflict, misunderstanding, miscommunication, and negative beliefs (Weber & Pargament, 2014). People who include spiritual solutions to physical or mental distress can, however, gain a sense of comfort and community support that aid in healing and lowering stress. Prayer can elicit the relaxation response (discussed later in this chapter), which is known to reduce stress physically and emotionally and to reduce stress on the immune system.

Figure 5-2 operationally defines the process of stress and the positive or negative results of attempts to relieve stress, and Box 5-1 identifies several stress busters that can be incorporated into our lives with little effort.

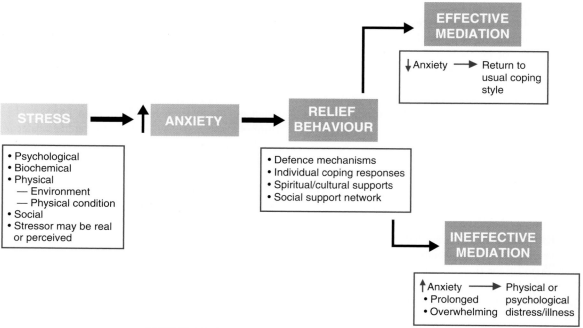

FIGURE 5-2 Stress and anxiety operationally defined.

BOX 5-1   EFFECTIVE STRESS BUSTERS

Sleep
- Chronically stressed people are often fatigued, so go to sleep 30 to 60 minutes early each night for a few weeks.
- If you are still fatigued, try going to bed another 30 minutes earlier.
- Sleeping later in the morning is not helpful and can disrupt body rhythms.

Exercise (Aerobic)
- Exercise:
  - Can dissipate chronic and acute stress
  - May decrease levels of anxiety, depression, and sensitivity to stress
  - Can decrease muscle tension and increase endorphin levels
- It is recommended that you exercise for at least 30 minutes three or more times a week.
- It is best to exercise at least 3 hours before bedtime.

Reduction or Cessation of Caffeine Intake

- Lowering or stopping caffeine intake can lead to more energy and fewer muscle aches and help you feel more relaxed.
- Slowly wean off coffee, tea, colas, and chocolate drinks.

Music (Classical or Soft Melodies of Choice)
- Listening to music increases your sense of relaxation.
- Increased healing effects may result.
- Therapeutically, music can:
  - Decrease agitation and confusion in older adults
  - Increase quality of life in hospice settings

Pets
- Pets can bring joy and reduce stress.
- They can be an important social support.
- Pets can alleviate medical problems aggravated by stress.

Massage
- Massage can slow the heart rate and relax the body.
- Alertness may actually increase.

NURSING MANAGEMENT OF STRESS RESPONSES

Measuring Stress

Health indicators are a range of measures that can facilitate comparisons across time and place at national, provincial, territorial, and regional levels. Since 1999, Statistics Canada and the Canadian Institute for Health Information have collaborated on developing and providing a broad range of indicators for health regions across Canada. Life satisfaction is a personal subjective assessment of global well-being, and in 2015, 93.2% of Canadians ages 12 and older, or roughly 27.3 million people, reported that they were satisfied or very satisfied with life, a rating that tends to decrease with age. Males and females ages 12 to 17 were the most likely to report being satisfied or very satisfied with life (97.8% of males and 97.6% of females) (Statistics Canada, 2016).

The Canadian Index of Wellbeing (CIW) also reports on key indicators that contribute to our understanding of the state of stress and resilience among Canadians. The 2016 CIW National Report titled *How Are Canadians Really Doing?* further highlights key stressors such as income inequality, time pressures, difficulties balancing commitments, poor sleep, less time with friends and at leisure, and poor self-reported health. Overall, Canadian reported conditions of increased stress and decreased life

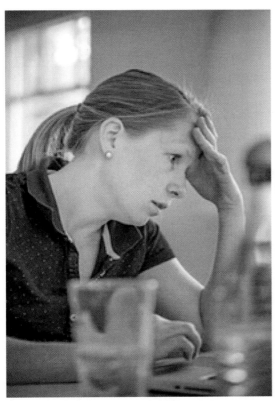

FIGURE 5-3 Canadians report high levels of stress and decreased life satisfaction. Source: Retrieved from https://pixabay.com/en/adult-annoyed-blur-burnout-1850268/

satisfaction in the reporting period (Canadian Index of Wellbeing, 2016). The report findings suggest the need for multiple levels of health promotion and stress-reduction interventions. The individual's level of stress illustrated in Figure 5-3 is expressed interpersonally, with family and friends, at work and community levels, and ultimately societally.

Take a few minutes to assess your stress level over the past 6 to 12 months using the Recent Life Changes Questionnaire (Table 5-2). Keep in mind that when you administer the questionnaire, you must take into account the following:

- Not all events are perceived to have the same degree of intensity or disruptiveness.
- Culture may dictate whether an event is stressful or how stressful it is.
- Different people may have different thresholds beyond which disruptions occur.
- The questionnaire equates change with stress.

Other stress scales that may be useful to nursing students have been developed. You might like to try the Perceived Stress Scale (Figure 5-4). Although there are no absolute scores, this scale measures how relatively uncontrollable, unpredictable, and overloaded you find your life. Try this scale in a clinical post-conference for comparison and discussion.

Assessing Coping Styles

People cope with life stressors in a variety of ways, and a number of factors can act as effective mediators to decrease stress in our lives. Rahe (1995) identified four discrete personal attributes (**coping styles**) people can develop to help manage stress:

1. Health-sustaining habits (e.g., medical compliance, proper diet, relaxation, adequate rest and sleep, pacing one's energy)
2. Life satisfactions (e.g., occasional escapism, reading, movie watching, work, family, hobbies, humour, spiritual solace, arts, nature)
3. Social supports (e.g., talk with trusted friends, family, counsellors, or support groups)
4. Effective and healthy responses to stress (e.g., work off anger through physical activity, go for a walk, dig in the garden, do yoga)

Examining these four coping categories can help nurses identify areas to target for improving their patients' responses to stress. Table 5-3 presents positive and negative responses to stress.

Managing Stress through Relaxation Techniques

Poor management of stress has been correlated with an increased incidence of a number of physical and emotional conditions, such as heart disease, poor diabetes control, chronic pain, and significant emotional distress (Thase, Wright, Friedman, et al., 2015). Psychoneuroimmunology provides the foundation for several integrative therapies, also referred to as mind–body therapies. There is now considerable evidence that many mind–body therapies can be used as effective adjuncts to conventional medical treatment for a number of common clinical conditions (Benson & Proctor, 2011). Chapter 35 offers a more detailed discussion of holistic, mind–body, and integrative care.

Nurses should be aware of a variety of stress and anxiety reduction techniques they can teach their patients. The following are some of the known benefits of stress reduction:

- Alters the course of certain medical conditions, such as high blood pressure, arrhythmias, arthritis, cancer, and peptic ulcers
- Decreases the need for medications such as insulin, analgesics, and antihypertensives
- Diminishes or eliminates the urge for unhealthy and destructive behaviours, such as smoking, addiction to drugs, insomnia, and overeating
- Increases cognitive functions such as learning and concentration and improves study habits
- Breaks up static patterns of thinking and allows fresh and creative ways of perceiving life events
- Increases the sense of well-being through endorphin release
- Reduces anxiety, increases comfort, and helps decrease sleep disturbances

Because no single stress-management technique is right for everyone, employing a mixture of techniques brings the best results. All are useful in a variety of situations for specific individuals. Essentially, there are stress-reducing techniques for every personality type, situation, and level of stress. Give them a try. Practising relaxation techniques will allow you not only to help your patients reduce their stress levels but also to manage your own physical responses to stressors. These techniques result in reduced heart and breathing rates, decreased blood pressure, improved oxygenation to major muscles, and reduced muscle tension. They also help manage subjective anxiety and improve appraisals of reality.

TABLE 5-2   RECENT LIFE CHANGES QUESTIONNAIRE

LIFE-CHANGING EVENT	LIFE CHANGE UNIT*	LIFE-CHANGING EVENT	LIFE CHANGE UNIT*
Health		To attend college	41
An injury or illness that:		Due to marriage	41
Kept you in bed a week or more or sent you to the hospital	74	For other reasons	45
		Change in arguments with spouse	50
Was less serious than above	44	In-law problems	38
Major dental work	26	Change in the marital status of your parents:	
Major change in eating habits	27	Divorce	59
Major change in sleeping habits	26	Remarriage	50
Major change in your usual type and/or amount of recreation	28	Separation from spouse:	
		Due to work	53
Work		Due to marital problems	76
Change to a new type of work	51	Divorce	96
Change in your work hours or conditions	35	Birth of grandchild	43
Change in your responsibilities at work:		Death of spouse	119
More responsibilities	29	Death of other family member:	
Fewer responsibilities	21	Child	123
Promotion	31	Brother or sister	102
Demotion	42	Parent	100
Transfer	32		
Troubles at work:		**Personal and Social**	
With your boss	29	Change in personal habits	26
With co-workers	35	Beginning or ending of school or college	38
With persons under your supervision	35	Change of school or college	35
Other work troubles	28	Change in political beliefs	24
Major business adjustment	60	Change in religious beliefs	29
Retirement	52	Change in social activities	27
Loss of job:		Vacation	24
Laid off from work	68	New close personal relationship	37
Fired from work	79	Engagement to marry	45
Correspondence course to help you in your work	18	Girlfriend or boyfriend problems	39
		Sexual differences	44
Home and Family		"Falling out" of a close personal relationship	47
Major change in living conditions	42	An accident	48
Change in residence:		Minor violation of the law	20
Move within the same town or city	25	Being held in jail	75
Move to a different town, city, or state	47	Death of a close friend	70
Change in family get-togethers	25	Major decision regarding your immediate future	51
Major change in health or behavior of family member	55	Major personal achievement	36
Marriage	50		
Pregnancy	67	**Financial**	
Miscarriage or abortion	65	Major change in finances:	
Gain of a new family member:		Increase in income	38
Birth of a child	66	Decrease in income	60
Adoption of a child	65	Investment and/or credit difficulties	56
A relative moving in with you	59	Loss or damage of personal property	43
Spouse beginning or ending work	46	Moderate purchase	20
Child leaving home:		Major purchase	37
		Foreclosure on a mortgage or loan	58

*One-year totals ≥500 life change units are considered indications of high recent life stress.

Source: Miller, M. A., & Rahe, R. H. (1997). Life changes scaling for the 1990s. *Journal of Psychosomatic Research, 43*(3), 279–292, Copyright 1997, with permission from Elsevier. doi:10.1016/S0022-3999(97)00118-9.

Relaxation Exercises

In 1938, Edmund Jacobson developed a rather simple procedure that elicits a relaxation response, which he coined progressive muscle relaxation (PMR) (Sadock & Sadock, 2017). This technique can be done without any external gauges or feedback and can be practised almost anywhere. The premise behind PMR is that since anxiety results in tense muscles, one way to decrease anxiety is to nearly eliminate muscle contraction. This muscle relaxation is accomplished by tensing groups of muscles

Instructions: The questions in this scale ask you about your feelings and thoughts during the last month. In each case, please indicate with a check how often you felt or thought a certain way.

1. In the last month, how often have you been upset because of something that happened unexpectedly?
   ___0 never ___1 almost never ___2 sometimes ___3 fairly often ___4 very often

2. In the last month, how often have you felt that you were unable to control the important things in your life?
   ___0 never ___1 almost never ___2 sometimes ___3 fairly often ___4 very often

3. In the last month, how often have you felt nervous and "stressed"?
   ___0 never ___1 almost never ___2 sometimes ___3 fairly often ___4 very often

4. In the last month, how often have you felt confident about your ability to handle your personal problems?
   ___0 never ___1 almost never ___2 sometimes ___3 fairly often ___4 very often

5. In the last month, how often have you felt that things were going your way?
   ___0 never ___1 almost never ___2 sometimes ___3 fairly often ___4 very often

6. In the last month, how often have you found that you could not cope with all the things that you had to do?
   ___0 never ___1 almost never ___2 sometimes ___3 fairly often ___4 very often

7. In the last month, how often have you been able to control irritations in your life?
   ___0 never ___1 almost never ___2 sometimes ___3 fairly often ___4 very often

8. In the last month, how often have you felt that you were on top of things?
   ___0 never ___1 almost never ___2 sometimes ___3 fairly often ___4 very often

9. In the last month, how often have you been angered because of things that were outside of your control?
   ___0 never ___1 almost never ___2 sometimes ___3 fairly often ___4 very often

10. In the last month, how often have you felt difficulties were piling up so high that you could not overcome them?
    ___0 never ___1 almost never ___2 sometimes ___3 fairly often ___4 very often

Perceived stress scale scoring
Items 4, 5, 7, and 8 are the positively stated items. PSS-10 scores are obtained by reversing the scores on the positive items—e.g., 0=4, 1=3, 2=2, etc.—and then adding all 10 items.

FIGURE 5-4 Perceived Stress Scale—10 Item (PSS-10). Source: Cohen, S., Kamarck, T., & Mermelstein, R. (1983). A global measure of perceived stress. *Journal of Health and Social Behavior*, *24*(4), Appendix A.

TABLE 5-3 POSITIVE AND NEGATIVE RESPONSES TO STRESS	
POSITIVE STRESS RESPONSES	**NEGATIVE STRESS RESPONSES**
Problem solving—figuring out how to deal with the situation	Avoidance—choosing not to deal with the situation, letting negative feelings and situations fester and continue to become chronic
Using social support—calling in others who are caring and may be helpful	Self-blame—faulting oneself, which keeps the focus on minimizing one's self-esteem and prevents positive action toward resolution or working through the feelings related to the event
Reframing—redefining the situation to see both positive and negative sides, as well as the way to use the situation to one's advantage	Wishful thinking—believing that things will resolve themselves and that "everything will be fine" (a form of denial)

Source: Adapted from Lazarus, R. S. (2012). Evolution of a model of stress, coping, and discrete emotions. In V. H. Rice (Ed.), *Handbook of stress, coping, and health: Implications for nursing research, theory, and practice* (2nd ed., pp. 199–225). Thousand Oaks, CA: Sage.

(beginning with the feet and ending with the face) as tightly as possible for 8 seconds and then suddenly releasing them. Considerable research supports the use of PMR as helpful for pain and a number of medical conditions, such as headaches and psychiatric disorders, especially those with anxiety components (Unger, Busse, & Yim, 2017). Many good PMR scripts are available online.

Herbert Benson (1975) expanded on Jacobson's work by incorporating a state of mind that is conducive to relaxation. His technique, influenced by Eastern practices, is achieved by adopting a calm and passive attitude and focusing on a pleasant mental image in a calm and peaceful environment. **Benson's relaxation technique** allows the patient to switch from the sympathetic mode of the autonomic nervous system (fight-or-flight response) to the parasympathetic mode (a state of relaxation). Follow the steps in Box 5-2 to practise the relaxation response. Benson's relaxation technique has been combined successfully with meditation and visual imagery to treat symptoms of numerous disorders, such as diabetes, high blood pressure, migraine headaches, cancer, and peptic ulcers.

Meditation

Meditation follows the basic guidelines described for the relaxation response. It is a discipline for training the mind to develop greater calm and then using that calm to bring penetrative insight

---

BOX 5-2 BENSON'S RELAXATION TECHNIQUE

- Choose any word or brief phrase that reflects your belief system, such as *love, unity in faith and love, joy, shalom, one God, peace.*
- Sit in a comfortable position.
- Close your eyes.
- Deeply relax all your muscles, beginning at your feet and progressing up to your face. Keep them relaxed.
- Breathe through your nose. Become aware of your breathing. As you breathe out, say your word or phrase silently to yourself. For example, breathe IN … OUT (phrase), IN … OUT (phrase), and so forth. Breathe easily and naturally.
- Continue for 10 to 20 minutes. You may open your eyes and check the time, but do not use an alarm. When you finish, sit quietly for several minutes, at first with your eyes closed and then with your eyes open. Do not stand up for a few minutes.
- Do not worry about whether you are successful in achieving a deep level of relaxation. Maintain a passive attitude, and permit relaxation to occur at its own pace. When distracting thoughts occur, try to ignore them by not dwelling on them, and return to repeating your word or phrase. With practice, the response should come with little effort. Practise the technique once or twice daily, but not within two hours after any meal, because the digestive process seems to interfere with the elicitation of the relaxation response.

Source: Benson, H. (1975). *The relaxation response.* New York: William Morrow & Company, Inc.

BOX 5-3 SCRIPT FOR GUIDED IMAGERY

- Imagine releasing all the tension in your body … letting it go.
- Now, with every breath you take, feel your body drifting down deeper and deeper into relaxation … floating down … deeper and deeper.
- Imagine a peaceful scene. You are sitting beside a clear, blue mountain stream. You are barefoot, and you feel the sun-warmed rock under your feet. You hear the sound of the stream tumbling over the rocks. The sound is hypnotic, and you relax more and more. You see the tall pine trees on the opposite shore bending in the gentle breeze. Breathe the clean, scented air, with each breath moving you deeper and deeper into relaxation. The sun warms your face.
- You are very comfortable. There is nothing to disturb you. You experience a feeling of well-being.
- You can return to this peaceful scene by taking time to relax. The positive feelings can grow stronger and stronger each time you choose to relax.
- You can return to your activities now, feeling relaxed and refreshed.

BOX 5-4 DEEP-BREATHING EXERCISE

- Find a comfortable position.
- Relax your shoulders and chest; let your body relax.
- Shift to relaxed, abdominal breathing. Take a deep breath through your mouth, expanding the abdomen. Hold it for 3 seconds and then exhale slowly through the nose; exhale completely, telling yourself to relax.
- With every breath, turn attention to the muscular sensations that accompany the expansion of the belly.
- As you concentrate on your breathing, you will start to feel focused.
- Repeat this exercise for 2 to 5 minutes.

---

into one's experience. Meditation can be used to help people reach their deep inner resources for healing, to calm the mind, and to operate more efficiently in the world. It can help people develop strategies to cope with stress, make sensible adaptive choices under pressure, and feel more engaged in life (Donnelly, 2013; Galante, Galante, Bekkers, et al., 2014).

Meditation elicits a relaxation response by creating a hypometabolic state of quieting the sympathetic nervous system. Some people meditate using a visual object or a sound to help them focus. Others may find it useful to concentrate on their breathing while meditating. There are many meditation techniques, some with a mindfulness or awareness base and some with a spiritual base, such as Siddha meditation or prayer. Meditation is easy to practise anywhere. Some students find that meditating on the morning of a test helps them to focus and lessens anxiety. Keep in mind that meditation, like most other skills, must be practised to produce the relaxation response.

Guided Imagery

Guided imagery is a process whereby a person is led to envision images that are both calming and health enhancing. It can be used in conjunction with Benson's relaxation technique. The content of the imagery exercises is shaped by the person helping with the imagery process. A person who has dysfunctional images can be helped to generate more effective and functional coping images to replace the depression- or anxiety-producing ones

(Bigham, McDannel, Luciano, et al., 2014). Often, audio recordings are made specifically for patients and their particular situations. However, many generic guided-imagery CDs, podcasts, and MP3s are available to patients and health care workers. An example of a script for guided imagery can be found in Box 5-3.

Breathing Exercises

Respiratory retraining, usually in the form of learning abdominal (diaphragmatic) breathing, has numerous merits in the modification of stress and anxiety reactions (Perciavalle, Blandini, Fecarotta, et al., 2017). Self-regulation of breathing through patterns or cycles of breathing as a yoga exercise to modulate the stress response has been studied (Jerath, Crawford, Barnes, et al., 2015). Another breathing exercise that has proved helpful for many patients with anxiety disorders has two parts: the first part focuses on abdominal breathing, while the second part helps patients to interrupt trains of thought, thereby quieting mental noise (Box 5-4). With increasing skill, breathing becomes a tool for dampening the cognitive processes likely to induce stress and anxiety reactions.

Physical Exercise

Physical exercise can lead to protection from the harmful effects of stress on both physical and mental states. In addition to its good effects for depression and anxiety, there is evidence to suggest that regular exercise and being physically fit can reduce stress levels generally. There are mixed results regarding the level of intensity (high or moderate exercise intensity) required to avoid stress, but aerobic exercise seems to have a better effect than strength training (Pedersen & Saltin, 2015). Yoga, an ancient form of exercise, has been found to be helpful for depression when used in conjunction with medication (Sharma, 2014). Spending time in forests (referred to as "forest bathing") and nature has been found to reduce blood pressure and heart rate, decrease stress hormone production, and improve overall feelings of well-being (Li, Kobayashi, Wakayama, et al., 2009). Other popular forms of exercise that show promise for stress reduction are walking, tai chi, dancing, drumming, cycling, aerobics, and water exercise. There are many considerations regarding motivation, energy, and other barriers, despite the benefits, particularly when patients are acutely unwell or struggling with serious and persistent anxiety, depression, or psychosis (Cooney, Dwan, Greig, et al., 2013). Although there are considerable benefits, motivating factors and barriers must also be addressed as nurses encourage physical exercise in the treatment and prevention of stress (Firth, Rosenbaum, Stubbs, et al., 2016).

Biofeedback

Through the use of sensitive instrumentation, biofeedback provides immediate and exact information about muscle activity, brain waves, skin temperature, heart rate, blood pressure, and other bodily functions. Indicators of the particular internal physiological process are detected and amplified by a sensitive recording device. An individual can achieve greater voluntary control over phenomena once considered to be exclusively involuntary if he or she knows instantaneously, through an auditory or visual signal, whether a somatic activity is increasing or decreasing.

Using biofeedback requires special training, and the technique is thought to be most effective for people with low to moderate hypnotic ability. For people with higher hypnotic ability, meditation, PMR, and other cognitive behavioural therapy techniques produce the most rapid reduction in clinical symptoms.

With increasing recognition of the role of stress in a variety of medical illnesses, including diseases affected by immune dysfunction, biofeedback has emerged as an effective strategy for stress management. The need to use the complex instrumentation required to detect minute levels of muscle tension or certain patterns of electroencephalographic activity is uncertain, but it has been confirmed that teaching people to relax deeply and apply these skills in response to real-life stressors can be helpful in lowering stress levels.

Cognitive Reframing

Cognitive reframing is a technique used to revise perceptions of a negative, distorted, or self-defeating belief with a goal of changing behaviours or improving well-being (Robson & Troutman-Jordan, 2014). The practice has been found to be positively correlated with greater positive affect and higher self-esteem. The goal of cognitive reframing is for an individual to change his or her perceptions of stress by reassessing a situation and replacing irrational beliefs ("I can't pass this course.") with more positive self-statements ("If I choose to study for this course, I will increase my chances of success."). We can learn from most situations by asking ourselves:

- What positive things came out of this situation or experience?
- What did I learn in this situation?
- What would I have done differently?

The desired result is to reframe a disturbing event or experience as less disturbing and to give the patient a sense of control over the situation. When the perception of the disturbing event is changed, there is less stimulation to the sympathetic nervous system, which in turn reduces the secretion of cortisol and catecholamines that destroy the balance of the immune system (Robson & Troutman-Jordan, 2014).

Cognitive distortions occur when our mind convinces us of something that is not really true. These incorrect thoughts help to reinforce negative thinking or emotions. These thoughts sound rational and accurate but really only reinforce the bad feeling we have about ourselves (Beck, 1976). They often include overgeneralizations ("He always …" or "I'll never …") and "should" statements ("I should have done better" or "He shouldn't have said that").

Table 5-4 shows some examples of cognitive reframing of anxiety-producing thoughts. Often cognitive reframing is used along with progressive muscle relaxation and guided imagery to reduce stress.

TABLE 5-4	COGNITIVE REFRAMING OF IRRATIONAL THOUGHTS
IRRATIONAL THOUGHT	**POSITIVE STATEMENTS**
"I have so many problems, I'll never find a partner who will accept me for who I am."	"If a potential partner doesn't seem to understand all of my issues and problems right away, that is fine, I can slowly help them to learn more."
	"If someone I seek as a partner rejects me in some way, that will seem unfortunate, but it is not the end of the world."
	"If a person I care for can't accept me, including my flaws, I can devote more time and energy to others who will."
	"If no one I care for fully accepts or appreciates me for me, I can still find enjoyment in friendships, family, hobbies, work, and in other things."
"Considering all I do for my partner, he should do more to appreciate me."	"I would like to be recognized when I go out of my way to support others. I don't support others simply for recognition, I get a good feeling by doing things for those I care about. I am free to make choices about where I spend my time and give of myself. If people take advantage of my generosity, I can redirect my acts of service to others."

Mindfulness

Mindfulness, a centuries-old form of meditation that has been dated back to Buddhist treatises, has received increased attention among health care providers. It is based on the premise that we are not aware of ourselves from moment to moment but operate on a sort of mental autopilot (Sharma & Rush, 2014). Mental activity often occurs unchecked; thoughts can become negative, untrue, and unrealistic and result in anxiety, depression, and lack of focus. Happiness or lack of happiness is not caused by outside forces but by our own perceptions and interpretations of reality.

Practitioners suggest that, to become mindful, we observe and monitor the content of our consciousness and recognize that thoughts are just thoughts. Negative interpretations ("Mowing the lawn is a hot, dirty, and exhausting job") can become positive ("Mowing the lawn is fantastic exercise") when mindfulness is practised.

This moment-to-moment awareness also extends to the outer world. Being mindful includes being in the moment by paying attention to what is going on around you—what you are seeing, feeling, and hearing. Imagine how much you miss during an ordinary walk to class if you spend it staring straight ahead as your mind wanders from one concern to the next. You miss the pattern of sunlight filtered through the leaves, the warmth of the sunshine on your skin, and the sounds of birds calling out to one another. By focusing on the here and now, rather than on the past and future, you are meditating and practising mindfulness.

Journaling

Journaling is an extremely useful yet simple method of identifying stressors. It is a technique that can ease worry and obsession, help identify hopes and fears, increase energy levels and confidence, and facilitate the grieving process (Pearson & Wilson, 2009). Keeping an informal diary of daily events and activities can reveal surprising information about sources of daily stress. Simply noting which activities put a strain on energy and time, which trigger anger or anxiety, and which precipitate a negative physical experience (e.g., headache, backache, fatigue) can be an important first step in stress reduction. Writing down thoughts and feelings is helpful not only in dealing with stress and stressful events but also in healing both physically and emotionally, providing a form of "emotional first aid" (Pearson & Wilson, 2009).

Humour

The use of humour as a cognitive approach is a good example of how a stressful situation can be "turned upside down." The intensity attached to a stressful thought or situation can be dissipated when it is made to appear absurd or comical. Essentially, the bee loses its sting.

■ KEY POINTS TO REMEMBER

- Stress is a universal experience and an important concept when caring for any patient in any setting.
- The body responds similarly whether stressors are real or perceived and whether the stressor is negative or positive.
- Physiologically, the body reacts to anxiety and fear by arousal of the sympathetic nervous system. Specific symptoms include rapid heart rate, increased blood pressure, diaphoresis, peripheral vasoconstriction, restlessness, repetitive questioning, feelings of frustration, and difficulty concentrating.
- Cannon introduced the fight-or-flight model of stress, and Selye, a Canadian endocrinologist, introduced the widely known general adaptation syndrome (GAS).
- The psychoneuroimmunology model describes the immune system's response to stress and its effect on neural pathways in the brain.
- Prolonged stress can lead to chronic psychological and physiological responses when not mitigated at an early stage (see Table 5-1).
- There are basically two categories of stressors: physical (e.g., heat, hunger, cold, noise, trauma) and psychological (e.g., death of a loved one, loss of job, schoolwork, humiliation).

- Age, gender, culture, life experience, and lifestyle all are important in identifying the degree of stress a person is experiencing.
- Lowering the effects of chronic stress can alter the course of many physical conditions; decrease the need for some medications; diminish or eliminate the urge for unhealthy and destructive behaviours such as smoking, insomnia, and drug addiction; and increase a person's cognitive functioning.
- Perhaps the most important factor for a nurse to assess is a person's support system. Studies have shown that high-quality social and intimate supports can go a long way toward minimizing the long-term effects of stress.
- Cultural differences exist in the extent to which people perceive an event as stressful and in the behaviours they consider appropriate to deal with a stressful event.
- Spiritual practices have been found to lead to an enhanced immune system and a sense of well-being.
- A variety of relaxation techniques are available to reduce the stress response and elicit the relaxation response, which results in improved physical and psychological functioning.

CRITICAL THINKING

1. Assess your level of stress using the Recent Life Changes Questionnaire found in Table 5-2, and evaluate your potential for illness in the coming year. Identify stress-reduction techniques you think would be useful to learn.

2. Teach a classmate the deep-breathing exercise identified in this chapter (see Box 5-4).

3. Assess a classmate's coping styles, and have that same classmate assess yours. Discuss the relevance of your findings.

4. Using Figure 5-1, explain to a classmate the short-term effects of stress on the sympathetic–adrenal medulla system, and identify three long-term effects if the stress is not relieved. How would you use this information to provide patient teaching? If your classmate were the patient, how would his or her response indicate that effective learning had taken place?

5. Using Figure 5-1, have a classmate explain to you the short-term effects of stress on the hypothalamus–pituitary–adrenal cortex

and the eventual long-term effects if the stress becomes chronic. Summarize to your classmate your understanding of what was presented. Using your knowledge of the short-term effects of stress on the hypothalamus–pituitary–adrenal cortex and the long-term effects of stress, develop and present to your clinical group a patient education model related to stress.

6. In clinical postconference, discuss a patient you have cared for who had one of the stress-related effects identified in Figure 5-1. See if you can identify some stressors in the patient's life and possible ways to lower chronic stress levels.

7. Assess the number of positive emotions, especially happiness, that you have experienced over the past week. Note the activities you were engaged in at the time. How might you increase the number of positive emotions in order to reduce your potential for illness in the coming year?

CHAPTER REVIEW

1. The nurse is caring for a patient who is experiencing a crisis. Which symptoms would indicate that the patient is in the stage of alarm?
   a. Constricted pupils
   b. Dry mouth
   c. Decrease in heart rate
   d. Sudden drop in blood pressure

2. If it is determined that a patient will benefit from guided imagery, what teaching should the nurse provide?
   a. Focus on a visual object or sound.
   b. Become acutely aware of your breathing pattern.
   c. Envision an image of a place that is peaceful.
   d. Develop deep abdominal breathing.

3. A patient is going to undergo biofeedback. Which patient statement requires further teaching by the nurse?
   a. "This will measure my muscle activity, heart rate, and blood pressure."
   b. "It will help me recognize how my body responds to stress."
   c. "I will feel a small shock of electricity if I tell a lie."
   d. "The instruments will know if my skin temperature changes."

4. A patient has told the nurse that she knows she is going to lose her job, which scares her because she needs to work to pay her bills. Which nursing response reflects the positive stress response of problem solving?
   a. "What are your plans to find a new job?"
   b. "Can you call your parents to support you during this time?"
   c. "Is it possible that this job loss is an opportunity to find a better-paying job?"
   d. "I'm sure everything will turn out just fine."

5. The nurse is caring for four patients. Which patient would be at highest risk for psychosocial compromise? The patient who has experienced:
   a. The death of a friend
   b. A divorce
   c. A recent job layoff
   d. The death of a spouse

evolve WEBSITE

Post-Test | interactive review

Visit the Evolve website for Chapter Review Answers and Rationales, Critical Thinking Answer Guidelines, and additional resources related to the content in this chapter: http://evolve.elsevier.com/Canada/Varcarolis/psychiatric/

REFERENCES

Ader, R., & Cohen, N. (1975). Behaviourally conditioned immunosuppression. *Psychosomatic Medicine, 37*(4), 333–340.

Anisman, H. (2015). *Stress and your health: From vulnerability to resilience.* Malden, MA.: Wiley Blackwell.

Bangasser, D. A. (2013). Sex differences in stress-related receptors: "Micro" differences with "macro" implications for mood and anxiety disorders. *Biology of Sex Differences, 4*(1), 2. doi:10.1186/2042-6410-4-2.

Beck, A. T. (1976). *Cognitive therapies and emotional disorders.* New York: New American Library.

Benson, H. (1975). *The relaxation response* (2nd ed.). New York: William Morrow & Company, Inc.

Benson, H., & Proctor, W. (2011). *Relaxation revolution: The science and genetics of mind body healing.* New York: Simon & Schuster.

Bigham, E., McDannel, L., Luciano, I., et al. (2014). Effect of a brief guided imagery on stress. *Biofeedback, 42*(1), 28.

Canadian Index of Wellbeing. (2016). *How are Canadians really doing? The 2016 CIW National Report.* Waterloo, ON: Canadian Index of Wellbeing and University of Waterloo. Retrieved from https://uwaterloo.ca/canadian-index-wellbeing/sites/ca.canadian-index-wellbeing/files/uploads/files/c011676-nationalreport-ciw_final-s_0.pdf.

Contrada, R. J., & Baum, A. (2011). *The handbook of stress science: Biology, psychology and health.* New York: Springer.

Cooney, G. M., Dwan, K., Greig, C. A., et al. (2013). Exercise for depression. *The Cochrane Database of Systematic Reviews,* (9), CD004366.

Donnelly, G. F. (2013). Health benefits of emptying the mind: Rediscovering meditation. *Holistic Nursing Practice, 27*(2), 57–58. doi:10.1097/HNP.0b013e3182837d64.

Firth, J., Rosenbaum, S., Stubbs, B., et al. (2016). Motivating factors and barriers towards exercise in severe mental illness: A systematic review and meta-analysis. *Psychological Medicine, 46*(14), 2869–2881. doi:10.1017/S0033291716001732.

Galante, J., Galante, I., Bekkers, M., et al. (2014). Effect of kindness-based meditation on health and well-being: A systematic review and meta-analysis. *Journal of Consulting and Clinical Psychology, 82*(6), 1101–1114. doi:10.1037/a0037249.

Jerath, R., Crawford, M. W., Barnes, V. A., et al. (2015). Self-regulation of breathing as a primary treatment for anxiety. *Applied Psychophysiology and Biofeedback, 40*(2), 107–115. doi:10.1007/s10484-015-9279-8.

Jones, C. E., & Monfils, M. (2016). Fight, flight, or freeze? The answer may depend on your sex. *Trends in Neurosciences, 39*(2), 51–53. doi:10.1016/j.tins.2015.12.010.

Kaiser, B. N., Haroz, E. E., Kohrt, B. A., et al. (2015). "Thinking too much": A systematic review of a common idiom of distress. *Social Science & Medicine (1982), 147,* 170–183. doi:10.1016/j.socscimed.2015.10.044.

Keller, A., Litzelman, K., Wisk, L. E., et al. (2012). Does the perception that stress affects health matter? The association with health and mortality. *Health Psychology: Official Journal of the Division of Health Psychology, American Psychological Association, 31*(5), 677–684. doi:10.1037/a0026743.

Koenig, H. G., King, D. E., & Carson, V. B. (2012). *Handbook of religion and health* (2nd ed.). New York: Oxford University Press.

Lazarus, R. S. (2012). Evolution of a model of stress, coping, and discrete emotions. In V. H. Rice (Ed.), *Handbook of stress, coping, and health: Implications for nursing research, theory, and practice* (2nd ed., pp. 199–225). Thousand Oaks, CA: Sage.

Li, Q., Kobayashi, M., Wakayama, Y., et al. (2009). Effect of phytoncide from trees on human natural killer cell function. *International Journal of Immunopathology and Pharmacology, 22*(4), 951–959. doi:10.1177/039463200902200410.

Lovallo, W. R. (2015). *Stress & health: Biological and psychological interactions* (3rd ed.). Thousand Oaks, CA: Sage Publications.

Newman, M. L., & Roberts, N. A. (2013). *Health and social relationships: The good, the bad, and the complicated* (1st ed.). Washington, DC: American Psychological Association.

Paquola, C., Bennett, M. R., Hatton, S. N., et al. (2017). Utility of the cumulative stress and mismatch hypotheses in understanding the neurobiological impacts of childhood abuse and recent stress in youth with emerging mental disorder. *Human Brain Mapping, 38*(5), 2709–2721. doi:10.1002/hbm.23554.

Pearson, M., & Wilson, H. (2009). *Using expressive arts to work with mind, body and emotions: Theory and practice.* Philadelphia: Jessica Kingsley Publishers.

Pedersen, B. K., & Saltin, B. (2015). Exercise as medicine—Evidence for prescribing exercise as therapy in 26 different chronic diseases. *Scandinavian Journal of Medicine & Science in Sports, 25*(S3), 1–72. doi:10.1111/sms.12581.

Perciavalle, V., Blandini, M., Fecarotta, P., et al. (2017). The role of deep breathing on stress. *Neurological Sciences, 38*(3), 451–458. doi:10.1007/s10072-016-2790-8.

Rahe, R. H. (1995). Stress and psychiatry. In H. I. Kaplan & B. J. Sadock (Eds.), *Comprehensive textbook of psychiatry/VI* (6th ed., Vol. 2, pp. 1545–1559). Baltimore: Williams & Wilkins.

Rahe, R. H., Veach, T. L., Tolles, R. L., et al. (2000). The stress and coping inventory: An educational and research instrument. *Stress Medicine, 16*(4), 199–208. doi:10.1002/1099-1700(200007)16:4<199::AID-SMI848>3.0.CO;2-D.

Robson, J. P., & Troutman-Jordan, M. (2014). A concept analysis of cognitive reframing. *Journal of Theory Construction & Testing, 18*(2), 55.

Sadock, V. A., & Sadock, B. J. (2017). *Kaplan and Sadock's concise textbook of clinical psychiatry* (4th ed.). Philadelphia: Wolters Kluwer Health/Lippincott Williams & Wilkins.

Selye, H. (1974). *Stress without distress.* Philadelphia: Lippincott.

Selye, H. (1993). History of the stress concept. In L. Goldberger & S. Breznitz (Eds.), *Handbook of stress: Theoretical and clinical aspects* (2nd ed., pp. 7–17). New York: Free Press.

Sharma, M. (2014). Yoga as an alternative and complementary approach for stress management: A systematic review. *Journal of Evidence-Based Complementary & Alternative Medicine, 19*(1), 59–67. doi:10.1177/2156587213503344.

Sharma, M., & Rush, S. E. (2014). Mindfulness-based stress reduction as a stress management intervention for healthy individuals: A systematic review. *Journal of Evidence-Based Complementary & Alternative Medicine, 19*(4), 271–286. doi:10.1177/2156587214543143.

Statistics Canada. (2016). *Perceived life stress.* Retrieved from http://www.statcan.gc.ca/pub/82-221-x/2013001/tblstructure/1hs/1wb/wb1pls-eng.htm.

Thase, M. E., Wright, J. H., Friedman, E. S., et al. (2015). Cognitive and behavioural therapies. In A. Tasman, J. Kay, & J. A. Lieberman (Eds.), *Psychiatry* (4th ed., pp. 1836–1858). West Sussex, UK: Wiley.

Underwood, P. (2012). Social support: The promise and reality. In V. H. Rice (Ed.), *Handbook of stress, coping, and health: Implications for nursing research, theory, and practice* (2nd ed., pp. 355–380). Thousand Oaks, CA: Sage.

Unger, C. A., Busse, D., & Yim, I. S. (2017). The effect of guided relaxation on cortisol and affect: Stress reactivity as a moderator. *Journal of Health Psychology, 22*(1), 29–38. doi:10.1177/1359105315595118.

Weber, S. R., & Pargament, K. I. (2014). The role of religion and spirituality in mental health. *Current Opinion in Psychiatry, 27*(5), 358.

Foundations for Practice

6. The Nursing Process and Standards of Care for Psychiatric Mental Health Nursing

7. Ethical Responsibilities and Legal Obligations for Psychiatric Mental Health Nursing Practice

8. Cultural Considerations for Psychiatric Mental Health Nursing

The Nursing Process and Standards of Care for Psychiatric Mental Health Nursing

Elizabeth M. Varcarolis
Adapted by Sonya L. Jakubec

KEY TERMS AND CONCEPTS

evidence-informed decision making
health teaching
mental status examination (MSE)
outcome criteria

psychosocial assessment
self-care activities
standards of nursing practice

OBJECTIVES

1. Compare the approaches you would consider when performing an assessment with a child, an adolescent, and an older adult.
2. Differentiate between the use of an interpreter and the use of a translator when performing an assessment with a non–English-speaking patient.
3. Understand the nursing process steps used in psychiatric mental health nursing.
4. Conduct a mental status examination (MSE).
5. Perform a psychosocial assessment, including brief cultural and spiritual components.

6. Explain three principles a nurse follows in planning actions to meet agreed-upon outcome criteria.
7. Construct a plan of care for a patient with a mental or emotional health problem.
8. Identify two advanced-practice psychiatric mental health nursing interventions.
9. Demonstrate basic nursing interventions and evaluation of care.
10. Compare and contrast *Nursing Interventions Classification (NIC)*, *Nursing Outcomes Classification (NOC)*, and evidence-informed practice.

℮volve WEBSITE

Visit the Evolve website for Flashcards, Case Studies, and additional testing resources related to the content in this chapter: *http://evolve.elsevier.com/Canada/Varcarolis/psychiatric/*

Pre-Test | interactive review

The nursing process is a six-step problem-solving approach intended to facilitate and identify appropriate, safe, culturally competent, developmentally relevant, and quality care for individuals, families, groups, or communities. The nursing process is not a linear but a continuous process of assessing, planning, implementing, and evaluating. Psychiatric mental health nursing practice bases nursing judgements and behaviours on this accepted practice framework (Figure 6-1). The most commonly used theoretical approaches to the framework are developmental, psychodynamic, systems, holistic, cognitive, and biological (refer to Chapter 4 to explore relevant theoretical approaches for practice).

Nursing care planning is a collaborative process undertaken with clients (individual patients, families, groups, or communities), working toward mutually agreed-upon definitions of problems, desired outcomes, and interventions. Engagement and collaboration in a client-centred, therapeutic relationship are fundamental to the practice of psychiatric mental health nursing (refer to Chapter 9 for more on relational practice and therapeutic relationships). Each step in the nursing process includes collaboration with the patient:

- *Data gathering* is a transparent process (the patient is aware of when, how, what, and why data are gathered about them, typically through interview or observation approaches).

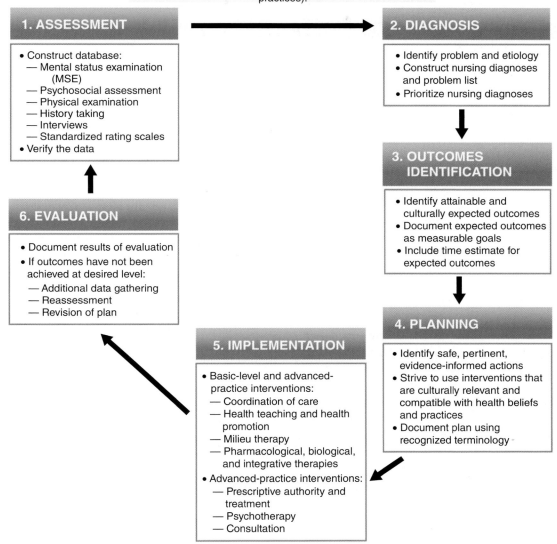

FIGURE 6-1 The nursing process in psychiatric mental health nursing.

- *Nursing diagnosis* is a process that includes the patient's definition of problems and patient education on the nursing perception of problems.
- *Outcome identification* is mutually negotiated and respects the patient's goals.
- *Planning* includes interventions to achieve goals and health teaching on best practice interventions.
- *Implementation* includes patient actions.
- *Evaluation* includes patient evaluation of progress toward goals.

Taken together, the process incorporates the arts of mental health nursing and recovery practice and the science of evidence-informed decision making (Varcarolis, 2017). See also Addiction and Mental Health Collaborative Project Steering Committee (2015) for a report on collaboration as inherent in evidence-informed practices aligned with recovery principles.

The use of the nursing process in psychiatric mental health nursing is aligned with **standards of nursing practice**, as outlined in the *Code of Ethics and Standards of Psychiatric Nursing Practice* (Registered Psychiatric Nurses of Canada, 2010) and *Canadian Standards for Psychiatric-Mental Health Nursing* (Canadian Federation of Mental Health Nurses, 2014). Regardless of practice area, standards of practice "guide the professional knowledge, skills and judgment needed to practise nursing safely" (College

They Told Us He Has Schizophrenia

My brother lived next door to my parents for years. After Dad died, Mom said it was nice to have my brother so close so he could help her with the yardwork. Although I knew that my brother had some strange ideas and had always been a loner, he seemed to be doing okay. It was really only after Mom died that I fully understood how much she had been helping him.

My brother had been afraid of the police and the spies that, he was convinced, were tracking him. He had piled up old papers and magazines in front of his windows so no one could look in. Although he had been prescribed medication to help reduce these fears, he was not taking it. Soon, my brother also stopped eating because of his belief that his food was being poisoned. He was admitted to hospital. After several weeks, he was discharged and came to live with me and my family. He was not happy about this arrangement, and, frankly, neither was I. We soon moved him into an apartment a few blocks from my home. As part of the hospital discharge plan, my brother and I saw a nurse at our local community mental health office. She met with us and helped us understand what schizophrenia is and how it would affect our lives. The question she asked that was most helpful was, "What action by your brother would let you know you didn't need to worry so much about him?" I told her his coming over for Sunday supper. My brother was surprised by my response. He thought that I was going to say his taking his medication. The nurse also helped my brother understand the purpose of the medication and how it would help reduce some of his worries, helped him get to his appointments, and helped him plan his meals. But most importantly, the nurse helped me reconnect with my brother as sister and brother rather than as caregiver and a person who needed care.

of Registered Nurses of Nova Scotia, 2017, p. 4). Both the code of ethics and the standards of practice are provided on the inside back cover of this book.

ASSESSMENT

A view of the individual as a complex blend of many parts is consistent with nurses' holistic approach to care. Nurses who care for people with physical illnesses ideally maintain a holistic view that involves an awareness of psychological, social, cultural, and spiritual issues. Likewise, nurses who work in the psychiatric mental health field need to assess or have access to reports on past and present medical history, a recent physical examination, and any physical complaints, as well as document any observable

physical conditions or behaviours (e.g., unsteady gait, abnormal breathing patterns, wincing as if in pain, doubling over to relieve discomfort). The assessment process begins with the initial patient encounter and continues throughout the duration of caring for the patient. To develop a basis for the plan of care and plan for discharge, every patient should have a thorough, formal nursing assessment upon entering treatment. Subsequent to the formal assessment, data are collected continually and systematically as the patient's condition changes and, it is to be hoped, improves. For example, a patient may have come into treatment actively suicidal, and the initial focus of care was on protection from injury; through regular assessment, it may be determined that although suicidal ideation has diminished, negative self-evaluation is still certainly a problem.

Assessments are conducted interprofessionally by a variety of practitioners, including nurses, psychiatrists, psychologists, social workers, recreation therapists, dietitians, and others. Building your confidence to conduct your assessment and to share your interpretations with the broad interprofessional team is essential to patient outcomes (Registered Nurses' Association of Ontario, 2013). Virtually all inpatient and outpatient health centres have standardized nursing assessment forms to aid in organization and consistency among reviewers. These forms may be paper or electronic versions, according to the resources and preferences of the institution. The time required for the nursing interview—a standard aspect of the formal nursing assessment—varies, depending on the assessment form and the patient's response pattern (e.g., speaks at great length or rambles, is prone to tangential thought, has memory disturbances, or gives markedly slow responses). Refer to Chapter 10 for sound guidelines on setting up and conducting a clinical interview.

Emergency situations may require immediate intervention based on a minimal amount of data and the emergency sharing of personal health information. However, health care workers are required to adhere to legislation regulating the collection of, use of, and access to patient information. Protection of personal health information is a provincial and territorial legislative responsibility, as mandated by the federal *Personal Information Protection and Electronic Documents Act* (Government of Canada, 2017); therefore, each province and territory has specific health information legislation (see Table 6-1).

The nurse's primary source for data collection is the patient; however, there may be times when it is necessary to supplement or rely completely on another for the assessment information. These secondary sources can be invaluable when caring for a patient experiencing psychosis, muteness, agitation, or catatonia. Such secondary sources may include members of the family, friends, neighbours, police, health care workers, and medical records. It may be appropriate to conduct a nursing family assessment with the patient and his or her significant others in order to understand more fully the resources, supports, and problems in the patient's life (Wright & Leahey, 2013).

The best atmosphere in which to conduct an assessment is one of minimal anxiety. Therefore, if an individual becomes upset, defensive, or embarrassed about any topic, the topic should be abandoned. The nurse can acknowledge that the subject makes the patient uncomfortable and suggest within the medical record

TABLE 6-1	PROVINCIAL AND TERRITORIAL HEALTH INFORMATION ACTS
PROVINCE OR TERRITORY	**WEBSITE LINK**
Alberta	http://www.health.alberta.ca/about/health-legislation.html
British Columbia	http://www.bclaws.ca/EPLibraries/bclaws_new/document/ID/freeside/00_03063_01
Manitoba	http://www.gov.mb.ca/health/phia/
New Brunswick	http://www2.gnb.ca/content/gnb/en/services/services_renderer.201227.Access_to_Personal_Health_Information.html
Newfoundland and Labrador	http://www.health.gov.nl.ca/health/PHIA/
Northwest Territories	http://www.priv.gc.ca/resource/prov/index_e.asp#006
Nova Scotia	http://novascotia.ca/dhw/phia/
Nunavut	http://www.priv.gc.ca/resource/prov/index_e.asp#008
Ontario	http://www.e-laws.gov.on.ca/html/statutes/english/elaws_statutes_04p03_e.htm
Prince Edward Island	http://www.healthpei.ca/index.php3?number=1020297&lang=E
Quebec	http://www.publicationsduquebec.gouv.qc.ca/fre/products/61184
Saskatchewan	http://www.qp.gov.sk.ca/documents/english/Statutes/Statutes/H0-021.pdf
Yukon	http://www.hss.gov.yk.ca/healthprivacy.php

that the topic be discussed when the patient feels more comfortable. It is important that the nurse not probe, pry, or push for information that is difficult for the patient to discuss. However, it should be recognized that increased anxiety about any subject is data in itself and should be noted in the assessment even without obtaining any further information.

Age Considerations
Assessment of Children
When assessing children, it is important to gather data from a variety of sources. Although the child is the best source for determining emotions, the caregivers (parents or guardians) often can best describe the behaviour, performance, and attitude of the child. Caregivers also are helpful in interpreting the child's words and responses. However, an interview separate from caregivers is advisable when an older child is reluctant to share information, especially in cases of suspected abuse (Arnold & Boggs, 2016).

Developmental levels should be considered in the evaluation of children. One of the hallmarks of psychiatric disorders in children is the tendency to regress (i.e., return to a previous level of development). Although it is developmentally appropriate for toddlers to suck their thumbs, such a gesture in an older child is unusual.

Age-appropriate communication strategies are perhaps the most important factor in establishing successful communication (Arnold & Boggs, 2016). Assessment of children should be accomplished by a combination of interview and observation. Watching children at play provides important clues to their functioning. From a psychodynamic view, supported play (play encouraged to a level with which the child is comfortable) is a safe way for the child to act out thoughts and emotions and to release pent-up emotions—for example, having a child act out his or her story (or family's story) with the use of anatomically correct dolls. Asking the child to tell a story, draw a picture, or engage in specific therapeutic games can be useful assessment tools in determining critical concerns and painful issues a child may have difficulty expressing. Usually, a clinician with special training in child and adolescent psychiatry works with young

BOX 6-1	THE HEADSSS PSYCHOSOCIAL INTERVIEW TECHNIQUE

H—Home environment (e.g., relationships with parents and siblings)
E—Education and employment (e.g., school performance)
A—Activities (e.g., sports participation, after-school activities, peer relations)
D—Drug, alcohol, or tobacco use
S—Sexuality (e.g., whether the patient is sexually active, practises safer sex, uses contraception)
S—Suicide risk or symptoms of depression or other mental health disorder
S—"Savagery" (e.g., violence or abuse in home environment or in neighbourhood)

children. Chapter 27 presents a more extensive overview of assessing children.

Assessment of Adolescents
Adolescents are especially concerned with confidentiality and may fear that anything they say to the nurse will be repeated to their parents. Lack of confidentiality can become a barrier of care with this population. Adolescents need to know that their records are private, and they should receive an explanation as to how information will be shared among the treatment team. The adolescent may be hesitant to answer questions related to such topics as substance use and sexual activity. Therefore, these must be asked in a nonjudgemental manner. If the answers to these questions do not indicate that the adolescent is at risk for harm, the answers may be handled confidentially (Arnold & Boggs, 2016). However, threats of suicide, homicide, sexual abuse, or behaviours that put the patient or others at risk for harm must be shared with other professionals, as well as with the parents. Because identifying risk factors is one of the key objectives when assessing adolescents, it is helpful to use a brief, structured interview technique such as the HEADSSS interview (Box 6-1). Chapter 27 offers more on assessment of adolescents.

Assessment of Older Adults

As we get older, our five senses (taste, touch, sight, hearing, and smell) and brain function begin to diminish, but the extent to which this affects each person varies. Your patient may be a spry and alert 80-year-old or a frail and confused 60-year-old. Therefore, it is important not to stereotype older adults or expect them to be physically or mentally deficient. For example, the tendency may be to jump to the conclusion that someone who is hard of hearing is cognitively impaired, an assumption that should be avoided. However, it is true that many older adults need special attention. The nurse needs to be aware of any physical limitations—for example, any sensory condition (difficulty seeing or hearing), motor condition (difficulty walking or maintaining balance), or medical condition (back pain, cardiac or pulmonary deficits)—that could cause increased anxiety, stress, or physical discomfort for the patient during assessment of mental and emotional needs. It is wise to identify any physical deficits at the onset of the assessment and make accommodations for them. If the patient is hard of hearing, speak a little more slowly in clear, louder tones (but not too loud) and seat the patient close to you without invading his or her personal space. Often, a voice that is lower in pitch is easier for older adults to hear, and a higher-pitched voice may convey anxiety to some.

Language Barriers

It is becoming more and more apparent that psychiatric mental health nurses can best serve their patients if they have a thorough understanding of the complex cultural and social factors that influence health and illness. Awareness of individual cultural beliefs and health care practices can help nurses minimize stereotyped assumptions that can lead to ineffective care and interfere with the ability to evaluate care. There are many opportunities for misunderstandings when assessing a patient from a different cultural or social background from your own, particularly if the interview is conducted in a language that is not the patient's primary language. To understand the patient's history and health care needs, health care providers often require translation and, at times, lay interpreters are used to communicate when there are language barriers. Such interpreters are often other staff or family members or friends who stand in to interpret back and forth from the patient to the mental health care team and vice versa. There are risks of these interpreters inserting their own understanding of what is being said, leading to potential misinterpretation and misunderstanding. There are further concerns related to confidentiality and ethics in this mode of interpretation (Elkington & Talbot, 2016). In this way, it is always preferred to use the services of trained translators, who are skilled in direct translation whenever possible.

Although there is no federal legislation mandating the use of trained translators for patients whose English or French proficiency is limited, Canadian health care organizations and providers recognize that language barriers compromise health and patient care and consider access to translators as a health care priority. Unfortunately, professional translators are not always readily available in many health care facilities.

Psychiatric Mental Health Nursing Assessment

The purposes of the psychiatric mental health nursing assessment are the following:

- Establish rapport
- Obtain an understanding of the current problem or chief complaint
- Review physical status and obtain baseline vital signs
- Assess for risk factors affecting the safety of the patient or others
- Perform a mental status examination
- Assess psychosocial status
- Identify mutual goals for treatment
- Formulate a plan of care

Gathering Data

Review of systems. The mind–body connection is significant in the understanding and treatment of psychiatric disorders. Many patients who are admitted for treatment of psychiatric conditions also are given a thorough physical examination by a primary care provider. Likewise, most nursing assessments include a baseline set of vital statistics, a historical and current review of body systems, and a documentation of allergic responses.

Martin (2016) points out that several medical conditions and physical illnesses may mimic psychiatric illnesses (Box 6-2). Therefore, physical causes of symptoms must be ruled out. Conversely, psychiatric disorders can result in physical or somatic symptoms such as stomach aches, headaches, lethargy, insomnia, intense fatigue, and even pain. When depression is secondary to a known physical medical condition, it often goes unrecognized and thus untreated. Therefore, all patients who come into the health care system need to have both a medical and a mental health evaluation to ensure correct diagnoses and appropriate care.

Individuals with certain physical conditions may be more prone to psychiatric disorders such as depression. It is believed, for example, that the disease process of multiple sclerosis or other autoimmune diseases may actually bring about depression. Other physical diseases typically associated with depression are coronary artery disease, diabetes, and stroke. Individuals need to be evaluated for any medical origins of their depression or anxiety.

When evidence suggests the presence of mental confusion or organic mental disease, a mental status examination (MSE), discussed below, should be performed.

Laboratory data. Hypothyroidism may have the clinical appearance of depression, and hyperthyroidism may appear to be a manic phase of bipolar disorder; a simple blood test can usually differentiate between depression and thyroid problems. Abnormal liver enzyme levels can explain irritability, depression, and lethargy. People who have chronic renal disease often suffer from the same symptoms when their blood urea nitrogen and electrolyte levels are abnormal. A toxicology screen for the presence of either prescription or illegal drugs also may provide useful information. Further information on the psychological needs of patients with medical conditions is found in Chapter 30.

BOX 6-2   SOME MEDICAL CONDITIONS THAT MAY MIMIC PSYCHIATRIC ILLNESS

Depression
Neurological disorders:
- Cerebrovascular accident (stroke)
- Alzheimer's disease
- Brain tumour
- Huntington's disease
- Epilepsy (seizure disorder)
- Multiple sclerosis
- Parkinson's disease

Infections:
- Mononucleosis
- Encephalitis
- Hepatitis
- Tertiary syphilis
- Human immunodeficiency virus (HIV)

Endocrine disorders:
- Hypothyroidism and hyperthyroidism
- Cushing's syndrome
- Addison's disease
- Parathyroid disease

Gastrointestinal disorders:
- Liver cirrhosis
- Pancreatitis

Cardiovascular disorders:
- Hypoxia
- Heart failure

Respiratory disorders:
- Sleep apnea

Nutritional disorders:
- Thiamine deficiency
- Protein deficiency
- B_{12} deficiency
- B_6 deficiency
- Folate deficiency

Collagen vascular diseases:
- Lupus erythematosus
- Rheumatoid arthritis

Cancer

Anxiety
Neurological disorders:
- Alzheimer's disease
- Brain tumour
- Stroke
- Huntington's disease

Infections:
- Encephalitis
- Meningitis

- Neurosyphilis
- Septicemia

Endocrine disorders:
- Hypothyroidism and hyperthyroidism
- Hypoparathyroidism
- Hypoglycemia
- Pheochromocytoma
- Carcinoid

Metabolic disorders:
- Low calcium
- Low potassium
- Acute intermittent porphyria
- Liver failure

Cardiovascular disorders:
- Angina
- Heart failure
- Pulmonary embolus

Respiratory disorders:
- Pneumothorax
- Acute asthma
- Emphysema

Drug effects:
- Stimulants
- Sedatives (withdrawal)

Lead, mercury poisoning

Psychosis
Medical conditions:
- Temporal lobe epilepsy
- Migraine headaches
- Temporal arteritis
- Occipital tumours
- Narcolepsy
- Encephalitis
- Hypothyroidism
- Addison's disease
- HIV

Drug effects:
- Marijuana
- Heroin/methadone
- Alcohol withdrawal
- Stimulants
- Cocaine
- Corticosteroids

Mental status examination. Fundamental to the psychiatric mental health nursing assessment is a **mental status examination (MSE)**. In fact, an MSE is part of the assessment in all areas of health care. The MSE in psychiatry is analogous to the physical examination in general medicine, and the purpose is to evaluate an individual's current cognitive, affective (emotional), and behavioural functioning. For acutely ill patients, it is not unusual for the mental health clinician to administer MSEs every day. It is the key assessment tool used by all members of the mental health team for ongoing assessment of the client and to establish treatment effectiveness, as well as certain aspects of recovery (Mental Health Commission of Canada, 2015). It is also the key assessment tool used to communicate assessment data across the interprofessional team (Registered Nurses Association of Ontario, 2013). Box 6-3 provides an example of the basic structure of and some descriptors for an MSE.

BOX 6-3   MENTAL STATUS EXAMINATION

A. Appearance (observed)

A person's appearance provides useful clues to their quality of self-care, lifestyle, and daily living skills. Assessment is observed in the following domains:

1. Grooming and dress
2. Level of hygiene
3. Pupil dilation or constriction
4. Facial expression
5. Height, weight, nutritional status
6. Presence of body piercing or tattoos, scars, etc.
7. Relationship between appearance and age

B. Behaviour (observed)

As well as noting what a person is actually doing during the examination, attention should be given to *nonverbal communication*, which reveal much about a person's emotional state and attitude.

1. Excessive or reduced body movements
2. Peculiar body movements (e.g., scanning of the environment, odd or repetitive gestures, mannerisms, balance and gait)
3. Abnormal movements (e.g., tardive dyskinesia, tremors)
4. Level of eye contact (keep cultural differences in mind; see Chapter 8)
5. Rapport (openness to the interview; e.g., resistive, open)

C. Speech (observed)

Speech can be a particularly revealing feature of a person's mental state and should be described behaviourally as well as having its content considered (see also "E. Thought"). Unusual speech is sometimes associated with mood and anxiety problems, schizophrenia, and organic pathology.

1. Rate (e.g., slow, rapid, pressured, normal)
2. Volume (e.g., loud, soft, normal)
3. Tonality (e.g., monotone, tremulous, varied)
4. Articulation (e.g., slurring, stuttering, mumbling)
5. Organization (e.g., disorganized, tongue-tied speech)
6. Quantity (e.g., poverty of speech, minimal, plentiful, voluminous)

D. Mood (observed and inquired)

The relationship of emotional affect and mood can be considered as being similar to that of the weather (affect) and the season (mood). Affect refers to immediate expressions of emotion (observed), whereas mood refers to emotional experience over a more prolonged period of time (inquired).

1. Affect (observed):
   - Range (e.g., restricted, blunted, flat, expansive)
   - Appropriateness (e.g., appropriate to conversation or setting, inappropriate, incongruous)
   - Stability (e.g., stable, labile)
2. Mood (inquired): sad, euphoric, duration, degree, stability
   - Tone (e.g., sad, euphoric, depressed, elevated, lowered)
   - Degree (e.g., extreme, moderate, mild, minor)
   - Irritability (e.g., explosive, irritable, calm)
   - Stability or duration (e.g., rapid, delayed)

E. Thought (observed and inquired)

Thinking is generally evaluated according to a person's thought *content* or *nature*, and thought *form* or *process*.

1. Thought content (e.g., delusions such as grandeur, jealousy, thought control/withdrawal/insertion; obsessions or preoccupations)
2. Thought process (e.g., disorganized, coherent, flight of ideas, neologisms, thought blocking, circumstantiality)

F. Perception (observed and inquired)

Assessment of perceptual disturbance is critical for detecting serious mental health problems like psychosis, severe anxiety, organic brain disorders, and mood disorders. It is also important in trauma or substance abuse. Perceptual disturbances are typically notable and may be disturbing or frightening. Consider the nature, timing, and triggers or precursors.

1. Hallucinations
   - Sensory involvement (e.g., auditory, visual, tactile, gustatory)
   - Content of auditory hallucination (e.g., conspiratory, command hallucinations telling a person to do something such as harm oneself or others)
   - Level of discernment of reality (e.g., questions the reality of the hallucination, hallucination is undistinguished from reality)
   - Level of associated distress (e.g., amused, distracted, fearful, extreme fear)
2. Illusions (similar to hallucinations but involving misperception of a real stimulus; e.g., perception of insects coming from pattern in wallpaper)
3. Dissociations (e.g., derealization, or feeling that the world or one's surroundings are not real; depersonalization, or feeling detached from oneself)

G. Cognition (inquired)

Cognitive assessment is in reference to a person's current capacity to process information. It is important because it is often sensitive (though in young people usually secondary) to mental health problems. Note that insight and judgement are particularly important in evaluating safety.

1. Orientation to reality (expressed as orientation to time, place, and person; e.g., awareness of the time/day/date, where they are, ability to provide personal details)
2. Level of consciousness (e.g., alert, drowsy, confused, clouded, stuporous, unconscious, comatose)
3. Memory functioning (e.g., immediate or short-term memory, memory for recent and remote information or events)
4. Fund of knowledge or intelligence (e.g., general knowledge as compared to the average person in a given society)
5. Language (e.g., naming objects, following instructions)
6. Abstraction (e.g., ability to describe similarity between two things—i.e., an apple and an orange; ability to explain the meaning of simple proverbs—i.e., "measure twice, cut once").
7. Attention and concentration: performance on serial sevens (counting down from 100 by increments of 7), serial threes (counting down from 20 by increments of 3), digit span tests (recalling in order a series of digits)
8. Visual or spatial processing (e.g., copying a diagram, drawing a bicycle, drawing a clock with the hands at 9 o'clock).
9. Insight (e.g., patient's acknowledgement and understanding of problems; potential pathological events—e.g., hallucinations, suicidal thoughts, and potential treatment. Evaluated by exploring questions such as "What do you believe is contributing

BOX 6-3	MENTAL STATUS EXAMINATION—cont'd

to the problems you are experiencing or that others are identifying?" "What might be the outcomes of the problems you are experiencing?")

10. Judgement (e.g., patient's general problem-solving ability. Evaluated by exploring recent decision making or by posing a practical dilemma such as "What would you do if you saw smoke coming out of a house?")

H. Ideas of Harming Self or Others (inquired)
Every mental status examination requires an assessment of thought content regarding self-harm and suicidal and homicidal ideation. Ideation, intent, and plan are all examined and explore the following (described in further detail in Chapter 22):

1. Target of ideation (e.g., the person—self or other, i.e., wife, boss, etc.)
2. Frequency of ideation (e.g., fleeting, constant, preoccupying)
3. Intent (an evaluation of whether the ideation is a reflection of wishing or thinking about death or harm versus an intent to kill oneself or another; e.g., general thoughts, presence of a plan)
4. Plan
   a. Level of specificity (e.g., vague, general, detailed, specific, secretive)
   b. Lethality of means (e.g., violent, lethal method)
   c. Means to carry out the plan (e.g., possesses a gun and ammunition, possesses a vehicle, has stockpiled medication)
   d. Opportunity to carry out the plan

The MSE, by and large, aids in collecting and organizing objective data of the here-and-now experience of the patient. The nurse both observes and asks directly about the patient's physical behaviour, nonverbal communication, appearance, speech patterns, mood and affect, thought content, perceptions, cognitive ability, and insight and judgement.

The MSE is much more than simply a means of gathering information, however; it is also a vehicle for relationship building and communication (see Chapters 9 and 10). Often a first or routine contact with a patient, the MSE sets the stage for your supportive care of a patient who may be agitated, depressed, suspicious, frightened, or angry. Choosing the time, place, and your approach to the MSE are all crucial to successful implementation (RNAO, 2017).

Psychosocial assessment. A psychosocial assessment (also called a mental health assessment) provides additional information from which to develop a plan of care. It may involve a more comprehensive assessment than the MSE and may involve collateral information from family or others (Coombs, Curtis, & Crookes, 2013). A comprehensive mental health assessment includes the following information about the patient:

- Central or chief complaint (in the patient's own words)
- History of violent, suicidal, or self-mutilating behaviours
- Alcohol or substance abuse
- Family psychiatric history
- Personal psychiatric treatment, including medications and complementary therapies
- Stressors and coping methods
- Quality of activities of daily living
- Personal background
- Social background, including support system
- Weaknesses, strengths, and goals for treatment
- Racial, ethnic, and cultural beliefs and practices
- Spiritual beliefs or religious practices

The patient's psychosocial history is most often the subjective part of the assessment. The focus of the history is the patient's perceptions and recollections of current lifestyle and life in general (family, friends, education, work experience, coping styles, and spiritual and cultural beliefs).

A psychosocial assessment elicits information about the person's social functioning and the systems in which a person operates. To conduct a mental health assessment, the nurse should have fundamental knowledge of growth and development, basic cultural and religious practices, pathophysiology, psychopathology, and pharmacology. Box 6-4 provides a basic psychosocial assessment tool.

Spiritual or religious assessment. Gomi and colleagues (2014) stress the importance of a spiritual or religious assessment to a holistic mental health assessment and for patient recovery. The idea that spirituality or religious involvement is recognized as an important influence on a person's health and behaviour has long been recognized. Spirituality and religious beliefs have the potential to exert a positive influence on patients' views of themselves and on how they interact with and respond to others (Chaze, Thomson, George, et al., 2015; Starnino, 2016).

Spirituality and religion are, however, quite different in their influences. *Spirituality* is more of an internal phenomenon, often understood as addressing universal human questions and needs (Anandarajab, 2008). Spirituality can be expressed as having three dimensions: (1) cognitive (beliefs, values, ideals, purpose, truth, wisdom), (2) experiential (love, compassion, connection, forgiveness, altruism), and (3) behavioural (daily behaviour, moral obligations, life choices, and medical choices) (Anandarajab, 2008). Spirituality can increase healthy behaviours, social support, and a sense of meaning, which are linked to decreased overall mental and physical illness (Starnino, 2016).

Religion, on the other hand, is an external system that includes beliefs, patterns of worship, symbols, and requirements of membership (Paniagua & Yamada, 2013). Although religion is often concerned with spirituality, religious groups are social entities and are often characterized by other goals as well (cultural, economic, political, social). Religious involvement is associated with better physical health, better mental health, and longer survival (Paniagua & Yamada, 2013). A religious community can provide support during difficult times, and prayer can be a source of hope, comfort, and support in healing.

Blazer (2009) notes that health care providers may be uncomfortable with assessing for or discussing spiritual and religious

BOX 6-4 PSYCHOSOCIAL ASSESSMENT

A. Previous hospitalizations
B. Educational background
C. Occupational background
   1. Employed? Where? What length of time?
   2. Special skills
D. Social patterns
   1. Describe family.
   2. Describe friends.
   3. With whom does the patient live?
   4. To whom does the patient go in times of crisis?
   5. Describe a typical day.
E. Sexual patterns
   1. Sexually active? Practises safer sex? Practises birth control?
   2. Sexual orientation?
   3. Sexual difficulties?
F. Interests and abilities
   1. What does the patient do in his or her spare time?
   2. What sport, hobby, or leisure activity is the patient good at?
   3. What gives the patient pleasure?
G. Substance use and abuse
   1. What medications does the patient take? How often? How much?
   2. What herbal or over-the-counter medications does the patient take (e.g., caffeine, anti-inflammatory or cough medicines, a herbal sleep aid or weight loss supplement)? How often? How much?
   3. What psychotropic medications does the patient take? How often? How much?

4. How many drinks of alcohol does the patient have per day? Per week?
5. What recreational drugs does the patient use (e.g., club drugs, marijuana, stimulants, heroin, steroids)? How often? How much?
6. Does the patient overuse prescription medications (benzodiazepines, pain medications)?
7. Does the patient identify the use of drugs as a problem?
H. Coping abilities
   1. What does the patient do when he or she gets upset?
   2. To whom can the patient talk?
   3. What usually helps to relieve stress?
   4. What did the patient try this time?
I. Spiritual assessment
   1. What importance does religion or spirituality have in the patient's life?
   2. Do the patient's religious or spiritual beliefs relate to the way the patient takes care of himself or herself or the illness? How does the patient's spiritual life contribute to recovery (meaning, purpose, joy, belonging, and so on)?
   3. Does the patient's faith help the patient in stressful situations?
   4. Whom does the patient see when he or she is medically ill? Mentally upset?
   5. Are there special health care practices within the patient's spiritual or cultural community that address his or her particular mental problem?

issues with patients, even though their proximity to patients and intimate patient needs gives them a unique opportunity to develop spiritual care theory and practices.

The following questions may be included in a spiritual or religious assessment:
- Who or what supplies you with strength and hope?
- Do you have a religious affiliation?
- Do you practise any spiritual activities (yoga, tai chi, meditation, prayer)?
- Do you participate in any religious activities?
- What role does religion or spiritual practice play in your life?
- Does your faith help you in stressful situations?
- Has your illness affected your religious or spiritual practices?
- Would you like to have someone from your church, synagogue, or temple or from our facility visit you?

Cultural and social assessment. Canada is rich in cultural diversity. Canada's official policy of multiculturalism means that cultural diversity is respected and the privilege of one culture over another is challenged. One consequence of Canadian multiculturalism is an increased responsibility of mental health professionals to concern themselves with the influence of culture on explanatory models of health and illness, expression of symptoms, coping styles, and willingness to seek treatment (Davis, 2013). The multicultural context requires a particular focus on Indigenous models of health and well-being and on addressing

the mental health needs of immigrants and refugees (Paniagua & Yamada, 2013), as well as a particular focus on spirituality and religion (Chaze, Thomson, George, et al., 2015). Chapter 8 offers a detailed discussion of the cultural implications for psychiatric mental health nursing and further information needed to conduct a cultural and social assessment in the Canadian context with a focus on Indigenous and refugee and immigrant mental health. Broadly, cultural assessment for mental health addresses language, history, cultural beliefs and understandings of the problem, social activities and relations within the culture, and supportive and coping practices established in the culture and community (Paniagua & Yamada, 2013).

Some questions that psychiatric mental health nurses can ask to help with a cultural and social assessment are:
- What is your primary language? Would you like a translator?
- How would you describe your cultural background and experiences that have been part of your history?
- Who are you close to?
- Who do you seek in times of crisis?
- How do people support one another at times of illness in your cultural, religious, or spiritual community?
- Who do you live with? How are activities at home organized in your cultural background?
- Who do you seek when you are medically ill? Mentally upset or concerned?

- What do you do to get better when you have physical problems?
- What are the attitudes toward emotional or social problems in your culture?
- How is your current problem viewed by your culture? Is it seen as a problem that can be fixed? A disease? A taboo? A fault or curse?
- Are there special foods that you eat?
- Are there special health care (or religious or spiritual) practices within your culture that address your particular mental or emotional health problem?
- Are there any special cultural beliefs about your experience that might help me understand and provide care for you?

After the cultural and social assessment, it is useful to summarize pertinent data with the patient. This summary provides patients with reassurance that they have been heard and gives them the opportunity to clarify any misinformation. The patient should be told what will happen next. For example, if the initial assessment takes place in the hospital, you should tell the patient who else he or she will be seeing. If you believe a referral is necessary, discuss this recommendation with the patient.

Validating the Assessment

To gain an even clearer understanding of your patient, it is helpful to look to outside sources. Emergency department records can be a valuable resource in understanding an individual's presenting behaviour and problems. Police reports may be available in cases in which hostility and legal altercations occurred. Old medical records, most now accessible by computer, are a great help in validating information you already have or in adding new information to your database. If the patient was admitted to a psychiatric unit in the past, information about the patient's previous level of functioning and behaviour gives you a baseline for making clinical judgements. Check with your provincial or territorial personal health information act to find out when signed consent of the patient or an appropriate relative is necessary to obtain access to records. All personal health information legislation requires nurses to obtain verbal consent from patients before discussing confidential information and treatment with their families; however, nurses have the skills and a responsibility to facilitate the involvement of families where appropriate.

Using Rating Scales

A number of standardized rating scales are useful for psychiatric evaluation and monitoring. Rating scales are often administered by a clinician, but many are self-administered. Table 6-2 lists some that are in common use. Many of the clinical chapters in this book include a rating scale.

NURSING DIAGNOSIS

A nursing diagnosis is a clinical judgement about a patient's response, needs, actual and potential psychiatric disorders, mental

TABLE 6-2	STANDARDIZED RATING SCALES*
USE	**SCALE**
Depression	Beck Inventory
	Brief Patient Health Questionnaire (Brief PHQ)
	Geriatric Depression Scale (GDS)
	Hamilton Depression Scale
	Zung Self-Report Inventory
	Patient Health Questionnaire–9 (PHQ-9)
Anxiety	Brief Patient Health Questionnaire (Brief PHQ)
	Generalized Anxiety Disorder–7 (GAD-7)
	Modified Spielberger State Anxiety Scale
	Hamilton Anxiety Scale
Substance use disorders	CAGE† (see Ewing, 1984; O'Brien, 2008)
	Addiction Severity Index (ASI)
	Recovery Attitude and Treatment Evaluator (RAATE)
	Brief Drug Abuse Screen Test (B-DAST)
Obsessive-compulsive behaviour	Yale-Brown Obsessive-Compulsive Scale (Y-BOCS)
Mania	Mania Rating Scale
Schizophrenia	Scale for Assessment of Negative Symptoms (SANS)
	Brief Psychiatric Rating Scale (BPRS)
Abnormal movements	Abnormal Involuntary Movement Scale (AIMS)
	Simpson Neurological Rating Scale
General psychiatric assessment	Brief Psychiatric Rating Scale (BPRS)
	Global Assessment of Functioning Scale (GAF)
Cognitive function	Mini-Mental State Examination (MMSE)
	St. Louis University Mental Status Examination (SLUMS)
	Cognitive Capacity Screening Examination (CCSE)
	Alzheimer's Disease Rating Scale (ADRS)
	Memory and Behavior Problem Checklist
	Functional Assessment Screening Tool (FAST)
	Global Deterioration Scale (GDS)
Family assessment	McMaster Family Assessment Device
Eating disorders	Eating Disorders Inventory (EDI)
	Body Attitude Test
	Diagnostic Survey for Eating Disorders

*These rating scales highlight important areas in psychiatric assessment. Because many of the answers are subjective, experienced clinicians use these tools as a guide when planning care and also draw on their knowledge of their patients and their patients' perception of their own experience.
†This acronym helps the clinician remember to ask questions about **c**utting down, **a**nnoyance by criticism related to substance use, feelings of **g**uilt related to substance use, and if the substance is needed to "get going" in the morning—the **e**ye opener.

health problems, and potential comorbid physical illnesses. A well-chosen and well-stated nursing diagnosis is the basis for selecting therapeutic outcomes and interventions (Herdman & Kamitsuru, 2014). Refer to Appendix B for a list of NANDA-I–approved nursing diagnoses.

A nursing diagnosis has three structural components:

1. Problem (unmet need)
2. Etiology (probable cause)
3. Supporting data (signs and symptoms)

The *problem*, or unmet need, describes the state of the patient at present. Problems that are within the nurse's domain to treat are termed *nursing diagnoses*. The nursing diagnostic title states what should change. Example: *Hopelessness.*

Etiology, or probable cause, is linked to the diagnostic title with the words *related to*. Stating the etiology or probable cause tells what needs to be addressed to effect the change and identifies causes the nurse can treat through nursing interventions. Example: *Hopelessness related to multiple losses.*

Supporting data, or signs and symptoms, state what the patient's condition is like at present. It may be linked to the diagnosis and etiology with the words *as evidenced by*. Supporting data (defining characteristics) that validate the diagnosis may include:

- The patient's statement (e.g., "It's no use; nothing will change.")
- Lack of involvement with family and friends
- Lack of motivation to care for self or environment

The complete nursing diagnosis might be *Hopelessness related to multiple losses, as evidenced by lack of motivation to care for self.*

OUTCOMES IDENTIFICATION

Outcome criteria are the hoped-for outcomes that reflect the maximal level of patient health that can realistically be achieved through nursing interventions. Whereas nursing diagnoses identify problems, outcomes reflect desired changes. The expected outcomes provide direction for continuity of care (American Nurses Association [ANA], American Psychiatric Nurses Association, & International Society of Psychiatric-Mental Health Nurses, 2014). Outcomes should take into account the patient's culture, values, ethical beliefs, and personal goals. Specifically, outcomes are stated in attainable and measurable terms and include a time estimate for attainment (ANA, American Psychiatric Nurses Association, & International Society of Psychiatric-Mental Health Nurses, 2014). Moorhead and colleagues (2013) have compiled a standardized list of nursing outcomes in the *Nursing Outcomes Classification*

(NOC) (see Chapter 1). *NOC* includes a total of 385 standardized outcomes that provide a mechanism for communicating the effect of nursing interventions on the well-being of patients, families, and communities. Each outcome has an associated group of indicators used to determine patient status in relation to the outcome. Whether nursing outcomes are derived from *NOC*, a psychiatric mental health nursing care plan text, best practice research, or other sources, it is important that criteria are individualized and documented as obtainable goals.

It is helpful to use long- and short-term outcomes, often stated as goals, when assessing the effectiveness of nursing interventions. The use of long- and short-term outcomes or goals is particularly helpful for teaching and learning purposes. It is also valuable in providing guidelines for appropriate interventions. The use of goals guides nurses in building incremental steps toward meeting the desired outcome. All outcomes (goals) are written in positive terms. Table 6-3 shows how specific outcome criteria might be stated for a suicidal individual with a nursing diagnosis of *Risk for suicide related to depression.*

PLANNING

The nurse considers the following specific principles when planning care:

- *Safe*—Interventions must be safe for the patient, as well as for other patients, staff, and family.
- *Compatible and appropriate*—Interventions must be compatible with other therapies and with the patient's personal goals and cultural values, as well as with institutional rules.
- *Realistic and individualized*—Interventions should be (1) within the patient's capabilities, given the patient's age, physical strength, condition, and willingness to change; (2) based on the number of staff available; (3) reflective of the actual available community resources; and (4) within the student's or nurse's capabilities.
- *Evidence-informed*—Interventions should be based on scientific evidence and principles when available.

In an evidence-informed practice model, the practitioner bases treatment decisions on a blend of information gleaned from empirical evidence, patient values, and practitioner expertise

TABLE 6-3 **EXAMPLES OF LONG- AND SHORT-TERM GOALS FOR A SUICIDAL PATIENT**	
LONG-TERM GOALS OR OUTCOMES	**SHORT-TERM GOALS OR OUTCOMES**
1. Patient will remain free from injury throughout the hospital stay.	a. Patient will state that he or she understands the rationale and procedure of the unit's protocol for suicide precautions shortly after admission.
	b. Patient will sign a "no-suicide" contract for the next 24 hours, renewable at the end of every 24-hour period (if approved for use by the mental health facility).
	c. Patient will seek out staff when feeling overwhelmed or self-destructive during hospitalization.
2. By discharge, patient will state that he or she no longer wishes to die and has at least two people to contact if suicidal thoughts arise.	a. Patient will meet with social worker to find supportive resources in the community before discharge and work on trigger issues (e.g., housing, job).
	b. By discharge, patient will state the purpose of medication, time and dose, adverse effects, and who to call with questions or concerns.
	c. Patient will have the written name and telephone numbers of at least two people to turn to if feeling overwhelmed or self-destructive.
	d. Patient will have a follow-up appointment to meet with a mental health professional by discharge.

| BOX 6-5 | USEFUL EVIDENCE-INFORMED DECISION MAKING AND NURSING PRACTICE WEBSITES AND LINKS |

- Canadian Best Practices Portal: http://cbpp-pcpe.phac-aspc.gc.ca/
- Canadian Nurses Association: Evidence-Informed Decision-Making: https://www.nurseone.ca/en/tools/evidence-based-practice
- Canadian Psychological Association: Evidence-Based Practice of Psychological Treatments: http://www.cpa.ca/docs/File/Practice/Report_of_the_EBP_Task_Force_FINAL_Board_Approved_2012.pdf
- National Collaborating Centre for Methods and Tools: http://www.nccmt.ca/
- Academic Center for Evidence-Based Practice (ACE): http://www.acestar.uthscsa.edu
- The Cochrane Collaboration: http://www.cochrane.org
- The Joanna Briggs Institute: http://joannabriggs.org

and skills (Jakubec & Astle, 2017). While empirical evidence is an important aspect of nursing practice, the Canadian Nurses Association promotes the use of the term **evidence-informed decision making** in nursing practice because it includes other elements that affect clinical decision making, such as professional clinical judgement, client preference, and collaboration with other key health stakeholders (Canadian Nurses Association, 2010). Certainly, there are elements within the nursing process for psychiatric mental health care whereby empirical evidence is simply not available, for example, in the area of spiritual and religious assessment and support (Blazer, 2009). Yet this does not mean that we cannot intervene appropriately and safely in the best interest of the patient. Box 6-5 lists several online resources for evidence-informed decision making and nursing practice. Keep in mind that whatever interventions are planned must be acceptable and appropriate to the individual patient, and that some care and interventions are outside the realm of empirical evidence. Psychiatric mental health nurses must also keep the principles of recovery, anchored by participation and choice (Baklien & Bongaardt, 2014; Mental Health Commission of Canada, 2015), front of mind when planning care. It is often this approach of "walking alongside" (Ness, Borg, Semb, et al., 2014) that facilitates more complete assessment and improves the outcomes of interventions, including outcomes of healthy risk taking and choices of patients (Higgins, Doyle, & Downes, et al., 2016).

The *Nursing Interventions Classification (NIC)* (Bulechek, Butcher, McCloskey, et al., 2013) is a research-based, standardized listing of 542 interventions reflective of current clinical practice that the nurse can use to plan care (see Chapter 1). Nurses in all settings can use *NIC* to support quality patient care and incorporate evidence-informed nursing actions. Although many safe and appropriate interventions may not be included in *NIC*, it is a useful guide for standardized care. Individualizing interventions to meet a patient's special needs, with patient input, should always be part of planning care.

When choosing nursing interventions from *NIC*, psychiatric nursing care plan texts, or other sources, the nurse uses not just those that fit the nursing diagnosis (e.g., risk for suicide) but also interventions that match the defining data. Although the outcome criteria might be similar or the same (e.g., suicide self-restraint), the safe and appropriate interventions may be totally different because of the defining data. For example, consider the nursing diagnosis *Risk for suicide related to feelings of despair, as evidenced by two recent suicide attempts and repeated statements that "I want to die."* The planning of appropriate nursing interventions might include the following:

- Initiate suicide precautions (e.g., ongoing observations and monitoring of the patient, provision of a protective environment) for the person who is at serious risk for suicide.
- Search the newly hospitalized patient and personal belongings for weapons or potential weapons during the inpatient admission procedure, as appropriate.
- Use protective interventions (e.g., area restriction seclusion, physical restraints) if the patient lacks the restraint to refrain from harming self, as needed.
- Assign the hospitalized patient to a room located near the nursing station for ease of observation, as appropriate.

However, if the defining data are different, the appropriate interventions will be as well—for example: *Risk for suicide related to loss of spouse, as evidenced by lack of self-care and statements evidencing loneliness.* The nurse might choose the following interventions for this patient's plan of care:

- Determine the presence and degree of suicide risk.
- Facilitate support of the patient by family and friends.
- Consider strategies to decrease isolation and opportunity to act on harmful thoughts.
- Assist the patient in identifying a network of supportive personnel and resources within the community (e.g., support groups, clergy, care providers).
- Provide information about available community resources and outreach programs.

Chapter 22 addresses assessment of and interventions for suicidal patients in more depth.

IMPLEMENTATION

The therapeutic interpersonal relationship is recognized as the first standard of practice by both the Registered Psychiatric Nurses of Canada (2010) and the Canadian Federation of Mental Health Nurses (2014), emphasizing the critical importance of this fundamental competency. The basic implementation skills are accomplished through the nurse–patient relationship and therapeutic interventions. The nurse implements the plan using evidence-informed practice whenever possible, uses community resources, and collaborates with nursing colleagues. Recent graduates and practitioners new to the psychiatric setting practise at the "entry to practice" level with the guidance and support of more experienced health care providers. The Registered Psychiatric Nurse Regulators of Canada (2014) outline that the level of education, experience, and context of employment all shape the characteristics of entry to practice expectations. Entry-level psychiatric mental health nurses enter practice working in a variety of practice settings, with diverse populations. They are responsible for practising within the context of their legislated scope of practice, the law, regulatory standards, employer policies, and their individual competence.

Basic-Level Interventions
Coordination of Care
The psychiatric mental health nurse coordinates the implementation of the plan and provides documentation.

Health Teaching and Health Promotion
Psychiatric mental health nurses use a variety of health teaching methods, which they adapt to the patient's needs (e.g., age, culture, ability to learn, readiness), integrating current knowledge and research and seeking opportunities for feedback and effectiveness of care. Health teaching includes identifying the health education needs of the patient and teaching basic principles of physical and mental health, such as giving information about coping, interpersonal relationships, social skills, mental health disorders, the treatments for such illnesses and their effects on daily living, relapse prevention, problem-solving skills, stress management, crisis intervention, and self-care activities. The last of these, self-care activities, assists the patient in assuming personal responsibility for activities of daily living (ADL) and focuses on improving the patient's mental and physical well-being.

Milieu Therapy
Milieu therapy requires managing the environment in which treatment takes place so that patients feel comfortable, safe, and respected (see Chapter 3). Milieu management includes orienting patients to their rights and responsibilities, selecting specific activities that meet patients' physical and mental health needs, and ensuring that patients are maintained in the least restrictive environment that safety permits. It also includes informing patients about the need for limits and the conditions necessary to set limits in a culturally competent manner (see Chapter 8).

Pharmacological, Biological, and Integrative Therapies
Nurses need to know the intended action, therapeutic dosage, adverse reactions, and safe blood levels of medications being administered and must monitor them when appropriate (e.g., blood levels for lithium). The nurse is expected to discuss and provide medication teaching tools to the patient and family regarding drug action, adverse effects, dietary restrictions, and drug interactions and to provide time for questions. The nurse's assessment of the patient's response to psychobiological interventions is communicated to other members of the multidisciplinary mental health team. Interventions are also aimed at alleviating untoward effects of medication. For more information on psychotropic drugs, refer to Chapter 11.

Advanced-Practice Interventions
Some registered nurses and registered psychiatric nurses are educationally and clinically prepared to conduct advanced interventions such as offering psychotherapy to individuals, couples, groups, and families and providing consultation to other disciplines using evidence-informed psychotherapeutic frameworks and nurse–patient therapeutic relationships. These assessment and intervention skills require advanced training and supervision (Rhoads & Murphy, 2014; Wheeler, 2014). Refer to Chapter 4 for an overview of various psychotherapies, Chapter 33 for a discussion of therapeutic groups, Chapter 34 for a discussion of family interventions, and Chapter 35 for a discussion of integrative therapies.

EVALUATION

Unfortunately, evaluation of patient outcomes is often the most neglected part of the nursing process. Evaluation of the individual's response to treatment should be systematic, ongoing, and criteria based. Supporting data are included to clarify the evaluation. Patient input is essential during the evaluation and establishment of next steps for the patient's recovery plan (Mental Health Commission of Canada, 2015). Simply asking the following is valuable in evaluation of patient outcomes: "How do you see things now?" "Have you observed any particular changes?" "Is there anything that you'd like to discuss about your recovery and plans?" Ongoing assessment of data allows for revisions of nursing diagnoses, changes to more realistic outcomes, or identification of more appropriate interventions when outcomes are not met.

DOCUMENTATION

Documentation could be considered the seventh step in the nursing process. Keep in mind that medical records are legal documents and may be used in a court of law. (Chapter 7 provides further information on the various purposes and guidelines for use of medical records.) Besides the evaluation of stated outcomes, the medical record should include changes in patient condition, informed consents (for medications and treatments), reaction to medication, documentation of symptoms (verbatim when appropriate), concerns of the patient, and any untoward incidents in the health care setting. Documentation of patient progress is the responsibility of the entire mental health team (Doenges, Moorhouse, & Murr, 2016).

Although communication among team members and coordination of services are the primary goals when choosing a system for documentation, practitioners in all settings must also consider professional standards, legal issues, and accreditation by regulatory agencies.

Information also must be in a format that is retrievable for quality-assurance monitoring, utilization management, peer review, and research. Electronic medical records are increasingly used in both inpatient and outpatient settings. Whatever format is used, documentation must be focused, organized, and pertinent and must conform to certain legal and other generally accepted principles (Box 6-6). The College and Association of Registered Nurses of Alberta (2013) and the Nurses Association of New Brunswick (2015) are among the provincial professional associations that have published nursing documentation guidelines.

BOX 6-6 LEGAL CONSIDERATIONS FOR DOCUMENTATION OF CARE

Do:
- Chart in a timely manner all pertinent and factual information.
- Be familiar with the nursing documentation policy in your facility, and make your charting conform to this standard. The policy generally states the method; frequency; and pertinent assessments, interventions, and outcomes to be recorded. If your employer's policies and procedures do not encourage or allow for quality documentation, bring the need for change to the administration's attention.
- Chart legibly in ink.
- Chart facts fully, descriptively, and accurately.
- Chart what you see, hear, feel, and smell.
- Chart pertinent observations: psychosocial observations, physical symptoms pertinent to the medical diagnosis, and behaviours pertinent to the nursing diagnosis.
- Chart follow-up care provided when a problem has been identified in earlier documentation. For example, if a patient has fallen and injured a leg, describe how the wound is healing.
- Chart fully the facts surrounding unusual occurrences and incidents.
- Chart all nursing interventions, treatments, and outcomes (including teaching efforts and patient responses) and safety and patient-protection interventions.
- Chart the patient's expressed subjective feelings.
- Chart each time you notify a physician, and record the reason for notification, the information that was communicated, the accurate time, the physician's instructions or orders, and the follow-up activity.

- Chart when nursing supervisors are consulted or informed about the patient, and record the reason for notification, information communicated, time, and any instructions or follow-up.
- Chart when family are notified of occurrences.
- Chart physicians' visits and treatments.
- Chart discharge medications and instructions given for use, as well as all discharge teaching performed, and note which family members were included in the process.

Don't:
- Do not chart opinions that are not supported by facts.
- Do not defame patients by calling them names or making derogatory statements about them (e.g., "an unlikeable patient who is demanding unnecessary attention").
- Do not chart before an event occurs.
- Do not chart generalizations, suppositions, or pat phrases (e.g., "patient in good spirits").
- Do not obliterate, erase, alter, or destroy a record. If an error is made, draw one line through the error, write "mistaken entry," record the date, and initial the clarification. Follow your employer's guidelines closely.
- Do not leave blank spaces for chronological notes. If you must chart out of sequence, chart "late entry." Identify the time and date of the entry and the time and date of the occurrence.
- If an incident report is filed, do not note in the chart that one was filed. This form is generally a privileged communication between the hospital and the hospital's attorney. Describing it in the chart may destroy the privileged nature of the communication.

KEY POINTS TO REMEMBER

- The nursing process is a six-step problem-solving approach to patient care.
- The primary source of assessment is the patient. Secondary sources of information include family members, neighbours, friends, police, and other members of the health care team.
- A professional translator often is needed to prevent serious misunderstandings during assessment, treatment, and evaluation with non–English- or non–French-speaking patients.
- The assessment interview includes gathering objective data (mental or emotional status) and subjective data (psychosocial assessment).
- Medical examination, history, and systems review round out a complete assessment.
- Assessment tools and standardized rating scales may be used to evaluate and monitor a patient's progress.
- Determination of the nursing diagnosis (NANDA-I) defines the practice of nursing, improves communication between staff members, and assists in accountability of care.
- A nursing diagnosis consists of (1) an unmet need or problem, (2) an etiology or probable cause, and (3) supporting data.
- Outcomes are variable, measurable, and stated in terms that reflect a patient's actual state. Planning involves determining desired outcomes.

- Behavioural goals support outcomes. Goals are short, specific, and measurable; indicate the desired patient behaviours; and include a set time for achievement.
- Planning nursing actions (using *NIC*, psychiatric nursing care plan texts, evidence-informed practice, or other sources) to achieve outcomes includes the use of specific principles. The plan should be (1) safe, (2) compatible with and appropriate for implementation with other therapies, (3) realistic and individualized, and (4) evidence informed whenever possible.
- Psychiatric mental health nursing practice includes four basic-level interventions: (1) coordination of care, (2) health teaching and health promotion, (3) milieu therapy, and (4) pharmacological, biological, and integrative therapies.
- Advanced-practice interventions (e.g., psychotherapy, consulting work) are carried out by a nurse with advanced education or experience.
- The evaluation of care is a continual process of determining to what extent the outcome criteria have been achieved. The plan of care may be revised based on the evaluation.
- Documentation of patient progress through evaluation of the outcome criteria is crucial. The medical record is a legal document and should accurately reflect the patient's condition, medications, treatment, tests, responses, and any untoward incidents.

CRITICAL THINKING

1. Martin Redbird, a 47-year-old Cree man, arrives by ambulance from a supermarket, where he had fallen. On his arrival to the emergency department (ED), his breath smells "fruity." He appears confused and anxious, saying that "they put a curse on me, they want me to die … they are yelling, they are yelling … no, no, I'm not bad. Oh God, don't let them get me!" Martin is from a reserve community 700 kilometres north of the city in which he is being treated. When his nephew (closest next of kin) is contacted by the ED by phone, he tells the staff that Martin has diabetes and a diagnosis of paranoid schizophrenia and that this happens when he doesn't take his medications or eat properly. In a group or in collaboration with a classmate, respond to the following:

   a. A number of nursing diagnoses are possible in this scenario. Given the above information, formulate at least two nursing diagnoses (problems); include *related to* and *as evidenced by* statements.
   b. For each of your nursing diagnoses, write one long-term outcome (the problem, what should change, etc.). Include a time frame, desired change, and three criteria that will help you evaluate whether the outcome has been met, not met, or partially met.
   c. What specific needs might you take into account when planning nursing care for Mr. Redbird?
   d. Formulate an initial nurse's note for Mr. Redbird.

CHAPTER REVIEW

1. The nurse is assessing a 6-year-old patient. When assessing a child's perception of a difficult issue, which methods of assessment are appropriate? Select all that apply.
   a. Engage the child in a specific therapeutic game.
   b. Ask the child to draw a picture.
   c. Provide the child with an anatomically correct doll to act out a story.
   d. Allow the child to tell a story.
2. Which are the purposes of a thorough mental health nursing assessment? Select all that apply.
   a. Establish a rapport between the nurse and patient.
   b. Assess for risk factors affecting the safety of the patient or others.
   c. Allow the nurse the chance to provide counselling to the patient.
   d. Identify the nurse's goals for treatment.
   e. Formulate a plan of care.
3. The nurse is performing a spiritual assessment on a patient. Which patient statement would indicate to the nurse that there is an experiential concern in the patient's spiritual life?
   a. "I really believe that my spouse loves me."
   b. "My sister will never forgive me for what I did."
   c. "I try to find time every day to pray, even though it's not easy."
   d. "I am happy with my life choices, even if my mother is not."

4. The nurse is caring for a patient who states that he has "given up on life." His wife left him, he was fired from his job, and he is four payments behind on his mortgage, meaning he will soon lose his house. Which nursing diagnosis is appropriate?
   a. *Anxiety related to multiple losses*
   b. *Defensive coping related to multiple losses*
   c. *Ineffective denial related to multiple losses*
   d. *Hopelessness related to multiple losses*
5. The nurse is documenting. Which statement is appropriate to include in the patient's chart?
   a. "Patient states, 'I am going to kill myself.'"
   b. "Patient is in good spirits today."
   c. "Patient has been nasty to the nursing staff this afternoon."
   d. "Patient is demanding and uncooperative."

Ǝvolve WEBSITE

Post-Test interactive review

Visit the Evolve website for Chapter Review Answers and Rationales, Critical Thinking Answer Guidelines, and additional resources related to the content in this chapter: http://evolve.elsevier.com/Canada/Varcarolis/psychiatric/

REFERENCES

Addiction and Mental Health Collaborative Project Steering Committee (2015). *Collaboration for addiction and mental health care: Best advice.* Ottawa: Canadian Centre on Substance Abuse. Retrieved from http://www.ccsa.ca/Resource%20Library/CCSA-Collaboration-Addiction-Mental-Health-Best-Advice-Report-2015-en.pdf.

American Nurses Association (ANA), American Psychiatric Nurses Association, & International Society of Psychiatric-Mental Health Nurses (2014). *Psychiatric–mental health nursing: Scope and standards of practice* (2nd ed.). Washington, DC: Nursebooks.org.

Anandarajab, G. (2008). The 3 H and BMSEST models for spirituality in multicultural whole-person medicine. *Annals of Family Medicine, 6*(5), 448–458.

Arnold, E. C., & Boggs, K. U. (2016). *Interpersonal relationships: Professional communication skills for nurses* (6th ed.). St. Louis, MO: Saunders.

Baklien, B., & Bongaardt, R. (2014). The quest for choice and the need for relational care in mental health work. *Medicine, Health Care, and Philosophy, 17*(4), 625–632. doi:10.1007/s11019-014-9563-z.

Blazer, D. G. (2009). Religion, spirituality, and mental health: What we know and why this is a tough topic to research. *The Canadian Journal of Psychiatry, 54*(5), 281–282. doi:10.1177/070674370905400501.

Bulechek, G. M., Butcher, H. K., McCloskey Dochterman, J. M., et al. (2013). *Nursing interventions classification (NIC)* (6th ed.). St. Louis, MO: Mosby.

Canadian Federation of Mental Health Nurses (2014). *Canadian standards for psychiatric-mental health nursing* (4th ed.). Toronto: Author. Retrieved from http://cfmhn.ca/positionpapers#1.

Canadian Nurses Association (2010). *Position statement: Evidence-informed decision-making and nursing practice.* Ottawa: Author.

Chaze, F., Thomson, M. S., George, U., et al. (2015). Role of cultural beliefs, religion, and spirituality in mental health and/or service utilization among immigrants in Canada: A scoping review. *Canadian Journal of Community Mental Health, 34*(3), 1–15. doi:10.7870/cjcmh-2015-015.

College and Association of Registered Nurses of Alberta. (2013). *Documentation standards for regulated members.* Retrieved from http://www.nurses.ab.ca/content/dam/carna/pdfs/DocumentList/Standards/DocumentationStandards_Jan2013.pdf.

College of Registered Nurses of Nova Scotia (2017). *Standards of practice for registered nurses 2017.* Halifax, NS: Author. Retrieved from http://crnns.ca/wp-content/uploads/2015/02/RNStandards.pdf.

Coombs, T., Curtis, J., & Crookes, P. (2013). What is the process of a comprehensive mental health nursing assessment? Results from a qualitative study: Process of mental health nursing assessment. *International Nursing Review, 60*(1), 96–102. doi:10.1111/j.1466-7657.2012.01036.x.

Davis, S. (2013). *Community mental health in Canada: Theory, policy, and practice* (rev. and expanded ed.). Vancouver: UBC Press.

Doenges, M. E., Moorhouse, M. F., & Murr, A. C. (2016). *Nursing diagnosis manual: Planning, individualizing, and documenting client care* (5th ed.). Philadelphia: F. A. Davis.

Elkington, E. J., & Talbot, K. M. (2016). The role of interpreters in mental health care. *South African Journal of Psychology, 46*(3), 364–375. doi:10.1177/0081246315619833.

Gomi, S., Starnino, V. R., & Canda, E. R. (2014). Spiritual assessment in mental health recovery. *Community Mental Health Journal, 50*(4), 447–453. doi:10.1007/s10597-013-9653-z.

Government of Canada. (2017). *Personal Information Protection and Electronic Documents Act.* Retrieved from http://laws-lois.justice.gc.ca/eng/acts/P-8.6/.

Herdman, T. H., & Kamitsuru, S. (Eds.), (2014). *NANDA international nursing diagnoses: Definitions and classification, 2015–2017.* Oxford, UK: Wiley-Blackwell.

Higgins, A., Doyle, L., Downes, C., et al. (2016). There is more to risk and safety planning than dramatic risks: Mental health nurses' risk assessment and safety-management practice. *International Journal of Mental Health Nursing, 25*(2), 159–170. doi:10.1111/inm.12180.

Jakubec, S. L., & Astle, B. J. (2017). *Research literacy for health and community practice.* Toronto: Canadian Scholars' Press.

Martin, C. T. (2016). The value of physical examination in mental health nursing. *Nurse Education in Practice, 17*, 91–96. doi:10.1016/j.nepr.2015.11.001.

Mental Health Commission of Canada (2015). *Recovery guidelines.* Ottawa: Author. Retrieved from http://www.mentalhealthcommission.ca/sites/default/files/2016-07/MHCC_Recovery_Guidelines_2016_ENG.PDF.

Moorhead, S., Johnson, M., Maas, M. L., et al. (2013). *Nursing outcomes classification (NOC)* (5th ed.). St Louis, MO: Mosby.

Ness, O., Borg, M., Semb, R., et al. (2014). "Walking alongside": Collaborative practices in mental health and substance use care. *International Journal of Mental Health Systems, 8*(1), 55. doi:10.1186/1752-4458-8-55.

Nurses Association of New Brunswick. (2015). *Standards for documentation.* Retrieved from http://www.nanb.nb.ca/media/resource/NANB-StandardsFor-Documentation-E.pdf.

Paniagua, F. A., & Yamada, A. M. (2013). *Handbook of multicultural mental health: Assessment and treatment of diverse populations* (2nd ed.). Amsterdam: Elsevier.

Registered Nurses' Association of Ontario (2013). *Developing and sustaining interprofessional health care: Optimizing patients/clients, organizational, and system outcomes.* Toronto: Author.

Registered Nurses' Association of Ontario. (2017). *Nursing best practice guidelines: Components of mental status assessment.* Retrieved from http://pda.rnao.ca/content/components-mental-status-assessment.

Registered Psychiatric Nurse Regulators of Canada. (2014). *Registered psychiatric nurse entry-level competencies.* Retrieved from http://www.rpnc.ca/sites/default/files/resources/pdfs/RPNRC-ENGLISH%20Compdoc%20(Nov6-14).pdf.

Registered Psychiatric Nurses of Canada (2010). *Code of ethics & standards of psychiatric nursing practice.* Edmonton: Author. Retrieved from http://www.rpnc.ca/.

Rhoads, J., & Murphy, P. J. M. (2014). *Clinical consult to psychiatric nursing for advanced practice.* New York: Springer.

Starnino, V. R. (2016). Conceptualizing spirituality and religion for mental health practice: Perspectives of consumers with serious mental illness. *Families in Society, 97*(4), 295–304. doi:10.1606/1044-3894.2016.97.36.

Varcarolis, E. M. (2017). *Essentials of psychiatric mental health nursing: A communication approach to evidence-based care.* Philadelphia: Elsevier.

Wheeler, K. (2014). *Psychotherapy for the advanced practice psychiatric nurse: A how-to guide for evidence-based practice* (2nd ed.). New York: Springer.

Wright, L. M., & Leahey, M. (2013). *Nurses and families: A guide to family assessment and intervention* (6th ed.). Philadelphia: F. A. Davis Company.

7

Ethical Responsibilities and Legal Obligations for Psychiatric Mental Health Nursing Practice

Cheryl L. Pollard

KEY TERMS AND CONCEPTS

abandonment
advance directives
assault
autonomy
battery
beneficence
bioethics
competency
confidentiality
consequentialist theory
conscientious objection
deontology
duty to protect
duty to warn
engagement
ethics
false imprisonment
guardianship
implied consent
informed consent

intentional torts
justice
malpractice
moral agent
moral distress
moral residue
moral resilience
moral uncertainty
negligence
nonmaleficence
relational ethics
respect for autonomy
right to privacy
right to refuse treatment
tort law
unintentional torts
utilitarianism
virtue ethics
virtues

OBJECTIVES

1. Identify the differences between ethical responsibilities and legal obligations within the practice of psychiatric mental health nursing.
2. Describe key elements of the common approaches that inform health care ethics.
3. Identify the ethical nursing responsibilities related to psychiatric mental health research.
4. Identify relevant legislation enacted to protect, promote, and improve the lives of Canadians with mental illness.
5. Describe the rights of the client in a psychiatric setting.
6. Discuss the meaning of standard care in a psychiatric setting.

⊖volve WEBSITE

Visit the Evolve website for Flashcards, Case Studies, and additional testing resources related to the content in this chapter: http://evolve.elsevier.com/Canada/Varcarolis/psychiatric/

Pre-Test interactive review

Every nurse will face dilemmas in which values, responsibilities, and obligations seem to conflict; in which there is no clear path to "doing good" or determining what is "most fitting." The purpose of this chapter is to help nurses think about the ethical responsibilities and the legal obligations of their practice. It is important to recognize that professional nursing ethical responsibilities and legal obligations are distinct areas, but they often have overlapping influences on clinical practice. Nursing ethics is unique in that it is an expression of the values and beliefs that guide nursing practice. Nurses must think about ethical issues on an individual level, professional level, and systems level as they respond to clinical questions.

In contrast, legislation, the foundation of legal obligations, is a means used within society to meet objectives and consolidate values. For example, provincial health protection acts define the scope of practice for health care professionals. Mental health legislation is designed to "protect, promote and improve the lives and mental well-being of citizens" (World Health Organization, 2005, p. 1). This legislation generally acknowledges the fundamental value of mental health and aims to ensure that the rights of individuals are protected. The type and form of legislative text varies from country to country and, within Canada, between jurisdictions. Jurisdictions may organize their laws related to the protection of rights for people with mental illness within a single statute or within a variety of different legislative measures. In Canada, the laws are dispersed within a variety of legislative measures, which include the *Canada Health Act*, the *Employment Equity Act*, and provincial or territorial legislation regarding social welfare and benefits, disability, guardianship, employment, housing, and involuntary admission and treatment of individuals with mental illness. Although the legislation that affects the social determinants of health for people with mental illness is important, the focus of the discussion of legal implications in this chapter relates to the involuntary admission and involuntary treatment of people with mental illness.

ETHICAL CONCEPTS

"Like other kinds of growth, moral development is more likely to occur in the right environment—one that provides models, mentors, heroes and antiheroes; support, guidance and correction; relevant experiences and time for healing, and reflection, and building" (Andre, 2000, p. 61).

Ethics are an expression of the values and beliefs that guide practice. Manitoba Provincial Health Ethics Network (2016) has developed a decision-making guide for patient care ethics (see Figure 7-1).

Three types of moral theories have traditionally been used as a foundation for the development of nursing ethics: deontological theory, consequentialist theory, and virtue theory. More recently, the developing theory of **relational ethics**—an ethical theory with the core elements of mutual respect, engagement, embodied knowledge, interdependent environment, and uncertainty (Bergum & Dosetor, 2004)—has also affected the application of ethics within nursing.

Deontology is a system of ethics with the central concepts of reason and duty: there is an obligation to act in accordance with particular rules and principles. The Canadian Nurses Association (CNA, 2008) code of ethics (Box 7-1), the Canadian Federation of Mental Health Nurses (2014) standards of practice (Box 7-2), and the Registered Psychiatric Nurses of Canada (RPNC, 2010) code of ethics and standards of practice (Box 7-3) are written from this perspective. Immanuel Kant (1724–1804), a prominent deontologist, believed that people were free to make choices and that those choices should be based not on emotion but on reason alone. Within the paradigm of deontology, Beauchamp and Childress (2013) outlined several fundamental principles that are irreducible and must be balanced in clinical situations (referred to as **bioethics**). The basic principles are as follows:

1. **Respect for autonomy**—respecting the rights of others to make their own decisions (e.g., acknowledging the patient's right to refuse medication).
2. **Nonmaleficence**—the duty to minimize harm and do no wrong to the patient (e.g., by maintaining expertise in nursing skill through nursing education).

BOX 7-1	CANADIAN NURSES' VALUES AND ETHICAL RESPONSIBILITIES

The ethical responsibilities of Canadian registered nurses are articulated through seven primary values. These seven primary values are as follows:
1. Providing safe, compassionate, competent, and ethical care
2. Promoting health and well-being
3. Promoting and respecting informed decision making
4. Honouring dignity
5. Maintaining privacy and confidentiality
6. Promoting justice
7. Being accountable

Source: Canadian Nurses Association. (2017). *Code of ethics for registered nurses.* Ottawa: Author. © Canadian Nurses Association. Reprinted with permission. Further reproduction prohibited.

BOX 7-2	CANADIAN FEDERATION OF MENTAL HEALTH NURSES STANDARDS OF PRACTICE

Psychiatric mental health nursing practice standards provide a guide for the evaluation of practice within a professional and ethical framework. Seven standards are used to evaluate ethical psychiatric mental health nursing practice:
1. Provides competent professional care through the development of a therapeutic relationship
2. Performs/refines client assessments through the diagnostic and monitoring function
3. Administers and monitors therapeutic interventions
4. Effectively manages rapidly changing situations
5. Intervenes through the teaching–coaching function
6. Monitors and ensures quality of health care practices
7. Practises within organizational and work-role structure

Source: Canadian Federation of Mental Health Nurses. (2014). *Canadian standards for psychiatric-mental health nursing practice* (4th ed.). Toronto: Author.

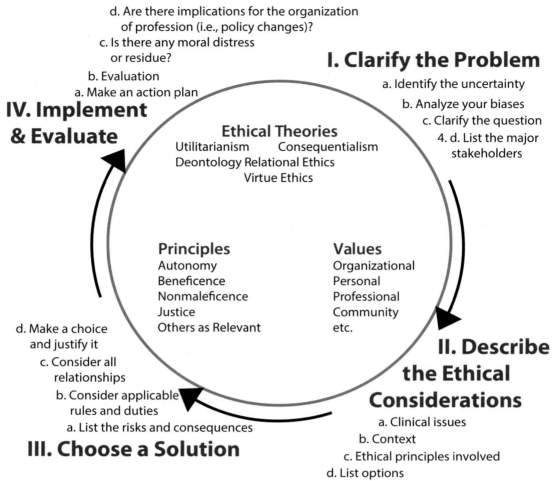

FIGURE 7-1 **Making ethical decisions.** Source: Manitoba Provincial Health Ethics Network. (2016). *Patient care ethics: Decision-making guide: Framework for clinical or patient-care issues.* Winnipeg: Author.

3. Beneficence—the duty to act to benefit or promote the good of others (e.g., spending extra time to help calm an extremely anxious patient).

4. Justice—the duty to distribute resources or care equally, regardless of personal attributes (e.g., an intensive care nurse devotes equal attention to someone who has attempted suicide as to someone who has suffered a brain aneurysm).

Other pluralistic deontologists have identified two other principles to consider when making ethical decisions in clinical settings. These additional principles are:

5. Principle of impossibility—the principle that a right or obligation that cannot be met within the current situation is no longer an obligation (e.g., a person does not have a right to receive magnetic resonance imaging [MRI] if MRI is not available, or a person does not have a right to be cured of schizophrenia when there are currently no permanent cures).

6. Principle of fidelity or best action—maintaining loyalty and commitment to the patient to perform your duty in the best manner possible (e.g., if a patient requires a dressing change, it is your duty to use the greatest skill and care possible).

The consequentialist theory is based on the belief that every person in society has the right to be happy and that we have an obligation to make sure happiness results from our actions. Within this theory, happiness is the maximization of pleasure and the minimization of pain. Accordingly, this theory's central concept relates to bringing about the greatest good and the least harm for the greatest number of people (called utilitarianism). John Stuart Mill (1806–1873) referred to this idea as the *principle of utility*. This type of approach is used when decisions are based on the outcomes of a cost–benefit analysis.

Critics of consequentialism argue that consequentialist theories fail to take into account how people are affected by actions. Elizabeth Anscombe (1919–2001) argued that consequentialism does not provide guidance on what ought to be done, and that it is through the use of virtues that decisions can be made. Virtues provide guidance on what one ought to do. Religiously based ethics, and more recently moral psychology, moral virtue, and facts of human nature, have been used by virtue ethicists to identify virtues relevant to ethical decision making.

Unlike deontology or utilitarianism theorists, who use duties and obligations to guide decision making, virtue theorists do

BOX 7-3 REGISTERED PSYCHIATRIC NURSES OF CANADA CODE OF ETHICS AND STANDARDS OF PRACTICE

Psychiatric nursing is regulated as a distinct profession in Canada by the provinces of Alberta, British Columbia, Manitoba, and Saskatchewan, as well as the territory of Yukon. Registered psychiatric nurses provide services relating to mental, physical, and developmental health and engage in various roles providing health care services to individuals, families, groups, and communities. The practice of psychiatric nursing occurs within the domains of direct practice, education, administration, and research.

The Code of Ethics
The code of ethics articulates four professional values that professional registered psychiatric nurses use to guide their practice:
1. Safe, competent, and ethical practice to ensure the protection of the public
2. Respect for the inherent worth, right of choice, and dignity of persons
3. Health, mental health, and well-being
4. Quality practice

Standards of Psychiatric Nursing Practice
The standards provide a guide to the knowledge, skills, values, judgement, and attitudes that psychiatric nurses need to practise safely. There are four standards of psychiatric nursing practice:
1. Registered psychiatric nurses establish professional, interpersonal, and therapeutic relationships with individual, groups, families, and communities.
2. Registered psychiatric nurses apply and integrate theory-based knowledge relevant to professional practice derived from psychiatric nursing education and continued lifelong learning.
3. Registered psychiatric nurses are accountable to the public for safe, competent, and ethical psychiatric nursing practice.
4. Registered psychiatric nurses understand, promote, and uphold the ethical values of the profession.

Source: Registered Psychiatric Nurses of Canada. (2010). *Code of ethics & standards of psychiatric nursing practice*. Edmonton: Author.

not. The ancient philosopher Aristotle believed that virtuous people would make decisions that would maximize their own and others' well-being. Similarly, the central premise of **virtue ethics** is that good people will make good decisions. **Virtues** are attitudes, dispositions, or character traits (e.g., honesty, courage, compassion, generosity, fidelity, integrity, fairness, self-control) that enable us to be and to act in ways that develop ethical potential and ensure ethical outcomes. The most prevalent and most valued virtues in health care are compassion and care. Just as the ability to run a marathon develops through much training and practice, so too does our capacity to be fair, to be courageous, and to be compassionate. Virtues, fostered through learning, practice, and self-discipline, enable us to use these attitudes and traits to guide decisions.

Relational ethics, an action-based ethics, requires nurses to appreciate the context in which an ethical issue arises. Context,

though, is not a mathematical equation to be figured out, nor is it a black-and-white phenomenon to be described. Context is a dynamic and fluid interaction of the participants, and it is this interaction that inspires (requires) responsibility (Olthuis, 1997). This responsibility, in turn, evokes ethical action. From the perspective of relational ethics, the fulcrum for action (how to be and how to act) is the relationship (Austin, Bergum, & Dossetor, 2003). When using a relational ethics approach, the core question to be answered in an ethical situation is "What action or decision is most fitting?" Understanding the relationship and the actions to be taken requires knowledge of traditions, universal principles, rationality, our subjectivity, and our interconnectedness (Rodney, Burgess, Phillips et al., 2012). As researchers explored relational ethics, they found five core elements that are cornerstones for ethical action (Austin, Bergum, & Dossetor, 2003):
1. Mutual respect—an intersubjective experience arising from a nonoppositional perception of difference. There is a recognition that individuals are affected by how others view and react to them as well as by their attitudes toward themselves and others.
2. Engagement—the connection between the self and another. It is through this connection that nurses can develop a meaningful understanding of another person's experience, perspective, and vulnerability.
3. Embodied knowledge—our understanding of the other, incorporated with a scientific body of knowledge. Nursing knowledge and compassion are given equal weight; therefore, emotions and feelings are viewed to be as important as physical signs and symptoms.
4. Interdependent environment—the recognition that we are not separate entities but that we exist as part of a larger community, society, and system. We are not merely affected by our environment; each action we take affects the environment, too.
5. Uncertainty or vulnerability—a recognition that ethical dilemmas exist and, furthermore, that ethical deliberation and contemplation are difficult and at times unpleasant.

From a relational ethics perspective, the consequences of uncertainty or vulnerability are ethical dilemmas. An ethical dilemma results when a choice must be made between two mutually exclusive courses of action, each of which has favourable and unfavourable consequences. How we respond to these dilemmas is based partly on our own morals (beliefs of right and wrong) and values. The nurse is a **moral agent** who has the power and capacity "to direct his or her motives and actions to some ethical end; essentially, doing what is good and right" (CNA, 2008, p. 26). Suppose you are caring for a pregnant woman with schizophrenia who wants to carry the baby to term but whose family insists she get an abortion. To promote fetal safety, her antipsychotic medication will need to be reduced, putting her at risk for exacerbation of the illness. Furthermore, there is a question as to whether she can safely care for the child. If you rely on the ethical principle of **autonomy** (the right to make decisions for oneself), you may conclude that she has the right to decide. Would other ethical principles be in conflict with autonomy in this case? At times, your personal values may be in conflict with the value system of the institution. This situation further complicates the decision-making process and necessitates careful consideration of the patient's desires. For example, you may experience a conflict of values in a setting where older adult patients are routinely tranquilized to a degree you are not comfortable with. Whenever one's value system is challenged, increased stress results.

Consequently, psychiatric mental health nurses may develop moral (or ethical) distress, moral uncertainty, moral residue, or a combination of these stressors. The CNA (2008) describes moral distress as arising "in situations where nurses know or believe they know the right thing to do, but for various reasons (including fear or circumstances beyond their control) do not or cannot take the right action or prevent a particular harm" (p. 6). This is in comparison to moral uncertainty, which occurs "when a nurse feels indecision or [has] a lack of clarity, or is unable to even know what the moral problem is, while at the same time feeling uneasy or uncomfortable" (CNA, 2008, p. 6). However, should nurses "seriously compromise themselves or allow themselves to be compromised" (CNA, 2008, p. 7), they will experience moral residue. "The moral residue that nurses carry forward from these kinds of situations can help them reflect on what they would do differently in similar situations in the future" (CNA, 2008, p. 7). Lachman (2016) has identified various means of coping with moral distress and moral residue—moral resilience. Moral resilience is the ability and willingness to speak and take the most fitting action in the presence of moral and ethical dilemmas (Lachman, 2016, p. 122). See Box 7-4 for strategies to develop moral resilience.

There may be particular times in nurses' careers when they are unable to align their own understanding of ethical principles, duties, or required virtues with those of their patients. In these situations, professional organizations and health care organizations may have policies that will help guide the nurse to balance professional obligations and personal values. Unfortunately, "where relevant policies exist in many Canadian provinces, there is much controversy and potential confusion, due to policy inconsistencies and terminological vagueness" (Shaw & Downie, 2014). Conscientious objection is the action a health care practitioner takes when his or her belief that the procedure requested by a patient or the employer is morally wrong. Most professional codes of conduct and organizational policies attempt to forge a means of compromising between individual conscience and professional responsibilities. However, if the health care provider is responsible for the patient's care, the provider must ensure that the patient's needs are met until another provider takes over responsibility for care provision (Wicclair, 2011).

The last area of ethical consideration to be discussed in this chapter is research ethics. The codes of ethics of the CNA (2008) and the RPNC (2010) outline ethical standards of practice, among them, for research. Actions and ethical responsibilities of the nurse can include ensuring that clients are informed of their rights with regard to research; however, the CNA code of ethics also contains rules and regulations to ensure that nursing research is conducted legally and ethically. These rules and regulations apply to all areas of nursing and parallel the *Tri-Council Policy Statement: Ethical Conduct for Research Involving Humans* (Canadian Institutes of Health Research, Natural Sciences and Engineering Research Council of Canada, & Social Sciences and Humanities Research Council of Canada, 2014) core principles of respect for persons, concern for welfare, and justice. Research within a mental health setting raises unique ethical considerations. People with a mental illness are potentially very vulnerable. "Vulnerability is often caused by limited decision-making capacity, or limited access to social goods, such as rights, opportunities and power" (Canadian Institutes of Health Research, Natural Sciences and Engineering Research Council of Canada, & Social Sciences and Humanities Research Council of Canada, 2014, p. 8). There is a strong research tradition in Canada. As nurses continue to transform their practices using evidence-informed knowledge, they must be aware of the consequences of not adhering to ethical standards. An example is included in the following Research Highlight.

MENTAL HEALTH LEGISLATION

Nurses must consider both the ethical and the legal dimensions of practice—which are distinct. Ideally, the system of law would be completely compatible with both the CNA's and the RPNC's codes of ethics; however, there may be times when nurses will need to collaborate with others to change a law or policy that is incompatible with ethical practice. When this occurs, the relevant codes of ethics can guide and support nurses' actions as they advocate for changes to law, policy, or practice. These "code[s] can be powerful political instrument[s] for nurses when they are concerned about being able to practice ethically" (CNA, 2008, p. 4).

Canada is a society that respects and cares for its people. As a result, legislation that protects vulnerable citizens has been

---

BOX 7-4 DEVELOPING MORAL RESILIENCE

1. Identify your beliefs and values.
2. Compare these to your professional code of ethics.
3. Compare these to your organizational values.
4. Identify if there are any differences.
   a. Identify potential responsibilities that may result in a conscientious objection.
   b. Articulate morally distressing concerns.
   c. Act as an advocate for resolution of these concerns.
5. Engage in ethical consultations.
6. Make a decision that balances your beliefs with professional responsibilities.
7. Identify emotional reactions after the decision has been made and an action has been taken.
8. Explore these reactions.
9. Explore the complexity of the situation.
10. Connect with others.

Source: Adapted from Lachman, V. D. (2016). Ethics, law, and policy. Moral resilience: Managing and preventing moral distress and moral residue. *MedSurg Nursing, 25*(2), 121–124. Retrieved from http://www.medsurgnursing.net/cgi-bin/WebObjects/MSNJournal.woa.

RESEARCH HIGHLIGHT

Moral Distress in Undergraduate Nursing Students: a Systematic Review

Problem

Nurses are faced with complex ethical situations. An increasing number of studies report that moral distress is common among health care professionals who face constraints that result in conflicting professional values or are perceived to compromise patient care. Moral distress also occurs in students when they perceive differences between the principles they learned in an academic setting and those they observe during their clinical experiences.

Purpose of Study

The aim of this review was to identify publications dealing with moral distress among undergraduate student nurses, to compare them, and to analyze and summarize their results. The questions that guided the review were as follows:
1. What ethical dilemmas and issues can cause moral distress in undergraduate nursing students during their clinical experience and their professional education?
2. Which environmental, relational, and organizational factors create situations of unease or of ethical dilemmas and issues that can give rise to moral distress in undergraduate nursing students?
3. During nurse education, what can be done to help students minimize moral distress?

Methods

A systematic review was completed on 157 articles published between 2004 and 2014. Articles relevant to the research topic were analyzed using a method developed by Hawker and colleagues to systematically appraise heterogeneous studies. Data were then extracted and synthesized from the relevant articles.

Key Findings

Four articles were found to be relevant to the research questions. These articles described one quantitative study and three qualitative studies conducted in the United Kingdom, United States, and Canada. Substantive findings identified that it was an important task for professional education to support students who encounter moral distress. This was especially true in the clinical areas of intensive care, gerontology, oncology, and psychiatry. Student nurses displayed a deep commitment to the ethical practice of nursing. However, they need greater support in developing relational and coping skills to help recognize and handle moral distress.

Implications for Nursing Practice

Moral distress is present in both clinical and academic settings. A knowledge gap exists related to understanding how moral distress is manifested and what educational experiences and factors can affect students most strongly. Evidence-informed strategies need to be developed to give future nurses the support they need in order to learn how to manage ethical dilemmas without experiencing moral distress, during both their educational experiences and their professional career.

Source: Sasso, L., Bagnasco, A., Bianchi, M., et al. (2016). Moral distress in undergraduate nursing students: A systematic review. *Nursing Ethics, 23*(5), 523–534. doi:10.1177/0969733015574926

developed. "People with mental disorders are, or can be, particularly vulnerable to abuse and violation of rights" (World Health Organization, 2005, p. 1). As a result, all provinces and territories have laws that protect the rights of people with mental illness and of others whose lives may be directly affected by another's mental illness.

Historically, in Canada, mental health legislation was developed to protect members of the public from so-called mentally deranged and dangerous patients. Legislation ensured that these "dangerous" individuals were isolated from the public, rather than ensuring that their rights as people and Canadian citizens were protected. Early legislation, when interpreted using today's societal values, allowed for violations of human rights. For example, there was legislation that permitted long-term custodial care for people who were deemed to be "a danger" and were unable to care for themselves. This type of legislation heightened the burden of stigma and discrimination faced by people with mental illness (World Health Organization, 2005). The Supreme Court of Canada has also recognized the disadvantages endured by people with mental illness. In *Battlefords and District Co-operative Ltd. v. Gibbs* (1996), the court recognized that it was discriminatory to differentiate between physical and mental disability. The court further recognized that individuals with mental illness are subjected to treatment that people with other illnesses are not and determined this treatment to be discriminatory (*Battlefords and District Co-operative Ltd. v. Gibbs*, 1996). Despite these historical legislative limitations, thoughtful and well-developed legislation "offers an important mechanism to ensure adequate and appropriate care and treatment, protection of human rights of people with mental disorders and promotion of the mental health of populations" (World Health Organization, 2005, p. 1). The United Nations Universal Declaration of Human Rights, written in 1948, and other international agreements provide the foundation for current mental health legislation. The fundamental basis for current mental health legislation is human rights, and the key rights and principles reflected are "equality and non-discrimination, the right to privacy and individual autonomy, freedom from inhuman and degrading treatment, the principle of least restrictive environment, and the rights to information and participation" (World Health Organization, 2005, p. 3). Many Canadian jurisdictions have used the *Mental Health Care Law: Ten Basic Principles* (World Health Organization, 1996) to guide the revision of old and the development of new mental health legislation. See Box 7-5.

Legislation consolidates fundamental principles, values, goals, and objectives of mental health policies and programs. It provides a legal framework to ensure that critical issues affecting the lives of people with mental disorders, in facilities and in the community, are addressed (World Health Organization, 1996). In Canada, there are 13 different mental health acts, all of which allow for the involuntary confinement of people with mental illness to protect them from themselves and others from them. Each of the provinces and territories has developed its mental health act from a perspective that prioritizes either the respect of persons (autonomy) or the concern for welfare (beneficence). As a result, the acts differ in many ways. However, there are three primary areas of difference: "(1) involuntary admission criteria, (2) the right to refuse treatment [including medication], and (3) who has the authority to authorize treatment" (Browne, 2010, p. 290). You are encouraged to review your province's or territory's act to better understand the legal climate in which you will practise (see Table 7-1). As you review the act relevant to your province, you will notice that there is different paperwork, or forms, required to enact various parts of the acts.

As people started to receive their psychiatric care while living in the community, provincial and territorial acts have changed to reflect a shift in emphasis from institutional care of people with mental illness to community-based care delivery models. Along with this shift in setting has come the more widespread use of psychotropic drugs in the treatment of mental illness—which has enabled many people to integrate more readily into the larger community—and an increasing awareness of the need to provide mentally ill patients with care that respects their human rights. However, the increased use of psychotropic drugs has resulted in more discussions, and debate, about the ethical use of medication.

BOX 7-5 | MENTAL HEALTH CARE LAW: TEN BASIC PRINCIPLES

These principles were developed from a comparative analysis of national mental health laws in 45 countries worldwide conducted by the World Health Organization. The selection of principles drew from the Principles for the Protection of Persons with Mental Illness and the Improvement of Mental Health Care adopted by the UN General Assembly Resolution 46/119 of December 17, 1991.

1. Promotion of mental health and prevention of mental disorders
2. Access to basic mental health care
3. Mental health assessments in accordance with internationally accepted principles
4. Provision of the least restrictive type of mental health care
5. Self-determination
6. Right to be assisted in the exercise of self-determination
7. Availability of review procedure
8. Automatic periodical review mechanism
9. Qualified decision-maker
10. Respect of the rule of law

Source: World Health Organization. (1996). *Mental health care law: Ten basic principles*. Geneva, Switzerland: Author.

ESTABLISHING BEST PRACTICE

Each province and territory provides a regulatory framework for the governance of health professions and gives professional bodies their mandates and powers. In many provinces this legislation is referred to as the Health Professions Act (HPA); however, a number of provinces continue to use legislation that is specific to each registering body, such as registered nurses, registered psychiatric nurses, or registered practical nurses. HPAs, or similar legislation, also authorize professional bodies to create and enforce bylaws, standards of practice, and professional ethics. This type of regulation also sets out reserved titles and scopes of practice for professional registrants, including restricted activities for general and certified registered or licensed nursing practice as well as for nurse practitioner practice. You are encouraged to review your province's or territory's legislation to better understand the legal climate in which you will practise (see Table 7-2).

Standards of Practice

The standards of practice determined by professional associations differ from the minimal qualifications set forth by provincial or territorial licensure for entry into the profession of nursing

---

TABLE 7-1 | PROVINCIAL AND TERRITORIAL MENTAL HEALTH ACTS

PROVINCE OR TERRITORY	WEBSITE LINK
Alberta	http://www.qp.alberta.ca/574.cfm?page=M13.cfm&leg_type=Acts&isbncln=0779748727
British Columbia	http://www.bclaws.ca/EPLibraries/bclaws_new/document/ID/freeside/00_96288_01
Manitoba	http://web2.gov.mb.ca/laws/statutes/ccsm/m110e.php
New Brunswick	http://laws.gnb.ca/en/ShowTdm/cs/M-10//
Newfoundland and Labrador	http://www.assembly.nl.ca/legislation/sr/statutes/m09-1.htm
Northwest Territories	https://www.justice.gov.nt.ca/en/files/legislation/mental-health/mental-health.a.pdf
Nova Scotia	http://novascotia.ca/dhw/mental-health/involuntary-psychiatric-treatment-act.asp
Nunavut	http://www.gov.nu.ca/sites/default/files/gnjustice2/justicedocuments/Consolidated%20Law/ Current/6350241081697764792-1835258198-consRSNWT1988cM-10.pdf
	(The Government of Nunavut is reviewing the *Mental Health Act* to ensure that amendments represent Inuit culture and knowledge and reflect the unique conditions of addressing mental illness in Nunavut; public consultations occurred in 2015 and 2016.)
Ontario	http://www.e-laws.gov.on.ca/html/statutes/english/elaws_statutes_90m07_e.htm
Prince Edward Island	http://www.gov.pe.ca/law/statutes/pdf/m-06_1.pdf
Quebec	http://legisquebec.gouv.qc.ca/fr/ShowDoc/cs/P-38.001
Saskatchewan	http://www.qp.gov.sk.ca/documents/English/Statutes/Statutes/M13-1.pdf
Yukon	http://www.hss.gov.yk.ca/mental_health_act.php

TABLE 7-2 PROVINCIAL AND TERRITORIAL HEALTH PROFESSIONS ACTS

PROVINCE OR TERRITORY	WEBSITE LINK
Alberta	http://www.qp.alberta.ca/documents/acts/h07.pdf
British Columbia	http://www.bclaws.ca/EPLibraries/bclaws_new/document/ID/freeside/00_96183_01
Manitoba	http://www.gov.mb.ca/health/rhpa/index.html
New Brunswick	http://www2.gnb.ca/content/gnb/en/departments/attorney_general/acts_regulations.html
Newfoundland and Labrador	http://www.assembly.nl.ca/legislation/sr/annualstatutes/2010/h01-02.c10.htm
Northwest Territories	http://www.assembly.gov.nt.ca/sites/default/files/15-02-25bill36_amended.pdf
Nova Scotia	http://www.novascotia.ca/just/regulations/index.htm
Nunavut	http://www.gov.nu.ca/sites/default/files/gnjustice2/justicedocuments/Consolidated%20Law/Original/ 633389069864062500-2131836274-type137.pdf
Ontario	https://www.ontario.ca/laws/statute/91r18?search=health+professions
Prince Edward Island	https://www.princeedwardisland.ca/en/legislation/regulated-health-professions-act
Quebec	https://professions-quebec.org/en/quebec-interprofessional-council/about-us/members/
Saskatchewan	http://www.publications.gov.sk.ca/deplist.cfm?d=13&c=1109#H
Yukon	http://www.gov.yk.ca/legislation/acts/hepr_c.pdf

because the primary purposes of each are different. The province's or territory's qualifications for practice provide consumer protection by ensuring that all practising nurses have successfully completed an approved nursing program and passed the national licensing examination, whereas the professional association's primary focus is to elevate the practice of its members by setting standards of excellence.

Standards of Care

Nurses are held to a basic standard of care that is based on what other nurses who possess the same degree of skill or knowledge would do in the same or similar circumstances. Psychiatric patients, whether in a large, small, rural, or urban facility, have a right to the standard of care recognized by professional bodies governing nursing. Nurses must participate in continuing education courses to stay current with existing standards of care.

Policies and Procedures

Hospital policies and procedures define institutional criteria for care, which may be introduced in legal proceedings to prove that a nurse met or failed to meet them. The weakness of individual institutions setting such criteria is that a particular hospital's policy may be substandard. Substandard institutional policies, however, do not absolve the individual nurse of responsibility to practise on the basis of professional standards of nursing care.

Traditional Practice Knowledge

Like hospital policies and procedures, traditional practice knowledge can be used as evidence of a standard of care. But using traditional practice knowledge to establish a standard of care may result in the same defect as using hospital policies and procedures: traditional practice knowledge may not comply with the laws, recommendations of the accrediting body, or other recognized standards of care. Traditional practice knowledge must be carefully and regularly evaluated to ensure that substandard routines have not developed.

GUIDELINES FOR ENSURING ADHERENCE TO STANDARDS OF CARE

Students or practising nurses may encounter situations in which they suspect negligence on the part of a peer. In most provinces and territories, nurses have a legal duty to report such risks for harm. It is also important for nurses to document the evidence clearly and accurately before making serious accusations against a peer. If you question any regulated health professional's orders or actions, it is wise to communicate these concerns directly to the person involved. If the risky behaviour continues, you have an obligation to communicate your concerns to a supervisor, who should then intervene to ensure that the patient's rights and well-being are protected.

If you suspect a peer of being chemically impaired or of practising irresponsibly, you have an obligation to protect not only the rights of the peer but also the rights of all patients who could be harmed by this person. If the danger persists after you have reported suspected behaviour of concern to a supervisor, you have a duty to report the concern to someone at the next level of authority. It is important to follow the channels of communication in an organization, but it is also important to protect the safety of the patients. To that end, if supervisors' actions or inactions do not rectify the dangerous situation, you have a continuing duty to report the behaviour of concern to the appropriate authority, such as the provincial or territorial nursing college or association.

The CNA, the RPNC, and the Canadian Federation of Mental Health Nurses have on their websites useful information related to standards of practice.

The issues become more complex when a professional colleague's conduct (including that of a student nurse) is criminally unlawful. Specific examples include the diversion of drugs from the hospital and sexual misconduct with patients. Increasing media attention and the recognition of substance abuse as an occupational hazard for health professionals have led to the establishment of substance abuse programs for health care workers in many provinces or territories. These programs provide appropriate treatment for impaired professionals to protect the public from harm and to rehabilitate the professional.

The problem of reporting impaired colleagues becomes a difficult one, particularly when no direct harm has occurred to any patients. Concern for professional reputations, damaged careers, and personal privacy has generated among health professionals a code of silence regarding substance abuse. Chapter 18 deals more fully with issues related to the chemically impaired nurse.

PATIENTS' RIGHTS UNDER THE LAW

Authorization of Treatment

Two models of decision making are supported by legislation. The first, the state model, is used to build a system wherein the psychiatrists make the decisions (paternalism). The premise of this model is that the education and experience of a psychiatrist enable him or her to make better treatment decisions than the patient's family members would make. Thus, treatment can be started immediately and without delay. The second is the private model. Within this model, the patient or his or her family member is viewed as the most appropriate authority for making treatment decisions. In Canada, in physical medicine, the private model is used exclusively, based on a civil liberties perspective (Browne, 2010). However, legislation regarding authorization of treatment of mental illnesses has been developed using either a state model or a private model, depending on the jurisdiction. Both models have consequences for the provision of mental health nursing care. Therefore, nurses need to reflect on the impact that the current legislation in use in their province or territory has on autonomy, beneficence, nonmaleficence, engagement, mutual respect, reciprocity, and an interdependent environment.

VIGNETTE

Elizabeth is a 50-year-old woman with a long history of admissions to psychiatric hospitals. During previous hospitalizations, she was diagnosed with paranoid schizophrenia. She has refused visits from her case worker and quit taking medication, and her young-adult children have become increasingly concerned about her behaviour. When they visit her, she is unkempt and smells bad, her apartment is filthy and filled with cats, and there is no food in the refrigerator except for ketchup and an old container of yogurt; as well, she is not paying her bills. Elizabeth accuses her children of spying on her and of being in collusion with the government to get at her secrets of mind control and oil-rationing plans. Elizabeth is making vague threats to the local officials, claiming that the people who have caused the problems need to be "taken care of." Her daughter contacts her psychiatrist with this information, and a decision is made to begin emergency involuntary admission proceedings.

Autonomy
Consent

The principle of **informed consent** is based on a person's right to self-determination and the ethical principle of autonomy.

Proper orders for specific therapies and treatments are required and must be documented in the patient's medical record. Consent for surgery, electroconvulsive treatment, or the use of experimental drugs or procedures must be obtained. Patients have the right to refuse participation in experimental treatments or research and the right to voice grievances and recommend changes in policies or services offered by the facility without fear of punishment or reprisal.

For consent to be effective, it must be informed. Generally, the informed consent of the patient must be obtained by the physician or other health care provider before a treatment or procedure is performed. Patients must be informed of the following:

- The nature of their problem or condition
- The nature and purpose of a proposed treatment
- The risks and benefits of that treatment
- The alternative treatment options
- The probability of success of the proposed treatment
- The risks of not consenting to treatment

It is important that psychiatric mental health nurses know that the presence of psychotic thinking does not mean that the patient is mentally incompetent or incapable of understanding; he or she is still able to provide or deny consent.

Competency is the capacity to understand the consequences of one's decisions. Patients must be considered legally competent until they have been declared incompetent through a legal proceeding. If found incompetent, the patient may be appointed a legal guardian or representative, who is legally responsible for giving or refusing consent for the patient while always considering the patient's wishes. Guardians are typically selected from among family members. The order of selection is usually (1) spouse, (2) adult children or grandchildren, (3) parents, (4) adult siblings, and (5) adult nieces and nephews. If a family member is either unavailable or unwilling to serve as guardian, the court may also appoint a court-trained and court-approved social worker, representing the province or territory, or a member of the community.

Many procedures nurses perform have an element of **implied consent** attached. For example, if you approach the patient with a medication in hand, and the patient indicates a willingness to receive the medication, implied consent has occurred. The fact that you may not have a legal duty to be the person to inform the patient of the associated risks and benefits of a particular medical procedure, however, does not excuse you from clarifying the procedure to the patient and ensuring his or her expressed or implied consent. When providing care, via implied consent, the nurse must be confident that the person understands, to the best of his or her abilities, the procedure, risks, and benefits.

The Right to Refuse Treatment

Admission to the hospital, whether voluntary or involuntary, is not synonymous with the commencement of treatment. "In some jurisdictions, treatment can begin as soon as admission is deemed appropriate, that is, after the confirmation by the second physician. In others, it cannot begin until all the appeals have been exhausted" (Browne, 2010, pp. 292–293). At the core of the **right to refuse treatment** is a person's ability to understand and appreciate his or her condition. The importance of this right was highlighted in 2003 in the case of *Starson v. Swayze*, discussed in Box 7-6.

Community treatment orders (CTOs) are "legal mechanisms by which individuals with mental illness and a history of non-compliance can be mandated against their will to undergo psychiatric treatment in an outpatient setting" (Snow & Austin, 2009, p. 177). There are several ethical implications related to the enactment of a CTO. The principles of respect for autonomy/paternalism, beneficence/nonmaleficence, and justice must be considered when working with an individual affected by a CTO. From a relational ethics perspective, this type of "forced treatment" or coercive relationship affects the power dynamics between the nurse and the person with mental illness. Therefore, special consideration needs to be given to the aspects of engagement, mutual respect, the environment, and uncertainty.

Beneficence and Nonmaleficence
Involuntary Admission Criteria
All provinces and territories have written legislation that enables the legally sanctioned violation of human rights for a person with mental illness. This violation occurs when an individual is involuntarily admitted to a mental health facility. Every mental health act in Canada specifies the data, assessment findings, or symptoms that must be present for an involuntary admission. For example, in Alberta, a person must be (1) suffering from a mental disorder, (2) likely to cause harm to himself or herself or others or to suffer substantial mental or physical deterioration or serious physical impairment, and (3) unsuitable for admission to a facility other than as a formal patient (*Mental Health Act*: Revised Statutes of Alberta, 2000, 2010). However, in all provinces and territories, coupled with the criteria for the original involuntary commitment are safeguards for inappropriately detaining a person in hospital by mandating the completion of an independent examination by a second physician before the person can be kept in hospital. Many jurisdictions stipulate that this physician must be a psychiatrist.

Provision of the Least Restrictive Type of Mental Health Care
As previously mentioned, the use of the least restrictive means of restraint for the shortest duration is always the general rule. Using verbal interventions such as asking the patient for cooperation is the first approach, and medications are considered if verbal interventions fail. Chemical interventions (i.e., medications) are usually considered less restrictive than physical or mechanical interventions (e.g., restraints, seclusion), but they can have a greater impact on the patient's ability to relate to the environment because medication alters our ability to think and produces other effects. However, when used judiciously, psychopharmacology is extremely effective and helpful as an alternative to physical methods of restraint.

The history of using mechanical restraints and seclusion is marked by abuse, overuse, and even a tendency to use restraint as punishment, especially prior to the 1950s, when there were no effective chemical treatments. Most mental health acts in Canada now legislate that clinicians attempting to bring under control people with a mental illness who are a danger to themselves or others are to use a minimal amount of force or treatment

---

BOX 7-6 FACTS: STARSON V. SWAYZE (2003)

Scott Starson (born Schutzman, 1956) was assessed with bipolar disorder with psychosis and was hospitalized many times from young adulthood onward. He had no formal education in physics but his interest in it led to co-publication of articles in the field. In the late 1990s he was arrested for uttering death threats, as he had done many times before. In 1998 he was found not criminally responsible for uttering more death threats and was once again arrested and taken to the Centre for Addiction and Mental Health in Toronto. There his treatment plan included neuroleptic medication, which he refused. Because Starson's physicians felt strongly that he needed this medication, the issue was taken to the Ontario Consent and Capacity Board and then to the courts above it. In January 1999, the Ontario Consent and Capacity Board found Starson incapable to refuse medication. Starson appealed the decision and, later that same year, won his case in the Superior Court of Ontario, which deemed him capable. The physicians appealed that ruling, taking the case first to the Ontario Court of Appeal (2001) and ultimately to the Supreme Court of Canada (SCC) (p. 53).

All of these decisions turned on how the board, and then the courts, interpreted Ontario's *Health Care Consent Act*, s. 4(1). Under that law, an individual is capable to refuse (in this case) treatment if s/he can understand information relevant to making a decision about treatment, and if s/he can appreciate that the information applies to the patient herself or himself and does not exist in the abstract or apply to a third party.

Decision of the Supreme Court of Canada
The SCC majority (six judges) interpreted the mental capacity test as being fairly low, or easy to pass. They found that Starson was capable to refuse treatment. They found that Starson's "enthusiasm" for (in Starson's words) his own "not normal" mental functioning was a sign that he was aware of the nature of the psychiatric diagnosis given to him, and that he simply disagreed with the medical treatment plan (pp. 67–68). By contrast, the SCC dissent (three judges) found that Starson's very enthusiasm for his condition was a sign that, despite obvious intelligence, he could neither understand nor appreciate the severity of his deteriorating condition and the need for treatment. The dissent found that the mental capacity test was not a general intelligence test but very specifically related to information tailored to the individual. Even a highly intelligent person can fail it (pp. 69-70).

Effects on Mr. Starson
With the SCC decision, Scott Starson continued to refuse treatment, and his condition declined markedly. He believed that his nonexistent son would be tortured if he ate or drank. He nearly died and was found without capacity in 2005. His mother became his substitute decision maker and allowed him to be treated with neuroleptic medication. His condition improved and he spent 2 years living in a community-based supportive housing setting while under a community treatment order. In April 2008, he appealed his incapacity finding. Treatment was suspended, his condition deteriorated, and he was again hospitalized involuntarily. Starson appealed his incapacity finding to the Ontario Superior Court. The court upheld the finding of incapacity (pp. 77–78).

Source: Dull, M. W. (2009). *Starson v. Swayze*, 2003–2008: Appreciating the judicial consequences. *Health Law Journal, 17*, 51–79.

BOX 7-7   CONTRAINDICATIONS TO SECLUSION AND RESTRAINT

- Psychological inability to tolerate the experience of confinement or isolation
- Physical condition that may be exacerbated by restraint application
- Desire for punishment of patient or convenience of staff

in order to protect the patient and others. Nurses must know under which circumstances the use of seclusion and restraints is contraindicated (Box 7-7).

When in restraints, the patient must be protected from all sources of harm. The behaviour leading to restraint or seclusion and the time the patient is placed in and released from restraint must be documented. The patient in restraint must be assessed at regular and frequent intervals (e.g., every 5 to 15 minutes) for physical needs (e.g., food, hydration, toileting), safety, and comfort, and these observations must also be documented. The patient must be removed from restraints when safer and quieter behaviour is observed.

Agencies have continued to revise their policies and procedures regarding restraint and seclusion, further limiting these practices after recent changes in laws.

Advance Directives

Since the 1960s, the public's desire to participate in decision making about health care has increased. Most provinces and territories have passed legislation that establishes the right of a person to provide directions (advance directives) for clinicians to follow in the event of a serious illness. Such a directive indicates preferences for the types of medical care or extent of treatment desired. The directive comes into effect should physical or mental incapacitation prevent the patient from making health care decisions. Health care institutions are required to (1) provide to each patient at the time of admission written information regarding his or her right to execute advance health care directives and (2) inquire if the patient has made such directives. The patient's admission records should state whether such directives exist.

Patients concerned that they may be subject to involuntary admission can prepare an advance directive document that will express their treatment choices. The advance directive for mental health decision making should be followed by health care providers when the patient is not competent to make informed decisions. This document can clarify the patient's choice of a surrogate decision maker and instructions about hospital choices, medications, treatment options, provider preferences, and emergency interventions.

Nursing responsibilities with advance directives. The nurse is often responsible for explaining the legal policies of the institution to both the patient and the family and can help them understand advance directives. The nurse serves as an advocate and knowledgeable resource for the patient and family and encourages the patient to verbalize thoughts and feelings during this sensitive time of decision making.

Nurses must be knowledgeable about both the provincial or territorial regulations on advance directives and the potential obstacles in completing the directives for the province or territory in which they practise. Maintaining an open and continuing dialogue among patient, family, nurse, and physician is of principal importance. The nurse supports any surrogates appointed to act on the patient's behalf and seeks consultation for ethical issues the nurse feels unprepared to handle.

Nurses must prepare themselves to deal with the legal, ethical, and moral issues involved when counselling about advance directives. The law does not specify who should talk with patients about treatment decisions, but in many facilities nurses are asked to discuss such issues with the patient. If the advance directive of a patient is not being followed, the nurse should intervene on the patient's behalf. If the problem cannot be resolved with the physician, the nurse must follow the facility's protocol providing for notification of the appropriate supervisor.

Although nurses may discuss options with their patients, they may not assist patients in writing advance directives because doing so is considered a conflict of interest. The existence of an advance directive serves as a guide to health care providers in advocating for the patient's rightful wishes in this process.

Guardianship

A guardianship is an involuntary trust relationship in which one party, the *guardian*, acts on behalf of an individual, the *ward*. The law regards the ward as incapable of managing his or her own person or affairs. Through investigation and an evaluation process, probate court determines if guardianship is warranted. A physician's expert opinion indicating incompetence is required to initiate the proceeding. Many people with mental illness, mental retardation, traumatic brain injuries, and organic brain disorders such as dementia have guardians. It is important that health care providers identify patients who have guardians and communicate with the guardians when health care decisions are being made.

Rights Regarding Confidentiality

Confidentiality (the right to privacy of information) of care and treatment is also an important right for all patients, particularly psychiatric patients. Any discussion or consultation involving a patient should be conducted discreetly and only with individuals who have a need and a right to know this privileged information.

The CNA (2008) asserts that it is a duty of the nurse to protect confidential patient information (see Box 7-1). The fundamental principle underlying the code on confidentiality is a person's right to privacy—the assurance that only those with a right to know will have access to privileged information. Failure to provide this protection may harm the nurse–patient relationship as well as the patient's well-being. However, the CNA's code of ethics clarifies that this duty is not absolute. In some situations, disclosure may be mandated to protect the patient, other persons, or public health. The following four situations warrant the violation of this right to privacy by the nurse:

1. There is the potential for suspected harm to another.
2. There is suspected harm to a child.

3. There is the potential for harm to the patient's self (suicide risk).
4. There is the presence of a reportable communicable disease.

Duty to Warn and Protect Third Parties

Although the following event occurred in the United States, it also had an impact in Canada. The California Supreme Court, in its 1974 landmark decision *Tarasoff v. Regents of the University of California*, ruled that a psychotherapist has a **duty to warn** a patient's potential victim of potential harm. A university student who was in counselling at the University of California was despondent over being rejected by Tatiana Tarasoff, whom he had once kissed. The psychologist notified police verbally and in writing that the young man might pose a danger to Tarasoff. The police questioned the student, found him to be rational, and secured his promise to stay away from his love interest. The student killed Tarasoff 2 months later.

The *Tarasoff* case acknowledged that generally there is no common-law duty to aid third persons, except when special relationships exist, and the court found the patient–therapist relationship sufficient to create a duty of the therapist to aid Ms. Tarasoff, the victim. It asserted that the duty to protect the intended victim from danger arises when the therapist determines—or, pursuant to professional standards, should have determined—that the patient presents a serious danger to another.

This case created much controversy and confusion in the psychiatric and medical communities over (1) breach of patient confidentiality and its impact on the therapeutic relationship in psychiatric care and (2) the ability of the therapist to predict when a patient is truly dangerous. Nevertheless, many jurisdictions have adopted or modified the California rule despite objections from the psychiatric community.

The California Supreme Court held a second hearing in 1976 in the case of *Tarasoff v. Regents of the University of California* (now known as *Tarasoff II*). It delivered a second ruling that broadened the earlier duty to warn: when a therapist determines that a patient presents a serious danger of violence to another, the therapist has the duty to protect that other person; in providing protection, it may be necessary for the therapist to call and warn the intended victim, the victim's family, or the police or to take whatever steps are reasonably necessary under the circumstances.

Most areas have similar laws regarding the duty to protect third parties of potential life threats. The **duty to protect** usually includes the following:

- Assessing and predicting the patient's danger of violence toward another
- Identifying the specific persons being threatened
- Taking appropriate action to protect the identified potential victims

As this trend toward the therapist's duty to warn third persons of potential harm continues to gain wider acceptance, it is important for nurses to understand its implications for nursing practice. Although none of these cases has dealt with nurses, it is fair to assume that in jurisdictions that have adopted the *Tarasoff* doctrine, the duty to warn third persons will be applied to advanced-practice psychiatric mental health nurses who engage in individual therapy in private practice. If a staff nurse—who is a member of a team of psychiatrists, psychologists, psychiatric social workers, and other nurses—does not report to other members of the team a patient's threats of harm against specified victims or classes of victims, this failure is considered substandard nursing care.

Failure to communicate and record relevant information from police, relatives, or the patient's old records may also be deemed negligent. Breach of patient–nurse confidentiality should not pose ethical or legal dilemmas for nurses in these situations, because a team approach to the delivery of psychiatric care presumes communication of pertinent information to other staff members to develop a treatment plan in the patient's best interest.

The nurse's assessment of the patient's potential for violence must be documented and acted on if it suggests legitimate concern about a patient discussing or exhibiting potentially violent behaviour. The psychiatric mental health nurse must communicate his or her observations to the medical staff when discharge decisions are being considered.

Collaboration of Treatment Team

Health care providers have a responsibility to communicate assessment findings and treatment plans to other members of the treatment team. For example, a health care provider who believes that a patient is going to try to kill himself or herself has a duty to try to mitigate the risk for that person. Strategies to mitigate this risk would include informing other treatment team members. The nurse working on an inpatient unit who has assessed a patient as acutely suicidal would, in consultation with the other team members, develop a plan of care to mitigate the potential for that person to commit suicide.

Documentation of care. The purposes of the medical record are to provide accurate and complete information about the care and treatment of patients and to give health care personnel a means of communicating with each other, supporting continuity of care. A record's usefulness is determined by its accuracy and thoroughness in portraying the patient's behavioural status at the time it was written. For example, if a psychiatric patient describes to a nurse a plan to harm himself or another person and that nurse fails to document the information—including the need to protect the patient or the identified victim—the information will be lost when the nurse leaves work. If the patient's plan is carried out, the harm caused could be linked directly to the nurse's failure to communicate this important information. Even though documentation takes time away from the patient, the importance of communicating and preserving the nurse's memory through the medical record cannot be overemphasized.

Patients have the right to see their medical records, but records belong to the institution. Patients must follow appropriate protocol to view their records.

Guidelines for electronic documentation. Electronic documentation, now common, has created new challenges for protecting the confidentiality of records of psychiatric patients. While ensuring the appropriate sharing of information, institutions must, at the same time, protect against intrusions into patient-record systems. Sensitive information regarding treatment for mental illness can adversely affect patients who are seeking employment, insurance, or credit (Meier, Csiernik, Warner et al, 2015).

Concerns for the privacy of patients' records have been addressed by provincial, territorial, and federal laws that provide guidelines for agencies that use electronic documentation. These guidelines include the recommendation that staff members be assigned individual passwords for entering patients' records to allow for the identification of persons who have accessed confidential information. Only health care providers who have a legitimate need for information about the patient are authorized to access a patient's electronic medical record. There are penalties, including termination of employment, for staff members who access a record without authorization. For this reason, it is important to keep your password private. You are responsible for all entries into records using your password. Various systems allow for specific time frames within which the nurse must make corrections if a documentation error is made.

Any documentation method that improves communication between health care providers should be encouraged. Courts assume that nurses and physicians read each other's notes on patient progress. Many courts take the attitude that if care is not documented, it did not occur. Your documentation also serves as a valuable memory refresher if the patient sues years after the care has been rendered. In providing complete and timely information on the care and treatment of patients, the medical record enhances communication among health care providers. Internal institutional audits of records can improve the quality of care rendered. Chapter 6 describes common documentation forms, provides examples, and gives the pros and cons of each.

Organizational use of medical records. The medical record has many uses aside from providing information on the course of the patient's care and treatment by health care providers. A retrospective medical record review can offer an organization valuable information on the quality of care given and on ways to improve that care. An organization may conduct reviews for risk-management purposes to determine areas of potential liability and to evaluate methods of reducing the organization's exposure to liability. For example, risk managers may review documentation of the use of restraints and seclusion for psychiatric patients, or a medical record may be used to evaluate care for quality assurance or peer review. Utilization review analysts use the medical record to determine appropriate use of hospital and staff resources consistent with reimbursement schedules. Insurance companies and other reimbursement agencies rely on the medical record in determining what payments they will make on the patient's behalf.

Medical records as evidence. From a legal perspective, the medical record is a recording of data and opinions made in the normal course of the patient's hospital care. It is deemed to be good evidence because it is presumed to be true, honest, and untainted by memory lapses. Accordingly, the medical record finds its way into a variety of legal cases for a variety of reasons. Some examples of its use include determining (1) the extent of the patient's damages and pain and suffering in personal injury cases, such as when a psychiatric patient attempts suicide while under the protective care of a hospital; (2) the nature and extent of injuries in child abuse or elder abuse cases; (3) the nature and extent of physical or mental disability in disability cases; and (4) the nature and extent of injury and rehabilitative potential in workers' compensation cases.

Medical records may also be used in police investigations, competency hearings, and involuntary-admission procedures. In provinces and territories that mandate mental health legal services or a patients' rights advocacy program, audits of medical records may be performed to determine the facility's compliance with provincial or territorial law or violation of patients' rights. Finally, medical records may be used in professional and hospital negligence cases.

During the initial, or discovery, phase of litigation, the medical record is a pivotal source of information for lawyers in determining whether a cause of action exists in a professional negligence or hospital negligence case. Evidence of the nursing care rendered will be found in what the nurse documented.

Reporting Suspected Child Abuse

All provinces and territories have enacted child abuse reporting legislation. Although these statutes differ among provinces and territories, they generally include a definition of *child abuse*, a list of persons required or encouraged to report abuse, and the governmental agency designated to receive and investigate these reports. Most statutes include the consequences of failure to report. Many provinces and territories specifically require nurses to report cases of suspected abuse. Refer to Box 7-8 for some guidelines on how to report abuse.

As incidents of abuse in society surface, some jurisdictions may require health care providers to report other kinds of abuse. A growing number of provinces and territories are enacting "protection for persons in care" legislation, which requires registered nurses and others to report cases of abuse of people who are receiving care or support services. Under most provincial or territorial law, a person who is required to report suspected abuse, neglect, or exploitation of a person in care and willfully does not do so is guilty of a misdemeanour crime. Most provincial or territorial legislation provides protection to anyone who makes a report in good faith, ensuring immunity from civil liability in connection with the report. Because provincial and territorial

---

BOX 7-8	HOW DOES A NURSE REPORT CHILD ABUSE?

Institutions usually have policies for reporting abuse. Often the responsibility goes to social workers who have expertise in these matters and know how to navigate the system. However, if you are caring for a child covered in old and new bruises or who has a broken bone or decaying teeth, and you suspect abuse, it is your legal and ethical responsibility to make a report to your province's or territory's child welfare agency. You should also let the child's parents or guardians know that you are filing the report. Whether the physician or your peers agree with you or not, if you report suspected child abuse in good faith, you will be protected from criminal or civil liability. More important, you may save a child from further suffering.

laws vary, students are encouraged to become familiar with the requirements of their province or territory.

Confidentiality and Communicable Diseases

All provinces and territories have enacted legislation that requires health care providers to report suspected or confirmed cases of selected communicable diseases. Examples of these are Creutzfeldt-Jakob disease, human immunodeficiency virus (HIV), syphilis, tuberculosis, and West Nile virus infections. In addition, some provinces and territories have enacted mandatory or permissive legislation that directs health care providers to warn a spouse if a partner tests positive for HIV. Nurses must understand the laws in their jurisdiction of practice regarding privileged communications and warnings of infectious disease exposure.

Confidentiality After Death

A person's reputation can be damaged even after death. Therefore, it is important after a person's death not to divulge information that you would not have been able to share legally before the person's death.

CIVIL OBLIGATIONS AND RESPONSIBILITIES

Legal issues common in psychiatric mental health nursing relate to the failure to protect the safety of patients (Table 7-3). Miscommunications and medication errors are common in all facets of nursing, including psychiatric care. Another common area of

liability in psychiatry is abuse of the therapist–patient relationship. Issues of sexual misconduct during the therapeutic relationship have become a source of concern in the psychiatric community. Diagnosing a patient—and avoiding misdiagnosing—also requires ethical, moral, and legal responsibility of the treatment team.

Tort Law

Tort law is a law developed from obligations to another. Although these laws are not based on nurses' professional codes of ethics, they have many similarities. Both describe the nurse's obligations and responsibilities to the patient. The difference is that tort laws have a much broader applicability. They apply to all Canadians.

Intentional Torts

Nurses in psychiatric settings may encounter provocative, threatening, or violent behaviour that may require the use of restraint or seclusion. However, such interventions must be carefully determined and used only in the most extreme situations. As discussed earlier in this chapter, restraint and seclusion historically were used with little regard to patients' rights, and overuse and abuses were common. Stories of patients restrained and left to lie in their own excrement or locked in seclusion for days for being annoying have resulted in strict laws. Accordingly, the nurse in the psychiatric setting should understand intentional torts, which are willful or intentional acts that violate another person's rights or property. Some examples of intentional torts are assault (reasonable belief that a person means to cause one harm), battery (offensive or harmful touching), and false

TABLE 7-3	COMMON LIABILITY ISSUES	
ISSUE	**EXAMPLES**
Patient safety	Failure to take notice of or take action on suicide risks
	Failure to use restraints properly or to monitor the restrained patient
	Miscommunication
	Medication errors
	Violation of boundaries (e.g., sexual misconduct)
	Misdiagnosis
Intentional torts	Voluntary acts intended to bring a physical or mental consequence
	Purposeful acts
	Recklessness
	Not obtaining patient consent
Negligence or malpractice	Carelessness
	Foreseeability of harm
Assault and battery	Reasonable belief that a person means to cause one harm (assault) through harmful or offensive touching (battery)
	Threat to use force, along with opportunity and ability to carry out threat
	Giving treatment without patient's consent
False imprisonment	Intent to confine to a specific area
	Indefensible use of seclusion or restraints
	Detention of voluntarily admitted patient, with no agency or legal policies to support detaining
Defamation of character:	Sharing private information with people who are not directly involved with care
• Slander (spoken)	Posting information on social media sites that identifies specific individuals or organizations and that has the potential
• Libel (written)	to damage their reputation
	Confidential documents shared with people who are not directly involved with care
Invasion of privacy	Taking a picture of your patient without permission
Supervisory liability (vicarious liability)	Inappropriate delegation of duties
	Lack of supervision of those supervising

imprisonment (detention of a patient with no agency or legal policies to support detention) (see Table 7-3).

Other types of intentional torts may hurt a person's sense of self or financial status. These include invasion of privacy and defamation of character. Invasion of privacy in health care has to do with breaking a person's confidences or taking photographs without explicit permission. Defamation of character includes slander (verbal), such as talking about patients on the elevator with others around, and libel (printed), such as sharing written information about the patient with people outside the professional setting.

Unintentional Torts

Unintentional torts are unintended acts that produce injury or harm to another person. Negligence (carelessness) is a general tort for which anyone may be found responsible. For example, if you do not shovel the snow from your driveway, and a visitor falls and breaks a hip, you may be found liable of negligence. Health care providers who fail to act in accordance with professional standards, or who fail to foresee consequences that other professionals with similar skills and education would foresee, can be found responsible as a result of professional negligence, or malpractice. Malpractice is an act or omission to act that breaches the duty of due care and results in or is responsible for a person's injuries. The five elements required to prove negligence are (1) duty, (2) breach of duty, (3) cause in fact, (4) proximate cause, and (5) damages. Foreseeability, or likelihood of harm, is also evaluated.

Duty. When nurses represent themselves as being capable of caring for psychiatric patients and accept employment, a duty of care has been assumed. As a psychiatric mental health nurse, you have the duty to understand the theory and medications used in the care of psychiatric patients, whether they are being treated in a community clinic, general practitioner's office, medical unit, or psychiatric treatment unit. The staff nurse who is responsible for care delivery must be knowledgeable enough to assume a reasonable or safe duty of care for the patients.

The nurse's duty of care includes a duty to intervene when the safety or well-being of the patient or another person is obviously at risk. For example, a nurse who knowingly follows an incorrect or possibly harmful order is responsible for any harm that results to the patient. If you have information that leads you to believe that the physician's orders need to be clarified or changed, it is your duty to intervene and protect the patient. It is important that you communicate the concern to the physician who has ordered the treatment. If the treating physician does not appear willing to consider your concerns, you should carry out your duty to intervene through other appropriate channels. The following vignette illustrates two possible outcomes of a nurse's intervention in a medication issue.

The duty to intervene on the patient's behalf poses legal and ethical dilemmas for nurses in the workplace. Institutions with a chain-of-command policy or other reporting mechanisms offer some assurance that the proper authorities in the administration are notified of nursing concerns. Most patient-care issues regarding physicians' orders or treatments can be settled fairly early in the process through the nurse discussing any concerns with

---

VIGNETTE

Monia is a new nurse on the crisis management unit. She completed the hospital and unit orientations 2 weeks ago and has begun to care for patients independently. As she prepares to give her 1700 hours medications, Monia notices that Greg Thorn, a 55-year-old man admitted after a suicide attempt, has been given a new order for the antidepressant sertraline (Zoloft). Monia remembers that Mr. Thorn had been taking phenelzine (Nardil) before his admission and seems to recall something unsafe about mixing these two medications. She looks up the antidepressants in her drug guide and realizes that Nardil is a monoamine oxidase inhibitor (MAOI) and that adding this second antidepressant within 2 weeks of discontinuing the Nardil could result in severe adverse effects and possibly a lethal response.

After clarifying with Mr. Thorn that he had been on Nardil and discussing the issue with another nurse, Monia realizes that she needs to put the medication on hold and contact Mr. Thorn's psychiatrist, Dr. Cruz. Monia phones him and begins by saying, "I see that Mr. Thorn has been ordered Zoloft. I am looking at his nursing admission assessment, and it says that he had been taking Nardil up until a few days ago. However, I don't see it listed on the medical assessment that was done by the resident."

First Possible Outcome
Dr. Cruz responds, "Thank you for calling that to my attention. When I make my rounds in the morning, I'll decide what to do with his medications. For now, please put a hold on the Zoloft." Monia clarifies what Dr. Cruz has said, writes the order, and documents what happened in the nurses' notes.

Second Possible Outcome
Dr. Cruz responds, "Are you telling me how to do my job? If it wasn't on the medical assessment, then he wasn't taking it. A nurse must have made a mistake—again. I wrote an order for Zoloft, so give him the Zoloft." He hangs up. Monia documents the exchange, determines that the safest and most appropriate response is to hold the medication for now, and contacts her nursing supervisor. The supervisor supports her decision and follows up with the chief of psychiatry.

---

the physician. However, if further intervention by the nurse is required to protect the patient, generally the nurse would notify his or her immediate nursing supervisor, who would discuss the problem with the physician and subsequently, if necessary, the chief of staff of a particular service until a resolution is reached. If there is no time to resolve the issue through the normal process because of a life-threatening situation, the nurse has no choice but to act to protect the patient's life. It is important to follow agency policies and procedures for reporting differences of opinion. If you fail to intervene and the patient is injured, you may be partly liable for the injuries that result because of your failure to use safe nursing practice and good professional judgement.

Breach of duty. Breach of duty is any conduct that exposes a patient to an unreasonable risk of harm, through either commission or omission of acts by the nurse. If you are not capable of providing the standard of care that other nurses would be expected to supply under similar circumstances, you have breached the duty of care. Or if you do not have the required education and experience to provide certain interventions, you have breached the duty by neglecting or omitting the provision of necessary care.

The legal concept of abandonment is another concern of nurses. When a nurse is given an assignment to care for a patient, he or she must provide the care or ensure that the patient is safely reassigned to another nurse, or abandonment occurs. Abandonment also takes place in the absence of accurate, timely, and thorough reporting and in the absence of follow-through of care on which the patient relies.

The same principles apply to the psychiatric mental health nurse working in a community setting. For example, if a suicidal patient refuses to go to the hospital for treatment, you must take the necessary steps to ensure the patient's safety. These actions may include enlisting the assistance of the law in involuntarily admitting the patient on a temporary basis.

Cause in fact, proximate cause, damages, and foreseeability. Cause in fact may be evaluated by asking, "Would this injury have occurred without the nurse's actions?" If the answer is no, the nurse is guilty of causing the injury.

Proximate cause, or legal cause, may be evaluated by determining whether any intervening actions or persons, other than the nurse, were, in fact, the cause of harm to the patient. If it is determined that the harm resulted from intervening persons or actions, the nurse is not guilty of proximate cause.

Damages include actual damages (e.g., loss of earnings, medical expenses, property damage), as well as pain and suffering. They also include incidental or consequential damages. For example, giving a patient the wrong medication may incur actual damage of a complicated hospital stay, but it also may result in permanent disability, which could require such needs as special education and special accommodations in the home. Furthermore, incidental damages may deprive others of the benefits of life with the injured person, such as losing a normal relationship with a husband or father.

Forseeability of harm evaluates the likelihood of the outcome under the circumstances. If the average, reasonable person could foresee that injury could result from the action or inaction, the injury was foreseeable.

KEY POINTS TO REMEMBER

- Deontology, consequentialist theory, virtue ethics, and relational ethics have provided the foundation for nursing ethics and nursing standards of practice.
- Psychiatric mental health nurses frequently encounter ethical dilemmas.
- The provinces and territories have enacted laws (mental health acts) for public health and safety and for the care of those unable to care for themselves. Within these acts are provisions for involuntary admissions to a psychiatric hospital or unit.
- The principle of respect of persons provides the foundation for a person's right to self-determination.
- Provincial, territorial, and federal legislation provides the framework for the development of mental health policies and programs.

- The nurse's privilege to practise carries with it the responsibility to practise safely, competently, and according to provincial, territorial, and federal laws.
- Best practices are determined by standards of practice, standards of care, policies and procedures, and the use of traditional practice knowledge.
- Knowledge of the law, nursing codes of ethics, and the standards of practice for psychiatric mental health nursing are essential for providing safe, effective psychiatric mental health nursing care and will serve as a framework for decision making.

CRITICAL THINKING

1. Noskye and Beth are nurses who have worked together on the psychiatric unit for 2 years. Beth confided to Noskye that her marital situation has become particularly difficult over the past 6 months. He expressed concern and shared his observation that she seems to be distracted and not as happy lately. Privately, Noskye concludes that this explains why Beth has become so irritable and distracted. As Noskye prepares the medication for the evening shift, he notices that two of his patients' medications are missing—both are bedtime lorazepam (Ativan). When he phones the pharmacy to request the missing medications, the pharmacist responds, "You people need to watch your carts more carefully because this has become a pattern." Shortly after, another patient complains to Noskye that he did not receive his 1700 hours alprazolam (Xanax). On the medication administration record, Beth has recorded that she has given the drugs. Noskye suspects that Beth may be diverting the drugs.

   a. What action, if any, should Noskye take? Should he confront Beth with his suspicions?

   b. If Beth admits that she has been diverting the drugs, should Noskye's next step be to report Beth to their supervisor or to the board of nursing?

   c. When Noskye talks to the nursing supervisor, should he identify Beth, or should he state his suspicions in general terms?

   d. How does the nature of the drugs affect your responses? That is, if the drugs were to treat a "physical" condition such as hypertension, would you be more concerned?

e. What does the nurse practice act in your province or territory mandate regarding reporting the illegal use of drugs by a nurse?

2. A 40-year-old man is admitted to the emergency department for a severe nosebleed and has both of his nostrils packed. Because of a history of alcoholism and the possibility for developing delirium tremens (withdrawal), the patient is transferred to the psychiatric unit. His physician has ordered a private room, restraints, continuous monitoring, and 15-minute checks of vital signs and other indicators. At the first 15-minute check, the nurse discovers that the patient has no pulse or respiration. He had apparently inhaled the nasal packing and suffocated.
   a. Does it sound as though the nurse was responsible for the patient's death?
   b. Was the order for the restraint appropriate for this type of patient?
   c. What factors did you consider in making your determination in (b)?

3. Assume that there are no mandatory-reporting laws for impaired or incompetent colleagues in the following clinical situation. A 15-year-old boy is admitted to a psychiatric facility voluntarily at the request of his parents because of violent, explosive behaviour. This behaviour began after his father's recent remarriage that followed his parents' divorce. In group therapy, he has become incredibly angry in response to a discussion about weekend passes for Mother's Day. "Everyone has abandoned me. No one cares!" he screamed. Several weeks later, on the day before his discharge, he convinces his nurse to keep his plan to kill his mother confidential. Consider the CNA code of ethics on patient confidentiality, the principles of psychiatric nursing, and the duty to warn third parties in answering the following questions:
   a. Did the nurse use appropriate judgement in promising confidentiality?
   b. Does the nurse have a legal duty to warn the patient's mother of her son's threat?
   c. Is the duty owed to the patient's father and stepmother?
   d. Would a change in the admission status from voluntary to involuntary (based on an assessment determining that he is a danger to himself or others, has a mental disorder, and is unwilling to voluntarily remain in hospital) protect the patient's mother without violating the patient's confidentiality?
   e. What nursing action, if any, should the nurse take after this disclosure by the patient?

4. Patients admitted to an inpatient psychiatric unit are being recruited for research on a new drug that is hoped to have an impact on the negative symptoms of schizophrenia. The attending psychiatrists are all involved in the research. One of the patients asks a nurse about the experimental medication.
   a. Does the nurse have a responsibility to explain the research to the patient?
   b. Why are the patients involved in this research considered vulnerable?
   c. How can the nurse advocate for vulnerable patients?
   d. What are the documentation responsibilities of the nurses when they observe a medication adverse effect in one of the patients involved in the research?

CHAPTER REVIEW

1. A patient with depression presents with her family in the emergency department. The family feels she should be admitted because "she might hurt herself." An assessment indicates moderate depression with no risk factors for suicide other than the depressed mood itself, and the patient denies any intent or thoughts of self-harm. The family agrees that the patient has not done or said anything to suggest that she might be a danger to herself. Which of the following responses is consistent with the concept of "least restrictive alternative" doctrine?
   a. Admit the patient as a temporary inpatient admission.
   b. Persuade the patient to agree to a voluntary inpatient admission.
   c. Admit the patient involuntarily to an inpatient mental health treatment unit.
   d. Arrange for an emergency outpatient counselling appointment the next day.

2. An advanced-practice nurse wishes to initiate treatment with an antipsychotic medication that, although very likely to benefit the patient, in a small percentage of patients may cause a dangerous adverse effect. The nurse explains the purpose, expected benefits, and possible risks of the medication. The patient readily signs a form accepting the medication, stating, "These pills will poison the demons inside of me." Although he has been informed of the risk for adverse effects, he is unable to state what these are and simply reports, "I won't have side effects because I am iron and cannot be killed." Which of the following responses would be most appropriate under these circumstances?
   a. Begin administration of the medications based on his signed permission because he has legally consented to treatment.
   b. Petition the court to appoint a guardian for the patient because he is unable to comprehend the proposed treatment.
   c. Administer the medications even though consent is unclear because the patient is clearly psychotic and in need of the medications.
   d. Withhold the medication until the patient is able to identify the benefits and risks of both consenting and refusing consent to the medications.

3. A patient incidentally shares with you that he has difficulty controlling his anger when around children because their play irritates him, leading to resentment and fantasies about attacking them. He has a history of impulsiveness and assault, escalates easily on the unit, and has a poor tolerance for frustration. This weekend he has an overnight pass, which he will use to see his sister and her family. As you meet with the patient and his sister just prior to his getting the pass, the sister mentions that she has missed her brother because he usually helps her watch the children, and she has to work this weekend and needs him to babysit. The patient becomes visibly apprehensive upon hearing this. Which of the following responses would best reflect appropriate nursing practice relative to the conflict this situation presents between safety and the patient's right to confidentiality?

a. Cancel the pass without explanation to the sister, and reschedule it for a time when babysitting would not be required of the patient.

b. Suggest that the sister make other arrangements for child care, but withhold the information the patient shared regarding his concerns about harming children.

c. Speak with the patient about the safety risk involved in babysitting, seeking his permission to share this information and advising against the pass if he declines to share the information.

d. Meet with the patient's sister, sharing with her the patient's disclosure about his anger toward children and the resultant risk that his babysitting would present.

4. Mrs. Fujiwara was admitted for treatment of depression with suicidal ideation triggered by marital discord. She has spoken with staff about her fears that the marriage will end, has indicated that she does not know how she could cope if her marriage ended, and has a history of suicide attempts when the marriage seemed threatened in the past. Her spouse visits one night and informs Mrs. Fujiwara that he has decided to file for divorce. Staff members, though aware of the visit and the husband's intentions regarding divorce, take no action, feeling that the 15-minute suicide checks Mrs. Fujiwara is already on are sufficient. Thirty minutes after the visit ends, staff make rounds and discover that Mrs. Fujiwara has hanged herself in her bathroom using hospital pyjamas she had tied together into a rope. Which of the following statements best describes this situation? Select all that apply.

a. The nurses have created liability for themselves and their employer by failing in their duty to protect Mrs. Fujiwara.

b. The nurses have breached their duty to reassess Mrs. Fujiwara for increased suicide risk after her husband's visit.

c. Given Mrs. Fujiwara's history, the nurses should have expected an increased risk for suicide after the husband's announcement.

d. The nurses correctly reasoned that suicides cannot always be prevented and did their best to keep Mrs. Fujiwara safe via the 15-minute checks.

e. The nurses are subject to a tort of professional negligence for failing to increase the suicide precautions in response to Mrs. Fujiwara's increased risk.

f. Had the nurses restricted Mrs. Fujiwara's movements or increased their checks on her, they would have been liable for false imprisonment and invasion of privacy, respectively.

℮volve WEBSITE

Post-Test interactive review

Visit the Evolve website for Chapter Review Answers and Rationales, Critical Thinking Answer Guidelines, and additional resources related to the content in this chapter: http://evolve.elsevier.com/Canada/Varcarolis/psychiatric/

REFERENCES

Andre, J. (2000). Humility reconsidered. In S. B. Rubin & L. Zoloth (Eds.), *Margin of error: The ethics of mistakes in the practice of medicine* (pp. 59–72). Hagerstown, MD: University Publishing Group.

Austin, W., Bergum, V., & Dossetor, J. (2003). Relational ethics. In V. Tshudin (Ed.), *Approaches to ethics* (pp. 45–52). Woburn, MA: Butterworth-Heinemann.

Battlefords and District Co-operative Ltd. v. Gibbs. (1996). 3 S.C.R. 566 (Supreme Court of Canada).

Beauchamp, T. L., & Childress, J. F. (2013). *Principles of biomedical ethics* (7th ed.). New York: Oxford University Press.

Bergum, V., & Dossetor, J. (2004). *Relational ethics: The full meaning of respect.* Hagerstown, MD: University Publishing Group.

Browne, A. (2010). Mental health acts in Canada. *Cambridge Quarterly of Healthcare Ethics, 19,* 290–298. doi:10.1017/S096318011000006X.

Canadian Federation of Mental Health Nurses (2014). *Canadian standards for psychiatric-mental health nursing* (4th ed.). Toronto: Author.

Canadian Institutes of Health Research, Natural Sciences and Engineering Research Council of Canada, & Social Sciences and Humanities Research Council of Canada. (2014). *Tri-council policy statement: Ethical conduct for research involving humans-2.* Retrieved from http://www.pre.ethics.gc.ca/pdf/eng/tcps2-2014/TCPS_2_FINAL_Web.pdf.

Canadian Nurses Association (CNA) (2008). *Code of ethics for registered nurses* (2008 centennial ed.). Ottawa: Author.

Lachman, V. D. (2016). Ethics, law, and policy. Moral resilience: Managing and preventing moral distress and moral residue. *Medsurg Nursing, 25*(2), 121–124. Retrieved from http://www.medsurgnursing.net/cgi-bin/WebObjects/MSNJournal.woa.

Manitoba Provincial Health Ethics Network (2016). *Patient care ethics: Decision-making guide: Framework for clinical or patient-care issues.* Winnipeg: Author.

Meier, A., Csiernik, R., Warner, L., et al. (2015). The stigma scale: A Canadian perspective. *Social Work Research, 39*(4), 213–222. doi:10.1093/swr/svv028.

Mental Health Act. (2010). Revised Statutes of Alberta 2000, Chapter M-13.

Olthuis, J. H. (1997). Face-to-face: Ethical asymmetry or the symmetry of mutuality? In J. H. Olthuis (Ed.), *Knowing other-wise: Philosophy at the threshold of spirituality* (pp. 131–158). New York: Fordham University Press.

Registered Psychiatric Nurses of Canada (RPNC) (2010). *Code of ethics & standards of psychiatric nursing practice.* Edmonton: Author.

Rodney, P., Burgess, M., Phillips, J. C., et al. (2012). Our theoretical landscape: A brief history of health care ethics. In J. Storch, R. Starzomski, & P. Rodney (Eds.), *Toward a moral horizon: Nursing ethics for leadership and practice* (2nd ed., pp. 77–97). Toronto: Pearson Education Canada.

Shaw, J., & Downie, J. (2014). Welcome to the wild, wild north: Conscientious objection policies governing Canada's medical, nursing, pharmacy, and dental professionals. *Bioethics, 28*(1), 33–46. doi:10.1111/bioe.12057.

Snow, N., & Austin, W. J. (2009). Community treatment orders: The ethical balancing act in community mental health. *Journal of Psychiatric and Mental Health Nursing, 16,* 177–186. doi:10.1111/j.1365-2850.2008.01363.x.

Tarasoff v. Regents of the University of California. (1974). 529 P.2d 553, 118 Cal Rptr 129.

Tarasoff v. Regents of the University of California. (1976). 551 P.2d 334, 131 Cal Rptr 14.

Wicclair, M. R. (2011). *Conscientious objection in health care: An ethical analysis.* New York: Cambridge University Press.

World Health Organization (1996). *Mental health care law: Ten basic principles.* Geneva, Switzerland: Author.

World Health Organization (2005). *WHO resource book on mental health, human rights and legislation.* Geneva, Switzerland: Author.

Cultural Considerations for Psychiatric Mental Health Nursing

Gwen Campbell McArthur, Sonya L. Jakubec

KEY TERMS AND CONCEPTS

acculturation
assimilation
colonization
cultural competence
cultural concepts of distress
cultural humility
cultural safety
culture
enculturation
ethnicity
ethnocentrism

Indigenous peoples
medicine wheel
multiculturalism
refugee
social determinants of health
somatization
stereotyping
trauma-informed practice
Western tradition
world view

OBJECTIVES

1. Consider the role of world view and cultural beliefs in Canada and their relation to mental health and mental illness.
2. Discuss the development of cultural safety and competence in the history of psychiatric mental health nursing.
3. Explore the cultural landscape of Canada.
4. Explain the unique mental health and mental illness issues of Indigenous, immigrant, and refugee peoples in Canada.
5. Identify barriers and facilitators to the provision of culturally safe nursing care.
6. Describe various cultural beliefs and practices that can affect mental health or illness.
7. Explain the nurse's role in assessing and working with patients of different cultural backgrounds.
8. Develop culturally sensitive nursing care plans for people from diverse cultures.

⊜volve WEBSITE

Visit the Evolve website for Flashcards, Case Studies, and additional testing resources related to the content in this chapter: *http://evolve.elsevier.com/Canada/Varcarolis/psychiatric/*

Pre-Test interactive review

Canadian psychiatric mental health nursing practice takes place within the rich Indigenous and multicultural contexts of the country. In these contexts, culturally safe practice is a goal and is anchored by approaches to relational inquiry (Hartrick Doane & Varcoe, 2015); broad, systemwide cultural competency (Dreachslin, Gilbert, & Malone, 2013); and trauma-informed practice (BC Provincial Mental Health

and Substance Use Planning Council, 2013). For further information, refer to Chapter 10 and 23. This chapter introduces the concepts of culture particular to the Canadian context, cultural influences on the conceptualization of mental health and illness, and, ultimately, culturally competent care of patients and families who may be experiencing mental illness or mental health problems.

UNDERSTANDING THE LANDSCAPE OF CULTURE IN MENTAL HEALTH

Culture, Race, Ethnicity, and the Social Determinants of Health

All nurses and their clients with mental illness, have a unique culture that influences their individual perspectives and choices. Culture comprises the shared beliefs, values, and practices that guide a group's members in patterned ways of thinking and acting, and includes factors such as religion, geography, socio-economic status, occupation, ability or disability, and sexual orientation. Culture can also be viewed as a blueprint for guiding actions that affect care, health, and well-being (Leininger, McFarland, & Wehbe-Alamah, 2015). *Cultural norms* define how group members make sense of the world and make decisions about how to relate and behave. Cultural norms prescribe what is "normal" and "abnormal" and influence the development of mental health and illness concepts. For example, in Western society, hearing voices and seeing visions is generally viewed as a sign of pathology and deviates from the cultural norms. In some Indigenous cultures, however, vision quests, the seeking of visions, is honoured and valued and would not be viewed as pathological.

Ethnicity refers to the sharing of common traits, customs, and race. Ethnic groups have a common heritage, history, and world view. A world view is a major paradigm used to explain the world and its mysteries, inclusive of beliefs about health, illness, and the hereafter. Three major world views explaining health and illness are magic and religion, empirical science, and holistic health (Andrews & Boyle, 2016). Nurses need to be aware that basic concepts of mental health and illness may differ among ethnic groups, may clash with their own world view, and may affect how nursing care is received and perceived by a patient.

All culture exists within a societal context that has the potential to affect the mental well-being of individuals and of groups. The social determinants of health influence culture and its effects on mental health and mental illness. These determinants are identified as economic status, genetics, job security, employment opportunities, access to safe and affordable housing, child care availability, food security, and inclusion or exclusion from society (World Health Organization, 2008).

Foundational theories derived from Western ideology have guided mental health service delivery and the formation of the Canadian mental health system. However, tensions exist between the divergent world views of the status quo delivering mental health services and those who use the services. Dr. Madeleine Leininger (1991), a nurse anthropologist, identified transcultural nursing as a theoretical approach to cultural skills education, an approach developed from largely Eurocentric perspectives. Cultural safety was later conceptualized by Irihapeti Ramsden, an Indigenous Maori nurse in New Zealand, in response to negative experiences in the health and nursing system. Cultural safety is concerned with power relations between health care professionals and clients and is an experience of particular importance in light of the Indigenous experience of colonization. Broadly, colonization is the invasion, dispossession, and subjugation of peoples. Awareness of cultural safety means that health care providers are aware of their privilege in this context of colonization; they recognize that they are in a powerful role as a health care provider and that their practice transfers that power to the client (Kurtz, Turner, Nyberg, et al., 2014). The history of colonization and abuses of power, experiences of discrimination, and structural barriers that can limit access to appropriate care for people from diverse backgrounds (Mental Health Commission of Canada, 2012) make cultural safety and trauma-informed practice a pivotal consideration in psychiatric mental health practice. Trauma-informed practice is an approach that recognizes the impacts of previous traumatic events on current health and mental health situations. The approach concentrates on relationship building; engagement and choice; awareness; and skills building across individual, interpersonal, and system levels of mental health service. A key aspect of trauma-informed practice is understanding how trauma can be experienced differently by immigrants and refugees, people with developmental disabilities, women, men, children and youth, Aboriginal peoples, and other populations (BC Provincial Mental Health and Substance Use Planning Council, 2013).

Cultural Views and Contexts Affecting Mental Health Care

All psychiatric mental health nursing theories and methods originate within cultural traditions. Psychiatric mental health nursing practice in Canada has historically been informed by borrowed theories from disciplines, such as psychology, that are grounded in the values and belief systems of the dominant Western culture (see Chapter 2). Nursing knowledge of psychology, human growth and development, and mental health and illness is based on traditions from Greek, Roman, and Judeo-Christian thought and the philosophy of Descartes's body–mind dualism. These predominant teachings often hinder nurses' understanding of other cultural groups' world views on mental health.

A group's world view outlines how its members explain and define their responses to life events, their position in the universe, and the phenomena of nature (Andrews & Boyle, 2016). World views shape perceptions about time, health and illness, rights and obligations in society, and acceptable ways of behaving in relation to others and to nature. Consider how your assumptions about personality development, emotional expression, ego boundaries, and interpersonal relationships were formed and how they affect your clinical judgements. Nursing care is designed to promote verbalization of feelings, teach individually focused coping skills, and assist with behavioural and emotional self-control—all consistent with Western cultural ideals. However, psychiatric mental health nurses come from diverse cultural backgrounds themselves and are likely to engage with people who have world views that differ from their own or from the dominant philosophical traditions of Western cultures. A diversity of world views will influence nursing assessments and interventions. Being open to the rich diversity of world views and their impact on mental health and illness is fundamental to culturally competent nursing care. Failing to consider or attempt to understand the world view of the patient and the family will lead to a loss of meaningful communication and an inability to establish trust, the cornerstone of psychiatric mental health nursing. As nurses begin to acknowledge that many of the concepts and interventions enshrined in psychiatric mental health nursing are based on beliefs different from those of many clients and families, they will progress toward culturally safe and competent practice. For highlights of some of the distinct values held within scientific, religious, and holistic world views, see Table 8-1.

In Western tradition (biomedical, scientific traditions), identity arises from one's individuality, and personal accomplishments are underscored by the much-valued autonomy and self-reliance. Mind and body, viewed as separate entities, are treated by different practitioners. Disease has a specific, measurable, and observable cause, and treatment focuses on curing and eliminating the cause. Time is linear, moving forward, and waiting for no one. Success in life is obtained by preparing for the future (Douglas, Pierce, Rosenkoetter, et al., 2011; Kirmayer, Simpson, & Cargo, 2007).

Some other traditions view the family as central to one's identity, and family interdependence and group decision making are the norm. Body–mind–spirit is seen as a single entity (Chan, Ng, Ho, et al., 2006). For example, such ideas predominate in Eastern world views, prevalent in Asia and among many Asian immigrants, and are based on the ancient beliefs of Chinese and Indian philosophers and the spiritual traditions of Confucianism, Buddhism, and Taoism (Chiu, Ganesan, Clark, et al., 2005). Time is circular and recurring, hence a belief in reincarnation. One is born into an unchangeable fate and has a duty to comply. Similarly, the magico-religious view perceives illness as imposed by the gods or fates and, therefore, beyond individual control.

The Indigenous world view of mental health acknowledges the connection between an individual and the collective. It is reflective of the balance that is achieved between physical, emotional, cognitive, and spiritual dimensions (Bellamy & Hardy, 2015). This world view is highlighted in Table 8-2.

The medicine wheel is an ancient symbol that can be interpreted in many ways: the four directions, the four grandfathers, the four components of human nature (physical, mental, spiritual, and emotional). The medicine wheel (see Figure 8-1) also represents a holistic world view of health and illness based on deep personal connections to the natural world and the collective. The four points of the compass, each with a guiding spirit, symbolize stages in the life journey.

While there is diversity among the many groups of Indigenous peoples, some key traditional world views, such as those outlined in Table 8-2, persist. However, Indigenous peoples in Canada, like other Indigenous groups in other parts of the world, have been subject to profound disruption of their traditional views and ways of life through contact with other cultures. For example, during precontact Indigenous societies valued the therapeutic use of herbs, and healing plants were used for treatment of illness (First Nations Health Authority [FNHA], 2011). Colonization has affected Indigenous peoples' practices of all kinds, practices that were traditionally situated on the land, the geography in which we work, play, and live (Vukic, Gregory, Martin-Misener, et al., 2011). Over time the geography and landscape have been

TABLE 8-1	WORLD VIEWS		
	SCIENTIFIC OR BIOMEDICAL	**RELIGIOUS**	**HOLISTIC**
General beliefs	Newest paradigm Belief in human manipulation of chemical and physical processes Reductionism: all life can be reduced to smaller components Determinism: cause and effect can explain everything Mechanism: life forms are viewed as parallel to machines	Belief in God or gods Supernatural controls fate, illness, and health	Ancient viewpoint Balance and harmony in individual and nature must be aligned for health Natural laws are important to uphold Concepts of the Aboriginal medicine wheel (Figure 8-1) and Chinese yin and yang—ideas of balance of natural forces to promote harmony
Dominant cultures	The Western world embraces the biomedical model's explanations of disease and health	Many Latino, African, Caribbean, and Middle Eastern cultures support this view	Indigenous and Asian peoples' traditional perspectives Increasingly accepted in the Western world
Responsibility for health	Individual has responsibility for his or her health	Sense of community: one person's actions may have caused the illness or health of an individual	Mind, body, and spirit are considered so united that there may not be words to indicate them as distinct entities
Explaining illness	Does not consider mystical explanations	A belief in sorcery, breaking of taboos, *mal de ojo* (evil eye), God's will; illness may be a gift whereby one is given responsibility to accept the illness; health is a blessing	Considers explanation of disharmony and imbalance in the cosmos, resulting in illness
Prevention and cure	Science will cure or treat the disease	Prayer alone may change the health of the ill person Techniques include laying on of hands and healing oils	Prevention and living well are the focus, not cure

Source: Derived from Andrews, M. M., & Boyle, J. S. (2016). *Transcultural concepts in nursing care* (7th ed.). Philadelphia: Wolters Kluwer.

TABLE 8-2	KEY CONCEPTS OF TRADITIONAL INDIGENOUS WORLD VIEWS	
WORLD VIEW CONCEPT	**INDIGENOUS**	**NON-INDIGENOUS**
Knowledge	Believe their ancestors are mostly right and thus value the preservation and use of ancestral knowledge. There can be many truths; truths are dependent on individual experiences.	Contemporary or futuristic knowledge valued over ancestral knowledge. Scientific, skeptical. Requiring proof as a basis of belief.
Time	Believe in expansive concepts of time that reach back and forward in time. For example, decisions should consider the impacts on "7 generations" of children to come.	Limited concepts of time usually confined to three generations. There is only one truth, based on science or Western-style law.
Connection	Indigenous peoples believe that they are part of the natural world and are interconnected across time to those who came before and those yet to come. Society operates in a state of relatedness. Everything and everyone is related. People, objects, and the environment are all believed to be connected. Law, kinship, and spirituality reinforce this connectedness. Identity comes from such connections.	Compartmentalized society, becoming more so. Non-Indigenous peoples believe that humans are apart from the natural world and do not perceive a fundamental interconnection to the past or future (with the possible exception of their children or grandchildren).
Health	Indigenous people believe that for a person, family, or community to be healthy, it must have balance between the physical, emotional, cognitive, and emotional aspects of health. All of these aspects of health are interconnected and thus any "treatment" must fully consider the whole person. They also believe that the land is sacred and is linked to culture and healing.	Non-Indigenous peoples believe that health care can be separated into specialized functions. Services to Non-Indigenous peoples tend to distinguish between physical health and mental well-being, with little interconnection between the two. Although there is a commitment to interdisciplinary health practice, the practical reality is that people get treated "one piece at a time."
Place in the world	Indigenous peoples view themselves as a link in a long chain of people who have come before and those who will follow. In this context, you are special to the extent that you live in a good way and pass along the information and values necessary to sustain your group across time.	Non-Indigenous peoples believe in individual as opposed to collective rights and give primacy to the generation that currently exists, with limited attention to the sustainability of their groups over time.

Source: Adapted from Blackstock, C. (2008). *Rooting mental health in an Aboriginal world view: Inspired by Many Hands, One Dream.* Ottawa: The Provincial Centre of Excellence for Child and Youth Mental Health at CHEO. Retrieved from http://www.excellenceforchildandyouth.ca/sites/default/files/position_aboriginal_world_view.pdf.

altered alongside a complex web of social changes and health epidemics like infectious diseases, extensive efforts of spiritual conversion, forced relocations and confinement to parcels of lands called reserves, sedentary lifestyles and prolonged forced absences of family from their traditional communities, and political marginalization. The effects of these historical and contemporary changes have been traumatic for communities, individuals, the collective identity, and the mental health of Indigenous peoples (Bourque-Bearskin & Jakubec, 2016; Kirmayer, Tait, & Simpson, 2009).

Although traumatic events happen to many people of any age or socioeconomic status, Indigenous communities have elevated rates of suicide, addictions, violence, mental illness, over-representation in the justice system, and pervasive demoralization that are consequences of the history of colonization (BC Provincial Mental Health and Substance Use Planning Council, 2013). When widespread trauma occurs—causing feelings of fear, horror, threats to the life of entire families and communities, helplessness, and psychological trauma—the impact of the events do not simply go away. These events have inextricably changed the way people view themselves; their children, parents, and leaders; and their relationship to society (Bellamy & Hardy, 2015; Kirmayer, Tait, & Simpson, 2009; Klinic Community Health, 2013).

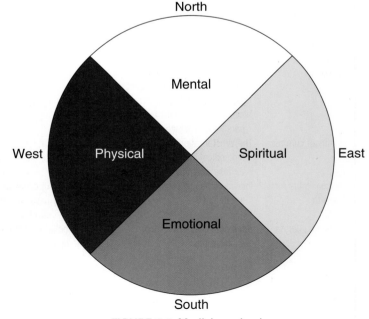

FIGURE 8-1 Medicine wheel.

Culture, Mental Health, and Mental Illness

Cultures are dynamic, changing, and adjusting in relation to their histories and influences from physical, social, historical, and political contexts. The pervasive experience of day-to-day cultural interactions shapes the mental health of both client and health care provider and influences how assessments and observations are conducted (Lo & Pottinger, 2007).

For all cross-cultural encounters, nurses must develop generic cultural competence inclusive of knowledge of the culture's values, locus of control, norms around emotional expression, and perspectives on time. Specific cultural competence is required to work with individual ethnocultural communities to ensure understanding of community norms (Lo & Pottinger, 2007). It is important to avoid stereotyping, the generalized conscious or unconscious conceptualization of a group of people that does not allow for individual differences within the group (Srivastava, 2007). For example, while many Indigenous people are reconnecting with their traditional roots, other Indigenous people may align themselves with Christian perspectives or have a mix of world views.

Diagnostic assessment of a mental illness is based on the interpretation of clinical behaviours and is guided by criteria from the *Diagnostic and Statistical Manual of Mental Disorders (DSM)*, which historically has undervalued sociocultural interpretations of mental health and mental illness. Due to globalization, migration, and the international use of the *DSM-IV*, the new *DSM-5* has broadened the sociocultural considerations within assessment and diagnoses (Alarcon, Becker, Lewis-Fernandez, et al., 2009). This effort addresses the critiques of insensitivity to the context

of people's lives and a lack of cultural awareness within previous editions (O'Mahony & Donnelly, 2007).

Understanding the cultural norms of ethnic groups is necessary to accurately assess behaviours, affect, and cognitions within the context of culture. For example, in Western culture, emotional expressiveness is valued, but some other cultures consider such expressiveness a sign of immaturity. In Western culture, independence and self-reliance are highly valued while the family interdependence valued by other cultures may be considered pathological enmeshment. Classic work by Kleinman (1980) and Kleinman, Eisenberg, and Good (1978) proposed that the environment and culture in which one lives determine the experience of health and illness and the value of treatment options. As such, nurses need to understand the perceptions and behaviours of patients and families within their cultural experience.

Each culture has different patterns of nonverbal communication (Table 8-3), etiquette norms (Box 8-1), beliefs, and values that shape the culture and influence how the culture understands health and illness.

Culture is transmitted to its members through a process called enculturation. Children learn from parents which behaviours, beliefs, values, and actions are "right" and which are "wrong." The culture outlines its acceptable range of options. Deviance from cultural expectations is problematic and frequently is labelled "illness." Mental health is perceived as the degree to which a person fulfills the expectations of the culture. The culture defines which differences are within the range of normal (mentally healthy) and which are outside the range of normal (mentally ill). The same thoughts and behaviours considered

TABLE 8-3 SELECTED NONVERBAL COMMUNICATION PATTERNS

NONVERBAL COMMUNICATION PATTERN	PREDOMINANT PATTERNS IN WESTERN SOCIETY	PATTERNS SEEN IN OTHER CULTURES
Eye contact	Associated with attentiveness, politeness, respect, honesty, and self-confidence	Associated with rudeness, arrogance, challenge, or sexual interest
Personal space	*Intimate space*: 0–0.5 m *Personal space*: 0.5–1 m Entering the intimate space of another person is perceived as aggressive, overbearing, and offensive. Staying more distant than expected is perceived as aloofness.	Personal space is significantly closer or more distant than in North American culture. *Closer*—Middle Eastern, Southern European, and Latin American cultures *Farther*—Asian cultures When closer is the norm, standing close indicates acceptance of the other.
Touch	Moderate touch indicates personal warmth and conveys caring. Often people will ask prior to touching an individual.	Touch norms vary. *Low-touch cultures*—Touch may be considered an overt sexual gesture, a way of "stealing the spirit," or a taboo between women and men. *High-touch cultures*—People frequently touch one another (e.g., linking arms when walking or holding a hand or arm when talking).
Facial expressions and gestures	A nod means "yes." Smiling and nodding means "I agree." Thumbs-up means "good job." Rolling one's eyes while another is talking is an insult.	Raising eyebrows or rolling the head from side to side means "yes." Smiling and nodding means "I respect you." Thumbs-up is an obscene gesture. Pointing one's foot at another is an insult.

Source: Adapted from Narayan, M. C. (2004). Cultural implications for psychiatric mental health nursing. In E. M. Varcarolis & M. J. Halter (Eds.), *Foundations of psychiatric mental health nursing: A clinical approach* (Table 6-3, p. 105). St. Louis: Saunders.

BOX 8-1 NORMS OF ETIQUETTE

Rules for polite behaviour vary greatly from one culture to another. Unless aware of cultural differences in etiquette norms, nurses can infer rudeness from patients who may believe their behaviour to be respectful. Norms of etiquette that vary across cultures include the following:

- Expectation and importance of promptness
- Formality in addressing others
- Which people deserve recognition and honour, and how respect is shown
- Forms of appropriate social touch—for example, shaking hands
- Wearing shoes in the home
- Appropriate dress to be "modest"
- The meaning of acceptance or rejection of hospitality, such as food or drink
- The importance of and length of time that should be given to "small talk" prior to the business at hand
- The directness or subtlety of communication
- The tone of voice and pace of the conversation
- Taboo topics
- The treatment of children in the home—for example, can they be touched and admired?

mentally healthy in one culture can be considered mentally ill in another. For example, many religious traditions view "speaking in tongues" as mentally healthy and as a gift from God, whereas a different cultural group might perceive this activity as psychosis and a sign of mental illness.

Cultural interpretation of behaviours creates challenges for the nurse in conducting appropriate assessments and treatments. Professional socialization and ethnocentrism may cause nurses to unintentionally impose their own cultural norms on members of other cultural groups (Leininger, McFarland, & Wehbe-Alamah, 2015). Ongoing self-awareness can provide clarity about personal and professional beliefs, and encouraging openness to alternative cultural explanations is a starting place to engaging sensitively with all people. Without specific intention, judgement may be imparted in nonverbal communication. The same nonverbal communication can be interpreted differently among cultures (Table 8-3). In North American culture, eye contact is a sign of respectful attention. In other cultures, it may be considered arrogant and intrusive. Dr. Clare Brandt, the first Indigenous psychiatrist in Canada, noted that often Indigenous children's behaviours were erroneously assessed as pathological when judged within the dominant cultural norms. In reality, these children's behaviours were culturally appropriate (Brandt, 1990). Norms of cultural etiquette are discussed in Box 8-1.

THE CULTURAL LANDSCAPE OF CANADA

Indigenous and Multicultural Contexts

All Canadians, with the exception of Indigenous peoples, entered this nation from other countries (British Columbia Public Service Agency, 2012). Indigenous peoples is a collective term that is used in this chapter to identify original peoples and their descendants living in Canada. In 2011, there were more than 1.8 million Indigenous people living in communities throughout the country (Statistics Canada, 2013). Though severely threatened, and in certain cases extinguished by colonial forces, Indigenous culture, language, and social systems have shaped the development of Canada and continue to grow and thrive despite extreme adversity (Parrott, 2015). More recently, the Truth and Reconciliation Commission of Canada (TRC, 2015) and the United Nations Declaration on the Rights of Indigenous Peoples (United Nations, 2007) have established awareness and recognition of Indigenous history and culture. Political pressures from Indigenous peoples and ethnic minorities prompted the recognition of Canadian multiculturalism.

Multiculturalism is a concept or philosophy that recognizes that all cultures have a value of their own and must be equally represented or recognized in the broader society for the worthwhile contributions made by those of diverse ethnic backgrounds (Douglas, Pierce, Rosenkoetter, et al., 2011). In July 1988, Canada became the first country to pass a multiculturalism law, the *Multiculturalism Act*, with the intent of honouring cultural diversity, decreasing discrimination, increasing cultural awareness, and formulating federal government decisions in a culturally sensitive manner (Library of Parliament, 2006). Table 8-4 lists key milestones in Canadian multicultural policy.

In Canada, multiculturalism is also a set of ideals, adopted at the federal, provincial, and municipal levels, celebrating the country's cultural diversity (Library of Parliament, 2006). Six of the ten Canadian provinces have policies on multiculturalism to ensure social justice and cohesion within the changing Canadian society. Census data from 2006 indicated that the percentage of foreign-born people in Canada had reached 19.6%, representing 1 in 5 Canadians (Natural Resources Canada, 2009). Immigration patterns have changed, with Asian and Middle Eastern immigrants composing 59.4% of recent immigrants to Canada; decreasing numbers of European immigrants, with the exception of Romanians; and an increase in African and South American immigrants. These rapid and massive shifts are concentrated in Toronto, Vancouver, and Montreal. Indigenous peoples constitute an increasing proportion of the Canadian population, with 4.4% of the Canadian population identifying some form of Indigenous ancestry (Library of Parliament, 2006). Table 8-5 highlights the countries of birth of recent immigrants to Canada. Their customs and unique perspectives are now more widely recognized and valued. This shifting Canadian demographic demands that nursing practice respond to cultural growth and a change within Canadian society as a whole and that culturally safe and competent care be practised.

Multiculturalism informs nursing practice and challenges nurses to educate themselves to deliver culturally sensitive, competent, holistic care, as required by nursing care standards at provincial and national governance levels. To meet this challenge, nurses must develop self-awareness, monitor their ethnocentrism (the perception that one's own values, beliefs, and behaviours are superior), and be open to diverse world views and conceptualizations of mental health and illness, which will increasingly become part of their practice (Registered Nurses' Association of Ontario, 2007).

TABLE 8-4	DEVELOPMENT OF MULTICULTURAL POLICY

YEARS	MULTICULTURALISM AS PUBLIC POLICY IN CANADA
1947	*Canadian Citizenship Act*: Previously, all citizens were British subjects with a focus on British identity
	Influx of post–World War II immigrants from Europe
1960s	Civil rights movements in the United States reflecting the growing dissatisfaction felt by Canadian racial minorities
	Assertiveness of the Canadian First Nations people to reclaim their rights
	Resentment of ethnic minorities related to their place in society
	Royal Commission on Bilingualism and Biculturalism recognized the contribution of ethnic groups to society
1970s	Beginning of an Integration Policy wherein cultural groups were given the right to identify with select elements of their cultural group
	Work began to incorporate diverse cultural groups into the institutions of Canada
1980s	Expanded multicultural policies; massive immigration; racist problems developed; anti-racism legislation was passed
	Canadian Charter of Rights and Freedoms passed to uphold multiculturalism
	Multiculturalism Act (1988) passed, honouring cultural identity and upholding equal participation in Canadian society
1990s	Formation of a Department of Multiculturalism and Citizenship, emphasizing cross-cultural understanding
	Review of multiculturalism policies with a renewed focus on identify, full participation in society, and social justice
2002	On November 13, 2002, the Government of Canada, by Royal Proclamation, designated June 27 of each year Canadian Multiculturalism Day.

Source: Dewing, M. (1994, updated 2009). *Canadian multiculturalism* (Publication no. PRB 09-20E). Retrieved from http://publications.gc.ca/collections/collection_2010/bdp-lop/prb/prb0920-eng.pdf. Reproduced with the permission of the Library of Parliament, 2013.

MENTAL HEALTH CONCERNS OF INDIGENOUS PEOPLES

Indigenous people disproportionately experience mental health problems, with suicide rates of Inuit people 11 times that of the general population and 4 times that of the general population for First Nations people (Parliament of Canada, 2014). Although all Indigenous populations in the world have undergone the process of colonization, the outcomes of legislation to eradicate certain practices and beliefs have had serious transgenerational consequences on the mental health and well-being of Indigenous peoples in Canada. It is important for psychiatric mental health nurses to be aware of how the history and context of Indigenous peoples and the social determinants of mental health have influenced mental health and illness for Indigenous peoples in Canada.

Intergenerational Trauma

For more than 500 years since first contact between the Indigenous peoples of Canada and dominant immigrant settler nations, Indigenous communities were displaced and disconnected from their traditional ways (Linklater & Mehl-Madrona, 2014). Consequent government policies and legislation signalled forced cultural genocide and attempts at assimilation of Indigenous peoples who had lived peacefully on the land for thousands of years prior to first contact with colonization and foreign settlers. The *Indian Act* of 1876 laid the foundation that would drastically change traditional Indigenous lives in Canada. Rather than remaining self-sufficient, "the Indian" became subjects of Canada considered inferior to their non-Indigenous counterparts and monitored by a system of constant surveillance (Government of Canada, 2016a, 2016b). The experience of colonization in Canada created a legacy of historical social and political injustices characterized by cultural oppression, displacement from traditional lands, incarceration of children in government-run Indian Residential Schools (IRSs), and removal of children by child

TABLE 8-5	TOP 10 COUNTRIES OF BIRTH OF RECENT IMMIGRANTS,* 1981 TO 2006				
RANK	2006 CENSUS	2001 CENSUS	1996 CENSUS	1991 CENSUS	1981 CENSUS
1	People's Republic of China	People's Republic of China	Hong Kong	Hong Kong	United Kingdom
2	India	India	People's Republic of China	Poland	Viet Nam
3	Philippines	Philippines	India	People's Republic of China	United States
4	Pakistan	Pakistan	Philippines	India	India
5	United States	Hong Kong	Sri Lanka	Philippines	Philippines
6	South Korea	Iran	Poland	United Kingdom	Jamaica
7	Romania	Taiwan	Taiwan	Viet Nam	Hong Kong
8	Iran	United States	Viet Nam	United States	Portugal
9	United Kingdom	South Korea	United States	Lebanon	Taiwan
10	Colombia	Sri Lanka	United Kingdom	Portugal	People's Republic of China

*"Recent immigrants" refers to landed immigrants who arrived in Canada within 5 years prior to a given census.
Source: Statistics Canada. (2008). *Censuses of population, 1981 to 2006.* Retrieved from http://www.statcan.gc.ca/pub/11-008-x/2008001/article/10556-eng.htm#2.

welfare authorities (Bourque-Bearskin & Jakubec, 2016; Legacy of Hope Foundation, 2010a, 2010b).

These experiences have resulted in intergenerational loss of traditional family values, leading to a breakdown of the nuclear family and community structures and, therefore, to social and economic challenges (Legacy of Hope Foundation, 2010a, 2010b). These traumatic experiences reverberate in subsequent generations as close-knit community networks cope with layers of psychic pain and disruptions in the social fabric (Campbell McArthur, 2009).

This legacy of colonization contributes to the elevated rates of alcoholism, suicide, domestic violence, and community demoralization, in addition to the social problems experienced in many communities (Kirmayer, Tait, & Simpson, 2009). For example, the Inuit people of Nunavut face tremendous social problems, with high incidences of suicide, domestic violence, and substance abuse, as well as overcrowding, unemployment, and legal difficulties. Societal changes, socioeconomic conditions, and interpersonal problems contribute to increased mental health needs (Law & Hutton, 2007).

Hopelessness and Suicide

Suicide and self-inflicted injuries are the leading causes of death for First Nations youth and adults up to 44 years of age. Approximately 55% of all Indigenous people are under 25 years of age. Suicide rates for Inuit youth are among the highest in the world, at 11 times the national average (Tempier, 2016). Between December 12, 2015, and March 16, 2016, six people, most of them youth, died by suicide in Pimicikamak Cree Nation. Dozens of others in this community of approximately 6 000 made attempts following these deaths, with more than 150 students—in a school of about 1 200—placed on a suicide watch list. During this time, band leaders declared a state of emergency, catapulting the crisis into the headlines and highlighting what the top Indigenous chief in Canada has deemed a national suicide epidemic that reaches well beyond Pimicikamak (Baum, 2016). The community of Attawapiskat in Northern Ontario reported a further 11 deaths by suicide in July 2016. Children as young as 10 years old reportedly died by suicide in other Indigenous communities in 2016. For more information on assessment of and intervention for suicide, refer to Chapter 22.

Family Violence and Separation and Community Violence

High rates of family violence, sexual abuse, incarceration, and emotional distress underscore the significance of historical trauma on the current mental health and societal problems facing many Indigenous peoples (Statistics Canada, 2013). The multiple traumas and revictimization that many Indigenous people endure are linked to complex trauma responses, which require strong, culturally sensitive intervention programs.

The intergenerational trauma is further exacerbated by family disunity as children are placed in the care of child welfare agencies. Mistrust and fear of these authorities resonates from the 1960s, when large numbers of children of Indigenous ancestry were removed from their families and placed for adoption (Duff, Bingham, Simo, et al., 2014). While Indigenous children continue to be over-represented in the child welfare system, women experience disproportionately higher levels of violence in terms of both incidence and severity and are disproportionately represented in the number of missing and murdered women across Canada (Oppal, 2012).

Relationship and community violence experienced among Indigenous communities has not been met with a thorough response by policing and legal systems (Carbone-Lopez, 2013; McCall & Lauridsen-Hoegh, 2014; Oppal, 2012). In 2016, a long-awaited inquiry into the root causes of the disproportionate rates of violent crime against Indigenous women and girls was initiated (Narine, 2016). For further discussion, see Chapter 25.

Substance Use

Although high proportions of mental health problems exist, most visible among them substance use issues (Assembly of First Nations, National Native Addictions Partnership Foundation, & Health Canada, 2011), mental health services are underused by Indigenous populations. Substance use disorders have reached epidemic proportions in many areas, and many Indigenous women become street involved in either sex or the drug trade (Native Women's Association of Canada, 2010).

As an integral part of the healing process, the National Native Alcohol and Drug Abuse Program (NNADAP) provides Indigenous-specific programs and inpatient, outpatient, and residential treatment for addictions. It provides direction and identifies opportunities to ensure that individuals, families, and communities have access to appropriate, culturally relevant services. There are approximately 53 Indigenous addiction treatment centres across the country that are not only used by Indigenous people but also open to other funding agencies. Barriers to access and cumbersome referral processes that require many pages of information and consents often hinder recovery. Like other specialist services, wait lists as long as 6 months and limited local detoxification resources continue to challenge many health authorities.

Need for Culturally Relevant and Appropriate Services

Colonization—the process whereby a people are overcome by a more powerful group, and the views, philosophies, values, and beliefs of the powerful group are imposed on the original inhabitants of the land—has left a legacy of grief for many Indigenous peoples who live with historical oppression, the effects of postcolonization, and a lack of culturally appropriate and sensitive mental health therapies. While general psychiatric treatment focuses on individuals, the problems affecting the mental health of many Indigenous people involve problems relating with others, including family members, social networks, their communities, and governmental structures (Kirmayer, Brass, & Valaskakis, 2009).

Recent theories of trauma indicate that those who have lived through traumatic events often experience shame due to feelings of powerlessness. Addressing trauma and resulting mental health and substance use problems can often be greatly feared and avoided, leading to secrecy and further embedding experiences of shame and stifling recovery (Duff, Bingham, Simo, et al., 2014; Klinic Community Health, 2013). Historical losses have created anger, discomfort, and mistrust of Western world views and practices (Kirmayer, Brass, & Valaskakis, 2009). The disease-focused paradigm of the biomedical model contrasts dramatically with the holistic model of Indigenous health and healing (Tang, Community Wellness Program, & Jardine, 2016). Consideration of the impact of the collective identity and political situations of Indigenous peoples is crucial for promoting healing (McCormick, 2009). However, most mental health services do not incorporate an Indigenous understanding of mental health, illness, and healing (Vukic, Rudderham, & Martin-Misener, 2009). Communities with higher levels of knowledge about traditional languages and in which Indigenous languages were widely spoken were among those that reported more than 50% fewer suicides than those that had lost their languages. Other dynamic influences that helped in creating more positive and healthier environments and resilience for both a community and its individual members are listed as protective factors; examples include "cultural continuity" (Chandler & Lalonde, 2008), self-government, control of land, control of education, command of police and fire services, cultural activities, and, most importantly, control and administration of health services (FNHA, 2011).

The establishment of the TRC in 1996 and reporting from that commission in 2015 have begun a process of formally documenting the truth about IRSs and how they have contributed to the mental health of and social conditions in Indigenous communities. Through this process, Indigenous communities have resumed greater ownership for health services. British Columbia has formed the First Nations Health Authority (FNHA), the first health authority of its kind in Canada (see Figure 8-2). In 2013, the FNHA assumed the programs, services, and responsibilities formerly handled by Health Canada's First Nations Inuit Health Branch—Pacific Region.

MENTAL HEALTH CONCERNS OF IMMIGRANTS

Eighteen percent of the Canadian population is made up of immigrants. Generally, immigrants to Canada are more physically and mentally healthy and use the health care system less than the Canadian-born population. This may be because of strong entry-screening measures. Immigrants' health issues and use of

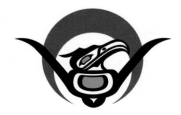

FIGURE 8-2 First Nations Health Authority logo. Health through wellness. Source: First Nations Health Authority. (2011). *Our history, our health.* Retrieved from http://www.fnha.ca/wellness/our-history-our-health.

the health care system align with those of the Canadian-born population as their length of residence increases (Statistics Canada, 2002).

While data on mental health problems and mental illness are sparse, certain factors may predispose immigrants to mental health problems. During their first 10 years in Canada, 30% of immigrants live in poverty, a known risk factor for developing mental health problems. Immigrants may experience acculturative stress in attempting to adapt to a new culture, negotiating new norms, and seeking meaningful employment (Samuel, 2009). For example, South Asian immigrant women in Atlantic Canada experienced acculturative stress in several ways: (1) self-perceived inability to adapt to the new country, (2) limited employment, (3) discrimination, (4) depression, and (5) interfamily and intergenerational conflicts (Samuel, 2009). In a study documenting the experiences of Chinese immigrant women in Canada, adverse life events related to employment and financial strain in the settlement period contributed to their sense of depression (Tang, Oatley, & Toner, 2007). Immigrant women are particularly vulnerable to mental illness and mental health problems due to their multiple social roles and limited autonomy (Reitmanova & Gustafson, 2009). In addition to assisting immigrants in a meaningful way, services need to be sensitive to language and culture and based on an understanding of the social context in which immigrants and refugees live (Chow, Law, & Andermann, 2009; Simich, Maiter, Moorlag, et al., 2009).

Immigrants and their families embark on a process of acculturation—learning and adopting the beliefs, values, and practices of their new cultural setting. Some immigrants adapt to the new culture quickly, absorbing the new world view, beliefs, values, and practices until these are more natural than the ones they learned in their homeland (assimilation). Others attempt to maintain their traditional cultural ways. Some become bicultural—able to move between their traditional culture and new culture, depending on where they are and with whom they associate. Some immigrants may suffer culture shock, finding the new norms disconcerting or offensive because they contrast so deeply with their traditional beliefs, values, and practices.

Children may assimilate into the new culture at a rapid pace while elders may maintain their traditional culture, predisposing families to intergenerational conflict. The hierarchical traditional status of elders may be challenged by children who are assimilating different values. Some children may feel caught between two cultures and unsure of where to place their cultural identity, similar to Indigenous youth who feel a disconnect between traditional ways of living and modern society (Iarocci, Root, & Burack, 2009).

For immigrant peoples, accessing mental health services may be problematic due to language barriers and stigma. Materials about mental illness and mental health care are needed in a variety of languages, in conjunction with strong outreach services (O'Mahony & Donnelly, 2007). Resources outside of formal medical services, such as social workers, health workers, and enhanced family support workers, may be better able to offer suitable services (Lai, 2007). Note that some Indigenous people who do not speak English as a first language experience some of the same issues related to accessing mental health services.

RESEARCH HIGHLIGHT

Mental Health and Well-Being of Recent Immigrants in Canada: Evidence From the Longitudinal Survey of Immigrants to Canada

Problem

According to the 2006 Census, the proportion of the foreign-born population in Canada is at the highest level it has been in 75 years. Therefore, the well-being of recent immigrants has powerful consequences for our current and future success as a nation. The process of immigration and settlement is inherently stressful, and the well-being of recent immigrants is of particular concern, primarily when migration is combined with additional risk factors such as unemployment and language barriers.

Purpose of Study

Canadian research on the mental health of recent immigrants, more specifically on the disparities among immigrant subgroups, is limited. While it is suggested that recent immigrants experience better mental health than other Canadians or immigrants who have resided longer in Canada, it is unclear whether this health advantage persists over time. This paper examines the different aspects related to mental health and well-being during the initial 4 years after landing. Specifically, this research explored the following questions:

1. What are the mental health outcomes of recent immigrants, specifically the incidence of emotional problems and stress, after arrival in Canada?
2. Are there differences between immigrant subgroups (e.g., refugee, family class immigrants, economic class immigrants) in terms of mental health outcomes after arrival in Canada?
3. What are the social, demographic, and economic factors that are associated with emotional problems and stress?

Methods

Using data from the Longitudinal Survey of Immigrants to Canada, this secondary statistical analysis used measures of incidence and prevalence with description examining different aspects related to mental health and well-being during the initial 4 years after landing, including prevalence of emotional problems, emotional help received, stress levels, and main sources of stress. Potential factors associated with the incidence of emotional problems and stress that were measured included sociodemographic, socioeconomic, social networking variables, and health utilization effects, and psychosocial variables were also explored through logistic regression.

Key Findings

Results showed that about 29% of immigrants reported having emotional problems and 16% reported high levels of stress. Descriptive and regression results suggested that females were more likely to report experiencing emotional problems. Immigration category (e.g., refugee, family immigration) was associated with the prevalence of emotional problems and stress. Refugees were significantly more likely to report experiencing emotional problems and high levels of stress compared to other immigrants. Region of origin was found to be associated with the prevalence of emotional problems. Immigrants from South and Central America were most likely to report experiencing emotional problems. Immigrants from North America, United Kingdom, and Western Europe were less likely to report experiencing emotional problems, compared to those from Asia and Pacific. Recent immigrants in the lowest income brackets were significantly more likely to report experiencing high levels of stress and emotional problems compared to those in the highest income quartile. Finally, it was found that recent immigrants' perceptions of the settlement process were related to emotional problems. Immigrants who were neutral or dissatisfied with the settlement process were more likely to report experiencing emotional problems than those who were satisfied.

Implications for Nursing Practice

These findings support the importance of mental health service provision to immigrants, which became an area of concentration for the Mental Health Commission of Canada. Strategies of community-based integrated mental health services that address social interventions in a preventive scope are gender and life stage sensitive and recognize both the challenges and the resilience of diverse groups of migrants. Further, this study has implications for focused policy and practice specifically concerned with immigrant women and with immigrants who arrive as refugees.

Source: Robert, A. M., & Gilkinson, T. (2012). Mental health and well-being of recent immigrants in Canada: Evidence from the Longitudinal Survey of Immigrants to Canada. Ottawa: Citizenship and Immigration Canada. Retrieved from http://www.cic.gc.ca/english/pdf/research-stats/mental-health.pdf.

MENTAL HEALTH CONCERNS OF REFUGEES

A refugee is a person who is seeking asylum in a new country due to threat of trauma or actual trauma and violation of human rights. Refugees in Canada have left their homeland to escape intolerable conditions. Refugee families, inclusive of their children, may require mental health assistance to adjust to their new surroundings and to feel a sense of safety and security. Many refugees from the Middle East, Southeast Asia, Central America, and Africa have been traumatized by war, genocide, torture, starvation, and other catastrophic events. Many have lost family members, a way of life, and a homeland to which they can never return. The mental health problems most commonly faced by refugees include anxiety, depression, grief responses, and, notably,

a risk for post-traumatic stress disorder related to their past experiences (Statistics Canada, 2006). The recent introduction of large numbers of refugees from government- and private-sponsored groups across Canada has highlighted the concerns of refugee mental health.

As discussed in Chapter 1, mental illness focuses on diagnosable patterns of behaviour or thinking that may need treatment. Although there is evidence of increased rates of post-traumatic stress disorder, depression, and adjustment problems among refugee children, it must be emphasized that only a very small number of refugees will develop a mental illness (Mental Health Commission of Canada, 2016). Even though a minority of refugees will develop problems, they are a high-risk group for mental health problems or illnesses, which can be complex.

Mental health promotion, resilience, the building of social support, and the prevention of mental illness through good planning of resettlement, education, and action on the social determinants of health are fundamental aspects of a good strategy. Trauma-informed practice approaches are crucial to culturally safe care and cultural competency for refugee populations (refer also to Chapters 22 and 24). In this type of care, most often nonclinical interventions (including a safe environment, food security, educational and employment opportunities, and social supports) related to resettlement are effective in treating symptoms (Hassan, Kirmayer, MekkiBerrada, et al., 2015). A focus on trauma-informed care with relationship building and social support so that refugees experience trust, comfort, and safety in sharing their traumatic experiences and psychological symptoms is often the most helpful approach, one that avoids pathologizing the normal response to abnormal and traumatic circumstances (Mental Health Commission of Canada, 2016; see also Chapter 22 for further discussion and psychiatric mental health nursing strategies).

BARRIERS AND FACILITATORS TO MENTAL HEALTH CARE IN A MULTICULTURAL CONTEXT

A multicultural context, such as in Canada, exposes many potential barriers to mental health care that must be attended to, including stigma and discrimination, communication barriers, client self-stigma about using mental health services or receiving a psychiatric diagnostic label, a lack of culturally safe and appropriate services (McCall & Lauridsen-Hoegh, 2014), misdiagnosis due to unrecognized cultural differences, and ethnic variations in pharmacodynamics, all of which influence the mental health status of Indigenous, immigrant, and refugee peoples and their use of health care services.

Stigma and Discrimination

The 10-year antistigma campaign Opening Minds, initiated by the Mental Health Commission of Canada in 2009, recognizes that stigma and discrimination are a reality that people with mental illness face (Corrigan & Wassel, 2008). Cultural beliefs, superstitions, and poor understanding of mental illness contribute to fear, stereotyping, and avoidance of people with mental illness. This stigma results in people concealing their illness and delaying or refusing treatment and follow-up care (Corrigan, Morris, Michaels, et al., 2012; Corrigan & Wassel, 2008). People with mental illness and their families face stigma and stigma by association because of mental illness. Stigma affects health determinants such as housing, since discrimination limits consumers' abilities to secure safe and affordable housing. People with comorbid mental illness and physical disability are doubly jeopardized by stigma from both society and health care professionals (Bahm & Forchuk, 2008).

The reality of recovery from mental illness is further complicated within many cultural contexts. Among cultural groups that emphasize the interdependence and harmony of the family, mental illness may be perceived as a failure of the family. Influenced by these values and perceptions, the pressures on both the person experiencing a mental illness and their family are increased since the illness is thought to reflect on the character of all family members. Stigma and shame can result in avoidance of the formal health care system; therefore, people from cultures where this shame predominates may enter the mental health care system only at an advanced stage of illness, when the family has exhausted its ability to cope with the problem (Na, Ryder, & Kirmayer, 2016). While great strides have been made through numerous campaigns and expanded global awareness, misunderstanding and stigmatization continue to be experienced on a number of personal, cultural, and institutional levels (Gaebel, Rössler, & Sartorius, 2017), warranting nursing care and community interventions related specifically to stigma.

Communication Barriers

Relational practice centred on listening to the stories of patients and families with humility (Anderson & Mitchell, 2016) requires deep listening and therapeutic communication, yet in the Canadian multicultural context, nurses and clients and families often do not speak the same language. In addition, emotional states can be difficult to accurately describe even in one's first language. In mental health nursing, communication and collateral data gathered from family members and loved ones are important methods used to understand a client's situation. When a language barrier prevents understanding of what is happening, problems are likely to occur: for the client, hesitancy to seek out mental health services, and for the nurse, a tendency to avoid or stereotype certain patients. O'Mahony and Donnelly (2007) found, for example, that Asian immigrants underused health care services due to language barriers and cultural beliefs about health and treatment options.

The use of translators is one strategy for overcoming communication barriers. Several cautions apply when a professional translator is used. The translator should be informed that his or her role is to translate what the client or family states, not to apply meaning to the client's communication (O'Mahony & Donnelly, 2007). The translator should be matched to the patient as closely as possible in gender, age, social status, and religion. The translator alerts the nurse to the meaning of cultural norms and thus acts as a cultural broker, interpreting both language and culture. Translators should not be relatives or friends of the patient, since the stigma of mental illness may prevent accurate portrayal of the situation (Srivastava, 2007). As well, informal translators may not have the language skills needed to meet the complex demands of translation in health care settings. Certain concepts may be so strongly culturally linked that an adequate translation is very difficult (Andrews & Boyle, 2016).

Nonverbal communication patterns are influenced by culture, so they also need to be interpreted within the context of the client's culture. For example, anecdotally, in some Indigenous languages there are no specific words or phrases about mental health or mental illness. Some clients may not know if their relatives experienced mental disorders, but they use a description of behaviours they may observe or sense. In these cases, assessments or interview questions may be met with extended silence. Although this might be mistaken as resistance, silence could make sense for the interaction. Silences in these cases may be employed as a pause, to listen with respect for the asker and to

BOX 8-2	COMMUNICATION TIPS FOR OVERCOMING LANGUAGE BARRIERS

- Avoid using complex words and jargon.
- Explain why you need to ask any questions.
- Always check that you understood the meaning of words the person has used and vice versa.
- Use diagrams, models, film/video and images to explain concepts, instructions and terms.
- Be cautious about using traditional languages or words unless you have excellent understanding.
- If required, seek help from local Indigenous resources like Elders, Band Office Health Staff of Indigenous health organizations in your area.

Source: Queensland Government. (2015). *Aboriginal and Torres Straight Islanders: Cultural capability.* Retrieved from https://www.health.qld.gov.au/__data/assets/pdf_file/0021/151923/communicating.pdf.

reflect on the appropriate response. Box 8-2 provides some general tips to overcome language barriers.

Misdiagnosis

One reason for misdiagnosis of mental illness in culturally diverse people is the use of culturally inappropriate psychometric instruments and diagnostic tools. Most available tools have been validated using subjects of European origin. For instance, Kim (2002) stated that although there are more than 40 validated depression scales, they tend to be "linguistically irrelevant and culturally inappropriate" (p. 110) for some groups. Kim argues that the current scales measure Western ways of expressing depression by focusing on the affective domain, whereas, for others, more attention needs to be given to the somatic domain. In cultures in which the body and mind are seen as one entity or in cultures in which there is a high degree of stigma associated with mental illness, people frequently *somatize* their feelings of psychological distress. With **somatization**, psychological distress is experienced as physical problems instead of being perceived as emotional or affective pain. For example, a Cambodian woman may describe feelings of back pain, fatigue, and dizziness and say nothing about feelings of sadness or hopelessness (Henderson, Yeung, Fan, et al., 2016). Many cross-cultural mental health experts are skeptical about using the criteria of the *DSM* for diagnosing mental illness because these criteria are based on studies that do not represent cultural diversity (Marsella, 2003). *DSM-5* has addressed some of these concerns.

The Glossary of Cultural Concepts of Distress in *DSM-5* was an attempt to recognize cultural presentations of illness. **Cultural concepts of distress** are sets of signs and symptoms that are common in a limited number of cultures but virtually nonexistent in most other cultural groups (Henderson, Yeung, Fan, et al., 2016; see Box 8-3). Better understanding of idioms of distress can assist in understanding and in communication from cultural (rather than pathologizing) perspectives (Kaiser, Haroz, Kohrt, et al., 2015).

Cultural concepts of distress or illnesses may seem foreign to Canadian-trained nurses, as these illnesses are poorly

BOX 8-3	EXAMPLES OF CULTURAL CONCEPTS OF DISTRESS

The following are examples of commonly recognized cultural concepts of distress:
- *Ataque de nervios*: Latin American. Characterized by a sudden attack of trembling, palpitations, dyspnea, dizziness, and loss of consciousness. Thought to be caused by an evil spirit and related to intolerable stress. Treated by an *espiritista* (spiritual healer) and by family and community support, which provides aid and considers the patient to be calling for help in a culturally acceptable way.
- **Ghost sickness:** Navajo. Characterized by "being out of one's mind," dyspnea, weakness, and bad dreams. Thought to be caused by an evil spirit. Treated by overcoming the evil spirit with a stronger spiritual force that the healer, a "singer," calls forth through a powerful healing ritual.
- **Being hit by bad medicine:** Indigenous. Characterized by feelings of malaise (emotional, physical, psychological, and spiritual) caused by deliberate use of bad medicine by another; believed to be able to cause death (E. G. McGillivary, personal communication, January 7, 2012).
- *Hwa-Byung*: Korean. Characterized by epigastric pain, anorexia, palpitations, dyspnea, and muscle aches and pains. Thought to be caused by a lack of harmony and suppressed anger. Treated by re-establishing harmony.
- **Neurasthenia:** Chinese. Characterized by somatic symptoms of depression (e.g., anorexia, weight loss, fatigue, weakness, trouble concentrating, insomnia), although feelings of sadness or depression are denied. Thought to be related to a lack of yin–yang balance.
- *Susto*: Latin American. Characterized by a broad range of somatic and psychological symptoms. Thought to be related to a traumatic incident or fright that caused the patient's soul to leave the body. Treated by an *espiritista* (spiritual healer).
- **Wind illness:** Chinese, Vietnamese. Characterized by a fear of cold, wind, or drafts. Derived from the belief that yin–yang and hot–cold elements must be in balance or illness occurs. Treated by keeping very warm and avoiding foods, drinks, and herbs that are considered to have a cold quality, as well as "cold" colours, emotions, and activities. Also treated by pulling the "cold wind" out of the patient by coining (vigorously rubbing a coin over the body) or cupping (applying a heated cup to the skin, creating a vacuum).

conceptualized in the Western biomedical perspective. However, these illnesses are well understood by the cultural group, which can name the problem, its etiology, its course, and its treatment. Accounts of illness are often told in a cultural narrative, a person's story that is well articulated and involves all significant psychosocial relationships and egocentric elements. When treated in corresponding culturally prescribed ways, the remedies are frequently effective. Kleinman's classic work serves as a guide to how culture is interlinked with health, illness, and health care. Kleinman (1980) suggested that three sectors of influence—professional, popular (family, community, social network), and folk—interact. Negotiations between the client, family, and health care provider are critical and must consider the culture, history, and environment of the client. Some of the cultural concepts of distress appear to be mental health problems that manifest in somatic ways. For example, *Hwa-Byung* and neurasthenia have many similarities to depression (Park, Kim, Kang, et al., 2001), but because the somatic complaints are prominent, and patients deny feelings of sadness or depression, the symptoms may not fit the *DSM-5* diagnostic criteria for depression.

Ataque de nervios and ghost sickness are characterized by abnormal behaviours culturally understood as illness and are culturally acceptable ways to express overwhelming stress. *Susto*, or "soul loss," occurs after a traumatic incident (Lim, 2006). From a Western perspective, the client may be experiencing depression, anxiety, or post-traumatic stress disorder, but the patient believes that he or she is experiencing the illness of soul loss. Similarly, some Indigenous people will strongly believe that their symptoms are caused by "bad medicine" deliberately sent to harm them. Some authors have suggested that anorexia nervosa and bulimia may be bound to European and North American cultural groups that place a high value on thinness (Marsella, 2003).

If culture is not considered in diagnosis and treatment, practitioners are more likely to see culturally normal behaviour as "abnormal" instead of merely different. For example, what some may view as delusional or hallucinatory behaviour may be part of a vision quest from an Indigenous perspective. Ross (1992) suggested that historical experiences of trauma were compounded by a loss of cultural traditions such as dance or song that would have helped Indigenous people to express and grieve their losses. Such historical experiences of many Indigenous peoples may have made them more attuned to their senses and receptive to alternative ways of being. Nurses often work in environments that are dominated by biomedical perspectives, which may dismiss other potential perspectives and subtly (or not so subtly) create barriers to cultural safety. Nurses require ongoing education to understand alternative explanations for illness and to develop cultural competence in their practice (Registered Nurses' Association of Ontario, 2007).

Ethnic Variation in Pharmacodynamics

There is a growing realization that the actions and effects of many drugs vary among diverse genetic–ethnic groups of people. For example, findings from drug studies performed with European-American subjects may not be valid for other ethnically diverse populations. Genetic variations in drug metabolism are documented for several drugs classifications, including anti-depressants and antipsychotics (Henderson, Yeung, Fan, et al., 2016). The relatively new field of ethnopharmacology investigates the genetic and ethnic variations in drug pharmacokinetics. Many drugs are metabolized in part by the more than 20 cytochrome P450 (CYP) enzymes present in human beings (Henderson, Yeung, Fan, et al., 2016). Genetic variations in enzymes, however, may alter drug metabolism and tend to be propagated through different racial and ethnic populations (Henderson, Yeung, Fan, et al., 2016). Some genetic variations result in rapid metabolism, resulting in minimization of the therapeutic effects; others may result in poor metabolism. With slow metabolism, serum levels become high, increasing intolerable adverse effects.

While science supports the genome theories, little has been written about Indigenous peoples' genetic variations. Much myth and stereotyping can be perpetuated without careful consideration.

For instance, the myth that Indigenous people have a genetic predisposition for alcohol intolerance or "addiction" is not supported by scientific evidence; rather, there is evidence that Indigenous people are more likely to abstain from alcohol or less frequently consume alcohol than non-Indigenous people. Despite these facts, assumptions are frequently made in health care settings, a form of discrimination and stereotyping that has a direct impact on Indigenous people's health and access to care (Ward, 2016). Current practice requires that nurses be critical, research literate, and aware of ethnic variations in drug metab-olism and monitor for unwanted adverse effects. Munoz and Hilgenberg (2005) have suggested the following interventions to minimize risk:

- Maintain a knowledge base on drugs likely to cause adverse responses in people from various ethnic groups.
- Monitor and document drug responses, and give the lowest possible safe dose.
- Carry out cultural assessments with all patients, avoiding stereotyping and myth.
- Incorporate cultural context in nursing education to client and family.

CULTURAL COMPETENCE IN PSYCHIATRIC MENTAL HEALTH NURSING

In a rapidly changing global health perspective, Canada has taken critical steps toward moving cultural safety into education. After the release of *Cultural Competency and Safety: A Guide for Health Care Administrators, Providers and Educators* (National Aboriginal Health Organization, 2008), which provides a working definition of culturally safe practice and programming, significant part-nerships were formed with the Association of Faculties of Medicine of Canada (AFMC), the Canadian Association of Schools of Nursing, the Canadian Nurses Association, the Indigenous Physicians Association of Canada (IPAC), and the Canadian Indigenous Nurses Association. These partnerships have generated frameworks for medical and nursing curricula to teach students and faculty how to build competency in cultural safety (Aboriginal Nurses Association of Canada, 2009; IPAC & AFMC, 2009). These efforts are focused on practices of cultural safety (Jefferies, 2016) and are supported by Health Canada, which has responsibility for administering and providing health care services to First Nations and Inuit communities.

CULTURALLY COMPETENT CARE

As discussed, nurses require cultural competence to assist patients and their families to maintain and achieve mental health and well-being. With the changing demographics of Canadian society, the recognition of the legacy of IRSs, and the effects of poverty, nurses in community and acute psychiatric care environments will routinely encounter patients whose lived experiences challenge nurses to examine ethnocentric views and be open to alternative explanations of behaviours. But how, exactly, are psychiatric mental health nurses to practise culturally competent care?

Cultural competence is the ability of nurses to apply knowledge and skill appropriately in cross-cultural situations (Srivastava,

2007). Having cultural sensitivity or awareness is an essential component of cultural competence. Culturally competent care goes beyond culturally sensitive care by adapting care to meet the patient's cultural needs and preferences (Narayan, 2006).

Campinha-Bacote (2007, 2008) constructed a model, the Process of Cultural Competence in the Delivery of Healthcare Services, to assist nurses in providing culturally competent care. This model requires nurses to view themselves as becoming culturally competent and as lifelong learners, open to learning from the immense cultural diversity of patients and families. The model consists of five constructs that promote the journey toward cultural competence:

1. Cultural awareness
2. Cultural knowledge
3. Cultural encounters
4. Cultural skill
5. Cultural desire

Cultural Awareness

The culturally aware nurse recognizes the enormous impact culture makes on patients' health values and practices, how and when patients decide they are ill and need care, and what treatments they will seek when illness occurs. Cultural awareness encourages nurses to practise self-awareness and recognize that the norms of their own ethnic and professional cultures seem "right" (ethnocentrism) but only because these norms are what they know. Cultural awareness guides the nurse to examine all beliefs, values, and practices to ascertain which are cultural and which may be universally held (Campinha-Bacote, 2007). The process of cultural awareness and cultural humility guides the nurse to recognize ethnocentricity and remain respectful of each patient's cultural norms.

Nurses who examine their cultural definitions and underlying assumptions of mental health and illness, "healthy" self-concept, "healthy" family, and the "right way" to behave in society are practising cultural awareness. Assumptions and expectations about how people express psychological distress require consideration in all assessments. Culturally biased assumptions may be the foundation of evidence-informed guidelines (derived from studies with dominant populations), so guidelines may thus require modification to address cultural diversity within nursing practice (Campinha-Bacote, 2007).

The Registered Nurses' Association of Ontario's (2007) document on cultural diversity suggests that four key concepts influence the delivery of culturally sensitive care within a culturally sensitive health care environment: globalization of society, human rights issues, workplace environment, and nursing shortages. Health care organizations are positively affected by a climate of diversity, group diversity (e.g., inclusion, communication, knowledge sharing), and individual characteristics related to cultural background, ethnicity, values, and beliefs.

Cultural Knowledge

Nurses can enhance their cultural knowledge by attending cultural events and programs, developing friendships with members of diverse cultural groups, and participating in events at which members of diverse groups speak. Cultural knowledge may also be obtained by studying resources designed for health care providers. Cultural knowledge increases our awareness of diverse world views and values, alerts us to cultural differences, and deepens our understanding of behaviours that might otherwise be misinterpreted. Cultural knowledge helps nurses to establish rapport, ask the right questions, avoid misunderstandings, and identify cultural variables that may need to be considered when planning nursing care (Narayan, 2002).

Cultural Encounters

Srivastava (2007) differentiates between stereotyping and the making of generalizations, noting that making generalizations that identify patterns of behaviour and knowledge related to a culture can be a helpful starting point for nurses. However, nurses need to be cautious about stereotyping people and acknowledge that there are individual variations within any culture. Individuals are a unique blend of the many ethnic, religious, socioeconomic, geographical, educational, and occupational cultures to which they belong. They have unique personalities, life experiences, and creative thoughts that contribute to their self-development and to the choices they make about which cultural norms to adopt or abandon.

Multiple cultural encounters enable nurses to personally experience diversity within cultural groups and help them understand that, although there are patterns that characterize a culture, individual members may adhere to the culture's norms in diverse ways. Through such encounters, nurses can develop confidence in cross-cultural interactions and skill at recognizing and avoiding the cultural pain that can occur when nursing care causes the patient discomfort or offence by failing to be culturally sensitive (Ehrmin, 2016). Nurses can become aware of signs of cultural pain (e.g., a patient's feeling of alienation) and recover trust and rapport by asking what has caused the offence, apologizing for insensitivity, and expressing willingness to provide culturally sensitive care.

Cultural Skill

Cultural skill is the ability to perform a cultural assessment in a sensitive way (Campinha-Bacote, 2008). A nurse's first step should be to establish meaningful rapport. If there is a language barrier, a professional medical translator should be engaged.

Many cultural clinical guidelines and assessment tools are available to guide psychiatric mental health nurses in multicultural practice. The voices of those who receive care should be incorporated in relational practice thoughout the psychiatric health care experienced (Baklien & Bongaardt, 2014; Canadian Federation of Mental Health Nurses, 2014). For example, Kleinman, Eisenberg, and Good (1978) proposed the following questions as a useful mental health assessment tool:

- Where are you from? (community, nation, Indigenous group)
- What do you call this illness? (diagnosis)
- When did it start? Do you know why it night have happened then? (onset)
- What do you think caused it? (etiology)

- How does the illness work? What does it do to you? (course)
- How long will it last? Is it serious? (prognosis)
- How have you treated the illness? How do you think it should be treated? (treatment)

These questions allow the patient to feel heard and understood and elicit information about cultural concepts of distress. They can be expanded to include questions such as the following:

- What are the chief problems this illness has caused you?
- What do you fear most about this illness? Do you think it is curable?
- Do you know others who have had this problem? What happened to them? Do you think this will happen to you?

A conversational approach is generally more effective than using a direct, formal approach. One indirect technique is to ask the patient, "What does your family think is wrong? Why do they think it started? What do they think you should do about it?" After the patient describes what the family thinks, the nurse can ask in a manner if the patient agrees.

Another technique for promoting openness is to make a declaratory statement before asking the questions. For instance, before asking about cultural treatments the patient has tried, the nurse can first say, "Everyone has remedies they find helpful when they are ill. Are there any special healers or treatments you have used or that you think might be helpful?"

Some areas that deserve special attention during an assessment interview are the following:

- Ethnicity, religious affiliation, and degree of acculturation to Western medical culture
- Spiritual practices important to preserving or regaining health
- Degree of proficiency in speaking and reading English
- Dietary patterns, including foods prescribed for sick people
- Attitudes about and experiences with pain in a Western medical setting
- Attitudes about and experience with Western medications
- Cultural remedies such as medicine people, intuitive healers, herbs, and practices the patient may find helpful
- Who the patient considers "family," who they are related to, who should receive health information, and how decisions are made
- Cultural customs the patient feels are essential and is fearful will be violated in the mental health care setting

The purpose of a culturally sensitive assessment is to develop a therapeutic plan that is mutually agreeable, culturally acceptable, and potentially productive of positive outcomes. While gathering assessment data, nurses should identify cultural patterns that may support or interfere with the patient's health and recovery process. Nursing knowledge then becomes integrated with the patient's cultural norms alongside the Western medical perspective.

The first Indigenous female psychiatrist in Canada, Corniela Wieman (2006), advised that Indigenous clients will need time and opportunity to develop trust in a helping relationship so that cultural strengths can blend together for improved mental health. Further, some people will prefer traditional ways of healing. A renegotiation of boundaries and the nurse honouring the helpful components of traditional ways together with Western theories can form the basis of a culturally sensitive approach

| BOX 8-4 | SOME CULTURAL CLINICAL GUIDELINES AND ASSESSMENT TOOLS |

- Giger and Davidhizar's Transcultural Assessment Model (in *Giger's Transcultural Nursing: Assessment and Intervention*, 7th edition, Elsevier.)
- Leininger's Inquiry Guide for Kinship and Social Factors (in *Transcultural Nursing: Concepts, Theories, Research and Practice*, 4th edition, page 137)
- Calgary Family Assessment Model: How to Apply in in Clinical Practice (http://www.familynursingresources.com/dvds.htm)
- First Nations Health Authority's Creating A Climate For Change (http://www.fnha.ca/wellness/cultural-humility)
- College of Nurses of Ontario's *Practice Guideline: Culturally Sensitive Care* (http://www.cno.org/Global/docs/prac/41040_CulturallySens.pdf)
- Aboriginal Nurses Association of Canada's *Cultural Competence and Cultural Safety in First Nations, Inuit and Métis Nursing Education* (https://www.uleth.ca/dspace/bitstream/handle/10133/720/An_Integrated_Review_of_the_Literature.pdf?sequence=1)
- Srivastava, R. (2012). *Developing health organizations for a culturally diverse society.* Toronto: Elsevier Canada. (http://www.ryerson.ca/content/dam/omh/pdfs/ktf_markhamstouffville_jan31.pdf).
- Aboriginal Relations Behavioural Competencies. (http://www2.gov.bc.ca/gov/content/careers-myhr/job-seekers/about-competencies/aboriginal-relations)
- New South Wales Government Australia. (2016). Transcultural Assessment Checklist (TAC): A practical guide for cultural assessment. http://www.dhi.health.nsw.gov.au/Transcultural-Mental-Health-Centre/Programs-and-Campaigns/GPs/Cultural-Resource-Kit/Assessment-Guidelines-and-Tools/default.aspx.
- Paniagua, F. A., & Yamada, A. M. (2013). *Handbook of multicultural mental health: Assessment and treatment of diverse populations* (2nd ed.). Amsterdam: Elsevier/Academic Press.
- Health Canada & Assembly of First Nations. (2014). *The First Nations Mental Wellness Continuum (the Continuum).* Retrieved from http://www.hc-sc.gc.ca/fniah-spnia/pubs/promotion/_mental/2014-sum-rpt-continuum/index-eng.php.

(Wieman, 2006). Including compatible culture-specific interventions assists nurses to build on the patient's coping and healing systems (Box 8-4). For example, First Nations people with substance abuse problems may find ceremonies such as sweat lodges, sharing circles, and medicine wheel concepts more appropriate to their therapeutic program than standardized interventions. Finally, when cultural patterns are determined harmful (e.g., if a patient is taking an herb that is contraindicated with the prescription medication), the nurse is responsible for alerting the patient and the mental health care team to these risks. Throughout this work, cultural humility is central to the therapeutic relationship and cultural assessment of the psychiatric mental health nurse. **Cultural humility** is a process of self-reflection and humbly recognizing oneself as a learner about the experience of another, with the responsibility to grow, and awareness that therapeutic relationships are reciprocal and formed, over time, with mutual respect (Anderson & Mitchell, 2016; Asbill, 2013). This approach to cultural assessment as a mutual learning process necessitates that the nurse engage in a process of self-reflection to understand personal and systemic biases and to develop and maintain respectful processes and relationships based on mutual trust (FNHA, 2016). Relational inquiry approaches (Refer to Chapters 9 and 10) are also instructive in this mutual learning process.

Cultural Desire

The final construct in Campinha-Bacote's (2008) cultural competence model for psychiatric mental health nurses is cultural desire. Cultural desire indicates that the nurse is not acting out of a sense of duty but out of a genuine concern for the patient's welfare. Nurses exhibit cultural desire through patience, consideration, and empathy. Cultural desire enables the nurse to achieve good outcomes with culturally diverse patients.

KEY POINTS TO REMEMBER

- *Culture* is the shared beliefs, values, and practices of a group that shape their thinking and behaviour in patterned ways. Cultural groups share their norms with new members of the group through enculturation.
- Mental health and illness are biological, psychological, social, and cultural phenomena.
- A group's culture influences its members' world view, nonverbal communication patterns, etiquette norms, and ways of viewing the person, the family, and the "right" way to think and behave in society.
- The concept of mental health is formed within a culture, and deviance from cultural expectations can be defined as "illness" by other group members.
- Psychiatric mental health nursing is based on personality and developmental theories advanced by Europeans and Americans and grounded in Western cultural ideals and values.
- Nurses are influenced by their own professional and ethnic cultures, as are patients. Nurses must guard against ethnocentric tendencies leading to cultural imposition.
- In the multicultural Canadian context, nurses will be caring for more people from diverse cultural groups.
- Nurses are challenged to deliver culturally competent care, inclusive of culturally congruent assessments and interventions.
- Barriers to quality mental health care include communication barriers, ethnic variations in psychotropic drug metabolism, and misdiagnoses caused by culturally inappropriate diagnostic tools.
- Colonization, including the residential school system and national assimilation policies, has resulted in intergenerational trauma of Indigenous peoples in Canada, significantly contributing to their social and mental health problems.
- Immigrants may experience acculturative stress related to resettlement. Refugees may develop post-traumatic stress because of past horrific experiences.
- Cultural competence consists of five constructs: cultural awareness, cultural knowledge, cultural encounters, cultural skill, and cultural desire.
- Through cultural awareness, nurses recognize their own cultural beliefs, values, and practices.
- Cultural knowledge is obtained by seeking cultural information from friends, attending cultural programs, immersing oneself in the culture, and consulting print and online sources.
- Cultural encounters help nurses to avoid stereotyping individuals.
- Cultural desire is a genuine interest in the patient's perspective; it enables nurses to provide flexible and respectful care to patients of all cultures.

CRITICAL THINKING

1. Describe the cultural factors that have influenced the development of Western psychiatric mental health nursing practice. Contrast these Western influences with the cultural factors that influence Indigenous ways of healing.
2. Discuss the impact of assimilation policies such as the residential school system on the current mental health and social problems of Indigenous peoples in Canada.
3. Analyze the effects that cultural competence (or incompetence) can have on psychiatric mental health nurses, their patients, and their patients' families.
4. How can barriers such as misdiagnosis and communication problems impede competent psychiatric mental health care? What can health care team members do to overcome such barriers?
5. Consider what types of programs might reinforce street youth's resilience and survival skills.

CHAPTER REVIEW

1. Mr. Yeung, a recent immigrant from China, has been admitted to the observation unit for investigation of unspecified physical malaise. His family tells the nurse that Mr. Yeung began to exhibit certain behaviours when his import business declined and his creditors demanded money. He has subsequently made vague physical complaints for the past 6 weeks. Which patient behaviour would alert the nurse to the potential for somatization?
   a. The patient states, "I am so sad that I don't know what to do."
   b. The patient shows the nurse bottles of medication used to treat anxiety.
   c. The patient presents with concerns involving back pain, dizziness, and fatigue.
   d. The patient states, "My doctor diagnosed me with bipolar disorder."

2. Mr. Oliva has been admitted to the psychiatric ward for depression and substance abuse, mainly of alcohol and recreational drugs. As you are explaining his diagnoses and the potential treatment plan to him, his wife and he state that the problem is "ghost sickness," which came about when his mother died. What is the most therapeutic nursing response?
   a. "I have no idea what 'ghost sickness' is."
   b. "Please explain what you mean by 'ghost sickness.'"
   c. "There is not a disorder known as 'ghost sickness.'"
   d. "Why do you believe in evil spirits?"

3. You are a nurse in an outpatient well-baby clinic. You are planning care for a young Cree mother and her infant. The young mother has been identified as at risk for postpartum depression. Which intervention is most appropriate?
   a. Assess whether the patient follows traditional Cree beliefs.
   b. Contact an elder from Indigenous Services.
   c. Discuss the medicine wheel concept of healing with the patient.
   d. Contact a "singer" to provide a healing ritual within 3 days of admission.

4. You are a nurse on a busy medical unit with a multicultural clientele. In your orientation to the unit, you learn that individualism is a concept closely aligned with North American values. When caring for clients with diverse cultural backgrounds, which general nursing action would be most appropriate?
   a. Maintain eye contact at all times.
   b. Assume that personal space is significantly closer than the nurse's personal space.
   c. State, "You can beat this diagnosis; you are in control of yourself."
   d. Ask if the family should be included in the decision-making process.

5. You are a flight nurse who is bringing a young Inuit man from Nunavut for psychiatric assessment in a Winnipeg hospital. You assess the client as acutely suicidal. Which goal is appropriate?
   a. Patient will visit with a cultural leader from the Inuit community.
   b. Patient will experience rebalance of yin–yang by discharge.
   c. Patient will identify sources that increase "cold wind" within 24 hours of admission.
   d. Patient will be put on suicidal observation and assessment.

⊖volve WEBSITE

| Post-Test | interactive review |

Visit the Evolve website for Chapter Review Answers and Rationales, Critical Thinking Answer Guidelines, and additional resources related to the content in this chapter: http://evolve.elsevier.com/Canada/Varcarolis/psychiatric/

REFERENCES

Aboriginal Nurses Association of Canada (2009). *Cultural competency and cultural safety in nursing education: A framework for First Nations, Inuit, and Métis nursing.* Ottawa: Author. Retrieved from https://cna-aiic.ca/~/media/cna/page-content/pdf-en/first_nations_framework_e.pdf.

Alarcon, R. D., Becker, A. E., Lewis-Fernandez, R., et al. (2009). Issues for DSM-V: The role of culture in psychiatric diagnosis. *The Journal of Nervous and Mental Disease, 197*(8), 559–560. doi:10.1097/NMD.0b013e3181b0cbff.

Anderson, B., & Mitchell, V. (2016). *The importance of story in cultural safety. Cultural Safety and Cultural Humility Webinar Action Series.* Retrieved from http://www.fnha.ca/Documents/FNHA-BCPSQC-Cultural-Safety-Webinar-3-Poster.pdf.

Andrews, M. M., & Boyle, J. S. (2016). *Transcultural concepts in nursing care* (7th ed.). Philadelphia: Wolters Kluwer.

Asbill, A. W. (2013). *Reflections on cultural humility.* Washington, DC: American Psychological Association. Retrieved from http://www.apa.org/pi/families/resources/newsletter/2013/08/cultural-humility.aspx.

Assembly of First Nations, National Native Addictions Partnership Foundation, & Health Canada (2011). *Honouring our strengths: A renewed framework to address substance use issues among First Nations people in Canada.* Ottawa: Government of Canada.

Bahm, A., & Forchuk, C. (2008). Interlocking oppressions: The effect of a comorbid physical disability on perceived stigma and discrimination among mental health consumers in Canada. *Health and Social Care in the Community, 17*(1), 63–70. doi:10.1111/j.1365-2524.2008.00799.x.

Baklien, B., & Bongaardt, R. (2014). The quest for choice and the need for relational care in mental health work. *Medicine, Health Care, and Philosophy, 17*(4), 625–632. doi:10.1007/s11019-014-9563-z.

Baum, K. B. (2016). *Manitoba community seeks answers as youth suicides soar.* The Globe and Mail, March 11. Retrieved from http://www.theglobeandmail.com/news/national/a-community-seeks-answers-as-youth-suicides-soar/article29199297/.

BC Provincial Mental Health and Substance Use Planning Council. (2013). *Trauma-informed practice guide.* Retrieved from http://bccewh.bc.ca/wp-content/uploads/2012/05/2013_TIP-Guide.pdf.

Bellamy, S., & Hardy, C. (2015). *Understanding depression in Aboriginal communities and families.* Prince George, BC: National Collaborating Centre for Aboriginal Health.

Bourque-Bearskin, L., & Jakubec, S. L. (2016). Indigenous health: Working with First Nations people, Inuit and Metis. In M. Stanhope, J. Lancaster, S. L. Jakubec, et al. (Eds.), *Community health nursing in Canada* (3rd ed., pp. 382–409). Toronto: Elsevier Canada.

Brandt, C. C. (1990). Native ethics and rules of behaviour. *Canadian Journal of Psychiatry*, 35(6), 534–539.

British Columbia Public Service Agency (2012). *Implementation guide: Aboriginal relations behavioural competencies.* Victoria: Province of British Columbia. Retrieved from http://www2.gov.bc.ca/gov/content/careers-myhr/job-seekers/about-competencies/aboriginal-relations.

Campbell McArthur, G. (2009). *Is the theory of historical trauma accepted by Canadian Aboriginal people? Providing voice for survivors of Indian Residential Schools.* Wagga Wagga, New South Wales, Australia: Charles Sturt University.

Campinha-Bacote, J. (2007). *The process of cultural competence in the delivery of healthcare services: The journey continues.* Retrieved from http://www.transculturalcare.net/Cultural_Competence_Model.htm.

Campinha-Bacote, J. (2008). Cultural desire: "Caught" or "taught"? *Contemporary Nurse*, 28(1–2), 141–148.

Canadian Federation of Mental Health Nurses (2014). *Canadian standards for psychiatric-mental health nursing* (4th ed.). Toronto: Author.

Carbone-Lopez, K. (2013). Across racial/ethnic boundaries: Investigating intimate violence within a national sample. *Journal of Interpersonal Violence*, 28(1), 3–24. doi:10.1177/0886260512448850.

Chan, C. L., Ng, S. M., Ho, R. T., et al. (2006). East meets West: Applying Eastern spirituality in clinical practice. *Journal of Clinical Nursing*, 15(7), 822–832. doi:10.1111/j.1365-2702.2006.01649.x.

Chandler, M. J., & Lalonde, C. E. (2008). Cultural continuity as a protective factor against suicide in First Nations youth. *Horizons—A Special Issue on Aboriginal Youth, Hope or Heartbreak: Aboriginal Youth and Canada's Future*, 10(1), 68–72.

Chiu, L., Ganesan, S., Clark, N., et al. (2005). Spirituality and treatment choices by South and East Asian women with serious mental illness. *Transcultural Psychiatry*, 24(4), 630–656. doi:10.1177/1363461505058920.

Chow, W., Law, S., & Andermann, L. (2009). ACT tailored for ethnocultural communities of metropolitan Toronto. *Psychiatric Services*, 60(6), 847. doi:10.1176/appi.ps.60.6.847.

Corrigan, P. W., Morris, S. B., Michaels, P. J., et al. (2012). Challenging the public stigma of mental illness: A meta-analysis of outcome studies. *Psychiatric Services*, 63(10), 963–973. doi:10.1176/appi.ps.005292011.

Corrigan, P. W., & Wassel, A. (2008). Understanding and influencing the stigma of mental illness. *Journal of Psychosocial Nursing and Mental Health Services*, 46(1), 42–48.

Douglas, M. K., Pierce, J. U., Rosenkoetter, M., et al. (2011). Standards of practice for culturally competent nursing care: 2011 update. *Journal of Transcultural Nursing*, 22(4), 317–333. doi:10.1177/1043659611412965.

Dreachslin, J. L., Gilbert, M. J., & Malone, B. (2013). *Diversity and cultural competence in health care: A systems approach.* San Francisco: John Wiley & Sons.

Duff, P., Bingham, B., Simo, A., et al. (2014). The "stolen generations" of mothers and daughters: Child apprehension and enhanced HIV vulnerabilities for sex workers of Aboriginal ancestry. *PLoS ONE*, 9(6), e99664. doi:10.1371/journal.pone.0099664.

Ehrmin, J. T. (2016). Transcultural perspectives in mental health nursing. In M. M. Andrews & J. S. Boyle (Eds.), *Transcultural concepts in nursing care* (5th ed., pp. 272–316). Philadelphia: Wolters.

First Nations Health Authority (FNHA). (2011). *Our history, our health.* Vancouver: Author. Retrieved from http://www.fnha.ca/wellness/our-history-our-health.

Gaebel, W., Rössler, W., & Sartorius, N. (2017). *The stigma of mental illness: End of the story?* Cham, Switzerland: Springer.

Government of Canada. (2016a). Indian Act. Ottawa: Minster of Justice. Retrieved from http://laws-lois.justice.gc.ca/PDF/I-5.pdf.

Government of Canada. (2016b). *Indigenous peoples and human rights in Canada.* Retrieved from http://www.canada.pch.gc.ca/eng/1448633333977.

Hartrick Doane, G. H., & Varcoe, C. (2015). *How to nurse: Relational inquiry with individuals and families in changing health care contexts.* Philadelphia: Wolters Kluwer/ Lippincott Williams & Wilkins.

Hassan, G., Kirmayer, L. J., MekkiBerrada, A., et al. (2015). *Culture, context and the mental health and psychosocial wellbeing of Syrians: A review for mental health and psychosocial support staff working with Syrians affected by armed conflict.* Geneva: United Nations High Commissioner for Refugees. Retrieved from http://www.unhcr.org/55f6b90f9.pdf.

Henderson, D. C., Yeung, A., Fan, X., et al. (2016). Culture and psychiatry. In T. A. Stern, J. F. Rosenbaum, M. Fava, et al. (Eds.), *Comprehensive clinical psychiatry* (pp. 907–916). Philadelphia: Mosby.

Iarocci, G., Root, R., & Burack, J. A. (2009). Social competence and mental health among Aboriginal youth: An integrative developmental perspective. In L. J. Kirmayer & G. Valaskakis (Eds.), *The mental health of Canadian Aboriginal peoples: Transformations of identity and community* (pp. 80–106). Vancouver: UBC Press.

Indigenous Physicians Association of Canada (IPAC) & Association of Faculties of Medicine Canada (AFMC). (2009). *First Nations, Inuit, Métis health core competencies: A curriculum framework for undergraduate medical education.* Retrieved from https://afmc.ca/pdf/CoreCompetenciesEng.pdf.

Jefferies, M. R. (2016). *Teaching cultural competence in nursing and health care: Inquiry, action, and innovation* (3rd ed.). New York: Springer Publishing Company, LLC.

Kaiser, B. N., Haroz, E. E., Kohrt, B. A., et al. (2015). "Thinking too much": A systematic review of a common idiom of distress. *Social Science & Medicine (1982)*, 147, 170–183. doi:10.1016/j.socscimed.2015.10.044.

Kim, M. (2002). Measuring depression in Korean Americans: Development of the Kim depression scale for Korean Americans. *Journal of Transcultural Nursing*, 13, 109–117. doi:10.1177/104365960201300203.

Kirmayer, L. J., Brass, G. M., & Valaskakis, G. G. (2009). Conclusion: Healing, intervention and tradition. In L. J. Kirmayer & G. G. Valaskakis (Eds.), *Healing traditions: The mental health of Aboriginal peoples in Canada* (pp. 440–480). Vancouver: UBC Press.

Kirmayer, L. J., Simpson, C., & Cargo, M. (2007). Healing traditions: Culture, community and mental health promotion with Canadian Aboriginal peoples. *Australasian Psychiatry*, 11(s1), S15–S23. doi:10.1046/j.1038-5282.2003.02010.x.

Kirmayer, L. J., Tait, C., & Simpson, C. (2009). The mental health of Aboriginal peoples in Canada: Transformations of identity and community. In L. J. Kirkmayer & G. G. Valaskakis (Eds.), *Healing traditions: The mental health of Aboriginal peoples in Canada* (pp. 3–35). Vancouver: UBC Press.

Kleinman, A. (1980). Major conceptual and research issues for cultural (anthropological) psychiatry. *Culture, Medicine and Psychiatry*, 4(1), 3–13.

Kleinman, A., Eisenberg, L., & Good, B. (1978). Culture, illness and care: Clinical lessons from anthropologic and cross-cultural research. *Annals of Internal Medicine*, 88, 251–258.

Klinic Community Health (2013). *Trauma-informed: The trauma toolkit* (2nd ed.). Winnipeg: Author.

Kurtz, D. L. M., Turner, D., Nyberg, J., et al. (2014). Social justice and health equity: Urban aborignal women's action for health forum. *The International Journal of Health, Wellness, and Society*, 3(4), 13–26.

Lai, D. W. L. (2007). For better or worse: Elderly Chinese immigrants living alone in Canadaz. *International Journal of Aging*, 92, 107–122.

Law, S., & Hutton, E. (2007). Community psychiatry in the Canadian Arctic: Reflections from a 1 year continuous consultation series in Iqaluit, Nunavut. *Canadian Journal of Community Mental Health*, 26(2), 123–140.

Legacy of Hope Foundation. (2010a). *About residential schools.* Retrieved from http://www.legacyofhope.ca.

Legacy of Hope Foundation. (2010b). *Where are the children?* Retrieved from http://www.legacyofhope.ca.

Leininger, M. (1991). *Culture care diversity and universality: A theory of nursing.* New York: National League for Nursing Press.

Leininger, M. M., McFarland, M., & Wehbe-Alamah, H. B. (2015). *Culture care diversity and universality: A worldwide nursing theory* (3rd ed.). Burlington, MA: Jones & Bartlett.

Library of Parliament. (2006). *Canadian multiculturalism.* Retrieved from http://www.parl.gc.ca/Content/LOP/ResearchPublications/prb0920-e.htm.

Lim, R. F. (2006). *Clinical manual of cultural psychiatry.* Arlington, VA: American Psychiatric Publishing.

Linklater, R., & Mehl-Madrona, L. (2014). *Decolonizing trauma work: Indigenous stories and stratgies*. Winnipeg: Fenwood Publishing.

Lo, H. T., & Pottinger, A. (2007). Mental health practice. In R. H. Srivastava (Ed.), *The health care professionals' guide to clinical cultural competence* (pp. 247–263). Toronto: Mosby Canada.

Marsella, A. J. (2003). Cultural aspects of depressive experience and disorders. In W. J. Lonner, D. L. Dinnel, S. A. Hayes, et al. (Eds.), *Online readings in psychology and culture* (Unit 9, Chapter 4). Retrieved from http://www.wwu.edu/culture/Vontress.htm.

McCall, J., & Lauridsen-Hoegh, P. (2014). Trauma and cultural safety: Providing quality care to HIV-infected women of Aboriginal descent. *The Journal of the Association of Nurses in AIDS Care, 25*(1S), S70–S78, doi. http://dx.doi.org/10.1016/j.jana.2013.05.005.

McCormick, R. (2009). Aboriginal approaches to counselling. In L. J. Kirkmayer & G. G. Valaskakis (Eds.), *Healing traditions: The mental health of Aboriginal peoples in Canada* (pp. 337–353). Vancouver: UBC Press.

Mental Health Commission of Canada (2012). *Changing directions, changing lives: The mental health strategy for Canada*. Calgary: Author. Retrieved from http://strategy.mentalhealthcommission.ca/download/.

Mental Health Commission of Canada. (2016). *Supporting the mental health of refugees to Canada*. Retrieved from http://www.mentalhealthcommission.ca/sites/default/files/2016-01-25_refugee_mental_health_backgrounder_0.pdf.

Munoz, C., & Hilgenberg, C. (2005). Ethnopharmacology. *The American Journal of Nursing, 105*(8), 40–48.

Na, S., Ryder, A. G., & Kirmayer, L. J. (2016). Toward a culturally responsive model of mental health literacy: Facilitating help-seeking among east Asian immigrants to North America. *American Journal of Community Psychology, 58*(1–2), 211–225. doi:10.1002/ajcp.12085.

Narayan, M. C. (2002). Six steps towards cultural competence: A clinician's guide. *Home Health Care Management and Practice, 14*, 378–386. doi:10.1177/1084822302014005010.

Narayan, M. C. (2006). Culturally relevant mental health nursing: A global perspective. In E. M. Varcarolis, V. B. Carson, & N. C. Shoemaker (Eds.), *Foundations of psychiatric mental health nursing: A clinical approach* (5th ed., pp. 99–113). Philadelphia: Saunders.

Narine, S. (2016). *Missing and murdered Indigenous women and girls: Commission has authority to conduct MMIWG inquiry as "they see fit"*. *Windspeaker*, August 3. Retrieved from http://www.ammsa.com/content/missing-and-murdered-indigenous-women-and-girls.

National Aboriginal Health Organization (2008). *Cultural competency and safety: A guide for health care administrators, providers and educators*. Ottawa: Author.

Native Women's Association of Canada. (2010). *Fact sheet: Missing and murdered Aboriginal women and girls*. Ottawa: Author. Retrieved from https://nwac.ca/wp-content/uploads/2015/05/Fact_Sheet_Missing_and_Murdered_Aboriginal_Women_and_Girls.

Natural Resources Canada. (2009). *The atlas of Canada*. Retrieved from http://atlas.nrcan.gc.ca/site/english/dataservices/wallmaps.html.

O'Mahony, J. M., & Donnelly, T. T. (2007). Health care providers' perspective of the gender influences on immigrant women's mental health care experiences. *Issues in Mental Health Nursing, 28*(10), 1171–1188. doi:10.1080/01612840701581289.

Oppal, W. (2012). *Forsaken: The report of the Missing Women Commission of Inquiry: Executive Summary*. Victoria: Government of British Columbia. Retrieved from http://www.missingwomeninquiry.ca/wp-content/uploads/2010/10/Forsaken-ES-web-RGB.pdf.

Park, Y., Kim, H., Kang, H., et al. (2001). A survey of Hwa-Byung in middle-age Korean women. *Journal of Transcultural Nursing, 12*, 115–122. doi:10.1177/104365960101200205.

Parliament of Canada. (2014). *Current issues in mental health in Canada: The mental health of First Nations and Inuit communities (in Brief)*. Publication no. 2014-02-E. Retrieved from http://www.lop.parl.gc.ca/content/lop/ResearchPublications/2014-02-e.pdf.

Parrott, Z. (2015). *Indigenous peoples. The encyclopedia Canada: Historica Canada*. Retrieved from http://www.thecanadianencyclopedia.ca/en/article/aboriginal-people/.

Registered Nurses' Association of Ontario. (2007). *Embracing cultural diversity in health care: Developing cultural competence*. Retrieved from http://rnao.ca/bpg/guidelines/embracing-cultural-diversity-health-care-developing-cultural-competence.

Reitmanova, S., & Gustafson, D. J. (2009). Mental health needs of visible minority immigrants in a small urban center: Recommendations for policy makers and service providers. *Journal of Immigrant Minority Health/Center for Minority Public Health, 11*, 46–56. doi:10.1007/s10903-008-9122-x.

Ross, R. (1992). *Dancing with a ghost: Exploring Indian reality*. Toronto: Reed Books.

Samuel, E. (2009). Acculturative stress: South Asian immigrant women's experiences in Canada's Atlantic provinces. *Journal of Immigrant & Refugee Studies, 7*, 16–34.

Simich, L., Maiter, S., Moorlag, E., et al. (2009). Taking culture seriously: Ethnolinguistic community perspectives on mental health. *Psychiatric Rehabilitation Journal, 30*, 208–214. doi:10.2975/32.3.2009.208.214.

Srivastava, R. H. (2007). *The health care professionals' guide to clinical cultural competence*. Toronto: Mosby Canada.

Statistics Canada. (2002). *Canadian community health survey: Mental health and well-being*. Retrieved from http://www.statcan.gc.ca/pub/82-617-x/index-eng.htm.

Statistics Canada. (2006). *Immigration in Canada: A portrait of the foreign-born population, 2006 census: Immigrants came from many countries*. Retrieved from http://www12.statcan.gc.ca/census-recensement/2006/as-sa/97-557/p6-eng.cfm.

Statistics Canada. (2013). *Aboriginal peoples reference guide, National Household Survey 2011*. Catalogue no. 99-011-X2011006. Ottawa: Author. Retrieved from http://www12.statcan.gc.ca/nhs-enm/2011/as-sa/99-011-x/99-011-x2011001-eng.pdf.

Tang, K. C., Community Wellness Program, & Jardine, C. G. (2016). Our way of life: Importance of Indigenous culture and tradition to physical activity practices. *International Journal of Indigenous Health, 11*(1), 211–227. doi:10.18357/ijih111201616018.

Tang, T. N., Oatley, K., & Toner, B. B. (2007). Impact of life events and difficulties on the mental health of Chinese immigrant women. *Journal of Immigrant and Minority Health, 9*(4), 281–290.

Tempier, R. (2016). Suicide among Aboriginals: A "burning" public health issue in need of solutions. *Canadian Journal of Psychiatry, 61*(11), 682–683.

Truth and Reconciliation Commission of Canada (TRC) (2015). *Honouring the truth, reconciling for the future: Summary of the final report of the Truth and Reconciliation Commission of Canada*. Ottawa: Author. Retrieved from www.trc.ca.

United Nations. (2007). *The United Nations declaration on the rights of Indigenous peoples*. Retrieved from http://www.un.org/esa/socdev/unpfii/documents/DRIPS_en.pdf.

Vukic, A., Gregory, D., Martin-Misener, R., et al. (2011). Aboriginal and Western conceptions of mental health and illness. *Pimatisiwin: A Journal of Aboriginal and Indigenous Community Health, 9*(1), 65–86. Retrieved from http://www.pimatisiwin.com/online/wp-content/uploads/2011/08/04VukicGregory.pdf.

Vukic, A., Rudderham, S., & Martin-Misener, R. (2009). A community partnership to explore gaps in mental health services in First Nations communities in Nova Scotia. *Canadian Journal of Public Health, 100*(6), 432–435. doi:10.17269/cjph.100.2096.

Ward, C. B. (2016). What is Indigenous cultural safety—and why should I care about it? *Visions, 11*(4), 29.

Wieman, C. (2006). Western medicine meets traditional healing: The experience of Six Nations mental health services. *Cross Currents, 10*(1), 10–11.

World Health Organization (2008). *Closing the gap in a generation: Health equity through action and the social determinants of health*. Geneva, Switzerland: Author. Retrieved from http://www.who.int/social_determinants/thecommission/finalreport/en/index.html.

Biopsychosocial Nursing Techniques

9. Therapeutic Relationships

10. Communication and the Clinical Interview

11. Psychotropic Drugs

Therapeutic Relationships

Elizabeth M. Varcarolis
Adapted by Cheryl L. Pollard

KEY TERMS AND CONCEPTS

clinical supervision
contract
empathy
genuineness
orientation phase
preorientation phase
rapport

social relationship
termination phase
therapeutic encounter
therapeutic relationship
therapeutic use of self
values
working phase

OBJECTIVES

1. Compare and contrast the three phases of the nurse–patient relationship and the dimensions of the helping relationship.
2. Compare and contrast a social relationship and a therapeutic relationship in terms of purpose, focus, communications style, and goals.
3. Identify at least four patient behaviours a psychiatric nurse may encounter in the clinical setting.
4. Explore qualities that foster a therapeutic nurse–patient relationship and qualities that contribute to a nontherapeutic psychiatric nursing interactive process.
5. Define and discuss the microcommunication skills of empathy, genuineness, and positive regard in a nurse–patient relationship.
6. Identify two attitudes and four actions that may reflect the nurse's positive regard for a patient.
7. Analyze what is meant by boundaries and the influence of transference and counter-transference on boundary blurring.
8. Understand the use of nonverbal behaviour or body language in the context of the psychiatric nurse–patient relationship of attending behaviours.
9. Discuss the influences of disparate values and cultural beliefs on the therapeutic relationship.

⊝volve WEBSITE

Visit the Evolve website for Flashcards, Case Studies, and additional testing resources related to the content in this chapter: http://evolve.elsevier.com/Canada/Varcarolis/psychiatric/

`Pre-Test` `interactive review`

Psychiatric mental health nurses practise in a variety of contexts, providing care to individuals, groups, families, and communities. Psychiatric nursing care is both an art and a science. Knowledge of anatomy, physiology, microbiology, and chemistry is the basis for providing safe and effective physiological nursing care. Knowledge of pharmacology—a medication's mechanism of action, indications for use, and adverse effects, based on evidence-informed studies and trials—is central to safe and competent psychiatric nursing practice. However, it is the nurse–patient relationship and the development of the interpersonal skills needed to enhance and maintain such a therapeutic relationship that comprise the art of psychiatric nursing.

Quinlan (1996) stated, "The development of that very human relationship allows a place for caring and healing to occur. This use of the essential humanness of the nurse as a person is the most critical part of the way nurses make themselves available to both patients and colleagues" (p. 7). Quinlan goes on to say that how this relationship is achieved remains the domain of the individual nurse.

⚙ HOW A NURSE HELPED ME

Dan's Story: "Our Friend Is Really a Well-Put-Together Guy!"

Our friend Dan was staying at our rural cottage for a long weekend. He had been increasingly stressed in his management job at an engineering firm in the city, where he was responsible for making big decisions that affected a number of employees. We knew Dan had not been sleeping or eating well and was finding his work increasingly difficult, so we offered our place as a sort of retreat while we were away.

When we returned on the Sunday afternoon, it was clear that Dan was in a very bad mental state. He recognized us, but he had not bathed or showered and could not really respond sensibly to any questions—it was almost as though he was speaking another language! My wife and I immediately drove Dan to our regional hospital's emergency department, where a psychiatric mental health nurse met with him. Dan could barely speak at this stage, so my wife and I were included in the interview. We had brought his belongings in with us and discovered he had been taking a strong herbal sleep aid that, in the end, was found to have contributed to the extreme changes—I guess it was a sort of drug reaction.

We were terribly frightened by the whole thing. We had never seen Dan like this before! Throughout the interview, the nurse paused often, spoke in a relaxed way, breathed,

and made sure we took breaks to eat at mealtimes. She asked Dan questions directly, even though he was not really taking it all in. When he was unable to answer, the nurse would invite my wife and me to think about our own possible responses. It was the most calming way of helping us all.

At the start of the interview, the nurse told us that "sometimes any number of things can create difficulties in the mood, behaviour, and thinking of people who are normally well put together." I remember my wife and I both spoke at the same time: "You are exactly right. Dan is normally the most well-put-together guy. This is something very out of the ordinary—please help sort it out!" This simple respect for Dan's dignity and acknowledgement of how seriously we took the situation allowed us to establish a good relationship with the nurse, helped get to the root of the problem, and started Dan's treatment in a way that made this complicated mess seem manageable. We felt Dan was in a good position to recover from the acute drug reaction and also his poor sleep and other stress-related troubles. Despite it being a very bad time for Dan—and us, as his friends—we will never forget how the nurse showed us all so much respect and dignity. What could have been an even more stressful as well as embarrassing experience for Dan ended up being okay.

CONCEPTS OF THE NURSE–PATIENT RELATIONSHIP

The nurse–patient relationship is the basis of all psychiatric mental health nursing care, regardless of the specific goals of patient care (Brown, 2015; Peplau, 1952). The very first connections between the psychiatric nurse and the patient are to establish an understanding that the nurse is safe, discreet, reliable, and consistent and that the relationship will be conducted within appropriate and clear boundaries (Badawi, 2016).

It is argued that many psychiatric disorders—for example, schizophrenia, bipolar disorder, and major depression—have strong biochemical and genetic elements of origin. However, many accompanying emotional problems, such as altered self-concept and self-image, low self-esteem, and difficulties with adherence to a treatment regimen, can be significantly improved through a therapeutic nurse–patient relationship (Kanera, Kivinen, & Lammintakanen, 2015). All too often, patients entering psychiatric treatment have exhausted their familial and social resources and find themselves isolated and in need of emotional and spiritual support.

The psychiatric nurse–patient relationship is a creative process unique to each nurse and patient. The notion of therapeutic use of self is rooted within one's individual, genuine ways of being with another person based on one's personal values and

beliefs of humanity and enhanced by the application of microcommunication skills (such as warmth, respect, and empathy) to guide the process of developing, maintaining, and terminating a therapeutic relationship. Travelbee (1971) defined therapeutic use of self as "the ability to use one's personality consciously and in full awareness in an attempt to establish relatedness and to structure nursing interventions" (p. 19). It is important to note that the efficacy of this therapeutic use of self has been scientifically substantiated as an evidence-informed intervention (Kim, Roth, & Wollburg, 2015).

Therapeutic success is thought to be as much a result of the quality and characteristics of the therapeutic relationship as of the particular medical treatment choices or processes (Kim, Roth, & Wollburg, 2015). Evidence suggests that psychotherapy (talk therapy) within a therapeutic relationship actually changes brain chemistry in much the same way as medication. Many therefore believe that the best treatment for most psychological stressors is a combination of medication and psychotherapy (less so in the case of psychotic disorders). Cognitive behavioural therapy, in particular, has met with great success in the treatment of depression, phobias, obsessive-compulsive disorders, and others.

Establishing a therapeutic relationship with a patient takes time. Competency in relationship building is developed from a basis in communication theory within the context of the

Narrative Descriptions of Miyo-mahcihoyãn (Physical, Emotional, Mental, and Spiritual Well-Being) From a Contemporary Néhiyawak (Plains Cree) Perspective

Problem

It is unclear why the health and mental status of Indigenous people continue to lag behind those of non-Indigenous people in Canada. The answer is embedded in the Indigenous/non-Indigenous historical relationship, specifically colonization.

Purpose of Study

The primary goal of this research project was to explore factors that improve the mental health and well-being of the néhiyawak from Thunderchild First Nation and what they perceived as necessary to attain optimal mental health and well-being. Second, the first author, an Indigenous woman, wanted to conduct research that was strength based and would give voice to contemporary Indigenous (Plains Cree) people from her community of Thunderchild First Nation, Saskatchewan.

Methods

Narrative inquiry was used to guide the research process, and thematic narrative analysis was used to analyze the data.

Key Findings

The researchers revealed four overarching themes that highlighted what positively affected mental health and well-being. These were (1) relationships, (2) spiritual beliefs and cultural practices, (3) tãnisî si wãpahtaman pimãtisiwin (world view), and (4) ēkwa ō hi kikwaya piko ka-ispayiki kī spin ka-nohtē-miyo-mahcihoyãn (these are the things that need to happen if I want to be healthy).

Implications for Nursing Practice

For Indigenous peoples, honouring Indigenous values and perspectives, which include interconnectedness, reciprocity, language, and ceremony, is the cornerstone of a collaborative therapeutic relationship. The insight gathered from an Indigenous perspective is essential for planning effective health care delivery strategies.

Source: Graham, H., & Martin, S. (2016). Narrative descriptions of miyo-mahcihoyãn (physical, emotional, mental, and spiritual well-being) from a contemporary néhiyawak (Plains Cree) perspective. *International Journal of Mental Health Systems, 10*(58), 1–12. doi:10.1186/s13033-016-0086-2.

nurse–patient relationship. With experience and mentoring from experts, nurses will develop expertise along the communication continuum from novice to expert (Benner, 2000).

Goals and Functions

The nurse–patient relationship is often loosely defined. However, a therapeutic relationship has specific goals and functions, including the following:

- Facilitating verbal expression of distressing thoughts and feelings
- Assisting patients to develop self-awareness and insight into their thoughts, feelings, and behaviours in order for them to better manage the activities of daily living

- Helping patients to examine self-defeating behaviours and test alternatives
- Promoting self-care and independence

Social Versus Therapeutic

A relationship is an interpersonal process that involves two or more people. Throughout life, we meet people in a variety of settings and share a variety of experiences. With some individuals, we develop long-term relationships; with others, the relationship lasts only a short time. Naturally, the kinds of relationships we enter vary from person to person and from situation to situation. Generally, relationships can be defined as intimate, social, or therapeutic. Intimate relationships occur between people who have an emotional commitment to each other. Within intimate relationships, mutual needs are met and intimate desires and fantasies are shared. For our purposes in this chapter, we limit our exploration to the aspects of social and therapeutic relationships.

Social Relationships

A social relationship can be defined as a relationship that is initiated primarily for the purpose of friendship, socialization, enjoyment, or accomplishment of a task. Mutual needs are met during social interaction (e.g., participants share ideas, feelings, and experiences). Communication skills may include giving advice, such as relationship advice, and, sometimes, meeting basic dependency needs, such as offering a listening ear or material support during a stressful time. Often the content of the communication remains superficial. During social interactions, roles may shift. Within a social relationship, there is little emphasis on the evaluation of the interaction, as seen in the following example of two friends at a shopping mall:

> *Friend A:* "Oh, gosh, I just hate to be alone. It's getting me down, and sometimes it hurts so much."
>
> *Friend B:* "I know just how you feel. I don't like it either. What I do is get a friend and go to a movie or something. Do you have someone to do that sort of stuff with?" (With this response, B is minimizing A's feelings and giving advice prematurely.)
>
> *Friend A:* "No, not really, but often I don't even feel like going out. I just sit at home feeling scared and lonely."
>
> *Friend B:* "Most of us feel like that at one time or another. Maybe if you took a class or joined a group, you could meet more people. I know of some great groups you could join. It's not good to be stuck in the house by yourself all the time." (Again, B is not "hearing" A's distress and is minimizing her pain and isolation. B goes on to give A unwanted and unhelpful advice, thus closing off A's feelings and experience.)

Therapeutic Relationships

In a therapeutic relationship, the psychiatric nurse maximizes his or her communication skills, understanding of human behaviours, and personal strengths to enhance the patient's growth. The focus of the relationship is on the patient's ideas, experiences, feelings, and personal issues introduced during the clinical interview, with the development of personal insight as a desired outcome. The nurse and the patient identify areas that need exploration and periodically evaluate the degree of change in the patient's understanding of the stressors and pinpoint strategies to manage them differently.

Although the psychiatric nurse may assume a variety of roles (e.g., teacher, counsellor, socializing agent, liaison), the relationship is consistently focused on the patient's problem and needs. The psychiatric nurse's needs must be met outside the relationship. When psychiatric nurses begin to want the patient to "like them," "do as they suggest," "be nice to them," or "give them recognition," the needs of the patient cannot be adequately met, and the interaction transitions from being therapeutic to being detrimental (nontherapeutic) to the patient.

Working under **clinical supervision** (i.e., being evaluated, receiving feedback, and gradually gaining autonomy and responsibility) is an excellent way for a psychiatric nurse's focus and boundaries to remain clear. Communication skills and knowledge of the stages and phenomena in a therapeutic relationship are critical tools in the formation and maintenance of the therapeutic relationship. Within the context of a therapeutic relationship, the following occur:

- The needs of the patient are identified and explored.
- Clear boundaries are established.
- Alternative problem-solving approaches are taken.
- New coping skills may be developed.
- Insight is developed, and behavioural change is encouraged.

Just like on-staff nurses, nursing students may struggle with the boundaries between social and therapeutic relationships initially because there is a fine line between the two. In fact, students often feel more comfortable "being a friend" because it is a more familiar role, especially with people close to their own age. However, before a social relationship takes root, the psychiatric nurse or student needs to make it clear (to himself or herself and to the patient) that the relationship is a therapeutic one. This does not mean that the nurse is not friendly toward the patient, and it does not mean that talking about everyday topics (television, weather, children's pictures) is forbidden. It does mean, however, that the nurse must follow the prior stated guidelines regarding a therapeutic relationship: essentially, the focus is on the patient, and the relationship is not designed to meet the psychiatric nurse's needs. The patient's problems and concerns are explored, potential solutions are discussed by both patient and psychiatric nurse, and solutions are implemented by the patient, as in the following example:

Patient: "Oh, gosh, I just hate to be alone. It's getting me down, and sometimes it hurts so much."

Nurse: "Loneliness can be painful. Tell me what is going on now that you are feeling so alone."

Patient: "Well, my mom died 2 years ago, and last month, my—oh, I am so scared." (Takes a deep breath, looks down, and looks as though she might cry)

Nurse: (Sits in silence while the patient recovers) "Go on … tell me more."

Patient: "My boyfriend left for Afghanistan. I haven't heard from him, and they say he's missing. He was my best friend, and we were going to get married, and if he dies, I don't want to live."

Nurse: "Have you thought of wanting to end your life?"

Patient: "Well, if he dies, I will. I can't live without him."

Nurse: "Have you ever felt like this before?"

Patient: "Yes, when my mom died. I was depressed for about a year until I met my boyfriend."

Nurse: "It sounds as though you are worried, scared, and uncertain whether your boyfriend is alive because you have not heard from him. Perhaps you and I can talk some more and come up with some ways for you to feel less anxious, scared, and overwhelmed. Let's take some time to talk more about this together."

The ability of the psychiatric nurse to engage in interpersonal interactions in a goal-directed manner to assist patients with their emotional, spiritual, or physical health needs is the foundation of the therapeutic psychiatric nurse–patient relationship. The following are necessary behaviours of health care workers, including nurses:

- Accountability—Psychiatric nurses assume responsibility for their conduct and the consequences of their actions.
- Focus on patient needs—The interest of the patient, rather than that of the nurse, other health care workers, or the institution, is given first consideration. The psychiatric nurse's role is that of patient advocate.
- Clinical competence—The criteria on which the nurse bases his or her conduct are principles of knowledge and the most appropriate actions for specific situations. This knowledge and action involve awareness and incorporation of the latest knowledge available from research (evidence-informed practice).
- Delaying judgement—Ideally, nurses refrain from judging patients and avoid inflicting their own values and beliefs on others.
- Supervision—Supervision by a more experienced clinician or team is essential to developing one's competence in establishing therapeutic psychiatric nurse–patient relationships.

Nurses interact with patients in a variety of settings: emergency departments, medical-surgical units, obstetric and pediatric units, clinics, community settings, schools, forensic milieus, correctional facilities, psychiatric assessment units, and patients' homes. Nurses who are empathic to patients' experiences and have effective holistic assessment and communication skills can significantly help patients confront current stressors and anticipate future choices.

Sometimes the type of relationship that occurs may be informal and short lived, such as when the psychiatric nurse and patient meet for only a few sessions. However, even though it is brief, the relationship may be substantial, useful, and important for the patient. This limited relationship is often referred to as a **therapeutic encounter**. When the nurse shows genuine concern for another's circumstances (empathy and compassion), even a short encounter can have a powerful effect.

At other times, the encounters may be longer and more formal, such as in inpatient settings, mental health units, crisis centres, and mental health facilities. This longer time span allows the therapeutic nurse–patient relationship to be more fully developed.

Relationship Boundaries

Establishing Boundaries

Health care professionals will discuss and negotiate boundaries very early in the therapeutic relationship as they use a patient-centred model to guide their practice. From a bioethical perspective, boundaries are necessary primarily to protect the patient from harm—nonmaleficence. Establishing and maintaining boundaries is an essential competency for psychiatric mental health nurses. Within therapeutic relationships, boundaries are commonly established to protect the space between the professional's power and the client's vulnerability. A trusting therapeutic relationship is based on clear boundaries that facilitate the sharing of the patient's ideas, thoughts, feelings, and behaviours, thus providing the opportunity to develop insight and explore barriers to achieving patient goals (Badawi, 2016). Boundaries are commonly established in the following three areas.

- Treatment planning and delivery: anticipated length of treatment or service delivery, limits of confidentiality, members of treatment team, etc.
- Personal space: physical space, emotional space, agreement between nurse and patient as to roles and responsibilities of all involved in the therapeutic relationship (nurse, patient, and family), and so forth.
- Location of service delivery: inpatient unit, community clinic, home visits, treatment room, conference room, and other such places.

Health professionals need to constantly assess the effectiveness of their boundaries. When there is a shift in the dynamics of the relationship related to power and vulnerability, the boundaries become blurred and the resulting shift in the psychiatric nurse–patient relationship may lead to nontherapeutic dynamics. Two common circumstances in which boundaries are blurred occur (1) when the relationship is allowed to slip into a social context and (2) when the psychiatric nurse's needs (for attention, affection, or emotional or spiritual support) are met at the expense of the patient's needs.

Blurring of Boundaries

The most egregious boundary violations are those related to physical or sexual abuse. These types of violations result in malpractice actions and may result in the loss of professional licensure on the part of the nurse. Other boundary issues are not as obvious. Table 9-1 illustrates some examples of patient and psychiatric nurse behaviours that reflect blurred boundaries.

Transference. Transference, originally identified by Sigmund Freud when he used psychoanalysis to treat patients, occurs when the patient unconsciously and inappropriately displaces (transfers) onto the nurse his or her feelings and behaviours related to significant figures in the patient's past (see Chapter 4). The patient may even say, "You remind me of my (mother, sister, father, brother, or so on)."

> *Patient:* "Oh, you are so high and mighty. Did anyone ever tell you that you are a cold, unfeeling machine, just like others I know?"
>
> *Nurse:* "Tell me about one person who is cold and unfeeling toward you." (In this example, the patient is experiencing the nurse in the same way he experienced a significant other or others during his formative years. In this case, the patient's mother was very aloof, leaving him with feelings of isolation, worthlessness, and anger.)

Although transference occurs in all relationships, it seems to be intensified in relationships of authority. One theory is that transference may occur in therapeutic relationships because parental figures were the original figures of authority. Physicians, nurses, and social workers are all potential objects of transference. This transference may be positive or negative. If a patient is motivated to work with you, completes assignments between sessions, and shares feelings openly, the patient may be experiencing positive transference (Wheeler, 2013).

Whereas positive transference does not need to be addressed with the patient, negative transference that threatens the nurse–patient relationship may need to be explored.

Common forms of transference include the desire for affection or respect and the gratification of dependency needs. Other transferential feelings are hostility, jealousy, competitiveness, and love.

Sometimes patients experience positive or negative thoughts, feelings, and reactions that are realistic and appropriate and not a result of transference onto the health care provider. For example, if a nurse makes promises to the patient that are not kept (e.g.,

---

TABLE 9-1	PATIENT AND NURSE BEHAVIOURS THAT REFLECT BLURRED BOUNDARIES	
WHEN THE PSYCHIATRIC NURSE IS OVERLY INVOLVED	**WHEN THE PSYCHIATRIC NURSE IS NOT INVOLVED**
More frequent requests for assistance by the patient, which causes increased dependency on the psychiatric nurse	Patient's increased verbal or physical expression of isolation (depression)
Inability of the patient to perform tasks that he or she is known to have been capable of prior to the psychiatric nurse's help, which causes regression	Lack of mutually agreed-upon goals
Unwillingness on the part of the patient to maintain performance or progress in the psychiatric nurse's absence	Lack of progress toward goals
Expressions of anger by other staff who do not agree with the psychiatric nurse's interventions or perceptions of the patient	Psychiatric nurse's avoidance of spending time with the patient
Psychiatric nurse's keeping of secrets about the psychiatric nurse–patient relationship	Failure of the psychiatric nurse to follow through on agreed-upon interventions

Source: Pilette, P. C., Berck, C. B., & Achber, L. C. (1995). Therapeutic management of helping boundaries. *Journal of Psychosocial Nursing and Mental Health Services, 33*(1), 40–47. Reprinted with permission from SLACK Incorporated.

not showing up for a scheduled meeting), the patient may feel resentment for and mistrust of the nurse.

Counter-transference. Counter-transference occurs when the nurse unconsciously and inappropriately displaces feelings and behaviours related to significant figures in his or her past onto the patient. Frequently, the patient's transference evokes counter-transference in the psychiatric nurse. For example, it is normal to feel angry when attacked persistently, annoyed when frustrated unreasonably, or flattered when idealized. A nurse might feel extremely important when depended on exclusively by a patient.

If the nurse does not recognize his or her own omnipotent feelings as counter-transference, he or she may minimize encouragement of independent growth in the patient; the therapeutic relationship may stall; and patients may be disempowered by the nurse's experience of them not as individuals but as extensions of themselves. Recognizing counter-transference, on the other hand, maximizes nurses' ability to empower patients. For example:

> *Patient:* "Yeah, well I decided not to go to that dumb group. 'Hi, I'm so-and-so, and I'm an alcoholic.' Who cares?" (Sits slumped in a chair chewing gum, nonchalantly looking around)
>
> *Nurse:* (In a very impassioned tone) "You always sabotage your chances. You need AA to get in control of your life. Last week you were going to go, and now you've disappointed everyone." (Here the nurse is reminded of his mother, who was an alcoholic. He had tried everything to get his mother into treatment and took it as a personal failure and deep disappointment that his mother never sought recovery. After the psychiatric nurse sorts out his thoughts and feelings and realizes that the frustration and feelings of disappointment and failure belonged with his mother and not the patient, he starts the next session with the following approach.)
>
> *Nurse:* "Look, I was thinking about last week, and I realize the decision to go to AA or find other help is solely up to you. It's true that I would like you to live a fuller and more satisfying life, but it's your decision. I'm wondering, however, what happened to change your mind about going to AA."

A nurse feeling either a strongly positive or a strongly negative reaction to a patient most often signals counter-transference. One common sign of counter-transference is overidentification with the patient. In this situation, the nurse may have difficulty recognizing or objectively seeing patient problems that are similar to his or her own problems. For example, a nurse who is struggling with an alcoholic family member may feel uninterested in, cold toward, or disgusted by an alcoholic patient. Other indicators of counter-transference are the nurse's becoming involved in power struggles, competition, or arguments with the patient. Table 9-2 lists some common counter-transference reactions.

Identifying and working through various transference and counter-transference issues is central to working therapeutically with the patient if we are to achieve professional and clinical growth and allow for positive change in the patient. Transference and counter-transference, as well as numerous other issues, are best dealt with through the use of supervision by either the peer group or the therapeutic team. Besides helping with boundary issues, supervision supplies practical and emotional support, education, and guidance regarding ethical issues. Regularly scheduled supervision sessions provide the psychiatric nurse with the opportunity to increase self-awareness, clinical skills, and growth, as well as allow for continued growth of the patient. No matter how objective clinicians may try to be in examining their interactions, professional support and help from an experienced supervisor are essential to good practice (Gonge & Buus, 2015).

Self-Check on Boundaries

It is useful for all of us to take time out to be reflective and aware of our thoughts and actions with patients, as well as with colleagues, friends, and family. Figure 9-1 is a helpful boundary self-test you can use throughout your career, no matter what area of nursing you choose.

VALUES, BELIEFS, AND SELF-AWARENESS

Values are abstract standards that represent an ideal, either positive or negative. It is crucial that we have an understanding of our own values and attitudes so we may become aware of the beliefs or attitudes we hold that may interfere with establishing positive therapeutic relationships with patient groups.

When working with patients, it is important for nurses to understand that their values and beliefs are not necessarily "right" and certainly are not right for everyone. It is helpful to realize that our values and beliefs (1) reflect our own culture or subculture, (2) are derived from a range of choices, and (3) are those we have chosen for ourselves from a variety of influences and role models. These chosen values (religious, cultural, societal) guide us in making decisions and taking actions that we hope will make our lives meaningful, rewarding, and fulfilling.

Interviewing others whose values, beliefs, cultures, or lifestyles are radically different from our own can be a challenge (Racine, 2014). Several topics that cause controversy in society in general—including religion, gender roles, abortion, war, politics, money, drugs, alcohol, sex, and corporal punishment—also can cause conflict between nurses and patients (Racine, 2014).

Although we emphasize that the patient and nurse should identify outcomes together, what happens when the psychiatric nurse's values, beliefs, and interpretive system are very different from those of a patient? Consider the following examples of possible conflicts:

- The patient wants an abortion, and abortion goes against the nurse's values.
- The psychiatric nurse believes that the patient, who was raped, should get an abortion, but the patient refuses.
- The patient engages in unsafe sex with multiple partners, which goes against the nurse's values.
- The psychiatric nurse cannot understand a patient who refuses medications on religious grounds.
- The patient puts material gain and objects far ahead of loyalty to friends and family, in direct contrast to the nurse's values.
- The nurse is deeply religious, whereas the patient is a nonbeliever who shuns organized religion.

TABLE 9-2	COMMON COUNTER-TRANSFERENCE REACTIONS

As a nurse, you will sometimes experience counter-transference feelings. Once you are aware of them, use them for self-analysis to understand those feelings that may inhibit productive nurse–patient communication.

REACTION TO PATIENT	BEHAVIOURS CHARACTERISTIC OF THE REACTION	SELF-ANALYSIS	SOLUTION
Boredom (indifference)	Showing inattention Frequently asking the patient to repeat statements Making inappropriate responses	Is the content of what the patient presents uninteresting? Or is it the style of communication? Does the patient exhibit an offensive style of communication? Have you anything else on your mind that may be distracting you from the patient's needs? Is the patient discussing an issue that makes you anxious?	Redirect the patient if he or she provides more information than you need or goes "off track" Clarify information with the patient Confront ineffective modes of communication
Rescue	Reaching for unattainable goals Resisting peer feedback and supervisory recommendations Giving advice	What behaviour stimulates your perceived need to rescue the patient? Has anyone evoked such feelings in you in the past? What are your fears or fantasies about failing to meet the patient's needs? Why do you want to rescue this patient?	Avoid secret alliances Develop realistic goals Do not alter the meeting schedule Let the patient guide interaction Facilitate patient problem solving
Overinvolvement	Coming to work early, leaving late Ignoring peer suggestions, resisting assistance Buying the patient clothes or other gifts Accepting the patient's gifts Behaving judgementally at family interventions Keeping secrets Calling the patient when off duty	What particular patient characteristics are attractive? Does the patient remind you of someone? Who? Does your current behaviour differ from your treatment of similar patients in the past? What are you getting out of this situation? What needs of yours are being met?	Establish firm treatment boundaries, goals, and nursing expectations Avoid self-disclosure Avoid calling the patient when off duty
Overidentification	Having a special agenda, keeping secrets Increasing self-disclosure Feeling omnipotent Experiencing physical attraction	With which of the patient's physical, emotional, cognitive, or situational characteristics do you identify? Recall similar circumstances in your own life. How did you deal with the issues now being created by the patient?	Allow the patient to direct issues Encourage a problem-solving approach from the patient's perspective Avoid self-disclosure
Misuse of honesty	Withholding information Lying	Why are you protecting the patient? What are your fears about the patient learning the truth?	Be clear in your responses and aware of your hesitation; do not hedge If you can provide information, tell the patient and give your rationale Avoid keeping secrets Reinforce the interdisciplinary nature of treatment
Anger	Withdrawing Speaking loudly Using profanity Asking to be taken off the case	What patient behaviours are offensive to you? What dynamic from your past may this patient be re-creating?	Determine the origin of the anger (nurse, patient, or both) Explore the roots of patient anger Avoid contact with the patient if you do not understand the roots of the anger
Helplessness or hopelessness	Feeling sadness	Which patient behaviours evoke these feelings in you? Has anyone evoked similar feelings in the past? Who? What past expectations were placed on you (verbally and nonverbally) by this patient?	Maintain therapeutic involvement Explore and focus on the patient's experience rather than on your own

Source: Aromando, L. (1995). *Mental health and psychiatric nursing* (2nd ed.). Springhouse, PA: Springhouse.

NURSING BOUNDARY INDEX SELF-CHECK

Please rate yourself according to the frequency with which the following statements reflect your behavior, thoughts, or feelings within the past 2 years while providing patient care.*

1. Have you ever received any feedback about your behavior being overly intrusive with patients and their families?	Never _____ Rarely _____ Sometimes _____ Often _____
2. Do you ever have difficulty setting limits with patients?	Never _____ Rarely _____ Sometimes _____ Often _____
3. Do you ever arrive early or stay late to be with your patient for a longer period?	Never _____ Rarely _____ Sometimes _____ Often _____
4. Do you ever find yourself relating to patients or peers as you might to a family member?	Never _____ Rarely _____ Sometimes _____ Often _____
5. Have you ever acted on sexual feelings you have for a patient?	Never _____ Rarely _____ Sometimes _____ Often _____
6. Do you feel that you are the only one who understands the patient?	Never _____ Rarely _____ Sometimes _____ Often _____
7. Have you ever received feedback that you get "too involved" with patients or families?	Never _____ Rarely _____ Sometimes _____ Often _____
8. Do you derive conscious satisfaction from patients' praise, appreciation, or affection?	Never _____ Rarely _____ Sometimes _____ Often _____
9. Do you ever feel that other staff members are too critical of "your" patient?	Never _____ Rarely _____ Sometimes _____ Often _____
10. Do you ever feel that other staff members are jealous of your relationship with your patient?	Never _____ Rarely _____ Sometimes _____ Often _____
11. Have you ever tried to "match-make" a patient with one of your friends?	Never _____ Rarely _____ Sometimes _____ Often _____
12. Do you find it difficult to handle patients' unreasonable requests for assistance, verbal abuse, or sexual language?	Never _____ Rarely _____ Sometimes _____ Often _____

*Any item that is responded to with "Sometimes" or "Often" should alert the nurse to a possible area of vulnerability. If the item is responded to with "Rarely," the nurse should determine whether it is an isolated event or a possible pattern of behavior.

FIGURE 9-1 Nursing Boundary Index Self-Check. Source: Pilette, P., Berck, C., & Achber, L. (1995). Therapeutic management. *Journal of Psychosocial Nursing and Mental Health Services, 33*(1), 45. Reprinted with permission from SLACK Incorporated.

- The patient's lifestyle includes taking illicit drugs, an action that goes against the nurse's values.

How can nurses develop working relationships and help patients solve problems when patients' values, goals, and interpretive systems are so different from their own? Self-awareness requires that we understand what we value and the beliefs that guide our own behaviour. It is critical that as nurses we not only understand and accept our own values and beliefs but also are sensitive to and accepting of the unique and different values and beliefs of others. Supervision by an experienced colleague can prove invaluable in helping us to develop this sensitivity.

PEPLAU'S MODEL OF THE NURSE–PATIENT RELATIONSHIP

Hildegard Peplau introduced the concept of the nurse–patient relationship in 1952 in her groundbreaking book *Interpersonal Relations in Nursing*. This model of the nurse–patient relationship is well accepted in the United States and Canada (Registered Nurses' Association of Ontario, 2002) and has become an important tool for all nursing practice. A professional nurse–patient relationship includes a nurse who has skills and expertise and a patient who wants to alleviate suffering, find solutions to problems, explore different avenues to an improved quality of life, find an advocate, or do any combination of the above (Racine, 2014).

Peplau (1952) proposed that the nurse–patient relationship "facilitates forward movement" for both the nurse and the patient (p. 12). This interactive nurse–patient process is designed to assist in the patient's boundary management, independent problem solving, and decision making that promotes autonomy (Haber, 2000).

Peplau (1952, 1999) described the nurse–patient relationship as evolving through distinct interlocking and overlapping phases, generally recognized as follows:

1. Orientation phase
2. Working phase
3. Termination phase

An additional preorientation phase, during which the nurse prepares for the orientation phase—for instance, by familiarizing himself or herself with the patient's background or engaging in self-reflection and other learning—has also since been identified.

Most likely, you will not have time to develop all phases of the nurse–patient relationship in a brief student practice experience. However, it is important to be aware of these phases in order to recognize and consciously engage in them in your nursing practice and in the patient's experience with the treatment team. It is also important to remember that any contact that is caring, respectful, and demonstrative of concern for the situation of another person can have an enormous positive impact, as illustrated by Dan's story earlier in this chapter (see How a Nurse Helped Me).

Preorientation Phase

Even before the first meeting, the psychiatric nurse may have many thoughts and feelings related to the first clinical session. Novice health care providers typically experience concerns and anxiety on their first practice days. These universal concerns include being afraid of people with psychiatric problems, saying "the wrong thing," and not knowing what to do in response to certain patient behaviours. Table 9-3 identifies common patient behaviours (e.g., crying, asking the nurse to keep a secret, threatening to commit suicide, giving a gift, wanting physical contact with the nurse) and gives examples of possible reactions by the nurse and suggested responses.

Talking with an instructor and participating in supervised peer group discussion will promote confidence and produce feedback and suggestions to prepare students for clinical practice. To prepare you for your first clinical day, your instructor will set the ground rules for safety. For example, do not go into a patient's room alone, know if there are any patients not to engage, stay in an open area where other people are around, and know the signs and symptoms of escalating anxiety. You should always trust your own instincts. If you feel uncomfortable for any reason, excuse yourself for a moment and discuss your feelings with your instructor or a staff member. In addition to getting reassurance and support, students can often provide valuable information about the patient's condition by sharing their perceptions.

Most experienced psychiatric mental health nursing faculty and staff are able to skillfully assess the unit atmosphere and behaviours that may indicate escalating tension. They are trained in crisis intervention, and formal security is often available on-site to give the staff support. There are actions a psychiatric nurse can take if a patient's anger begins to escalate, many of which are presented in Table 9-4. Chapter 23 offers a more detailed discussion of maintaining personal safety, recognizing potential agitation, and intervening with angry or aggressive patients. Refer to Chapter 10 for a detailed discussion of communication strategies used in clinical practice.

Orientation Phase

The orientation phase can last for a few meetings or extend over a longer period. It marks the first time the nurse and the patient meet and is the phase during which the nurse conducts the initial interview (see Chapter 10). When strangers meet, they interact according to their own backgrounds, standards, values, and experiences. The fact that each person has a unique frame of reference underlies the need for self-awareness on the part of the nurse. The initial interview includes the following aspects:

- An atmosphere is established in which rapport can grow.
- The nurse's role is clarified, and the responsibilities (parameters) of both the patient and the nurse are defined.
- The contract containing the time, place, date, and duration of the meetings is discussed.
- Confidentiality is discussed and assumed.
- The terms of termination are introduced (these are also discussed throughout the orientation phase and beyond).
- The nurse becomes aware of transference and counter-transference issues.
- Patient problems are articulated, and mutually agreed-upon goals are established.

Establishing Rapport

A major emphasis during the first few encounters with the patient is on providing an atmosphere in which trust and understanding, or rapport, can grow. As in any relationship, **rapport** can be nurtured by demonstrating genuineness and empathy, developing positive regard, showing consistency, and offering assistance in problem solving and providing support.

Parameters of the Relationship

The patient needs to know about the psychiatric mental health nurse (who the nurse is and the nurse's background) and the purpose of the meetings. For example, a student might provide the following information:

> *Student:* "Hello, Mrs. Almodovar. I am Jim Thompson from the university. I am in my psychiatric rotation and will be coming here for the next six Thursdays. I would like to spend time with you each Thursday while you are here. I'm here to be a support person for you as you work on your treatment goals."

Formal or Informal Contract

A contract emphasizes the patient's participation and responsibility because it shows that the psychiatric nurse does something *with* the patient rather than *for* the patient. The **contract**, either stated or written, contains the place, time, date, and duration of the meetings. During the orientation phase, the patient may begin to express thoughts and feelings, identify problems, and discuss realistic goals. Mutual agreement about those goals is also part of the contract. Students also make this contract with patients they interact with.

> *Student:* "Mrs. Almodovar, we will meet at 10 o'clock each Thursday in the consultation room at the clinic for 45 minutes. We can use that time for further discussion of your feelings of loneliness and anger and explore some strategies you could use to make the situation better for yourself."

Confidentiality

The patient has a right to know (1) that specific information may be shared with others on the treatment team and (2) who else will be given the information (e.g., a clinical supervisor, the physician, the staff, or, if the nurse is in training, other students in conference). The patient also needs to know that the information will not be shared with relatives, friends, or others outside

TABLE 9-3   **COMMON PATIENT BEHAVIOURS, POSSIBLE NURSE REACTIONS, AND SUGGESTED NURSE RESPONSES**

POSSIBLE REACTIONS	USEFUL RESPONSES
If the Patient Threatens Suicide ...	
The nurse may feel overwhelmed or responsible for "talking the patient out of it." The nurse may pick up some of the patient's feelings of hopelessness.	The nurse assesses whether the patient has a plan and the lethality of the plan. The nurse tells the patient that this situation is serious, that the nurse does not want harm to come to the patient, and that this information needs to be shared with other staff: "This is very serious, Mr. Lamb. I don't want any harm to come to you. I'll have to share this with the other staff." The nurse can then discuss with the patient the feelings and circumstances that led to this decision. (Refer to Chapter 22 for strategies for suicide intervention.)
If the Patient Asks the Nurse to Keep a Secret ...	
The nurse may feel conflict because he or she wants the patient to share important information but is unsure about making such a promise.	The nurse cannot make such a promise. The information may be important to the health or safety of the patient or others: "I cannot make that promise. It might be important for me to share the information with other staff." The patient then decides whether to share the information
If the Patient Asks the Nurse a Personal Question ...	
The nurse may think that it is rude not to answer the patient's question. A new psychiatric nurse might feel relieved to put off having to start the interview. The nurse may feel put on the spot and want to leave the situation. New nurses are often manipulated by a patient into changing roles, thereby keeping the focus off the patient and preventing the building of a relationship.	The nurse may or may not answer the patient's query. If the nurse decides to answer a natural question, he or she answers in a word or two, then returns the focus to the patient: *Patient:* Are you married? *Nurse:* Yes. Do you have a spouse? *Patient:* Do you have any children? *Nurse:* This time is for you. Tell me about yourself. *Patient:* You can just tell me if you have any children. *Nurse:* This is your time to focus on your concerns. Tell me something about your family.
If the Patient Makes Sexual Advances ...	
The nurse feels uncomfortable but may feel conflicted about "rejecting" the patient or making him or her feel "unattractive" or "not good enough."	The nurse needs to set clear limits on expected behaviour: "I'm not comfortable having you touch (kiss) me. This time is for you to focus on your problems and concerns." Frequently restating the nurse's role throughout the relationship can help maintain boundaries. If the patient does not stop the behaviour, the nurse might say: "If you can't stop this behaviour, I'll have to leave. I'll be back at [time] to spend time with you then." Leaving gives the patient time to gain control. The nurse returns at the stated time.
If the Patient Cries ...	
The nurse may feel uncomfortable and experience increased anxiety or feel somehow responsible for making the person cry.	The nurse should stay with the patient and reinforce that it is all right to cry. Often, it is at that time that feelings are closest to the surface and can be best identified: "You seem ready to cry." "You are still upset about your brother's death." "Tell me what are you thinking right now." The psychiatric nurse offers tissues when appropriate.
If the Patient Leaves Before the Session Is Over ...	
The nurse may feel rejected, thinking it was something that he or she did. The nurse may experience increased anxiety or feel abandoned by the patient.	Some patients are not able to relate for long periods without experiencing an increase in anxiety. Some patients may be testing the nurse: "I'll wait for you here for 15 minutes, until our time is up." During this time, the nurse does not engage in conversation with any other patient or even with the staff. When the time is up, the nurse approaches the patient, says the time is up, and restates the day and time of their next meeting.
If the Patient Does Not Want to Talk ...	
The nurse new to this situation may feel rejected or ineffectual.	At first, the nurse might say something to this effect: "It's all right. I would like to spend time with you. We don't have to talk." The nurse might spend short, frequent periods (e.g., 5 minutes) with the patient throughout the day: "Our 5 minutes is up. I'll be back at 10 o'clock and stay with you 5 more minutes." This response gives the patient the opportunity to understand that the nurse means what he or she says and consistently returns on time. It also gives the patient time between visits to assess how he or she feels, to formulate thoughts about the nurse, and perhaps to feel less threatened.

TABLE 9-3	COMMON PATIENT BEHAVIOURS, POSSIBLE NURSE REACTIONS, AND SUGGESTED NURSE RESPONSES—cont'd	
POSSIBLE REACTIONS	**USEFUL RESPONSES**	

If the Patient Gives the Nurse a Present ...

The nurse may feel uncomfortable when offered a gift.	Possible guidelines:
The meaning needs to be examined. Is the gift (1) a way of getting better care, (2) a way to maintain self-esteem, (3) a way of making the nurse feel guilty, (4) a sincere expression of thanks, or (5) a cultural expectation?	If the gift is expensive, the only policy is to graciously refuse. If it is inexpensive, then (1) if it is given at the end of hospitalization when a relationship has developed, graciously accept; (2) if it is given at the beginning of the relationship, graciously refuse and explore the meaning behind the present: "Thank you, but it is our job to care for our patients. Are you concerned that some aspect of your care will be overlooked?" If the gift is money, it is always graciously refused.

If Another Patient Interrupts During Time With Your Current Patient ...

The nurse may feel a conflict: he or she does not want to appear rude. Sometimes the nurse tries to engage both patients in conversation.	The time the nurse had contracted with a selected patient is that patient's time. By keeping his or her part of the contract, the nurse demonstrates commitment and conviction that the sessions are important: "I am with Mr. Rob for the next 20 minutes. At 10 o'clock, after our time is up, I can talk to you for 5 minutes."

TABLE 9-4	GUIDELINES FOR MAINTAINING SAFETY WHEN A PATIENT'S ANGER ESCALATES	
NURSING INTERVENTION	**RATIONALE**	

Pay attention to angry and aggressive behaviour. Respond as early as possible.	Minimization of angry behaviours and ineffective limit setting are the most frequent factors contributing to the escalation of violence.
Assess for and provide for personal safety. Pay attention to the environment: • Leave door open or use hallway. Interact with the patient in a quiet place that is visible to staff. • Have a quick exit available. The more angry the patient, the more space he or she will need to feel comfortable. Never turn your back on an angry patient. Leave immediately if there are signs that behaviour is escalating out of control or if you are uncomfortable. State, "I am leaving now. I will be back in 10 minutes," and seek out your clinical instructor or another staff member right away.	Exercising basic caution is essential to protecting yourself. Although the risk for violence may be minimal, it is easier to prevent a problem than to get out of a bad situation. These precautions are similar to using universal precautions (gloves, masks, gowns, etc.) on medical floors.
Appear calm and in control.	The perception that someone is in control can be comforting and calming to an individual whose anxiety is beginning to escalate.
Speak softly in a nonprovocative, nonjudgemental manner.	When tone of voice is low and calm and the words are spoken slowly, anxiety levels in others may decrease.
Demonstrate genuineness and concern.	Even the most psychotic individual with schizophrenia may respond to nonprovocative interpersonal contact and expressions of concern and caring.
If patient is willing, both the psychiatric nurse and the patient should sit at a 45-degree angle. Do not tower over or stare at the patient.	Sitting at a 45-degree angle puts you both on the same level but allows for frequent breaks in eye contact. Towering over or staring at someone can be interpreted as threatening or controlling by paranoid individuals.
When patient begins to talk, listen. Use clarification techniques.	Active listening allows the patient to feel heard and understood, helps build rapport, and can productively channel energy.

the treatment team, except in extreme situations. Extreme situations include (1) child or elder abuse, (2) threats of self-harm or of harm to others, and (3) intention not to follow through with the treatment plan.

If information must be shared with others, it is usually the physician who will share it, according to legal guidelines (see Chapter 7). The psychiatric nurse must be aware of the patient's right to confidentiality and must not violate that right. Safeguarding the privacy and confidentiality of patients is not only

an ethical obligation but a legal responsibility as well (Wong, Lavoie, Browne, et al., 2015). For example, a student may say the following:

> **Student:** "Mrs. Almodovar, I will be sharing some of what we discuss with my nursing instructor, and at times I may discuss certain concerns with my peers in conference or with the staff. However, I will not be sharing this information with your husband or any other members of your family or anyone outside the hospital without your permission."

Planning for Terms of Termination

Termination is that last phase in Peplau's model, but planning for termination actually begins in the orientation phase. It also may be mentioned, when appropriate, during the working phase if the nature of the relationship is time limited (e.g., six or nine sessions). The date of the termination should be clear from the beginning. In some situations, the nurse–patient contract may be renegotiated once the termination date has been reached. In other situations, when the therapeutic psychiatric nurse–patient relationship is an open-ended one, the termination date is not known.

> **Student:** "Mrs. Almodovar, as I mentioned earlier, our last meeting will be on October 25. We will have three more meetings after today."

Working Phase

The development of a strong working relationship can provide support and safety for the patient, who may experience increased levels of anxiety and demonstrate dysfunctional behaviours while trying out new and more adaptive coping behaviours. In 1988, Moore and Hartman identified specific tasks of the working phase of the nurse–patient relationship that remain relevant in current practice:

- Maintain the relationship.
- Gather further data.
- Promote the patient's problem-solving skills, self-esteem, and use of language.
- Facilitate behavioural change.
- Overcome resistance behaviours.
- Evaluate problems and goals, and redefine them as necessary.
- Promote practice and expression of alternative adaptive behaviours.

During the working phase, the psychiatric nurse and patient together identify and explore areas that are causing problems in the patient's life. Often the patient's present ways of handling situations stem from earlier means of coping devised to survive in a chaotic and dysfunctional family environment. Although certain coping methods may have worked for the patient at an earlier age, they now interfere with the patient's interpersonal relationships and prevent attainment of current goals. The patient's dysfunctional behaviours and basic assumptions about the world are often defensive, and the patient is usually unable to change the dysfunctional behaviour at will. Therefore most of the problem behaviours or thoughts continue because of unconscious motivations and needs that are beyond the patient's awareness.

The psychiatric nurse can work with the patient to identify unconscious motivations and assumptions that keep the patient from finding satisfaction and reaching his or her potential. Describing, and often re-experiencing, old conflicts generally awakens high levels of anxiety. Patients may use various defences against anxiety and displace their feelings onto the nurse. Therefore, during the working phase, intense emotions such as anxiety, anger, self-hate, hopelessness, and helplessness may surface. Defence mechanisms, such as acting out anger inappropriately, withdrawing, intellectualizing, manipulating, and denying are to be expected.

During the working phase, the patient may unconsciously transfer strong feelings about or for significant others from the past into the present and onto the nurse (transference). The emotional responses and behaviours of the patient may also awaken strong counter-transference feelings in the psychiatric nurse. The nurse's awareness of these personal feelings and of reactions to the patient are vital for effective interaction with the patient.

Termination Phase

The termination phase is the final, integral phase of the nurse–patient relationship. Termination is discussed during the first interview and again during the working stage at appropriate times. Termination occurs when the patient is discharged. The tasks of termination are as follows:

- Summarize the goals and objectives achieved in the relationship.
- Discuss ways for the patient to incorporate into daily life any new coping strategies learned.
- Review situations that occurred during the nurse–patient relationship.
- Exchange memories, which can help validate the experience for both the nurse and the patient and facilitate closure of the relationship.

Termination can stimulate strong feelings in both the nurse and the patient. Termination of the relationship signifies a loss for both, although the intensity and meaning of termination may be different for each. If a patient has unresolved feelings of abandonment, loneliness, being unwanted, or rejection, these feelings may be reawakened during the termination process. This process can be an opportunity for the patient to express these feelings, perhaps for the first time.

Important reasons for the nurse to engage consciously in the termination phase of the therapeutic relationship include the following:

- Feelings are aroused in both the patient and the nurse about the experience they have had; when these feelings are recognized and shared, patients learn that it is acceptable to feel sadness and loss when someone they care about leaves.
- Termination can be a learning experience; patients can learn that they are important to at least one person, and psychiatric nurses learn continually from each clinical experience and patient encounter.
- By sharing the termination experience with the patient, the psychiatric nurse demonstrates genuineness and caring for the patient.
- This encounter may be the first successful termination experience for the patient.

If a psychiatric nurse has been working with a patient for a while, it is important for the nurse to bring into awareness any feelings or reactions the patient may be experiencing related to separations. If a patient denies that the termination is having an effect (assuming that the nurse–patient relationship was strong), the nurse may say something like "Goodbyes are difficult for people. Often they remind us of other goodbyes. Tell me about another separation in your past." If the patient appears to be displacing anger, either by withdrawing or by being overtly angry at the nurse, the nurse may use generalized statements such as "People may experience anger when saying goodbye. Sometimes they are angry with the person who is leaving. Tell me how you feel about my leaving."

New practitioners and students in a psychiatric nursing setting need to give serious thought to their final clinical experience with a patient and work with their supervisor or instructor to facilitate communication during this time. A common response of beginning practitioners and of students is feeling guilty about terminating the relationship. These feelings may, in rare cases, be manifested by the student's giving the patient his or her telephone number, making plans to get together for coffee after the patient is discharged, continuing to see the patient afterward, or exchanging emails or other communications. Often such actions are in response to the student's need to feel less guilty for using the patient to meet learning needs, to maintain a feeling of being important to the patient, or to sustain the illusion that the student is the only one who understands the patient, among other student-centred rationales. Maintaining contact with a patient after discharge, however, is not acceptable and is in opposition to the goals of a therapeutic relationship.

Indeed, part of the termination process may be to explore—after discussion with the patient's case manager—the patient's plans for the future: where the patient can go for help, which agencies to contact, and which people may best help the patient find appropriate and helpful resources.

WHAT HINDERS AND WHAT HELPS THE NURSE–PATIENT RELATIONSHIP

Not all nurse–patient relationships follow the classic phases outlined by Peplau. Some start in the orientation phase and move to a mutually frustrating phase and finally to mutual withdrawal (Figure 9-2).

Forchuk and colleagues (2000) conducted a qualitative study of the nurse–patient relationship. They examined the phases of both therapeutic and nontherapeutic relationships. From this study, they identified certain behaviours that were beneficial to the progression of the nurse–patient relationship, as well as those that hampered its development. The study emphasized that consistent, regular, and private interactions with patients are essential to the development of a therapeutic relationship. Nurses in this study stressed the importance of consistency, pacing, and listening. Specifically, the study found evidence that the following factors enhanced the nurse–patient relationship, allowing it to progress in a mutually satisfying manner:

- Consistency—ensuring that a nurse is always assigned to the same patient and that the patient has a regular routine for activities. Interactions are facilitated when they are frequent and regular in duration, format, and location. The importance of consistency extends to the nurse's being honest and consistent (congruent) in what is said to the patient.
- Pacing—letting the patient set the pace and letting the pace be adjusted to fit the patient's moods. A slow approach helps reduce pressure; at times, it is necessary to step back and realize that developing a strong relationship may take a long time.
- Listening—letting the patient talk when needed. The nurse becomes a sounding board for the patient's concerns and issues. Listening is perhaps the most important skill for nurses to master. Truly listening to another person (i.e., attending to what is behind the words) is a learned skill.
- Initial impressions, especially positive initial attitudes and preconceptions, are significant considerations in how the relationship will progress. Preconceived negative impressions and feelings toward the patient (e.g., the nurse's feeling that the patient is "interesting" or a "challenge") usually bode poorly for the positive growth of the relationship. In contrast, an inherent positive regard for the patient as a person is usually a favourable sign for the developing therapeutic relationship.
- Promoting patient comfort and balancing control usually reflect caring behaviours. *Control* refers to keeping a balance in the relationship: not too strict and not too lenient.
- Patient factors that seem to enhance the relationship include trust on the part of the patient and the patient's active participation in the nurse–patient relationship.

In relationships that did not progress to therapeutic levels, there seemed to be two major factors that hampered the development of positive relationships: inconsistency and unavailability (e.g., lack of contact, infrequent meetings, meetings in the hallway) on the part of the nurse, patient, or both. When nurse and patient are reluctant to spend time together, and meeting times become sporadic or superficial, the term *mutual avoidance* is used. This is clearly a lose–lose situation.

The nurse's personal feelings and lack of self-awareness are major elements that contribute to the lack of progression toward a positive relationship. Negative preconceived ideas and feelings (e.g., discomfort, dislike, fear, avoidance) about the patient seem to be a constant in relationships that end in frustration and mutual withdrawal. Sometimes these feelings are known, and sometimes the nurse is only vaguely aware of them.

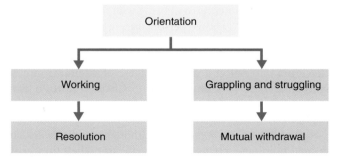

FIGURE 9-2 Phases of therapeutic and nontherapeutic relationships. Source: Forchuk, C., Westwell, J., Martin, M., et al. (2000). The developing nurse–client relationship: Nurses' perspectives. *Journal of the American Psychiatric Nurses Association, 6*(1), 3–10, copyright © 2000 by SAGE Publications. Reprinted by Permission of SAGE Publications. doi:10.1177/107839030000600102.

FACTORS THAT ENCOURAGE AND PROMOTE PATIENTS' GROWTH

Rogers and Truax (1967) identified three personal characteristics of the nurse that help promote change and growth in patients—factors still valued today as vital components for establishing a therapeutic relationship: genuineness, empathy, and positive regard. These are some of the intangibles that are at the heart of the art of nursing.

Genuineness

Genuineness, or self-awareness of one's feelings as they arise within the relationship and the ability to communicate them when appropriate, is a key ingredient in building trust. When a person is genuine, one gets the sense that what the person displays is congruent with his or her internal processes. Genuineness is conveyed by listening to and communicating with patients without distorting their messages and being clear and concrete in communications. Being genuine in a therapeutic relationship implies the ability to use therapeutic communication tools in an appropriately spontaneous manner, rather than rigidly or in a parrotlike fashion.

Empathy

Empathy is a complex multidimensional concept in which the helping person attempts to understand the world from the patient's perspective. It does not mean that the nurse condones or approves of the patient's actions but rather is nonjudgemental or uncritical of the patient's choices (Hsiao, Lu, & Tsai, 2015). Essentially, it means "temporarily living in the other's life, moving about in it delicately without making judgments" (Rogers, 1980, p. 142).

In the past, empathy has been thought of as the nurse accurately perceiving the patient's situation, perspective, and feelings; however, as relational ways of caring are further developed, the concept of empathy is shifting to include the idea of care and responsiveness that supports people's health and healing (Doane & Varcoe, 2010). The ability to empathize is developed through practising relational competencies related to understanding the meaning and complexity of experience. There is a relationship intersubjectivity that is developed between the patient and the nurse. It is that relationship that becomes the foundation of being, knowing, and doing.

Empathy Versus Sympathy

There is much confusion regarding empathy versus sympathy. A simple way to distinguish them is to recognize that in empathy, we *understand* the feelings of others; in sympathy, we *feel* the feelings of others. When a helping person is feeling sympathy for another, objectivity is lost, and the ability to assist the patient in solving a personal problem ceases. Furthermore, sympathy is associated with feelings of pity and commiseration. Although these are considered nurturing human traits, they may not be particularly useful in a therapeutic relationship. When people express sympathy, they express agreement with another, which in some situations may discourage further exploration of a person's thoughts and feelings.

The following examples are given to clarify the distinction between empathy and sympathy. A friend tells you that her mother was just diagnosed with inoperable cancer. Your friend then begins to cry and pounds the table with her fist.

Sympathetic response: "I feel so sorry for you. I know exactly how you feel. My mother was hospitalized last year, and it was awful. I was so depressed. I still get upset just thinking about it." (You go on to tell your friend about the incident.)

Sometimes when psychiatric nurses try to be sympathetic, they are apt to project their own feelings onto the patient's, which can limit the patient's range of responses. A more useful response might be as follows:

Empathic response: "It sounds as though you are feeling upset and angry having learned about your mother's inoperable cancer diagnosis. Tell me what thoughts and feelings you are having." (You continue to stay with your friend and listen to his or her thoughts and feelings.)

Empathy is not a technique but rather an attitude that conveys respect, acceptance, and validation of the patient's strengths. In the practice of psychotherapy or counselling, empathy is one of the most important factors in building a trusting and therapeutic relationship (Wheeler, 2013).

Positive Regard

Positive regard implies respect. It is the ability to view another person as being worthy of being cared about and as someone who has strengths and achievement potential. Positive regard is usually communicated indirectly by attitudes and actions rather than directly by words.

Attitudes

One attitude through which a nurse might convey positive regard, or respect, is willingness to work with the patient. That is, the nurse takes the patient and the relationship seriously. The experience is viewed not as a job, part of a course, or time spent talking but as an opportunity to work with patients to help them develop personal resources and actualize more of their potential in living.

Actions

Some actions that manifest an attitude of respect are attending, suspending value judgements, calling the individual by his or her first or last name, and helping patients develop their own resources.

Attending. Attending behaviour is the foundation of interviewing. To be effective, psychiatric nurses must pay attention to their patients in culturally and individually appropriate ways (Racine, 2014). *Attending* is a special kind of listening that refers to an intensity of presence, or of being with the patient. At times, simply being with another person during a painful time can make a difference.

Posture, eye contact, and body language are nonverbal behaviours that reflect a person's degree of attending and are highly influenced by culture. Refer to Chapter 10 for a more detailed discussion of the cultural implications of the clinical interview.

Suspending value judgements. Although we will always have personal opinions, nurses are more effective when they guard against using their own value systems to judge patients' thoughts, feelings, or behaviours. For example, if a patient is taking drugs or is involved in risky sexual behaviour, the nurse may recognize that these behaviours are hindering the patient from living a more satisfying life, posing a potential health threat, or preventing the patient from developing satisfying relationships. However, labelling these activities as bad or good is not useful. Rather, the nurse should focus on exploring the behaviour and work toward identifying the thoughts and feelings that influence this behaviour. Judgement on the part of the nurse will most likely interfere with further exploration.

The first steps in eliminating judgemental thinking and behaviours are to (1) recognize their presence, (2) identify how or where you learned these responses to the patient's behaviour, and (3) construct alternative ways to view the patient's thinking and behaviour. Denying judgemental thinking will only compound the problem.

> *Patient:* "I guess you could consider me an addictive personality. I love to gamble when I have money and spend most of my time in the casino. It seems as though I'm hooking up with a different woman every time I'm there, and it always ends in sex. This has been going on for at least 3 years."

A judgemental response would be:

> *Nurse A:* "So your compulsive gambling and promiscuous sexual behaviours really haven't brought you much happiness, have they? You're running away from your problems and could end up with sexually transmitted infections and no money."

A more helpful response would be:

> *Nurse B:* "So your sexual and gambling activities are part of the picture also. You make it sound as though these activities are not making you happy."

In this example, nurse B focuses on the patient's behaviours and the possible meaning they might have to the patient. This nurse does not introduce personal value statements or prejudices regarding promiscuous behaviour, as nurse A does. Empathy and positive regard are essential qualities in a successful nurse–patient relationship.

Helping patients develop resources. The nurse becomes aware of patients' strengths and encourages patients to work at their optimal level of functioning. This support can be seen as one form of collaboration with the patient. The psychiatric nurse does not act for patients unless absolutely necessary, and then only as a step toward helping them to act on their own. It is important that patients remain as independent as possible to develop new resources for problem solving. The following are examples of helping the patient to develop independence:

> *Patient:* "This medication makes my mouth so dry. Could you get me something to drink?"
>
> *Nurse:* "There is juice in the refrigerator. I'll wait here for you until you get back" *or* "I'll walk with you while you get some juice from the refrigerator."
>
> *Patient:* "Could you ask the doctor to let me have a pass for the weekend?"
>
> *Nurse:* "Your doctor will be on the unit this afternoon. I'll let her know that you want to speak with her."

Consistently encouraging patients to use their own resources helps minimize the patients' feelings of helplessness and dependency and validates their potential for change.

KEY POINTS TO REMEMBER

- The nurse–patient relationship is well defined, and the roles of the nurse and the patient must be clearly stated.
- It is important that the nurse be aware of the differences between a therapeutic relationship and a social or intimate relationship. In a therapeutic psychiatric nurse–patient relationship, the focus is on the patient's needs, thoughts, feelings, and goals. The psychiatric nurse is expected to meet personal needs outside this relationship.
- Although the boundaries and roles of the nurse–patient relationship generally are clearly defined, they can become blurred; this blurring can be insidious and may occur on an unconscious level. Usually transference and counter-transference phenomena are operating when boundaries are blurred.

- It is important to have a grasp of common counter-transferential feelings and behaviours and of the psychiatric nursing actions to counteract these phenomena.
- Supervision aids in promoting both the professional growth of the psychiatric nurse and the psychiatric nurse–patient relationship, allowing the patient's goals to be worked on and met.
- The phases of the psychiatric nurse–patient relationship include preorientation, orientation, working, and termination.
- Genuineness, empathy, and positive regard are personal strengths of effective helpers who are able to foster growth and change in others.

CRITICAL THINKING

1. On your first clinical day, you are assigned to work with an older adult, Mrs. Schneider, who is depressed. Your first impression is, "Oh my, she looks like my nasty aunt Helen. She even sits like her." You approach her with a vague feeling of uneasiness and say hello. Mrs. Schneider responds, "Who are you, and how can you help me?" You answer by providing your name and telling her that you are a nursing student and will be working with her today. She tells you that "a student" could never understand what she is going through. She then says, "If you really want to help me, you would get me a good job after I leave here."

   a. Identify transference and counter-transference issues in this situation. What is your most important course of action?

   b. How could you best respond to Mrs. Schneider's question about who you are? What other information will you give her during this first clinical encounter? Be specific.

c. What are some useful responses you could give Mrs. Schneider regarding her legitimate questions about ways you could be of help to her?

d. Analyze Mrs. Schneider's request that you find her a job. Keeping in mind the aim of Peplau's interactive nurse–patient process, describe some useful ways you could respond to this request.

e. Consider how your response and ongoing discussions with Mrs. Schneider can convey key characteristics of a therapeutic relationship: respect, positive regard, genuineness, and empathy.

2. You are interviewing Tom Stone, a 17-year-old who was admitted to a psychiatric unit after a suicide attempt. How would you best respond to each of the following patient requests and behaviours?

a. "I would feel so much better if you would sit closer to me and hold my hand."

b. "I will tell you if I still feel like killing myself, but you have to promise not to tell anyone else. If you do, I just can't trust you, ever."

c. "I don't want to talk to you. I have absolutely nothing to say."

d. "I will be going home tomorrow, and you have been so helpful and good to me. I want you to have my watch to remember me by."

e. Tom breaks down and starts sobbing.

CHAPTER REVIEW

1. Which of the following actions best represents the basis or foundation of all other psychiatric nursing care?
   a. The nurse assesses the patient at regular intervals.
   b. The nurse administers psychotropic medications.
   c. The nurse spends time sitting with a withdrawn patient.
   d. The nurse participates in team meetings with other professionals.

2. A male patient frequently inquires about the female student nurse's boyfriend, social activities, and school experiences. Which of the following initial responses by the student best addresses the issue raised by this behaviour?
   a. The student requests assignment to a patient of the same gender as the student.
   b. The student points out to the patient that he is making social inquiries and explores this behaviour.
   c. The student tells the patient that she cannot talk about her personal life and returns the focus to his issues.
   d. The student explains that if the patient persists in focusing on her, she cannot work with him.

3. Mary, a patient in the psychiatric unit, had a very rejecting and abusive father and a difficult childhood, but from age 10 on was raised by a very warm and supportive grandmother who recently passed away. Mary frequently comments on how hard her nurse, Jessa, works and on how other staff do not seem to care as much about their patients as Jessa does. Jessa finds herself agreeing with Mary and appreciating her insightfulness, recalling to herself that except for her former head nurse, other staff do not seem to appreciate how hard she works and seem to take her for granted. Jessa enjoys the time she spends with Mary and seeks out opportunities to interact with her. What phenomenon is occurring here, and which response by Jessa would most benefit her and the patient?
   a. Mary is experiencing transference; Jessa should help Mary to understand that she is emphasizing in Jessa those qualities that were missing in her father.

b. Jessa is idealizing Mary, seeing in her strengths and abilities that Mary does not really possess; Jessa should temporarily distance herself somewhat from Mary.

c. Mary is overidentifying with Jessa, seeing similarities that do not in reality exist; Jessa should label and explore this phenomenon in her interactions with Mary.

d. Jessa is experiencing counter-transference in response to Mary's meeting Jessa's needs for greater appreciation; Jessa should seek clinical supervision to explore these dynamics.

4. Which of the following statements would be appropriate during the orientation phase of the nurse–patient relationship? Select all that apply.
   a. "My name is Sarah, and I am a student nurse here to learn about mental health."
   b. "I will be here each Thursday from 8 a.m. until noon if you would like to talk."
   c. "Tell me about what you think would best help you to cope with the loss of your wife."
   d. "Let's talk today about how our plan for improving your sleep has been working."
   e. "We will meet weekly for 1 hour, during which we will discuss how to meet your goals."
   f. "Being home alone while your wife was hospitalized must have been very difficult for you."

5. A student nurse exhibits the following behaviours or actions while interacting with her patient. Which of these is appropriate as part of a therapeutic relationship?
   a. Sitting attentively in silence with a withdrawn patient until the patient chooses to speak.
   b. Offering the patient advice on how he or she could cope more effectively with stress.
   c. Controlling the pace of the relationship by selecting topics for each interaction.
   d. Limiting the discussion of termination issues so as not to sadden the patient unduly.

Evolve WEBSITE

Post-Test   interactive review

REFERENCES

Badawi, A. (2016). Boundaries in therapeutic practice. *Journal of the Australian Traditional-Medicine Society*, 22(2), 90–93. Retrieved from http://www.atms.com.au/page.php?id=11.

Benner, P. (2000). *From novice to expert: Excellence and power in clinical nursing practice (commemorative ed.).* Upper Saddle River, NJ: Prentice-Hall.

Brown, B. (2015). Towards a critical understanding of mutuality in mental healthcare: Relationships, power and social capital. *Journal of Psychiatric & Mental Health Nursing*, 22(10), 829–835. doi:10.1111/jpm.12269.

Doane, G. H., & Varcoe, C. (2010). Boundaries and the culture of theorizing in nursing. *Nursing Science Quarterly*, 23(2), 130–137. doi:10.1177/0894318410362544.

Forchuk, C., Westwell, J., Martin, M., et al. (2000). The developing nurse–client relationship: Nurses' perspectives. *Journal of the American Psychiatric Nurses Association*, 6(1), 3–10. doi:10.1177/107839030000600102.

Gonge, H., & Buus, N. (2015). Is it possible to strengthen psychiatric nursing staff's clinical supervision? RCT of meta-supervision intervention. *Journal of Advanced Nursing*, 71(4), 909–921. doi:10.1111/jan.12569.

Haber, J. (2000). Hildegard E. Peplau: The psychiatric nursing legacy of a legend. *Journal of the American Psychiatric Nurses Association*, 6(2), 56–62. doi:10.1067/mpn.2000.104556.

Hsiao, C., Lu, H., & Tsai, Y. (2015). Factors influencing mental health nurses' attitudes towards people with mental illness. *International Journal of Mental Health Nursing*, 24(3), 272–280. doi:10.1111/inm.12129.

Kanera, A., Kivinen, T., & Lammintakanen, J. (2015). Communication elements supporting patient safety in psychiatric inpatient care. *Journal of Psychiatric and Mental Health Nursing*, 22(5), 298–305. doi:10.1111/jpm.12187.

Kim, S., Roth, W. T., & Wollburg, E. (2015). Effects of therapeutic relationship, expectancy, and credibility in breathing therapies for anxiety. *Bulletin of the Menninger Clinic*, 79(2), 116–130. doi:10.1521/bumc.2015.79.2.116.

Moore, J. C., & Hartman, C. R. (1988). Developing a therapeutic relationship. In C. K. Beck, R. P. Rawlins, & S. R. Williams (Eds.), *Mental health–psychiatric nursing.* St. Louis: Mosby.

Peplau, H. E. (1952). *Interpersonal relations in nursing: A conceptual frame of reference for psychodynamic nursing.* New York: Putnam.

Peplau, H. E. (1999). *Interpersonal relations in nursing: A conceptual frame of reference for psychodynamic nursing.* New York: Springer.

Quinlan, J. C. E. (1996). *Co-creating personal and professional knowledge through peer support and peer approval in nursing* (Doctorial dissertation). Retrieved from http://people.bath.ac.uk/mnspwr/doc_theses_links/j_quinlan.html.

Racine, L. (2014). The enduring challenge of cultural safety. *Canadian Journal of Nursing Research*, 46(2), 6–9. Retrieved from http://www.mcgill.ca/cjnr/.

Registered Nurses' Association of Ontario (2002). *Nursing best practice guidelines: Establishing therapeutic relationships.* Toronto: Author. Retrieved from http://rnao.ca/bpg/guidelines/establishing-therapeutic-relationships.

Rogers, C. R. (1980). *A way of being.* Boston: Houghton Mifflin.

Rogers, C. R., & Truax, C. B. (1967). The therapeutic conditions antecedent to change: A theoretical view. In C. R. Rogers (Ed.), *The therapeutic relationship and its impact.* Madison, WI: University of Wisconsin Press.

Travelbee, J. (1971). *Interpersonal aspects of nursing* (2nd ed.). Philadelphia: F. A. Davis Co.

Wheeler, K. (2013). *Psychotherapy for the advanced practice psychiatric nurse* (2nd ed.). St. Louis: Mosby.

Wong, S. T., Lavoie, J. G., Browne, A. J., et al. (2015). Patient confidentiality within the context of group medical visits: Is there cause for concern? *Health Expectations*, 18(5), 727–739. doi:10.1111/hex.12156.

10

Communication and the Clinical Interview

Elizabeth M. Varcarolis
Adapted by Sonya L. Jakubec

KEY TERMS AND CONCEPTS

active listening
closed-ended questions
cultural filters
debriefing
double messages
double-bind messages
feedback

nontherapeutic communication techniques
nonverbal behaviours
nonverbal communication
open-ended questions
therapeutic communication skills and strategies
verbal communication

OBJECTIVES

1. Identify three personal and two environmental factors that can impede communication.
2. Discuss the differences between verbal and nonverbal communication, and identify five examples of nonverbal communication.
3. Identify two attending behaviours the psychiatric nurse might focus on to increase communication skills.
4. Compare and contrast the range of verbal and nonverbal communication of different cultural groups in the areas of communication style, eye contact, and touch.
5. Relate problems that can arise when nurses are insensitive to cultural aspects of patients' communication styles.
6. Demonstrate the use of four techniques that can enhance communication, highlighting what makes them effective.
7. Demonstrate the use of four techniques that can obstruct communication, highlighting what makes them ineffective.
8. Identify and give rationales for suggested setting, seating, and methods for beginning the psychiatric nurse–patient interaction.
9. Explain the importance of clinical supervision.

⊖volve WEBSITE

Visit the Evolve website for Flashcards, Case Studies, and additional testing resources related to the content in this chapter: http://evolve.elsevier.com/Canada/Varcarolis/psychiatric/

Pre-Test   interactive review

Humans have a built-in need to relate to others, and our advanced ability to communicate contributes to the substance and meaning in our lives. Our need to express ourselves to others is powerful; it is the foundation on which we form happy and productive relationships in our adult lives. At the same time, stress and negative feelings within a relationship are often the result of ineffective communication. All of our actions, words, and facial expressions convey meaning to others. It has been said that we cannot not communicate. Even silence can convey acceptance, anger, or thoughtfulness.

In the provision of psychiatric nursing care, communication takes on a new emphasis. Just as social relationships are different from therapeutic relationships (see Chapter 9), *basic communication* is different from professional, patient-centred, goal-directed, and scientifically based *therapeutic communication*.

The ability to form therapeutic relationships is fundamental and essential to effective psychiatric nursing care, and therapeutic communication is central to the formation of a therapeutic relationship. Determining levels of pain in the postoperative patient; listening as parents express feelings of fear concerning their child's diagnosis; or understanding, without words, the needs of the intubated patient in the intensive care unit are essential skills in providing quality nursing care.

Research about psychiatric patients' perspectives on their therapeutic relationships with nurses revealed that the nurses' verbal and nonverbal communication shaped the development or deterioration of these relationships (Coatsworth-Puspoky, Forchuk, & Ward-Griffin, 2006). Ideally, therapeutic communication is a professional skill you learn and practise early in your nursing curriculum. But in psychiatric mental health nursing, communication skills take on a different and new emphasis. Psychiatric disorders cause not only physical responses (fatigue, loss of appetite, insomnia) but also emotional responses (sadness, anger, hopelessness, euphoria) that affect a patient's ability to relate to others.

It is often during a psychiatric nursing practice experience that students discover the utility of therapeutic communication and begin to rely on techniques they once considered artificial. For example, restating may seem like a funny thing to do. Using it in a practice session between students ("I felt sad when my dog ran away." "You felt sad when your dog ran away?") can derail communication and end the seriousness with laughter. Yet in the clinical setting, restating can become a powerful and profound communication strategy in building a therapeutic alliance:

> **Patient:** "At the moment they told me my daughter would never be able to walk like her twin sister, I felt as though I couldn't go on."
>
> **Nurse:** (After a short silence) "You felt uncertain that you could go on when you learned your daughter would never be able to walk like her twin sister."

The technique, and the empathy it conveys, is appreciated in such a situation. Developing therapeutic communication skills takes time, and with continued practice, you will develop your own style and rhythm. Eventually these communication skills and strategies will become a part of the way you instinctively communicate with others in the clinical setting and in your personal life as you integrate them into your way of being with others.

Beginning psychiatric practitioners are often concerned that they may say the wrong thing, especially when learning to apply therapeutic techniques. Will you say the wrong thing? Yes, you probably will, but that is how we all learn to find more useful and effective ways of helping individuals to reach their goals. The challenge is to recover from your mistakes and use them for learning and growth (Sommers-Flanagan & Sommers-Flanagan, 2013).

One of the most common concerns students have is that they will say the one thing that will "push the patient over the edge" or maybe even be the cause for the patient to give up on living. This is highly unlikely. Consider that behaviours associated with psychiatric disorders, such as irritability, agitation, negativity, disinterest in communication, and being hypertalkative, often frustrate and alienate friends and family. It is likely that the interactions the patient has had to date have not always been pleasant and supportive. Patients often see a well-meaning person who conveys genuine acceptance, respect, empathy, and concern for their well-being as a gift. Even if mistakes in communication are made or the "wrong thing" is said, there is little chance that the comments will do actual harm. With reflection and supervision, mistakes in communication can be corrected and repaired. When a nurse explains his or her errors in communication and repairs the miscommunication, this show of humility and genuineness may even strengthen the therapeutic relationship.

THE COMMUNICATION PROCESS

Communication is an interactive process between two or more people who send and receive messages to one another. The following is a simplified model of communication (Berlo, 1960):

1. One person has a need to communicate with another (*stimulus*) for information, comfort, or advice.
2. The person sending the message (*sender*) initiates interpersonal contact.
3. The *message* is the information sent or expressed to another. The clearest messages are those that are well organized and expressed in a manner familiar to the receiver.
4. The message can be sent through a variety of media, including auditory (hearing), visual (seeing), tactile (touch), smell, or any combination of these.
5. The person receiving the message (*receiver*) then interprets the message and responds to the sender by providing feedback (communication of impressions of and reactions to the sender's actions or verbalizations). Validating the accuracy of the sender's message is extremely important. The nature of the feedback often indicates whether the meaning of the message sent has been correctly interpreted by the receiver. An accuracy check may be obtained by simply asking the sender, "Is this what you mean?" or "I notice you turn away when we talk about your going back to college. Is there a conflict there?"

Figure 10-1 shows this simple model of communication, along with some of the many factors that affect it.

Effective communication in therapeutic relationships depends on nurses knowing what they are trying to convey (the purpose of the message), communicating to the patient what is really meant, and comprehending the meaning of what the patient intentionally or unintentionally conveys (Arnold & Boggs, 2016). A systematic review of Peplau (1952) identified two main principles that can guide the communication process during the nurse–patient interview (discussed in detail later in this chapter): (1) clarity, which ensures that the meaning of the message is accurately understood by both parties in an ongoing mutual effort, and (2) continuity, which promotes the connections among relevant ideas and encourages a shared understanding of the activities, emotions, and context of those ideas. Maintaining this clarity and continuity requires particular concentration and attention when patients are acutely mentally ill and possibly experiencing symptoms impairing their communication.

FACTORS THAT AFFECT COMMUNICATION

Personal Factors

Personal factors that can impede accurate transmission or interpretation of messages include emotional factors (e.g., mood,

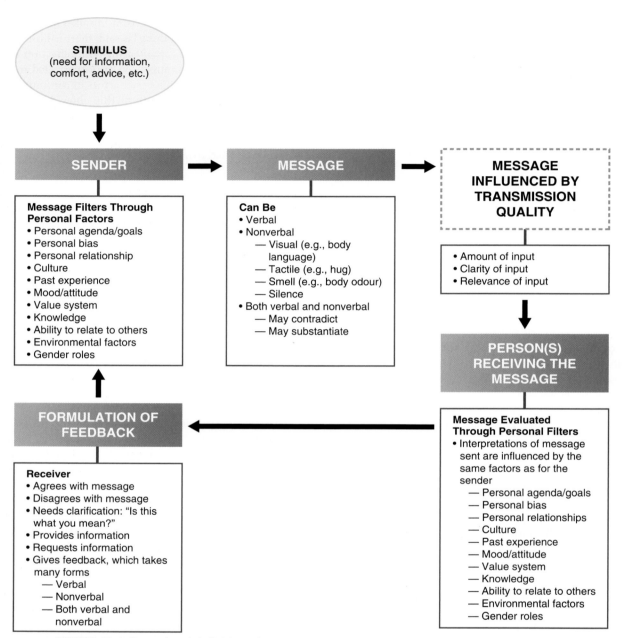

FIGURE 10-1 Operational definition of *communication*. Source: Data from Ellis, R., & McClintock, A. (1990). *If you take my meaning.* London, UK: Arnold.

responses to stress, personal bias), social factors (e.g., previous experience, cultural differences, language differences), and cognitive factors (e.g., problem-solving ability, knowledge level, language use).

Environmental Factors

Environmental factors that may affect communication include physical factors (e.g., background noise, lack of privacy, uncomfortable accommodations) and societal determinants (e.g., sociopolitical, historical, and economic factors; the presence of others; expectations of others).

Relationship Factors

Relationship factors refer to the status of individuals in terms of social standing, power, roles, responsibilities, age, and so on. Communication is influenced by all of these factors. Consider how you would describe your day in the clinical setting to your instructor, compared to how you would describe it to your friend. The fact that your instructor has more education than you and is in an evaluative role would likely influence how much you share and your choice of words.

Now think about the relationship between you and your patient. Your patient may be older or younger than you are,

RESEARCH HIGHLIGHT

Supplementing Goal Setting for Families Using Motivational Interviewing

Problem

Communication with and for families around healthy eating and behaviours can be challenging, and it is unclear what kind of interviewing will be most effective to support change in food choices and habits of family meals.

Purpose of Study

The purpose of the study was to describe how motivational interviewing (a style of communication that prepares people for change through questions and interviewing to enhance intrinsic motivation, building confidence for change) can be used to support parents to facilitate health behaviour change, particularly around healthy eating, family meals, and obesity prevention.

Methods

A motivational interviewing (MI) intervention (focused on healthy homes and meals) was part of a randomized controlled trial that included 81 families (children 8 to 12 years old and their parents) in the intervention group. The intervention included 10 monthly 2-hour group sessions and 5 bimonthly motivational or goal-setting phone calls. Data were collected for intervention families only at each of the goal-setting calls, and a behaviour change assessment was administered at the tenth and final group session.

Key Findings

Descriptive statistics were used to analyze the MI call data and behaviour assessment. Overall group attendance was high (68% attending ≥7 sessions). Motivational or goal-setting phone calls were well accepted by parents, with an 87% average completion rate. More than 85% of the time, families reported meeting their chosen goal between calls. Families completing the behavioural assessment reported the most change in having family meals more often and improving home food healthfulness.

Implications for Nursing Practice

A combination of delivery methods using MI may be useful when implementing behaviour change programs for families to promote goal setting.

Source: Draxten, M., Flattum, C., & Fulkerson, J. (2016). An example of how to supplement goal setting to promote behavior change for families using motivational interviewing. *Health Communication, 31*(10), 1276–1283. doi:10.1080/10410236.2015.1062975.

more or less educated, richer or poorer, successful at work or unemployed. These factors play into the dynamics of the communication, whether at a conscious or an unconscious level, and recognizing their influence is important. It may be difficult for you to work with a woman your mother's age or one your own age, or you may feel impatient with a patient who is unemployed and abuses alcohol.

It is sometimes difficult for students to grasp or remember that patients, regardless of these relationship factors, are in a position of vulnerability. Wearing a hospital identification band or stepping through the door of a community mental health clinic formally indicates a need for care, and as a caregiver, you are viewed to be in a role of authority. Part of the art of therapeutic communication is finding a balance between your role as a professional and your role as a human being who has been socialized into complex patterns of interactions based, at least in part, on status.

Students sometimes fall back into time-tested and comfortable roles. As such, one of the most common responses of nursing students to nurse–patient relationships is treating the patient as a buddy. Imagine a male nursing student walking onto the unit, seeing his assigned patient, and saying, "Hey, how's it going today?" while giving the patient a high-five. Or consider the female nursing student assigned to a 60-year-old woman who used to work as a registered nurse. This relationship has the potential to become unbalanced and nontherapeutic if the patient shifts the focus away from his or her own concerns and onto the student nurse's interests and concerns (see Chapter 9).

VERBAL AND NONVERBAL COMMUNICATION

Verbal Communication

Verbal communication consists of all the words a person speaks. We live in a society of symbols, and our main social symbols are words. Talking is our most common activity. It is our public link to one another, the primary instrument of instruction, a need, an art, and one of the most personal aspects of our private lives. When we speak, we:

- Communicate our beliefs and values
- Communicate perceptions and meanings
- Convey interest and understanding or insult and judgement
- Convey messages clearly or convey conflicting or implied messages
- Convey clear, honest feelings or disguised, distorted feelings

Words are culturally perceived; therefore clarifying the intent of certain words is very important. Even if the nurse and patient have a similar cultural background, the mental image that each has for a given word may not be exactly the same. Although they believe they are talking about the same thing, the nurse and patient may actually be talking about two quite different things. While they produce mental images, words are also symbols for emotions.

Nonverbal Communication

Nonverbal communication (often called *cues*) are those messages expressed through directly observable behaviours such as physical appearance, facial expressions, body posture, amount of eye contact, eye cast (i.e., emotion expressed in the eyes), hand gestures, sighs, fidgeting, and yawning. A person's tone of voice, emphasis on certain words, and pacing of speech are also examples of **nonverbal behaviours**. Sometimes these behaviours operate outside of the awareness of the person exhibiting the behaviours— or unconsciously. It is often said that "it's not what you say but how you say it." In other words, it is the nonverbal behaviours that may be communicating the "real" message (see Table 10-1). Nonverbal behaviours must be observed and interpreted in light of a person's culture, class, gender, age, sexual orientation, and spiritual beliefs. Cultural influences on communication are addressed later in this chapter.

TABLE 10-1   NONVERBAL BEHAVIOURS

BEHAVIOUR	POSSIBLE NONVERBAL CUES	EXAMPLE
Body behaviours	Posture, body movements, gestures, gait	The patient is slumped in a chair, puts her face in her hands, and occasionally taps her right foot.
Facial expressions	Frowns, smiles, grimaces, raised eyebrows, pursed lips, licking of lips, tongue movements	The patient grimaces when speaking to the nurse; when alone, he smiles and giggles to himself.
Eye cast	Angry, suspicious, and accusatory looks	The patient's eyes harden with suspicion.
Voice-related behaviours	Tone, pitch, level, intensity, inflection, stuttering, pauses, silences, fluency	The patient talks in a loud singsong voice.
Observable autonomic physiological responses	Increase in respirations, diaphoresis, pupil dilation, blushing, paleness	When the patient mentions discharge, she becomes pale, her respirations increase, and her face becomes diaphoretic.
Personal appearance	Grooming, dress, hygiene	The patient is dressed in a wrinkled shirt, his pants are stained, his socks are dirty, and he is unshaven.
Physical characteristics	Height, weight, physique, complexion	The patient is grossly overweight, and his muscles appear flabby.

Interaction of Verbal and Nonverbal Communication

Shawn Shea (2017), a nationally renowned psychiatrist and communication workshop leader, suggests that communication is roughly 10% verbal and 90% nonverbal. Our interpretation of feelings and attitudes may account for the high percentage of communication attributed to nonverbal behaviours. While it would be difficult to watch a foreign film and understand 90% of its meaning based solely on body language and vocal tones, nonverbal behaviours and cues do influence communication to a surprising degree in nurse–patient interactions. Communication thus involves two radically different but highly interdependent kinds of symbols: verbal and nonverbal.

Spoken words can be straightforward or may distort, conceal, deny, or disguise true feelings. Whereas spoken words represent our public selves, nonverbal behaviours (e.g., how a person listens and uses silence and sense of touch) can convey important information about the private self that is not available from conversation alone, especially in consideration of cultural norms.

Some elements of nonverbal communication, such as facial expressions, seem to be inborn and are similar across cultures. Matsumoto and Hwang (2011) cited studies that found a high degree of agreement in spontaneous facial expressions or emotions across 10 different cultures. However, some cultural groups (e.g., Japanese) may control their facial expressions in public. Other types of nonverbal behaviours, such as how close people stand to each other when speaking, depend on cultural conventions. Some nonverbal communication is formalized and has specific meanings (e.g., the military salute, the Japanese bow).

Messages are not always simple; they can appear to be one thing when, in fact, they are another (Shea, 2017). Often people have greater conscious awareness of their verbal messages than of their nonverbal behaviours. The verbal message is sometimes referred to as the *content* of the message (what is said), and the nonverbal behaviour is called the *process* of the message (nonverbal cues a person gives to substantiate or contradict the verbal message—or how it is said). When the content is congruent with the process, the communication is more clearly understood and is considered healthy. For example, a student saying "It's important

that I get good grades in this class" is content. The student buying the required books, taking good notes, and working with a study buddy is process. The content and process in this example are congruent and straightforward, and there is a "healthy" message. If, however, the verbal message is not reinforced or is in fact contradicted by the nonverbal behaviour, the message is confusing. For example, the student not buying the books, skipping several classes, and not studying is also process, but in this case the student is sending two different messages.

Messages are sent to create meaning but also can be used defensively to hide what is actually going on, create confusion, and attack relatedness (Shea, 2017). Conflicting messages are known as **double messages** or *mixed messages*. One way a nurse can respond to verbal and nonverbal incongruity is to reflect and validate the patient's feelings. For example, the nurse could say to the student, "You say you are upset you did not pass this semester, but I notice you look more relaxed and less conflicted than you have all term. What do you see as some of the pros and cons of not passing the course this semester?"

Bateson and colleague (1956) coined the term **double-bind messages**. A double-bind message is a contradictory mix of content and process that communicates both nurturing and hurtful expressions. The following vignette gives an example of a double-bind message.

VIGNETTE

A 21-year-old female who lives at home with her chronically ill mother wants to go out for an evening with her friends. She is told by her frail but not helpless mother: "Oh, go ahead, have fun. I'll just sit here by myself, and I can always call 911 if I don't feel well, but you go ahead and have fun." The mother says this while looking sad, eyes downcast, slumped in her chair, and letting her cane drop to the floor.

The recipient of this double-bind message is caught inside contradictory statements, so she cannot decide what is right. If she goes, the implication is that she is being selfish by leaving her sick mother alone. But if she stays, the mother could say, "I told you to go have fun." If she does go, the chances are she will not have much fun because of concern for her mother. The daughter is trapped in a no-win situation of which she may not be fully aware.

With experience, nurses become increasingly aware of patients' verbal and nonverbal communication and compare the two to gain important clues about the real message. What individuals do may either express and reinforce or contradict what they say. So, as in the saying "Actions speak louder than words," actions often reveal the true meaning of a person's intent, whether the intent is conscious or unconscious.

COMMUNICATION SKILLS FOR NURSES

Therapeutic Communication Strategies

Peplau emphasized the art of communication to highlight the importance of nursing interventions in facilitating achievement of quality patient care and quality of life (Haber, 2000). The nurse must establish and maintain a therapeutic relationship in which the patient will feel safe and hopeful that positive change is possible.

Once a therapeutic relationship is established, specific needs and problems can be identified, and the nurse can work with the patient on increasing self-awareness, developing insight and problem-solving skills, learning new coping behaviours, and experiencing more appropriate and satisfying ways of relating to others. To do this, the nurse must have a sound knowledge of communication theory and skills. Therefore nurses must become more aware of their own interpersonal methods, eliminating obstructive, nontherapeutic communication techniques and strategies and developing additional responses that maximize the nurse–patient interactions and increase the use of therapeutic communication skills and strategies (i.e., skills such as warmth, respect, and empathy and strategies such as using silence, recognizing strengths, and making observations). Helpful tools for nurses when communicating with their patients are silence, active listening, and clarifying techniques.

Silence

Silence can sometimes intimidate both interviewers and patients (Sommers-Flanagan & Sommers-Flanagan, 2013). In Canada, there is an emphasis on action and a high level of verbal activity. Students and practising nurses alike may find that when the flow of words stops, they become uncomfortable. They may rush to fill the void with "questions or chatter," thus cutting off potentially important thoughts and feelings the patient might be taking time to think about before articulating. Silence is not the absence of communication but a specific channel for transmitting and receiving messages; therefore the practitioner needs to understand that silence is a significant means of influencing and being influenced by others.

Talking is a highly individualized practice. Some people find phone calls a nuisance, whereas others believe they cannot live without speaking on the phone and having their phone available at all times. In the initial interview, patients may be reluctant to speak because of the newness of the situation; the fact that the nurse is a stranger; or feelings of distrust, self-consciousness, embarrassment, or shyness. The nurse must recognize and respect individual differences in styles and tempos of responding. People who are quiet, those who have a language barrier or speech disorder, older adults, and those who lack confidence in their ability to express themselves may communicate a need for support and encouragement through their silence.

Although there is no universal rule concerning how much silence is too much, silence has been said to be worthwhile only as long as it is serving some function and not frightening the patient. Knowing when to speak during the interview depends largely on one's perception about what is being conveyed through the silence. Icy silence may be an expression of anger and hostility; being ignored or given "the silent treatment" is recognized as an insult and is a particularly hurtful form of communication.

Silence may provide meaningful moments of reflection for both participants, giving an opportunity to contemplate thoughtfully what has been said and felt, weigh alternatives, formulate new ideas, and gain a new perspective on the matter under discussion. If the nurse waits to speak and allows the patient to break the silence, the patient may share thoughts and feelings that would otherwise have been withheld. Nurses who feel compelled to fill every void with words often do so because of their own anxiety, self-consciousness, and embarrassment. This action, however, prioritizes the nurse's need for comfort over the needs of the patient.

It is crucial to recognize that for some individuals living with a psychiatric disorder, such as major depression or schizophrenia, medications may cause an overall slowing of thought processes. This slowing may be so severe that it may seem like an eternity before the patient responds. Patience and gentle prompting (e.g., "You were saying that you would like to get a pass this weekend to visit your niece") can help patients gather their thoughts.

Silence is not always therapeutic. Prolonged and frequent silences by the psychiatric nurse may hinder an interview that requires verbal articulation. Although a less talkative nurse may be comfortable with silence, this mode of communication may make the patient feel like a fountain of information to be drained dry. Moreover, without feedback, patients have no way of knowing whether what they said was understood. In addition, children and adolescents in particular tend to feel uncomfortable with silence.

Active Listening

People want more than just a physical presence in human communication. Most people want the other person to be there for them psychologically, socially, emotionally, and spiritually. Active listening in the nurse–patient relationship includes the following aspects:

- Observing the patient's nonverbal behaviours
- Understanding and reflecting on the patient's verbal message
- Understanding the patient in the context of the social setting of the patient's life
- Detecting "false notes" (e.g., inconsistencies or things the patient says that need more clarification)
- Providing constructive feedback about the patient of which he or she might not be aware

Effective interviewers learn to become active listeners not only when the patient is talking but also when the patient becomes silent. During active listening, psychiatric nurses carefully note verbal and nonverbal patient responses and monitor their own nonverbal responses. Using silence effectively and learning to listen actively—both to the patient and to your own thoughts and reactions—are key ingredients in effective communication. Both skills take time to develop but can be learned; you will become more proficient with guidance and practice.

Some important principles of active listening include the following (Mohl & Carr, 2015):
- The answer is always inside the patient.
- Objective truth is never as simple as it seems.
- Everything you hear is modified by the patient's filters.
- Everything you hear is modified by your own filters.
- It is okay to feel confused and uncertain.
- Listen to yourself, too.

Active listening helps strengthen the patient's ability to solve problems. By giving the patient undivided attention, the nurse communicates that the patient is not alone. This kind of intervention enhances self-esteem and encourages the patient to direct energy toward finding ways to deal with problems. Serving as a sounding board, the nurse listens as the patient tests thoughts by voicing them aloud. This form of interpersonal interaction often enables the patient to clarify thinking, link ideas, and tentatively decide what should be done and how best to do it.

Listening with empathy. Wheeler (2014) identifies empathy as the most important element in therapeutic communication. Research indicates that the connectedness that results from empathy actually improves brain function by increasing brain plasticity. Wheeler describes the empathic process as the nurse entering and feeling the patient's world, the patient perceiving his or her own understanding of the world, and the patient experiencing acceptance and confirmation of himself or herself.

It is not enough for the nurse to feel empathy; an important part of this process is the communication of empathy to the patient. Egan (2013) suggested that the communication of empathy is achieved by connecting to the emotions, experiences, and thoughts of our patients and, to this end, proposed two forms of empathic statements, demonstrated through these examples:

1. "You feel _____ (name the emotion) because _____ (describe the *experiences*, thoughts, and behaviours)."
2. "Your _____ (name the emotion) is an outcome of _____ (describe the *context* of the experiences)."

If we plug in a scenario to the first statement, emphasizing the experience, it could sound something like this: "You feel like a failure because you have let your father down by joining the Canadian Armed Forces rather than becoming a lawyer." Now, try composing an empathic statement for the same scenario that encompasses the emotion in light of a particular context.

It is not always easy to be empathic and communicate a connection to the experiences, emotions, thoughts, behaviours, and contexts of our patients. Patients may describe experiences of brutal physical or sexual abuse, feelings of torment watching a loved one die, hate and anger toward another person, or acts of violence or hurtful inconsideration they have committed.

When people are self-pitying, critical, angry, sarcastic, or demeaning, the nurse's ability to connect to these experiences and communicate empathy may also be challenged. Chapter 9 offers a more detailed discussion of empathy.

Clarifying Techniques

Understanding depends on clear communication, which is aided by the nurse's verifying his or her interpretation of the patient's messages. The nurse can request feedback on the accuracy of the message received from verbal and nonverbal cues. The use of clarifying techniques helps both participants identify major differences in their frame of reference, giving them the opportunity to correct misperceptions before they cause any serious misunderstandings. The patient who is asked to elaborate on or clarify vague or ambiguous messages needs to know that the purpose is to promote mutual understanding.

Paraphrasing. To clarify, the nurse might use *paraphrasing*, or explaining in different (often fewer) words the basic content of a patient's message (Sommers-Flanagan & Sommers-Flanagan, 2013). Using simple, precise, and culturally relevant terms, the nurse may readily confirm interpretation of the patient's previous message before the interview proceeds. By prefacing statements with a phrase such as "I'm not sure I understand" or "In other words, you seem to be saying…," the nurse helps the patient form a clearer perception of what may be a bewildering mass of details. After paraphrasing, the nurse must validate the accuracy of the restatement and its helpfulness to the discussion. The patient may confirm or deny the perceptions through nonverbal cues or by direct response to a question from the nurse, such as "Was I correct in saying … ?" As a result, the patient is made aware that the interviewer is actively involved in the search for understanding.

Restating. In *restating*, the nurse mirrors the patient's overt and covert messages, so the technique may be used to echo feeling as well as content or context. Restating differs from paraphrasing in that it involves repeating the same key words the patient has just spoken. If a patient remarks, "My life is empty … it has no meaning," additional information may be gained by restating, "Your life has no meaning?" The purpose of this technique is to explore more thoroughly subjects that may be significant.

Too frequent and indiscriminate use of restating, however, may be interpreted by patients as inattention or disinterest. It is easy to overuse this tool so that its application becomes mechanical. As well, parroting or mimicking what another has said may be perceived as poking fun at the person; therefore the use of this nondirect approach can become a definite barrier to communication. To avoid overuse of restating, the nurse can combine restatements with direct questions that encourage descriptions: "What is lacking in your life?" "What are you missing in your life?" "Describe a day in your life that felt empty to you."

Reflecting. *Reflection* is a means of assisting people to better understand their own thoughts and feelings. Reflecting may take the form of a question or a simple statement that conveys the nurse's observations of the patient when sensitive issues are being discussed. The nurse might then describe briefly to the patient the apparent meaning of the emotional tone of the patient's verbal and nonverbal behaviour. For example, to reflect a patient's feelings about his or her life, a good beginning might be, "You sound as if you have had many disappointments."

Sharing observations with a patient shows that you accept him or her and that the patient has your full attention. When you reflect, you make the patient aware of inner feelings and encourage the patient to own them. For example, you may say to a patient, "You look sad." Perceiving your concern may allow the patient to spontaneously share feelings. The use of a question in response to the patient's question is another reflective technique (Arnold & Boggs, 2016). For example:

Patient: "Nurse, do you think I really need to be hospitalized?"

Nurse: "What do you think, Jane?"

Patient: "I don't know—that's why I'm asking you."

Nurse: "I'll be willing to share my impression with you at the end of this first session. However, you've probably thought about hospitalization and have some feelings about it. I wonder what they are."

Exploring. A technique that enables the nurse to examine important ideas, experiences, or relationships more fully is *exploring.* For example, if a patient tells you he does not get along well with his wife, you will want to further explore this area. Possible openers include:

"*Tell me more* about your relationship with your wife."

"*Describe* your relationship with your wife."

"*Give me an example* of how you and your wife don't get along."

Asking for an example can greatly clarify a vague or generic statement made by a patient.

Patient: "No one likes me."

Nurse: "Give me an example of one person who doesn't like you."

or

Patient: "Everything I do is wrong."

Nurse: "Give me an example of one thing you do that you think is wrong."

Table 10-2 lists more examples of therapeutic communication techniques.

Asking Questions and Eliciting Patient Responses

Open-ended questions. Many of the questions cited as examples above and in Table 10-2 are open-ended. Open-ended questions and comments encourage lengthy responses and facilitate expression of thoughts, feelings, and information about experiences, perceptions, or responses to a situation. For example:

- "What do you perceive as your biggest problem right now?"
- "Give me an example of some of the stresses you are under right now."
- "Tell me more about your relationship with your wife."

Since open-ended questions are not intrusive and do not put the patient on the defensive, they help the clinician elicit information, especially at the beginning of an interview or when a patient is guarded or resistant to answering questions. They are particularly useful when establishing rapport with a person.

Closed-ended questions. Nurses are usually urged to ask open-ended questions to elicit more than a "yes" or "no" response. However, closed-ended questions, when used sparingly, can give you specific and needed information. Closed-ended questions (those requiring only a "yes" or "no" response) are most useful during an initial assessment or intake interview, to obtain concrete responses to specific assessment data such as a suicide risk assessment, or to determine outcomes of interventions (e.g., "Are the medications helping you?" "When did you start hearing voices?" "Did you seek therapy after your first suicide attempt?"). Care needs to be exercised with this technique. Frequent use of closed-ended questions with a patient leaves the patient feeling interrogated and can close down an interview rapidly, especially in the case of patients who are guarded or resist engaging in interactions.

Nontherapeutic Communication Techniques

Although people may use "nontherapeutic," or ineffective, communication techniques in their daily lives, these techniques can cause problems for nurses because they tend to impede or shut down nurse–patient interaction. Table 10-3 describes nontherapeutic communication techniques and suggests more helpful responses.

Excessive Questioning

Excessive questioning—asking multiple questions (particularly closed-ended questions) consecutively or very rapidly—casts the nurse in the role of an interrogator who demands information without respect for the patient's willingness or readiness to respond. This approach conveys a lack of respect for and sensitivity to the patient's needs. Excessive questioning controls the range and nature of the responses, can easily result in a therapeutic stall, or may completely shut down an interview. It is a controlling tactic and may reflect the interviewer's lack of security in letting the patient tell his or her own story. It is better to ask more open-ended questions and follow the patient's lead. For example:

Excessive questioning: "Why did you leave your wife? Did you feel angry at her? What did she do to you? Are you going back to her?"

More therapeutic approach: "Tell me about the situation between you and your wife."

Giving Approval or Disapproval

"You look great in that dress." "I'm proud of the way you controlled your temper at lunch." "That's a great quilt you made." What could be bad about giving someone a pat on the back once in a while? Nothing, if it is done without conveying a positive or negative judgement. We often give our friends and family approval when they do something well. However, in a nurse–patient relationship, giving praise and approval becomes much more complex.

A patient may be feeling overwhelmed, experiencing low self-esteem, feeling unsure of where his or her life is going, or desperately seeking recognition, approval, and attention. Yet when people are feeling vulnerable, a value comment may be misinterpreted. For example, the nurse may say, "You did a great job in group telling John just what you thought about how rudely he treated you." This message implies that the nurse was pleased by the manner in which the patient talked to John. The patient then sees such a response as "doing the right thing" and as a way

TABLE 10-2 THERAPEUTIC COMMUNICATION TECHNIQUES

THERAPEUTIC TECHNIQUE	DESCRIPTION	EXAMPLE
Using silence	Gives the person time to collect thoughts or think through a point	Encouraging a person to talk by waiting for the answers
Accepting	Indicates that the person has been understood; an accepting statement does not necessarily indicate agreement but it is nonjudgemental (The nurse should not imply understanding when he or she does not understand.)	"Yes." "Uh-huh." "I follow what you say."
Giving recognition	Indicates awareness of change and personal efforts; does not imply good or bad, right or wrong	"Good morning, Mr. James." "You've combed your hair today." "I see you've eaten your whole lunch."
Offering self	Offers presence, interest, and a desire to understand; is not offered to get the person to talk or behave in a specific way	"I would like to spend time with you." "I'll stay here and sit with you awhile."
Offering general leads	Allows the other person to take direction in the discussion; indicates interest in what comes next	"Go on." "And then?" "Tell me about it."
Giving broad openings	Clarifies that the lead is to be taken by the patient; however, the nurse discourages pleasantries and small talk	"Where would you like to begin?" "What are you thinking about?" "What would you like to discuss?"
Placing the events in time or sequence	Puts events and actions in better perspective; notes cause-and-effect relationships and identifies patterns of interpersonal difficulties	"What happened before?" "When did this happen?"
Making observations	Calls attention to the person's behaviour (e.g., trembling, nail biting, restless mannerisms); encourages patient to notice the behaviour and describe thoughts and feelings for mutual understanding; helpful with mute and withdrawn people	"You appear tense." "I notice you're biting your lips." "You appear nervous whenever John enters the room."
Encouraging description of perception	Increases the nurse's understanding of the patient's perceptions; talking about feelings and difficulties can lessen the need to act them out inappropriately	"Tell me, what do these voices seem to be saying?" "What is happening now?" "Tell me when you feel anxious."
Encouraging comparison	Brings out recurring themes in experiences or interpersonal relationships; helps the person clarify similarities and differences	"Has this ever happened before?" "Is this how you felt when … ?" "Was it something like … ?"
Restating	Repeats the main idea expressed; gives the patient an idea of what has been communicated; if the message has been misunderstood, the patient can clarify it	**Patient:** "I can't sleep. I stay awake all night." **Nurse:** "You have difficulty sleeping?" or **Patient:** "I don't know … he always has some excuse for not coming over or keeping our appointments." **Nurse:** "You think he no longer wants to see you?"
Reflecting	Directs questions, feelings, and ideas back to the patient; encourages the patient to accept his or her own ideas and feelings; acknowledges the patient's right to have opinions and make decisions and encourages the patient to think of self as a capable person	**Patient:** "What should I do about my husband's affair?" **Nurse:** "What do you think you should do?" or **Patient:** "My brother spends all of my money and then has the nerve to ask for more." **Nurse:** "You feel angry when this happens?"
Focusing	Concentrates attention on a single point; especially useful when the patient jumps from topic to topic; if a person is experiencing a severe level of anxiety, the nurse should not persist until the anxiety lessens	"This point you are making about leaving school seems worth looking at more closely." "You've mentioned many things. Let's go back to your thinking of 'ending it all.'"
Exploring	Examines certain ideas, experiences, or relationships more fully; if the patient chooses not to elaborate by answering no, the nurse does not probe or pry but instead respects the patient's wishes	"Tell me more about that." "Would you describe it more fully?" "Could you talk about how you learned your mom was dying of cancer?"
Giving information	Makes available facts the person needs; supplies knowledge from which decisions can be made or conclusions can be drawn—for example, the patient needs to know the role of the nurse; the purpose of the nurse–patient relationship; and the time, place, and duration of the meetings	"My purpose for being here is …" "This medication is for …" "The test will determine … "

TABLE 10-2	THERAPEUTIC COMMUNICATION TECHNIQUES—cont'd	
THERAPEUTIC TECHNIQUE	**DESCRIPTION**	**EXAMPLE**
Seeking clarification	Helps patients clarify their own thoughts and maximizes mutual understanding between nurse and patient	"I am not sure I follow you." "What would you say is the main point of what you just said?" "Give an example of a time you thought everyone hated you."
Presenting reality	Indicates what is real; the nurse does not argue or try to convince the patient but just describes personal perceptions or facts in the situation	"That was Dr. Todd, not a man from the Mafia." "That was the sound of a car backfiring." "Your mother is not here; I am a nurse."
Voicing doubt	Undermines the patient's beliefs by not reinforcing the exaggerated or false perceptions	"Isn't that unusual?" "Really?" "That's hard to believe."
Seeking consensual validation	Clarifies that both the nurse and the patient share mutual understanding of communications; helps the patient see more clearly what he or she is thinking	"Tell me whether my understanding agrees with yours."
Verbalizing the implied	Puts into concrete terms what the patient implies, making the patient's communication more explicit	***Patient:*** "I can't talk to you or anyone else. It's a waste of time." ***Nurse:*** "Do you perceive that no one understands?"
Encouraging evaluation	Aids the patient in considering people and events from the perspective of the patient's own set of values	"How do you feel about … ?" "What did it mean to you when he said he couldn't stay?"
Attempting to translate into feelings	Responds to the feelings expressed, not just the content; often termed *decoding*	***Patient:*** "I am dead inside." ***Nurse:*** "Are you saying that you feel lifeless? Does life seem meaningless to you?"
Suggesting collaboration	Emphasizes working with the patient, not doing things for the patient; encourages the view that change is possible through collaboration	"Perhaps you and I can discover what produces your anxiety." "Perhaps by working together, we can come up with some ideas that might improve your communications with your spouse."
Summarizing	Brings together important points of discussion to enhance understanding; also allows the opportunity to clarify communications so that both nurse and patient leave the interview with the same ideas in mind	"Have I got this straight?" "You said that …" "During the past hour, you and I have discussed …"
Encouraging formulation of a plan of action	Allows the patient to identify alternative actions for interpersonal situations the patient finds disturbing (e.g., when anger or anxiety is provoked)	"What could you do to let anger out harmlessly?" "The next time this comes up, what might you do to handle it?" "What are some other ways you can approach your boss?"

Source: Adapted from Hays, J. S., & Larson, K. (1963). *Interacting with patients.* New York: Macmillan.

to please the nurse. To continue to please the nurse (and get approval), the patient may continue the behaviour. The behaviour may indeed be useful for the patient, but when done to please another person, it is not coming from the individual's own volition or conviction. Also, when the person the patient needs to please is not around, the motivation for the new behaviour may not be either. Thus, the new response really is not a change in behaviour as much as a ploy to win approval and acceptance from another.

Giving approval also cuts off further communication. A more therapeutic approach may be to say, "I noticed that you spoke up to John in group yesterday about his rude behaviour. How did it feel to be more assertive?" This response opens the way for finding out if the patient was scared, was comfortable, wants to work more on assertiveness, and so on. It also suggests that this behaviour was a self-choice made by the patient. While the patient is recognized for the change in behaviour, the topic is also opened for further discussion.

Giving disapproval (e.g., "You really should not cheat, even if you think everyone else is doing it") implies that the nurse has the right to judge the patient's thoughts or feelings. Again, an observation should be made instead (e.g., "Can you give me

two examples of how cheating could negatively affect your goal of graduating?").

Giving Advice

Although we ask for and give advice all the time in daily life, giving advice to a patient is rarely helpful. Often when we ask for advice, our real motive is to discover whether we are thinking along the same lines as someone else or if they would agree with us. When a nurse gives advice or offers solutions to a patient, the nurse is interfering with the patient's ability to make personal decisions. The patient may eventually begin to think the nurse does not view him or her as capable of making effective decisions. People often feel inadequate when they are given no choices over decisions in their lives. Not only can giving advice to patients undermine the patient's sense of competence and adequacy, it can also foster dependency ("I'll have to ask the nurse what to do about …").

However, people do need information and time to reflect in order to make informed decisions. Often you can help a patient define a problem and identify what information might be needed to come to an informed decision. A useful approach would be to ask, "What do you see as some possible actions you can take?"

TABLE 10-3 NONTHERAPEUTIC COMMUNICATION TECHNIQUES

NONTHERAPEUTIC TECHNIQUE	DESCRIPTION	EXAMPLE	MORE HELPFUL RESPONSE
Giving premature advice	Assumes the nurse knows best and the patient can't think for self; inhibits problem solving and fosters dependency	"Get out of this situation immediately."	*Encouraging problem solving:* "What are the pros and cons of your situation?" "What were some of the actions you thought you might take?" "What are some of the ways you have thought of to meet your goals?"
Minimizing feelings	Indicates that the nurse is unable to understand or empathize with the patient; the patient's feelings or experiences are being belittled, which can cause the patient to feel small or insignificant and devalued	*Patient:* "I wish I were dead." *Nurse:* "Everyone gets down in the dumps." "I know what you mean." "You should feel happy you're getting better." "Things get worse before they get better."	*Empathizing and exploring:* "You must be feeling very upset. Are you thinking of hurting yourself?"
Falsely reassuring	Under-rates a person's feelings and belittles a person's concerns; may cause the patient to stop sharing feelings if he or she expects to be ridiculed or not taken seriously	"I wouldn't worry about that." "Everything will be all right." "You will do just fine—you'll see."	*Clarifying the patient's message:* "What specifically are you worried about?" "What do you think could go wrong?" "What are you concerned might happen?"
Making value judgements	Prevents problem solving; can make the patient feel guilty, angry, misunderstood, not supported, or anxious to leave	"Why do you still smoke when your wife has lung cancer?"	*Making observations:* "I notice you are still smoking even though your wife has lung cancer. Is this a problem?"
Asking "why" questions	Implies criticism; often has the effect of making the patient feel a need to justify behaviour and leaves the patient feeling defensive	"Why did you stop taking your medication?"	*Asking open-ended questions; giving a broad opening:* "Tell me some of the events that led up to your not taking your medications."
Asking excessive questions	Results in the patient not knowing which question to answer and possibly being confused about what is being asked	*Nurse:* "How's your appetite? Are you losing weight? Are you eating enough?" *Patient:* "No."	*Clarifying:* "Tell me about your eating habits since you've been depressed."
Giving approval, agreeing	Implies the patient is doing the right thing—and that not doing it is wrong; may lead the patient to focus on pleasing the nurse or clinician; denies the patient the opportunity to change his or her mind or decision	"I'm proud of you for applying for that job." "I agree with your decision."	*Making observations:* "I noticed that you applied for that job. What factors might contribute to your choice one way or the other?" *Asking open-ended questions; giving a broad opening:* "What led to that decision?"
Disapproving; disagreeing	Can make a person defensive	"You really should have shown up for the medication group." "I disagree with that."	*Exploring:* "What was going on with you when you decided not to come to your medication group?" "That's one point of view. How did you arrive at that conclusion?"
Changing the subject	May invalidate the patient's feelings and needs; can leave the patient feeling alienated and isolated and increase feelings of hopelessness	*Patient:* "I'd like to die." *Nurse:* "Did you go to Alcoholics Anonymous like we discussed?"	*Validating and exploring:* *Patient:* "I'd like to die." *Nurse:* "This sounds serious. Have you thought of harming yourself?"

Source: Adapted from Hays, J. S., & Larson, K. (1963). *Interacting with patients.* New York: Macmillan.

It is much more respectful and ultimately constructive to encourage problem solving by the patient than simply to provide solutions. Sometimes, though, you might suggest several alternatives a patient could consider (e.g., "What are your thoughts on telling your friend about the incident?"). When you open up the conversation in this way, the patient is free to express his or her thoughts and feelings about such a disclosure, giving the nurse an opportunity to explore other potential alternatives and to support the patient in his or her decision.

Asking "Why" Questions

"Why did you come late?" "Why didn't you go to the funeral?" "Why didn't you study for the exam?" Very often, "why" questions imply criticism. We may ask our friends or family such questions, and in the context of a solid relationship, the "why" may be understood more as "What happened?" With people we do not know—especially those who may be anxious or overwhelmed—a "why" question from a person in authority (e.g., nurse, psychiatrist, teacher) can be perceived as intrusive and judgemental, serving only to make the person feel the need to justify behaviour and respond defensively.

It is much more useful to ask *what* is happening than *why* it is happening. Questions that focus on who, what, where, and when often elicit important information that can facilitate problem solving and further the communication process. See Table 10-3 for additional ineffective communication techniques, as well as statements that would better facilitate interaction and patient comfort.

Cultural Considerations

Canada is becoming increasingly culturally diverse, and health care providers need to be familiar with the verbal and nonverbal communication characteristics of a multicultural national population. The nurse's awareness of cultural meanings of certain verbal and nonverbal communications in initial face-to-face encounters with a patient can lead to the formation of a positive therapeutic relationship (Ehrmin, 2015).

Unrecognized differences in cultural identities can result in assessment and interventions that are not optimally respectful of the patient and can be inadvertently biased or prejudiced. Health care workers need to have not only knowledge of various patients' cultures but also awareness of their own cultural identities. Especially important are nurses' attitudes and beliefs about those from cultures other than their own, because these will affect their relationships with patients (Ehrmin, 2015). Four areas that may prove problematic for the nurse trying to interpret specific verbal and nonverbal messages of the patient are:
1. Communication style
2. Use of eye contact
3. Perception of touch
4. Cultural filters

Further information about working with people of various cultures is presented in Chapter 8.

Communication Style

People may communicate in an intense and highly emotional manner. Some may consider it normal to use dramatic body language when describing emotional problems, and others may perceive such behaviour as being out of control or reflective of some degree of pathology. For example, within the Hispanic community, intensely emotional styles of communication often are culturally appropriate and expected (Ehrmin, 2015). Similarly, French and Italian Canadians typically use animated facial expressions and expressive hand gestures during communication, which can be misinterpreted by others.

In other cultures, a calm façade may mask severe distress. For example, in many South Asian cultures, expression of positive or negative emotions is a private affair, and open expression of them is considered to be in bad taste and possibly a weakness. A quiet smile by a South Asian Canadian may express joy, an apology, stoicism, or even anger. German and British Canadians also tend to value highly the concept of self-control and may show little facial emotion in the presence of great distress or emotional turmoil.

Eye Contact

The presence or absence of eye contact should not be used to assess attentiveness, judge truthfulness, or make assumptions about the degree of engagement one has with a patient. Cultural norms often dictate a person's comfort or lack of comfort with direct eye contact. Some cultures consider direct eye contact disrespectful and improper. For example, Indigenous individuals have traditionally been taught to avoid eye contact with authority figures, including nurses, physicians, and other health care providers; avoidance of direct eye contact is seen as a sign of respect to those in authority, but it could be misinterpreted as a lack of interest or even as a lack of respect.

In Japanese culture, making direct eye contact is also considered a lack of respect and a personal affront; the preference is for shifting or downcast eyes or a focus on the speaker's neck. For many Chinese people, gazing around and looking to one side when listening to another is considered polite. In some Middle Eastern cultures, a woman making direct eye contact with a man may imply a sexual interest or even promiscuity. On the other hand, most Canadians of European descent maintain eye contact during conversation and may interpret avoidance of eye contact by another person as a lack of interest, a show of dishonesty, or avoiding the sharing of important information.

Touch

The therapeutic use of touch is a basic aspect of the nurse–patient relationship and is generally considered a gesture of warmth and friendship; however, the degree to which a patient is comfortable with the use of touch is often culturally determined. People from some cultures—Indigenous people, for example—are accustomed to frequent physical contact. Holding an Indigenous patient's hand in response to a distressing situation or giving the patient a reassuring pat on the shoulder may be experienced as supportive and thus facilitate openness (Ehrmin, 2015). People from Italian or French backgrounds may also be accustomed to frequent touching during conversation, and in the Russian culture touch is an important part of nonverbal communication used freely with intimate and close friends (Giger, 2017).

However, in other cultures, personal touch within the context of an interview may be perceived as an invasion of privacy or as patronizing, intrusive, aggressive, or sexually inviting. Among German, Swedish, and British Canadians, touch practices are infrequent, although a handshake may be common at the beginning and end of an interaction. Chinese Canadians may not like to be touched by strangers.

Even among people from similar cultures, the use of touch has different interpretations and rules regarding gender and class. Nurses and nursing students are urged to find out if their facility has a "no touch" policy, particularly with adolescents and children who have experienced inappropriate touch and may not know how to interpret therapeutic touch from the health care provider.

Cultural Filters

It is important to recognize that it is impossible to listen to people in an unbiased way. In the process of socialization, we develop cultural filters through which we listen to ourselves, others, and the world around us (Egan, 2013). Cultural filters are a form of cultural bias or cultural prejudice that determine what we pay attention to and what we ignore. Egan (2013) stated that we need these cultural filters to provide structure for our lives and help us interpret and interact with the world. However, these cultural filters also unavoidably introduce various forms of bias into our communication, because they are bound to influence our personal, professional, familial, and sociological values and interpretations.

We all need a frame of reference to help us function in our world, but at the same time we must understand that other people use other frames of reference to help them function in their worlds. Acknowledging that everyone views the world differently and understanding that these various views affect each person's beliefs and behaviours can go a long way toward minimizing our personal distortions in listening. Building acceptance and understanding of cultural diversity is a skill that can be learned. Chapter 8 has a more in-depth discussion of cultural considerations in nursing.

Assertive Communication

Openness and patient-centred communication has been introduced and likely practised to date. Another aspect of communication for psychiatric mental health nursing that must be emphasized is *assertive communication*. Assertive communication means clearly expressing what you need, with respectful language and behaviour (Balzer-Riley, 2017). Psychiatric mental health nurses must face anger and depression, psychosis and dementia, intense elation and despair, and behaviour that may be bizarre or at time self-destructive. In this work nurses hear and witness some of the worst experiences of people's lives, and assertive communication is important to maintain clarity of purpose to meet goals of empathy while also addressing immediate needs for information, care, and safety.

At times assertive communication will mean challenging patients who may be inhibiting their own success or in denial of the problems they are facing. Assertive communication may be necessary to de-escalate the agitation a patient is experiencing and to avoid aggression. At other times, assertive communication will establish an avenue for thought-provoking or alternative viewpoints for families or colleagues in a team meeting.

Working as advocates—and as part of interprofessional teams, where not everyone shares the same priorities, goals or views—psychiatric mental health nurses must routinely practise assertive communication. Psychiatric mental health nurses must be assertive to maintain clarity; to ask the right questions; and to respect themselves and the dignity of their patients, families, and colleagues. Finally, psychiatric mental health nurses must draw on assertive communication to communicate their own needs and to establish balance in their lives (Balzer-Riley, 2017).

Assertiveness for these purposes can be accomplished with a calm mind, careful thought, and attention to maintaining therapeutic and professional relationships with the utmost respect for all concerned. Asking questions in a humble inquiry (e.g., asking "Have you thought about …" or "What might happen if we took _____ approach?") can be an effective part of assertive communication (Schein, 2014).

Evaluation of Communication Skills

After you have had some introductory clinical experience, you may find the facilitative skills checklist in Figure 10-2 useful for evaluating your progress in developing interviewing and assessment skills. Note that some of the items might not be relevant for some of your patients (e.g., numbers 11 through 13 may not be possible when a patient is experiencing psychosis [disordered thought, delusions, or hallucinations]). Self-evaluation of clinical skills is a way to focus on therapeutic improvement. Role-playing can help prepare you for clinical experience and provide practice in using effective and professional communication skills.

THE CLINICAL INTERVIEW

Ideally, the content and direction of the clinical interview are decided and led by the patient. The nurse uses communication skills and active listening to better understand the patient's situation.

Preparing for the Interview
Pace

Helping a person with an emotional or medical problem is rarely a straightforward task, and the goal of assisting a patient to regain psychological or physiological stability can be difficult to achieve. Extremely important to any kind of counselling is permitting the patient to set the pace of the interview, no matter how slow or halting the progress may be (Arnold & Boggs, 2016).

Setting

Effective communication can take place almost anywhere. However, the quality of the interaction—whether in a clinic, a clinical unit, an office, or the patient's home—depends on the degree to which the nurse and patient feel safe; establishing a setting that enhances feelings of security is important to the therapeutic relationship. A health care setting, a conference room, or a quiet part of the unit that has relative privacy but is within view of others is ideal, but when the interview takes place in the patient's home, the nurse has a valuable opportunity to assess the patient in the context of everyday life.

Facilitation Skills Checklist

The following list identifies several different facilitation skills. Think about a clinical experience in which you were trying to facilitate a conversation or discussion. Place a check mark by each of the skills you believe you did well. Circle the ones you would like to improve.

Communication
_____Invites quiet participants to contribute.
_____Asks open questions to stimulate discussion.
_____Paraphrases ideas and suggestions.
_____Maintains open, balanced and clear communication.

Keeping on Track
_____Allows time to address process issues.
_____Keeps group on track to achieve objectives in given time frame.
_____Establishes and reminds group members of norms for meeting behaviour.

Goals and Roles
_____Clarifies goals and objectives of interaction or discussion.
_____Checks and ensures common understanding of goals.
_____Provides time to discuss, clarify, or modify or negotiate goals.
_____Ensures roles are assigned and understood.

Conflict Management
_____Steers conflict away from personalities and toward task-related issues.
_____Summarizes opposing or differing positions.
_____Determines when members are suppressing their ideas to avoid conflict.
_____Determines whether conflict is constructive and task-related.

FIGURE 10-2 Facilitative Skills Checklist.

Seating

In all settings, chairs should be arranged so that conversation can take place in a normal tone of voice and eye contact can be comfortably maintained or avoided. A nonthreatening physical environment for both nurse and patient involves:
- Assuming the same height, either both sitting or both standing
- Avoiding a face-to-face stance when possible; a 90- to 120-degree angle or side-by-side position may be less intense, and the patient and nurse can look away from each other without discomfort
- Providing safety and psychological comfort in terms of exiting the room—the patient should not be positioned between the nurse and the door, nor should the nurse be positioned in such a way that the patient feels trapped in the room
- Avoiding a desk barrier between the nurse and the patient

Introductions

In the orientation phase, nurses introduce themselves to their patients, describe the purpose of the meeting, and explain for how long and at what times they will be meeting with the patient. This introduction process sets an important tone and is crucial to later interventions and outcomes (Wright & Leahy, 2013). The issue of confidentiality is brought up during the initial interview. Remember that all health care providers must respect the private, personal, and confidential nature of the patient's communication, except in the specific situations outlined earlier (e.g., harm to self or others, child abuse, elder abuse). What is discussed with fellow staff and your clinical group in conference should not be discussed outside with others, no matter who they are (e.g., patient's relatives, news media, friends). The patient needs to know that whatever is discussed will stay confidential unless permission is given for it to be disclosed. Refer to Chapter 9 to review the nurse's responsibilities in the orientation phase.

Ask the patient how he or she would like to be addressed. This question conveys respect and gives the patient direct control over an important ego issue. Some patients like to be called by their last names; others prefer being on a first-name basis with the nurse (Arnold & Boggs, 2016).

Initiating the Interview

Once introductions have been made, you can turn the interview over to the patient by using one of a number of open-ended questions or statements:
- "Where should we start?"
- "Tell me a little about what has been going on with you."
- "What are some of the stresses you have been coping with recently?"
- "Tell me a little about what has been happening in the past couple of weeks."
- "Perhaps you can begin by letting me know what some of your concerns have been recently."
- "Tell me about your difficulties."

Communication can be facilitated by appropriately offering leads (e.g., "Go on"), making statements of acceptance (e.g., "Uh-huh"), or otherwise conveying interest.

Tactics to Avoid

Certain behaviours are counterproductive and should be avoided. For example:

Do Not ...	Try To ...
Argue with, minimize, or challenge the patient	Keep the focus on facts and the patient's perceptions
Give false reassurance	Make observations of the patient's behaviour (e.g., "Change is always possible.")
Interpret situations for the patient or speculate on interpersonal dynamics	Listen attentively, use silence, and try to clarify the patient's problems
Question or probe patients about sensitive topics they do not wish to discuss	Pay attention to nonverbal communication; strive to keep the patient's anxiety to a minimum
Try to sell the patient on accepting treatment	Encourage the patient to look at pros and cons
Join in attacks that patients launch on their mates, parents, friends, or associates	Focus on facts and the patient's perceptions; be aware of nonverbal communication
Participate in criticism of another nurse or any other staff member	Focus on facts and the patient's perceptions; check out serious accusations with the nurse or staff member; have the patient meet with the nurse or staff member in question in the presence of a senior staff member and clarify perceptions

Helpful Guidelines

Meier and Davis (2010) offer some guidelines for conducting the initial interview:
- Speak briefly.
- When you do not know what to say, say nothing.
- When in doubt, focus on feelings.
- Avoid giving advice.
- Avoid relying on questions.
- Pay attention to nonverbal cues.
- Keep the focus on the patient.

Attending Behaviours: The Foundation of Interviewing

Engaging in attending behaviours and actively listening are two key principles of counselling on which almost everyone can agree (Sommers-Flanagan & Sommers-Flanagan, 2013). Positive attending behaviours serve to open up communication and encourage free expression, whereas negative attending behaviours are more likely to inhibit expression. All behaviours must be evaluated in terms of cultural patterns and past experiences of both the interviewer and the interviewee. There are no universals; however, there are guidelines that students can follow.

Eye Contact

As previously discussed, cultural and individual variations influence a patient's comfort with eye contact. For some patients and interviewers, sustained eye contact is normal and comfortable.

For others, it may be more comfortable and natural to make brief eye contact but look away or down much of the time. Sommers-Flanagan and Sommers-Flanagan (2013) state that in most situations, it is appropriate for nurses to maintain more eye contact when the patient speaks and less constant eye contact when the nurse speaks.

Body Language

Body language involves two elements: kinesics and proxemics. *Kinesics* is associated with physical characteristics, such as body movements and postures. Facial expressions; eye contact or lack thereof; the way someone holds the head, legs, and shoulders; and so on convey a multitude of messages. A person who slumps in a chair, rolls the eyes, and sits with arms crossed in front of the chest can be perceived as resistant and unreceptive to what another wants to communicate. On the other hand, a person who leans in slightly toward the speaker, maintains a relaxed and attentive posture, makes appropriate eye contact, makes hand gestures that are unobtrusive and smooth while minimizing the number of other movements, and whose facial expressions match his or her feelings or the patient's feelings can be perceived as open to and respectful of the communication.

Proxemics refers to the study of personal space and the significance of the physical distance between individuals. Proxemics takes into account that these distances may be different for different cultural groups. Intimate distance in Canada is 0 to 45 centimetres and is reserved for those we trust most and with whom we feel most safe. Personal distance (45 to 120 centimetres) is for personal communications, such as those with friends or colleagues. Social distance (120 to 360 centimetres, or approximately 3.5 metres) applies to strangers or acquaintances, often in public places or formal social gatherings. Public distance (3.5 metres) relates to public space (e.g., public speaking). In public space, one may hail another, and the parties may move about while communicating.

Vocal Quality

Vocal quality, or paralinguistics, encompasses voice loudness, pitch, rate, and fluency. Sommers-Flanagan and Sommers-Flanagan (2013) report that vocal qualities can improve rapport, demonstrate empathy and interest, and add emphasis to words or concepts. Speaking in soft and gentle tones is apt to encourage a person to share thoughts and feelings, whereas speaking in a rapid, high-pitched tone may convey anxiety and create it in the patient. Consider, for example, how tonal quality can affect communication in a simple sentence like "I will see you tonight."

1. "*I* will see you tonight." (I will be the one who sees you tonight.)
2. "I *will* see you tonight." (No matter what happens, or whether you like it or not, I will see you tonight.)
3. "I will see *you* tonight." (Even though others are present, it is you I want to see.)
4. "I will see you *tonight*." (It is definite—tonight is the night we will meet.)

Verbal Tracking

Verbal tracking is just that: tracking what the patient is saying. Individuals cannot know if you are hearing or understanding what they are saying unless you provide them with cues. Verbal tracking offers neutral feedback in the form of simply restating or summarizing what the patient has already said without personal or professional opinions, judgements, or comments (Sommers-Flanagan & Sommers-Flanagan, 2013). For example:

Patient: "I don't know what the fuss is about. I smoke marijuana to relax, and everyone makes a fuss."

Nurse: "Do you see the use of marijuana as a problem for you?"

Patient: "No, I don't. It doesn't affect my work ... well, most of the time, anyway. I mean, of course, if I have to think things out and make important decisions, then obviously it can get in the way. But most of the time, I'm cool."

Nurse: "So when important decisions have to be made, then it interferes; otherwise, you don't see it affecting your functioning."

Patient: "Yeah, well, most of the time, I'm cool."

Meier and Davis (2010) stated that verbal tracking involves checking one's understanding with the patient by restating—as much as possible, in one's own words—in order to confirm the patient's speech content (as well as to clarify the meaning of speech volume and tone, as discussed earlier). It can be difficult to know which leads to follow if the patient introduces many topics at once. When this happens, the nurse can summarize what he or she has heard; reflect the emotions, experiences, thoughts, and contexts as much as possible; and help the patient focus on and explore a specific topic or goal. "With everything going on in your life recently, you must really feel overwhelmed. You're $2 000 in debt and don't have a job, you've gained 15 kilograms in 6 months, and your wife is frustrated with your drinking. Let's talk more about what is going on with your wife and her concerns about alcohol."

Clinical Supervision

Communication and interviewing techniques are acquired skills. You will learn to improve these abilities through practice and clinical supervision. With clinical supervision, the focus is on the nurse's behaviour in the nurse–patient relationship; the nurse and supervisor have opportunities to examine and analyze the nurse's feelings and reactions to the patient and the way they affect the relationship. Clinical supervision for students in psychiatric mental health practice can occur in a one-to-one conversation or as part of a group discussion in postconference. The rationale for and importance of clinical supervision is stressed in Chapter 9.

An increasingly popular method of providing clinical supervision is through debriefing. According to the National League for Nursing (2015), debriefing is such an excellent learning method that it should be incorporated into all clinical experiences. Debriefing refers to a critical conversation and reflection regarding an experience that results in growth and learning. Debriefing supports essential learning along a continuum of "knowing what" to "knowing how" and "knowing why" (Varcarolis, 2017).

The opportunity to examine interactions, obtain insights, and devise alternative strategies for dealing with various clinical issues enhances clinical growth and minimizes frustration and burnout. Clinical supervision and debriefing are necessary professional activities that foster professional growth and curiosity and help minimize the development of nontherapeutic nurse–patient relationships.

Process Recordings

The best way to improve communication and interviewing skills is to review your clinical interactions exactly as they occur. This process offers the opportunity to identify themes and patterns in both your own and your patients' communications. As students, clinical review helps you learn to deal with the variety of situations that arise in the clinical interview.

Process recordings are written records of a segment of the nurse–patient session that reflect as closely as possible the verbal and nonverbal behaviours of both patient and nurse. Process recordings have some disadvantages because they rely on memory and are subject to distortions. However, they can be a useful tool for identifying communication patterns. Sometimes an observing clinician takes notes during the interview, but this practice also has disadvantages in that it may be distracting for both interviewer and patient. Some patients (especially those with a paranoid disorder) may resent or misunderstand the observer's intent.

It is usually best to write notes verbatim (word for word) in a private area immediately after the interaction has taken place. You can carefully record your words and the patient's words, identify whether your responses are therapeutic, and recall your thinking and emotions at the time.

Videotaped simulations with professional actors or in role-play may also provide students with an opportunity to analyze their communication skills through the use of a process recording.

Table 10-4 gives an example of a process recording.

TABLE 10-4   EXAMPLE OF A PROCESS RECORDING

NURSE	PATIENT	COMMUNICATION TECHNIQUE	NURSE'S THOUGHTS AND FEELINGS
"Good morning, Mr. Long."		**Therapeutic.** Giving recognition. Acknowledging a patient by name can enhance self-esteem and communicates that the nurse views the patient as an individual.	I was feeling nervous. He had attempted suicide, and I didn't know if I could help him. Initially I was feeling somewhat overwhelmed.
	"Who are you, and where the devil am I?" (Gazes around with a confused look on his face—quickly sits on the edge of the bed)		
"I am Ms. Rossi. I am your nurse, and you are at St. Paul's Hospital. I would like to spend some time with you today."		**Therapeutic.** Giving information. Informing the patient of facts needed to make decisions or come to realistic conclusions. **Therapeutic.** Offering self. Making oneself available to the patient.	
	"What am I doing here? How did I get here?" (Spoken in a loud, demanding voice)		I felt a bit intimidated when he raised his voice.
"You were brought in by your wife last night after swallowing a bottle of aspirin. You had to have your stomach pumped."		**Therapeutic.** Giving information. Giving needed facts so that the patient can orient himself and better evaluate his situation.	
	"Oh … yeah." (Silence for 2 minutes; shoulders slumped, Mr. Long stares at the floor and drops his head and eyes)		I was uncomfortable with the silence, but since I didn't have anything useful to say, I stayed with him in silence for the 2 minutes.
"You seem upset, Mr. Long. What are you thinking about?"		**Therapeutic.** Making observations. **Therapeutic.** Giving broad openings in an attempt to get at his feelings.	I began to feel sorry for him; he looked so sad and helpless.
	"Yeah, I just remembered…. I wanted to kill myself." (Said in a low tone almost to himself)		
"Oh, Mr. Long, you have so much to live for. You have such a loving family."		**Nontherapeutic.** Defending **Nontherapeutic.** Introducing an unrelated topic.	I felt overwhelmed. I didn't know what to say—his talking about killing himself made me nervous. I could have said, "You must be very upset" (verbalizing the implied) or "Tell me more about this" (exploring).
	"What do you know about my life? You want to know about my family? My wife is leaving me, that's what." (Faces the nurse with an angry expression on his face and speaks in loud tones)		Again, I felt intimidated by his anger, but now I linked it with his wife's leaving him, so I didn't take it as personally as I did the first time.
"I didn't know. You must be terribly upset by her leaving."		**Therapeutic.** Reflective. Observing the angry tone and content of the patient's message and reflecting the patient's feelings.	I really felt for him, and now I thought that encouraging him to talk more about this could be useful for him.

KEY POINTS TO REMEMBER

- Knowledge of communication and interviewing techniques is the foundation for development of any nurse–patient relationship. Goal-directed professional communication is referred to as *therapeutic communication.*
- Communication is a complex process. Berlo's (1960) communication model has five parts: stimulus, sender, message, medium, and receiver.
- Feedback is a vital component of the communication process for validating the accuracy of the sender's message.
- A number of factors can minimize, enhance, or otherwise influence the communication process: culture, language, knowledge level, noise, lack of privacy, presence of others, and expectations.
- There are verbal and nonverbal elements in communication; the nonverbal elements often play the larger role in conveying a person's message. Verbal communication consists of all words a person speaks. Nonverbal communication consists of the behaviours displayed by an individual, outside the actual content of speech.
- Communication has two levels: the content level (verbal speech) and the process level (nonverbal behaviour). When content is congruent with process, the communication is said to be healthy. When the verbal message is not reinforced by the communicator's actions, the message is ambiguous and incongruent; this is called a double (or mixed) message.

- Cultural background (as well as individual differences) has a great deal to do with what nonverbal behaviour means to different individuals. The degree of eye contact and the use of touch are two nonverbal behaviours that can be misunderstood by individuals of different cultures.
- There are a number of therapeutic communication techniques nurses can use to enhance their nursing practices (see Table 11-2).
- There are also a number of nontherapeutic communication techniques that nurses can learn to avoid to enhance their effectiveness in therapeutic relationships (see Table 11-3).
- Most nurses are most effective when they use nonthreatening and open-ended communication techniques.
- Effective communication is a skill that develops over time and is integral to the establishment and maintenance of a therapeutic relationship.
- The clinical interview is a key component of psychiatric mental health nursing, and the nurse must establish a safe setting and plan for appropriate seating, introductions, and initiation of the interview.
- Attending behaviours (e.g., eye contact, body language, vocal qualities, verbal tracking) are key elements in effective communication.
- A meaningful therapeutic relationship is facilitated when values and cultural influences are considered. It is the nurse's responsibility to seek to understand the patient's perceptions.

CRITICAL THINKING

1. Keep a written log of a conversation you have with a patient. In your log, identify the therapeutic and nontherapeutic techniques you noticed yourself using. Then rewrite the nontherapeutic communications using statements that would better facilitate discussion of thoughts and feelings. Share your log and discuss the changes you are working on with one classmate.
2. Role-play with a classmate at least five nonverbal communications, and have your partner identify the message he or she received.

3. With the other students in your class watching, plan and role-play a nurse–patient conversation that lasts about 3 minutes. Use both therapeutic and nontherapeutic techniques. When you are finished, have your other classmates try to identify the techniques you used. Discuss ways in which a reliance on colleagues or other subtle institutional concerns might factor in to the communication.
4. Demonstrate how the nurse would use touch and eye contact when working with patients from three different cultural groups.

CHAPTER REVIEW

1. You have been working closely with a patient for the past month. Today, he tells you he is looking forward to meeting with his new psychiatrist but frowns and avoids eye contact while reporting this to you. Which of the following responses would most likely be therapeutic?
   a. "A new psychiatrist is a chance to start fresh. I'm sure it will go well for you."
   b. "You say you look forward to the meeting, but you appear anxious or unhappy."
   c. "I notice that you frowned and avoided eye contact just now—don't you feel well?"
   d. "I get the impression you don't really want to see your psychiatrist—can you tell me why?"

2. Which behaviour is consistent with therapeutic communication?
   a. Offering your opinion when asked in order to convey support
   b. Summarizing the essence of the patient's comments in your own words
   c. Interrupting periods of silence before they become awkward for the patient
   d. Telling the patient he did well when you approve of his statements or actions

3. Which statement about nonverbal behaviour is accurate?
   a. A calm expression means that the patient is experiencing low levels of anxiety.
   b. Patients respond more consistently to therapeutic touch than to verbal interventions.
   c. The meaning of nonverbal behaviours varies with cultural and individual differences.
   d. Eye contact is a reliable measure of the patient's degree of attentiveness and engagement.

4. A nurse stops in to interview a patient on a medical unit and finds the patient lying supine in her bed with the head elevated at 10 degrees. Which initial response would most enhance the chances of achieving a therapeutic interaction?
   a. Apologize for the differential in height and proceed while standing to avoid delay.
   b. If permitted, raise the head of the bed and, with the patient's permission, sit on the bed.
   c. If permitted, raise the head of the bed to approximate the nurse's height while standing.
   d. Sit in whatever chair is available in the room to convey informality and increase comfort.

5. A patient with schizophrenia approaches staff arriving for the day shift and anxiously reports, "Last night, demons came to my room and tried to rape me." Which response would be most therapeutic?
   a. "There are no such things as demons; what you saw were hallucinations."
   b. "It is not possible for anyone to enter your room at night; you are safe here."
   c. "You seem very upset; please tell me more about what you experienced last night."
   d. "That must have been very frightening, but we'll check on you at night, and you'll be safe."

⊖volve WEBSITE

Post-Test   interactive review

Visit the Evolve website for Chapter Review Answers and Rationales, Critical Thinking Answer Guidelines, and additional resources related to the content in this chapter: http://evolve.elsevier.com/Canada/Varcarolis/psychiatric/

REFERENCES

Arnold, E. C., & Boggs, K. U. (2016). *Interpersonal relationships: Professional communication skills for nurses* (7th ed.). St. Louis: Saunders.

Balzer-Riley, J. W. (2017). *Communication in nursing* (8th ed.). St. Louis: Elsevier.

Bateson, G., Jackson, D., Haley, J., et al. (1956). Toward a theory of schizophrenia. *Behavioural Sciences, 1,* 251–264.

Berlo, D. K. (1960). *The process of communication.* San Francisco: Reinhart Press.

Coatsworth-Puspoky, R. R., Forchuk, C. C., & Ward-Griffin, C. C. (2006). Nurse–client processes in mental health: Recipients' perspectives. *Journal of Psychiatric and Mental Health Nursing, 13*(3), 347–355. doi:10.1111/j.1365-2850.2006.00968.x.

Egan, G. (2013). *The skilled helper: A problem-management approach and opportunity-development approach to helping* (10th ed.). Belmont, CA: Brooks/Cole, Cengage Learning.

Ehrmin, J. T. (2015). Transcultural perspectives in mental health nursing. In M. M. Andrews & J. S. Boyle (Eds.), *Transcultural concepts in nursing care* (7th ed., pp. 272–316). Philadelphia: Lippincott Williams & Wilkins.

Giger, J. N. (2017). *Transcultural nursing: Assessment and intervention* (7th ed.). St. Louis: Mosby.

Haber, J. (2000). Hildegard E. Peplau: The psychiatric nursing legacy of a legend. *Journal of the American Psychiatric Nurses Association, 6,* 510–562. doi:10.1067/mpn.2000.104556.

Matsumoto, D., & Hwang, H. S. (2011). Reading facial expressions of emotion. *Psychological Science Agenda,* May. Retrieved from http://www.apa.org/science/about/psa/2011/05/facial-expressions.aspx.

Meier, S. T., & Davis, S. R. (2010). *The elements of counseling* (7th ed.). Pacific Grove, CA: Brooks/Cole.

Mohl, P. C., & Carr, R. B. (2015). Listening to the patient. In A. Tasman, J. Kay, J. A. Lieberman, et al. (Eds.), *Psychiatry* (4th ed., pp. 1–19). Chichester, UK: Wiley. doi:10.1002/9781118753378.ch1.

National League for Nursing. (2015). *Debriefing across the curriculum.* Retrieved from http://www.nln.org/docs/default-source/about/nln-vision-series-(position-statements)/nln-vision-debriefing-across-the-curriculum.pdf?sfvrsn=0.

Peplau, H. E. (1952). *Interpersonal relations in nursing: A conceptual frame of reference for psychodynamic nursing.* New York: Putnam.

Schein, E. H. (2014). *Humble inquiry: The gentle art of asking instead of telling.* San Francisco: Berrett-Koehler.

Shea, S. C. (2017). *Psychiatric interviewing: The art of understanding* (3rd ed.). Philadelphia: Elsevier.

Sommers-Flanagan, J., & Sommers-Flanagan, R. (2013). *Clinical interviewing* (5th ed.). Hoboken, NJ: Wiley.

Varcarolis, E. M. (2017). *Essentials of psychiatric mental health nursing: A communication approach to evidence-based care.* Philadelphia: Elsevier.

Wheeler, K. (2014). *Psychotherapy for the advanced practice psychiatric nurse: A how-to guide for evidence-based practice* (2nd ed.). New York: Springer.

Wright, L. M., & Leahey, M. (2013). *Nurses and families: A guide to family assessment and intervention* (6th ed.). Philadelphia: F. A. Davis Company.

Psychotropic Drugs

Martin Davies, Paul M. Kerr

KEY TERMS AND CONCEPTS

agonist

antagonist

antianxiety (anxiolytic) drugs

anticholinesterase drugs

biopsychiatry

circadian rhythms

first-generation antipsychotic drugs

hypnotic

limbic system

lithium carbonate

metabolites

monoamine oxidase inhibitors (MAOIs)

mood stabilizer

neurons

neurotransmitters

pharmacodynamics

pharmacogenetics

pharmacokinetics

receptors

reticular activating system (RAS)

reuptake

second-generation antipsychotic drugs

selective serotonin reuptake inhibitors (SSRIs)

serotonin–norepinephrine reuptake inhibitor (SNRI)

synapse

therapeutic index

tricyclic antidepressants (TCAs)

OBJECTIVES

1. Identify the functions of the brain and discuss how these functions can be altered by psychotropic drugs.
2. Describe how a neurotransmitter functions as a chemical messenger.
3. Identify the functions of the three major areas of the brain.
4. Explain how specific brain functions are altered in mental health disorders such as depression, anxiety, bipolar disorder, and schizophrenia.
5. Describe how imaging techniques are used to study brain structure and function in individuals with mental health disorders.
6. Describe the result of blockage of muscarinic receptors and α_1-adrenergic receptors by drugs used to treat psychosis.
7. Identify the main neurotransmitters affected by the following psychotropic drugs and their subgroups:
   a. Antianxiety drugs
   b. Sedative–hypnotic drugs
   c. Antidepressant drugs
   d. Mood stabilizers
   e. Antipsychotic drugs
   f. Anticholinesterase drugs
8. Discuss dietary and drug restrictions for a patient taking a monoamine oxidase inhibitor.
9. Identify specific cautions for a patient taking natural health products and psychotropic drugs.
10. Explore the relevance of pharmacogenetics (i.e., variations in effects and therapeutic actions of medications among different ethnic groups) in the use of psychotrophic drugs.

⊜volve WEBSITE

Visit the Evolve website for Flashcards, Case Studies, and additional testing resources related to the content in this chapter: http://evolve.elsevier.com/Canada/Varcarolis/psychiatric/

Pre-Test | interactive review

One in every five Canadians will have a mental health problem at some point in their lives.

Biopsychiatry, sometimes referred to as the *biological approach*, is a theoretical approach to understanding mental health disorders as biological malfunctions of the nervous system. Implied in this approach is the idea that brain function is related to, and can be affected by, several factors; these include genetics, neurodevelopmental factors, drugs, infection, and psychosocial experience, either alone or in combination with one another. Clinicians using this approach believe that abnormal changes in a patient's behaviour and in mental and emotional experiences are caused by disturbances in normal brain function. For example, when the brain is not working as it should, the way it produces and responds to neurotransmitters, the "chemical messengers" of the nervous system, changes. These changes can, in turn, result in symptoms of depression, anxiety, post-traumatic stress disorder, or any other combination of behavioural, emotional, or mental disorders.

The primary goal of drug therapy is to restore "balance" to a malfunctioning brain. During recent years, there has been an explosion of information about the efficacy of psychotropic drugs (medication to treat mental illness); however, a full understanding of how these drugs improve symptoms continues to elude investigators. Early theories, such as the dopamine theory of schizophrenia and the monoamine theory of depression, are currently seen as overly simplistic because a large number of other neurotransmitters, hormones, and coregulators are now thought to play important and complex roles. Indeed, evidence suggests that some clinically useful drugs may be working by additional pathways at the genetic level that lead to long-term changes in brain structure and function. Current research, therefore, is focused on refining our understanding of how drugs can be used to alter the brain's responses to neurotransmitters, hormones, and coregulators, either by making more of the chemical available in the brain or by making the brain more sensitive to the chemical that is already there. In addition, as our understanding of these drugs grows, research is focusing more and more on how they bring about long-term changes in neuronal survival and connectivity via effects at the genetic level.

Included in this chapter is an overview of the major drugs used to treat mental health disorders and an explanation of how they work. Additional and detailed information regarding adverse and toxic effects, dosage, nursing implications, and teaching tools is presented in the appropriate clinical chapters (see Chapters 12 to 20).

Despite new knowledge about complex brain functions, there is still much to be clarified in understanding the ways in which the brain carries out its normal functions, is altered during disease, and is improved by pharmacological intervention. After reading this chapter, you should have a neurobiological framework into which you can place existing, as well as future, information about mental illness and its treatment.

STRUCTURE AND FUNCTION OF THE BRAIN

Functions and Activities of the Brain

Regulating behaviour and carrying out mental processes are two of the many important responsibilities of the brain. Some of

 HOW A NURSE HELPED ME

When the Adverse Effects Are Too Much to Take

A patient with a mental health disorder faces numerous challenges during the search for the correct medication and treatment regimen. At 19, my brother was hearing voices and felt that others were talking about him or trying to watch him through windows. A number of factors were thought to contribute to his strange behaviours, among them, his being stressed over a recent breakup with a girlfriend and using marijuana. However, he was diagnosed with paranoid schizophrenia. It was an extremely stressful time for my family, which had difficulty understanding and coping with his seemingly irrational and illogical behaviours.

He was admitted to hospital and started on first-generation antipsychotics. After a psychiatric nurse met my parents, she assessed that they needed assistance in understanding my brother's illness. Specifically, she explained that my brother's behaviours were symptoms of his illness and also how the medications would help ease his symptoms. She also outlined the common adverse effects that he might experience as a consequence of taking the medication. As well, she listened to my parents' worries about the future.

My brother was started on fluphenazine decanoate, a medication administered by injection, and his symptoms improved. The drug was administered for 2 years, but then he stopped taking it because of the adverse effects he was experiencing. We learned that restlessness, dry mouth, fatigue, tremors, and dizziness are not uncommon for people who are being treated with this kind of medication. It has been 40 years now since my brother's diagnosis, and he has not been on any medications for treatment since. Unfortunately, without any medication, he has been homeless for many years.

If my brother resumes psychopharmacological treatment in the future, the nurse will need to identify what factors will affect his decision to continue to take the prescribed medication. The nurse will need to listen to my brother's preferences about when he takes the medication, and his level of tolerance for various adverse effects will need to be considered when making decisions about possible interventions. The treatment team will also have to examine ways to predict how my brother will respond to the medication so as to optimize initial treatment selections. It will be important to select the medication that will have the best effect on his schizophrenia and the one with the fewest adverse effects, because they may get only one more chance.

BOX 11-1   FUNCTIONS OF THE BRAIN

- Monitor changes in the external world
- Monitor the composition of body fluids
- Regulate the contractions of skeletal muscles
- Regulate the internal organs
- Initiate and regulate the basic drives: hunger, thirst, sex, aggressive self-protection
- Mediate conscious sensation
- Store and retrieve memories
- Regulate mood (affect) and emotions
- Think and perform intellectual functions
- Regulate the sleep cycle
- Produce and interpret language
- Process visual and auditory data

the major functions and activities of the brain are summarized in Box 11-1. Because these brain functions are carried out by similar mechanisms (interactions between neurons) and often in similar locations, mental health disturbances are often associated with alterations in other brain functions, and the drugs used to treat mental disturbances can interfere with other activities of the brain.

Maintenance of Homeostasis

The brain serves as the coordinator and director of the body's response to both internal and external changes. Appropriate responses require a constant monitoring of the environment, interpretation and integration of the incoming information, and control over the appropriate organs of response. The goal of these responses is to maintain homeostasis and thus to maintain life.

Information about the external world is relayed from various sense organs to the brain by the peripheral nerves. This information, at first received as stimuli such as light, sound, or touch, must ultimately be interpreted into a picture, a train whistle, or a hand on the back. Interestingly, a component of major psychiatric disturbance (e.g., schizophrenia) is an alteration of sensory experience. Thus, the patient may experience a sensation that does not originate in the external world. For example, people with schizophrenia may hear voices talking to them (auditory hallucination).

To respond to external changes, the brain has control over the skeletal muscles. This control involves the ability not only to initiate contraction (e.g., to contract the biceps and flex the arm) but also to fine-tune and coordinate contraction so a person can, for example, guide the fingers to the correct keys on a piano. Unfortunately, both psychiatric disease and the treatment of psychiatric disease with psychotropic drugs are associated with movement disturbances. It is important to remember that the skeletal muscles controlled by the brain include the diaphragm, essential for breathing, and the muscles of the throat, tongue, and mouth, essential for speech. Therefore, drugs that affect brain function can, for example, stimulate or depress respiration or lead to slurred speech.

The brain not only makes sense of the external world but also keeps a close watch on internal functions. Information about

blood pressure, body temperature, blood gases, and the chemical composition of body fluids is continuously received by the brain, allowing it to send the responses required to maintain homeostasis. Adjustments to changes within the body require that the brain exert control over the various internal organs. For example, if blood pressure drops, the brain must direct the heart to pump more blood and the smooth muscle cells of arterioles to constrict. This increase in cardiac output and vasoconstriction allows the body to return blood pressure to its normal level.

Regulation of the Autonomic Nervous System and Endocrine System

The autonomic nervous system and the endocrine system serve as the communication links between the brain and the internal organs of the body (Figure 11-1). If the brain needs to stimulate the heart, it must activate the sympathetic nerves to the sinoatrial node and the ventricular myocardium. If the brain needs to bring about vasoconstriction, it must activate sympathetic nerves that innervate the smooth muscle cells of arterioles.

The linkage between the brain and the internal organs that allows for the maintenance of homeostasis may also serve to translate mental health disturbances, such as anxiety, into alterations of internal function. For example, anxiety in some people can cause inappropriate activation of parasympathetic nerves to the digestive tract, leading to hypermotility and diarrhea. Likewise, anxiety can activate the sympathetic nerves innervating cardiac muscle, leading to a pounding, fast heart rate, and arterioles, leading to vasoconstriction and hypertension.

The brain also exerts influence over the internal organs by regulating hormonal secretions of the pituitary gland, which in turn regulates other glands. The hypothalamus is involved in several functions of the brain. It secretes hormones that act on the pituitary gland to stimulate or inhibit the synthesis and release of pituitary hormones. Once in the general circulation, these hormones influence various internal activities. For example, when gonadotropin-releasing hormone is secreted by the hypothalamus at puberty, this hormone stimulates the release of two gonadotropins—follicle-stimulating hormone and luteinizing hormone—by the pituitary gland, which consequently activate the ovaries or testes.

The relationship between the brain, the pituitary gland, and the adrenal glands is particularly important in determining normal and abnormal mental function. Specifically, the hypothalamus secretes corticotropin-releasing hormone (CRH), which stimulates the pituitary to release corticotropin, which in turn stimulates the cortex of each adrenal gland to secrete the hormone cortisol. This system is activated as part of the normal response to a variety of mental and physical stresses. Among many other actions, all three hormones—CRH, corticotropin, and cortisol—influence the functions of the nerve cells of the brain. There is considerable evidence that in both anxiety and depression this system is overactive and does not respond properly to negative feedback.

Control of Biological Drives and Behaviour

Apart from the many higher cognitive tasks in which the brain engages, it is also responsible for the basic drives such as sex and hunger that play a strong role in moulding behaviour.

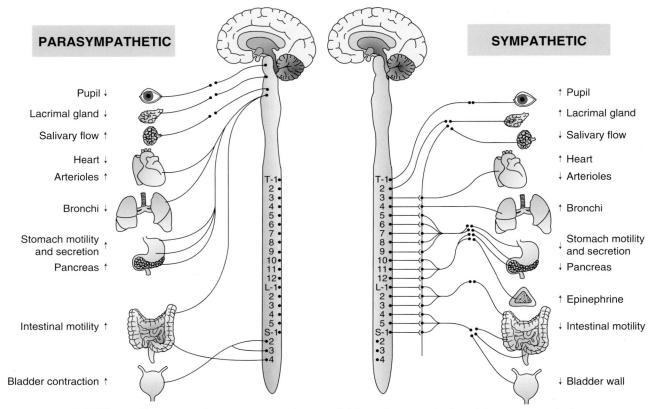

FIGURE 11-1 The autonomic nervous system has two divisions: the sympathetic and the parasympathetic. The sympathetic division is dominant in stressful situations such as those that incite fear or anger—known as the *fight-or-flight response*.

Disturbances in these drives, which may be manifested as eating disorders or loss of sexual interest, can be an indication of an underlying mental health disorder such as depression. By understanding why these disturbances occur, we may start to unravel the underlying pathology of these illnesses and establish a rational framework from which to approach treatment.

Cycle of sleep and wakefulness. The entire cycle of sleep and wakefulness, as well as the intensity of alertness while the person is awake, is regulated and coordinated by various regions of the brain. Although the true homeostatic function of sleep is not well understood, sleep is known to be essential for both physiological and psychological well-being. Assessment of sleep patterns is part of what is required to determine a diagnosis of a mental health disorder.

Unfortunately, many of the drugs used to treat mental health problems interfere with the normal regulation of sleep and alertness. Drugs with a sedative–hypnotic effect can blunt the degree to which a person feels alert and focused and can cause drowsiness. Because of the sedative–hypnotic effect, caution is necessary in using these drugs while engaging in activities that require a great deal of attention, such as driving a car or operating machinery. One way of minimizing the danger is to take such drugs at night just before bedtime.

Circadian rhythms. The cycle of sleep and wakefulness is only one aspect of circadian rhythms, the fluctuation of various physiological and behavioural parameters over a 24-hour cycle.

Other variations include changes in body temperature, secretion of hormones such as corticotropin and cortisol, and secretion of neurotransmitters—chemicals that transmit signals from one neuron to another across a synapse—such as norepinephrine and serotonin. Both norepinephrine and serotonin are thought to be involved in mood, and daily fluctuations of mood may be related in part to circadian variations in these neurotransmitters. There is evidence that the circadian rhythm of neurotransmitter secretion is altered in mental health disorders, particularly in those that involve mood.

Conscious Mental Activity

All aspects of conscious mental experience and sense of self originate from the neurophysiological activity of the brain. Conscious mental activity can be a basic, meandering, stream-of-consciousness flow among thoughts of future responsibilities, memories, fantasy, and so on. Conscious mental activity can also be much more complex when it is applied to problem solving and the interpretation of the external world. Both the random stream of consciousness and the complex problem solving and interpretation of the environment can become distorted in mental health disorders. For instance, a person with schizophrenia may have chaotic and incoherent speech and thought patterns (e.g., a jumble of unrelated words known as *word salad*, unconnected phrases and topics known as *looseness of association*) and delusional interpretations of personal interactions (e.g., beliefs about people or events that are not supported by data or reality).

Memory

Memory, the ability to retain and recall past experience, is a crucial component of mental activity. From both an anatomical and a physiological perspective, there is thought to be a major difference in the processing of short- and long-term memory. This can be seen dramatically in some forms of cognitive mental health disorders such as dementia, in which a person has no recall of the events of the previous 10 minutes but may have vivid recall of events that occurred decades earlier.

Social Skills

An important and often neglected aspect of brain functioning involves the social skills that make interpersonal relationships possible. In almost all types of mental health disorders, from mild anxiety to severe schizophrenia, difficulties in interpersonal relationships is an important characteristic, and improvements in these relationships are important gauges of progress. The connection between brain activity and social behaviour is an area of intense research and is believed to be influenced by a combination of genetic makeup and individual experience.

Cellular Composition of the Brain

The brain is composed of approximately 100 billion **neurons**, nerve cells that conduct electrical impulses, as well as other types of cells that surround the neurons. Most functions of the brain, from regulation of blood pressure to the conscious sense of self, are thought to result from the actions of individual neurons and the interconnections between them. Although neurons come in a great variety of shapes and sizes, all carry out the same three types of physiological actions: (1) they respond to stimuli; (2) they conduct electrical impulses; and (3) they release chemicals called *neurotransmitters*.

An essential feature of neurons is their ability to conduct an electrical impulse (action potential) from one end of the cell to the other. The action potential consists of a change in membrane permeability that first allows the inward flow of sodium ions and then the outward flow of potassium ions. The inward flow of sodium ions changes the polarity of the membrane potential from negative to positive with respect to the outside. Movement of potassium ions out of the cell re-establishes the negative membrane potential readying the cell to generate the next action potential. Because these electrical charges are self-propagating, a change at one end of the cell is conducted along the membrane until it reaches the other end (Figure 11-2). The functional significance of this propagation is that the electrical impulse serves as a means of communication between one part of the body and another.

Once action potentials reach the end of a neuron, neurotransmitter is released. Neurotransmitters are released from storage compartments called vesicles in the axon terminal of the *presynaptic neuron* (the term for the neuron from which the neurotransmitter is released). This neurotransmitter then diffuses across a space, or **synapse**, to an adjacent *postsynaptic neuron* (the neuron receiving the neurotransmitter), where it binds to

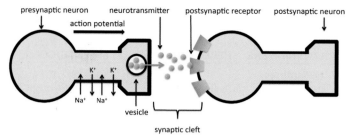

FIGURE 11-2 Activities of neurons. Conduction of an action potential along a neuron involves the inward movement of sodium ions (Na⁺) followed by the outward movement of potassium ions (K⁺). When the action potential reaches the end of the neuron, neurotransmitter is released from vesicles (storage compartments). The neurotransmitter crosses the synapse and binds to a receptor on the postsynaptic cell. The interaction of neurotransmitter and receptor either stimulates or inhibits the postsynaptic cell.

receptors (protein molecules embedded in a cell membrane). A postsynaptic neuron may have a variety of receptors that allow for multiple neurotransmitters to affect its function. This communication between neurons by way of neurotransmitter–receptor interaction allows the activity of one neuron to influence the activity of other neurons. Depending on the chemical structure of the neurotransmitter and the specific type of receptor to which it binds, the postsynaptic cell will be rendered either more or less likely to initiate an action potential. The interaction between neurotransmitter and receptor is a major target of drugs used to treat mental health disorders. Important neurotransmitters and the types of receptors to which they bind are identified in Table 11-1. Also identified are the mental health disorders associated with an increase or decrease in these neurotransmitters.

The signal from the presynaptic to postsynaptic neuron is terminated by a reduction in the amount of neurotransmitter in the synapse. There are two basic mechanisms by which this is achieved: (1) Some neurotransmitters, such as acetylcholine are degraded by specific enzymes in the synapse. Acetylcholinesterase is the enzyme that destroys acetylcholine. (2) Other neurotransmitters, such as norepinephrine, are taken back into the presynaptic neuron from which they were originally released, a process called cellular **reuptake**. The neurotransmitters are then either reused or degraded by intracellular enzymes. In the case of the monoamine neurotransmitters (e.g., norepinephrine, dopamine, serotonin), the degrading enzyme is called *monoamine oxidase* (MAO). The processes of neurotransmitter removal are described further in Box 11-2.

As a means of fine control of communication between neurons, the amount of neurotransmitter released from presynaptic nerve terminals can be regulated by presynaptic neurotransmitter receptors. Autoreceptors are presynaptic receptors that bind to the very neurotransmitter that the nerve ending is releasing, and their activation typically inhibits further neurotransmitter release. On the other hand, some presynaptic receptors respond to different neurotransmitters released from adjacent neurons, and their activation can inhibit or stimulate further neurotransmitter release.

Researchers have found that in many cases, neurons release more than one chemical at the same time. Neurotransmitters

TABLE 11-1   TRANSMITTERS AND RECEPTORS

TRANSMITTERS	RECEPTORS	EFFECTS/COMMENTS	ASSOCIATION WITH MENTAL HEALTH DISORDERS
Monoamines			
Dopamine (DA)	D_1, D_2, D_3, D_4, D_5	Involved in fine muscle movement Involved in integration of emotions and thoughts Involved in decision making Stimulates hypothalamus to release hormones (sex, thyroid, adrenal)	*Decreases:* Parkinson's disease Depression *Increases:* Schizophrenia Mania
Norepinephrine (NE) (noradrenaline)	α_1, α_2, β_1, β_2	Causes changes in mood Causes changes in attention and arousal Stimulates sympathetic branch of autonomic nervous system for fight or flight in response to stress	*Decreases:* Depression *Increases:* Mania Anxiety states Schizophrenia
Serotonin (5-HT)	5-HT$_1$, 5-HT$_2$, 5-HT$_3$, 5-HT$_4$	Plays a role in sleep regulation, hunger, mood states, and pain perception Alters hormonal activity Plays a role in aggression and sexual behaviour	*Decreases:* Depression *Increases:* Anxiety states
Histamine	H_1, H_2	Involved in alertness Involved in inflammatory response Stimulates gastric secretion	*Decreases:* Sedation Weight gain
Amino Acids			
Gamma-aminobutyric acid (GABA)	GABA$_A$, GABA$_B$	Plays a role in inhibition; reduces aggression, excitation, and anxiety May play a role in pain perception Has anticonvulsant and muscle-relaxing properties May impair cognition and psychomotor functioning	*Decreases:* Anxiety disorders Schizophrenia Mania Huntington's disease *Increases:* Reduction of anxiety
Glutamate	*N*-methyl-D-aspartate (NMDA), α-amino-3-hydroxy-5-methyl-4-isoxazolepropionic acid (AMPA)	Is excitatory AMPA plays a role in learning and memory	*Decreases (NMDA):* Psychosis *Increases (NMDA):* Prolonged increased state can be neurotoxic Neurodegeneration in Alzheimer's disease *Increases (AMPA):* Improvement of cognitive performance in behavioural tasks
Cholinergics			
Acetylcholine (ACh)	Nicotinic, muscarinic (M_1, M_2, M_3)	Plays a role in learning, memory Regulates mood, mania, sexual aggression Affects sexual and aggressive behaviour Stimulates parasympathetic nervous system	*Decreases:* Alzheimer's disease Huntington's disease Parkinson's disease *Increases:* Depression
Peptides (Neuromodulators)			
Substance P (SP)	SP	Has antidepressant and antianxiety effects in depression Promotes and reinforces memory Enhances sensitivity of pain receptors	Involved in regulation of mood and anxiety Plays a role in pain management
Somatostatin (SRIF)	SRIF	Alters cognition, memory, and mood	*Decreases:* Alzheimer's disease Decreased levels of SRIF in spinal fluid of some depressed patients *Increases:* Huntington's disease
Neurotensin (NT)	NT	Has endogenous antipsychotic-like properties	Decreased levels in spinal fluid of schizophrenic patients

BOX 11-2 REDUCTION OF NEUROTRANSMITTERS IN THE SYNAPSE

A full explanation of the various ways in which psychotropic drugs alter neuronal activity requires a brief review of the manner in which neurotransmitter levels are reduced in the synapse to avoid continuous and prolonged action on the postsynaptic cell.

Following release of neurotransmitter from vesicles in the presynaptic neuron, the neurotransmitter is dealt with in one of two ways.

1. Degradation of the neurotransmitter in the synapse. An example of this method of destruction is the action of the enzyme acetyl-cholinesterase (AChE) on the neurotransmitter acetylcholine. AChE is located on the pre- and postsynaptic membrane and breaks down acetylcholine.

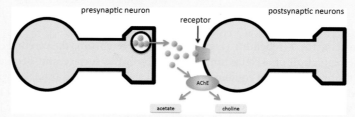

2. Neurotransmitter is taken back into the presynaptic neuron. Following release of neurotransmitter into the synapse, it re-enters the presynaptic neuron via a transporter in the cell membrane. This process, referred to as *reuptake*, is a target for many drugs. Once inside the presynaptic neuron, the neurotransmitter is either recycled into vesicles or inactivated by an enzyme within the cell. The monoamine neurotransmitters norepinephrine, dopamine, and serotonin are all inactivated in this manner by the enzyme monoamine oxidase (MAO).

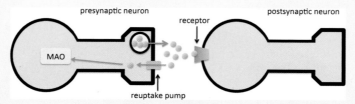

such as norepinephrine or acetylcholine—which have immediate effects on postsynaptic neurons—are often accompanied by larger molecules, neuropeptides, that may initiate long-term changes in the postsynaptic neurons. These changes may involve basic cell functions, such as genetic expression, and lead to modifications of cell shape and responsiveness to stimuli. Ultimately, this means that the action of one neuron on another affects not only the immediate response of that neuron but also its sensitivity to future influence. The long-term implications of this for neural development, normal and abnormal mental health, and the treatment of mental health disorders are being investigated.

The communication between neurons at a synapse is not unidirectional. *Neurotrophic factors*—proteins and even simple gases, such as carbon monoxide and nitric oxide—are released by postsynaptic cells and influence the growth, shape, and activity of presynaptic cells. These factors are thought to be particularly important during the development of the fetal brain, guiding the growing brain to form the proper neuronal connections. However, it is now apparent that the brain retains anatomical plasticity throughout life and that internal and external influences can alter synaptic networks of the brain. The role of altered genetic expression or environmental trauma in the action of these factors and the negative and positive consequences of these changes on mental function and psychiatric disease are areas of much research.

The development and responsiveness of neurons is dependent not only on chemicals released by other neurons but also on chemicals, particularly the steroid hormones, carried to the brain in the blood. Estrogen, testosterone, and cortisol can bind to receptors in neurons, where they can cause short- and long-term changes in neuronal activity. A clear example of this is seen in the psychosis that can sometimes result from the hypersecretion of cortisol in Cushing's disease or from the use of prednisone in high doses to treat chronic inflammatory disease.

Organization of the Brain

Brainstem

The brainstem is responsible for such vital functions as the regulation of internal organs, blood gases, and blood pressure. It also serves as a crucial psychosomatic link between higher brain activities, such as thought and emotion, and the functioning of the internal organs. The brainstem also functions as an initial processing centre for sensory information that is then sent on to the cerebral cortex. Through projections of the **reticular activating system (RAS)**, the brainstem regulates the entire cycle of sleep and wakefulness and the ability of the cerebrum to carry out conscious mental activity.

Other ascending pathways, referred to as *mesolimbic* and *mesocortical pathways*, seem to play a strong role in modulating the emotional value of sensory material. These pathways project to those areas of the cerebrum—the hypothalamus, amygdala, and hippocampus, collectively known as the **limbic system**—that play a crucial role in emotional status and psychological function. The hypothalamus, a small area in the ventral superior portion of the brainstem, plays a vital role in such basic drives as hunger, thirst, and sex. The pathways use norepinephrine, serotonin, and dopamine as their neurotransmitters. Much attention has been paid to the role of these pathways in normal and abnormal mental activity. For example, it is thought that the release of dopamine from the *ventral tegmental pathway* plays a role in psychological reward and substance dependence. The neurotransmitters released by the neurons in the mesolimbic and mesocortical pathways are major targets of the drugs used to treat mental health disorders.

Cerebellum

Located posteriorly to the brainstem, the cerebellum (Figure 11-3) is primarily involved in the regulation of skeletal muscle coordination and contraction and the maintenance of equilibrium. It plays a crucial role in coordinating contractions so that movement is accomplished in a smooth and directed manner.

Cerebrum

The human brainstem and cerebellum are similar in both structure and function to these same structures in other mammals. The development of a much larger and more elaborate cerebrum is what distinguishes human beings from the rest of the animal kingdom.

The cerebrum, situated on top of and surrounding the brainstem, is responsible for mental activities and a conscious sense of being, including our conscious perception of the external world and our own body, emotional status, memory, and control of skeletal muscles that allows willful direction of movement. It is also responsible for language and the ability to communicate.

The cerebrum (the cerebral cortex and basal ganglia) consists of both the surface and deep areas of undulating grey matter and the connecting tracts of white matter that link these areas with each other and the rest of the nervous system. The cerebral cortex, which forms the outer layer of the brain, is responsible for conscious sensation and the initiation of movement. Specific areas of the cortex are responsible for specific sensations: the parietal cortex for touch, the temporal cortex for sound, the occipital cortex for vision, and so on. The initiation of skeletal

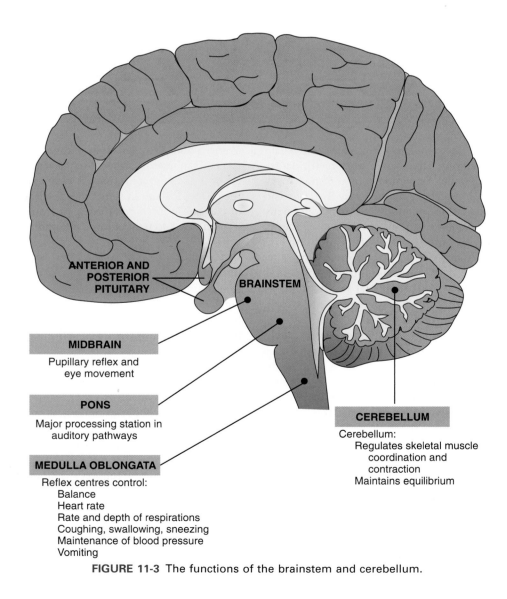

ANTERIOR AND POSTERIOR PITUITARY

BRAINSTEM

MIDBRAIN
Pupillary reflex and eye movement

PONS
Major processing station in auditory pathways

MEDULLA OBLONGATA
Reflex centres control:
  Balance
  Heart rate
  Rate and depth of respirations
  Coughing, swallowing, sneezing
  Maintenance of blood pressure
  Vomiting

CEREBELLUM
Cerebellum:
  Regulates skeletal muscle coordination and contraction
  Maintains equilibrium

FIGURE 11-3 The functions of the brainstem and cerebellum.

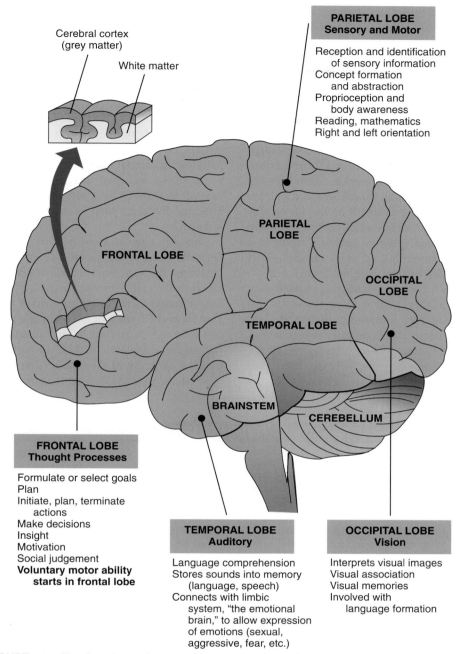

Cerebral cortex (grey matter)

White matter

PARIETAL LOBE
Sensory and Motor

Reception and identification
of sensory information
Concept formation
and abstraction
Proprioception and
body awareness
Reading, mathematics
Right and left orientation

PARIETAL LOBE

FRONTAL LOBE

OCCIPITAL LOBE

TEMPORAL LOBE

BRAINSTEM

CEREBELLUM

FRONTAL LOBE
Thought Processes

Formulate or select goals
Plan
Initiate, plan, terminate
actions
Make decisions
Insight
Motivation
Social judgement
Voluntary motor ability
starts in frontal lobe

TEMPORAL LOBE
Auditory

Language comprehension
Stores sounds into memory
(language, speech)
Connects with limbic
system, "the emotional
brain," to allow expression
of emotions (sexual,
aggressive, fear, etc.)

OCCIPITAL LOBE
Vision

Interprets visual images
Visual association
Visual memories
Involved with
language formation

FIGURE 11-4 The functions of the cerebral lobes: frontal, parietal, temporal, and occipital.

muscle contraction is controlled by a specific area of the frontal cortex. All areas of the cortex are interconnected to enable an appropriate picture of the world to be formed and, if necessary, linked to a proper response (Figure 11-4).

Specialized areas of the cerebral cortex are responsible for language in both its sensory and its motor aspects. Sensory language functions include the ability to read, understand spoken language, and know the names of objects perceived by the senses. Motor functions involve the physical ability to use muscles properly for speech and writing. In both neurological and psychological dysfunction, the use of language may become compromised or distorted. A change in linguistic ability may be a factor in determining a diagnosis.

The basal ganglia are located deep within the grey matter of the cerebrum; they are involved in the regulation of movement. Other structures, the amygdala and hippocampus, are involved in emotions, learning, memory, and basic drives. Significantly, there is an overlap of these various areas both anatomically and in the types of neurotransmitters employed. One consequence of this overlap is that drugs used to treat emotional disturbances may cause movement disorders, and drugs used to treat movement disorders may cause emotional changes.

Visualizing the Brain

Various noninvasive imaging techniques can be used to visualize brain structure, function, and biological activity. Some common brain imaging techniques and preliminary findings as they relate to psychiatry are identified in Table 11-2. There are basically two types of information that can be obtained using neuroimaging techniques: structural and functional. By obtaining structural information from people with a specific disease and comparing it to those free of the disease, investigators can determine whether differences in the structure or volume of specific brain regions may be tied to the disease (Lui, Zhou, Sweeney, et al. 2016). Techniques such as computed tomography (CT) and magnetic resonance imaging (MRI) are often used in these types of studies. Functional information can reveal whether people suffering from psychiatric illness display changes in communication between different brain regions, alterations in blood flow and glucose metabolism, or differences in the function of specific neurotransmitter systems. For these types of studies, positron emission tomography (PET) and single-photon emission computed tomography (SPECT) are commonly used, as is a variant of MRI called functional magnetic resonance imaging (fMRI).

PET scans are particularly useful in identifying physiological and biochemical changes as they occur in living tissue. Usually a radioactive "tag" is used to trace compounds such as glucose. Because neurons rely on glucose as their primary energy source, the tagged glucose can be followed to see which parts of the brain are most active. For example, in patients with untreated schizophrenia, PET scans may show a decreased use of glucose in the frontal lobes. Figure 11-5 shows lower brain activity in the frontal lobe of a twin diagnosed with schizophrenia than in that of the asymptomatic twin. The area affected in the frontal cortex of the twin with schizophrenia is an area associated with reasoning skills, which are greatly impaired in people with schizophrenia. Scans such as these suggest a location in the frontal cortex as the site of functional impairment in people with schizophrenia.

In one study of people with obsessive-compulsive disorder (OCD), PET scans revealed abnormally high activity in certain parts of the frontal cortex. This is illustrated in Figure 11-6, which shows increased use of glucose in these regions in an individual with OCD when compared with a control. This indicates that these parts of the brain are working harder than is usual.

Similarly, changes in activity in discrete brain regions have been shown in people diagnosed with depression. Figure 11-7 illustrates findings from a PET study with depressed people showing decreased glucose use (and therefore lower activity) in the prefrontal cortex and other areas of the brain. Finally, Figure 11-8 shows PET scans of the brain of a patient with Alzheimer's disease at age 56 and age 58. In this study, investigators used a radioactive chemical (^{11}C-PIB) to tag β-amyloid, the protein that is a hallmark of the disease. The scans indicate increased amounts of β-amyloid in various brain regions as the patient

TABLE 11-2   COMMON BRAIN IMAGING TECHNIQUES

TECHNIQUE	DESCRIPTION	DETECTION	PSYCHIATRIC RELEVANCE AND PRELIMINARY FINDINGS
Structural: Show Gross Anatomical Details of Brain Structures			
Computed tomography (CT)	A series of X-ray images of the brain is taken, and computer analysis produces "slices," providing a precise 3D-like reconstruction of each segment	Lesions Abrasions Areas of infarct Aneurysm	*Schizophrenia:* Cortical atrophy Third ventricle enlargement *Cognitive disorders:* Abnormalities
Magnetic resonance imaging (MRI)	A magnetic field is applied to the brain; nuclei of hydrogen atoms absorb and emit radio waves that are analyzed by computer, providing 3D visualization of the brain's structure in sectional images	Brain edema Ischemia Infection Neoplasm Trauma	*Schizophrenia:* Enlarged ventricles Reduction in temporal lobe and prefrontal lobe
Functional magnetic resonance imaging (fMRI)	Functional imaging approach avoids exposure to ionizing radiation	(See MRI)	(See MRI)
Functional: Show Some Activity of the Brain			
Positron emission tomography (PET)	Radioactive substance (tracer) injected, travels to the brain, and shows up as bright spots on the scan; data collected by detectors are relayed to a computer, which produces images of the activity and 3D visualization of CNS	Oxygen use Glucose metabolism Blood flow Neurotransmitter–receptor interaction	*Schizophrenia:* Increased D_2, D_3 receptors in caudate nucleus Abnormalities in limbic system *Mood disorders:* Abnormalities in temporal lobes *Adult ADHD:* Decreased use of glucose (See PET)
Single-photon emission computed tomography (SPECT)	Similar to PET but uses radionuclides that emit gamma radiation (photons); measures various aspects of brain functioning and provides images of multiple layers of the CNS (as does PET)	Circulation of cerebrospinal fluid Similar functions to PET	

3D, Three-dimensional; ADHD, attention-deficit/hyperactivity disorder; CNS, central nervous system.

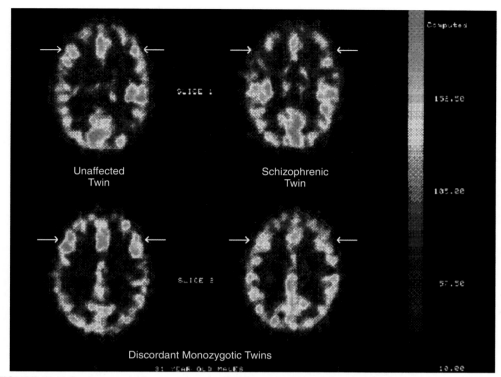

FIGURE 11-5 Positron emission tomography (PET) scans of blood flow in identical twins, one of whom has schizophrenia, illustrate that individuals with this illness have reduced brain activity in the frontal lobes when asked to perform a reasoning task that requires activation of this area. Patients with schizophrenia perform poorly on the task. This suggests a site of functional impairment in schizophrenia. (From Karen Berman, MD, courtesy National Institute of Mental Health, Clinical Brain Disorders Branch.)

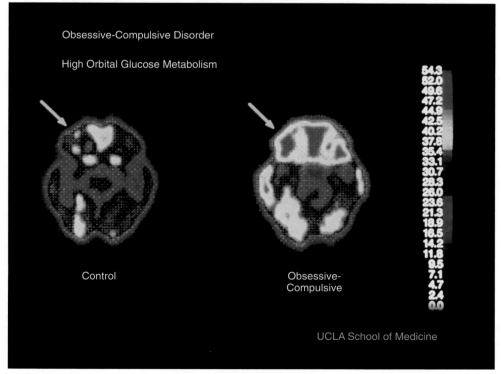

FIGURE 11-6 Positron emission tomography (PET) scans show increased brain metabolism (brighter colours), particularly in the frontal cortex, in a patient with obsessive-compulsive disorder, compared with a control. This suggests altered brain function in OCD. (From Lewis Baxter, MD, University of California, Los Angeles.)

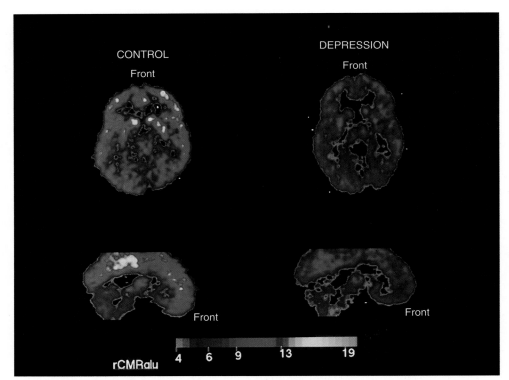

FIGURE 11-7 Positron emission tomography (PET) scans of a patient with depression (*right*) and a person without depression (*left*) reveal reduced brain activity (darker colours) in depression, especially in the prefrontal cortex. A form of radioactively tagged glucose was used as a tracer to visualize levels of brain activity. (From Mark George, MD, courtesy National Institute of Mental Health, Biological Psychiatry Branch.)

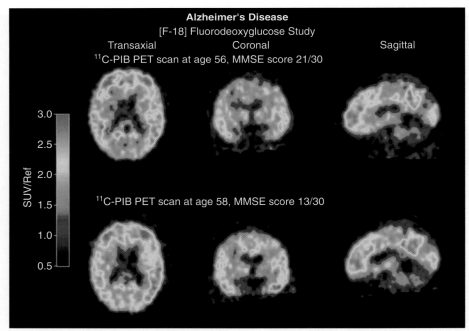

FIGURE 11-8 Positron emission tomography (PET) scan of a patient with Alzheimer's disease demonstrates the retention of ^{11}C-PIB, a marker for amyloid protein. Scans of the same patient at ages 56 and 58 show a consistently high amyloid load in various brain regions. Note that as the disease progresses, a drop in her cognitive abilities is reflected in a lower score in the mini-mental standard evaluation (MMSE). (From Kadir, A., Marutle, A., Gonzalez, D., et al. [2011]. Positron emission tomography imaging and clinical progression in relation to molecular pathology in the first Pittsburgh Compound B positron emission tomography patient with Alzheimer's disease. *Brain, 134,* 301–317. By permission of Oxford University Press.)

ages, and this was associated with diminished cognitive performance as assessed by a mini-mental state examination (MMSE). In a separate experiment, this study also showed that there was a strong correlation between a decrease in MMSE scores and a decrease in cerebral glucose metabolism as assessed by PET. Modern imaging techniques have also become important tools in assessing molecular changes in mental health disorders and in marking the receptor sites of drug action. It is important to be able to understand which brain areas are associated with psychopathology and which biological functions are altered in psychiatric disease states in order to develop new therapies as well as to improve the use of those currently available. While these imaging techniques have greatly increased our understanding of psychiatric diseases, they still cannot be used in isolation to diagnose these diseases. However, it is hoped that as these techniques mature and become more sophisticated, they can be used in the early diagnosis of various conditions and to monitor changes that occur in response to pharmacotherapy in order to personalize drug treatment. In conjunction with other validated diagnostic tools, this could lead to a powerful new approach to disease management (Fu & Costafreda, 2013)

Disturbances of Mental Function

The origin of most mental health dysfunction is unknown. Among known causes are drugs (e.g., lysergic acid diethylamide [LSD]), long-term use of prednisone, unusually high levels of hormones (e.g., thyroxine, cortisol), infection (e.g., encephalitis, acquired immunodeficiency syndrome [AIDS]), and physical trauma. However, even when the cause is known, the mechanistic link between the causative factor and the mental health dysfunction is far from understood.

Evidence suggests that many people with psychiatric disorders are genetically predisposed to them. The incidence of both thought and mood disorders is higher in relatives of people with these diseases than in the general population. Evidence has also shown a strong concordance among identical twins, even when they are raised apart. *Concordance* refers to how often one twin will be affected by the same illness as the other. Psychosocial stress, either in the family of origin or in contacts with society at large, increases the likelihood of mental health problems, as does physical disease. Genetics and environment interact in complex ways so that some people are better able to cope with stress than others (Amstadter, Myers, & Kendler, 2014).

Researchers ultimately want to be able to understand mental health dysfunction in terms of altered activity of neurons in specific areas of the brain. The hope is that such an understanding will lead to better treatments and possible prevention of mental disorders. Current interest is focused on certain neurotransmitters and their receptors, particularly those in the limbic system: norepinephrine, dopamine, serotonin, gamma-aminobutyric acid (GABA), and glutamate.

As shown in Figure 11-9, dysfunction of these neurotransmitter systems may be due to a deficiency in neurotransmitter release by the presynaptic cell or an inability of postsynaptic receptors to respond to neurotransmitters. Changes in neurotransmitter release and receptor response can be both a cause and a consequence of disease states, and it has proven to be difficult to

determine which happens first. Thought disorders such as schizophrenia are associated physiologically with excess transmission of the neurotransmitter dopamine, among other changes. As illustrated in Figure 11-10, this change in dopamine transmission may be due to either an excess release of neurotransmitter or an increase in receptor responsiveness.

The neurotransmitter GABA plays a central role in modulating neuronal excitability. Abnormalities in GABA-related neurotransmission have been linked to anxiety. Not surprisingly, many antianxiety (anxiolytic) drugs act by increasing the effectiveness of this neurotransmitter, primarily by increasing receptor responsiveness.

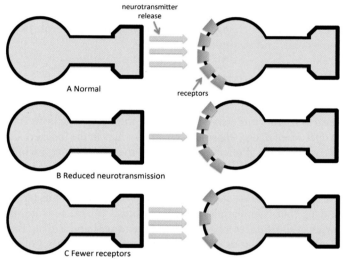

FIGURE 11-9 A, Normal neurotransmission can be affected by both how much neurotransmitter is released and the number of receptors to which it binds. Deficiency in neurotransmission may be due to a decrease in neurotransmitter release, as shown in **B**, or to a reduction in the number of postsynaptic receptors, as shown in **C**.

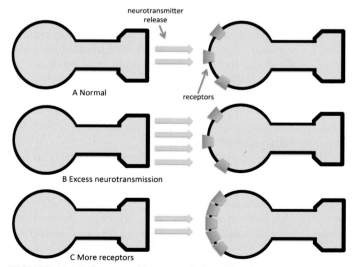

FIGURE 11-10 Causes of increased signalling between neurons. Increased neurotransmission may be due to excess release of neurotransmitter, as shown in **B**, or to increased numbers of receptors, as shown in **C**.

It is important to keep in mind that the various areas of the brain are interconnected structurally and functionally by a vast network of neurons. This network serves to integrate the many and varied activities of the brain. A limited number of neurotransmitters are used in the brain, and thus a particular neurotransmitter is often used by different neurons and neuronal circuits to carry out quite different activities. For example, dopamine is used by neuronal circuitry involved not only in mood and reward but also in the regulation of movement. Because one neurotransmitter can mediate multiple brain functions, alterations in its activity due to a mental disturbance or to the drugs used to treat the disturbance can produce multiple effects that at first glance may seem unrelated to one another. In other words, alterations in one particular aspect of brain function, whether arising from disease or from medication, are often accompanied by changes in basic drives, sleep patterns, body movement, and autonomic functions.

USE OF PSYCHOTROPIC DRUGS

The concepts of pharmacodynamics and pharmacokinetics are central to the understanding of the therapeutic actions and properties of drugs. Pharmacodynamics refers to the biochemical and physiological effects of drugs on the body, which include the mechanisms of drug action and its effect. When discussing the pharmacodynamics of a drug, the terms agonist and antagonist may be used to describe the actions of the drug at its target. A drug that is an agonist is one that binds to and activates its target and produces a response. On the other hand, a drug that is an antagonist binds to, but does not activate, its target. Rather, antagonists typically prevent other molecules such as neurotransmitters from binding to and activating the target protein. Antagonists produce no measurable effect by themselves. Pharmacokinetics refers to the actions of the body on the drug and involves four key aspects: (1) absorption (how much of the drug enters the circulation following administration); (2) distribution of an administered drug to body tissues; (3) metabolism of the drug (chemical change of the drug by the body); and (4) excretion of the drug or its metabolites (the products of metabolism). The major organ responsible for drug metabolism is the liver, and the major route of excretion is via urine produced by the kidneys. Ultimately, pharmacokinetics determines the change in blood level of a drug with time and is used to guide the dosage schedule. It is also used to determine the appropriate characteristics and doses of drugs that can safely be used in patients with liver and kidney disease.

The processes of pharmacokinetics and pharmacodynamics play an extensive role in how genetic factors give rise to variations in drug response among individuals and among ethnic groups. Pharmacogenetics is an approach to treatment that takes into consideration individual genetic differences when determining which and how much medication to prescribe (see Considering Culture box).

An ideal psychiatric drug would relieve the mental health disturbance of the patient without inducing additional cerebral (mental) or somatic (physical) effects. Unfortunately, in psychopharmacology—as in most areas of pharmacology—no

CONSIDERING CULTURE
Pharmacogenetics

Pharmacogenetic researchers are attempting to explain how genetic variations lead to clinical differences in drug responses for different individuals and ethnic groups (Zhang & Nebert, 2017). For example, different metabolizer phenotypes have significant differences in drug metabolism rates due to variations in the genes that code for their cytochrome P450 (CYP450) liver enzymes (Bertilsson, 2007). Of the more than 50 different CYP450 enzymes identified in humans, seven metabolize greater than 90% of the clinically most important drugs. For example, CYP2D6 alone is involved in the metabolism of 25% to 30% of all prescribed drugs, including those used to treat depression and schizophrenia (Lewis, 2004). Because of this, variations in any of the genes that code for these seven enyzmes can have significant effects on drug metabolism, which, in turn, affects circulating levels of the drug. There are variations in the CYP2D6 enzyme within any given population that result in some people being poor metabolizers of some drugs while others are so-called ultra-metabolizers because they metabolize certain drugs more rapidly than expected (Gaedigk, 2013). Poor metabolizers may experience adverse effects due to higher than expected circulating levels of the drug, whereas ultra-metabolizers may receive fewer therapeutic benefits than expected due to lower circulating levels of the drug (Teh & Bertilsson, 2012). The differences in genes that influence drug response are the key to the idea of personalized medicine, the goal of which is to tailor drug treatments (specific drugs, and doses) to the particular genetic makeup of individuals in order for them to receive the maximum benefit from any therapeutic treatment plan. Although the costs of obtaining genetic information of individuals continue to fall and the techniques used to obtain the information become more powerful, we are probably still far away from achieving a genetics-based approach to therapy (Zhang & Nebert, 2017).

In addition to adverse effects related to genetic factors, many other factors influence adherence to a medical regimen. For example, cultural and ethnic beliefs surrounding mental health disorders, attitudes toward the mental health system, and the cultural practices of an ethnic group all greatly affect a patient's degree of engagement with and adherence to the medical regimen. Cultural factors are discussed more fully in Chapter 8.

Sources: Bertilsson, L. (2007). Metabolism of antidepressant and neuroleptic drugs by cytochrome P450s: Clinical and interethnic aspects. *Clinical Pharmacology and Therapeutics, 82*(5), 606–609. doi:10.1038/sj.clpt.6100358; Gaedigk, A. (2013). Complexities of CYP2D6 gene analysis and interpretation. *International Review of Psychiatry, 25*(5), 534–553. doi.org/10.3109/09540261.2013.825581; Lewis, D. F. (2004). 57 varieties: The human cytochromes P450. *Pharmacogenomics, 5*(3), 305–318. doi:10.1517/phgs.5.3.305.29827; Teh, L. K., & Bertilsson, L. (2012). Pharmacogenomics of CYP2D6: Molecular genetics, interethnic differences and clinical importance. *Drug Metabolism and Pharmacokinetics, 27*(1), 55–67; and Zhang, G., & Nebert, D. W. (2017). Personalized medicine: Genetic risk prediction of drug response. *Pharmacology and Therapeutics.* doi.org/10.1016/j.pharmthera.2017.02.036.

drugs are both fully effective and free of unwanted effects. Nevertheless, researchers are working toward developing medications that target the symptoms while producing no or few adverse effects.

The development of new drugs or treatment protocols with existing drugs that minimize adverse effects are important goals, as experiencing adverse effects is frequently listed as a reason why many patients stop taking their psychotropic medications. Nonadherence to medications (i.e., primarily medication non-persistence and the lack of consistency in adhering to the prescribed regimen) is a significant barrier to the successful treatment of mental health disorders. For example, a systematic review of adherence to antipsychotic medications in schizophrenia reveals adherence rates ranging from 47% to 95% (Sendt, Tracy, & Bhattacharyya, 2015). Similarly, adherence to medications for the treatment of depression is often poor, resulting in an increased risk of relapse and hospitalization (Ho, Chong, Chaiyakunapruk, et al., 2016). Nonadherence is typically due to a combination of the patient experiencing adverse effects and a lack of efficacy (Leucht, Cipriani, Spineli, et al., 2013).

Because all functions of the brain involve activity of neurons, neurotransmitters, and receptors, these are the targets of pharmacological intervention. Most psychotropic drugs act by either increasing or decreasing the activity of certain neurotransmitter–receptor systems. It is generally agreed that the dysfunctional neurotransmitter–receptor systems differ depending on a person's mental health condition. These differences offer more specific targets for drug action. In fact, much of what is known about the relationship between specific neurotransmitters and specific disturbances has been derived from knowledge of the pharmacology of the drugs used to treat these conditions. For example, most drugs that are effective in reducing the delusions and hallucinations of schizophrenia block D_2 dopamine receptors. Therefore we can infer that delusions and hallucinations result from overactivity of dopamine pathways in the brain. In turn, this type of understanding subsequently leads to the development of drugs that are more selective for these targets.

Drugs Used to Treat Anxiety and Insomnia

Gamma-aminobutyric acid (GABA) is the major inhibitory (calming) neurotransmitter in the central nervous system (CNS). There are three major types of GABA receptors: $GABA_A$, $GABA_B$, and $GABA_C$ receptors. The family of $GABA_A$ receptors contains several different subtypes (versions) of receptor, each with its own particular drug recognition properties. Specific members of the $GABA_A$ receptor family are the targets of benzodiazepines, barbiturates, and alcohol. Drugs that enhance the actions of GABA at $GABA_A$ receptors exert a sedative–hypnotic action on brain function. The most commonly used antianxiety drugs are the benzodiazepines and, more recently, the selective serotonin reuptake inhibitors and serotonin–norepinephrine reuptake inhibitors, which were originally introduced for the treatment of depression.

Benzodiazepines

Benzodiazepines enhance the actions of GABA by binding to a specific location on the $GABA_A$ receptor complex. They only

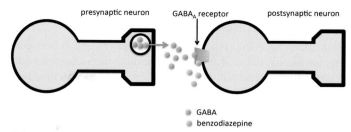

FIGURE 11-11 Action of benzodiazepines. Drugs in this group bind to a site that is part of the $GABA_A$ receptor complex to which gamma-aminobutyric acid (GABA) itself binds. Clinically useful benzodiazepines enhance the inhibitory effects of GABA. Benzodiazepines do not produce an inhibitory effect in the absence of GABA. Both must simultaneously bind to the receptor for any clinical effect to occur.

have an effect if GABA is also bound to its binding sites on the receptor complex. This interaction decreases the probability that the neuron on which the receptors are found will depolarize and thus leads to an overall decrease in neuronal excitability. As shown in Figure 11-11, benzodiazepines, such as diazepam (Valium), clonazepam (Rivotril), and alprazolam (Xanax), bind to $GABA_A$ receptors. The receptors are common in the limbic system, the brain's emotional centre, and enhanced GABA activity is important for decreasing anxiety.

At higher doses, all benzodiazepines can cause sedation. There are six benzodiazepines used in Canada for treatment of insomnia—lorazepam (Ativan), nitrazepam (Mogadon), oxazepam (Serax), temazepam (Restoril), triazolam (Halcion), and flurazepam (Dalmane)—with a predominantly **hypnotic** (sleep-inducing) effect. Used at lower doses, lorazepam (Ativan) and alprazolam (Xanax) can reduce anxiety without being as *soporific* (sleep producing).

The fact that the benzodiazepines promote the ability of GABA to decrease neuronal excitability probably accounts for their efficacy in the treatment of seizures and for their ability to reduce the neuronal overexcitement that is characteristic of alcohol withdrawal. While being efficacious at treating seizures and convulsions, benzodiazepines cannot be used prophylactically due to their tendency to quickly induce tolerance in those that use them. When used in the absence of other CNS depressant agents, even at high dosages, these drugs rarely inhibit the brain to the degree that respiratory depression, coma, and death result, and so they are considered relatively safe drugs. However, when combined with other CNS depressants, such as alcohol, opioids, or tricyclic antidepressants (TCAs), the inhibitory actions of the benzodiazepines can lead to life-threatening respiratory and CNS depression.

Any drug that inhibits electrical activity in the brain can interfere with motor ability, attention, and judgement. A patient taking benzodiazepines must be cautioned about engaging in activities that could be dangerous if reflexes and attention are impaired, including specialized activities such as working in construction and more common activities such as driving a car. In older adults, the use of benzodiazepines may contribute to falls and broken bones. Ataxia is a common adverse effect secondary to the abundance of GABA receptors in the cerebellum.

Short-Acting Sedative–Hypnotic Sleep Drugs

Zopiclone (Imovane) is a member of a newer class of benzodiazepine-like hypnotics. It, along with the other benzodiazepine-like drugs, zaleplon and zolpidem, has been grouped together into a class colloquially called the *Z-drugs*. Structurally, zopicline is not a true benzodiazepine; however, zopiclone displays similar actions as the true benzodiazepines at GABA$_A$ receptors. Thus its use also results in a decrease in neuronal excitability. As a result, zopiclone has sedative effects as well as hypnotic, anxiolytic, anticonvulsant, and muscle-relaxant effects. The onset of action is faster than that of most benzodiazepines. It is important to inform patients taking nonbenzodiazepine hypnotic drugs about the quick onset and advise them to take the drug only when they are ready to go to sleep.

Zopiclone reaches peak plasma concentration within 2 hours and has a short half-life (the amount of time it takes the body to eliminate half of the drug). Zopiclone also has the unique adverse effect of an unpleasant bitter taste upon awakening. Severe drowsiness or impaired coordination are signs of drug intolerance or excessive doses. Because of the potential for misuse, zopiclone should not be taken for more than 7 to 10 consecutive days and should be used with caution in those who misuse alcohol and other substances. All of the benzodiazepines are categorized as schedule IV to the *Controlled Drugs and Substances Act (CDSA)* and to the Benzodiazepines and Other Targeted Substances Regulations and require a prescription for use. Zopiclone is on the Prescription Drug List under the *Food and Drugs Act*, meaning that a prescription is required for its use.

Buspirone

Buspirone (Bustab) is an anxiolytic drug that is useful for bringing about the short-term relief of excessive anxiety without producing strong sedative–hypnotic effects. Because this drug does not leave the patient sleepy or sluggish, it is often much better tolerated than the benzodiazepines. It is not a CNS depressant, and so the danger of it interacting with other CNS depressants such as alcohol is minimal. Also, there is not the potential for dependence that exists with benzodiazepines.

Although, at present, the mechanism of action of buspirone is not clearly understood, one possibility is illustrated in Figure 11-12. Buspirone is a partial agonist (a drug that is unable to fully activate a receptor) at 5-HT$_{1A}$ receptors. These receptors are known to modulate the release of a number of neurotransmitters, including serotonin and dopamine. Buspirone may also enhance dopamine release from nerve endings via its action as an antagonist at presynaptic dopamine D$_2$ autoreceptors.

Refer to Chapter 12 for a discussion of adverse reactions, dosages, nursing implications, and patient and family teaching related to the drugs used to treat anxiety and related disorders.

Treating Anxiety Disorders With Antidepressant Drugs

The symptoms, neurotransmitters, and circuits associated with anxiety disorders overlap extensively with those of depressive disorders (see Chapter 13), and many drugs used to treat depression have proven to be effective treatments for anxiety disorders (Curtis, Andrews, Davis, et al., 2017). **Selective serotonin**

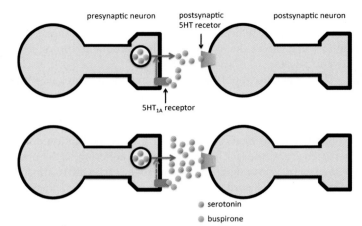

FIGURE 11-12 Proposed mechanism of action of buspirone. *Top,* In a normal state, excessive serotonin release is prevented when serotonin binds to the presynaptic 5-HT$_{1A}$ autoreceptors. The inhibitory effect of these autoreceptors on release is indicated by the red arrow. *Bottom,* Feedback inhibition by serotonin is blocked when buspirone binds and occupies 5-HT$_{1A}$ receptors, leading to a loss of inhibition on serotonin release from the presynaptic cell as indicated by the dashed red line. This leads to an increase in serotonin levels in the synaptic cleft.

reuptake inhibitors (SSRIs), medications that preferentially act to increase serotonin levels in the synapse, are often used to treat obsessive-compulsive disorder (OCD), social anxiety disorder (SAD), generalized anxiety disorder (GAD), panic disorder (PD), and post-traumatic stress disorder (PTSD). The **serotonin–norepinephrine reuptake inhibitor (SNRI)** venlafaxine (Effexor XR) is used to treat GAD, SAD, and PD. Duloxetine (Cymbalta), another SNRI, is approved for GAD.

Drug Treatment for Depression

Understanding of the neurophysiological basis of depression is far from complete. However, some theories have been proposed to explain why this disease occurs. The monoamine theory of depression suggests that depression occurs as a result of a deficit in the monoamine neurotransmitters serotonin (sometimes called 5-hydroxytryptamine and abbreviated as 5-HT) and norepinephrine. This theory arose from the findings that drugs used to treat various disease states that had the adverse effect of altering monoamine levels also affected mood. Further investigation revealed that by deliberately decreasing monoamine neurotransmitter levels, mood could be depressed, with the opposite effect occurring when monoamine levels were deliberately elevated. Thus arose the idea that depressed mood is tied to deficits in monoamine neurotransmitter signalling. These findings ultimately led to the development of various types of drugs whose mode of action was to elevate serotonin or norepinephrine in the brain through a number of different mechanisms. Figure 11-13 identifies the effects these drugs produce via interactions with a variety of drug targets that are responsible for both therapeutic and nontherapeutic effects. Figure 11-14 illustrates the processes of normal release, reuptake, and degradation of the monoamine neurotransmitters. A grasp of this underlying physiology is essential for understanding the mechanisms by which the antidepressant drugs are thought to act.

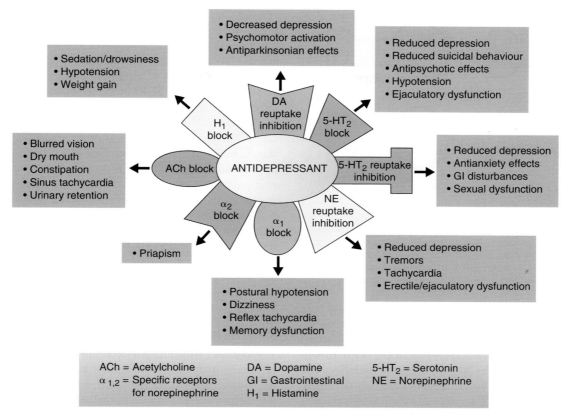

FIGURE 11-13 Potential receptor interactions of drugs used to treat depression. Note that the therapeutic targets of these drugs (e.g., 5-HT$_2$ receptors and 5-HT transporters) may be involved in both wanted and unwanted effects of these drugs. This diagram reflects all possible interactions and resulting side effects; most drugs will manifest only a limited number of these.

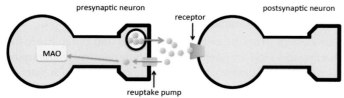

FIGURE 11-14 The cycle of release, reuptake, and degradation of the monoamine neurotransmitters. Neurotransmitter release occurs when vesicles containing neurotransmitter fuse with the membrane of the nerve ending. The neurotransmitter is released into the synaptic cleft where it can bind to postsynaptic receptors. To terminate this process, the monoamine is removed from the synaptic cleft by a reuptake protein. The neurotransmitter can then be degraded by monoamine oxidase (MAO).

Tricyclic Antidepressants

Tricyclic and heterocyclic antidepressants were widely used prior to the development of SSRIs. TCAs are no longer considered first-line treatment for depression since they have more adverse effects, take longer to reach an optimal dose, and have a greater potential for lethality when taken in overdose situations. They have more recently found a place in the treatment of neuropathic pain. The tricyclic antidepressants (TCAs) are thought to act primarily by blocking the reuptake of serotonin and norepinephrine.

TCAs that contain a secondary amine in their structure (e.g., nortriptyline [Aventyl, Norventyl]) primarily block the reuptake of norepinephrine, whereas those that possess a tertiary amine in their structure (e.g., amitriptyline [Elavil, Levate], imipramine [Impril]) can block the reuptake of both norepinephrine and serotonin. As shown in Figure 11-15, this block of reuptake processes results in the accumulation of neurotransmitter in the synapse.

Many of the tricyclic drugs produce adverse effects by acting as antagonists at muscarinic acetylcholine receptors. Acetylcholine, as mentioned, is the neurotransmitter released by postganglionic neurons of the parasympathetic nervous system. Through its binding to muscarinic acetylcholine receptors on internal organs, it serves to help regulate many important physiological functions. Antagonism of muscarinic receptors by tricyclic drugs as well as a wide variety of other psychotropic drugs, can lead to a constellation of untoward effects, which are predictable based on knowledge of which physiological systems are regulated by the parasympathetic nervous system. These adverse effects usually involve blurred vision, dry mouth, constipation, and urinary hesitancy. Because of the central role of acetylcholine in memory and cognition, these drugs can also result in deficits in these processes. These adverse effects can be troubling to patients and may limit their adherence to the regimen.

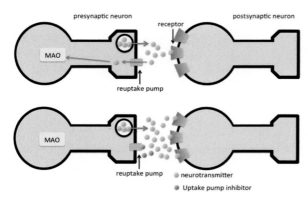

FIGURE 11-15 Drugs that block the reuptake process increase neurotransmitter levels in the synaptic cleft. *Top,* In the undrugged state, neurotransmitter is removed from the synaptic cleft by reuptake proteins into the presynaptic terminal, where it can then be degraded by monoamine oxidase (MAO). *Bottom,* In the presence of an uptake inhibitor, this process is interrupted and the neurotransmitter can no longer be removed, thus leading to greater availability in the synaptic cleft.

Depending on the individual drug, these drugs can also act as antagonists at histamine (H_1) receptors in the brain. Antagonism of these receptors by any drug causes sedation and drowsiness, an unwelcome adverse effect in daily use (see Figure 11-13). People taking the TCAs often have compliance issues because of these issues. TCA overdose can be fatal, secondary to cardiac conduction disturbances from excessive sodium channel and calcium channel blockade.

Selective Serotonin Reuptake Inhibitors

The selective serotonin reuptake inhibitors (SSRIs) were introduced in hopes of providing a useful tool in the treatment of depression that would display fewer adverse effects than the TCAs. As the name implies, SSRIs such as fluoxetine (Prozac), paroxetine (Paxil), citalopram (Celexa), escitalopram (Cipralex), and fluvoxamine (Luvox) preferentially block the reuptake of serotonin from the synaptic cleft. Sertraline (Zoloft) inhibits the neuronal reuptake of serotonin but to a lesser degree also inhibits norepinephrine and dopamine neuronal reuptake. SSRIs bind more poorly to acetylcholine muscarinic and H_1 receptors than the TCAs and so tend to have fewer adverse effects in comparison. They seem to show comparable efficacy in treating depression without the anticholinergic and sedating adverse effects that limit patient adherence to other drug regimens. However, SSRIs have other adverse effects: inappropriate stimulation of various serotonin receptors due to increased serotonin levels may lead to insomnia, low libido and failure of orgasm, and nausea or vomiting (Rang, Ritter, Flower, et al., 2016). See Figure 11-13. While much less likely to cause cardiotoxicity in comparison to TCAs in overdose situations, SSRIs in high doses can cause ventricular arrhythmias that can lead to death.

Serotonin–Norepinephrine Reuptake Inhibitors

Serotonin–norepinephrine reuptake inhibitors (SNRIs) are medications that increase both serotonin and norepinephrine levels in the brain. Venlafaxine (Effexor XR) and desvenlafaxine (Pristiq) are effective inhibitors of neuronal serotonin and norepinephrine reuptake and weak inhibitors of dopamine reuptake. Thus these neurotransmitters will accumulate in the synapse. Venlafaxine has the dual mechanism of working as an SSRI at lower doses (75 mg/day), affecting the reuptake of serotonin, and as an SNRI at higher doses (150–225 mg/day), affecting the reuptake of both serotonin and norepinephrine.

Duloxetine (Cymbalta) affects norepinephrine and serotonin reuptake equally. Thus it has a greater noradrenergic effect than does venlafaxine at lower doses. This SNRI is indicated for acute and maintenance treatment of major depressive disorder, for acute treatment of generalized anxiety disorder, for managing fibromyalgia, and for managing neuropathic pain associated with diabetic peripheral neuropathy. In fact, many SNRIs, as with the TCAs, have therapeutic effects on neuropathic pain. The common underlying mechanism of *neuropathic pain* is nerve injury or dysfunction. The mechanism by which TCAs and SNRIs reduce neuropathic pain is through activation of the descending norepinephrine and serotonin pathways to the spinal cord, thereby limiting pain signals ascending to the brain.

Serotonin Modulator and Stimulator

Vortioxetine (Trintellix) is a serotonin modulator and stimulator. It affects many different serotonin receptors by inhibiting serotonin reuptake like the SSRIs, activating 5-HT_{1A} receptors like buspirone, acting as a partial agonist at 5-HT_{1B} receptor, and blocking 5-HT_3, 5-HT_{1D}, and 5-HT_7 receptors. Geriatric patients may experience an improvement of cognitive deficits independent of its antidepressant properties. Common adverse effects include constipation, nausea, and vomiting. More serious side effects are hyponatremia and, rarely, induction of hypomania or mania.

Serotonin and Norepinephrine Disinhibitors

The class of drugs described as serotonin and norepinephrine disinhibitors (SNDIs) is represented by only one drug, mirtazapine (Remeron). This unique drug increases norepinephrine, dopamine, and serotonin transmission by acting as an antagonist at central presynaptic α_2-adrenergic receptors. The normal function of these receptors is to inhibit neurotransmitter release when norepinephrine binds to them. Thus any drug that prevents noradrenaline from binding to these receptors will potentiate neurotransmitter release. This is why this drug is called a disinhibitor. Mirtazapine tends to have a more rapid onset of effect than do single neurotransmitter antidepressant drugs, and this may be because it can simultaneously affect several neurotransmitter systems. Mirtazapine is a potent antagonist of 5-HT_{2C} receptors, which may account for its antianxiety and antidepressant effects, as these receptors, when activated by serotonin, typically inhibit norepinephrine and dopamine release. In addition, this drug acts as an antagonist at 5-HT_{2A} and 5-HT_3 receptors, activation of which are thought to mediate sexual dysfunction and nausea. Thus these effects are less likely to occur, and this is an advantage compared to other drugs used in depression. Mirtazapine is also a potent H_1-receptor antagonist, which accounts for drowsiness and increased appetite resulting in weight gain being the most common adverse effects. Patients may also experience orthostatic hypotension and the occasional occurrence of anticholinergic adverse effects. When discontinuing use of any antidepressant drug, but particularly SSRIs or SNRIs, patients should be weaned gradually over several weeks rather than abruptly due to the risk of discontinuation symptoms such as dizziness, agitation, anxiety, sleeping difficulties, nausea, excessive sweating, and fatigue. These symptoms do not indicate that an addiction has developed. Most people taking antidepressant drugs never develop a "craving" or feel the need to increase the dose. What these symptoms do indicate is that the brain has adapted to drug-induced changes in neurotransmitter levels. These symptoms typically resolve within 4 to 6 weeks after discontinuation of the drug. However, if the symptoms persist beyond this time frame, there is the potential that depression is still present and that the drugs are still needed.

Monoamine Oxidase Inhibitors

Monoamine oxidase inhibitors (MAOIs) are a group of drugs used to treat depression that prevent the destruction of monoamines by inhibiting the action of monoamine oxidase. MAOIs illustrate the principle that drugs can have a desired and beneficial effect in the brain, while at the same time having possibly dangerous effects elsewhere in the body. To understand the action of these drugs, keep in mind the following definitions:

- *Monoamines* are a type of organic compound and include the neurotransmitters norepinephrine, epinephrine, dopamine, and serotonin, as well as many different food substances and drugs.
- *Monoamine oxidase (MAO)* is an enzyme that degrades monoamines and is located in the nerve endings that release dopamine, serotonin, and noradrenaline.
- *Monoamine oxidase inhibitors (MAOIs)* inhibit the action of MAO and thereby prevent the degradation of monoamines.

The monoamine neurotransmitters, as well as any monoamine food substance or drug, are destroyed by the enzyme MAO, which is located in neurons and in the liver. Antidepressant drugs such as phenelzine (Nardil), tranylcypromine (Parnate), and selegiline (Anipryl) are MAOIs that act by inhibiting the enzyme and interfering with the degradation of the monoamine neurotransmitters. This action, in turn, increases the presynaptic availability of the neurotransmitters, which leads to the neurotransmitter leaking out of the nerve endings and into the synaptic cleft. This is the mechanism by which synaptic levels of neurotransmitters are increased and by which the antidepressant effects of these drugs are thought to occur (Figure 11-16).

The use of MAO-inhibiting drugs is complicated by the fact that MAO is also present in the liver and is responsible for destroying monoamines that enter the body via food or drugs. Of particular importance is the monoamine tyramine, which is present in many food substances, such as aged cheeses, pickled or smoked fish, chocolate, many types of beans, and beer and wine. Tyramine, which is normally metabolized by liver and gut MAO and so never reaches a concentration in the blood high enough to cause any issues, poses a threat of hypertensive crisis when MAO is inhibited. The displacement of norepinephrine from neuronal storage vesicles by elevated tyramine levels and the resulting increase in norepinephrine availability is thought

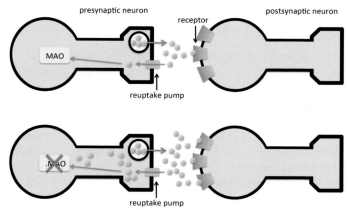

FIGURE 11-16 Monoamine oxidase inhibitors (MAOIs) prevent the breakdown of monoamines and increase the availability of neurotransmitter in the presynaptic nerve terminal. This increased availability leads to an increase in neurotransmitter concentrations in the synaptic cleft.

to cause an increase in blood pressure (pressor response). In severe cases, a hypertensive crisis can occur.

A substantial number of drugs are chemically monoamines. The dosages of these drugs are determined by the rate at which they are metabolized by MAO in the liver. In a patient taking MAOIs, the blood level of monoamine drugs can reach high levels and cause serious toxicity. Therefore MAOIs are contraindicated with concurrent use of any other antidepressant or sympathomimetic drugs (those that affect the sympathetic nervous system). Concurrent use with some over-the-counter products with sympathomimetic properties (e.g., oral decongestants) should also be avoided.

Because of the serious dangers that result from inhibition of hepatic MAO, patients taking MAOIs *must* be given a list of foods high in tyramine and drugs that must be avoided. Chapter 13 contains a list of these foods, along with nursing measures and instructions for patient teaching.

Other Drugs Used to Treat Depression

Bupropion is effective both as a treatment for depression and as a smoking cessation aid. It seems to act as a dopamine–norepinephrine reuptake inhibitor and also as an antagonist at nicotinic acetylcholine receptors. Since bupropion has no serotonergic action, it does not cause sexual dysfunction. Adverse effects include insomnia, tremor, anorexia, and weight loss. Bupropion is contraindicated in patients with a seizure disorder, in patients with a current or prior diagnosis of bulimia or anorexia nervosa, and in patients undergoing abrupt discontinuation of alcohol or sedatives (including benzodiazepines), owing to the increased seizure risk.

Trazodone (Oleptro, Trazodone, Trazorel) is a serotonin antagonist and reuptake inhibitor (SARI) and is not a first choice for treatment of depression. Its antidepressant effects are seen only at high therapeutic doses. An adverse effect of trazadone is sedation, which arises from its ability to act as a potent H_1-receptor antagonist. However, this can prove to be useful in those patients who suffer from insomnia. Another common adverse effect is orthostatic hypotension due to α_1-adrenergic receptor antagonism. Its potent blockade of these receptors can lead to rare cases of priapism (painful, prolonged penile erection).

Is the Monoamine Theory of Depression Still Valid?

The monoamine theory of depression served as a useful lens through which to view the underlying pathology leading to depression. Indeed, it resulted in many clinically useful drugs whose main mechanism of action was to elevate monoamine neurotransmitter release in brain tissue being brought to market. However, physicians noted an interesting phenomenon in patients prescribed these drugs. There was a delay of several weeks before the patients experienced a relief in symptoms. Drugs such as the SSRIs will block serotonin reuptake almost immediately after entering the brain, so why the delay in clinical response? This question led scientists to explore the idea that mechanisms occurring after the initial drug effect or separate from the proposed mechanism of the drug were bringing about their clinical efficacy. A reinvestigation of these drugs revealed that their therapeutic benefit may be a result of their ability to increase levels of brain-derived neurotrophic factor (BDNF), a peptide that is essential for the survival and growth of neurons (Castren & Kojima, 2017). The concentration of this peptide is low in people with depression and increases in those who receive antidepressant drug therapy. The time scale of this effect fits better with the alleviation of depressive symptoms due to antidepressant drug treatment. In addition, BDNF supports the growth of new neurons in the hippocampus. A number of lines of evidence suggest that depressed people have lower levels of hippocampal neurogenesis compared to nondepressed people (Wilner, Scheel-Kruger, & Belzung, 2013). In addition, animal models have revealed that antidepressant drugs can promote neurogenesis and lessen behaviours associated with depression (Castren & Kojima, 2017).

Another explanation for the delay in symptom relief is that clinical efficacy is not due to the initial increase in monoamine levels that most of these drugs provide, but rather due to this effect bringing about a loss of neurotransmitter receptor responsiveness over time, a process called receptor desensitization (Rang, Ritter, Flower, et al., 2016). For example 5-HT$_{1A}$ receptors can act as presynaptic autoreceptors to inhibit serotonin release. Therefore, once desensitized by high levels of serotonin, there will be less inhibitory action on further serotonin release, and the overall levels of this neurotransmitter will increase. Again, the timeline of this type of effect correlates better with the onset of clinical relief brought about by these drugs.

Suicide Risk and Antidepressant Drugs

There is concern that antidepressant drug use results in an increased risk of suicide. Since first reported, many studies have investigated this relationship. The results of these studies have often been contradictory or inconclusive and have been difficult to reconcile with one another. This is partly because these events are rare and also because of inconsistency in how these events are reported. However, the evidence thus far suggests that suicide risk in adults is likely not increased, and the data are most consistent in showing an increased risk in children and adolescents (Brent, 2016; Sharma, Guski, Freund, et al., 2016),

although even this relationship has been questioned (Dubicka, Cole-King, Reynolds, et al., 2016; Garland, Kutcher, Virani, et al., 2016). Health Canada requires a warning on drug labels for users of all ages but specifically for SSRIs and SNRIs. In addition, a warning about being aware of potentially dangerous changes in behaviour must be included in drug information sheets and labels.

Drug Treatment for Bipolar Disorders
Lithium Carbonate

Although the efficacy of lithium carbonate (Carbolith, Lithane, Lithmax) as a "mood stabilizer" in patients with bipolar disorders has been established for many years ("Lithium is still …," 2010), its mechanism of action is still far from understood. While it was originally believed to exert its clinical effects via a nonspecific disruption of neurotransmission, recent evidence suggests that it may be enhancing neuroprotective pathways and decreasing neuronal injury and death (Forlenza, De-Paula, & Diniz, 2014). One target that may play a key role in mediating the effects of lithium is glycogen synthase kinase 3ß (GSK3ß). This enzyme can affect a number of neuroprotective pathways, and its inhibition by lithium appears to trigger those that bring about a clinical response. In addition, lithium appears to increase levels of BDNF, which is thought to be neuroprotective. Another target affected by lithium is inositol monophosphatase 1, an enzyme involved in the phosphatidylinositol second messenger pathway. Lithium has been shown to inhibit inositol monophosphatase activity, resulting in a disruption of the entire signalling pathway. This is thought to lead to less intracellular signalling from receptor activation and to lessen the risk of neuronal cell death by improving mitochondrial health. Lastly, there is evidence that lithium decreases excitatory neurotransmission by decreasing glutamate release and acting as an antagonist at certain glutamate receptors. Excessive glutamate release can lead to neuronal injury and death, and so these effects are thought to prevent neuronal harm that may arise from excessive glutamatergic activity (Malhi & Outhred, 2016).

While it is not known exactly how lithium works, many of its adverse effects are thought to arise from the fact that it mimics the role of sodium in neurons and thus alters the electrical properties of neuronal membranes. By altering electrical conductivity, lithium represents a potential threat to all body functions regulated by electrical currents. Foremost among these functions is cardiac contraction; lithium can induce, although not commonly, sinus bradycardia. Overdose causes extreme alteration of cerebral conductivity, which can lead to convulsions. Changes in nerve and muscle conduction can commonly lead to tremor at therapeutic doses or to more extreme motor dysfunction with overdose.

Lithium commonly induces polyuria (the output of large volumes of urine) as a consequence of decreasing the effectiveness of vasopressin on renal function. Long-term use of lithium can result in thyroid gland enlargement (goiter) and, possibly, hypothyroidism in some patients. In addition, hyponatremia can increase the risk of lithium toxicity because increased kidney reabsorption of sodium leads to increased reabsorption of lithium as well.

TABLE 11-3	ADVERSE AND TOXIC EFFECTS OF LITHIUM
SYSTEM	**ADVERSE AND TOXIC EFFECTS**
Nervous and muscular	Tremor, ataxia, confusion, convulsions
Digestive	Nausea, vomiting, diarrhea
Cardiac	Arrhythmias
Fluid and electrolyte	Polyuria, polydipsia, edema
Endocrine	Goiter and hypothyroidism

Primarily because of its effects on electrical conductivity, lithium has a low therapeutic index. The therapeutic index is a measure of overall drug safety with respect to the risk for overdose or toxicity. It can be expressed as the ratio between the median lethal dose and the median effective dose. A low therapeutic index means that the dose of the drug that can cause death is not that much greater than the dose required for therapeutic effectiveness. This risk mandates that the blood level of lithium be monitored on a regular basis to ensure that the drug is not accumulating and rising to dangerous levels. See Table 11-3 for a list of some of the adverse and toxic effects of lithium. Chapter 14 contains a more in-depth discussion of lithium carbonate treatment and specific dose-related adverse and toxic effects, nursing implications, and the patient teaching plan.

Other Drugs Used to Treat Bipolar Disorders

While lithium has played a central role in the pharmacological management of bipolar depression for many years, drugs that were once used primarily to treat seizure disorders have also emerged as useful therapeutic agents (Corrado & Walsh, 2016). These drugs work through several different mechanisms but all share the common property of decreasing neuronal excitability. The major modes of action for these drugs include (1) inhibition of sodium channel activity, (2) inhibition of calcium channel activity, (3) enhancement of GABAergic neurotransmission pathways, and (4) inhibition of glutamatergic neurotransmission pathways. Although some drugs work almost exclusively via a single one of these mechanisms, a number of the drugs in this group work through a combination of these effects. Three drugs used in the treatment of seizure disorders, valproate, carbamazepine, and lamotrigine, have displayed efficacy in the treatment of bipolar disorder and, in the context of this disease, are considered to be mood stabilizers. It is thought that their ability to re-establish a balance between excitatory and inhibitory neuronal pathways has a stabilizing effect on mood. More recent evidence suggests that, much like lithium, these drugs that are efficacious in treating bipolar disorders are also able to inhibit GSK3B activity.

Carbamazepine

The primary mechanism of action of carbamazepine is to inhibit neuronal sodium channels during depolarization events, hence reducing neuronal excitability. Interestingly, this blocking action is greater in neurons that fire frequently and repetitively, and so the drug is effective at reducing inappropriate excitability. Because of this mechanistic characteristic, carbamazepine does not have as strong of an effect on neurons that are behaving normally and is therefore less likely to affect normal neuronal function. Common adverse effects include anticholinergic effects (e.g., dry mouth, constipation, urinary retention, blurred vision), orthostatic hypotension, sedation, and ataxia. Rash may occur in 10% of patients (Sadock, Sadock, & Ruiz, 2015). Recommended baseline laboratory work includes liver function tests, complete blood count (CBC), electrocardiogram, and electrolyte levels. Blood levels are monitored to avoid toxicity, but there are no established therapeutic blood levels for carbamazepine in the treatment of bipolar disorder.

Valproate

As with carbamazepine, valproate also displays efficacy in treating bipolar disorders. Valproate works through a number of the mechanisms listed above. It blocks both sodium and calcium channels and may elevate GABA levels by inhibiting the enzyme that normally degrades this neurotransmitter. Common adverse effects include tremor, weight gain, and sedation. More rarely occurring but serious adverse effects include thrombocytopenia, pancreatitis, and hepatic failure. In addition, this drug has been demonstrated to be a potent teratogen. Because of its potential to cause hepatotoxicity, baseline levels are established for liver function indicators and a CBC is obtained before an individual is started on this medication. These measurements are then repeated periodically. In addition, the level of the drug in the blood is monitored to ensure that it stays within the recommended therapeutic range.

Lamotrigine

Lamotrigine (Lamictal) is perhaps the most effective drug for maintenance therapy of bipolar disorder, but it is not as effective in acute mania (Preston, O'Neal, & Talaga, 2013). Lamotrigine is best known for its ability to treat the depressive phase of bipolar disorder, with less risk of causing a switch into mania when compared to antidepressant drugs (Prabhavalkar, Poovanpallil & Bhatt, 2015). It inhibits neuronal sodium and calcium channels and modulates the release of the excitatory neurotransmitters glutamate and aspartate. Patients should promptly report any rashes, which could be a sign of life-threatening Stevens–Johnson syndrome. This risk can be minimized by slow titration to therapeutic doses.

Other Antiseizure Drugs

Because these drugs work by inhibiting neuronal excitability, they have found a home in the treatment of other disorders. Along with their use with bipolar disorders (as discussed above), some of these drugs show efficacy in treating neuropathic pain, anxiety, and migraines.

Other antiseizure drugs used as mood stabilizers are gabapentin (Neurontin), topiramate (Topamax), and oxcarbazepine (Trileptal). None of them have Health Canada approval as mood stabilizers, and studies have not provided strong support for their use as primary treatments for bipolar disorders. However, they are used for their calming effects during mania. Chapter 14 offers a more detailed discussion of these medications.

Drugs Used To Treat Psychosis

First-Generation (Conventional) Antipsychotic Drugs

First-generation antipsychotic drugs, introduced into clinical practice in the 1950s and also referred to as conventional or typical antipsychotic drugs, are antagonists or weak partial agonists at the D_2 type of dopamine receptors. By binding to these receptors and therefore preventing dopamine from doing so, these drugs reduce dopaminergic neurotransmission. It has been postulated that an overactivity of the dopamine system in certain areas of the mesolimbic system may be responsible for at least some of the symptoms of schizophrenia; thus antagonism of certain dopamine receptors should reduce these symptoms—particularly the "positive" symptoms of schizophrenia, such as delusions (e.g., paranoid and grandiose ideas) and hallucinations (e.g., hearing or seeing things not present in reality). While these drugs are relatively selective for certain types of dopamine receptors, as with many therapeutic agents, they can interact with other receptors such as those for acetylcholine, α_1-adrenergic receptors to which norepinephrine binds, and H_1 receptors. It is not clear if any of these interactions leads to a clinical benefit, but many of the adverse effects associated with the use of first-generation antipsychotic drugs come from these interactions. See Chapter 15 for a more detailed discussion of schizophrenia and its symptoms.

The proposed mechanism of action of the first generation of antipsychotic drugs—which includes the phenothiazines (e.g., chlorpromazine), thioxanthenes (e.g., thiothixene), butyrophenones (e.g., haloperidol), and pharmacologically related drugs—is illustrated in Figure 11-17. As summarized in Figure 11-18, many of the untoward adverse effects of these drugs can be understood as a logical extension of their receptor antagonism profile, which varies from drug to drug. Because dopamine in the basal ganglia plays a major role in the regulation of movement, it is not surprising that inhibition of dopamine signalling through its receptors can lead to acute drug-induced motor abnormalities (extrapyramidal side effects [EPS]) such as parkinsonism, akinesia, akathisia, dyskinesia, and delayed EPS (tardive dyskinesia). The extent of the EPS varies between drugs. While chlorpromazine and haloperidol are equally effective in treating the symptoms of psychosis, haloperidol is associated with a greater risk of developing acute EPS. Risks of tardive dyskinesia are the same for all first-generation drugs. Normally there is a balance between dopamine and acetylcholine signalling in the striatum. Dopamine antagonists upset this balance and allow acetylcholine signalling to predominate, thus leading to EPS. With this in mind, muscarinic acetylcholine receptor antagonists, such as benztropine, are often prescribed to prevent or treat these antipsychotic drug–induced extrapyramidal symptoms. Nurses and physicians often monitor patients for evidence of involuntary movements after administration of the first-generation antipsychotic drugs. One commonly used scale is the Abnormal Involuntary Movement Scale (AIMS). See Chapter 15 for an example of AIMS and a discussion of the clinical use of antipsychotic drugs, adverse effects, specific nursing interventions, and patient teaching strategies.

An important physiological function of dopamine is to act as the hypothalamic factor that inhibits the release of prolactin from the anterior pituitary gland. A blockade of dopaminergic neurotransmission can lead to increased pituitary secretion of prolactin. In women, this drug-induced hyperprolactinemia can result in amenorrhea (absence of the menses) or galactorrhea (breast milk flow); in men, it can lead to gynecomastia (development of the male mammary glands).

Many of first-generation drugs act as antagonists at muscarinic receptors that are normally activated by acetylcholine. This leads to typical anticholinergic effects such as blurred vision, dry mouth, tachycardia, urinary retention, and constipation.

In addition to blocking dopamine and muscarinic receptors, many first-generation antipsychotic drugs act as antagonists at α_1-adrenergic receptors. These receptors are found on smooth muscle cells that contract in response to norepinephrine released from sympathetic nervous system neurons. In blood vessels, for example, antagonism of these receptors can bring about vasodilation and a consequent drop in blood pressure and provoke orthostatic hypotension.

α_1-Adrenergic receptors are also found on the vas deferens and are responsible for the propulsive contractions leading to ejaculation. Antagonism of these receptors can lead to a failure to ejaculate. Finally, many of these first-generation antipsychotic drugs, as well as a variety of other psychiatric drugs, block the histamine H_1 receptors. The two most significant adverse effects of blocking these receptors are sedation and substantial weight gain. The sedation may be beneficial in severely agitated patients.

It is believed that patient compliance is negatively affected due to the numerous and sometimes severe adverse effects of the first-generation drugs used in the treatment of psychosis. A quest for efficacious drugs to treat psychosis with fewer adverse effects led to the development of the second generation of antipsychotic drugs.

Second-Generation Antipsychotic Drugs

Introduced in the 1990s, second-generation antipsychotic drugs (or *atypicals*) used to treat psychosis target both the positive and possibly the negative symptoms of schizophrenia (see Chapter 15) and may produce fewer extrapyramidal side effects. They are thought to differ from the first generation of drugs because of a difference in their pharmacological profile. While, like the first-generation drugs, they act as dopamine D_2 receptor antagonists, they also act as antagonists at a type of serotonin receptor

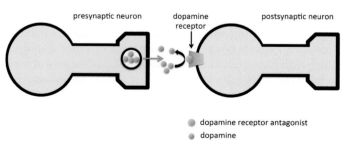

FIGURE 11-17 The first generation of drugs to show efficacy in treating psychosis work, at least in part, by acting as antagonists at dopamine D_2 receptors. These drugs bind to the receptors but do not activate them. Rather, they prevent dopamine from binding to and activating these receptors.

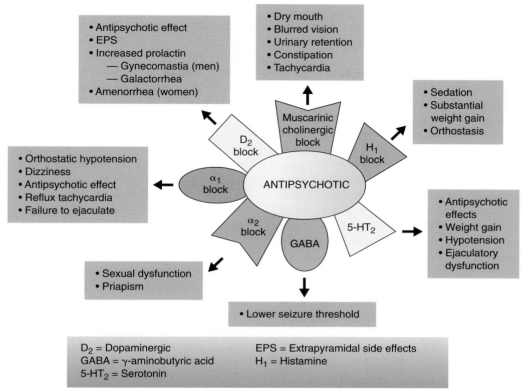

FIGURE 11-18 Potential receptor interactions of the second-generation drugs used in the treatment of psychosis. Note that drug interaction with the D_2 and 5-HT_2 receptors is necessary for symptomatic relief, but it can also result in unpleasant or dangerous side effects. While these drugs are relatively selective for D_2 and 5-HT_2 receptors, they still interact with a number of other receptors. These nonselective interactions are often the source of additional side effects. Also note that use of most of these drugs will result in only a limited number of the potential side effects illustrated here. Sources: Lehne, R. A. (2001). *Pharmacology for nursing care* (4th ed.). Philadelphia: Saunders; Varcarolis, E. (2002). *Foundations of psychiatric mental health nursing* (4th ed.). Philadelphia: WB Saunders; and Keltner, N. L., & Folks, D. G. (2001). *Psychotropic drugs* (3rd ed.). St. Louis: Mosby.

that can regulate neurotransmitter release. This interaction may alleviate the negative symptoms, as well as the cognitive and memory effects of schizophrenia. In addition, it is the antagonism of these receptors that is believed to result in fewer extrapyramidal side effects (Li, Snyder & Vanover, 2016). These newer drugs are often chosen as first-line treatment over the first generation of antipsychotic drugs because of a lower risk of EPS (Leucht, Corves, Arbter, et al., 2009).

However, several of the available second-generation drugs can increase the risk for a metabolic syndrome, resulting in increased weight, elevated blood glucose, and elevated levels of triglycerides. This is, again, due in part to the fact that while selective for their therapeutic targets, these drugs will still interact with other neurotransmitter receptors. The simultaneous blockade of muscarinic, 5-HT, and H_1 receptors is associated with weight gain due to increased appetite stimulation via the hypothalamic eating centres. Strong antimuscarinic properties on pancreatic beta cells may cause insulin resistance, leading to hyperglycemia. The mechanism leading to elevated triglycerides is currently unknown (Stahl, 2013). Clozapine and olanzapine use has a high risk of causing metabolic syndrome, whereas aripiprazole and ziprasidone use has a lower risk (De Hert, Detraux, van Winkel, et al., 2012).

Clozapine. Clozapine (Clozaril), the first of the second-generation drugs to be developed, is relatively free of extrapyramidal motor disturbances. It is thought that clozapine preferentially blocks the dopamine receptors in the mesolimbic system, rather than those in the nigrostriatal area. This pattern of selectivity allows clozapine to exert an antipsychotic action while minimizing EPS. In addition, clozapine is an antagonist at serotonin 5-HT_{2A} receptors. Although people who take clozapine are more likely to adhere to their medication regimen than those who are taking other antipsychotic drugs, it has the potential to suppress bone marrow and induce agranulocytosis. Because any deficiency in white blood cells renders a person prone to serious infection, regular measurement of white blood cell count is required. As a result of these risks, all patients taking clozapine must have cell counts weekly for the first 6 months, every other week for the next 6 months, and monthly thereafter. To ensure that these blood tests are completed, clozapine is dispensed at these same intervals. Due to the significant risk of agranulocytosis and seizure (in 5% of patients) associated with its use, clozapine should be limited to patients with treatment-resistant schizophrenia who are nonresponsive to, or intolerant of, other antipsychotic drugs.

Caution should be used when introducing other drugs that can increase the concentration of clozapine. There is also a potential for myocarditis that should be monitored, and for fever, but the most common adverse effects of clozapine are drowsiness and sedation, hypersalivation, reflex tachycardia, constipation, and dizziness and vertigo.

Risperidone. Risperidone (Risperdal) acts at D_2 receptors and is also a potent antagonist at $5\text{-}HT_{2A}$ receptors. This drug has a low potential for inducing agranulocytosis or convulsions. However, high therapeutic doses (greater than 6 mg/day) may lead to motor-related complications. It has the highest risk of EPS among the second-generation antipsychotic drugs and may increase prolactin release, which may lead to sexual dysfunction. Risperidone can cause orthostatic hypotension that can lead to falls, a serious problem among older adults. Weight gain, sedation, and sexual dysfunction are adverse effects that may affect adherence to the medication regimen and should be discussed with patients. It is notable that risperidone is the first of the second-generation antipsychotic drugs available as a long-acting depot injection. Risperdal Consta, administered every 2 weeks, provides an alternative to the depot injection of first-generation antipsychotic drugs. A rare but serious adverse effect is an increased risk of stroke and transient ischemic attacks in older adults with dementia who are being treated for agitation (Lee, Gill, Freedman, et al., 2004).

Quetiapine. Quetiapine (Seroquel) has a broad receptor-binding profile. Along with its ability to act as an antagonist at D_2 receptors, it is a potent antagonist of both $5\text{-}HT_{1A}$ and $5\text{-}HT_{2A}$ receptors. Its strong antagonism of H_1 receptors accounts for its ability to induce sedation. The combination of H_1 and serotonin receptor antagonism leads to the weight gain associated with use of this drug and also to a moderate risk for metabolic syndrome. Due to its antagonism of α_1-adrenergic receptors, it can cause orthostatic hypotension, dizziness, and syncope. Patients taking quetiapine have a low risk for EPS or prolactin elevation. Studies investigating how quetiapine interacts with D_2 receptors show that it dissociates rapidly and therefore does not occupy the binding site for dopamine for long periods of time. This characteristic is thought to be the reason why quetiapine tends to produce few EPS and prolactin-related adverse effects.

Other second-generation antipsychotic drugs.
- Olanzapine (Zyprexa) is similar to clozapine in chemical structure. Adverse effects include sedation, weight gain, hyperglycemia with new-onset type 2 diabetes, and higher risk for metabolic syndrome.
- Ziprasidone (Zeldox) binds to a variety of dopamine and 5-HT receptors and is also a serotonin–norepinephrine reuptake inhibitor. The main adverse effects are dizziness and moderate sedation. Ziprasidone is contraindicated in patients with a known history of QT interval prolongation, recent acute myocardial infarction, or uncompensated heart failure.
- Aripiprazole (Abilify) is a unique antipsychotic drug known as a *dopamine system stabilizer*. Its unique profile is thought to be due to the fact that, rather than acting as a D_2 antagonist, this drug is actually a partial agonist. This means that at low dopamine levels, the drug will partially activate D_2 receptors. However, at high levels, the drug will prevent excess dopamine from activating the receptor but still provide some degree of receptor activation itself. In this way, it tends to prevent extreme fluctuations in D_2 receptor activation that may occur with other drugs that are antagonists. It induces little sedation or weight gain. Adverse effects include insomnia and akathisia.
- Paliperidone (Invega) is the major active metabolite of risperidone. It has similar adverse effects to risperidone, such as EPS and prolactin elevation. Additional adverse effects are orthostasis and sedation. It is also available as a prolonged-release injectable suspension.
- Lurasidone (Latuda) has high affinity for $5\text{-}HT_{2A}$ and D_2 receptors in addition to other serotonergic receptors such as $5\text{-}HT_{1A}$. Lurasidone has similar pharmacological properties to the tetracyclic antidepressant mirtazapine. Lurasidone has high affinity for serotonergic (such as $5\text{-}HT_{2A}$ and $5\text{-}HT_{2C}$), noradrenergic, and dopaminergic receptors (D_3 and D_4). There is minimal muscarinic receptor antagonism.
- Asenapine (Saphris) is unique among antipsychotic drugs as being administered in a sublingual formulation. Thus it avoids much of the hepatic metabolism that restricts its availability when administered orally. Bioavailability of asenapine is reduced from 35% with sublingual administration to less than 2% with oral administration. Patients should avoid food and water for 10 minutes after sublingual administration (Zacher & Holmes, 2012). It has a higher affinity for $5\text{-}HT_{2A}$ receptors than D_2 receptors. It also has antagonistic activity at α_1-adrenergic receptors, which accounts for the orthostatic hypotension, and H_1 antagonistic activity, which causes sedation.

Traditionally, the drugs that are used to treat psychosis have been grouped together based on the order in which they were introduced into clinical practice (first or second generation) or by comparison of effects between groups (typical versus atypical). However, given the often overlapping range of pharmacological targets and adverse effect profiles of the members of these groups, the usefulness of such categorization is limited. Consideration of each drug on an individual basis would seem to be a more informative way of assessing the suitability of a drug (Leucht, Cipriani, Spineli, et al., 2013).

The antipsychotic drugs are discussed in detail in Chapter 15, including the indications for use, adverse effects, nursing implications, and patient and family teaching.

Drug Treatment for Attention-Deficit/Hyperactivity Disorder

Children and adults with attention-deficit/hyperactivity disorder (ADHD) show symptoms of short attention span, impulsivity, and overactivity. Paradoxically, the mainstay of treatment for this condition in children—and increasingly in adults—is the administration of psychostimulant drugs. Both methylphenidate (Biphentin, Concerta, Ritalin) and amphetamines such as amphetamine (Adderall XR) seem to show efficacy in treating these conditions. They block the reuptake of norepinephrine and dopamine into the presynaptic neuron and increase the concentration of these monoamines in the synaptic cleft. Thus they potentiate the signalling pathways of these neurotransmitters. How this translates into clinical efficacy is far from understood, but it is thought that the monoamines may inhibit an overactive part of the limbic system to prolong periods of concentration and focus on tasks.

Among many concerns with the use of these drugs are the adverse effects of agitation, exacerbation of psychotic thought processes, hypertension, and long-term growth suppression, as well as their potential for misuse and abuse. One medication that is not classified as a stimulant and is available for the treatment of ADHD is atomoxetine (Strattera), a selective norepinephrine reuptake inhibitor approved for use in children 6 years and older, adolescents, and adults. Common adverse effects include decreased appetite and weight loss, fatigue, and dizziness. Refer to Chapter 27 for more details on these drugs.

Drug Treatment for Alzheimer's Disease

The insidious and progressive loss of memory and other higher executive brain functions brought about by Alzheimer's disease is a tremendous individual, family, and social tragedy. Because the disease seems to involve progressive structural degeneration of the brain, there are two major pharmacological directions in its treatment. The first is to attempt to prevent or slow the structural degeneration. Although actively pursued, this approach has been unsuccessful so far. The second is to attempt to maintain normal brain function for as long as possible.

Much of the memory loss in this disease has been attributed to dysfunction of neurons that use acetylcholine as a neurotransmitter. The anticholinesterase drugs (also called *cholinesterase inhibitors*) show some efficacy in slowing the rate of memory loss and, in some patients, may even improve memory. The drugs work by interfering with the action of acetylcholinesterase, an enzyme that normally degrades acetylcholine. Inhibition of this enzyme leads to reduced breakdown of acetylcholine and therefore to a higher concentration in the synapse. Three of the four drugs approved for the treatment of mild to moderate Alzheimer's disease in Canada are acetylcholinesterase inhibitors: donepezil (Aricept), galantamine (Reminyl), and rivastigmine (Exelon). The fourth drug is memantine (Ebixa), an *N*-methyl-D-aspartate (NMDA) receptor antagonist. The glutamatergic neurotransmitter system plays an important role in memory formation. Amyloid plaques in the brain that form during the course of the disease can lead to glutamatergic dysfunction. When glutamate binds to NMDA receptors in a healthy brain, it opens calcium channels and calcium flows into the neurons. Excessive stimulation of these receptors by high concentrations of glutamate can lead to something called excitotoxicity. This is a phenomenon whereby too much calcium enters a neuron and may lead to neuronal damage and death. Memantine acts to prevent glutamate from binding to the NMDA receptor and activating the calcium channel. Memantine is used in treatment of moderate to severe Alzheimer's disease.

Refer to Chapter 17 for a more detailed discussion of these drugs, as well as their nursing considerations and patient and family teaching.

Natural Health Products

The growing interest in natural health products is driven by a variety of factors. Many people think that these products are safer either because they are "natural" or because they believe they have fewer adverse effects than conventional medications.

Natural health products, such as kava kava and St. John's wort, have been studied in clinical trials to determine safety and clinical efficacy (Sarris & Kavanagh, 2009). Some natural health products have been found to lack any therapeutic efficacy (Leach & Page, 2015), while others have been shown to potentially be deadly if taken over long periods of time or in combination with other chemical substances and prescription drugs (Brown, 2016; Gurley, Fifer, & Gardner, 2012). For example, the risk of bleeding may be increased in patients taking the natural product ginkgo biloba in combination with warfarin (a drug that inhibits blood clotting), and taking the natural product kava kava by itself may increase the risk of hepatotoxicity at doses over 240 mg/day.

Among the major concerns of health care providers are the potential long-term effects of some natural health products (nerve, kidney, and liver damage) and the possibility of adverse chemical reactions when natural health products are taken in conjunction with other substances, especially conventional medications (Gurley, Fifer, & Gardner, 2012).

St. John's wort can have serious interactions with a number of conventional medications (Hoffman, Howland, Lewin, et al., 2015). For example, St. John's wort when taken with other serotonergic drugs (e.g., SSRIs, triptans) can cause serotonin syndrome. This is a potentially life-threatening reaction that occurs when there is excessive 5-HT neurotransmission in the CNS. Symptoms include agitation, overactive reflexes (hyperreflexia), tremors, excessive sweating, racing heart, rapid changes in blood pressure, nausea, and loss of coordination (ataxia). St. John's wort may also reduce the effectiveness of other medications by increasing their rate of metabolism and reducing blood levels of these medications. This is because St. John's wort is a CYP3A4 enzyme inducer. The levels of any medications that are metabolized by CYP3A4 (e.g., hormonal contraceptives, human immunodeficiency virus [HIV] protease inhibitors, HIV non-nucleoside reverse transcriptase inhibitors, the immunosuppressant drugs cyclosporine and tacrolimus, the antineoplastic drugs irinotecan and imatinib) may drop to subtherapeutic levels, as their metabolism will be increased (Alpert, 2016). Drugs with a narrow therapeutic index should be monitored more closely when St. John's wort is added or discontinued or when its dosage is changed.

Another key concern regarding the use of natural health products is how they are regulated. Health Canada provides information on natural health products via the Licensed Natural Health Products Database. Any product authorized by Health Canada carries an eight-digit number. This means that it has been authorized for sale in Canada and meets the safety and efficacy guidelines of Health Canada (Health Canada, 2017a). Health care providers, especially nurses, need to stay current, using unbiased sources of product information and passing this information to patients who are contemplating using alternative remedies. Recalls and warnings to stop use of certain brands are available at MedEffect Canada (Health Canada, 2017b). It should be noted that there is often little to no substantive scientific evidence that natural health products are therapeutically effective. It is important that nurses and other health care providers explore the patient's use of natural health products in a nonjudgemental manner by asking, "What over-the-counter medications or natural health products do you take to help your symptoms? Do they help? How much are you taking? How long have you been taking them?" Individuals taking medications or other natural health products should be made aware of drug or substance interactions and product safety. Such discussion should be part of the initial and ongoing interviews with patients. Complementary and integrative therapies are covered in more detail in Chapter 35.

KEY POINTS TO REMEMBER

- All actions of the brain—sensory, motor, and intellectual—are carried out physiologically through the interactions of neurons. These interactions involve impulse conduction, neurotransmitter release, and receptor activation and response. Alterations in these basic processes can lead to mental disturbances and physical manifestations.
- In particular, it seems that overactivity of dopamine-related signalling pathways underlies the thought disturbances of schizophrenia, and that deficiencies in pathways involving norepinephrine, serotonin, or both underlie depression and anxiety. Insufficient GABA-related signalling may play a role in anxiety.
- Pharmacological treatment of mental health disturbances is directed at suspected neurotransmitter–receptor problems. Antipsychotic drugs ameliorate dopamine signalling;

antidepressant drugs alter neurotransmission by norepinephrine, serotonin, or both; and antianxiety drugs enhance the actions of GABA, 5-HT, norepinephrine, or all three.
- Because the immediate target activity of a drug can result in many downstream alterations in neuronal activity, drugs with a variety of chemical actions may show efficacy in treating the same clinical condition. Thus newer drugs with novel mechanisms of action are being used in the treatment of schizophrenia, depression, and anxiety.
- Unfortunately, drugs used to treat mental health disease can cause various undesired effects. Prominent among these can be sedation or excitement, motor disturbances, anticholinergic effects, α_1-adrenergic receptor antagonism, sexual dysfunction, and weight gain. There is a continuing effort to develop new drugs that are effective, safe, and well tolerated.

CRITICAL THINKING

1. No matter where you practise psychiatric mental health nursing, individuals under your care will be taking psychotropic drugs. Consider the importance of understanding normal brain structure and function as they relate to mental disturbances and psychotropic drugs by answering the following questions:
   a. How can you use the knowledge of normal brain function (control of peripheral nerves, skeletal muscles, the autonomic nervous system, hormones, and circadian rhythms) to better understand how a patient can be affected by psychotropic drugs or psychiatric illness?
   b. What information from the various brain imaging techniques can you use to understand and treat patients with mental disorders and to provide support to their families? How might you use that information for patient and family teaching?

2. Based on your understanding of symptoms that may occur when the following components of neurotransmission are altered, what specific information would you include in medication teaching?
   a. Dopamine D_2 (as with use of antipsychotic drugs)
   b. Muscarinic receptors (as with use of phenothiazines and other drugs)
   c. α_1-Adrenergic receptors (as with use of phenothiazines and other drugs)
   d. Histamine receptors (as with use of phenothiazines and other drugs)
   e. Monoamine oxidase (MAO) (as with use of a monoamine oxidase inhibitor [MAOI])
   f. Gamma-aminobutyric acid (GABA) (as with use of benzodiazepines)
   g. Serotonin (as with use of selective serotonin reuptake inhibitors [SSRIs] and other drugs)
   h. Norepinephrine (as with use of serotonin–norepinephrine reuptake inhibitors [SNRIs])

CHAPTER REVIEW

1. Which patient statement would the nurse attribute to a neurobiological basis of mental disease?
   a. "I like to eat all day long."
   b. "I sleep 7 hours nightly."
   c. "I have a number of close friends."
   d. "I enjoy solving word puzzles."

2. Which of the following medication orders would the nurse question?
   a. Buspirone hydrochloride—take in the morning
   b. Temazepam—take at bedtime
   c. Zopiclone—take early in the morning
   d. Flurazepam—take at bedtime

3. Which patient statement would require the nurse to provide further teaching?
   a. "I should report any unusual bleeding when I take gingko biloba."
   b. "I should not take St. John's wort with sertraline hydrochloride."
   c. "Natural health products are safe because they are made with all-natural ingredients."
   d. "I will tell my doctor that I am taking a natural health product."

4. The nurse is caring for a patient who is taking lithium. Which adverse effect would the nurse anticipate?
   a. Oliguria
   b. Confusion
   c. Constipation
   d. Hyperthyroidism

5. The nurse understands that norepinephrine is involved with the stimulation of which bodily process?
   a. The fight-or-flight response to stress
   b. The hypothalamus to release hormones
   c. Involvement in the inflammatory response
   d. The parasympathetic nervous system

⊖volve WEBSITE

Post-Test interactive review

Visit the Evolve website for Chapter Review Answers and Rationales, Critical Thinking Answer Guidelines, and additional resources related to the content in this chapter: http://evolve.elsevier.com/Canada/Varcarolis/psychiatric/

REFERENCES

Alpert, J. E. (2016). Drug–drug interactions in psychopharmacology. In T. A. Stern, J. F. Rosenbaum, M. Fava, et al. (Eds.), *Comprehensive clinical psychiatry* (pp. 552–566). Philadelphia: Elsevier.

Amstadter, A. B., Myers, J. M., & Kendler, K. S. (2014). Psychiatric resilience: Longitudinal twin study. *The British Journal of Psychiatry, 205*(4), 275–280.

Brent, D. A. (2016). Antidepressants and suicidality. *Psychiatric Clinics of North America, 39,* 503–512.

Brown, A. C. (2016). Liver toxicity related to herbs and dietary supplements: Online table of case reports: Part 3 of 6. *Food and Chemical Toxicology : An International Journal Published for the British Industrial Biological Research Association.* pii:S0278-6915(16)30221-6. doi:10.1016/j.fct.2016.07.001.

Castren, E., & Kojima, M. (2017). Brain-derived neurotrophic factor in mood disorders and antidepressant treatments. *Neurobiology of Disease, 97,* 119–126.

Corrado, A. C., & Walsh, J. P. (2016). Mechanisms underlying the benefits of anticonvulsants over lithium in the treatment of bipolar disorder. *Neuroreport, 27*(3), 131–135. doi:10.1097/WNR.0000000000000510.

Curtis, J., Andrews, L., Davis, M., et al. (2017). A meta-analysis of pharmacotherapy for social anxiety disorder: An examination of efficacy, moderators, and mediators. *Expert Opinion on Pharmacotherapy, 18,* 243–251.

De Hert, B., Detraux, J., van Winkel, R., et al. (2012). Metabolic and cardiovascular adverse effects associated with antipsychotic drugs. *Nature Reviews. Endocrinology, 8*(2), 114–126.

Dubicka, B., Cole-King, A., Reynolds, S., et al. (2016). Paper on suicidality and aggression during antidepressant treatment was flawed and the press release was misleading. *British Medical Journal, 352,* i911. doi:10.1136/bmj.i911.

Forlenza, O. V., De-Paula, V. J. R., & Diniz, B. S. O. (2014). Neuroprotective effects of lithium: Implications for the treatment of Alzheimer's disease and related neurodegenerative disorders. *ACS Chemical Neuroscience, 5*(6), 443–450. doi:10.1021/cn5000309.

Fu, C. H., & Costafreda, S. G. (2013). Neuroimaging-based biomarkers in psychiatry: Clinical opportunities of a paradigm shift. *Canadian Journal of Psychiatry, 58*(9), 499–508.

Garland, E. J., Kutcher, S., Virani, A., et al. (2016). Update on the use of SSRIs and SNRIs with children and adolescents in clinical practice. *Journal of the Canadian Academy of Child and Adolescent Psychiatry, 25*(1), 4–10.

Gurley, B. J., Fifer, E. K., & Gardner, Z. (2012). Pharmacokinetic herb-drug interactions (part 2): Drug interactions involving popular botanical dietary supplements and their clinical relevance. *Planta Medica, 78*(13), 1490–1514.

Health Canada. (2017a). *Licensed Natural Health Database (LNHPD).* Retrieved from http://www.hc-sc.gc.ca/dhp-mps/prodnatur/applications/licen-prod/lnhpd-bdpsnh-eng.php.

Health Canada. (2017b). *MedEffect Canada: Adverse reaction reporting.* Retrieved from http://www.hc-sc.gc.ca/dhp-mps/medeff/report-declaration/index-eng.php.

Ho, S. C., Chong, H. Y., Chaiyakunapruk, N., et al. (2016). Clinical and economic impact of non-adherence to antidepressants in major depressive disorder: A systematic review. *Journal of Affective Disorders, 193,* 1–10.

Hoffman, R. S., Howland, M. A., Lewin, N. A., et al. (2015). *Goldfrank's toxicologic emergencies* (10th ed.). Toronto: McGraw Hill.

Leach, M. J., & Page, A. T. (2015). Herbal medicine for insomnia: A systematic review and meta-analysis. *Sleep Medicine Reviews, 24,* 1–12. doi:10.1016/j.smrv.2014.12.003.

Lee, P. E., Gill, S. S., Freedman, M., et al. (2004). Atypical antipsychotic drugs in the treatment of behavioural and psychological symptoms of dementia: Systematic review. *British Medical Journal, 329,* 75. doi:10.1136/bmj.38125.465579.55.

Leucht, S., Cipriani, A., Spineli, L., et al. (2013). Comparative efficacy and tolerability of 15 antipsychotic drugs in schizophrenia: A multiple-treatment meta-analysis. *Lancet, 382,* 951–962.

Leucht, S., Corves, C., Arbter, D., et al. (2009). Second-generation versus first-generation antipsychotic drugs for schizophrenia: A meta-analysis. *Lancet, 373*(9657), 31–41.

Li, P., Snyder, G., & Vanover, K. E. (2016). Dopamine targeting drugs for the treatment of schizophrenia: Past, present and future. *Current Topics in Medicinal Chemistry, 16*(29), 3385–3403.

(2010). Lithium is still a first-line option in the treatment of patients with bipolar disorder. *Drugs & Therapy Perspectives, 26*(3), 9–14.

Lui, S. L., Zhou, X. J., Sweeney, J. A., et al. (2016). Psychoradiology: The frontier of neuroimaging in psychiatry. *Radiology, 281*(2), 357–372.

Malhi, G. S., & Outhred, T. (2016). Therapeutic mechanisms of lithium in bipolar disorder: Recent advances and current understanding. *CNS Drugs, 30*(1), 931–949. doi:10.1007/s40263-016-0380-1.

Prabhavalkar, K. S., Poovanpallil, N. B., & Bhatt, L. K. (2015). Management of bipolar depression with lamotrigine: An antiepileptic mood stabilizer. *Frontiers in Pharmacology, 6,* 242. doi:10.3389/fphar.2015.00242.

Preston, J. D., O'Neal, J. H., & Talaga, M. C. (2013). *Handbook of clinical psychopharmacology for therapists* (7th ed.). Oakland, CA: New Harbinger.

Rang, H. P., Ritter, J. M., Flower, R. J., et al. (2016). *Rang and Dales's pharmacology* (8th ed.). London, UK: Churchill Livingstone.

Sadock, B. J., Sadock, V. A., & Ruiz, P. (2015). *Kaplan and Sadock's synopsis of psychiatry: Behavioral science/clinical psychiatry* (11th ed.). Kingston upon Thames, UK: Wolters Kluwer.

Sarris, J., & Kavanagh, D. J. (2009). Kava and St. John's wort: Current evidence for use in mood and anxiety disorders. *Journal of Alternative & Complementary Medicine, 15*(8), 827–836.

Sendt, K., Tracy, D. K., & Bhattacharyya, S. (2015). A systematic review of factors influencing adherence to antipsychotic medication in schizophrenia-spectrum disorders. *Psychiatry Research, 225*, 14–30.

Sharma, T., Guski, L. S., Freund, N., et al. (2016). Suicidality and aggression during antidepressant treatment: Systematic review and meta-analyses based on clinical study reports. *British Medical Journal, 352*, i65. doi:10.1136/bmj.i65.

Stahl, S. W. (2013). *Stahl's essential psychopharmacology: Neuroscientific basis and practical applications* (4th ed.). New York: Cambridge University Press.

Wilner, P., Scheel-Kruger, J., & Belzung, C. (2013). The neurobiology of depression and antidepressant action. *Neuroscience and Biobehavioral Reviews, 37*, 2331–2371.

Zacher, J. L., & Holmes, J. C. (2012). Second-generation antipsychotics: A review of recently-approved agents and drugs in the pipeline. *Formulary (Cleveland, Ohio), 47*, 106–121.

Psychobiological Disorders

12. Anxiety and Related Disorders

13. Depressive Disorders

14. Bipolar Disorders

15. Schizophrenia Spectrum and Other Psychotic Disorders

16. Eating and Feeding Disorders

17. Neurocognitive Disorders

18. Psychoactive Substance Use and Treatment

19. Personality Disorders

20. Sleep–Wake Disorders

12

Anxiety and Related Disorders

Margaret Jordan Halter
Adapted by Cheryl L. Pollard

KEY TERMS AND CONCEPTS

acute stress disorder
agoraphobia
alternate personality (alter)
anxiety
compulsions
conversion disorder
dissociative amnesia
dissociative disorders
dissociative fugue
dissociative identity disorder (DID)
fear
flashbacks
generalized anxiety disorder (GAD)
illness anxiety disorder
la belle indifférence
mild anxiety

moderate anxiety
normal anxiety
obsessions
panic
panic attack
panic disorder (PD)
post-traumatic stress disorder (PTSD)
secondary gains
selective inattention
severe anxiety
social phobia
somatic symptom disorders
specific phobias
subpersonality
substance-induced anxiety disorder

OBJECTIVES

1. Compare and contrast the four levels of anxiety in relation to perceptual field, ability to learn, and physical and other defining characteristics.
2. Identify defence mechanisms and consider one adaptive and one maladaptive use of each.
3. Compare and contrast foundational characteristics of anxiety, obsessive-compulsive, post-traumatic stress, somatic symptom, and dissociative disorders.
4. Identify genetic, biological, psychological, and cultural factors that may contribute to anxiety and related disorders.
5. Describe feelings that may be experienced by nurses caring for patients with anxiety disorders.
6. Identify essential assessment components for anxiety, somatic symptom, and dissociative disorders.

7. Formulate four appropriate nursing diagnoses that can be used in providing care to a person with an anxiety or related disorder.
8. Propose realistic outcome criteria for a patient with (a) generalized anxiety disorder, (b) panic disorder, and (c) post-traumatic stress disorder.
9. Identify nursing interventions for patients with anxiety, obsessive-compulsive, post-traumatic stress, somatic symptom, and dissociative disorders.
10. Discuss three classes of medications appropriate for the treatment of anxiety and related disorders.
11. Describe basic-level and advanced-practice interventions for anxiety and related disorders.

⊖volve WEBSITE

Visit the Evolve website for Flashcards, Case Studies, and additional testing resources related to the content in this chapter: http://evolve.elsevier.com/Canada/Varcarolis/psychiatric/

Pre-Test | interactive review

HOW A NURSE HELPED ME

I Am Not the Only One

I am in my mid-fifties now, but when I was a young girl I lived a secret life. I was always a quiet girl, preferring to play dolls by myself or with Judy, my best and only friend, rather than with a group of girls. I was especially uncomfortable with the boys. I don't know what it was; I just didn't feel comfortable with them. I often felt as though others were judging me and making comments about me. I never told anyone how being around a group of people made me feel: I felt embarrassed and stupid. My parents called me "the quiet one" of the family, and I lived up to that label. I struggled through school, constantly feeling on edge and worrying that a teacher would ask me a question.

I know it seems silly, but one of my greatest fears was having to introduce myself in a group. I would start sweating, my heart pounded, I felt like I was going to die, and I was petrified that I might stutter. I became good at managing this situation by always volunteering to go first. You see, if I introduced myself first, then I could relax. I was very pleased with myself when I made this discovery. But other situations that caused even greater anxiety began to crop up. When I had to do a presentation in front of the class, I would pretend that I was ill, and my mother would let me stay home. I found that when I was extremely anxious, I would have difficulty breathing. This led to another strategy for getting out of embarrassing situations: I was diagnosed with childhood asthma, and I very quickly learned how to bring on an asthma attack to get out of going to school. My fear of being found out was always present, and I hated lying to my parents, but I was too ashamed to tell them that I was afraid of sweating, dying, or stuttering in public.

When I went on to university, I would force myself to step out of my comfort zone. I always had a sense of doom and a fear that I was going to die of embarrassment. It was not so much the situation that caused me anxiety; it was more the fear of doing something to embarrass myself that caused me anxiety. It was as if I feared the fear.

My adult years have been lonely. I wanted to talk with people and have fun, but I couldn't get over my anxiety. Then, 5 years ago, I met a nurse who works in psychiatry. He asked me how long I had been struggling with social anxiety disorder (social phobia). "You mean the way I feel is a disorder? I am not the only one?" He arranged for me to see a psychiatrist, who ordered a low dose of medication and enrolled me in 20 cognitive behavioural therapy classes (in a group, of course). The change in me has been

remarkable. I still get anxious in some situations, but I am able to reframe my thoughts and move on. I no longer feel as if I am going to die of embarrassment.

A therapist could be many things, but the following points describe the nurse who was able to help me with my anxiety disorder:

1. *Was kind, compassionate, and easy to talk to*
2. *Conversed with me to get a feel for how strong or resilient my character is*
3. *Was able to "walk a mile in my shoes," so to speak*
4. *Was willing to research the problem on the Internet and in books, as needed*
5. *Considered my feelings and offered constructive yet gentle criticism*
6. *Suggested tangible ways that I could try to advance my position and rectify my problem one step at a time*
7. *Offered positive self-esteem–enhancing comments during the process as, more than likely, these were lacking in my life*
8. *Encouraged me to be proud of myself for my accomplishments*
9. *Challenged me occasionally so that I could continue to move forward*
10. *Realized when I was emotionally and physically well or exhausted or overwhelmed and in need of rest*
11. *Helped me recognize coping strategies for relapse prevention or maintenance of my current level of coping*
12. *Helped me better understand my illness and the types of evidence-informed treatments available*
13. *Helped to educate me about my medication and to monitor for adverse effects*
14. *Unmasked the real problem in my core before attempting to rectify the manifestation of my condition, which is probably very obvious*
15. *Took time during appointments to "read between the lines" of what I say*
16. *Was available if I really needed to speak with him*
17. *Asked questions, especially if he was unsure of what I meant*
18. *Gave me some homework*
19. *Kept the therapy on point for both of us*
20. *Engaged in a truly well-rounded therapeutic relationship with me*
21. *Learned from me as I learned from him*
    Being positive and being interested—it is a tall order!

Source: Holly, a client with an anxiety disorder.

For most people, stress and anxiety is an everyday part of life: "I was really stressed when I couldn't find a parking space just before my final exam. I think I would have done better without that worry." For some people, however, anxiety-related symptoms become severely debilitating and interfere with normal functioning: "Today I was so worried that I wouldn't find a parking space before the final exam, I stayed home." Imagine being so incapacitated by anxiety, you live in dread of germs to the point that handwashing has become the focal point of your day (obsessive-compulsive disorder). Consider repeatedly feeling the immediate terror of emotionally reliving a horrific event in your life, such as hydroplaning on the highway and finding yourself facing oncoming traffic in the wrong lane. You may refuse to drive when it rains (post-traumatic stress disorder). Or when you get into a car, it seems as if your surroundings are foggy, dreamlike—visually distorted (depersonalization/derealization disorder). Anxiety can also affect individuals through physical symptoms, such as fatigue, pain, or numbness. Imagine thinking about your somatic symptoms all the time. This causes you significant distress, and you try to talk with your doctor and the nurse every day. If the doctor is away, you will go to the hospital emergency department. You are unable to maintain friendships because there is no time left after you have attended all your appointments, and you have spent most of your money on various therapies that are not covered by your health plan (somatic symptom disorder).

This chapter examines disorders with a common phenomenology of fear and anxiety. The concept of anxiety and defences against anxiety are described. A brief overview of anxiety disorders, obsessive-compulsive disorders, dissociative disorders, and somatic symptom disorders is provided. There are many commonalities in treatment approaches and associated nursing care strategies for these illnesses that may be used by nurses who work in either a psychiatric or a medical setting.

ANXIETY

Anxiety is a universal human experience and is the most basic of emotions. It can be defined as a feeling of apprehension, uneasiness, uncertainty, or dread resulting from a real or perceived threat. Whereas anxiety is a vague sense of dread related to an unspecified or unknown danger, fear is a reaction to a real or perceived specific danger. Another important distinction between anxiety and fear is that anxiety affects us at a deeper level: it invades the central core of the personality and erodes feelings of self-esteem and personal worth. Physiologically, however, the body reacts to anxiety and fear in similar ways.

Normal anxiety is a healthy reaction necessary for survival. It provides us with energy to carry out everyday tasks and strive toward goals; motivates us to make and survive change; and prompts constructive behaviours, such as studying for an examination, being on time for a job interview, preparing for a presentation, and working toward a promotion.

An understanding of the levels of anxiety and of the defensive patterns used in response to anxiety is fundamental to psychiatric mental health nursing care. With this understanding and practice, you will become skilled at identifying levels of anxiety,

recognizing the defences used to alleviate anxiety, evaluating the possible stressors that contribute to increased anxiety, and planning interventions to lower anxiety levels (including one's own) effectively.

People with anxiety-related disorders will often use rigid and ineffective behaviours repetitively to try to control their anxiety. The common element of such disorders is that those affected experience a degree of anxiety so high that it interferes with personal, occupational, or social functioning. Recent studies also suggest that the presence of chronic anxiety disorders may increase the number of cardiovascular system–related deaths (Chauvet-Gelinier & Bonin, 2017). All anxiety-related disorders tend to be persistent and are often disabling.

LEVELS OF ANXIETY

As discussed in Chapter 4, Hildegard Peplau had a profound role in shaping the specialty of psychiatric mental health nursing. She identified anxiety as one of the most important concepts and developed an anxiety model that consists of four levels: mild, moderate, severe, and panic (Peplau, 1968). The boundaries between these levels are not distinct, and the behaviours and characteristics of individuals experiencing anxiety can and often do overlap. Identification of a patient's specific level of anxiety is essential because interventions are based on the degree of the anxiety.

Mild Anxiety

Mild anxiety, which occurs in the normal experience of everyday living, allows an individual to perceive reality in sharp focus. A person experiencing a mild level of anxiety sees, hears, and grasps more information, and problem solving becomes more effective. Physical symptoms may include slight discomfort, restlessness, irritability, or mild tension-relieving behaviours (e.g., nail biting, foot or finger tapping, fidgeting, wringing of hands).

Moderate Anxiety

As anxiety increases, the perceptual field narrows, and some details are excluded from observation. The person experiencing moderate anxiety sees, hears, and grasps less information and may demonstrate selective inattention, in which only certain things in the environment are seen or heard unless they are pointed out. While the person's ability to think clearly is hampered, learning and problem solving can still take place, although not at an optimal level. Physical symptoms of moderate anxiety include tension, pounding heart, increased pulse and respiratory rate, perspiration, and mild somatic symptoms (gastric discomfort, headache, urinary urgency). Voice tremors and shaking may be noticed. Mild or moderate anxiety levels can be constructive because anxiety may signal that something in the person's life needs attention or is dangerous.

Severe Anxiety

The perceptual field of a person experiencing severe anxiety is greatly reduced. A person with severe anxiety may focus on one particular detail or many scattered details and have difficulty noticing his or her environment, even when it is pointed out by another. Learning and problem solving are not possible at this level, and the person may be dazed and confused. Behaviour becomes automatic (e.g., wringing hands, pacing) and is aimed at reducing or relieving anxiety. Somatic symptoms such as headache, nausea, dizziness, and insomnia often increase; trembling and a pounding heart are common; and the person may hyperventilate and experience a sense of impending doom or dread (see Case Study and Nursing Care Plan 12-1).

Panic

Panic, the most extreme level of anxiety, results in noticeably disturbed behaviour. Someone in a state of panic is unable to process what is going on in the environment and may lose touch with reality, even experiencing hallucinations, or false sensory perceptions (e.g., seeing people or objects not really there). Physical manifestations may include pacing, running, shouting, screaming, or withdrawal, and actions may become erratic, uncoordinated, and impulsive. These sorts of automatic behaviours are used to reduce or relieve anxiety, although such efforts may be ineffective. Acute panic may lead to exhaustion.

Table 12-1 distinguishes among the levels of anxiety in regard to their (1) effects on perceptual field, (2) effects on the ability to learn, and (3) physical and other defining characteristics.

DEFENCES AGAINST ANXIETY

Dysfunctional behaviour (e.g., compulsions, stress headaches, detachment) is a result of *defence mechanisms* (automatic coping styles that protect people from anxiety and maintain self-image by blocking feelings, conflicts, and memories). When behaviour is recognized as dysfunctional, nurses can initiate interventions to reduce anxiety. As anxiety decreases, dysfunctional behaviour will frequently decrease, although initially, as dysfunctional behaviour decreases, anxiety may actually increase until the individual learns to cognitively restructure thoughts. Therefore nurses must be

TABLE 12-1 LEVELS OF ANXIETY

MILD	MODERATE	SEVERE	PANIC
Perceptual Field			
May have heightened perceptual field	Has narrow perceptual field	Has greatly reduced perceptual field	Is unable to focus on the environment
	Grasps less of what is going on	Focuses on details or one specific detail	
		Attention is scattered	
Is alert and can see, hear, and grasp what is happening in the environment	Can attend to more if pointed out by another (selective inattention)	May not be able to attend to events in environment even when pointed out by another	Experiences the utmost state of terror and emotional paralysis
			Feels he or she "ceases to exist"
Can identify things that are disturbing and are producing anxiety		Completely absorbed with self	May have hallucinations or delusions that take the place of reality
		In severe to panic levels of anxiety, the environment is blocked out. It is as if these events are not occurring.	
Ability to Learn			
Able to work effectively toward a goal and examine alternatives	Able to solve problems but not at optimal ability	Unable to see connections between events or details	May be mute or have extreme psychomotor agitation, leading to exhaustion
	Benefits from guidance of others	Has distorted perceptions	Shows disorganized or irrational reasoning
Mild and moderate levels of anxiety can alert the person that something is wrong and can stimulate appropriate action.		*Severe and panic levels prevent problem solving and discovery of effective solutions. Unproductive relief behaviours are called into play, thus perpetuating a vicious cycle.*	
Physical or Other Characteristics			
Slight discomfort	Voice tremors	Feelings of dread	Feeling of terror
Attention-seeking behaviours	Change in voice pitch	Ineffective functioning	Immobility or severe hyperactivity, fight-or-flight or freeze
Restlessness, irritability, or impatience	Difficulty concentrating	Confusion	Dilated pupils
	Shakiness	Purposeless activity	
Mild tension-relieving behaviour (e.g., foot or finger tapping, lip chewing, fidgeting)	Repetitive questioning	Sense of impending doom	Unintelligible communication or inability to speak
	Somatic complaints (e.g., urinary frequency and urgency, headache, backache, insomnia)	More intense somatic complaints (e.g., dizziness, nausea, headache, sleeplessness)	Severe shakiness
	Increased respiration rate	Hyperventilation	Sleeplessness
	Increased pulse rate	Tachycardia	Severe withdrawal
	Increased muscle tension	Withdrawal	Hallucinations or delusions—likely out of touch with reality
	More extreme tension-relieving behaviour (e.g., pacing, banging hands on table)	Loud and rapid speech	
		Threats and demands	

available to help support alternative coping strategies as the individual learns to restructure his or her thinking patterns.

Sigmund Freud and his daughter, Anna Freud, outlined most of the defence mechanisms we recognize today. Although they operate all the time, defence mechanisms are not always apparent to the individual using them. The *adaptive use* of defence mechanisms helps people lower their anxiety to achieve goals in acceptable ways. The excessive application of defence mechanisms, however, results in their *maladaptive use* and is particularly problematic when immature defences are called upon. Figure 12-1 operationally defines anxiety and illustrates how defences come into play.

With the exception of sublimation and altruism, which are always healthy coping mechanisms, all defence mechanisms can be used in both healthy and unhealthy ways. Most people use a variety of defence mechanisms but not always at the same level. Keep in mind that evaluating whether the use of defence mechanisms is adaptive or maladaptive is determined, for the most part, by their frequency, intensity, duration of use, and effect on relationships. Table 12-2 describes defence mechanisms and their adaptive and maladaptive uses.

CLINICAL PICTURE

Anxiety exerts a powerful influence on the mind and body. The experience of anxiety is an underlying factor in several disorders, including:
- Acute stress disorder
- Anxiety disorder not otherwise specified
- Anxiety due to medical conditions
- Depersonalization/derealization disorder
- Generalized anxiety disorder
- Obsessive-compulsive disorder and related disorders
- Panic disorders

- Phobias
- Post-traumatic stress disorder
- Somatic symptom disorder
- Substance-induced anxiety disorder

ANXIETY DISORDERS

The following disorders share symptoms related to excessive fear and anxiety that result in behavioural changes or disturbances. Fear is a response to an imminent threat. Anxiety is related to the perception of a future threat.

Panic Disorder

Panic disorder (PD) is an anxiety disorder characterized by recurring severe panic attacks. It may also effect significant behavioural changes lasting at least a month and ongoing worry about having other attacks. A panic attack is the sudden onset

> **VIGNETTE**
> Sophia, a 30-year-old pharmacist, began to experience tension, irritability, and sleep disturbances after her mother's death from heart disease. On several occasions, Sophia has awakened gasping for breath. Her heart pounds and she feels a tight sensation like a band around her chest. Her pulse typically increases to more than 110 beats per minute, and she experiences dizziness. She fears that she is going to die. The symptoms come on within 10 minutes (sudden onset) and then dissipate. On these occasions, Sophia telephones a friend to come over. The friend typically finds Sophia wringing her hands, moaning, and appearing totally disorganized. In each instance, the friend takes Sophia to the emergency department, where Sophia remains overnight for observation and tests. All diagnostic test results are normal. Because the physician finds no apparent organic basis for the episodes, she suggests that they are likely panic attacks.

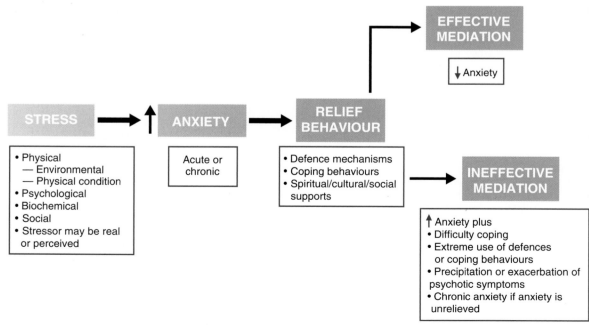

FIGURE 12-1 Anxiety operationally defined.

TABLE 12-2 ADAPTIVE AND MALADAPTIVE USES OF DEFENCE MECHANISMS

DEFENCE MECHANISM	ADAPTIVE USE	MALADAPTIVE USE
Altruism is dedicating oneself to meeting the needs of others as a means of diffusing potentially anxious situations.	A man who is worried that his boss is angry at him will go out of his way and try to be helpful.	*The use of altruism is always constructive.*
Compensation is used to make up for perceived deficiencies and to cover up shortcomings related to these deficiencies to protect the conscious mind from recognizing them.	A shorter-than-average man becomes assertively verbal and excels in business.	An individual drinks alcohol when self-esteem is low to temporarily diffuse discomfort.
Conversion is the unconscious transformation of anxiety into a physical symptom with no organic cause. Often the symptom functions to gain attention or to provide an excuse.	A student is unable to take a final examination because of a terrible headache.	A man becomes blind after seeing his wife flirt with other men.
Denial involves escaping unpleasant, anxiety-causing thoughts, feelings, wishes, or needs by ignoring their existence.	A man reacts to news of the death of a loved one by saying, "No, I don't believe you. The doctor said he was fine."	A woman whose husband died 3 years earlier still keeps his clothes in the closet and talks about him in the present tense.
Displacement is the transference of emotions associated with a particular person, object, or situation to another nonthreatening person, object, or situation.	A patient criticizes a nurse after his family fails to visit.	A child who is unable to acknowledge fear of his father becomes fearful of animals.
Dissociation is a disruption in the usually integrated functions of consciousness, memory, identity, or perception of the environment. It may result in a separation between feeling and thought. Dissociation can also be manifested by compartmentalizing uncomfortable or unpleasant aspects of oneself.	A nursing student is able to mentally separate herself from the noisy environment in the gymnasium as she writes her final exam.	As the result of an abusive childhood and the need to separate from its realities, a woman finds herself perpetually in a world where she feels disconnected from reality. She feels like an outside observer to her thoughts, feelings, and body sensations.
Identification is attributing to oneself the characteristics of another person or group, which may be done consciously or unconsciously.	An 8-year-old girl dresses up like her teacher and puts together a pretend classroom for her friends.	A young boy thinks a neighbourhood gang leader with money and drugs is someone to look up to.
Intellectualization is the process of analyzing events based on remote, cold facts (i.e., without passion), rather than incorporating feeling into the processing.	Despite the fact that a man has lost his farm to a tornado, he analyzes his options and leads his child to safety.	A man responds to the death of his wife by focusing on the details of day care and operating the household, rather than processing the grief with his children.
Introjection is the process by which the outside world is incorporated or absorbed into a person's view of the self.	After his wife's death, a man has transient complaints of chest pains and difficulty breathing—the symptoms his wife had before she died.	A woman whose parents overcriticized and belittled her as a child grows up thinking that she is no good. She has taken on her parents' evaluation of her as part of her self-image.
Projection refers to the unconscious rejection of emotionally unacceptable features and the transfer of them onto other people, objects, or situations. You can remember this defence through the childhood retort of "What you say is what you are."	A man who is unconsciously attracted to other women teases his wife about being attracted to other men.	A woman who has repressed an attraction toward other women refuses to socialize. She fears another woman will make homosexual advances toward her.
Rationalization consists of justifying illogical or unreasonable ideas, actions, or feelings by developing acceptable explanations that satisfy the teller as well as the listener.	An employee says, "I didn't get the raise because the boss doesn't like me."	A man who thinks his son was fathered by another man excuses his malicious treatment of the boy by saying, "He is lazy and disobedient," when that is not the case.
Reaction formation occurs when unacceptable feelings or behaviours are controlled and kept outside of awareness by developing the opposite behaviour or emotion.	A recovering alcoholic constantly preaches about the evils of drink.	A woman who has an unconscious hostility toward her daughter is overprotective and hovers over her to protect her from harm, interfering with her normal growth and development.
Regression is the reversion to an earlier, more primitive, and childlike pattern of behaviour that may or may not have been previously exhibited.	A 4-year-old boy with a new baby brother starts sucking his thumb and wanting a bottle.	A man who loses a promotion starts complaining to others, hands in sloppy work, misses appointments, and comes in late for meetings.
Repression is a first-line psychological defence against anxiety. It is the unconscious temporary or long-term exclusion of unpleasant or unwanted experiences, emotions, or ideas from conscious awareness.	A man forgets his wife's birthday after a marital fight.	A woman is unable to enjoy sex after having pushed out of awareness a traumatic sexual incident from childhood.

Continued

TABLE 12-2　ADAPTIVE AND MALADAPTIVE USES OF DEFENCE MECHANISMS—cont'd

DEFENCE MECHANISM	ADAPTIVE USE	MALADAPTIVE USE
Splitting is the inability to integrate the positive and negative qualities of oneself or others into a cohesive image. Aspects of the self and of others tend to alternate between opposite poles—for example, either good, loving, worthy, and nurturing, or bad, hateful, destructive, rejecting, and worthless.	A toddler views her parents as superhuman and wants to be like them.	A 26-year-old woman has difficulty maintaining close relationships. Although she can initially find many positive qualities about new acquaintances, eventually she becomes disillusioned when they turn out to be flawed.
Sublimation is an unconscious process of substituting mature, constructive, and socially acceptable activity for immature, destructive, and unacceptable impulses. Often these impulses are sexual or aggressive.	A woman who is angry with her boss writes a short story about a heroic woman.	*The use of sublimation is always constructive.*
Suppression is the conscious denial of a disturbing situation or feeling.	A businessman who is preparing to make an important speech later in the day is told by his wife that morning that she wants a divorce. Although visibly upset, he puts the incident aside until after his speech, when he can give the matter his total concentration.	A woman who feels a lump in her breast shortly before leaving for a 3-week vacation puts the information in the back of her mind until after returning from her vacation.
Undoing, most commonly seen in children, is atoning for an act or communication.	After flirting with her male assistant, a woman brings her husband tickets to a concert he wants to see.	A man with rigid, moralistic beliefs and repressed sexuality is driven to wash his hands to gain composure when around attractive women.

of extreme apprehension or fear, usually associated with feelings of impending doom. The feelings of terror present during a panic attack are so severe that normal function is suspended, the perceptual field is extremely limited, severe personality disorganization is evident, and misinterpretation of reality may occur. The following vignette gives an example of a patient with signs and symptoms of a panic attack.

People experiencing panic attacks may believe that they are losing their minds or having a heart attack since the attacks are often accompanied by highly uncomfortable physical symptoms such as palpitations, chest pain, breathing difficulties, nausea, a choking feeling, chills, and hot flashes. Typically, panic attacks occur within 10 minutes "out of the blue" (i.e., suddenly and not necessarily in response to stress), are extremely intense, last a matter of minutes, and then subside. Table 12-3 outlines a generic nursing care plan for PD (see also Case Study and Nursing Care Plan 12-1).

Agoraphobia

When individuals actively avoid situations from which escape might be difficult or embarrassing or in which help might not be available if panic-like symptoms were to occur, they may be diagnosed with agoraphobia. Agoraphobia without a history of

panic attacks occurs only rarely and early in the patient's history. Over time, panic attacks usually develop over the course of this illness. Situations that are commonly avoided by people with agoraphobia include being outside alone; waiting in line at a grocery store; travelling in a car, bus, or airplane; being on a bridge; riding in an elevator; or going to a movie theatre. These types of feared places are avoided in an effort to control anxiety. Avoidance behaviours, however, can be debilitating and life constricting. Consider the effect on a father whose agoraphobia renders him unable to leave home and prevents him from seeing his child's high school graduation, or on the businesswoman whose avoidance of flying prevents her from attending distant business conferences.

Phobias

A *phobia* is a persistent, irrational fear of a specific object, activity, or situation that leads to a desire for avoidance or to actual avoidance of the object, activity, or situation despite the awareness and reassurance that it is not dangerous. Specific phobias, which are more intense, cause impaired daily functioning and last at least half a year. They are characterized by the experience of high levels of anxiety or fear in response to specific objects or situations, such as dogs, spiders, heights, storms, water, blood, closed spaces, tunnels, and bridges. Specific phobias are common and usually do not cause sufferers much difficulty because they

> **VIGNETTE**
> Dmitri is a 28-year-old man who suffers from panic attacks with agoraphobia. He once lived a very active life, often participating in thrill-seeking activities like bungee jumping and skydiving. Dmitri's father, who had severe cardiovascular disease, died 2 years previously on his way to work one day. Since then, Dmitri has become increasingly fearful of the outdoors. He has gradually stopped leaving the family home because he experiences panic attacks, fearing he will die if he goes out.

> **VIGNETTE**
> Abdi developed a morbid fear of elevators after being trapped in one for 3 hours during a power outage. As his fear and anxiety intensified, it became necessary for him to use only stairs or escalators. Abdi even became anxious if he had to enter closets or small storage rooms. He had developed claustrophobia, a fear of closed spaces.

TABLE 12-3 GENERIC CARE PLAN FOR PANIC DISORDER

Nursing diagnosis: *Anxiety* as evidenced by sudden onset of fear or sense of impending doom, increased pulse and respirations, shortness of breath, possible chest pain, dizziness, abdominal distress, and panic attacks.

Outcome: Panic attacks will become less intense, and time between episodes will lengthen so that patient can function comfortably at the usual level.

SHORT-TERM GOAL	INTERVENTION	RATIONALE
1. Patient's anxiety will decrease to moderate by (date).	1a. If hyperventilation occurs, encourage patient to take slow, deep breaths. Breathing with the patient may be helpful.	1a. Focus is shifted away from distressing symptoms. Slow, deep breathing triggers a relaxation response.
	1b. Keep expectations minimal and simple.	1b. Anxiety limits ability to attend to complex tasks.
2. Patient will gain mastery over panic episodes by (date).	2a. Help patient connect feelings before attack with onset of attack: "What were you thinking about just before the attack?" "Can you identify what you were feeling just before the attack?"	2a. Physiological symptoms of anxiety usually appear first as the result of a stressor. They are immediately followed by automatic thoughts, such as "I'm dying" or "I'm going crazy," which are distorted assessments.
	2b. Help patient recognize symptoms as resulting from anxiety, not from a catastrophic physical problem. Examples: Explain physical symptoms of anxiety. Discuss the fact that anxiety causes sensations similar to those of physical events, such as a heart attack.	2b. Factual information and alternative interpretations can help patient recognize distortions in thought.
	2c. Identify effective therapies for panic episodes.	2c. Cognitive behavioural treatment is highly effective. Antianxiety medication is appropriate.
	2d. Teach patient abdominal breathing.	2d. Breathing breaks the cycle of escalating symptoms of anxiety.
	2e. Teach patient to reframe anxiety by using positive self-talk, such as "I can control my anxiety."	2e. Cognitive restructuring is an effective way to replace negative self-talk.
	2f. Teach patient and family about any medication ordered for patient's panic attacks.	2f. Patient and family need to know what the medication can do, the adverse effects and toxic effects, and when to offer medication to the patient.

TABLE 12-4 CLINICAL NAMES FOR COMMON PHOBIAS

CLINICAL NAME	FEARED OBJECT OR SITUATION
Acrophobia	Heights
Agoraphobia	Open spaces
Apiphobia	Bees
Astraphobia	Electrical storms
Claustrophobia	Closed spaces
Glossophobia	Talking
Hematophobia	Blood
Hydrophobia	Water
Monophobia	Being alone
Mysophobia	Germs or dirt
Nyctophobia	Darkness
Pyrophobia	Fire
Social phobia	Fear of a social or performance situation
Triskaidekaphobia	Fear of the number 13
Zoophobia	Animals

Characteristically, phobic individuals experience overwhelming and crippling anxiety when faced with the object or situation provoking the phobia. Phobic people go to great lengths to avoid the feared object or situation. A phobic person may not be able to think about or visualize the object or situation without becoming severely anxious. The life of a phobic person becomes increasingly restricted as activities are given up in order to avoid the phobic object. All too frequently, complications ensue when people try to decrease anxiety through self-medication with alcohol or drugs.

> **VIGNETTE**
>
> David, a 22-year-old musical theatre major, has developed a fear of performing on stage. He suffers severe anxiety attacks whenever he is scheduled to appear in a student production. Recently, he has become severely anxious when faced with giving classroom readings or singing solo in music class. He is thinking about changing his major.

can contrive to avoid the feared object. See Table 12-4 for clinical names for common phobias.

Social phobia, also called *social anxiety disorder (SAD)*, is characterized by severe anxiety or fear provoked by exposure to a social or performance situation (e.g., fear of being scrutinized, saying something that sounds foolish in public, not being able to answer questions in a classroom, eating in public, performing on stage). Fear of public speaking is the most common social phobia.

Generalized Anxiety Disorder

Generalized anxiety disorder (GAD) is an anxiety reaction characterized by persistent and exaggerated apprehension and tension. Worry is the major concern in GAD. The individual's beliefs about worry are then linked to beliefs about himself or herself, such as having the inability to control anxiety and fear, that if he or she worries significantly about an upcoming issue it will be prevented, or that worrying is a valued part of his or her personal identity (Macaulay, Angus, Khattra, et al., 2017). The individual with GAD also displays many of the following symptoms:

- Restlessness
- Fatigue
- Poor concentration
- Irritability
- Tension
- Sleep disturbance

The individual's anxiety is out of proportion to the true impact of the event or situation about which he or she worries. Examples of concerns typical of GAD include inadequacy in interpersonal relationships, job responsibilities, finances, the health of family members, household chores, and lateness for appointments. Sleep disturbance is common because the individual pores over the day's events and real or imagined mistakes, reviews past problems, and anticipates future difficulties. Decision making becomes difficult, owing to poor concentration and dread of making a mistake. Refer to Table 12-5 for a generic care plan for GAD.

VIGNETTE

Jane is a 49-year-old legal secretary. She comes to the clinic complaining of feeling "so anxious I could jump out of my skin." She is shaky and diaphoretic; she has dilated pupils, an elevated pulse, and a quivering voice. She tells the nurse, "It was probably foolish to come here. Nobody understands me." Jane's only daughter is expecting her first child. Although the pregnancy is going well, Jane worries that something is wrong with the baby. "What if it's premature? What if it's deformed?"

Jane describes herself as tense and irritable. She has difficulty initiating sleep and cannot concentrate at her job. She worries about making mistakes at work, about being fired from her position, and about the financial problems that could result. She often says, "I just can't cope." Her daughter has begun calling several times a day to reassure her that all is well with the pregnancy and to try to decrease Jane's worry over other matters. The daughter has also begun shopping and housecleaning for Jane "to help her get some rest."

TABLE 12-5   GENERIC CARE PLAN FOR GENERALIZED ANXIETY DISORDER

Nursing diagnosis: *Ineffective coping* related to persistent anxiety as evidenced by fatigue and irritability.
Outcome: Patient will maintain role performance.

SHORT-TERM GOAL	INTERVENTION	RATIONALE
1. Patient will state that immediate distress is decreased by end of session.	1a. Stay with patient.	1a. Conveys acceptance and ability to give help
	1b. Speak slowly and calmly.	1b. Conveys calm and promotes security
	1c. Use short, simple sentences.	1c. Promotes comprehension
	1d. Assure patient that you are in control and can assist him or her.	1d. Counters feeling of loss of control that accompanies severe anxiety
	1e. Give brief directions.	1e. Reduces indecision; conveys belief that patient can respond in a healthy manner
	1f. Decrease excessive stimuli; provide quiet environment.	1f. Reduces need to focus on diverse stimuli; promotes ability to concentrate
	1g. After assessing level of anxiety, administer appropriate dose of anxiolytic agent if warranted.	1g. Reduces anxiety and allows patient to use coping skills
	1h. Monitor and control own feelings.	1h. Avoids transmission of anxiety (which is transmissible); displays of negative emotion can cause patient anxiety
2. Patient will be able to identify source of anxiety by (date).	2a. Encourage patient to discuss preceding events.	2a. Promotes future change through identification of stressors
	2b. Link patient's behaviour to feelings.	2b. Promotes self-awareness
	2c. Teach cognitive therapy principles: • Anxiety is the result of a dysfunctional appraisal of a situation. • Anxiety is the result of automatic thinking.	2c. Provides a basis for behavioural change
	2d. Ask questions that clarify and dispute illogical thinking: • "What evidence do you have?" • "Explain the logic in that." • "Are you basing that conclusion on fact or feeling?" • "What's the worst thing that could happen?"	2d. Helps promote accurate cognition
	2e. Have patient give an alternative interpretation.	2e. Broadens perspective; helps patient think in a new way about problem or symptom
3. Patient will identify strengths and coping skills by (date).	3a. Have patient identify what has provided relief in the past.	3a. Provides awareness of self as individual with some ability to cope
	3b. Have patient write assessment of strengths.	3b. Increases self-acceptance
	3c. Reframe situation in ways that are positive.	3c. Provides a new perspective and converts distorted thinking

Substance-Induced Anxiety Disorder

Substance-induced anxiety disorder is characterized by symptoms of anxiety, panic attacks, obsessions, and compulsions that develop with the use of a substance or within a month of discontinuing use of the substance. For a diagnosis of substance-induced anxiety disorder, the patient's history, physical examination, or laboratory findings must reveal evidence of the use of a psychoactive substance (e.g., alcohol, cocaine, heroin, hallucinogens) (Canadian Network for Mood and Anxiety Treatments, 2013a).

Anxiety Due to Nonpsychiatric Medical Conditions

In anxiety due to a medical condition, the individual's symptoms of anxiety are a direct physiological result of a medical condition, such as hyperthyroidism, pulmonary embolism, or cardiac dysrhythmias. Determining such a source of anxiety symptoms requires a careful and comprehensive assessment of multiple factors. Once again, evidence must be present in the history, physical examination, or laboratory findings for a diagnosis of anxiety due to a medical condition. Table 12-6 lists medical disorders that may contribute to anxiety symptoms.

TABLE 12-6	COMMON NONPSYCHIATRIC MEDICAL CAUSES OF ANXIETY
SYSTEM	**DISORDERS**
Respiratory	Chronic obstructive pulmonary disease
	Pulmonary embolism
	Asthma
	Hypoxia
	Pulmonary edema
Cardiovascular	Angina pectoris
	Arrhythmias
	Congestive heart failure
	Hypertension
	Hypotension
	Mitral valve prolapse
Endocrine	Hyperthyroidism
	Hypoglycemia
	Pheochromocytoma
	Carcinoid syndrome
	Hypercortisolism
Neurological	Delirium
	Essential tremor
	Complex partial seizures
	Parkinson's disease
	Akathisia
	Otoneurological disorders
	Postconcussion syndrome
Metabolic	Hypercalcemia
	Hyperkalemia
	Hyponatremia
	Porphyria

EPIDEMIOLOGY

Anxiety disorders are one of the most common forms of psychiatric disorders in Canada. In 2014, the Public Health Agency of Canada reported that 11.6% of Canadians over the age of 18 years reported symptoms of mood or anxiety disorder in the previous 12 months. *Report from the Canadian Chronic Disease Surveillance System: Mood and Anxiety Disorders In Canada, 2016* indicates that the prevalence for these disorders is increasing in children and youth. The highest relative increase in prevalence was seen among those ages 5 to 10 years.

COMORBIDITY

Clinicians and researchers have clearly demonstrated that anxiety disorders frequently co-occur with other psychiatric problems (Goodwin, 2015; Meng & D'Arcy, 2015). Anxiety-related disorders occur so frequently with depressive disorders that the treatments for both disorders are similar due to shared neurobiology, symptom similarities, and abnormalities of emotional processing.

SOMATIC SYMPTOM AND RELATED DISORDERS

In contrast to nonpsychiatric medical conditions causing anxiety, somatic symptoms may also cause anxiety, fear, and worry. Somatic symptom disorders (*soma* is the Greek word for "body") are a complex spectrum of physical and emotional signs and symptoms. Health care professionals working in traditional medical settings are more likely to see individuals experiencing a psychiatric illness with predominantly somatic symptoms than are those working within a psychiatric setting. Individuals with these disorders will have physical symptoms and abnormal alterations in thoughts, feelings, and behaviours directly related to the physical symptoms experienced. There may, or may not be, a nonpsychiatric medical diagnosis made related solely to the physical symptoms. These illnesses are often misunderstood and mislabelled. For example, in the Middle Ages, a person who exhibited physical symptoms for no known cause was said to have a "disease of the soul." It was often women who had these "diseases," and many believed they were bewitched or possessed by the devil (Soltis-Jarrett, 2010, p. 183). Freud later used the term *hysteria*, the Greek term meaning "uterus," to refer to somatic and "histrionic" behaviours—behaviours that were attention seeking, emotionally over-reactive, and often inappropriately seductive.

Somatization, the expression of psychological stress through physical symptoms, can affect women, men, and children (Silber, 2011); in fact, somatic symptom disorder symptoms account for nearly 25% of primary care clinic visits (Landa, Peterson, & Fallon, 2012). Anxiety, depression, and trauma exert a powerful influence on the mind and may lead to a variety of clinical conditions—both mental and physical. When psychiatric disorders are present along with general medical conditions, increased health care costs and lengths of stay may result. They also can negatively affect outcomes and increase morbidity and mortality (Konnopka, Löbner, Luppa, et al., 2012).

CLINICAL PICTURE

The somatic disorders include the following:

- Somatic symptom disorder (SSD)
- Illness anxiety disorder (previously *hypochondriasis*)
- Conversion disorder (also called *functional neurological symptom disorder*)
- Psychological factors affecting medical condition
- Factitious disorder

Somatic Symptom Disorder

Somatic symptom disorder manifests itself through distress or a significant disruption in quality of life related to physical symptoms or health concerns that are disproportionate to the seriousness of the symptoms. Often the patient has a comorbid psychiatric disorder such as depression, anxiety, or a personality disorder. Young women, ages 16 to 25, are more likely to receive a somatic diagnosis than men or older individuals (Huang & McCarron, 2011). It has been proposed that women are more aware of their body sensations, have different health-seeking behaviours when faced with physical and psychological distress, and use more health care services than men (Matthew, 2015). Included in the most common symptoms that prompt visits to primary care providers are chest pain, fatigue, dizziness, headache, swelling, back pain, shortness of breath, insomnia, abdominal pain, and numbness. Health-related quality of life is frequently severely impaired, and patients appraise their body symptoms as unduly troublesome, threatening, or harmful, often fearing the worst about their health. Some patients feel that their medical assessment and treatment have been inadequate.

Providers tend to use less patient-centred communication with these patients as compared to those with straightforward symptoms, even though somatic symptom visits require more time (Huang & McCarron, 2011). Patient personality can contribute to an inadequate workup: for example, a "difficult" patient may receive a somatic diagnosis more readily than a "pleasant" patient. In fact, studies show that the strongest predictor of misdiagnosing somatic disorders is the primary care provider's dissatisfaction with the clinical encounter (Huang & McCarron, 2011) (see Case Study and Nursing Care Plan 12-2).

Illness Anxiety Disorder

Previously known as *hypochondriasis*, **illness anxiety disorder** results in the misinterpretation of physical sensations as evidence of a serious illness. Illness anxiety can be quite obsessive as thoughts about illness may be intrusive and hard to dismiss even when patients realize that their fears are unrealistic (MacDonald, 2011). People with this disorder experience extreme worry and fear about the possibility of having a disease. Even normal body changes, such as a change in heart rate or abdominal cramps, can be seen as red flags for serious illness and imminent death. Frequent exposure to media messages reminding us to seek regular medical screenings may also contribute to fears about health (MacDonald, 2011).

In response to a patient's symptoms, primary care providers may suggest a consultation with a mental health professional, but the suggestion typically is refused. The course of the illness is chronic and relapsing, with symptoms becoming amplified during times of increased stress. Furthermore, depressive symptoms may be a catalyst for the diagnosis of illness anxiety (Dols, Rhebergen, Eikelenboom, et al., 2012).

Overall, a patient with illness anxiety disorder uses 41% to 78% more health care services, excluding laboratory tests and X-rays prescribed in primary care, per year than patients with well-defined medical conditions (Fink, 2010). Because illness anxiety disorder is so prevalent, it is important that clinicians achieve basic skills in treating and identifying this disorder. Addressing patient health concerns at an early stage may prevent repeated consultations, multiple trials of medications, and medical examinations (Fink, 2010).

Conversion Disorder

Conversion disorder (also known as *functional neurological symptom disorder*) manifests itself as neurological symptoms in the absence of a neurological diagnosis (Feinstein, 2011). Conversion disorder is marked by the presence of deficits in voluntary motor or sensory functions, including paralysis, blindness, movement disorder, gait disorder, numbness, paresthesia (tingling or burning sensations), loss of hearing, or seizures resembling epilepsy.

Conversion disorder is a clinical problem that requires the application of multiple perspectives—biological, psychological, and social—to fully understand the symptoms of individual patients. Patients with conversion disorder symptoms may be found to have "no neurological disorder" by the neurologist and "no psychiatric disorder" by the psychiatrist, thus adding to the complexity of treatment planning (Yakobov, Jurcik, & Sullivan, 2017).

Conversion disorder is attributed to the channelling of emotional conflicts or stressors into physical symptoms; however, some magnetic resonance imaging (MRI) studies suggest that patients with conversion disorder have an abnormal pattern of cerebral activation (Feinstein, 2011). While some patients become quite distressed about their symptoms, many show a lack of emotional concern about them (*la belle indifférence*). Imagine someone casually discussing sudden blindness. Care providers should assume an organic cause for the symptoms until physical pathology has been ruled out. Patients truly believe in the presence of the symptoms; they are not fabricated or under voluntary control.

Experiences of childhood physical or sexual abuse are common among patients with conversion disorder, and comorbid psychiatric conditions include depression, anxiety, post-traumatic stress disorder, other somatic disorders, and personality disorders. There are also cases in which a comorbid medical or neurological condition exists, and the conversion disorder is an exaggeration of the physical problem (Nicholson, Stone, & Kanaan, 2011).

The course of the disorder is related to its acuity and the length of symptom durations. In cases of acute onset during stressful events, remission rate is high; in cases of a more gradual onset, the disorder is not as readily treatable (Yakobov, Jurcik, & Sullivan, 2017).

VIGNETTE

Gerald is a 63-year-old, married real estate agent who was recently hospitalized for heart failure. Because of insomnia, lack of appetite, and some anger problems toward his wife, his primary care provider has referred him for a mental health consultation. During this consultation, Gerald complains of waking up at night obsessing about possibly losing his job, his lack of retirement savings, and providing for his wife in case he dies. He states, "I am very scared, and I worry about my health and being forced to retire. I don't know where I would get the money to live. I am too old to start another career." These observations were reported to the nurse practitioner. After a thorough assessment and medical workup, it is determined that Gerald is experiencing depression and severe anxiety, which precipitated increased symptoms of heart failure. Gerald has responded well to couples therapy and a men's support group. His blood pressure has decreased, and his mood is improved. Gerald has been able to return to work.

EPIDEMIOLOGY

Specific prevalence rates for somatic symptom disorders in the general population are unknown. Instead, the literature describes their occurrence in the population of individuals who seek medical care but do not have an underlying physiological cause for their symptoms. In the latest edition of the *Diagnostic and Statistical Manual of Mental Disorders (DSM)*, the requirement for no underlying psychological cause for their symptoms was removed. As a result, there is very limited current information on the prevalence of this disorder based on the new diagnostic criteria.

COMORBIDITY

A thorough psychosocial history is also required to confirm a somatic symptom disorder diagnosis, as well as any comorbid psychiatric disorders. People with this type of illness will also have a depressive, psychotic, or anxiety disorder.

Both the medical and the mental health communities recognize the interrelationships between psychiatric and medical illnesses (Shidhaye, Mendenhall, Sumathipala, et al., 2013). This relationship was first introduced by Hans Selye (1956). Selye's description of the *general adaptation syndrome* (see Chapter 5) and Cannon's 1914 identification of the *fight-or-flight response* (see Chapter 23) provided insight into the biological and molecular reactions to stressors in the sympathetic nervous system, the hypothalamic-pituitary–adrenocortical axis, and the immune system. Extensive studies have left little doubt that psychosocial stress affects the course and severity of illness (Table 12-7). Psychological factors may present a risk for a medical disease, or they may magnify or adversely affect a nonpsychiatric medical condition. For example, researchers are consistently providing evidence demonstrating links between mental disorders and cardiovascular disease (Charlson, Stapelberg, Baxter, et al., 2011) and cancer (Deimling, Albitz, Monnin, et al., 2017).

OBSESSIVE-COMPULSIVE DISORDERS

Obsessions are defined as thoughts, impulses, or images that persist and recur and cannot be dismissed from the mind.

Obsessions often seem senseless to the individual who experiences them (*ego-dystonic*), and their presence causes severe anxiety.

Compulsions are ritualistic behaviours or thoughts an individual feels compelled to perform in an attempt to reduce anxiety. Performing the compulsive act temporarily reduces high levels of anxiety. Primary gain is achieved by compulsive rituals, but because the relief is only temporary, the compulsive act must be repeated again and again until it feels "just right" (Haase, 2002).

Although obsessions and compulsions can exist independently of each other, they most often occur together (Table 12-8). Common types of obsessions include losing control, harm, contamination, perfectionism, sexual, and religious. There are also common categories of compulsions: washing and cleaning, checking, repeating, and mental compulsions. Obsessive-compulsive behaviour exists along a continuum. "Normal" individuals may experience mildly obsessive-compulsive behaviour. For example, nearly everyone has had the experience of having a tune run persistently through the mind despite attempts to push it away. Many people have had nagging doubts as to whether a door is locked or not. These doubts may require people to go back to check the door once, but then they can carry on with their day. Compulsive superstitions such as touching a lucky charm or avoiding a black cat are not harmful, and mild compulsions about timeliness, orderliness, and reliability are, in fact, valued traits in Canadian society.

At the pathological end of the continuum are obsessive-compulsive symptoms that typically involve issues of contamination, fear of losing control, need for symmetry, unwanted thoughts of a sexual nature, and recurrent feelings of doubt. Pathological obsessions or compulsions cause marked distress to individuals, who often feel humiliation and shame for these behaviours. The rituals are time consuming and interfere with normal routines, social activities, and relationships with others. Severe obsessive-compulsive disorder (OCD) consumes so much of the individual's mental processes that the performance of cognitive tasks may be impaired.

The fifth edition of the *Diagnostic and Statistical Manual of Mental Disorders (DSM-5)* (American Psychiatric Association, 2013) includes a new chapter on obsessive-compulsive and related disorders to reflect the increasing evidence of these disorders' relatedness to one another and their distinction from other anxiety

---

VIGNETTE

Scott is a 23-year-old university student who is having difficulty handing in assignments on time, and his marks are suffering because of it. He is spending hours on assignments. Each page needs to be perfect. When the assignments are handwritten there needs to be no erasure marks, no cross-outs, and no white-out; all the ink needs to be exactly the same shade; and all margins need to be exactly 4 centimetres. If he hasn't stayed up all night to complete an assignment, he tries to sleep, but only after his bedtime rituals of checking all electrical appliances for fear that he had started a fire, all faucets for fear that he had left them running, and all door locks for fear that he had left them open. These checks are done three times before he can retire to bed. These checks require approximately 2 hours to complete.

TABLE 12-7   COMMON MEDICAL CONDITIONS NEGATIVELY AFFECTED BY STRESS

MEDICAL CONDITION	INCIDENCE	GENETIC AND BIOLOGICAL CORRELATES	COMMON PRECIPITATING FACTORS	POTENTIAL HOLISTIC THERAPIES USED IN ADDITION TO MEDICAL MANAGEMENT
Cardiovascular disease (e.g., coronary heart disease)	Rates higher in Caucasian males until age 60 years	Risk factors: family history of cardiac disease, hypertension, increased serum lipid levels, obesity, sedentary lifestyle, cigarette smoking Psychosocial risk factors: stress, depression, loneliness High anxiety risk in patient with prior cardiac events	Sudden stress preceded by a period of losses, frustration, and disappointments (often resulting in myocardial infarction)	Relaxation training, stress management, group social support, and psychosocial intervention Support groups for type A personalities
Peptic ulcer (caused by *Helicobacter pylori* infection)	Occurs in 12% of men, 6% of women (more prevalent in industrialized societies)	Infection with *H. pylori* is associated with 95% to 99% of peptic ulcers Both peptic and duodenal ulcers cluster in families, but separately from each other	Periods of social tension and increased life stress Losses Postmenopause	Biofeedback to alter gastric acidity Cognitive behavioural approaches to reduce stress (stress management)
Cancer	Men: most common in lung, prostate, colon, and rectum Women: most common in breast, uterus, colon, and rectum Death rate higher in men than in women	Genetic evidence suggesting dysfunction of cellular proliferation Familial patterns of breast cancer, colorectal cancer, stomach cancer, melanoma	Prolonged and intensive stress Stressful life events (e.g., separation from or loss of significant other 2 years before diagnosis) Feelings of hopelessness, helplessness, and despair (depression)	Relaxation (e.g., meditation, autogenic training, self-hypnosis) Visualization Psychological counselling Support groups Massage therapy Stress management
Tension headache	Occurs in 80% of population when under stress Begins at end of workday or early evening		Associated with anxiety and depression	Psychotherapy for chronic tension headaches Learning to cope or avoiding tension-creating situations or people Relaxation and stress-management techniques Cognitive restructuring techniques
Essential hypertension	Rates higher in males until age 60 years	Risk factors: family history of cardiac disease and hypertension	Life changes and traumatic life events Stressful job (e.g., air traffic controller)	Behavioural feedback, stress reduction techniques, meditation, yoga, hypnosis *Note:* Pharmacological treatment considered primary for treatment of hypertension.

disorders, as well as to help clinicians better identify and treat individuals suffering from these disorders. Disorders in this chapter of *DSM-5* include OCD, body dysmorphic disorder, and trichotillomania (hair-pulling disorder), as well as two new disorders: hoarding disorder and excoriation (skin-picking) disorder. For further information, visit http://www.dsm5.org/psychiatrists/practice/dsm.

EPIDEMIOLOGY

OCD is the fourth most common psychiatric illness. Everyone on occasion will obsess about something. However, only 1% to 3% of people will spend more than an hour a day having obsessive thoughts. The typical age of onset is bimodal (10 years and 21 years) (Grant, 2014). Males generally will have an earlier onset than females. Childhood OCD is diagnosed almost three times as frequently in boys than in girls. However, by adulthood OCD occurs with approximately equal frequency in women and men.

COMORBIDITY

Other psychiatric conditions with common symptoms of rumination (mood disorder) and worry (anxiety disorder) commonly occur with OCD. Psychotic disorders may also occur, however; people with only OCD are able to recognize that their thoughts are irrational but that they cannot control them.

TABLE 12-8 COMMON OBSESSIONS AND COMPULSIONS

TYPE OF OBSESSION	EXAMPLE	ACCOMPANYING COMPULSION
Losing control	Fear of acting on an impulse to harm oneself	Praying to prevent harm to oneself
	Fear of violent or horrific images in one's mind	Thinks about something else when horrific images come to mind
		Praying to get rid of the images
Harm	Fear of being responsible for something terrible happening	Checking that nothing terrible happened
		Checking that you did not make a mistake
	Fear of harming others because of not being careful enough (e.g., dropping something on the ground will cause another person to fall and break an arm)	Praying to prevent harm to prevent terrible consequences.
		Checking that you did not or will not harm others
Perfectionism	Need for symmetry—concern about evenness	Rereading or rewriting
		Putting things in order or arranging things until it "feels right"
	Inability to decide whether to keep or discard things	Collecting items that results in significant clutter in the home (hoarding)
Contamination	Environmental contaminants (radiation, oil, or lead)	Cleaning household items in a certain way to remove contaminants
	Germs or viruses	Washing hands excessively
Unwanted sexual thoughts	Forbidden or perverse sexual thoughts or images	Telling, asking, or confessing to get reassurance
	Obsessions about aggressive sexual behaviour toward others	Avoiding situations that might trigger your obsessions
Religious obsessions	Concern with offending God	Praying to seek forgiveness
		Repeatedly touching or kissing religious objects
	Excessive concern with morality	Replaying interactions with others and repeatedly reviewing every remark to determine if you said anything wrong
Other obsessions	Concern about getting a disease, such as cancer, colitis, or diabetes	Checking some parts of your physical condition or body
	Superstitious ideas	Repeating activities in "multiples" (e.g., doing a task three times because three is a "good," "right," or "safe" number)

 RESEARCH HIGHLIGHT

"On My Own, but Not Alone"—Adolescents' Experiences of Internet-Delivered Cognitive Behavioural Therapy for Obsessive-Compulsive Disorder

Problem

Obsessive-compulsive disorder (OCD) can effectively be treated with cognitive behavioural therapy (CBT). However, many people with this illness do not have access to a health professional who is experienced in delivering this treatment.

Purpose of Study

The purpose of this study was to describe the experience of adolescents with OCD who had received Internet-provided CBT. This treatment was delivered via a secure Internet platform that enabled age-appropriate presentation of different treatment content to pediatric patients.

Methods

Participants in this study were a subset of participants who were in a research project that evaluated the effectiveness and efficiency of Internet-provided CBT to adolescents. The Internet-provided CBT content is presented in chapters, much like chapters in a self-help book.

The chapters contain psychoeducative texts, films, and CBT exercises, such as exposure exercises and cognitive interventions. Patients have regular contact with an experienced clinician via messages that can be sent inside the treatment platform (resembling email). The clinician can also directly comment on exercises that the patient has been working on and can therefore give specific feedback and support and motivate the patient. In this way, a patient usually has contact with his or her treating clinician several times a week.

Key Findings

The effectiveness and efficiency portion of this research program indicated that the Internet could be used effectively and efficiently to provide CBT to adolescents. In this study, participants described the ability to work independently with the treatment material and, through that, have some degree of control over the therapy process. In addition, several participants also reported advantages of being able to choose when and where to work. Participants were willing to communicate information about themselves, such as thoughts, feelings, doubts, failures, successes, and fears, and at the same time felt secure about doing so.

Implications for Nursing Practice

Service accessibility is an issue for many people in Canada. This study supports the use of alternate delivery formats as a means of supporting patient recovery. This type of alternate service delivery model allowed for a relationship to develop between the patient and service provider in a manner that promoted patient autonomy.

Source: Lenhard, F., Vigerland, S., Engberg, H., et al. (2016). "On my own, but not alone"—Adolescents' experiences of internet-delivered cognitive behavior therapy for obsessive-compulsive disorder. *PLoS ONE, 11*(10), e0164311. doi:10.1371/journal.pone.0164311.

TRAUMA- AND STRESSOR-RELATED DISORDERS

ACUTE STRESS DISORDER

Acute stress disorder occurs within 1 month of a highly traumatic event, such as those that precipitate post-traumatic stress disorder. To be diagnosed with acute stress disorder, the individual must display at least three dissociative symptoms either during or after the traumatic event, including a subjective sense of numbing, detachment, or absence of emotional responsiveness; a reduction in awareness of surroundings; derealization (a sense of unreality related to the environment); depersonalization (a sense of unreality or self-estrangement); or dissociative amnesia (loss of memory) (Canadian Network for Mood and Anxiety Treatments, 2013b). By definition, acute stress disorder resolves within 4 weeks.

> **VIGNETTE**
>
> Olivia, a 22-year-old university student, is sexually assaulted by a family friend. In the emergency department, she describes feeling detached from her body and being unaware of her surroundings during the assault, "as though it took place in a vacuum." She displays virtually no affect (i.e., she does not cry or appear anxious, angry, or sad). Olivia finds it difficult to concentrate on the examiner's questions. Three days later, Olivia still feels as though her mind is detached from her body; she reports having difficulty sleeping, not being able to concentrate, and startling whenever anyone touches her. When she sees the nurse 4 weeks after the event, Olivia expresses feelings of anger and sadness over the assault, displays the ability to concentrate, and states that she no longer feels as though her mind and body are detached. She reports being able to sleep better and not being so jittery and easily startled.

POST-TRAUMATIC STRESS DISORDER

Post-traumatic stress disorder (PTSD) is included in a new chapter in the *DSM-5* on trauma- and stressor-related disorders. Post-traumatic stress disorder (PTSD) is an acute emotional response to a traumatic event or situation involving severe environmental stress (*Mosby's Dictionary of Medicine*, 2012).

The individual with PTSD persistently re-experiences a traumatic event that involved threatened or actual death or serious injury to self or others, and to which the person responded with intense fear, helplessness, or horror. PTSD may present after any traumatic event that is outside the range of usual experience, such as military combat, detention as a prisoner of war, natural disasters (e.g., floods, tornadoes, earthquakes), human disasters (e.g., plane and train accidents), crime-related events (e.g., sexual abuse, bombing, assault, mugging, rape, being taken hostage), or diagnosis of a life-threatening illness.

Due to the traumatic events faced by members of the Canadian Armed Forces, it has been estimated that nearly 20% of Canadian Armed Forces veterans have an operational stress injury (OSI) such as PTSD, addiction, or another mental health problem (Pearson, Zamorski, & Janz, 2014). PTSD symptoms often begin within 3 months of the trauma, but a delay of several months or years is not uncommon.

The major features of PTSD are:

- Persistent re-experiencing of the trauma through recurrent intrusive recollections of the event, dreams about the event, and flashbacks—dissociative experiences during which the event is relived (i.e., the person behaves as though he or she is experiencing the event in the present)
- Persistent avoidance of stimuli associated with the trauma, causing the individual to avoid talking about the trauma or avoid activities, people, or places that rouse memories of the trauma
- Persistent numbing of general responsiveness, as evidenced by the individual's feeling empty inside or feeling disconnected from others
- Persistent symptoms of increased arousal, as evidenced by irritability, difficulty sleeping, difficulty concentrating, hypervigilance, or exaggerated startle response

Difficulty with interpersonal, social, or occupational relationships nearly always accompanies PTSD, and trust is a common issue of concern. Child and spousal abuse may be associated with hypervigilance and irritability, and chemical abuse may begin as an attempt to self-medicate to relieve anxiety (see Case Study and Nursing Care Plan 12-3).

DISSOCIATIVE DISORDERS

Dissociative disorders are a group of disorders precipitated by significant adverse experiences or traumas and resulting in the unconscious altering of mind–body connections. Dissociation is an unconscious defence mechanism that protects the individual against overwhelming anxiety and stress through an emotional separation; however, this separation results in disturbances in memory, consciousness, self-identity, and perception.

Patients with dissociative disorders are able to assess a situation realistically, rather than for what they want it to be or fear that it might be. They do not have hallucinations or delusions (meaning that they have "intact reality testing"), but they may have flashbacks or see images that are triggered by current events that are related to the past trauma. Mild, fleeting dissociative experiences are relatively common to all of us; for example, we may be listening to someone and suddenly realize that we have not heard part or all of what was said. These common experiences are distinctly different from the processes of pathological dissociation.

Pathological dissociation is involuntary and results in failure of control over one's mental processes and the integration of conscious awareness (Spiegel, Loewenstein, Lewis-Fernandez, et al., 2011). With pathological dissociation, pieces of a memory become fragmented. For example, normally, when people remember an experience, they can recall the people who were there, maybe a significant smell (like cooking turkey), maybe singing, and maybe an uncle who wore a bright red suit. However, when memories become fragmented, as in pathological dissociation, a person may recall a sound or smell but not be able to link these sensations to the actual event, instead feeling as though there is something familiar about the smell or sound but not knowing why. If the pieces of memory are associated with a traumatic experience, the fragments can leave the person fearful, confused, or both. If the memory was very traumatic, the fragments may cause the person to re-enact, as well as re-experience, trauma without consciously knowing why.

Symptoms of dissociation may be either *positive* or *negative*. Positive symptoms refer to unwanted additions to mental activity, such as flashbacks; negative symptoms refer to deficits, such as memory problems or the inability to sense or control different parts of the body. It is thought that dissociation decreases the immediate subjective distress of the trauma (a self-protective mechanism) and also continues to protect the individual from full awareness of the disturbing event. Continued dissociative symptoms, however, can interfere with activities of daily living and relationships.

In the case of abused or neglected children, dissociation can be interpreted as somewhat protective, allowing the child to continue to be attached to abusive or neglectful caretakers. This instinctive mechanism highlights the importance of attachments and relationships in allowing the child to grow socially, intellectually, and cognitively. If abuse or neglect has occurred, memories of it become compartmentalized and often do not intrude into awareness until later in life during a stressful situation or in trying to develop another significant relationship.

All of the dissociative disorders affect both the patient and the patient's family. For example, people with depersonalization disorder are often fearful that others may perceive their appearance as distorted and may avoid being seen in public. If they exhibit consistently high levels of anxiety, the family is likely to find it difficult to keep relationships stable. By comparison, people who experience fugue states often function adequately in their new identities by choosing simple, undemanding occupations and having few intimate social interactions. Patients with amnesia, in contrast to those with fugue, may be more dysfunctional. Their perplexity often renders them unable to work, and their memory loss impairs normal relationships. Families often direct considerable attention toward the patient but may exhibit concern over having to assume roles that were once assigned to the patient. Finally, patients with dissociative identity disorder often have both family and work problems. Families find it difficult to accept the seemingly erratic behaviours of the patient. Employers dislike the lost time that may occur when alternate identities are in control.

CLINICAL PICTURE

Dissociative disorders include (1) depersonalization/derealization disorder, (2) dissociative amnesia, and (3) dissociative identity disorder.

Depersonalization/Derealization Disorder

Depersonalization/derealization disorder may cause a person to feel mechanical, dreamy, or detached from the body. Some people suffer episodes of these problems that come and go, while others have episodes that begin with stressors and eventually become constant. People with this disorder may experience episodes of depersonalization or derealization or both. When experiencing depersonalization, individuals feel as though they are observers of their own body or mental processes—there is an internal feeling of disconnect. Similarly, with derealization, there is a recurring feeling that one's surroundings are unreal or distant—an external or outside feeling of disconnect. These feelings are not consciously controlled by the patients with dissociative disorders and are reported to be very distressing to those who experience them.

VIGNETTE

Marguerite describes becoming very troubled by perceived changes in her appearance when she looks in a mirror. She thinks that her image looks wavy and indistinct. Soon after, she describes feeling as though she is floating in a fog, with her feet not actually touching the ground. Questioning reveals that Marguerite's son has recently confided to her that he tested positive for human immunodeficiency virus (HIV) and that she is extremely worried about him.

Dissociative Amnesia

Dissociative amnesia is marked by the inability to recall important autobiographical information, often of a traumatic or stressful nature, that is too pervasive to be explained by ordinary forgetfulness. While autobiographical memory is available (i.e., stored within the brain), the information is not accessible (i.e., the memory cannot be retrieved). When memories are stored, information about the situation (*retrieval cues*) is also stored. This additional information can be about the environment (smell, place, colour) or about a feeling (happy, sad, mad) or about an activity at the time (walking, crying, sitting, studying). Seeing or thinking about these retrieval cues helps us recall the memory. For example, have you ever got up from watching television and gone into the kitchen to do something but then forgotten what you were going to do once you got to the kitchen? But then you go back and sit down in front of the television and you remember? You have just accessed a memory using a retrieval cue.

In contrast, a patient with generalized amnesia is unable to recall information about his or her entire lifetime. The generalized amnesia may be *localized* (the patient is unable to remember all events in a certain period) or *selective* (the patient is able to recall some but not all events in a certain period). For the person with generalized amnesia, the information is neither available nor accessible, contrary to dissociative amnesia.

A subtype of dissociative amnesia, also usually precipitated by a traumatic event, is dissociative fugue. This disorder is characterized by sudden, unexpected travel away from the customary locale and an inability to recall one's identity and information about some or all of the past. The word *fugue* comes from the Latin word for *flight*. In rare cases, an individual with dissociative fugue assumes a whole new identity. During a fugue state (individuals are in a different location, unable to recall personal information about themselves or their past), individuals show no signs of illness and tend to lead rather simple lives, rarely calling attention to themselves. Only the memories tied to their identities are lost. If the person experiencing the fugue state knows how to drive, use the computer, make meals, and use a public transit system, he or she retains that knowledge. After a few weeks to a few months, the person may become confused about his or her identity or remember the former identity and then become amnesic for the time spent in the fugue state.

Dissociative Identity Disorder

The essential feature of dissociative identity disorder (DID) is the presence of two or more distinct personality states that alternately and recurrently take control of behaviour. It is believed that severe sexual, physical, or psychological trauma in childhood predisposes an individual to the development of DID. Each alternate personality (alter), or subpersonality, has its own pattern of perceiving, relating to, and thinking about the self and the environment. Each alter is a complex unit with its own memories, behaviour patterns, and social relationships that dictate how the person acts when that personality is dominant. If the original or primary personality is religious and moralistic, the subpersonality or subpersonalities are often pleasure seeking and nonconforming. The alters may also behave as individuals of a different sex, race, or religion.

Dissociative identity disorder appears to be associated with two dissociative identity states (alternate personalities): (1) a state in which the individual blocks access and responses to traumatic memories so as to be able to function daily and (2) a state fixated on traumatic memories. The primary personality, or *host*, is usually not aware of the subpersonalities and is perplexed by lost time and unexplained events. Experiences such as finding unfamiliar clothing in the closet, being called a different name by a stranger, and not having childhood memories are characteristic of DID. Subpersonalities are often aware of the existence of each other to some degree. Transition from one personality to another occurs during times of stress and may range from a dramatic to a barely noticeable event. Some patients experience the transition when awakening. Shifts may last from minutes to months, although shorter periods are more common.

EPIDEMIOLOGY

Although mental health care providers in Canada believe that dissociative disorders are rare, depersonalization disorder prevalence rates range from about 1% to 3%, which is comparable to disorders such as schizophrenia, bipolar disorder, and obsessive-compulsive disorder (Spiegel, Loewenstein, Lewis-Fernandez, et al., 2011).

COMORBIDITY

Psychiatric comorbidities are extremely common for people with dissociative disorders. Patients with dissociative disorders usually seek treatment for another problem such as anxiety or depression (International Society for the Study of Trauma and Dissociation, 2012; Spiegel, Loewenstein, Lewis-Fernandez, et al., 2011).

ETIOLOGY OF ANXIETY-RELATED DISORDERS

There is no longer any doubt that biological factors predispose some individuals to develop pathological emotional and mental states (e.g., generalized anxiety, phobias, panic attacks, dissociation, somatization). However, traumatic life events, psychological factors, and sociocultural factors are also etiologically significant for all the disorders identified in this chapter. Regardless of the age at which symptoms start, their purpose is to reduce disturbing feelings and protect the person from the effects of the trauma.

BIOLOGICAL FACTORS

Genetic

Numerous studies substantiate that anxiety disorders tend to cluster in families. Twin studies demonstrate the existence of a genetic component to panic disorder, obsessive-compulsive disorder, and conversion disorder (Pauls, 2010). First-degree biological relatives of those with OCD or phobias have a higher frequency of these disorders than exists in the general population, and relatives of people with a somatic symptom disorder are more likely to have chronic pain, depressive disorder, and alcohol dependence. Although genetic variability is thought to play a role in stress reactivity, dissociation is thought to be largely due to extreme stress or environmental factors.

Neurobiological

Certain anatomical pathways in the midbrain (the limbic system) provide the transmission structure for the electrical impulses that occur when anxiety-related responses are sent or received. Neurons release chemicals (neurotransmitters) that convey these messages. The neurochemicals that regulate anxiety-related disorders include epinephrine, norepinephrine, dopamine, serotonin, gamma-aminobutyric acid (GABA), and endogenous opioids. Repeated trauma or stress not only alters the release of neurotransmitters but also changes the anatomy of the brain. Animal studies show that early, prolonged emotional detachment from the caretaker negatively affects the development of the limbic system, which is where traumatic memories are processed; therefore trauma negatively interferes with the normal development of the limbic system. Studies suggest that the stress response of the hypothalmic–pituitary–adrenal system is abnormal in patients with PTSD. In addition, individuals with dissociative disorders have increased activation of the orbital frontal cortex, which inhibits activation of the amygdala and insular cortex as well as the hippocampal areas, where traumatic memories are stored (Spiegel, Loewenstein, Lewis-Fernandez, et al., 2011). Any abnormality in the structure of the brain or the function of the neurotransmitters can lead to a misinterpretation of ordinary events. For example, the brain may misunderstand (or amplify the significance of) a stimulus, such as identifying a minor gas pain as a serious abdominal injury (somatization). The brain may also over-react in its analysis of the stimulus, deciding that the same minor gas pain is a sign of colon cancer (illness anxiety) and then hope that death comes quickly.

PSYCHOLOGICAL FACTORS

Psychodynamic Theories

Psychodynamic theories about the development of anxiety disorders centre on the idea that unconscious childhood conflicts are the basis for symptom development. Sigmund Freud suggested that anxiety results from the threatened breakthrough of repressed ideas or emotions from the unconscious into consciousness. Freud also suggested that the individual uses ego defence mechanisms to keep anxiety at manageable levels (see Chapter 4). The use of defence mechanisms results in behaviour that is not wholly adaptive because of its rigidity and repetitive nature.

Harry Stack Sullivan (1953) believed that anxiety is linked to the emotional distress caused when early needs go unmet or disapproval is experienced (interpersonal theory). He also suggested that anxiety is "contagious," being transmitted to the infant from the mother or caregiver. Thus the anxiety experienced early in life becomes the prototype for anxiety experienced when unpleasant events occur later in life.

Since the late nineteenth century, psychoanalytic theory has dominated medical thinking about conversion disorder (Stone, Vuilleumier, & Friedman, 2010). Psychoanalytic theorists believe that psychosomatic complaints of pain, illness, or loss of physical function are related to repression of a conflict or unwelcome experiences (usually of an aggressive or sexual nature) and that the transformation of anxiety into a physical symptom is symbolically related to the conflict (Nicholson, Stone, & Kanaan, 2011). For example, in conversion disorder, conversion symptoms permit the individual to communicate a need for special treatment or consideration from others.

Illness anxiety disorder is considered by many clinicians to have psychodynamic origins. These clinicians suggest that anger, aggression, or hostility that had its source in past losses or disappointments are expressed as a need for help and concern from others. Other clinicians suggest that illness anxiety is a defence against guilt or low self-esteem (van Dijke, 2012). In the view of many patients, the somatic symptoms serve as deserved punishment.

Behavioural Theory

Behavioural theories suggest that anxiety is a learned response to specific environmental stimuli (*classical conditioning*). Anxiety may also be learned through the modelling of parents or peers. For example, a mother who is fearful of thunder and lightning and hides in closets during storms may transmit her anxiety to her children, who adopt her behaviour into adulthood. Such individuals can unlearn this behaviour by observing others who react normally to a storm, perhaps by lighting candles and telling stories.

Behaviourists suggest that people with somatic symptoms learn methods of communicating helplessness. These "helpless" behaviours are used to get their needs met. The symptoms become more intense when they are reinforced by attention from others. Behaviourists also identify potential secondary gains from many disorders. Secondary gains are those benefits derived from the symptoms alone; for example, in the sick role, the patient is not able to perform the usual family, work, and social functions and receives extra attention from loved ones. Other potential benefits include avoiding activities the individual considers distasteful, obtaining financial benefit, and gaining some advantage in interpersonal relationships due to the symptom.

Cognitive Theory

Cognitive theorists believe that anxiety disorders are caused by distortions in an individual's thoughts and perceptions. Because individuals with such distortions may believe that any mistake will have catastrophic results, they experience acute anxiety. In contrast, patients with somatic symptoms focus on body sensations, misinterpret their meaning, and then become excessively alarmed by them.

Learning Theory

Dissociation is one of the most primitive ego defence mechanisms. The pattern of avoidance occurs when an individual deals with an unpleasant event by consciously deciding not to think about it. The more anxiety provoking the event is, the greater is the need to avoid thinking about it. As the individual increasingly depends on this coping strategy, dissociation becomes easier, and it becomes more likely that this defence mechanism will be the individual's predominant means of reacting to stress. Thus learning theory suggests that dissociative disorders can be explained as learned methods for avoiding stress and anxiety.

ENVIRONMENTAL FACTORS

The environmental factors related to a person developing an anxiety-related disorder are exposures to traumatic events, including any experience that is overwhelming to the person, such as a motor vehicle accident, combat experience, emotional or verbal abuse, incest, neglectful or abusive caregivers, and imprisonment. We know that adverse childhood events result in lifelong problems, including post-traumatic stress disorder, anxiety disorders, dissociative disorders, and somatic disorders (van Dijke, 2012). The Adverse Childhood Experiences (ACE) Study (Fuller-Thomson, Sulman, Brennenstuhl, et al., 2011) surveyed more than 16 000 adults and discovered that childhood trauma exposure accounted for negative outcomes across a variety of diagnoses in later life, including multiple somatic symptoms of diabetes, heart disease, cancer, gastrointestinal conditions, and immune functioning.

SOCIOCULTURAL FACTORS

Reliable data on the incidence of anxiety disorders are sparse, but sociocultural variation in symptoms of anxiety disorders has been noted. In some cultures, most individuals express anxiety through somatic symptoms, whereas in other cultures, cognitive symptoms predominate. Panic attacks in Latin Americans and Northern Europeans often involve sensations of choking, smothering, numbness, or tingling, as well as fear of dying. In some other cultural groups, panic attacks involve fear of magic or witchcraft. Physical symptoms are believed to result from the casting of spells. Spellbound individuals often seek the help of traditional healers in addition to modern medical staff. The medical health care provider may diagnose a non–life-threatening somatic symptom disorder, whereas the traditional healer may offer an entirely different explanation and prognosis. The individual might not show improvement until the traditional healer removes the spell.

The type and frequency of psychosomatic symptoms vary across cultures as well (Brown & Lewis-Fernandez, 2011). The sensation of burning hands and feet, worms in the head, or ants under the skin is more common in Africa and southern Asia than in North America. Fainting is a symptom commonly associated with culture-specific religious and healing rituals.

Somatic symptom disorder, which is rarely seen in men in North America, is often reported in Greek and Puerto Rican men, suggesting that cultural customs permit these men to somatize as an acceptable approach to dealing with life stress. Somatization related to post-traumatic stress and depression was the most prevalent psychiatric symptom in North Korean defectors to South Korea (Kim, Lee, Kim, et al., 2011). West Indians (Caribbean) attribute somatic symptoms to chronic overwork and the irregularity of daily living, citing symptoms such as dizziness, fatigue, joint pain, and muscle tension.

Culture-Bound Syndromes

Up to 175 culture-bound syndromes have been identified. Culture-bound syndromes express distress about a range of personal and social problems in a culture and do not necessarily indicate psychopathology (e.g., heat in the head, heart-squeezed, bored). Some, such as trance, possession states, and fainting or seizure-like episodes, may in Western thinking be assessed as pathological (e.g., delusions or hallucinations) but are accepted expressions of distress in other cultures. In addition, cultural idioms of distress encompass explanatory mechanisms for behaviours or symptoms (e.g., evil eye, witchcraft, extreme emotion that upsets hot–cold balance) (Flaskerud, 2009).

🌐 CONSIDERING CULTURE

Evidence-Based Practice and Cultural Adaptations

When delivering treatment for anxiety guided by an evidenced-based practice guideline, the clinician must become aware of the cultural assumptions of the research on which the guidelines have been developed. Usually, implementing an evidence-based practice guideline is an opportunity to improve the effectiveness and efficiency of nursing care. However, most evidence-based practice guidelines are developed from research using data collected from the dominant cultural group. This results in shortfalls in understanding the responsiveness of interventions within minority cultural groups. The guidelines identify the determinants of effective treatment. However, is it reasonable to assume that all cultural groups define effective treatment for anxiety in the same way? As a result, clinicians need to question the universal applicability of evidence-based practice guidelines and determine whether sociocultural differences necessitate different forms of interventions and how cultural factors affect the impact of the guideline. Once it is determined whether a guideline requires cultural adaptation the dimensions of language—metaphors, symbols, and sayings—the language of the intervention, cultural values of the community, and unique context of the individual are reviewed prior to treatment initiation.

Rather than listing various culture-bound syndromes the *DSM-5* provides a cultural formulation interview guide to help mental health practitioners assess information about the cultural features of an individual's mental health, history, and social context. Nurses need to show acceptance of and respect for culture-bound syndromes. However, showing acceptance and respect does not mean that the patient is not offered antipsychotics or other medications. Depending on the results of a thorough assessment, medication may be used to help alleviate a patient's distress. The Considering Culture box discusses factors relevant to the intersection of cultural adaptation of the implementation of evidence-based practices. Review Chapter 8 for more discussion of cultural issues.

APPLICATION OF THE NURSING PROCESS

ASSESSMENT

General Assessment

People with anxiety disorders rarely need hospitalization unless they are in extreme distress, suicidal, or have compulsions that cause injury (e.g., cutting self, banging a body part). When assessing any patient, it is essential that all aspects of patient safety are considered. Most patients prone to anxiety disorders are encountered in non–mental health settings. A common example is someone taken to an emergency department to rule out a heart attack when, in fact, the individual is experiencing a panic attack. It is essential for clinicians to determine whether the anxiety is secondary to another source (medical condition or substance) or is the primary problem, as in an anxiety disorder.

Rating Scales

The Hamilton Anxiety Rating Scale is a popular tool for measuring anxiety (Table 12-9). High scores may indicate GAD or PD, although it is important to note that high anxiety scores may also be a symptom of major depressive disorder. Keep in mind that although the Hamilton Anxiety Rating Scale highlights important areas in the assessment of anxiety, it is intended for use by experienced clinicians as a guide for planning care and not as a method of self-diagnosis.

Goodman, Price, and Rasmussen (1989) developed the Yale-Brown Obsessive Compulsive Scale (YBOCS). To review this scale, you may access it at https://psychology-tools.com/yale-brown-obsessive-compulsive-scale/. The YBOCS has become the preferred measurement tool for OCD. It is important to note that the YBOCS is not a diagnostic tool. Rather, it is a scale used to gauge the severity and nature of OCD symptoms. Foa and colleagues (1998) developed the Obsessive-Compulsive Inventory (OCI) with the following subscales: washing, checking, doubting, ordering, obsessions, hoarding, and neutralizing. The Panic Disorder Severity Scale (PDSS) is a clinician-administered questionnaire developed to measure the severity of panic disorder and to monitor treatment outcome (Shear, Brown, Barlow, et al., 1997). The PDSS consists of seven items: panic frequency, distress during panic, panic-focused anticipatory anxiety, phobic avoidance of situations, phobic avoidance of physical sensations, impairment in work functioning, and impairment in social functioning.

ASSESSMENT GUIDELINES

Anxiety Disorders

1. Ensure that a sound physical and neurological examination is performed to help determine whether the anxiety is primary or secondary to another psychiatric disorder, medical condition, or substance use.
2. Assess for substance use (i.e., prescription and nonprescription medication, alcohol consumption, nicotine and caffeine consumption).
3. Determine current level of anxiety (mild, moderate, severe, or panic).
4. Assess for potential for self-harm and suicide; people suffering from high levels of intractable anxiety may become desperate and attempt suicide.
5. Perform a psychosocial assessment. Always ask the person, "What is going on in your life that may be contributing to your anxiety?" The patient may identify a problem that should be addressed by counselling (e.g., stressful marriage, recent loss, stressful job or school situation).
6. Remember that culture can affect how anxiety is manifested.

A useful assessment tool to understand the degree of somatization is the Patient Health Questionnaire–15 (PHQ), a somatic symptom severity scale for the purpose of diagnosis (Figure 12-2). The questionnaire inquires about 15 somatic symptoms (stomach pain, back pain, headache, chest pain, dizziness, fainting, palpitations, shortness of breath, bowel complaints, nausea, fatigue, sleep problems, pain in joints or limbs, menstrual pain, and problems during sexual intercourse) that account for more than 90% of physical complaints reported in the primary care setting by asking patients to rate the severity of symptoms during the previous 4 weeks on a three-point scale (Korber, Frieser, Steinbrecher, et al., 2011). In addition, information should be sought about the patient's ability to meet his or her own basic needs. Rest, comfort, activity, and hygiene needs may be altered as a result of patient problems such as fatigue, weakness, insomnia, muscle tension, pain, and avoidance of diversional activities (hobbies). Safety and security needs may be threatened by patient experiences of blindness, deafness, loss of balance, and anaesthesia of various parts of the body. During assessment, it is important to determine whether symptoms are under the patient's voluntary control. Somatic symptoms *are not* under the individual's voluntary control. Although the relationship between symptoms and interpersonal conflicts may be obvious to others, the patient is not aware of it.

TABLE 12-9 **HAMILTON ANXIETY RATING SCALE**

The symptom inventory provides scaled information that classifies anxiety behaviours and assists the clinician in targeting behaviours and achieving outcome measures. Provide a rating for each indicator based on the following scale: 0 = none; 1 = mild; 2 = moderate; 3 = disabling; 4 = severe, grossly disabling.

ITEM	SYMPTOMS	RATING
1. Anxious mood	Worry, anticipation of the worst, fearful anticipation, irritability	_____
2. Tension	Feelings of tension, fatigability, startle response, moved to tears easily, trembling, feelings of restlessness, inability to relax	_____
3. Fear	Fearful of dark, strangers, being left alone, animals, traffic, crowds	_____
4. Insomnia	Difficulty in falling asleep, broken sleep, unsatisfying sleep and fatigue on waking, dreams, nightmares, night terrors	_____
5. Intellectual (cognitive) manifestations	Difficulty in concentrating, poor memory	_____
6. Depressed mood swings	Loss of interest, lack of pleasure in hobbies, depression, early waking, diurnal	_____
7. Somatic (sensory) symptoms	Tinnitus, blurring of vision, hot and cold flushes, feelings of weakness, picking sensation	_____
8. Somatic (muscular) symptoms	Pains and aches, twitching, stiffness, myoclonic jerks, grinding of teeth, unsteady voice, increased muscular tone	_____
9. Cardiovascular symptoms	Tachycardia, palpitations, skipped beats, pain in chest, throbbing of vessels, fainting feelings	_____
10. Respiratory symptoms	Pressure of constriction in chest, choking feelings, sighing, dyspnea	_____
11. Gastrointestinal symptoms	Difficulty in swallowing, flatulence, abdominal pain, burning sensations, abdominal fullness, nausea, vomiting, borborygmi, looseness of bowels, loss of weight, constipation	_____
12. Genitourinary symptoms	Frequency of urination, urgency of urination, amenorrhea, menorrhagia, development of frigidity, premature ejaculation, loss of libido, impotence	_____
13. Autonomic symptoms	Dry mouth, flushing, pallor, tendency to sweat, giddiness, tension headache, raising of hair	_____
14. Behaviour at interview	Fidgeting, restlessness or pacing, tremor of hands, furrowed brow, strained face, sighing or rapid respiration, facial pallor, swallowing, belching, brisk tendon jerks, dilated pupils, exophthalmos	_____

Scoring:
14–17 = Mild anxiety
18–24 = Moderate anxiety
25–30 = Severe anxiety

Source: Adapted from Hamilton, M. (1959). The assessment of anxiety states by rating. *British Journal of Medical Psychology, 32*, 50–55. doi:10.1111/j.2044-8341.1959.tb00467.x. Copyright © 2011, John Wiley and Sons.

During the past four (4) days how much have you been bothered by . . .		Not bothered at all	Bothered a little	Bothered a lot
1.	Stomach pain	0	1	2
2.	Back pain	0	1	2
3.	Pain in your arms, legs, or joints	0	1	2
4.	Menstrual cramps or other problems with your periods (women)	0	1	2
5.	Headaches	0	1	2
6.	Chest pain	0	1	2
7.	Dizziness	0	1	2
8.	Fainting spells	0	1	2
9.	Feeling your heart pound or race	0	1	2
10.	Shortness of breath	0	1	2
11.	Pain or problems during sexual intercourse	0	1	2
12.	Constipation, loose bowels, or diarrhea	0	1	2
13.	Nausea, gas, or indigestion	0	1	2
14.	Feeling tired or having no energy	0	1	2
15.	Trouble sleeping	0	1	2

Scores of 5 or less indicate mild somatization, 10 or less are moderate somatization, and 15 or more are considered severe indications of somatization.

FIGURE 12-2 Patient Health Questionnaire Somatic Symptom—Short Form (PHQ-SSS) Source: Adapted from Kroenke, K., Spitzer, R. L., Williams, J. B. W., et al. (2010). The patient health questionnaire somatic, anxiety, and depressive symptom scales: A systematic review. *General Hospital Psychiatry, 32*(4), 345–359. doi:10.1016/j.genhosppsych.2010.03.006. Copyright 2010, with permission from Elsevier.

ASSESSMENT GUIDELINES

Somatic Symptom Disorders

1. Assess for nature, location, onset, characteristics, and duration of the symptom(s).
2. Assess the patient's ability to meet basic needs.
3. Assess risks to the safety and security needs of the patient as a result of the symptom(s).
4. Determine whether the symptoms are under the patient's voluntary control.
5. Identify any secondary gains the patient is experiencing from symptom(s).
6. Explore the patient's cognitive style and ability to communicate feelings and needs.
7. Assess the type and amount of medication the patient is using.

Several scales have been developed to assess dissociation, including the Dissociative Experiences Scale (DES) (Bernstein & Putnam, 1986), the Structured Clinical Interview for Dissociative Disorders (SCID-D) (Schlozman & Nonacs, 2008), the Somatoform Dissociation Questionnaire (SDQ) (available at http://www.enijenhuis.nl/sdq/), and the Dissociative Disorders Interview Schedule (DDIS) (available at http://www.rossinst.com/downloads/DDIS-DSM-5.pdf). For a diagnosis of a dissociative disorder to be made, other medical and neurological illnesses, substance use, and other coexisting (comorbid) psychiatric disorders must be ruled out as the cause of the patient's symptoms. Specific information about identity, memory, consciousness, life events, mood, suicide risk, and the impact of the disorder on the patient and the family is important to assess. The assessment should include objective data from physical examination, electroencephalography, imaging studies, and specific questions to identify dissociative symptoms. Assessment tools are important because a psychiatric interview will often miss the presence of dissociation because the individual does not know what he or she does not know—that is, by definition, dissociative periods involve lapses of memory of which the person may not even be aware.

ASSESSMENT GUIDELINES
Dissociative Disorders

1. Assess identity and memory.
   a. Assess for signs of dissociation.
      - Can you remember recent and past events?
      - Is your memory clear and complete or partial and fuzzy?
      - Are you aware of gaps in memory (e.g., lack of memory for events such as a graduation or a wedding)?
      - Do your memories place you with a family, in school, or in an occupation?
      - Do you ever lose time or have blackouts?
      - Do you find yourself in places with no idea how you got there?
   b. Assess for a history of a similar episode in the past with benign outcomes.
      - Have you ever found yourself wearing clothes you cannot remember buying?
   - Have you ever had strange people greet and talk to you as though they were old friends?
   - Does your ability to engage in things such as athletics, artistic activities, or mechanical tasks seem to change?
   - Do you have differing sets of memories about childhood?
2. Determine if there are comorbid medical conditions.
   - Have you sustained a recent injury, such as a concussion?
   - Do you have a history of epilepsy, especially temporal lobe epilepsy?
3. Establish whether the person suffered abuse, trauma, or loss as a child.
4. Evaluate mood and level of anxiety.
5. Identify support systems through a psychosocial assessment.
6. Identify relevant psychosocial distress issues by performing a basic psychosocial assessment.
7. Assess for safety for self and others.

Psychosocial Factors

Psychosocial factors are relevant to anxiety-related symptoms, and the way a patient thinks and feels can have a profound effect on recovery. For example, strong emotions such as fear, anger, sadness, confusion, and guilt can affect a patient's physical, emotional, and spiritual recovery. Patients may feel overwhelmed and alone, and friends and family members may feel helpless and at a loss emotionally. Thus the nurse must complete a psychosocial assessment in tandem with a thorough physical workup and mental status examination (Table 12-10).

Coping Skills

Assessing how a patient has dealt with adversity in the past provides information about the availability of coping skills. Health care workers can also support the patient in gaining additional coping skills that may help him or her better manage.

Spirituality and Religion

Nurses and other health care workers are becoming increasingly aware of the role spirituality or religion plays in many patients' lives and its importance as a source of peace. Support from a priest, pastor, rabbi, imam, or other religious leader may be indicated, especially in a case of spiritual distress. Religious beliefs and practices are forces that can promote resilience. Practising healthy coping depends on the capacity to create meaning from life experiences.

Secondary Gains

The nurse should try to identify secondary gains the patient may be receiving from the symptoms. If a patient derives personal benefit from the symptoms, giving up the symptoms is more difficult unless the patient can achieve the same benefits through healthier avenues, such as learning to communicate more adaptively and to connect with others—skills the clinician can

help the patient learn. One approach to identifying the presence of secondary gains is to ask the patient questions such as the following:
- What are you unable to do now that you used to be able to do?
- How has this problem affected your life?

Self-Assessment

As a nurse working with an individual with an anxiety-related disorder, you may experience uncomfortable personal reactions. You may have feelings of frustration or anger while working with a patient, especially if the symptoms seem to be a matter of choice or under personal control. For example, the rituals of the patient with OCD may hinder your ability to accomplish certain nursing tasks within the usual time. Communicating with such patients can be difficult since patients with a phobia may acknowledge that the fear is exaggerated and unrealistic yet continue to practise avoidant behaviour, which may bewilder the nurse.

It is natural for nurses to experience feelings of scepticism while caring for patients who are diagnosed with dissociative disorders. Believing in the authenticity of the symptoms the patient is displaying can be difficult, and feeling confused and bewildered by the presence of dissociative symptoms is not unusual. Some nurses even experience feelings of fascination and get caught up in the intrigue of caring for a patient with dissociative symptoms.

Unlike the patient who just needs a dressing changed several times a week, the patient with an anxiety-related disorder requires "emotional bandaging" much more often, and behavioural change is often accomplished slowly. When rapid progress is not made, nurses can become impatient. Most people with dissociative disorders have experienced a significant trauma or have been in relationships in which trust was betrayed. As a result, developing a therapeutic relationship with these patients can be a slower

TABLE 12-10   PSYCHOSOCIAL ASSESSMENT OF PATIENTS

AREAS TO ASSESS	SPECIFIC QUESTIONS TO ASK
Social Supports and Cultural Issues	
Family	What were the effects of the patient's illness, treatments, and recovery on the family in the past?
Friends	Who can the patient share painful feelings with?
	Does the patient have friends to joke and laugh with?
	Are there people the patient believes would stand by him or her?
Religious or spiritual beliefs	Does the patient find comfort and support in spiritual practices?
	Is the patient a member of a spiritual or religious group in the community (e.g., church, temple, other place of worship)?
	Does the patient find inner peace and strength in religious or spiritual practices?
	The following statements may be used in performing a spiritual assessment of a patient:
	• I [often/sometimes/seldom] believe that life has value, meaning, and direction.
	• I [often/sometimes/seldom] feel a connection with the universe.
	• I [often/sometimes/seldom] believe in a power greater than myself.
	• I [often/sometimes/seldom] believe that my actions make a difference.
	• I [often/sometimes/seldom] believe that my actions express my true self.
Cultural beliefs	Does the patient use specific culture-oriented treatments or remedies for his or her condition?
	Do the patient's cultural beliefs allow for adequate treatment by Western medical standards?
Work	Are there colleagues at work that the patient can count on for support?
	Have there been any work-related changes or sudden stressful events or occurrences?
Coexisting Physical Conditions Affecting Psychosocial Well-Being	
Physical pain	Is the patient in pain?
	How does the patient cope with the pain?
	Is the pain disabling?
	Are there pain-reducing techniques that might help?
Major illness	Does the patient have a co-occurring major illness that will negatively affect his or her current condition?
	Is the patient undergoing treatments that are affecting daily life more than expected?
	Are there interventions that would help the patient better cope with the sequelae of the illness and treatments?
	Has the patient been hospitalized in the past?
	How many times?
	For what?
	How did the patient cope?
Addictions and mental health	Does the patient have a co-occurring mental health problem (e.g., depression, anxiety, compulsions)?
	Has the patient suffered a mental illness in the past?
	Does the patient participate in any compulsive behaviour (e.g., smoking, overworking, excessive spending, gambling, cybersex)?
	Does the patient abuse substances (e.g., alcohol, drugs [illicit, over-the-counter, prescription])?

process than with patients who have other mental illnesses. Nurses may therefore feel inadequate and frustrated by their efforts. At the very least, they are likely to experience increased tension and fatigue from mental strain. They may also feel anger or frustration and, as a consequence, may withdraw from the patient emotionally and physically. Such negative feelings are easily transmitted to the patient, who then feels increasingly anxious and may also withdraw.

Therefore patience, the ability to provide clear structure, and empathy are important assets when working with patients with anxiety and related disorders. Staging outcomes in small, attainable steps can help prevent the nurse from feeling overwhelmed by the patient's slow progress and help the patient gain a sense of control.

By having a clear understanding of the emotional pitfalls of working with patients who have anxiety and related disorders, a nurse is better prepared to minimize and avoid the guilt associated with strong negative feelings. It is important, then, to examine your personal feelings so you can better understand their origin and respond objectively and constructively.

DIAGNOSIS

The North American Nursing Diagnosis Association International (NANDA-I) provides many nursing diagnoses that can be considered for patients experiencing anxiety and anxiety-related disorders. The "related to" component will vary with the individual patient. Table 12-11 identifies potential nursing diagnoses for the patient experiencing anxiety, Table 12-12 for patients experiencing somatic symptom disorders, Table 12-13 for patients experiencing dissociative disorders, and signs and symptoms that might be found upon assessment to support the diagnosis are included.

OUTCOMES IDENTIFICATION

The *Nursing Outcomes Classification (NOC)* identifies desired outcomes for patients with anxiety or anxiety-related disorders (Moorhead, Johnson, Maas, et al., 2012). Each outcome contains a definition and rating scale to measure the severity of the symptom or the frequency of the desired response. This rating

TABLE 12-11 POTENTIAL DIAGNOSES FOR ANXIETY DISORDERS

SIGNS AND SYMPTOMS	NURSING DIAGNOSES
Concern that a panic attack will occur	Anxiety (moderate, severe, panic)
Exposure to phobic object or situation	Fear
Presence of obsessive thoughts	
Recurrent memories of traumatic event	
Fear of panic attacks	
High levels of anxiety that interfere with the ability to work, disrupt relationships, and change ability to interact with others	Ineffective coping
	Deficient diversional activity
Avoidance behaviours (phobia, agoraphobia)	Social isolation
Hypervigilance after a traumatic event	Ineffective role performance
Inordinate time taken for obsession and compulsions	
Difficulty with concentration	Ineffective health maintenance
Preoccupation with obsessive thoughts	
Disorganization associated with exposure to phobic object	
Intrusive thoughts and memories of traumatic event	Post-trauma syndrome
Excessive use of reason and logic associated with overcautiousness and fear of making a mistake	Decisional conflict
Disruption in sleep related to intrusive thoughts, worrying, replaying of a traumatic event, hypervigilance, fear	Insomnia
	Sleep deprivation
	Fatigue
Feelings of hopelessness, inability to control one's life, low self-esteem related to inability to have some control in one's life	Hopelessness
	Chronic low self-esteem
	Spiritual distress
Inability to perform self-care related to rituals	Self-care deficit
Skin excoriation related to rituals of excessive washing or excessive picking at the skin	Impaired skin integrity
Inability to eat because of constant ritual performance	Imbalanced nutrition: less than body requirements
Feeling of anxiety or excessive worrying that overrides appetite and the need to eat	
Excessive overeating to appease intense worrying or high anxiety levels	Imbalanced nutrition: more than body requirements

TABLE 12-12 POTENTIAL NURSING DIAGNOSES FOR SOMATIC SYMPTOM DISORDERS

SIGNS AND SYMPTOMS	NURSING DIAGNOSES
Inability to meet occupational, family, or social responsibilities because of symptoms	Ineffective coping
Inability to participate in usual community activities or friendships because of psychogenic symptoms	Ineffective role performance
	Impaired social interaction
Dependence on pain relievers	Powerlessness
Distortion of body functions and symptoms	Disturbed body image
Presence of secondary gains by adoption of sick role	Pain, acute or chronic
Inability to meet family role function and need for family to assume role function of the somatic individual	Interrupted family processes
	Ineffective sexuality pattern
Assumption of some of the roles of the somatic parent by the children	Impaired parenting
Shifting of the sexual partner's role to that of caregiver or parent and of the patient's role to that of recipient of care	Risk for caregiver role strain
Feeling of inability to control symptoms or understand why he or she cannot find help	Chronic low self-esteem
Development of negative self-evaluation related to losing body function, feeling useless, or not feeling valued by significant others	Spiritual distress
Inability to take care of basic self-care needs related to conversion symptoms (paralysis, seizures, pain, fatigue)	Self-care deficit
Inability to sleep due to psychogenic pain	Disturbed sleep pattern

scale enables you to evaluate outcomes in the nursing care plan. Some of the *NOC*-recommended outcomes related to anxiety include *Anxiety self-control*, *Anxiety level*, *Stress level*, *Coping*, *Social interaction skills*, and *Symptom control*. Refer to Table 12-14 for examples of intermediate and short-term indicators related to *NOC* outcomes.

Because shared decision making promotes goal attainment, patients should participate in identifying desired outcomes. Outcome criteria must be realistic and attainable. Structuring outcomes in small steps helps the patient and the nurse see concrete evidence of progress. The following are examples of possible outcomes for a patient with a somatic symptom disorder (Ackley, Ladwig, & Makic, 2017):

- Patient will exhibit sensitivity to self-needs and needs of others.
- Patient will resume performance of work, family, and social role behaviours.
- Patient will identify ineffective coping patterns.

- Patient will make realistic appraisal of strengths and weaknesses.
- Patient will assertively verbalize feelings such as anger, shame, or guilt.

PLANNING

Planning for the delivery of specific nursing care is influenced by both the setting (community or inpatients) and the presenting problem. A top priority stated in the report *Changing Directions, Changing Lives: The Mental Health Strategy for Canada* (Mental Health Commission of Canada, 2012) is to identify and integrate mental health needs into primary care settings. Anxiety disorders are encountered in all health care settings. Nurses care for people with coexisting anxiety disorders in medical-surgical units, as well as in homes, day programs, and clinics. Patients with anxiety disorders usually do not require admission to inpatient psychiatric units, so planning for their care may involve selecting interventions that can be implemented in a community setting.

Whenever possible, the patient should be encouraged to participate actively in planning. By including the patient in decision making, you increase the likelihood of positive outcomes. Shared planning is especially appropriate for someone with mild or moderate anxiety. When experiencing severe levels of anxiety, a patient may be unable to participate in planning, and the nurse may be required to take a more directive role.

One of the many advantages of integrating mental health services into primary health care settings is less stigmatization of treatment for mental illness and of people with mental disorders. Because primary health care services are not associated with any specific health conditions, this level of care seems far more "acceptable," and therefore accessible, for most users and families (World Health Organization, 2007). Many primary care centres have psychiatric mental health nurses as part of the regular treatment team, as these nurses can bring a strong perspective in terms of managing both physical and mental health needs in integrated care settings.

Establishing a therapeutic relationship is the first step in delivering effective nursing care. Six key recommendations have been made for developing effective relationships with and treatment for patients with somatic symptom disorders (Kenny & Egan, 2011):

1. Provide continuity of care.
2. Avoid unnecessary tests and procedures.
3. Provide frequent, brief, and regular office visits.
4. Always conduct a physical examination.
5. Avoid making disparaging comments such as "Your symptoms are all in your head."

TABLE 12-13	POTENTIAL NURSING DIAGNOSES FOR DISSOCIATIVE DISORDERS
SIGNS AND SYMPTOMS	**NURSING DIAGNOSES**
Amnesia or fugue related to a traumatic event	*Disturbed personal identity* *Disturbed body image*
Symptoms of depersonalization; feelings of unreality or body-image distortions	
Alterations in consciousness, memory, or identity	*Ineffective coping* *Ineffective role performance*
Abuse of substances related to dissociation	
Disorganization or dysfunction in usual patterns of behaviour (absence from work, withdrawal from relationships, changes in role function)	
Disturbances in memory and identity	*Interrupted family processes* *Impaired parenting*
Interrupted family processes related to amnesia or erratic and changing behaviour	
Feeling of being out of control of memory, behaviours, and awareness	*Anxiety* *Spiritual distress*
Inability to explain actions or behaviours when in altered state	*Risk for other-directed violence* *Risk for self-directed violence*

TABLE 12-14	*NOC* OUTCOMES FOR ANXIETY DISORDERS		
NURSING OUTCOME AND DEFINITION	**INTERMEDIATE INDICATORS**	**SHORT-TERM INDICATORS**
Anxiety self-control: Personal actions to eliminate or reduce feelings of apprehension, tension, or uneasiness from an unidentifiable source	Controls anxiety response Maintains role performance	Monitors intensity of anxiety Uses relaxation techniques to decrease anxiety Decreases environmental stimuli when anxious Maintains adequate sleep
Coping: Personal actions to manage stressors that tax an individual's resources	Identifies multiple coping strategies Modifies lifestyle as needed	Reports decrease in physical symptoms of stress Identifies ineffective coping patterns Verbalizes need for assistance Seeks information concerning illness and treatment
Self-esteem: Personal judgement of self-worth	Describes pride in self Describes success in social groups	Maintains eye contact Maintains grooming and hygiene Accepts self-limitations Accepts compliments from others
Knowledge: Disease process: Extent of understanding conveyed about a specific disease process	Describes usual disease course	Describes signs and symptoms Describes cause or contributing factors Describes signs and symptoms of complications Describes precautions to prevent complications

Source: Moorhead, S., Johnson, M., Maas, M., et al. (2012). *Nursing outcomes classification (NOC)* (5th ed.). St. Louis: Mosby.

6. Set reasonable therapeutic goals such as maintaining function despite ongoing pain.

A phase-oriented treatment model is recommended for individuals with a dissociative disorder for any setting and includes the following (International Society for the Study of Trauma and Dissociation, 2012):

Phase 1: Establishing safety, stabilization, and symptom reduction

Phase 2: Confronting, working through, and integrating traumatic memories

Phase 3: Integrating identity and rehabilitating

The nurse will most often encounter the patient in times of crisis (i.e., when the patient is suicidal or expressing homicidal behaviour), and in times of crisis the care plan will focus on Phase 1 strategies to ensure safety and crisis intervention. Basic nursing interventions should be implemented. Phases 2 and 3 are advanced interventions, so clinicians using these interventions require special training.

IMPLEMENTATION

Determining Levels of Distress

When working with patients with anxiety disorders, you must first determine what level of distress they are experiencing. A general framework for anxiety interventions can then be built on a solid foundation of understanding.

Mild to Moderate Levels of Anxiety

A person experiencing a mild to moderate level of anxiety is still able to solve problems; however, the ability to concentrate decreases as anxiety increases. A patient can be helped to focus and solve problems when you use specific nursing communication techniques, such as asking open-ended questions, giving broad openings, and exploring and seeking clarification. Closing off topics of communication and bringing up irrelevant topics can increase a person's anxiety, making the nurse, but not the patient, feel better.

Reducing the patient's anxiety level and preventing escalation to more distressing levels can be aided by providing a calm presence, recognizing the anxious person's distress, and being willing to listen. Evaluation of effective past coping mechanisms is also useful. Often you can help the patient consider alternatives to problematic situations and offer activities that may temporarily relieve feelings of inner tension. Table 12-15 identifies interventions useful in assisting people experiencing mild to moderate levels of anxiety.

Severe to Panic Levels of Anxiety

A person experiencing a severe to panic level of anxiety is unable to solve problems and may have a poor grasp of what is happening in the environment. Unproductive relief behaviours may take over, and the person may not be in control of his or her actions. Extreme regression and aimless running about are behavioural manifestations of a person's intense psychic pain.

Appropriate nursing interventions are to provide for the safety of the patient and others and to meet physical needs (e.g., fluids, rest) to prevent exhaustion. Anxiety reduction measures may take the form of removing the person to a quiet environment (seclusion room) with minimal stimulation and providing gross motor activities to drain some of the tension. The use of medications may have to be considered, but both medications and a seclusion room should be used only after other more personal

TABLE 12-15 INTERVENTIONS FOR MILD TO MODERATE LEVELS OF ANXIETY	
Nursing diagnosis: *Anxiety (moderate)* related to situational event or psychological stress, as evidenced by increase in vital signs, moderate discomfort, narrowing of perceptual field, and selective inattention	
INTERVENTION	**RATIONALE**
Help the patient identify anxiety: "Are you comfortable right now?"	It is important to validate observations with the patient, name the anxiety, and start to work with the patient to lower anxiety.
Anticipate anxiety-provoking situations.	Escalation of anxiety to a more disorganizing level is prevented.
Use nonverbal language to demonstrate interest (e.g., lean forward, maintain eye contact, nod your head).	Verbal and nonverbal messages should be consistent. The presence of an interested person provides a stabilizing focus.
Encourage the patient to talk about his or her feelings and concerns.	When concerns are stated aloud, problems can be discussed and feelings of isolation decreased.
Avoid closing off avenues of communication that are important for the patient. Focus on the patient's concerns.	When staff anxiety increases, changing the topic or offering advice is a common temptation, but this action isolates the patient.
Ask questions to clarify what is being said: "I'm not sure what you mean. Give me an example."	Increased anxiety results in scattering of thoughts. Clarifying helps the patient identify thoughts and feelings.
Help the patient identify thoughts or feelings before the onset of anxiety. "What were you thinking right before you started to feel anxious?"	The patient is assisted in identifying thoughts and feelings, and problem solving is facilitated.
Encourage problem solving with the patient.*	Encouraging patients to explore alternatives increases sense of control and decreases anxiety.
Assist in developing alternative solutions to a problem through role-play or modelling behaviours.	The patient is encouraged to try out alternative behaviours and solutions.
Explore behaviours that have worked to relieve anxiety in the past.	The patient is encouraged to mobilize successful coping mechanisms and strengths.
Provide outlets for working off excess energy (e.g., walking, playing Ping-Pong, dancing, exercising).	Physical activity can provide relief of built-up tension, increase muscle tone, and increase endorphin levels.

*Patients experiencing mild to moderate anxiety levels can problem-solve.

and less restrictive interventions have failed to decrease anxiety to safer levels. Although a patient's communication may be scattered and disjointed, feeling understood can reduce anxiety and decrease the overwhelming sense of isolation.

Because individuals experiencing severe to panic levels of anxiety are unable to solve problems, the techniques suggested for communicating with people with mild to moderate levels of anxiety may not be effective at more severe levels. These patients are out of control, so they need to know they are safe from their own impulses. Firm, short, and simple statements are useful. Reinforcing what is observable in the environment (e.g., the door, the painting) and pointing out reality when there are distortions can also be useful interventions for severely anxious people. Table 12-16 suggests some basic nursing interventions for patients with severe to panic levels of anxiety.

Anxiety management and reduction are primary concerns when working with patients who have anxiety disorders, but these patients may have a variety of other needs as well. When developing a plan of care, psychiatric mental health nurses can refer to the appropriate standards of practice for their governing body. The *Nursing Interventions Classification (NIC)* offers pertinent interventions in the behavioural and safety domains (Bulechek, Butcher, & Dochterman, 2013) (Box 12-1).

The following are basic nursing interventions:
1. Identify community resources that can offer the patient specialized, effective treatment.
2. Identify community support groups for people with specific anxiety disorders and their families.
3. Use counselling, milieu therapy, promotion of self-care activities, and psychobiological and health teaching interventions as appropriate.

Psychosocial Interventions

People who have distressing symptoms are vulnerable to a variety of psychosocial stresses. How they cope with these stresses may make the difference between living with an acceptable quality of life and experiencing despair, withdrawal, helplessness, hopelessness, and suicidal ideation. Nurses are in a position to assess and understand patients' psychosocial stressors, identify needed coping skills, and teach stress-management techniques. Nurses can play an important role not only in managing patients' immediate care but also in helping patients improve their ability to cope and increase their quality of life during the course of their illness.

Effective coping skills that can be taught are many and varied (e.g., assertiveness training, cognitive reframing, problem-solving skills, social supports). A nurse is in a key position to assess, educate, or provide referrals to a patient to enable healthier ways of looking at and dealing with illness. Consider referring the patient for instruction in relaxation techniques such as reiki, meditation, guided imagery, breathing exercises, and others, or teach the patient some techniques yourself. Behavioural techniques, such

TABLE 12-16	INTERVENTIONS FOR SEVERE TO PANIC LEVELS OF ANXIETY
Nursing diagnosis: *Anxiety (severe, panic)* related to severe threat (biochemical, environmental, psychosocial), as evidenced by verbal or physical acting out, extreme immobility, sense of impending doom, inability to differentiate reality (possible hallucinations or delusions), and inability to problem-solve	
INTERVENTION	**RATIONALE**
Maintain a calm manner.	Anxiety is communicated interpersonally. The quiet calm of the nurse can serve to calm the patient. The presence of anxiety can escalate anxiety in the patient.
Always remain with the person experiencing an acute severe to panic level of anxiety.	Alone with immense anxiety, a person feels abandoned. A caring face may be the patient's only contact with reality when confusion becomes overwhelming.
Minimize environmental stimuli. Move to a quieter setting and stay with the patient.	A quieter setting helps minimize further escalation of anxiety.
Use clear and simple statements and repetition.	A person experiencing a severe to panic level of anxiety has difficulty concentrating and processing information.
Use a low-pitched voice; speak slowly.	A high-pitched voice can convey anxiety. A low pitch can decrease anxiety.
Reinforce reality if distortions occur (e.g., seeing objects that are not there or hearing voices when no one is present).	Anxiety can be reduced by focusing on and validating what is going on in the environment.
Listen for themes in communication.	In severe to panic levels of anxiety, verbal communication themes may be the only indication of the patient's thoughts or feelings.
Attend to physical and safety needs (e.g., warmth, fluids, elimination, pain relief, family contact) when necessary.	High levels of anxiety may obscure the patient's awareness of physical needs.
Because safety is an overall goal, physical limits may need to be set. Speak in a firm, authoritative voice: "You may not hit anyone here. If you can't control yourself, we will help you."	A person who is out of control is often terrorized. Staff must offer the patient and others protection from destructive and self-destructive impulses.
Provide opportunities for exercise (e.g., walk with nurse, punching bag, Ping-Pong game).	Physical activity helps channel and dissipate tension and may temporarily lower anxiety.
When a person is constantly moving or pacing, offer high-calorie fluids.	Dehydration and exhaustion must be prevented.
Assess need for medication or seclusion after other interventions have been tried but have not been successful.	Exhaustion and physical harm to self and others must be prevented.

BOX 12-1 *NIC* INTERVENTIONS FOR ANXIETY DISORDERS

Coping Enhancement

Definition of coping enhancement: Assistance provided to a patient in adapting to perceived stressors, changes, or threats that interfere with meeting life demands and roles.

Activities*:
- Provide an atmosphere of acceptance.
- Encourage verbalization of feelings, perceptions, and fears.
- Acknowledge the patient's spiritual or cultural background.
- Discourage decision making when the patient is under severe stress.

Hope Inspiration

Definition of hope inspiration: Enhancement of the belief in one's capacity to initiate and sustain actions.

Activities*:
- Assist the patient to identify areas of hope in life.
- Demonstrate hope by recognizing the patient's intrinsic worth and viewing the patient's illness as only one facet of the individual.
- Avoid masking the truth.
- Help the patient expand the spiritual self.

Self-Esteem Enhancement

Definition of self-esteem enhancement: Assistance provided to a patient in increasing his or her personal judgement of self-worth.

Activities*:
- Make positive statements about the patient.
- Monitor frequency of self-negating verbalizations.
- Explore previous achievements.
- Explore reasons for self-criticism or guilt.

Relaxation Therapy

Definition of relaxation therapy: The use of techniques to encourage and elicit relaxation for the purpose of decreasing undesirable signs and symptoms such as pain, muscle tension, or anxiety.

Activities*:
- Demonstrate and practise the relaxation technique with the patient.
- Provide written information about preparing and engaging in relaxation techniques.
- Anticipate the need for the use of relaxation.
- Evaluate and document the response to relaxation therapy.

*Partial list.
Source: Bulechek, G. M., Butcher, H. K., & Dochterman, J. M. (2013). *Nursing interventions classification (NIC)* (6th ed.). Toronto: Elsevier.

as progressive muscle relaxation and biofeedback (which nurses can get special training to perform), are also useful. Relaxation techniques, stress-management skills, and supportive education should be part of patient care, regardless of the comorbid conditions.

The following interventions have all been shown to positively affect a patient's recovery:
- Educating the patient about specific treatments
- Referring the patient to community support groups (or systems)
- Teaching patients more effective coping skills that take into consideration patients' values, preferences, and lifestyle
- Focusing on a patient's strengths and reinforcing coping skills that work (e.g., prayerfulness, participation in hobbies, relaxation techniques)

To be successful, therapeutic interventions must address patient needs. The primary goal is to help patients identify ways to get their needs met without using harmful defence mechanisms or having pathological behaviour reinforced. The secondary gains derived from illness behaviours become less important to the patient when underlying needs can be met directly. Table 12-17 provides basic-level interventions for somatic symptom disorders. *Reattribution treatment*, an advanced nursing treatment approach also used with the treatment of somatization (Box 12-2), helps toward this goal.

Refer to Table 12-18 for examples of basic-level interventions for individuals experiencing a dissociative disorder.

Counselling

Psychiatric mental health nurses use counselling to reduce anxiety, enhance coping and communication skills, and intervene in crises.

From a behaviourist perspective, when appropriate, relaxation training would occur during the counselling session. The training would include teaching relaxation exercises used to relax breathing or muscle groups. The relaxation response is the opposite of the stress response and results in a reduced heart rate, slower breathing, and relaxed muscles. Refer to Chapter 5 for a description of different approaches to relaxation training. When psychiatric mental health nurses begin to practise from a cognitive therapy perspective, they will help patients identify that what they think is linked with what they feel.

Health Teaching and Health Promotion

Health teaching is a significant nursing intervention for patients with anxiety disorders. Patients may conceal symptoms for years before seeking treatment and often come to the attention of health care providers because of a co-occurring problem. Three out of every five individuals with an anxiety disorder do not consult a health care provider about their disorder (Public Health Agency of Canada, 2016). And those who do often wait years before getting medical attention.

Teaching about the specific disorder and available effective treatments is a major step toward improving the quality of life for those with anxiety disorders. Whether in a community or hospital setting, nurses can teach patients about signs and symptoms of anxiety disorders, presumed causes or risk factors (especially substance abuse), medications, the use of relaxation techniques, and the benefits of psychotherapy. When patients request or prefer to use integrative therapies, the nurse performs assessment and teaching as appropriate.

Some patients who somatize as a way of coping with anxiety may benefit from education about body functions. The type and

TABLE 12-17   BASIC-LEVEL INTERVENTIONS FOR SOMATIC SYMPTOM DISORDERS

INTERVENTION	RATIONALE
Offer explanations and support during diagnostic testing.	Reduces anxiety while ruling out organic illness
After physical complaints have been investigated, avoid further reinforcement (e.g., do not take vital signs each time patient complains of palpitations).	Directs focus away from physical symptoms
Spend time with patient at times other than when patient summons nurse to voice physical complaint.	Rewards non–illness-related behaviours and encourages repetition of desired behaviour
Observe and record frequency and intensity of somatic symptoms. (Patient or family can give information.)	Establishes a baseline and later enables evaluation of effectiveness of interventions
Do not imply that symptoms are not real.	Acknowledges that psychogenic symptoms are real to the patient
Shift focus from somatic complaints to feelings or to neutral topics.	Conveys interest in patient as a person rather than in patient's symptoms; reduces need to gain attention via symptoms
Assess secondary gains "physical illness" provides for patient (e.g., attention, increased dependency, distraction from another problem).	Allows these needs to be met in healthier ways and thus minimizes secondary gains
Use matter-of-fact approach to patient exhibiting resistance or covert anger.	Avoids power struggles; demonstrates acceptance of anger and permits discussion of angry feelings
Have patient direct all requests to primary nurse.	Reduces manipulation
Help patient look at effect of illness behaviour on others.	Encourages insight; can help improve family relationships
Show concern for patient while avoiding fostering dependency needs.	Shows respect for patient's feelings while minimizing secondary gains from "illness"
Reinforce patient's strengths and problem-solving abilities.	Contributes to positive self-esteem; helps patient realize that needs can be met without resorting to somatic symptoms
Teach assertive communication.	Provides patient with a positive means of getting needs met; reduces feelings of helplessness and need for manipulation
Teach patient stress-reduction techniques, such as meditation, relaxation, and mild physical exercise.	Provides alternative coping strategies; reduces need for medication

TABLE 12-18   NURSING INTERVENTIONS FOR DISSOCIATIVE DISORDERS

INTERVENTION	RATIONALE
Ensure patient safety by providing safe, protected environment and frequent observation.	Patient's sense of bewilderment may lead to inattention to safety needs
Provide undemanding, simple routine.	Reduces anxiety
Confirm identity of patient and orientation to time and place.	Supports reality and promotes ego integrity
Encourage patient to do things for self and make decisions about routine tasks.	Enhances self-esteem by reducing sense of powerlessness and reduces secondary gain associated with dependence
Assist with other decision making until memory returns.	Lowers stress and prevents patient from having to live with the consequences of unwise decisions
Support patient during exploration of feelings surrounding the stressful event.	Helps lower the defence of dissociation used by patient to block awareness of the stressful event
Do not flood patient with data regarding past events.	Memory loss serves the purpose of preventing severe to panic levels of anxiety from overtaking and disorganizing the individual
Allow patient to progress at own pace as memory is recovered.	Prevents undue anxiety and resistance
Provide support during disclosure of painful experiences. Do not force the patient to disclose.	Can be healing, while minimizing feelings of isolation Forced disclosure can retraumatize the patient
Help patients see consequences of using dissociation to cope with stress.	Increases insight and helps patient understand own role in choosing behaviours
Accept patient's expression of negative feelings.	Conveys permission to have negative or unacceptable feelings
Teach stress-reduction methods.	Provides alternatives for anxiety relief
If patient does not remember significant others, work with involved parties to re-establish relationships.	Helps patient experience satisfaction and relieves sense of isolation

depth of teaching is determined by the information the patient already understands. Others may know extensively about their physical. In these situations, the teaching would focus on accurately assessing and interpreting the body's responses to digestion, stress, fatigue, and excitement.

Stress management and coping skills are important areas of health education for people with dissociative disorders. Normalizing experiences by explaining that symptoms are adaptive responses to past overwhelming events is important. Often the victim of childhood trauma feels as if he or she is a bad person

BOX 12-2	REATTRIBUTION TREATMENT TO LINK PHYSICAL COMPLAINTS AND PSYCHOLOGICAL DISTRESS: AN EXAMPLE OF AN ADVANCED-LEVEL INTERVENTION

Reattribution treatment is a structured intervention designed to provide a simple explanation of somatic symptoms to patients. Health care providers with reattribution skills help patients feel understood and help them make the link between physical complaints and psychological distress.

Reattribution has four stages:

Stage 1: Feeling Understood
The health care provider uses empathetic listening skills in taking the history of physical, emotional, spiritual, and social factors of the presenting symptoms, including patient beliefs about and perceptions of the cause of illness, times when it is worse, and what helps improve symptoms. This stage includes a brief, focused physical examination.

Stage 2: Broadening the Agenda
The health care provider gives feedback of assessment findings, discusses the implications of the findings, and acknowledges the patient's distress.

Stage 3: Making the Link
The health care provider uses empowering explanations for symptoms—for example, "You may have a heightened sensitivity to particular stressors that is affected by genetics, your personal experiences, and the environment." This comment is patient centred and does not blame the patient for the symptoms (Fuller-Thomson, Sulman, Brennenstuhl, et al., 2011).

Stage 4: Negotiating Further Treatment
The health care provider and the patient collaboratively create a treatment plan that includes regular follow-up visits and short-term and long-term goals.

Source: Adapted from Walters, P., Tylee, A., Fisher, J., et al. (2007). Teaching junior doctors to manage patients who somatise: Is it possible in an afternoon? *Medical Education, 41*, 995–1001. doi:10.1111/j.1365-2923.2007.02833.x. Copyright © 2007, John Wiley and Sons.

and grows up with the false negative belief that the abuse was deserved punishment.

Another important intervention strategy is to teach grounding techniques that help the person focus on the present and help to counter dissociative symptoms. Examples of grounding techniques include stomping one's feet on the ground, taking a shower, holding an ice cube, exercising, breathing deeply, counting beads, and touching fabric or upholstery on a chair. Patients can also be taught to keep a daily journal to increase their awareness of feelings and to identify triggers of their dissociative symptoms. If a patient has never written a journal, the nurse should suggest beginning with 5 to 10 minutes of daily writing.

Milieu Therapy

As mentioned earlier, most patients with anxiety disorders can be treated successfully as outpatients. Hospital admission is necessary only if severe anxiety or symptoms interfere with the individual's health or if the individual is suicidal. When hospitalization is necessary, providing a safe environment is fundamental. Other characteristics of a therapeutic milieu that can be especially helpful to the patient are:

- Structuring the daily routine to offer physical safety and predictability, thus reducing anxiety over the unknown
- Providing daily activities to promote sharing and cooperation
- Providing therapeutic interactions, including one-on-one nursing care and behaviour contracts
- Including the patient in decisions about his or her own care

Promotion of Self-Care Activities

Patients with anxiety disorders are usually able to meet their own basic physical needs. Individuals with a somatic symptom disorder may require more assistance with self-care activities due to the physical limitations of their illness. Self-care activities that are most likely to be affected are discussed in the following sections.

Nutrition and Fluid Intake

Patients who engage in ritualistic behaviours may be too involved with their rituals to take time to eat and drink. Some phobic patients may be so afraid of germs, they cannot eat. In general, nutritious diets with snacks should be provided. Adequate intake should be firmly encouraged, but a power struggle should be avoided. Weighing patients frequently (e.g., three times a week) is useful in assessing whether nutrition needs are being met.

Personal Hygiene and Grooming

Some patients, especially those with OCD and phobias, may be excessively neat and engage in time-consuming rituals associated with bathing and dressing. Hygiene, dressing, and grooming may take several hours. Maintenance of skin integrity may become a problem when the rituals involve excessive washing and skin becomes excoriated and infected.

Some patients are indecisive about bathing or about what clothing should be worn. For the latter, limiting choices to two outfits is helpful. In the event of severe indecisiveness, simply presenting the patient with the clothing to be worn may be necessary. You may also need to remain with the patient to give simple directions: "Put on your shirt. Now put on your slacks." Matter-of-fact support is effective in assisting patients to perform as much of a task as possible independently. Encourage patients to express thoughts and feelings about self-care. This communication can provide a basis for later health teaching or for ongoing dialogue about the patient's abilities.

Elimination

Patients with OCD may be so involved with the performance of rituals that they may suppress the urge to void and defecate, sometimes resulting in constipation or urinary tract infections. Interventions may include creating a regular schedule for taking the patient to the bathroom.

✎ DRUG TREATMENT OF PATIENTS WITH ANXIETY DISORDERS

GENERIC (TRADE)	HEALTH CANADA–APPROVED USES	OFF-LABEL USES
Antidepressants		
Selective Serotonin Reuptake Inhibitors		
Citalopram hydrobromide (Celexa)		Panic disorder Social anxiety disorder Obsessive-compulsive disorder Generalized anxiety disorder Post-traumatic stress disorder
Escitalopram oxalate (Cipralex)	Generalized anxiety disorder	Panic disorder Social anxiety disorder Obsessive-compulsive disorder Post-traumatic stress disorder
Fluoxetine hydrochloride (Prozac)	Obsessive-compulsive disorder	Social anxiety disorder Generalized anxiety disorder Panic disorder Post-traumatic stress disorder
Fluvoxamine maleate (Luvox)	Obsessive-compulsive disorder Social anxiety disorder	Panic disorder Generalized anxiety disorder Post-traumatic stress disorder
Paroxetine hydrochloride (Paxil)	Panic disorder Social anxiety disorder Obsessive-compulsive disorder Generalized anxiety disorder Post-traumatic stress disorder	
Sertraline hydrochloride (Zoloft)	Panic disorder Social anxiety disorder Obsessive-compulsive disorder Post-traumatic stress disorder	Generalized anxiety disorder
Selective Serotonin–Norepinephrine Reuptake Inhibitors		
Duloxetine hydrochloride (Cymbalta)	Panic disorder Generalized anxiety disorder	Obsessive-compulsive disorder Post-traumatic stress disorder
Venlafaxine hydrochloride (Effexor XR)	Generalized anxiety disorder Social anxiety disorder Panic disorder	Obsessive-compulsive disorder Post-traumatic stress disorder
Tricyclics		
Amitriptyline hydrochloride (Elavil)		Panic disorder Generalized anxiety disorder Post-traumatic stress disorder
Clomipramine hydrochloride (Anafranil)	Obsessive-compulsive disorder	Panic disorder Generalized anxiety disorder Post-traumatic stress disorder
Desipramine hydrochloride (Norpramin)		Panic disorder Generalized anxiety disorder Post-traumatic stress disorder
Doxepin hydrochloride (Adapin, Sinequan)		Panic disorder Generalized anxiety disorder Post-traumatic stress disorder
Imipramine hydrochloride (Tofranil)		Panic disorder Generalized anxiety disorder Post-traumatic stress disorder
Nortriptyline hydrochloride (Aventyl, Norventyl)		Panic disorder Generalized anxiety disorder Post-traumatic stress disorder

DRUG TREATMENT OF PATIENTS WITH ANXIETY DISORDERS—cont'd

GENERIC (TRADE)	HEALTH CANADA–APPROVED USES	OFF-LABEL USES
Monoamine Oxidase Inhibitors		
Phenelzine sulphate (Nardil)		Panic disorder
		Social anxiety disorder
		Generalized anxiety disorder
		Post-traumatic stress disorder
Tranylcypromine sulphate (Parnate)		Panic disorder
		Social anxiety disorder
		Generalized anxiety disorder
		Post-traumatic stress disorder
Antianxiety Agents		
Benzodiazepines		
Alprazolam (Xanax)	Panic disorder	Social anxiety disorder
	Generalized anxiety disorder	
Chlordiazepoxide hydrochloride (Librax)		Panic disorder
		Social anxiety disorder
		Generalized anxiety disorder
Clonazepam (Rivotril)	Panic disorder	Generalized anxiety disorder
		Social anxiety disorder
Diazepam (Valium)	Generalized anxiety disorder	Panic disorder
		Social anxiety disorder
Lorazepam (Ativan)		Panic disorder
		Social anxiety disorder
		Generalized anxiety disorder
Oxazepam (Serax)		Panic disorder
		Social anxiety disorder
		Generalized anxiety disorder
Nonbenzodiazepines		
Buspirone hydrochloride (Bustab)	Generalized anxiety disorder	Social anxiety disorder
		Obsessive-compulsive disorder
Other Classes		
Antihistamines		
Hydroxyzine hydrochloride (Atarax)		Generalized anxiety disorder
Hydroxyzine pamoate (Vistaril)		Generalized anxiety disorder
Beta Blockers		
Atenolol (Tenormin)		Social anxiety disorder
Propranolol (Inderal)		Social anxiety disorder
Anticonvulsants		
Carbamazepine (Tegretol)		Post-traumatic stress disorder
		Panic disorder
Gabapentin (Neurontin)		Panic disorder
		Social anxiety disorder
		Generalized anxiety disorder
		Post-traumatic stress disorder
Valproic acid (Depakote)		Panic disorder
		Social anxiety disorder
		Generalized anxiety disorder
		Post-traumatic stress disorder

Sources: Health Canada. (2016). *Drug product database (DPD)*. Retrieved from http://www.hc-sc.gc.ca/dhp-mps/index-eng.php; and Schatzberg, A. F. (2017). *Textbook of psychopharmacology* (*DSM-5* ed.). Arlington, VA: American Psychiatric Association Publishing.

Sleep

Patients experiencing anxiety frequently have difficulty sleeping. They may perform rituals to the exclusion of resting and sleeping, causing physical exhaustion. Those with GAD, PTSD, and acute stress disorder often experience sleep disturbance from nightmares. Teaching patients ways to promote sleep (e.g., warm bath, warm milk, relaxing music) and monitoring sleep through a sleep record are useful interventions. Chapter 20 offers an in-depth discussion of sleep disturbances.

Pharmacological Interventions

Several classes of medications have been found to be effective in the treatment of anxiety disorders. The Drug Treatment box identifies medications approved by Health Canada for the treatment of anxiety, as well as medications that do not have specific approval but are commonly used "off-label" for anxiety-related disorders. Review Chapter 11 for more detailed explanations of the actions of psychotropic medications.

Researchers are currently investigating the effectiveness of medications for the treatment of somatic symptom disorders. Medication trials with antidepressants (including serotonin–norepinephrine reuptake inhibitors (SNRIs), such as venlafaxine (Effexor XR) and duloxetine (Cymbalta), and a noradrenergic and specific serotonergic antidepressant, such as mirtazapine (Remeron), have been effective in reducing the somatic symptoms, but further controlled trials are needed to determine the most effective antidepressants (Garcia-Martin, Miranda-Vicario, & Soutullo, 2012). Patients may also benefit from short-term use of antianxiety medication, which must be monitored carefully because of the risk for dependence.

There are no specific medications used to treat patients with dissociative disorders, but medications are often prescribed for the presenting symptoms (International Society for the Study of Trauma and Dissociation, 2012). In the acute care setting, intravenous benzodiazepines may be used to decrease intense anxiety; subsequently, the nurse may witness dramatic memory retrieval in patients with dissociative amnesia or fugue. Other medications sometimes prescribed are antidepressants, anxiolytics, and antipsychotics. As is the case whenever medications are prescribed, substance use disorders and potential suicidal risk must be assessed carefully prior to selecting a safe and appropriate medication.

Antidepressants

Antidepressants prescribed for anxiety have the secondary benefit of treating comorbid depressive disorders. Selective serotonin reuptake inhibitors (SSRIs) are the first-line treatment for acute stress disorders and PTSD (Schatzberg, 2017). Some of the SSRIs, however, exert more of an "activating" effect than others and therefore may increase anxiety. Sertraline (Zoloft) and paroxetine (Paxil) seem to have a more calming effect than do other SSRIs. SSRIs are preferable to the tricyclic antidepressants (TCAs) because they have a more rapid onset of action and fewer problematic adverse effects.

Monoamine oxidase inhibitors (MAOIs) are reserved for treatment-resistant conditions because of the risk for life-threatening hypertensive crisis in patients who do not follow dietary restrictions (e.g., to not eat foods containing tyramine). The risk for hypertensive crisis also makes the use of MAOIs contraindicated in patients with comorbid substance abuse.

Antianxiety Drugs

Antianxiety drugs (also called anxiolytics) are often used to treat the somatic and psychological symptoms of anxiety disorders (Schatzberg, 2017). When moderate or severe anxiety is reduced, patients are better able to participate in treatment of any underlying problems. Benzodiazepines are most commonly used because they have a quick onset of action. However, due to the potential for dependence, these medications ideally should be used for short periods, only until other medications or treatments reduce symptoms. An important nursing intervention is to monitor for adverse effects of the benzodiazepines, including sedation, ataxia, and decreased cognitive function. Benzodiazepines are not recommended for patients with a known substance abuse problem and should not be given to women during pregnancy or breastfeeding. Other important information for patients and their families is outlined in the Patient and Family Teaching box.

🖐 PATIENT AND FAMILY TEACHING
Antianxiety Medications

1. Caution the patient:
   - Not to increase dose or frequency of ingestion without prior approval of doctor
   - That these medications reduce the ability to handle mechanical equipment (e.g., cars, machinery)
   - Not to drink alcoholic beverages or take other antianxiety drugs, because depressant effects of both would be potentiated
   - To avoid drinking beverages containing caffeine, because they decrease the desired effects of the drug
2. Recommend that the patient taking benzodiazepines avoid becoming pregnant, because these drugs increase the risk of congenital anomalies.
3. Advise the patient not to breastfeed while taking benzodiazepines, because these drugs are excreted in the milk and would have adverse effects on the infant.
4. Teach a patient who is taking monoamine oxidase inhibitors the details of a tyramine-restricted diet.
5. Teach the patient that:
   - Cessation of benzodiazepines after 3 to 4 months of daily use may cause withdrawal symptoms such as insomnia, irritability, nervousness, dry mouth, tremors, convulsions, and confusion
   - Medications should be taken with or shortly after meals or snacks to reduce gastrointestinal discomfort
   - Drug interactions can occur: antacids may delay absorption; cimetidine interferes with metabolism of benzodiazepines, causing increased sedation; central nervous system depressants, such as alcohol and barbiturates, cause increased sedation; serum phenytoin concentration may build up because of decreased metabolism

Buspirone (BuSpar) is an alternative antianxiety medication that does not cause dependence, but 2 to 4 weeks are required for it to reach full effect. The drug may be used for long-term treatment and should be taken regularly.

Other Classes of Medications

Other classes of medications sometimes used to treat anxiety disorders include beta blockers, antihistamines, and anticonvulsants. These agents are often added if the first course of treatment is ineffective. Beta blockers block the nerves that stimulate the heart to beat faster and have been used to treat social anxiety disorder (SAD). Anticonvulsants have shown some benefit in the management of GAD, PD, PTSD, and SAD (Schatzberg, 2017). Antihistamines are a safe, nonaddictive alternative to benzodiazepines to lower anxiety levels, and again are helpful in treating patients with substance abuse problems.

Another therapeutic strategy may come in a most unusual form: D-cycloserine, an antibiotic used to treat tuberculosis, has also been demonstrated to enhance learning. D-cycloserine binds with N-methyl-D-aspartate (NMDA) receptors in the amygdala, the area of the brain that mediates fears and phobic responses, and may help patients unlearn fear responses more quickly. Administering this drug to a patient undergoing cognitive behavioural therapy actually promotes fear extinction, not just fear conditioning, in phobic individuals. It has also been useful when combined with extinction-based exposure therapy in the treatment of OCD and SAD (Rodrigues, Figueira, Lopes, et al., 2014).

Integrative Therapy

Chapter 35 identifies a number of complementary practices or integrative therapies that people use to cope with stress in their lives. Herbal and complementary therapy is popular in Canada; however, herbs and dietary supplements are not subject to the same rigorous testing as prescription medications. Also, herbs and dietary supplements are not required to be uniform, and there is no guaranteed bioequivalence of the active compound among preparations.

Problems that can occur with the use of psychotropic herbs include toxic adverse effects and herb–drug interactions. Nurses and other health care providers do well to improve their knowledge of these products so that discussions with their patients provide informed and reliable information. The Integrative Therapy box discusses kava kava, an herb often used for its sedative and antianxiety effects.

Advanced Interventions

Advanced-practice nurses may use various types of psychotherapy or provide consultation to primary care providers who treat patients with anxiety and related disorders. Because nursing has as a major focus viewing the patient in a holistic way, the advanced-practice nurse can lead the health care team in assessing each patient's unique biological, environmental, psychological, spiritual, and sociocultural needs to develop the most comprehensive, individualized plan of care to alleviate the distress of symptoms. Advanced-practice nurses build on basic nursing interventions and use more complex cognitive and behavioural

⚙ INTEGRATIVE THERAPY

Kava Kava

Kava kava is prepared from a South Pacific plant (*Piper methysticum*) and is marketed as an herbal sedative with antianxiety effects. Prior to seeking psychiatric treatment, patients with anxiety disorders may try kava kava in the belief that herbs are safer than medications, but it may have a darker side.

Kava kava is known to dramatically inhibit a liver enzyme (P450) necessary for the metabolism of many medications. This inhibition could result in liver failure, especially when taken along with alcohol or other medications such as central nervous system depressants (antianxiety agents fall into this category). This potentially dangerous interaction highlights the need for the nurse to ask about all medications the patient is taking—both prescribed and over-the-counter—before administering medications to those with anxiety disorders. Several countries have actually taken kava kava off the market, but some researchers believe that the benefits of this drug may outweigh the risks, compared to other medications used to treat anxiety.

The bottom line is that kava kava is considered to be beneficial for short-term use for mild to moderate anxiety. However, as with any drug, it should be used carefully.

Source: Chua, H. C., Christensen, E. T., Hoestgaard-Jensen, K., et al. (2016). Kavain, the major constituent of the anxiolytic kava extract, potentiates GABAA receptors: Functional characteristics and molecular mechanism. *PLoS ONE, 11*(6), e0157700. doi:10.1371/journal. pone.0157700.

treatment strategies, including modelling, systematic desensitization, flooding, response prevention, and thought stopping.

Managing both psychiatric and physical symptoms can be a challenge for general medical nurses. Psychiatric liaison nurses, a subspecialty of psychiatric mental health nursing initiated in the early 1960s, can bridge that gap. Usually the psychiatric liaison nurse has a master's degree and a background in psychiatric and medical-surgical nursing. He or she functions as a consultant assisting other nurses in managing psychiatric symptoms and as a clinician working directly to help the patient deal more effectively with physical and emotional problems. The psychiatric liaison nurse first meets with the nurse who initiated the consultation and then reviews the patient's medical records, talks with the physicians, and interviews the patient. After the patient interview, the liaison nurse discusses the assessment and suggestions with the referring nurse. If a psychiatric consultation is warranted, the psychiatric liaison nurse initiates the consultation by contacting the patient's physician. The liaison nurse will support general practice nurses to learn how to deliver more advanced intervention. A case conference is sometimes needed to enhance communication and consistency in the care of a particular patient.

Behavioural Therapy

Beyond basic interventions there are several forms of behavioural therapy currently used to decrease anxious or avoidant behaviour:

- **Modelling**—The therapist or significant other acts as a role model to demonstrate appropriate behaviour in a feared situation, and then the patient imitates it. For example, the role model rides in an elevator with a claustrophobic patient.

- **Systematic desensitization**—The patient is gradually introduced to a feared object or experience through a series of steps, from the least frightening to the most frightening (graduated exposure). The patient is taught to use a relaxation technique at each step when anxiety becomes overwhelming. For example, a patient with agoraphobia would start with opening the door to the house to go out on the steps and advance to attending a movie in a theatre. The therapist may start with imagined situations in the office before moving on to in vivo (real-life) exposures.
- **Flooding**—Unlike systematic desensitization, flooding exposes the patient to a large amount of an undesirable stimulus in an effort to extinguish the anxiety response. The patient learns through prolonged exposure that survival is possible and that anxiety diminishes spontaneously. For example, an obsessive patient who usually touches objects with a paper towel may be forced to touch objects with a bare hand for 1 hour. By the end of that period, the anxiety level is lower.
- **Response prevention**—Patients with compulsive behaviour are not allowed to perform the compulsive ritual (e.g., handwashing), and the patient learns that anxiety subsides even when the ritual is not completed. After trying this activity in the office, the patient learns to set time limits at home to gradually lengthen the time between rituals until the urge fades away.
- **Thought stopping**—With this technique, a negative thought or obsession is interrupted. The patient may be instructed to say "Stop!" out loud when the idea comes to mind or to snap a rubber band worn on the wrist. This distraction briefly blocks the automatic undesirable thought and cues the patient to select an alternative, more positive idea. (After learning the exercise, the patient gives the command silently.)

Cognitive Therapy

Advanced forms of cognitive therapy will build on the basic intervention of establishing that our thoughts have a link to our emotions. For example, "I have to be perfect or my boyfriend will not love me." Through a process called *cognitive restructuring*, the therapist helps the patient to (1) identify automatic negative beliefs that cause anxiety, (2) explore the basis for these thoughts, (3) re-evaluate the situation realistically, and (4) replace negative self-talk with supportive ideas.

Cognitive Behavioural Therapy

Cognitive behavioural therapy (CBT) is the most consistently supported treatment for the full spectrum of anxiety and related disorders. CBT combines cognitive therapy with specific behavioural therapies to reduce the anxiety responses and distress. CBT includes a combination of cognitive restructuring, psycho-education, breathing, muscle relaxation, teaching of self-monitoring for symptoms, and in vivo (real-life) exposure to feared objects or situations. Refer to Chapter 4 for a more complete explanation of CBT.

Somatic Therapy

Verbal and body psychotherapies are seen as complementary interventions. Dance movement therapists work with traumatized dissociative patients in emotional recovery (Koch & Harvey, 2012). A specific type of somatic psychotherapy, sensorimotor psychotherapy, combines talking therapy with body-centred interventions and movement to address the dissociative symptoms inherent in trauma (Ogden & Fisher, 2015). This type of therapy is integrated into phase-oriented trauma treatment to facilitate symptom reduction and stability, to integrate the traumatic memory, and to restore the person's ability to stay in the present moment. This therapy is based on the premise that the body, mind, emotions, and spirit are interrelated, and that a change at one level results in changes at the others. Being aware, focusing on the present, and recognizing touch as a means of communicating are some of the principles of this therapy. During psychotherapy sessions, the patient is asked to describe physical sensations he or she is experiencing. The goal is to safely disarm the pathological defence mechanism of dissociation and replace it with other resources, especially body awareness and mindfulness.

EVALUATION

Evaluation of patients with anxiety-related disorders is a simple process when measurable behavioural outcomes have been written clearly and realistically. Each *NOC* outcome has a built-in rating scale that helps the nurse measure improvement. In general, evaluation of outcomes for patients with anxiety disorders deals with questions such as the following:

- Has patient safety been maintained?
- Is the patient experiencing a reduced level of anxiety or distress?
- Does the patient recognize symptoms as anxiety related?
- Does the patient continue to display obsessions, compulsions, phobias, worrying, or other symptoms of anxiety disorders? If still present, are they more or less frequent? More or less intense?
- Is the patient able to use newly learned behaviours to manage their symptoms?
- Can the patient adequately perform self-care activities?
- Can the patient maintain satisfying interpersonal relations?
- Can the patient assume usual roles?

CASE STUDY AND NURSING CARE PLAN 12-1

Severe Level of Anxiety

The following case study describes a man experiencing a severe level of acute anxiety. See if you can match his signs and symptoms with those in Table 12-1.

Ted Silvestri, a 63-year-old man, comes into the emergency department (ED) with his wife, Julie, who has taken an overdose of sleeping pills and antidepressant medications. Ten years earlier, Julie's mother died, and since that time Julie has suffered several episodes of severe depression with suicide attempts. She has needed hospitalization during these episodes. Julie had been released from the hospital 2 weeks earlier after treatment for depression and threatened suicide.

Ted has a long-established routine of giving his wife her antidepressant medications in the morning and her sleeping medication at night and keeping the bottles hidden when he is not at home. Today he had forgotten to hide the medications before he went to work. His wife had taken the remaining pills from both bottles with large quantities of alcohol. When Ted returned home for lunch, Julie was comatose. In the ED, Julie suffers cardiac arrest and is taken to the intensive care unit (ICU).

Ted appears very jittery. He moves about the room aimlessly. He drops his hat, a medication card, and his keys. His hands are trembling, and he looks around the room, bewildered. He appears unable to focus on any one thing. He says over and over, in a loud, high-pitched voice, "Why didn't I hide the bottles?" He is wringing his hands and begins stomping his feet, saying, "It's all my fault. Everything is falling apart."

Other people in the waiting room appear distracted and alarmed by his behaviour. Ted seems to be oblivious to his surroundings.

ASSESSMENT

Jean Gautier, the psychiatric nurse working in the ED, comes into the waiting room and assesses Ted's behaviour as indicative of a severe anxiety level. After talking with Ted briefly, Jean believes that nursing intervention is indicated, based on the following assessment of the patient:

Objective Data	**Subjective Data**
Unable to focus on anything	"Everything is falling apart."
Engaging in purposeless activity (walking around aimlessly)	"Why didn't I hide the bottles?"
Oblivious to his surroundings	"It's all my fault."
Showing unproductive relief behaviour (stomping, wringing hands, dropping things)	

DIAGNOSIS

1. *Anxiety (severe)* related to the patient's perception of responsibility for his wife's coma and possible death

Supporting Data
- Inability to focus
- Confusion
- The feeling that "everything is falling apart"

OUTCOMES IDENTIFICATION

Patient will demonstrate effective coping strategies.

PLANNING

Jean thinks that if he can lower Ted's anxiety to a moderate level, he can work with Ted to get a clear picture of his situation and place the events in a more realistic perspective. He also thinks Ted needs to talk to someone and share some of his pain and confusion to help sort out his feelings. Jean identifies two short-term goals:
1. Patient's anxiety will decrease from severe to moderate by 1600 hours.
2. Patient will verbalize his feelings and a need for assistance by 1600 hours.

IMPLEMENTATION

Jean takes Ted to a quiet room in the back of the ED. He introduces himself and comments that he notices that Ted is upset. He says, "I will stay with you." At first, Ted finds it difficult to sit down and continues pacing around the room. Jean sits quietly and calmly while listening to Ted's self-recriminations. He attends carefully to what Ted is saying—and what he is not saying—to identify themes.

After a while, Ted becomes calmer and is able to sit next to Jean. Jean offers him orange juice, which he accepts and holds tightly.

Jean speaks calmly, using simple, clear statements. He uses communication tools that are helpful to Ted in sorting out his feelings and naming them.

Continued

CASE STUDY AND NURSING CARE PLAN 12-1—cont'd

Severe Level of Anxiety

Dialogue	Therapeutic Tool or Comment
Ted: "Yes … yes … I forgot to hide the bottles. She usually tells me when she feels bad. Why didn't she tell me?"	
Nurse: "You think that if she had told you she wanted to kill herself, you would have hidden the pills?"	Jean asks for clarification of Ted's thinking.
Ted: "Yes, if I had only known, this wouldn't have happened."	
Nurse: "It sounds as if you believe you should have known what your wife was thinking without her telling you."	Here, Jean clarifies Ted's expectations that he should be able to read his wife's mind.
Ted: "Well, yes … when you put it that way … I just don't know what I'll do if she dies."	

When Jean thinks that Ted has discussed his feelings of guilt sufficiently, he asks Ted to clarify his thinking about his wife's behaviour. Ted is able to place his feelings of guilt in a more realistic perspective. Next, Jean brings up another issue—the question of whether Ted's wife will live or die.

Dialogue	Therapeutic Tool or Comment
Nurse: "You said that if your wife dies, you don't know what you will do."	Jean reflects Ted's feelings back to him.
Ted: "Oh, God" (he begins to cry) "I can't live without her. She's all I have in the world."	
Silence	
Nurse: "She means a great deal to you."	Jean reflects Ted's feelings back to him.
Ted: "Everything. Since her mother died, we are each other's only family."	
Nurse: "What would it mean to you if your wife died?"	Jean asks Ted to evaluate his feelings about his wife.
Ted: "I couldn't live by myself, alone. I couldn't stand it." (Starts to cry again.)	
Nurse: "It sounds as if being alone is very frightening to you."	Jean restates in clear terms Ted's experience and feelings.
Ted: "Yes, I don't know how I'd manage by myself."	
Nurse: "A change like that could take time to adjust to."	Jean validates that Ted's wife dying would be very painful for Ted. At the same time, he implies hope that Ted could work through the death in time.
Ted: "Yes … it would be very hard."	

Again, Jean gives Ted a chance to sort out his feelings and fears. Jean helps him focus on the reality that his wife may die and encourages him to express fears related to her possible death. After a while, Jean offers to go to the ICU with Ted to see how his wife is doing. When they arrive they learn that, although Julie is still comatose, her condition has stabilized and she is breathing on her own.

After his arrival at the ICU, Ted starts to worry about whether he remembered to lock the door at home. Jean suggests that he call neighbours and ask them to check the door. Ted is now able to focus on everyday things. Jean makes arrangements to see Ted the next day when he comes in to visit his wife.

The next day, Julie has regained consciousness. She is discharged 1 week later. At the time of her discharge, Ted and Julie Silvestri are considering family therapy once a week with a nurse in the outpatient psychiatry department.

EVALUATION

The first short-term goal is to lower Ted's anxiety level from severe to moderate. Jean can see that Ted has become more visibly calm: his trembling, wringing of hands, and stomping of feet have ceased, and he is able to focus on his thoughts and feelings with Jean's help.

The second short-term goal established for Ted is that he will verbalize his feelings and his need for assistance. Ted is able to identify and discuss with Jean his feelings of guilt and fear of being left alone in the world if his wife should die. Both of these feelings are overwhelming him. He is also able to state that he needs assistance in coping with these feelings in order to make tentative plans for the future.

CASE STUDY AND NURSING CARE PLAN 12-2

Somatic Symptom Disorder

Cara, age 49, a recently divorced mother of twin teenage daughters, works as a copy editor for a local newspaper and has been trying to sell her house in order to downsize after her daughters graduate from high school next year. She has a 2-year history of numerous physical complaints—insomnia, fatigue, muscle aches, irritable bowel syndrome, and occasional paroxysmal atrial tachycardia (PAT); she feels "nervous most of the time"; and she leaves the house only to go to work or to do grocery shopping. She attends work regularly but has no real social life, as she is often "too tired to go out."

She has been referred to a variety of specialists, but there continues to be no evidence of organic origins of her ailments. Today, she presented in the local emergency department with tachycardia and shortness of breath. All diagnostic tests were normal.

Cara agreed to attend an outpatient mental health intensive outpatient program (IOP) three mornings each week. After attending IOP for 2 days, she has not made much progress and states concern about a possible job loss if she does not return to work as soon as possible. She says that she feels happy at times when at home but is very frustrated that her fatigue and physical symptoms are continuing. She says that nothing seems to help her, that she is not sure what she is doing here, and that her future looks bleak. Most staff members have reported frustration that Cara is helpful with other patients but not actively engaged in working on any of her own issues and that she continually states that her mood is fine but her body is a "major problem."

ASSESSMENT

Self-Assessment

Ms. Silverthorn, a registered nurse, has 3 years of experience in this IOP. She recognizes that she has mixed feelings toward Cara. On the one hand, the patient is interesting, talkative, and charming as she discusses her happy childhood. On the other, she refuses to identify any psychological concerns and consistently prods staff to see if she can "graduate" from this program and go back to work. Staff members feel that Cara negates all of their suggestions. Ms. Silverthorn realizes that she has to carefully monitor her emotional reactions to Cara and adopt a persistent matter-of-fact approach to encourage the patient to be more assertive, self-aware, and independent. Ms. Silverthorn plans to actively support Cara in creating her discharge plan.

Objective Data	Subjective Data
• Results of all diagnostic tests are negative. • Onset of symptoms coincides with her divorce and impending loss of daughters as their high school graduations are approaching. • There is no prior history of somatic or psychiatric disorders.	• "I don't know what I'm doing here." • She says her mood is fine, but her body is a "major problem."

DIAGNOSIS

1. *Complicated grieving* related to loss of significant other (spouse) and anticipatory losses of children and home

Supporting Data
  • Patient has difficulty communicating needs or emotions.
  • Patient reports recent and impending losses with lack of emotion or concern.

2. *Social isolation* related to fatigue and pain

Supporting Data
  • Patient has minimal support system.
  • Patient reports frequent fatigue and loss of social interests.

OUTCOMES IDENTIFICATION

Long-term goal: Patient will identify and express emotions without physical symptoms.

PLANNING

The initial plan is to encourage Cara to explore feelings related to recent and impending losses and develop a support system.

Continued

CASE STUDY AND NURSING CARE PLAN 12-2—cont'd
Somatic Symptom Disorder

IMPLEMENTATION

The personalized plan for Cara is as follows:

Short-Term Goal	Intervention	Rationale	Evaluation
1. Patient will identify levels of anxiety in at least three situations and encounters with other patients and staff.	1. Develop a relationship with the patient that includes a mutually agreed-upon contract that details expected changes in behaviours.	1. A contract provides a concrete means to keep track of patient's actions and enhances self-direction and independent actions.	1. After spending 3 weeks in the intensive outpatient mental health program, Cara developed a trusting relationship with one staff member and two patients.
2. Patient will seek support from staff and patients when feelings of anxiety become difficult to handle or physical symptoms increase.	2. Educate the patient about sharing feelings of loss with staff, friends, and family members.	2. Communication and expression of feelings with family and friends helps to alleviate stress and often provides a more supportive environment.	2a. Ms. Silverthorn made several attempts to engage Cara in discussion of feelings, losses, and conflicts to no avail until she arranged for a family meeting with Cara, her daughters, and her former husband. Cara was able to express her anxiety and occasional anger about the loss of her role as wife and the impending loss of her daughters when they attend university away from home.
			2b. Cara also became more active in expressing her grief, particularly in the assertiveness and anger-management classes, and actively sought out Ms. Silverthorn on three occasions to discuss her feelings.
3. Patient will make a list with contacts and phone numbers of community resources of interest to her and make plans to attend a community event within a week.	3. Identify available support systems.	3. Patients are more successful handling stressful life events if they have adequate support.	3. Cara decided to take piano lessons and also enrolled in some of her town's adult-education classes.
4. Patient will remain free of injury throughout the hospitalization.	4. Assess for suicidal ideation.	4. Suicidal ideation may occur in response to depression or hopelessness over medical conditions.	4. Cara made no attempts to self-injure while in the hospital.

EVALUATION

Many of Cara's symptoms have decreased; in particular, there have been no further episodes of tachycardia. However, Cara states that she is still hindered by some fatigue and muscle pain but much less so than previously. She admits she has not fully adhered to her exercise and healthy-eating plan, and occasionally she still feels furious with herself for not coping as well as she would like in social situations. Cara feels that the assertiveness training was particularly helpful to her, as she has realized how her passivity and bottled-up anger could have contributed to her physical symptoms and distress. Cara will continue to see her nurse therapist weekly to work on assertiveness skills, identification of and expression of feelings, and living a healthier lifestyle.

CASE STUDY AND NURSING CARE PLAN 12-3

Post-Traumatic Stress Disorder

Mr. Charbonneau, age 46, is brought to the emergency department by his very distraught wife after she finds him writing a suicide note and planning to shoot himself in the woods with a handgun. He had written: "I don't deserve to live. I should have died with the others." Mr. Charbonneau is subdued and shows minimal affect, and his breath has the distinct odour of alcohol. When asked about suicidal thoughts, he states that he is worthless and that his wife and family would be better off if he were dead. The decision is made to hospitalize him to protect him from danger to himself.

Mr. Charbonneau's wife gives further history. Her husband is a construction contractor who served in the Canadian Armed Forces during the War in Afghanistan. He lost half of his squad in a roadside bombing. He walks with a permanent limp due to a leg injury acquired during this attack. Upon returning home, he showed no signs of anxiety and refused offers of crisis treatment, stating, "I was in a war—I can handle stress." But 6 months later, Mrs. Charbonneau noticed that her husband had trouble sleeping, his mood was irritable or withdrawn, he avoided news reports on television, and he started drinking daily. He complained of nightmares but would not talk to her about his fears. He agreed to go to the psychiatrist only to request sleeping medication.

Mr. Charbonneau was admitted to the psychiatric unit and his care was assigned to Ms. Dawson, a dually educated nurse. She observes that, as he is oriented to the unit, Mr. Charbonneau is quiet and passive but that he looks around vigilantly and is easily startled by sounds on the unit.

ASSESSMENT

Self-Assessment

Ms. Dawson initially feels sympathy for Mr. Charbonneau, and he reminds her of her uncle James, who served in World War II. She is concerned because his suicide plan was lethal and he is guarded in his speech, not revealing his thoughts or feelings. She realizes that as she implements suicide precautions, she must demonstrate an attitude of hope and acceptance to encourage him to develop trust. Also, she must stay neutral and not convey any pity or sympathy.

Objective Data	Subjective Data
Sleep difficulty, nightmares	"I don't deserve to live. I should have died with the others."
Hypervigilance	
Alcohol use	
Irritability	
Withdrawn mood	
Constricted range of affect	
Feels estranged from wife and children	
Avoidance of news coverage with potential for emergency reports	
Refusal of treatment and safety contract	
Plan for suicide	

DIAGNOSIS

1. *Risk for suicide* related to anger and hopelessness due to severe trauma, as evidenced by suicidal plan and verbalization of intent

Supporting Data

- Lethal plan with weapon
- Refusal to agree to a safety plan—that is, to speak to staff when experiencing suicidal ideation
- Emotional withdrawal from wife, as evidenced by his refusal to talk to her about his fears

OUTCOMES IDENTIFICATION

Patient will consistently refrain from attempting suicide.

PLANNING

The initial plan is to maintain safety for Mr. Charbonneau while encouraging him to express feelings and recognize that his situation is not hopeless.

Continued

CASE STUDY AND NURSING CARE PLAN 12-3—cont'd

Post-Traumatic Stress Disorder

IMPLEMENTATION

Mr. Charbonneau's plan of care is personalized as follows:

Short-Term Goal	Intervention	Rationale	Evaluation
1. Patient will speak to staff whenever experiencing self-destructive thoughts.	1a. Administer medications with mouth checks. 1b. Provide ongoing surveillance of patient and environment. 1c. Agrees to safety plan, to talk with staff when experiencing suicidal ideation 1d. Use direct, nonjudgemental approach in discussing suicide. 1e. Provide teaching about PTSD.	1a. Addresses risk of hiding medications 1b. Provides one-to-one monitoring for safety 1c. Encourages increased self-control 1d. Shows acceptance of patient's situation with respect 1e. Offers reality of treatment	**GOAL MET** After 8 hours, patient agrees to safety plan every shift and starts to discuss feelings of self-harm.
2. Patient will express feelings by the third day of hospitalization.	2a. Interact with patient at regular intervals to convey caring and openness and to provide an opportunity to talk. 2b. Use silence and listening to encourage expression of feelings. 2c. Be open to expressions of loneliness and powerlessness. 2d. Share observations or thoughts about patient's behaviour or response.	2a. Encourages development of trust 2b. Shows positive expectation that patient will respond 2c. Allows patient to voice these uncomfortable feelings 2d. Directs attention to here-and-now treatment situation	**GOAL MEG** By second day, patient occasionally answers questions about feelings and admits to anger and grief.
3. Patient will express will to live by discharge from unit.	3a. Listen to expressions of grief. 3b. Encourage patient to identify own strengths and abilities. 3c. Explore with patient previous methods of dealing with life problems. 3d. Assist in identifying available support systems. 3e. Refer patient to spiritual advisor of his choice.	3a. Supports patient and communicates that such feelings are natural 3b. Affirms patient's worth and potential to survive 3c. Reinforces patient's past coping skills and ability to problem-solve now 3d. Addresses fact that anxiety has narrowed patient's perspective, distorting reality about loved ones. 3e. Allows patient opportunity to explore spiritual values and self-worth	**GOAL MET** By fifth day, patient becomes tearful and states that he does not want to hurt his wife and daughter.

EVALUATION

See individual outcomes and evaluation within the care plan.

KEY POINTS TO REMEMBER

- Anxiety has an unknown or unrecognized source, whereas fear is a reaction to a specific threat.
- Peplau operationally defined four levels of anxiety: mild, moderate, severe, and panic. The patient's perceptual field, ability to learn, and physical and other characteristics are different at each level (see Table 12-1).
- Defences against anxiety can be adaptive or maladaptive. Table 12-2 provides adaptive and maladaptive examples of the more common defence mechanisms.
- Anxiety, somatic symptom, or dissociative disorders frequently co-occur with mood disorders or substance use and addictive disorders.
- Research has identified genetic and biological factors in the etiology of anxiety and related disorders.
- Psychological theories and cultural influences are also pertinent to the understanding of anxiety and related disorders.
- People with anxiety disorders suffer from panic attacks, irrational fears, excessive worrying, uncontrollable rituals, or severe reactions to stress.

- Dissociative disorders involve a disruption in consciousness with a significant impairment in memory, identity, or perceptions of self.
- Nursing interventions include counselling, milieu therapy, promotion of self-care activities, psychobiological intervention, health teaching, and behavioural and cognitive behavioural therapies.
- Because these patients may not seek psychiatric treatment, the nurse does not usually see them in the acute psychiatric setting, except during a period of crisis such as suicidal risk.
- The nursing assessment is especially important to clarify the history and course of past symptoms, as well as to obtain a complete picture of the current physical and mental status.
- Although these patients do respond to crisis intervention, they usually require referral for longer-term treatment to attain sustained improvement in level of functioning.

CRITICAL THINKING

1. Ethan is in his final year of university and is taking his examinations for an engineering course. The professor catches him copying from the examination of his willing partner, Jessica, and takes his exam away. Ethan's heart immediately begins to pound, his pulse and respiration rates increase, and he has to wipe perspiration from his hands and face several times. He feels as if he needs to vomit and has a throbbing in his head. When talking with the professor after the examination, he initially has difficulty focusing; when he starts to speak, his voice trembles. Ethan says that Jessica convinced him that cheating was done all the time—in fact, it was her idea. Ethan goes on to say that this "silly little exam" does not mean anything anyway, that he already passed the important courses. He tells the professor, "I thought you were the greatest, and now I see that you're a fool." The professor remains calm and explains that regardless of Ethan's thoughts on this matter, Ethan was caught cheating, he will have to take responsibility for his actions, and the choice to cheat was his. The professor will have Ethan go before the disciplinary board, which is the well-known procedure when one is caught cheating. When Ethan realizes that this incident could affect his graduating on time, he begins to yell at the professor and call him offensive names. Another professor walking past the classroom witnesses this encounter.

   a. Identify the level of anxiety Ethan was experiencing once he was caught cheating, and describe the signs and symptoms that helped you determine this level.
   b. Identify and define five defence mechanisms Ethan used to lessen his anxiety.
   c. Given the circumstances, once Ethan was caught, how could he have reacted using healthier coping defences in a manner that would have reflected more self-responsibility?

2. Ms. Halevy, a patient with OCD, washes her hands until they are cracked and bleeding. Your nursing goal is to promote healing of her hands. What interventions will you plan?

3. A patient with suspected somatic symptom disorder has been admitted to the medical-surgical unit after an episode of chest pain with possible electrocardiographic changes. She frequently complains of palpitations, asks the nurse to check her vital signs, and begs staff to stay with her. Some nurses take her pulse and blood pressure when she asks. Others evade her requests. Most staff members try to avoid spending time with her.

   a. How would you feel as a nurse in this situation? Consider why staff might wish to avoid her.
   b. Design interventions to cope with the patient's behaviours. Give rationales for your interventions.

4. How would you assess for anxiety in an adolescent who has repeated attacks of asthma prior to examinations at school?

CHAPTER REVIEW

1. Since learning that he will have a trial pass to a new group home tomorrow, Bill's behaviour has changed. He has started to pace rapidly, has become very distracted, and is breathing rapidly. He has trouble focusing on anything other than the group home issue and complains that he suddenly feels very nauseated. Which initial nursing response is most appropriate for Bill's level of anxiety?

   a. "You seem anxious. Would you like to talk about how you are feeling?"

b. "If you do not calm down, I will have to give you medicine to calm you."

c. "Bill, slow down. Listen to me. You are safe. Take a nice, deep breath."

d. "We can delay the visit to the group home if that would help you calm down."

2. A patient who seems to be angry when his family again fails to visit as promised tells the nurse that he is fine and that the visit was not important to him anyway. When the nurse suggests that perhaps he might be disappointed or even a little angry that the family has again let him down, the patient responds that it is his family who is angry, not him, or else they would have visited. Which of the following defence mechanisms is this patient using to deal with his feelings?

   a. Rationalization
   b. Introjection
   c. Regression
   d. Dissociation

3. John, a construction worker, is on duty when a wall under construction suddenly falls, crushing a number of co-workers. Shaken initially, he seems to be coping well with the tragedy but later begins to experience tremors, nightmares, and periods during which he feels numb or detached from his environment. He finds himself frequently thinking about the tragedy and feeling guilty that he was spared while many others died. Which statement about this situation is most accurate?

   a. John is experiencing post-traumatic stress disorder (PTSD) and requires therapy.
   b. John has acute stress disorder and should be treated with antianxiety medications.

   c. John is experiencing anxiety and grief and should be monitored for PTSD symptoms.
   d. John is experiencing mild anxiety and a normal grief reaction; no intervention is needed.

4. A patient states that she has been ill for several months with stomach pain, headache, and dizziness. A review of her records shows that she has been tested repeatedly for various conditions, She has been diagnosed with dyspepsia and vertigo. She states that her pain is "10 out of 10" on a scale of 1 to 10. She has been treated in the past for anxiety and depression. Which condition should the nurse anticipate?

   a. Illness anxiety disorder
   b. Somatic symptom disorder
   c. Dissociation disorder
   d. Generalized anxiety disorder

5. An older adult in the outpatient internal medicine clinic complains of feeling a sense of dread and fearfulness without apparent cause. It has been growing steadily worse and is to the point that it is interfering with the patient's sleep and volunteer work. After a brief interview and cursory physical exam, the nurse diagnoses the patient with generalized anxiety disorder and suggests a referral to the mental health clinic. Which responses by the medical clinic nurse would be the priority response?

   a. Complete the referral to the mental health clinic.
   b. Meet with the patient's family to discuss treatment options for generalized anxiety disorder.
   c. Instruct the client in deep-breathing and basic cognitive behavioural techniques for coping with worry.
   d. Suggest that a battery of blood tests, including a complete blood count (CBC), be ordered and reviewed.

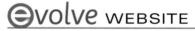 **WEBSITE**

Post-Test   interactive review

Visit the Evolve website for Chapter Review Answers and Rationales, Critical Thinking Answer Guidelines, and additional resources related to the content in this chapter: http://evolve.elsevier.com/Canada/Varcarolis/psychiatric/

REFERENCES

Ackley, B., Ladwig, G., & Makic, B. F. (2017). *Nursing diagnosis handbook: An evidence-based guide to planning care* (11th ed.). St. Louis: Mosby/Elsevier.

American Psychiatric Association (2013). *Diagnostic and statistical manual of mental disorders* (5th ed.). Arlington, VA: Author.

Bernstein, E. M., & Putnam, F. W. (1986). Development, reliability, and validity of a dissociation scale. *Journal of Nervous and Mental Disorders*, 174(12), 727–735. doi:10.1097/00005053-198612000-00004.

Brown, R. J., & Lewis-Fernandez, R. (2011). Culture and conversion disorder: Implications for *DSM-5*. *Psychiatry: Interpersonal & Biological Processes*, 74(3), 187–206. doi:10.1521/psyc.2011.74.3.187.

Bulechek, G. M., Butcher, H. K., & Dochterman, J. M. (2013). *Nursing interventions classification (NIC)* (6th ed.). Toronto: Elsevier.

Canadian Network for Mood and Anxiety Treatments. (2013a). *Anxiety: Diagnosing substance-induced anxiety disorder.* Retrieved from http://www.canmat.org/cme-anxiety-substance-induced-anxiety-disorder.php.

Canadian Network for Mood and Anxiety Treatments. (2013b). *Disorder information: Acute stress disorder.* Retrieved from http://www.canmat.org/di-anxiety-acute-stress-disorder.php.

Charlson, F. J., Stapelberg, N. J. C., Baxter, A. J., et al. (2011). Should global burden of disease estimates include depression as a risk factor for coronary heart disease? *BMC Medicine*, 9(47), doi:10.1186/1741-7015-9-47.

Chauvet-Gelinier, J., & Bonin, B. (2017). Stress, anxiety and depression in heart disease patients: A major challenge for cardiac rehabilitation. *Annals of Physical and Rehabilitation Medicine*, 60(1), 6–12. doi:10.1016/j.rehab.2016.09.002.

Deimling, G. T., Albitz, C., Monnin, K., et al. (2017). Personality and psychological distress among older adult, long-term cancer survivors. *Journal of Psychosocial Oncology*, 35(1), 17–31. doi:10.1080/07347332.2016.1225145.

Dols, A., Rhebergen, D., Eikelenboom, P., et al. (2012). Hypochondriacal delusion in an elderly woman recovers quickly with electroconvulsive therapy. *Clinical and Practice*, 2(11), 21–22. doi:10.4081/cp.2012.e11.

Feinstein, A. (2011). Conversion disorder: Advances in our understanding. *Canadian Medical Association Journal*, 183(8), 915–920. doi:10.1503/cmaj.110490.

Fink, P. (2010). The outcome of health anxiety in primary care: A two-year follow up study on health care costs and self-rated health. *PLoS ONE*, *5*(3), doi:10.1371/journal.pone.0009873.

Flaskerud, J. H. (2009). What do we need to know about culture-bound syndromes? *Issues in Mental Health Nursing*, *30*, 406–407. doi:10.1080/01612840902812947.

Foa, E. B., Kozak, M. J., Salkovskis, P. M., et al. (1998). The validation of a new obsessive compulsive disorder scale: The Obsessive Compulsive Inventory (OCI). *Psychological Assessment*, *10*, 206–214.

Fuller-Thomson, E., Sulman, J., Brennenstuhl, S., et al. (2011). Functional somatic syndromes and childhood physical abuse in women: Data from a representative community-based sample. *Journal of Aggression, Maltreatment and Trauma*, *20*, 445–469.

Garcia-Martin, I., Miranda-Vicario, E. M., & Soutullo, C. A. (2012). Duloxetine in the treatment of adolescents with somatoform disorders: A report of two cases. *Actas espanolas de psiquiatra*, *20*(3), 165–168.

Goodman, W. K., Price, L. H., & Rasmussen, S. A. (1989). The Yale-Brown Obsessive Compulsive Scale. *Archives of General Psychiatry*, *46*, 1006–1011.

Goodwin, G. M. (2015). The overlap between anxiety, depression, and obsessive-compulsive disorder. *Dialogues in Clinical Neuroscience*, *17*(3), 249–260. Retrieved from http://www.dialogues-cns.org/.

Grant, J. E. (2014). Obsessive-compulsive disorder. *The New England Journal of Medicine*, *371*(7), 646–653. doi:10.1056/NEJMcp1402176.

Haase, M. (2002). Uncommon experiences: Living with obsessive compulsive disorder. In M. van Manen (Ed.), *Writing in the dark: Phenomenological studies in interpretive inquiry* (pp. 62–83). London, ON: Althouse Press.

Huang, H., & McCarron, R. M. (2011). Medically unexplained symptoms: Evidence-based interventions. *Current Psychiatry*, *10*(7), 17.

International Society for the Study of Trauma and Dissociation. (2012). Guidelines for treating dissociative identity disorder in adults (3rd rev.). *Journal of Trauma and Dissociation*, *12*(2), 115–187. doi:10.1080/15299732.2011.537247.

Kenny, M., & Egan, J. (2011). Somatization disorder: What clinicians need to know. *The Psychologist*, *37*(4), 93–96.

Kim, H. H., Lee, Y. J., Kim, H. K., et al. (2011). Prevalence and correlates of psychiatric symptoms in North Korean defectors. *Psychiatry Investigation*, *8*(3), 179–185.

Koch, S. C., & Harvey, S. (2012). Dance/movement therapy with traumatized dissociative patients. In S. C. Koch, T. Fuchs, M. Summa, et al. (Eds.), *Body memory, metaphor and movement* (pp. 369–386). Philadelphia: John Benjamins Publishing.

Konnopka, A., Löbner, M., Luppa, M., et al. (2012). Psychiatric comorbidity as predictor of costs in backpain patients undergoing disc surgery: A longitudinal observational study. *BioMed Central Musculoskeletal Disorders*, *13*, 165. doi:10.1186/1471-2474-13-165.

Korber, S., Frieser, D., Steinbrecher, N., et al. (2011). Classification characteristics of Patient Health Questionnaire-15 Screening for somatoform disorders in a primary care setting. *Journal of Psychosomatic Research*, *71*, 142–147.

Landa, A., Peterson, B., & Fallon, B. (2012). Somatoform pain: A developmental theory and translational research review. *Psychosomatic Medicine*, *74*(7), 717–727. doi:10.1097/PSY.0b013e3182688e8b.

Macaulay, C., Angus, L., Khattra, J., et al. (2017). Client retrospective accounts of corrective experience in motivational interviewing integrated with cognitive behavioral therapy for generalized anxiety disorder. *Journal of Clinical Psychology*, *73*(2), 168–181. doi:10.1002/jclp.22430.

MacDonald, P. (2011). Dealing with health anxiety. *Practice Nurse*, *41*(16), 38.

Matthew, M. J. (2015). Gaps in knowledge: Tracking and explaining gender differences in health information seeking. *Social Sciences & Medicine*, *128*, 151–158. doi:10.1016/j.socscimed.2015.01.028.

Meng, X., & D'Arcy, C. (2015). Comorbidity between lifetime eating problems and mood and anxiety disorders: Results from the Canadian community health survey of mental health and well-being. *European Eating Disorders Review*, *23*(2), 152–162. doi:10.1002/erv.2347.

Mental Health Commission of Canada. (2012). *Changing directions, changing lives: The mental health strategy for Canada*. Retrieved from strategy.mentalhealthcommission.ca/pdf/strategy-images-en.pdf.

Moorhead, S., Johnson, M., Maas, M., et al. (2012). *Nursing outcomes classification (NOC)* (5th ed.). St. Louis: Mosby.

Mosby's dictionary of medicine, nursing & health professions (9th ed.). (2012). St. Louis: Mosby.

Nicholson, T., Stone, J., & Kanaan, R. A. A. (2011). Conversion disorder: A problematic diagnosis. *Journal of Neurology, Neurosurgery, and Psychiatry*, *82*, 1267–1273.

Ogden, P., & Fisher, J. (2015). *Sensorimotor psychotherapy: Interventions for trauma and attachment*. New York: Norton.

Pauls, D. L. (2010). The genetics of obsessive-compulsive disorder: A review. *Dialogues in Clinical Neuroscience*, *12*(2), 149–163.

Pearson, C., Zamorski, M., & Janz, T. (2014). *Health at a glance: Mental health of the Canadian Armed Forces*. Ottawa: Statistics Canada.

Peplau, H. E. (1968). A working definition of anxiety. In S. F. Burd & M. A. Marshall (Eds.), *Some clinical approaches to psychiatric nursing* (pp. 323–327). New York: Macmillan.

Public Health Agency of Canada (2016). *Report from the Canadian chronic disease surveillance system: Mood and anxiety disorders in Canada, 2016*. Ottawa: Author.

Rodrigues, H., Figueira, I., Lopes, A., et al. (2014). Does D-cycloserine enhance exposure therapy for anxiety disorders in humans? A meta-analysis. *PLoS ONE*, *9*(7), e93519. doi:10.1371/journal.pone.0093519.

Schatzberg, A. F. (2017). *Textbook of psyhopharmacology* (DSM-5 ed.). Arlington, VA: American Psychiatric Association Publishing.

Schlozman, S. C., & Nonacs, R. M. (2008). Dissociative disorders. In T. A. Stern, J. F. Rosenbaum, M. Fava, et al. (Eds.), *Massachusetts General Hospital comprehensive clinical psychiatry* (pp. 481–486). St. Louis: Mosby.

Selye, H. (1956). What is stress. *Metabolism: Clinical and Experimental*, *5*(5), 525–530. Retrieved from http://www.metabolismjournal.com.

Shear, M. K., Brown, T. A., Barlow, D. H., et al. (1997). Multicenter collaborative panic disorder severity scale. *American Journal of Psychiatry*, *154*(11), 1571–1575. doi:10.1176/ajp.154.11.1571.

Shidhaye, R., Mendenhall, E., Sumathipala, K., et al. (2013). Association of somatoform disorders with anxiety and depression in women in low and middle income countries: A systematic review. *International Review of Psychiatry*, *259*(1), 65–76. doi:10.3109/09540261.2012.748651.

Silber, T. J. (2011). Somatization disorders: Diagnosis, treatment and prognosis. *Pediatrics in Review*, *32*(2), 56–64. doi:10.1542/pir.32-2-56.

Soltis-Jarrett, V. M. (2010). His-story or her-story: Deconstruction of the concepts of somatization towards a new approach in advanced nursing practice care. *Perspectives in Psychiatric Care*, *47*(4), 183–193. doi:10.1111/j.1744-6163.2010.00288.x.

Spiegel, D., Loewenstein, R., Lewis-Fernandez, R., et al. (2011). Dissociative disorders in DSM-5. *Depression and Anxiety*, *28*, 824–852. doi:10.1002/da.20874.

Stone, J., Vuilleumier, P., & Friedman, J. H. (2010). Conversion disorder: Separating the "how" from "why.". *Neurology*, *74*, 190–191.

Sullivan, H. S. (1953). *The interpersonal theory of psychiatry*. New York: W. W. Norton.

van Dijke, A. (2012). Dysfunctional affect regulation in borderline personality disorder and in somatoform disorder. *European Journal of Psychotraumatology*, *3*, doi:10.3402/ejpt.v3i0.19566.

World Health Organization (2007). *Integrating mental health services into primary health care. Mental Health Policy, Planning and Service Development Sheet*. Geneva, Switzerland: Author.

Yakobov, E., Jurcik, T., & Sullivan, M. L. (2017). Conversion disorder. In M. A. Budd, S. Hough, S. T. Wegener, et al. (Eds.), *Practical psychology in medical rehabilitation* (pp. 277–285). Cham, Switzerland: Springer International Publishing.

13

Depressive Disorders

Margaret Jordan Halter, Mallie Kozy
Adapted by Cheryl L. Pollard

KEY TERMS AND CONCEPTS

affect
anergia
anger
anhedonia
Beck's cognitive triad
depressive disorder due to another medical condition
diathesis–stress model of depression
disruptive mood dysregulation disorder
electroconvulsive therapy (ECT)
hypersomnia
learned helplessness
light therapy

major depressive disorder (MDD)
mood disorders
persistent depressive disorder
premenstrual dysphoric disorder
psychomotor agitation
psychomotor retardation
serotonin syndrome
substance/medication-induced depressive disorder
suicidal ideation
transcranial magnetic stimulation (TMS)
vagus nerve stimulation (VNS)
vegetative signs of depression

OBJECTIVES

1. Compare and contrast major depressive disorder and persistent depressive disorder (dysthymia).
2. Discuss the origins of depression.
3. Assess behaviours in a patient with depression with regard to each of the following areas: (a) affect, (b) thought processes, (c) feelings, (d) physical behaviour, and (e) communication.
4. Formulate five nursing diagnoses for a patient with depression, and include outcome criteria.
5. Name unrealistic expectations a nurse may have while working with a patient with depression, and compare them to your own personal thoughts.

6. Demonstrate six principles of communication useful in working with patients with depression.
7. Identify major classifications of antidepressants and general advantages and disadvantages of each.
8. Develop a medication teaching plan for a patient taking an antidepressant, including adverse effects, toxic reactions, and other drugs or foods that can trigger an adverse reaction.
9. Write a nursing care plan incorporating the recovery model of mental health.
10. Discuss nonpharmaceutical interventions for major depressive disorder such as electroconvulsive therapy (ECT).

⊖volve WEBSITE

Visit the Evolve website for Flashcards, Case Studies, and additional testing resources related to the content in this chapter: http://evolve.elsevier.com/Canada/Varcarolis/psychiatric/

Pre-Test   interactive review

No textbook chapter can adequately convey the personal pain and suffering experienced by the individual with depression, not to mention the pain, helplessness, and frustration felt by the affected individual's friends and loved ones. However, it is essential for nursing students to gain a fundamental understanding of this group of mood disorders. Mood disorders (also called affective disorders) are a group of psychiatric disorders including depression and bipolar disorder. People of all ethnicities, cultures, ages, socioeconomic groups, education levels, and geographic areas are susceptible to depressive episodes, but some individuals are more susceptible than others. Virtually all nurses will come into contact with patients with depression or whose primary condition is complicated by depression. This chapter includes basic information and therapeutic tools that will facilitate the care of patients with depression.

 HOW A NURSE HELPED ME

Diagnosed but Not Forgotten

After months of my not having any interest in doing anything and withdrawing from friends and family, my husband took me to the hospital emergency department, where I was admitted to the hospital's mental health unit and diagnosed with major depressive disorder (MDD). While major depression is common, I believed that this diagnosis would change my life. During my 2 weeks in hospital, psychiatric nurses helped me to understand the distorted beliefs I had about myself and others. Outside of the one-on-one time with the nurses, they taught me how to incorporate yoga and exercise in my treatment plan. Initially, because of my fear of gaining weight, I wanted to stop taking my venlafaxine (Effexor XR), but the nurses taught me about the importance of taking my medications even once I was feeling better. The nurses also helped me to identify a support system. My husband and girlfriend help me along when I want to give up. I also attend a monthly depression group, and if I feel as though I am slipping back into a depression, I know I can call the mental health clinic or speak to the psychiatric nurse in the emergency department. It has been 10 years since I was diagnosed with major depression, and there are still times when I need help; however, I know that my life has changed and is not over.

CLINICAL PICTURE

Major depressive disorder (MDD) is one of the most common psychiatric disorders. Almost 1 in 8 adults (12.6%) have identified symptoms that met the criteria for a mood disorder at some point during their lifetime (Pearson, Janz, & Ali, 2013). Major depressive disorder, or major depression, is characterized by a persistently depressed mood lasting for a minimum of 2 weeks. The length of a depressive episode may be 5 to 6 months (McInnis, Riba, & Greden, 2014). About 20% of cases become chronic (i.e.,

lasting more than 2 years). While depression begins with a single occurrence, most people experience recurrent episodes. People experience a recurrence within the first year about 50% of the time and within a lifetime up to 85% of the time. The full criteria for major depressive disorder are listed in DSM-5: Diagnostic Criteria for Major Depressive Disorder.

The diagnosis for MDD may include one of the following specifiers to describe the most recent episode of depression:
- **Psychotic features.** Indicates the presence of disorganized thinking, delusions (e.g., delusions of guilt or of being punished for sins, somatic delusions of horrible disease or body rotting, delusions of poverty or going bankrupt), or hallucinations (usually auditory, voices berating person for sins).
- **Melancholic features.** This outdated term indicates a severe form of endogenous depression (not attributable to environmental stressors) characterized by severe apathy, weight loss, profound guilt, symptoms that are worse in the morning, early morning awakening, and often suicidal ideation.
- **Atypical features.** Refers to dominant vegetative symptoms (e.g., overeating, oversleeping). Onset is younger, psychomotor activities are slow, and anxiety is often an accompanying problem, which may cause misdiagnosis.
- **Catatonic features.** Marked by nonresponsiveness, extreme psychomotor retardation (may seem paralyzed), withdrawal, and negativity.
- **Postpartum onset.** Indicates onset within 4 weeks after childbirth. It is common for psychotic features to accompany this depression. Severe ruminations or delusional thoughts about the infant signify increased risk of harm to the infant.
- **Seasonal features (seasonal affective disorder [SAD]).** Indicates that episodes mostly begin in fall or winter and remit in spring. These patients have reduced cerebral metabolic activity. SAD is characterized by anergia (lack of energy or passivity), hypersomnia (excessive daytime sleep), overeating, weight gain, and a craving for carbohydrates; it responds to light therapy.

While the focus in this chapter is major depressive disorder, you should also be aware of several other depressive disorders:
- Disruptive mood dysregulation disorder
- Persistent depressive disorder (dysthymia)
- Premenstrual dysphoric disorder
- Substance/medication-induced depressive disorder
- Depressive disorder due to another medical condition

Disruptive Mood Dysregulation Disorder

Disruptive mood dysregulation disorder is a disorder characterized by severe and recurrent temper outbursts that are inconsistent with developmental level. This disorder was introduced in 2013 in response to an alarming number of children and adolescents being diagnosed with bipolar disorder. A bipolar diagnosis resulted in exposure to powerful medications that probably were not helping and a lifelong label of serious mental illness. Perhaps the most compelling reason to change this diagnostic practice was that most of the young people who received a diagnosis of bipolar disorder did not go on to exhibit classic bipolar symptoms as adults. In fact, most children and adolescents once diagnosed with bipolar disorder actually

DSM-5

Diagnostic Criteria for Major Depressive Disorder

A. Five (or more) of the following symptoms have been present during the same 2-week period and represent a change from previous functioning; at least one of the symptoms is either (1) depressed mood or (2) loss of interest of pleasure.
Note: Do not include symptoms that are clearly attributable to another medical condition.
1. Depressed mood most of the day, nearly every day, as indicated by either subjective report (e.g., feels sad, empty, hopeless) or observation made by others (e.g., appears tearful). (**Note:** In children and adolescents, it can be irritable mood.)
2. Markedly diminished interest or pleasure in all, or almost all, activities most of the day, nearly every day (as indicated by either subjective account or observation).
3. Significant weight loss when not dieting or weight gain (e.g., a change of more than 5% of body weight in a month) or decrease or increase in appetite nearly every day. (**Note:** In children, consider failure to make expected weight gain.)
4. Insomnia or hypersomnia nearly every day.
5. Psychomotor agitation or retardation nearly every day (observable by others, not merely subjective feelings of restlessness or being slowed down).
6. Fatigue or loss of energy nearly every day.
7. Feelings of worthlessness or excessive or inappropriate guilt (which may be delusional) nearly every day (not merely self-reproach or guilt about being sick).
8. Diminished ability to think or concentrate or indecisiveness nearly every day (either by subjective account or as observed by others).
9. Recurrent thoughts of death (not just fear of dying), recurrent suicidal ideation without a specific plan, or a suicide attempt or a specific plan for suicide.

B. The symptoms cause clinically significant distress or impairment in social, occupational, or other important areas of functioning.
C. The episode is not attributable to the physiological effects of a substance or to another medical condition.
Note: Criteria A through C represent a major depressive episode.
Note: Responses to a significant loss (bereavement, financial ruin, losses from a natural disaster, a serious medical illness or disability) may include the feelings of intense sadness, rumination about the loss, insomnia, poor appetite, and weight loss as noted in Criterion A, which may resemble a depressive episode. Although such symptoms may be understandable or considered appropriate to the loss, the presence of a major depressive episode in addition to the normal response to a significant loss should also be carefully considered. This decision inevitably requires the exercise of clinical judgment based on the individual's history and the cultural norms for the expression of distress in the context of loss.
D. The occurrence of the major depressive episode is not better explained by schizoaffective disorder, schizophrenia, schizophreniform disorder, delusional disorder, or other specified and unspecified schizophrenia spectrum and other psychotic disorders.
E. There has never been a manic or a hypomanic episode.
Note: This exclusion does not apply to all of the manic-like or hypomanic-like episodes that are substance-induced or are attributable to the physiological effects of another medical condition.

Source: American Psychiatric Association. (2013). *Diagnostic and statistical manual of mental disorders* (5th ed.). Arlington, VA: Author.

converted to major depressive disorder or an anxiety disorder in adulthood.

The basic symptoms of disruptive mood dysregulation disorder are constant and severe irritability and anger in individuals between the ages of 6 and 18. Onset is before age 10. Temper tantrums with verbal or behavioural outbursts out of proportion to the situation occur at least three times a week. Sometimes children and adolescents with this problem can maintain control in certain settings such as school. To be diagnosed with disruptive mood dysregulation disorder, individuals need to exhibit the irritability, anger, and temper tantrums in at least two of these settings: home, school, and with peers.

The prevalence rate for disruptive mood dysregulation disorder is believed to fall in the range of 2% to 5%. It is more common in males than females, and it is more common in children than adolescents.

There is little information available on the treatment of disruptive mood dysregulation disorder. Sadock and colleagues (2015) suggest a symptom-based approach. If the disorder resembles major depression, antidepressants may be considered. If the disorder is accompanied by attention-deficit/hyperactivity

disorder (ADHD), medications for that condition could be tried. Antidepressants may be used to address irritability. The second-generation antipsychotics risperidone (Risperdal) and aripiprazole (Abilify) have approval from Health Canada for irritability in autism and are sometimes used for disruptive mood dysregulation disorder.

Psychosocial interventions such as cognitive behavioural therapy (CBT) are essential considering the degree of turmoil this disorder brings about. Parent training helps parents to interact with a child in such a way to predict and reduce aggression and irritability through consistency and rewarding appropriate behaviour. There is some evidence that these young people may be misperceiving others' facial expressions as angry. Computer-based training can help them become more aware of the meaning of facial expressions.

Persistent Depressive Disorder

Persistent depressive disorder (dysthymia) is diagnosed when feelings of depression occur most of the day, for the majority of days. These low-level depressive feelings last at least 2 years in adults and 1 year in children and adolescents. In addition to depressed mood, individuals with this disorder have at least two of the following: decreased appetite or overeating, insomnia or hypersomnia, low energy, poor self-esteem, difficulty thinking, and hopelessness.

The symptoms are difficult for the patient to live with and bring about social and occupational distress, but they are usually not severe enough to require hospitalization. Because the onset of persistent depressive disorder usually occurs in teenage years, patients frequently express that they have "always felt this way" and that being depressed seems like a normal way of functioning. It is not uncommon for people with this low-level depression to also have periods of full-blown major depressive episodes.

The prevalence of persistent depressive disorder ranges from 0.5% to 1.5%. The problem tends to have an early onset and, as the name suggests, it is a chronic illness.

Treatment for this disorder is similar to that for MDD, which we discuss in more depth later in this chapter. Psychotherapy, particularly CBT, is quite useful in managing symptoms. Antidepressants such as selective serotonin reuptake inhibitors (SSRIs), serotonin–norepinephrine reuptake inhibitors (SNRIs), and tricyclics are the other main treatments.

Premenstrual Dysphoric Disorder

Premenstrual dysphoric disorder is a relatively new addition to the diagnostic system for psychiatry. It refers to a cluster of symptoms that occur in the last week before the onset of a woman's period. Premenstrual dysphoric disorder causes problems severe enough to interfere with the ability of a woman to work or interact with others. Symptoms include mood swings, irritability, depression, anxiety, feeling overwhelmed, and difficulty concentrating. Other physical manifestations include lack of energy, overeating, hypersomnia or insomnia, breast tenderness, aching, bloating, and weight gain. Symptoms decrease significantly or disappear with the onset of menstruation.

The prevalence of premenstrual dysphoric disorder is about 2% to 6% of menstruating women. Symptoms cease after menopause, although they may return with hormone replacement therapy.

Treatment for this disorder includes regular exercise, particularly aerobic exercise. Other recommendations include eating food rich in complex carbohydrates and getting sufficient sleep. Acupuncture, light therapy, and relaxation therapy have also been used to reduce symptoms.

Several drugs have Health Canada approval for treatment of this disorder. A drosperinone and ethinyl estradiol combination (Yaz) is a contraceptive that improves symptoms. SSRIs have been used successfully and three have FDA approval. They are fluoxetine (Prozac, Serafem), sertraline (Zoloft), and controlled-release paroxetine (Paxil CR). Diuretics may be useful in reducing bloating and weight gain brought on by water retention.

Substance/Medication-Induced Depressive Disorder

Substance/medication-induced depressive disorder is a depressive disorder, such as MDD, that is a result of prolonged use of or withdrawal from drugs and alcohol. The depressive symptoms last longer than the expected length of physiological effects, intoxication, or withdrawal of the substance. The person with this diagnosis would not experience depressive symptoms in the absence of drug or alcohol use or withdrawal. Symptoms appear within 1 month of use. Once the substance is removed, depressive symptoms usually remit within a few days to several weeks.

The lifetime prevalence rate is fairly low—about 0.25%. Medications associated with depressive symptoms include antiviral agents, cardiovascular drugs, retinoic acid derivatives, antidepressants, anticonvulsants, antimigraine agents, antipsychotics, hormonal agents, smoking cessation agents, and immunological agents.

Depressive Disorder Due to Another Medical Condition

Depressive disorder due to another medical condition may be caused by disorders that affect the body's systems or from long-term illnesses that cause ongoing pain. The depressive symptoms are the same as the diagnostic criteria for the depressive disorders. It is important to review medications being used for the medical condition to rule out them being the causative agents.

There are clear associations, along with neuroanatomical changes, with some disease states. The prevalence rate of depression in people who have suffered a cerebrovascular accident (stroke) is high—30% to 50%—in the first year (Flaster, Sharma, & Rao, 2013). Parkinson's disease, Huntington's disease, Alzheimer's disease, and traumatic brain injury are also clearly associated with depressive disorders. Neuroendocrine conditions such as Cushing's disease and hypothyroidism are also commonly accompanied by depression. Arthritis, back pain, metabolic conditions (e.g., vitamin B_{12} deficiency), human immunodeficiency virus (HIV), diabetes, infection, cancer, and autoimmune problems may also contribute to depressions. Table 13-1 summarizes medical problems and substances that are associated with major depression.

Depression and Grieving

People who experience a significant loss can exhibit feelings and behaviours similar to depression. They may cry, feel hopeless about the future, have disruptions in eating and sleeping, and lose pleasure in everyday activities. They may even experience a lack interest in caring for themselves and neglect normal hygiene. At what point does grief become pathological? This is a controversial question and one that is not easily answered.

Until recently, clinicians were advised against diagnosing a person with depression in the first 2 months following a significant loss. This was called the bereavement exclusion. The rationale for avoiding a psychiatric diagnosis follows:
1. Normal mourning could be labelled pathological.
2. A psychiatric diagnosis could result in a lifelong label.
3. Unnecessary medications might be prescribed.

Although controversial, a diagnosis of depression can now be given in the first 2 months following death of a loved one or other loss. The reason for the change is that grief, like other stressors, can result in depression. For some people, waiting 2 months for an official diagnosis of major depression may delay treatment and adversely affect prognosis. Further research about grief may clarify diagnostic categories and prevent overdiagnosis of depression in the presence of grief.

CONSIDERING CULTURE

Suicide and Suicide Prevention Among Inuit in Canada

Inuit in Canada have among the highest suicide rates in the world, and suicide occurs primarily among their youth. Risk factors include known ones such as depression, substance use, a history of abuse, and knowing others who have made attempts or have killed themselves; however, of importance are the negative effects of colonialism. Multiple generations are affected by historical trauma. The origins of this trauma took place for Inuit primarily during the government era starting in the 1950s, when Inuit were moved from their family-based land camps to crowded settlements run by white men, and children were removed from their parents and placed in residential or day schools. This caused more disorganization than reorganization within their family-based collectivist culture. The most negative effect of this rapid culture change brought about by colonialism and imperialism for Inuit has been on their relationships. There have been changes in parenting practices, domestic violence rates, and language loss. Many Inuit youth feel alone and rejected. Their relational bond, ungajuk, or sense of belonging, ilagijauttiarniq, has been disrupted.

Suicide prevention programs that include the involvement of elders and connecting with the land through family-focused activities have been the most successful. Connecting with their family members and friends has been identified as an important factor in building resilience among Inuit youth. Western suicide prevention programs, when used without integrating Indigenous knowledge, have not been effective, as suicide rates continued to rise when these programs were used. Canada's National Aboriginal Youth Suicide Prevention Strategy, which was developed in partnership with Indigenous organizations, has supported the Indigenous reclamation of control over their lives.

Mental health factors for Indigenous peoples are often cultural. It is recommended that health care practitioners work with the community and with Indigenous organizations. Empowered communities can be healing through identifying individual responsibility and acknowledging historical and current injustices.

Source: Kral, M. J. (2016). Suicide and suicide prevention among Inuit in Canada. *The Canadian Journal of Psychiatry, 61*(11), 688–695. doi:10.1177/0706743716661329.

EPIDEMIOLOGY

Depression is the leading cause of disability in the world. The lifetime prevalence of a major depressive episode or the total number of adults in Canada who will experience the disorder within their lifetime is 11.3% (Pearson, Janz, & Ali, 2013). The average age of MDD onset is between 15 and 45 years of age. Studies find that mood disorders are more common in women than men (Pearson, Janz, & Ali, 2013). See Figure 13-1 for rates of depression in Canada. Several Canadian studies found that MDD tends to have higher prevalence rates in lower-income or unemployed populations and in unmarried or divorced people.

Children and Adolescents

Children as young as 3 years of age have been diagnosed with depression; however, the prevalence is relatively low, with little

TABLE 13-1	MEDICAL CONDITIONS AND SUBSTANCES OR MEDICATIONS ASSOCIATED WITH MAJOR DEPRESSIVE DISORDER
Substances or Medication	
Central nervous system depressants	Alcohol, barbiturates, benzodiazepines, clonidine
Central nervous system medications	Amantadine, bromocriptine, levodopa, phenothiazines, phenytoin
Psychostimulants	Amphetamines
Systemic medications	Corticosteroids, digoxin, diltiazem, enalapril, ethionamide, isotretinoin, mefloquine, methyldopa, metoclopramide, quinolones, reserpine, statins, thiazides, vincristine
Medical Conditions	
Neurological	Epilepsy, Parkinson's disease, multiple sclerosis, Alzheimer's disease, Huntington's disease, traumatic brain injury, cerebrovascular accident
Infectious or inflammatory	Neurosyphilis, human immunodeficiency virus (HIV)
Cardiac disorders	Ischemic heart disease, cardiac failure, cardiomyopathies
Endocrine	Hypothyroidism, diabetes mellitus, vitamin deficiencies, parathyroid disorders
Inflammatory disorders	Collagen vascular diseases, irritable bowel syndrome, chronic liver disorders
Neoplastic disorders	Central nervous system tumours, paraneoplastic syndromes

difference between boys and girls. Levels rise in the early teen years, more sharply among girls than boys (Maughan, Collishaw, & Stringaris, 2013). This is especially troubling since a youth onset carries a high recurrence rate, setting the stage for lifelong periods of depression. In the last edition of the *Diagnostic and Statistical Manual of Mental Disorders (DSM-5)*, disruptive mood dysregulation disorder was added to represent the presentation of irritability and frequent episodes of uncontrolled behaviour in an attempt to deal with the potential of children being misdiagnosed with schizophrenia, a personality disorder, or bipolar disorder (American Psychiatric Association, 2013).

Older Adults

Although depression in older adults is common, it is *not* a normal result of aging. The risk for depression in the elderly increases as health deteriorates. About 1% to 5% of older adults who live in the community have depression. This statistic rises to 11.5% for hospitalized older adults and 13.5% for those requiring home care (National Institute of Mental Health [NIMH], 2012). A disproportionate number of older adults with depression are likely to die by suicide.

Many older adults suffer from *subsyndromal depression* in which they experience many, but not all, of the symptoms of a major depressive episode. These individuals have an increased risk of eventually developing major depression. Sometimes the

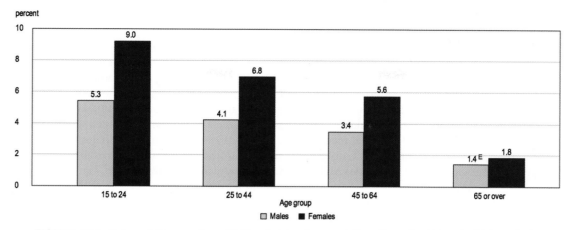

FIGURE 13-1 Rates of Depression, 12-Month,[1] by Age and Sex, Canada, Household Population 15 and Older, 2012 Use with caution (these data have a coefficient variation from 1.6.6 to 33.3%) [1]Respondents were classified with depression if they met the criteria for this condition in the 12 months prior to the survey. Source: Statistics Canada. (2013). Canadian Community Health Survey: Mental health, 2012. Ottawa: Author.

psychomotor slowing and cognitive effects of depression lead others to believe that the older adult is developing a neurocognitive disorder such as Alzheimer's disease. This condition is referred to as pseudodementia, a problem that can be reversed when the underlying depression is treated and eliminated.

COMORBIDITY

A depressive syndrome frequently accompanies other psychiatric disorders, such as anxiety disorders, schizophrenia, substance abuse, eating disorders, and schizoaffective disorder. People with anxiety disorders (e.g., panic disorder, generalized anxiety disorder, obsessive-compulsive disorder) commonly present with depression, as do people with personality disorders (particularly borderline personality disorder), adjustment disorder, and brief depressive reactions.

The combination of anxiety and depression is perhaps one of the most common psychiatric presentations. Symptoms of anxiety occur in an average of 70% of cases of major depression. Some clinicians believe that mixed anxiety and depression should be a stand-alone diagnosis and be treated as a distinct entity.

ETIOLOGY

Although many theories attempt to explain the cause of depression, many psychological, biological, and cultural variables make identification of any one cause difficult; furthermore, it is unlikely that there is a single cause of depression. The high variability in symptoms, response to treatment, and course of the illness support the supposition that depression results from a complex interaction of causes. For example, genetic predisposition to the illness combined with childhood stress may lead to significant changes in the central nervous system (CNS) that result in depression. However, there seem to be several common risk factors for depression, listed in Box 13-1.

BOX 13-1 RISK FACTORS FOR DEPRESSION

- Female gender
- Early childhood trauma
- Stressful life events
- Family history of depression, especially in first-degree relatives
- High levels of neuroticism (a negative personality trait characterized by anxiety, fear, moodiness, worry, envy, frustration, jealousy, and loneliness)
- Other disorders such as substance use, anxiety, and personality disorders
- Chronic or disabling medical conditions

Biological Factors
Genetic

Twin studies consistently show that genetic factors play a role in the development of depressive disorders. The concordance rate for MDD among monozygotic (identical) twins is nearly 50%. That is, if one twin is affected, the second has about a 50% chance of being affected as well. It is likely that multiple genes are involved, each one having a small but substantial role in the development and severity of depression. For instance, certain genetic markers seem to be related to depression when accompanied by early childhood maltreatment or a history of stressful life events. In this case, there is no gene directly related to the development of the mood disorder. There is a genetic marker associated with depression in the context of stressful life events.

One of the more important aspects of understanding the role of genetics in relation to mental illness such as major depression may be in pharmacological treatments. Understanding genetic influences on the role of the transport of certain neurotransmitters, such as serotonin, across synapses will make it much easier to prescribe effective medical treatment of depression based on individual genetic patterns.

Biochemical

The brain is a highly complex organ that contains billions of neurons. There is much evidence to support the concept that many CNS neurotransmitter abnormalities may cause clinical depression. These neurotransmitter abnormalities may be the result of genetic or environmental factors or other medical conditions, such as cerebral infarction, Parkinson's disease, hypothyroidism, acquired immunodeficiency syndrome (AIDS), or drug use.

Two of the main neurotransmitters involved in mood are serotonin (5-hydroxytryptamine [5-HT]) and norepinephrine. Serotonin is an important regulator of sleep, appetite, and libido. Therefore serotonin circuit dysfunction can result in sleep disturbances, decreased appetite, low sex drive, poor impulse control, and irritability. Norepinephrine modulates attention and behaviour. It is stimulated by stressful situations, which may result in overuse and a deficiency of norepinephrine. A deficiency, an imbalance as compared with other neurotransmitters, or an impaired ability to use available norepinephrine can result in apathy, reduced responsiveness, or slowed psychomotor activity.

Research suggests that depression results from the dysregulation of a number of neurotransmitter systems beyond serotonin and norepinephrine. For example, glutamate is a common neurotransmitter that increases the ability of a nerve fibre to transmit information. A deficit in glutamate can interfere with normal neuron transmission in the areas of the brain that affect mood, attention, and cognition.

Stressful life events, especially losses, seem to be a significant factor in the development of depression. Norepinephrine, serotonin, and acetylcholine play a role in stress regulation. When these neurotransmitters become overtaxed through stressful events, neurotransmitter depletion may occur. Research indicates that stress is associated with a reduction in neurogenesis, which is the ability of the brain to produce new brain cells.

At this time, no single mechanism of depressant action has been found. The relationships among the serotonin, norepinephrine, dopamine, acetylcholine, gamma-aminobutyric acid (GABA), and glutamate systems are complex and need further assessment and study. However, treatment with medication that helps regulate these neurotransmitters has proven to be empirically successful in the treatment of many patients. Figure 13-2 shows a positron emission tomography (PET) scan of the brain of a woman with depression before and after taking medication.

Hormonal

The neuroendocrine characteristic most widely studied in relation to depression has been hyperactivity of the hypothalamic–pituitary–adrenal axis. People with major depression have increased urine cortisol levels and elevated levels of corticotrophin-releasing hormone. Dexamethasone, an exogenous steroid that suppresses cortisol, is used in the dexamethasone suppression test (DST) for depression. Results of this test are abnormal in about 50% of people with depression, which indicates hyperactivity of the hypothalamic–pituitary–adrenal axis.

Depression rates are almost equal for males and females in the years preceding puberty and in older adults. This has led to more research into the effect of hormones on depression in women (Ryan & Ancelin, 2012). Recent studies have found that estradiol, a form of estrogen, affects receptors sensitive to serotonin in the areas of the brain responsible for mood in rats. As the relationships between sex hormones such as estrogen in women and testosterone in males are better understood, more effective therapies may be developed.

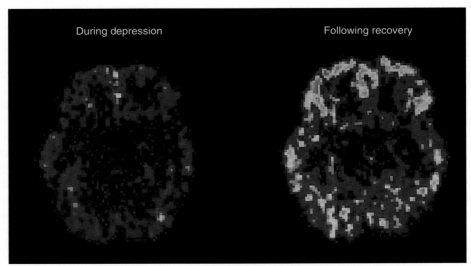

During depression   Following recovery

FIGURE 13-2 Positron emission tomography (PET) scans of a 45-year-old woman with recurrent depression. The scan on the left was taken when the patient was on no medication and very depressed. The scan on the right was taken several months later when the patient was well, after she had been treated with medication for her depression. Note that her entire brain, particularly the left prefrontal cortex, is more active when she is well. Source: Courtesy Mark George, MD, Biological Psychiatry Branch, National Institute of Mental Health.

Inflammation

Inflammation is the body's natural defence to physical injury. There is growing evidence that inflammation may be the result of psychological injury as well. Researchers have focused on two important blood components related to inflammation, C-reactive protein and interleukin-6. In young females with a history of adversity, depression is accompanied by elevations in these blood components, but this elevation does not occur in children without a history of adversity (Miller & Cole, 2012). Adversity in life may compromise resilience and place children at risk for depression and other disorders.

While we do not believe that inflammation causes depression, research indicates that it does play a role (Krishnadas & Cavanagh, 2012). Support for this belief includes the finding that about a third of people with major depression have elevated inflammatory biomarkers in the absence of a physical illness. Also, people who have inflammatory diseases have increased risk for major depression. Finally, people treated with cytokines to enhance immunity during cancer treatment develop major depression at a high rate.

Diathesis–Stress Model

The diathesis–stress model of depression takes into account the interplay of biology and life events in the development of depressive disorders. It is believed that psychosocial stressors and interpersonal events trigger neurophysical and neurochemical changes in the brain. Early life trauma may result in long-term hyperactivity of the CNS corticotropin-releasing factor (CRF), which releases the cortisol hormone, and norepinephrine systems, with a consequent neurotoxic effect on the hippocampus, which leads to overall neuronal loss. These changes could cause sensitization of the CRF circuits to even mild stress in adulthood, leading to an exaggerated stress response (Gillespie & Nemeroff, 2007).

Some people may be born with a predisposition toward depression, which is then triggered by a stressful life event. The experience of depression further alters the neurological connections in the brain, further increasing the predisposition toward depression. The result is a vicious cycle of recurrent depressive disorder. Early, effective treatment is needed to break the cycle.

Psychological Factors

Cognitive Theory

In cognitive theory, the underlying assumption is that a person's thoughts will result in emotions. If a person looks at his or her life in a positive way, the person will experience positive emotions, but negative interpretation of life events can result in sorrow, anger, and hopelessness. Cognitive theorists believe that people may acquire a psychological predisposition to depression due to early life experiences. These experiences contribute to negative, illogical, and irrational thought processes that may remain dormant until they are activated during times of stress (Beck & Rush, 1995). Beck and Rush (1995) found that people with depression process information in negative ways, even in the midst of positive factors. He believed that automatic, negative, repetitive, unintended, and not readily controllable thoughts

perpetuate depression. Three thoughts constitute Beck's cognitive triad:

1. A negative, self-deprecating view of self
2. A pessimistic view of the world
3. The belief that negative reinforcement (or no validation for the self) will continue in the future

Realizing that one has an ability to interpret life events in positive ways provides an element of control over emotions and, therefore, over depression.

Learned Helplessness

An older but still plausible theory of depression is that of learned helplessness. Seligman (1973) stated that although anxiety is the initial response to a stressful situation, it is replaced by depression if the person feels no control over the outcome of a situation. A person who believes that an undesired event is his or her fault and that nothing can be done to change it is prone to depression. The theory of learned helplessness has been used to explain the development of depression in certain social groups, such as older adults, people living in impoverished areas, and women.

APPLICATION OF THE NURSING PROCESS

ASSESSMENT

Major depressive disorder often goes unrecognized and underdiagnosed, yet early treatment can result in improved outcomes. Nurses at both the generalist and advanced-practice level are frequently in the position to screen and assess for signs of depression, thereby facilitating early and appropriate treatment.

General Assessment

Assessment Tools

Numerous standardized depression screening tools that help assess the type of depression are available, including the Beck Depression Inventory, the Hamilton Depression Rating Scale, the Zung Self-Rating Depression Scale, and the Geriatric Depression Scale.

The Patient Health Questionnaire-9 (PHQ-9), a short inventory that highlights predominant symptoms of depression, is presented here because of its ease of use (Figure 13-3). Many clinicians also use the mnemonic SIGECAPS (sleep, interest, guilt, energy, concentration, appetite, psychomotor activity, and suicidal thoughts) to guide their assessment.

The website http://heretohelp.bc.ca/screening/online/, sponsored by the BC Partners for Mental Health and Addictions Information, enables people to take an online confidential screening test for depression and anxiety and find reliable information on the illness.

Assessment of Suicide Potential

Suicidal Ideation

The most dangerous aspect of MDD is a preoccupation with death. A patient may fantasize about her funeral or experience recurring dreams about death. Beyond these passive fantasies are thoughts of wanting to die. As a whole, all of these nihilistic thoughts are referred to as suicidal ideation. These thoughts

PATIENT HEALTH QUESTIONNAIRE-9 (PHQ-9)

Over the <u>last 2 weeks</u>, how often have you been bothered by any of the following problems?	Not at all	Several days	More than half the days	Nearly every day
1. Little interest or pleasure in doing things	0	1	2	3
2. Feeling down, depressed, or hopeless	0	1	2	3
3. Trouble falling or staying asleep, or sleeping too much	0	1	2	3
4. Feeling tired or having little energy	0	1	2	3
5. Poor appetite or overeating	0	1	2	3
6. Feeling bad about yourself — or that you are a failure or have let yourself or your family down	0	1	2	3
7. Trouble concentrating on things, such as reading the newspaper or watching television	0	1	2	3
8. Moving or speaking so slowly that other people could have noticed? Or the opposite — being so fidgety or restless that you have been moving around a lot more than usual	0	1	2	3
9. Thoughts that you would be better off dead or of hurting yourself in some way	0	1	2	3

<u> 0 </u> + <u>   </u> + <u>   </u> + <u>   </u>

=Total score: <u>   </u>

If you checked off <u>any</u> problems, how <u>difficult</u> have these problems made it for you to do your work, take care of things at home, or get along with other people?

Not difficult at all	Somewhat difficult	Very difficult	Extremely difficult
☐	☐	☐	☐

I confirm this information is accurate.	Patient's/Subject's initials:	Date:

A

PHQ-9 SCORING CARD FOR SEVERITY DETERMINATION

for healthcare professional use only

Scoring—add up all checked boxes on PHQ-9

Total Score	Depression Severity
0-4	None
5-9	Mild
10-14	Moderate
15-19	Moderately severe
20-27	Severe

B

FIGURE 13-3 A, Patient Health Questionnaire-9 (PHQ-9). **B,** Scoring the PHQ-9. Source: © 2005 Pfizer, Inc. Developed by Drs. Robert L. Spitzer, Janet B. Williams, Kurt Kroenke, and colleagues.

may be relatively mild and fleeting, or persistent and involve a plan. Suicidal ideation, especially that in which the patient has a plan for suicide and the means to carry the plan out, represents an emergency requiring immediate intervention (refer to Chapter 22). Suicidal thoughts are a major reason for hospitalization for patients with major depression.

Patients diagnosed with MDD should always be evaluated for suicidal ideation. Risk for suicide is increased when depression is accompanied by hopelessness, substance use problems, a recent loss or separation, a history of past suicide attempts, or acute suicidal ideation. The following statements and questions help set the stage for assessing suicide potential:

- You have said you are depressed. Tell me what that is like for you.
- When you feel depressed, what thoughts go through your mind?

- Have you gone so far as to think about taking your own life?
- Do you have a suicide plan?
- Do you have the means to carry out your plan?
- Is there anything that would prevent you from carrying out your plan?

Refer to Chapter 22 for a detailed discussion of suicide, critical risk factors, warning signs, and strategies for suicide prevention. Also see Case Study and Nursing Care Plan 13-1.

Key Assessment Findings

A depressed mood and anhedonia (loss of ability to experience joy or pleasure in living) are the key symptoms of depression. Almost 97% of people with depression have anhedonia. Anxiety, a common symptom in depression, is seen in about 60% to 90% of patients with depression. Psychomotor agitation may be evidenced by constant pacing and wringing of hands. The slowed movements of psychomotor retardation, however, are more common. Somatic complaints (e.g., headaches, malaise, backaches) are also common. Vegetative signs of depression—alterations in those activities necessary to support physical life and growth (e.g., change in bowel movements and eating habits, sleep disturbances, lack of interest in sex)—are universally present.

Areas to Assess

Affect

Affect is the outward presentation of a person's internal state of being. It is reported as an objective finding based on the nurse's assessment. A person who has depression sees the world through grey-coloured glasses. Posture is poor, and the patient may look older than his or her stated age. Facial expressions convey sadness and dejection, and the patient may have frequent bouts of weeping. Conversely, the patient may say that he or she is unable to cry. Feelings of worthlessness, guilt, anger, helplessness, hopelessness, and despair are readily reflected in the person's affect. For example, the patient may not make eye contact, may speak in a monotone, may show little or no facial expression (flat affect), and may make only "yes" or "no" responses. Some individuals can be very depressed yet present as the "smiling depressed."

Thought Processes

During a depressive episode, the person's ability to solve problems and think clearly is negatively affected. Judgement is poor, and indecisiveness is common, largely because thinking is slow and memory and concentration are poor. People with depression also dwell on and exaggerate their perceived faults and failures and are unable to focus on their strengths and successes. They may experience delusions of being punished for doing bad deeds or being a terrible person. Common statements of delusional thinking are "I have committed unpardonable sins," "God wants me dead," and "I am wicked and should die."

Mood

Mood is the patient's subjective experience of sustained emotions or feelings. People, when asked to describe their mood, will describe how they are feeling. Should a client describe a feeling when asked about their mood, the clinician needs to follow-up with a question asking about how long they have felt this way. Mood is about feelings that last over several days, weeks, or months.

Feelings

Feelings frequently reported by those with depression include worthlessness, guilt, helplessness, hopelessness, and anger. Feelings of worthlessness range from feeling inadequate to having an unrealistically negative evaluation of self-worth. These feelings reflect the low self-esteem that is a painful partner to depression. Statements such as "I am no good" or "I'll never amount to anything" are common. Anhedonia (an "without" + hedone "pleasure" = inability to feel happy) refers to the absence of happiness or pleasure in aspects of life that once made the patient happy.

Guilt is a nearly universal accompaniment to depression. A person may ruminate over present or past failings: "I was never a good parent," or "it's my fault that project at work failed." These thoughts tend to occur again and again and are difficult for the patient to stop. These negative ruminations fill in the hours of lost sleep.

Cognitive Changes

Helplessness is demonstrated by a person's inability to solve problems in response to common concerns. In severe situations, helplessness may be evidenced by the inability to carry out the simplest tasks (e.g., grooming, doing housework, working, caring for children) because they seem too difficult to accomplish. With feelings of helplessness come feelings of hopelessness, which are particularly correlated with suicidality. Even though most depressive episodes are time limited, people experiencing them believe that things will never change. This feeling of utter hopelessness can lead people to view suicide as a way out of constant mental pain. Hopelessness includes the following attributes:

- Negative expectations for the future
- Loss of control over future outcomes
- Passive acceptance of the futility of planning to achieve goals
- Emotional negativism, as expressed in despair, despondency, or depression

Anger is a strong feeling of displeasure or hostility. It is a natural outcome of profound feelings of helplessness. Anger in depression is often expressed inappropriately through hurtful verbal attacks, physical aggression toward others, or destruction of property, and anger may be directed toward the self in the form of suicidal or otherwise self-destructive behaviours (e.g., alcohol abuse, substance abuse, overeating, smoking). These behaviours often reinforce feelings of low self-esteem and worthlessness.

Physical Behaviour

Lethargy and fatigue may result in psychomotor retardation, in which movements are extremely slow, facial expressions are decreased, and the gaze is fixed. The continuum of psychomotor retardation may range from slowed and difficult movements to complete inactivity and incontinence. Psychomotor agitation, in which patients constantly pace, bite their nails, smoke, tap their fingers, or engage in some other tension-relieving activity, may also be observed. At these times, patients commonly feel fidgety and unable to relax.

Vegetative signs of depression refer to alterations in those activities necessary to support physical life and growth (e.g., eating, sleeping, elimination, sex). Appetite changes vary in individuals experiencing depression. Appetite loss is common, and sometimes patients can lose up to 5% of their body weight in less than a month. Other patients find they eat more often and complain of weight gain.

Change in sleep pattern is a cardinal sign of depression. Often people experience insomnia, wake frequently, and have a total reduction in sleep, especially deep-stage sleep. Waking at 3 or 4 a.m. and then staying awake is common, as is sleeping for short periods only. The light sleep of a person with depression tends to prolong the agony of depression over a 24-hour period. For some, sleep is increased (hypersomnia) and provides an escape from painful feelings. In any event, sleep is rarely restful or refreshing.

Grooming, dressing, and personal hygiene may be markedly neglected. People who usually take pride in their appearance and dress may allow themselves to look shabby and unkempt. They may neglect to bathe, change clothes, or engage in other basic self-care activities.

Sexual interest declines (loss of libido) during depression. Some men experience impotence, and a declining interest in sex often occurs among both men and women, which can further complicate marital and social relationships.

Changes in bowel habits are common. Constipation is seen most frequently in patients with psychomotor retardation. Diarrhea occurs less frequently, often in conjunction with psychomotor agitation or anxiety.

Communication

A person with depression may speak and comprehend very slowly. The lack of an immediate response by the patient to a remark does not necessarily mean the patient has not heard or chooses not to reply; the patient may need more time to comprehend what was said and then compose a reply. In extreme depression, however, a person may become mute.

Religious Beliefs and Spirituality

Many studies have found a negative correlation between relational spiritual factors and depression. Specifically, it seems to be spiritual instability and a disappointment in a higher power that are predictors of depression (Paine & Sandage, 2017). In addressing spirituality, nurses must assess patients' spiritual strengths, whether peace focused, meaning, or religious. Addressing spiritual issues is not the domain of one discipline. Encouraging a connection with religious or spiritual practices that have brought the patient comfort in the past may be therapeutic.

Age Considerations
Assessment of Children and Adolescents

As children grow and develop, they may display a wide range of mood and behaviour, making it easy to overlook signs of depression. The core symptoms of depression in children and adolescents are the same as for adults, which are sadness and loss of pleasure. What differs is how these symptoms are displayed. For example, a very young child may cry, a school-aged child might withdraw, and a teenager may become irritable in response to feeling sad or hopeless. Younger children may suddenly refuse to go to school while adolescents may engage in substance abuse or sexual promiscuity and be preoccupied with death or suicide.

Assessment of Older Adults

Because older adults are more likely to complain of physical illness than emotional concerns, depression might be overlooked. Older patients actually do have comorbid physical problems, and it is difficult to determine whether fatigue, pain, and weakness are the result of an illness or depression. The Geriatric Depression Scale is a 30-item tool that is both valid and reliable in screening for depression in the older adult (Sheikh & Yesavage, 1986). Its "yes" or "no" format makes this scale easier to administer with patients with cognitive deficits. It can be helpful in determining suicidality in this population.

Self-Assessment

Patients with depression often reject the advice, encouragement, and understanding of the nurse and others, and they often appear not to respond to nursing interventions and seem resistant to change. When this occurs, the nurses may experience feelings of frustration, hopelessness, and annoyance. These problematic responses can be altered in the following ways:

- Recognizing any unrealistic expectations for yourself or the patient
- Identifying feelings that originate with the patient
- Understanding the roles that biology and genetics play in the precipitation and maintenance of a depressed mood

Unrealistic Expectations of Self

Nursing students and others new to caring for individuals with depression may have unrealistic expectations of themselves and their patients, and problems result when these expectations are not met. Unmet expectations usually result in a nurse feeling anxious, hurt, angry, helpless, or incompetent. Unrealistic expectations of self and others may be held even by experienced health care workers, a phenomenon that contributes to staff burnout. Many of your nursing expectations may not be conscious, but when these expectations are made conscious and are worked through with peers and more experienced clinicians (supervisors), more realistic expectations can be formed and attainable outcomes identified. Realistic expectations of self and the patient can decrease feelings of helplessness and increase a nurse's self-esteem and therapeutic potential.

Feeling What the Patient Is Feeling

It is not uncommon for nurses and other health care providers to experience intense anxiety, frustration, annoyance, hopelessness, and helplessness while caring for individuals with depression; nurses empathically sense what the patient is feeling. Novice nurses may interpret these emotions as personal reactions to the patient with whom they are working. However, these feelings can be important diagnostic clues to the patient's experience. You can discuss feelings of annoyance, hopelessness, and helplessness with peers and supervisors to separate personal feelings

RESEARCH HIGHLIGHT

Describing the Population Health Burden of Depression

Problem

Few studies have evaluated the impact of depression in terms of losses to both premature mortality and health-related quality of life (HRQOL) on the overall population.

Purpose of Study

The objective of the study was to estimate period life expectancy (LE) and health-adjusted life expectancy (HALE) of Canadian adults (ages 20 years and older) according to depression status. HALE is a summary measure of population health that combines both morbidity and mortality into a single summary statistic that describes the current health status of a population.

Methods

National Population Health Survey (NPHS) participants 20 years and older (n = 12 373) were followed for mortality outcomes from 1994 to 2009, based on depression status. Depression was defined as having likely experienced a major depressive episode in the previous year as measured by the Composite International Diagnostic Interview Short Form. Life expectancy was estimated by building period abridged life tables by sex and depression status using the relative risks of mortality from the NPHS and mortality data from the Canadian Chronic Disease Surveillance System (2007–2009). The Canadian Community Health Survey (2009/10) provided estimates of depression prevalence, and the Health Utilities Index was used as a measure of HRQOL. Using the combined mortality, depression prevalence, and HRQOL estimates,

HALE was estimated for the adult population according to depression status and by sex.

Key Findings

- Men and women in Canada who have depression live a substantially higher proportion of their life in an unhealthy state compared to their counterparts without depression.
- This gap in healthy life expectancy between Canadians with and without depression is primarily associated with losses in quality of life.
- Emotional state, cognitive state, and pain are the key attributes associated with losses in quality of life for Canadians experiencing a recent major depressive episode.
- Based on observations from past studies of the Canadian household population, the burden of depression on healthy life expectancy at a population level appears to be greater than that associated with other chronic conditions such as diabetes, hypertension, and obesity.

Implications for Nursing Practice

The population of adult men and women with depression in Canada has a substantially lower healthy life expectancy than those without depression. Reducing hopelessness and increasing positive future anticipation are factors associated with improving quality of life for people who experience depression. Nurses will need to consider using a future-directed therapy.

Source: Steensma, C., Loukine, L., Orpana, H., et al. (2016). Describing the population health burden of depression: Health-adjusted life expectancy by depression status in Canada. *Maladies Chroniques et Blessures au Canada, 36*(10), 205–213. Retrieved from http://www.phac-aspc.gc.ca/publicat/hpcdp-pspmc/index-fra.php.

from those originating with the patient. If personal feelings are not recognized, named, and examined, the nurse is likely to withdraw.

People instinctively avoid situations and other people that arouse feelings of frustration, annoyance, or intimidation. If the nurse also has unresolved feelings of anger and depression, the complexity of the situation is compounded. There is no substitute

VIGNETTE

Velma is working with Aleks, a patient with depression who is living at a homeless shelter after losing his job and being evicted from his apartment. Aleks expresses a lot of hopelessness about his future and believes that he will never get another job or be able to live on his own. During clinical conference, Velma states that she is feeling threatened and frustrated because Aleks rejects her suggestions and her attempts to help. She confesses that she thinks Aleks is not trying to feel better or improve his situation. Velma spends time reviewing the illness of depression, common behaviours, and patient needs. She also reviews the recovery model of mental illness. In subsequent visits, she refocuses on Aleks and stops giving him suggestions. After 4 weeks, Aleks has worked out a plan to live with relatives while he undergoes vocational training. He thanks Velma for listening and not making him "feel like a failure."

 ASSESSMENT GUIDELINES

Depression

1. Always evaluate the patient's risk for harm to self or others. Overt hostility is highly correlated with suicide (see Chapter 22).
2. Depression is a mood disorder that can be secondary to a host of medical or other psychiatric disorders, as well as to medications. A thorough medical and neurological examination helps determine if the depression is primary or secondary to another disorder. Essentially, evaluate whether:
   - The patient is psychotic
   - The patient has taken drugs or alcohol
   - Medical conditions are present
   - The patient has a history of a comorbid psychiatric syndrome (eating disorder, borderline or anxiety disorder)
3. Assess the patient's past history of depression, what past treatments worked and did not work, and any events that may have triggered this episode of depression.
4. Assess support systems, family, significant others, and the need for information and referrals.

for competent and supportive supervision to facilitate growth, both professionally and personally. Being supervised by a more experienced clinician and sharing with peers help minimize feelings of confusion, frustration, and isolation and can increase your therapeutic potential and self-esteem while you care for individuals with depression.

DIAGNOSIS

Depression is a complex disorder, and individuals with depression have a variety of needs; therefore nursing diagnoses are many. However, a high priority for the nurse is determining the risk for suicide, and the nursing diagnosis of *Risk for suicide* is always considered. Refer to Chapter 22 for assessment guidelines and interventions for suicidal individuals. Other key targets for nursing interventions are represented by the diagnoses of *Hopelessness*, *Ineffective coping*, *Social isolation*, *Spiritual distress*, and *Self-care deficit* (bathing, dressing, feeding, toileting). Table 13-2 identifies signs and symptoms commonly experienced in depression and offers potential nursing diagnoses.

OUTCOMES IDENTIFICATION

The Recovery Model

In 1993, Dr. William Anthony changed the focus of mental health to recovery from mental illness rather than treatment of it. The recovery model emphasizes that individuals with mental illnesses, including depression, can learn to live with their disease. It is individuals who define who they are, not their diseases. Recovery is attained through partnership with health care providers who focus on the patient's strengths. Treatment goals are mutually developed based on the patient's personal needs and values, and interventions are evidence informed. The recovery model is consistent with the focus on patient-centred care, which is a key component of safe, quality health care.

Remember that MDD can be a recurrent and chronic illness. Care should be directed not only at resolution of the acute phase but also at long-term management. The nurse and the patient identify realistic outcome criteria and formulate concrete, measurable short-term and intermediate indicators. Each patient is a unique individual, and indicators should be selected according to individual needs.

Table 13-3 presents some outcome criteria from the *Nursing Outcomes Classification (NOC)* (Moorhead, Johnson, Maas, et al., 2012). Indicators for the outcomes of the vegetative or physical signs of depression (e.g., reports adequate sleep) are formulated to show, for example, evidence of weight gain, return to normal bowel activity, sleep duration of 6 to 8 hours per night, or return of sexual desire.

PLANNING

The planning of care for patients with depression is geared toward the patient's phase of depression, particular symptoms, and personal goals. At all times during the care of a person with depression, nurses and members of the health care team must

TABLE 13-2 POTENTIAL NURSING DIAGNOSES FOR DEPRESSION	
SIGNS AND SYMPTOMS	**POTENTIAL NURSING DIAGNOSES**
Previous suicide attempts, putting affairs in order, giving away prized possessions, suicidal ideation (has plan, ability to carry it out), overt or covert statements regarding killing self, feelings of worthlessness, hopelessness, helplessness	*Risk for suicide* *Risk for self-mutilation* *Risk for self-harm*
Lack of judgement, memory difficulty, poor concentration, inaccurate interpretation of environment, negative ruminations, cognitive distortions	*Altered thought processes*
Difficulty with simple tasks, inability to function at previous level, poor problem solving, poor cognitive functioning, verbalizations of inability to cope	*Ineffective coping* *Interrupted family processes* *Risk for impaired attachment* *Ineffective role performance*
Difficulty making decisions, poor concentration, inability to take action	*Decisional conflict*
Feelings of helplessness, hopelessness, powerlessness	*Hopelessness* *Powerlessness*
Questioning the meaning of life and own existence, inability to participate in usual religious practices, conflict over spiritual beliefs, anger toward spiritual deity or religious representatives	*Spiritual distress* *Impaired religiosity* *Risk for impaired religiosity*
Feelings of worthlessness, poor self-image, negative sense of self, self-negating verbalizations, feeling of being a failure, expressions of shame or guilt, hypersensitivity to slights or criticism	*Chronic low self-esteem* *Situational low self-esteem*
Withdrawal, noncommunicativeness, monosyllabic speech, avoidance of contact with others	*Impaired social interaction* *Social isolation* *Risk for loneliness*
Vegetative signs of depression: changes in sleeping, eating, grooming and hygiene, elimination, sexual patterns	*Self-care deficit (bathing, dressing, feeding, toileting)* *Imbalanced nutrition: less than body requirements* *Disturbed sleep pattern* *Constipation* *Sexual dysfunction*

TABLE 13-3	*NOC* OUTCOMES RELATED TO DEPRESSION	
NURSING OUTCOME AND DEFINITION	**INTERMEDIATE INDICATORS**	**SHORT-TERM INDICATORS**
Depression self-control: Personal actions to minimize melancholy and maintain interest in life events	Reports improved mood Adheres to therapy schedule Takes medication as prescribed Follows treatment plan	Monitors intensity of depression Identifies precursors of depression Plans strategies to reduce effects of precursors Reports changes in symptoms to health care provider

Source: Moorhead, S., Johnson, M., Maas, M., et al. (2012). *Nursing outcomes classification (NOC)* (5th ed.). St. Louis: Mosby.

be cognizant of the potential for suicide; therefore assessment of risk for self-harm (or harm to others) is ongoing. A combination of therapy (cognitive, behavioural, and interpersonal) and psychopharmacology is an effective approach to the treatment of depression across all age groups.

Be aware that the vegetative signs of depression (e.g., changes in eating, sleeping, and sexual satisfaction), as well as changes in concentration, activity level, social interaction, care for personal appearance, and so on, often need targeting. The planning of care for a patient with depression is based on the individual's symptoms and goals, and it attempts to encompass a variety of areas in the person's life. Safety is always the highest priority.

IMPLEMENTATION

There are three phases in treatment of and recovery from major depression:

1. The *acute phase* (6 to 12 weeks) is directed at reduction of depressive symptoms and restoration of psychosocial and work function. Hospitalization may be required.
2. The *continuation phase* (4 to 9 months) is directed at prevention of relapse through pharmacotherapy, education, and depression-specific psychotherapy.
3. The *maintenance phase* (1 year or more) of treatment is directed at prevention of reoccurrences of depression.

It is important to keep in mind that the primary goal of both the continuation and the maintenance phases is keeping the patient a functional and contributing member of the community after recovery from the acute phase.

Counselling and Communication Techniques

Some patients with depression may be so withdrawn that they are unwilling or unable to speak. Nurses often experience some difficulty communicating with patients without talking; just sitting with them in silence may seem like a waste of time or be uncomfortable. As anxiety increases, the nurse may start daydreaming, feel bored, remember something that "must be done now," and so on. It is important to be aware, however, that this time can be meaningful, especially for the nurse who has a genuine interest in learning about the patient with depression.

Determining when a withdrawn patient will be able to respond is difficult. However, certain techniques are known to be useful in guiding effective nursing interventions. Some communication techniques to use with a severely withdrawn patient are listed in Guidelines for Communication: Communicating With Severely Withdrawn People. Counselling guidelines for use with patients

◆ GUIDELINES FOR COMMUNICATION
Communicating With Severely Withdrawn People

Intervention	Rationale
When a patient is mute, use the technique of making observations: "There are many new pictures on your wall." "You are wearing your new shoes." "You ate some of your breakfast."	When a patient is not ready to talk, direct questions can raise the patient's anxiety level and frustrate the nurse. Pointing to commonalities in the environment draws the patient into and reinforces reality.
Use simple, concrete words.	Slowed thinking and difficulty concentrating impair comprehension.
Allow time for the patient to respond.	Slowed thinking necessitates time to formulate a response.
Listen for covert messages and ask about suicide plans.	People often experience relief and a decrease in feelings of isolation when they share thoughts of suicide.
Avoid platitudes such as "Things will look up," "Everyone gets down once in a while," or "Tomorrow will be better."	Platitudes tend to minimize the patient's feelings and can increase feelings of guilt and worthlessness, because the patient cannot "look up" or "snap out of it."

with depression are offered in Guidelines for Communication: Counselling People With Depression.

Health Teaching and Health Promotion

One basic premise of the recovery model of mental illness is that each person controls his or her treatment based on individual goals. Within this model, health teaching is especially important because it allows patients to make informed choices. Health teaching is also an avenue for providing hope to the patient and should include the following information:

- Depression is an illness that is beyond a person's voluntary control.
- Although it is beyond voluntary control, depression can be managed through medication and lifestyle.
- Illness management depends in large part on understanding personal signs and symptoms of relapse.
- Illness management depends on understanding the role of medication and possible adverse effects of medication.
- Long-term management is best assured if the patient undergoes psychotherapy along with taking medication.
- Identifying and coping with the stress of interpersonal relationships—whether they are familial, social, or occupational—is a key to illness management.

GUIDELINES FOR COMMUNICATION
Counselling People With Depression

Intervention	Rationale
Help the patient question underlying assumptions and beliefs and consider alternative explanations for problems.	Reconstructing a healthier and more hopeful attitude about the future can alter depressed mood.
Work with the patient to identify cognitive distortions that encourage negative self-appraisal. For example: a. Overgeneralizations b. Self-blame c. Mind reading d. Discounting of positive attributes	Cognitive distortions reinforce a negative, inaccurate perception of self and world. a. The patient takes one fact or event and makes a general rule out of it ("He always …"; "I never…"). b. The patient consistently blames self for everything perceived as negative. c. The patient assumes others do not like him or her without any real evidence that assumptions are correct. d. The patient focuses on the negative.
Encourage activities that can raise self-esteem. Identify need for (a) problem-solving skills, (b) coping skills, and (c) assertiveness skills.	Many people with depression, especially women, are not taught a range of problem-solving and coping skills. Increasing social, family, and job skills can change negative self-assessment.
Encourage exercise, such as running or weight lifting.	Exercise can improve self-concept and potentially shift neurochemical balance.
Encourage formation of supportive relationships, such as through support groups, therapy, and peer support.	Such relationships reduce social isolation and enable the patient to work on personal goals and relationship needs.
Provide information referrals, when needed, for religious or spiritual information (e.g., readings, programs, tapes, community resources).	Spiritual and existential issues may be heightened during depressive episodes; many people find strength and comfort in spirituality or religion.

- Including the family in discharge planning is also important and helps the patient in the following ways:
  - Increases the family's understanding and acceptance of the family member and helps family recognize the importance of medication adherence during the aftercare period.
  - Increases the patient's use of aftercare facilities in the community.
  - Contributes to higher overall adjustment in the patient after discharge.

Promotion of Self-Care Activities

In addition to feelings of hopelessness, despair, and physical discomfort, signs of physical neglect may be apparent, in which case nursing measures for improving physical well-being and promoting adequate self-care are initiated. Some effective interventions targeting physical needs are listed in Table 13-4. Nurses in the community can work with family members to encourage a family member with depression to perform and maintain his or her self-care activities.

Milieu Management: Teamwork and Safety

Safe, quality inpatient care requires the skills of a well-coordinated team. Treating a patient with depression requires the skills of nurses and prescribers. Other members of the team include mental health technicians, pharmacists, dietitians, social workers, and the patient's significant others.

Safety becomes the most important issue facing a team that cares for people with depression who may be at high risk for suicide. Suicide precautions are usually instituted and include the removal of all harmful objects such as "sharps" (e.g., razors, scissors, nail files), strangulation risks (e.g., belts), and medication that can be used to overdose. Some patients with severe depression may need to have someone check on them frequently, perhaps every 15 minutes, or even have one-to-one observation.

Pharmacological Interventions

At the cellular level, mood disorders are caused by problems with neurotransmitters. It follows that medications that alter brain chemistry are an important component in their treatment. Refer to Figure 13-4 for a brief description of the neurobiology of depression. Antidepressant therapy is an effective strategy for most cases of MDD, particularly in severe cases. A combination of psychotherapies and antidepressant therapy is superior to either psychotherapy or psychopharmacological treatment alone (de Roten, Ambresin, Herrera, et al., 2017).

Antidepressant Drugs

Antidepressant drugs can positively alter poor self-concept, degree of withdrawal, vegetative signs of depression, and activity level. Target symptoms include the following:
- Sleep disturbance
- Appetite disturbance (decreased or increased)
- Fatigue
- Decreased sex drive
- Psychomotor retardation or agitation
- Diurnal variations in mood (often worse in the morning)
- Impaired concentration or forgetfulness
- Anhedonia

A drawback of antidepressant drugs is that improvement in mood may take 1 to 3 weeks or longer. If a patient is acutely suicidal, electroconvulsive therapy (discussed in detail later in this chapter) can be a reliable and effective alternative.

The goal of antidepressant therapy is the complete remission of symptoms. Often the first antidepressant prescribed is not the one that will ultimately bring about remission; aggressive treatment helps in finding the proper treatment. An adequate trial for the treatment of depression is 3 months. Individuals experiencing their first depressive episode are maintained on antidepressants for 6 to 9 months after symptoms of

TABLE 13-4 INTERVENTIONS TARGETING THE VEGETATIVE SIGNS OF DEPRESSION

INTERVENTION	RATIONALE
Nutrition—Anorexia	
Offer small, high-calorie and high-protein snacks frequently throughout the day and evening.	Low weight and poor nutrition render the patient susceptible to illness. Small, frequent snacks are more easily tolerated than large plates of food when the patient is anorexic.
Offer high-protein and high-calorie fluids frequently throughout the day and evening.	These fluids prevent dehydration and can minimize constipation.
When possible, encourage family or friends to remain with the patient during meals.	This strategy reinforces the idea that someone cares, can raise the patient's self-esteem, and can serve as an incentive to eat.
Ask the patient which foods or drinks he or she likes. Offer choices. Involve the dietitian.	The patient is more likely to eat the foods provided.
Weigh the patient weekly and observe the patient's eating patterns.	Monitoring the patient's status gives the information needed for revision of the intervention.
Sleep—Insomnia	
Provide periods of rest after activities.	Fatigue can intensify feelings of depression.
Encourage the patient to get up and dress and to stay out of bed during the day.	Minimizing sleep during the day increases the likelihood of sleep at night.
Encourage the use of relaxation measures in the evening (e.g., tepid bath, warm milk).	These measures induce relaxation and sleep.
Reduce environmental and physical stimulants in the evening—provide decaffeinated coffee, soft lights, soft music, and quiet activities.	Decreasing caffeine and epinephrine levels increases the possibility of sleep.
Self-Care Deficits	
Encourage the use of toothbrush, washcloth, soap, makeup, shaving equipment, and so forth.	Being clean and well groomed can temporarily increase self-esteem.
When appropriate, give step-by-step reminders such as "Wash the right side of your face; now the left."	Slowed thinking and difficulty concentrating make organizing simple tasks difficult.
Elimination—Constipation	
Monitor intake and output, especially bowel movements.	Many patients with depression are constipated. If the condition is not checked, fecal impaction can occur.
Offer foods high in fibre, and provide periods of exercise.	Roughage and exercise stimulate peristalsis and help evacuation of fecal material.
Encourage the intake of fluids.	Fluids help prevent constipation.
Evaluate the need for laxatives and enemas.	These measures prevent fecal impaction.

depression remit. Some people may have multiple episodes of depression or may have a chronic form (similar to the chronicity of diabetes) and benefit from indefinite antidepressant therapy.

Antidepressants may precipitate a psychotic episode in a person with schizophrenia or a manic episode in a patient with bipolar disorder. Patients with bipolar disorder often receive a mood-stabilizing drug along with an antidepressant.

Choosing an antidepressant. All antidepressants work to increase the availability of one or more of the neurotransmitters, serotonin, norepinephrine, or dopamine. All antidepressants work equally well; however, a variety of antidepressants or a combination of antidepressants may need to be tried before the most effective regimen is found for an individual patient. Each of the antidepressants has different adverse effects, costs, safety issues, and maintenance considerations. Selection of the appropriate antidepressant is based on the following considerations:
- Adverse-effect profile (e.g., sexual dysfunction, weight gain)
- Ease of administration
- History of past response
- Safety and medical considerations

Drug Treatment of Patients with Major Depression provides an overview of antidepressants used in Canada.

Selective serotonin reuptake inhibitors. The selective serotonin reuptake inhibitors (SSRIs) are recommended as first-line therapy for most types of depression. Essentially, the SSRIs selectively block the neuronal uptake of serotonin (e.g., 5-HT, 5-HT$_1$ receptors), which increases the availability of serotonin in the synaptic cleft. Refer to Chapter 11 for a more detailed discussion of how the SSRIs work.

SSRI antidepressant drugs have a relatively low adverse-effect profile compared with the older antidepressants (tricyclics—discussed later in this chapter); blurred vision, or urinary retention, making it easier for patients to take these medications as prescribed. Adherence to the medication regimen is a crucial step toward recovery or remission of symptoms. The SSRIs are effective in depression with anxiety features and in depression with psychomotor agitation.

Because the SSRIs cause relatively few adverse effects and have low cardiotoxicity, they are less dangerous than older antidepressants when taken in overdose. The SSRIs, selective serotonin–norepinephrine reuptake inhibitors (SNRIs), and

▶ Neurobiology of Depression and the Effect of Antidepressants

Imbalance of certain neurotransmitters (serotonin and norepinephrine) contribute to depression in certain parts of the brain.
Prefrontal cortex: regulates role in executive functions and emotional control and memory.

Limbic system: regulates activities such as emotions, physical and sexual drives, and the stress response, as well as processing, learning, and memory (amygdala, hypothalamus, hippocampus).

Anterior cingulate cortex: regulates heart rate and blood pressure. Other functions include decision making, emotional regulation, error detection, preparation for tasks, and executive functions.

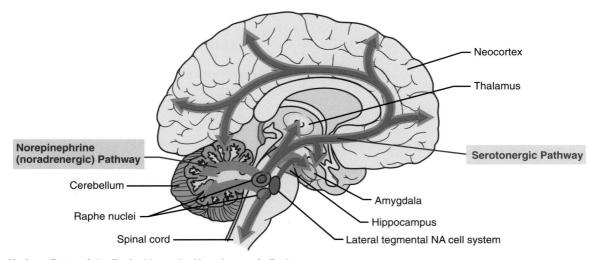

Various Parts of the Brain Along the Noradrenergic Pathway
The axons of these neurons project upward through the forebrain to the cerebral cortex, the limbic system, the thalamus, and the hippocampus.

Norepinephrine (NE) and the Noradrenergic System: plays a major role in mood and emotional behaviour as well as energy, drive, anxiety, focus, and metabolism.

Various Parts of the Brain Along the Serotonergic Pathway
The axons of serotonergic neurons originate in the raphe nuclei of the brainstem and project to the cerebral cortex, the limbic system, cerebellum, and spinal cord.

Serotonin (5-HT) and the Serotonergic System: involved in the regulation of pain, depression, pleasure, anxiety, panic arousal, sleep cycle, carbohydrate craving, and premenstrual syndrome.

Medications for Depression
Medications for depression include the selective serotonin reuptake inhibitors (**SSRIs**), serotonin–norepinephrine reuptake inhibitors (**SNRIs**), serotonin antagonist and reuptake inhibitors (**SARIs**), norepinephrine–dopamine reuptake inhibitor (**NDRI**), noradrenergic and specific serotonergic antidepressants (**NaSSAs**), tricyclic antidepressants (**TCAs**), and monoamine oxidase inhibitors (**MAOIs**).
They all work equally well and are chosen by their safety profile and side effects.* All have a delayed response, a discontinuation syndrome, and a Black Box Warning for suicide.

Patient's Problem*	Side-Effect Profile*	Example of Drug*
Fatigue	Stimulates the CNS	Fluoxetine (SSRI)
Insomnia	Substantial sedation	Mirtazapine (NaSSA)
Sexual dysfunction	Enhances libido	Bupropion (NDRI)
Chronic pain	Relieves pain	TCAs or duloxetine (SNRI)

*Adapted from Burchum, J. R.,& Rosenthal, L. D.(2016). *Lehne's pharmacology for nursing care* (9th ed.). St. Louis: Elsevier.

FIGURE 13-4 Neurobiology of depression.

DRUG TREATMENT OF PATIENTS WITH MAJOR DEPRESSION

GENERIC (TRADE)	ACTION	NOTES	ADVERSE EFFECTS	WARNINGS
Selective Serotonin Reuptake Inhibitors (SSRIs)				
Citalopram (Celexa) Fluoxetine (Prozac) Fluvoxamine (Luvox) Paroxetine (Paxil) Sertraline (Zoloft) Escitalopram (Cipralex)	Blocks the reuptake of serotonin	First-line treatment for major depression Some SSRIs activate and others sedate; choice depends on patient symptoms Risk of lethal overdose minimized with SSRIs	Agitation, insomnia, headache, nausea and vomiting, sexual dysfunction, hyponatremia	Discontinuation syndrome—dizziness, insomnia, nervousness, irritability, nausea, and agitation—may occur with abrupt withdrawal (depending on half-life); taper slowly Contraindicated in people taking MAOIs
Serotonin–Norepinephrine Reuptake Inhibitors (SNRIs)				
Venlafaxine (Effexor) Duloxetine (Cymbalta)	Blocks the reuptake of serotonin and norepinephrine	Effexor is a popular next-step strategy after trying SSRIs Cymbalta has the advantage of decreasing neuropathic pain	Hypertension (venlafaxine), nausea, insomnia, dry mouth, sweating, agitation, headache, sexual dysfunction	Monitor blood pressure with Effexor, especially at higher doses and with a history of hypertension Hypertension may be particularly noted in the diastolic measurement Discontinuation syndrome (see SSRIs above) Contraindicated in people taking MAOIs
Norepinephrine Reuptake Inhibitors (NRIs)				
Venlafaxine (Effexor XR) Duloxetine (Cymbalta)	Blocks the reuptake of norepinephrine and enhances its transmission	Antidepressant effects similar to SSRIs and TCAs Useful with severe depression and impaired social functioning	Insomnia, sweating, dizziness, dry mouth, constipation, urinary hesitancy, tachycardia, decreased libido	Contraindicated in people taking MAOIs
Norepinephrine–Dopamine Reuptake Inhibitors (NDRIs)				
Bupropion (Wellbutrin)	Blocks the reuptake of norepinephrine and dopamine Not indicated for patients under 18 years of age	Stimulant action may reduce appetite May increase sexual desire Used as an aid to quit smoking	Agitation, insomnia, headache, nausea and vomiting, seizures (0.4%)	Contraindicated in people taking MAOIs High doses increase seizure risk, especially in people who are predisposed to seizures
Serotonin–Norepinephrine Disinhibitors (SNDIs)				
Mirtazapine (Remeron)	Blocks α_1-adrenergic receptors that normally inhibit norepinephrine and serotonin	Antidepressant effects equal SSRIs and may occur faster	Weight gain, sedation, dizziness, headache; sexual dysfunction is rare	Drug-induced somnolence exaggerated by alcohol, benzodiazepines, and other CNS depressants Contraindicated in people taking MAOIs
Tricyclic Antidepressants (TCAs)				
Amitriptyline (Elavil) Clomipramine (Anafranil) Nortriptyline (Aventyl)	Inhibits the reuptake of serotonin and norepinephrine Antagonizes adrenergic, histaminergic, and muscarinic receptors	Therapeutic effects similar to SSRIs, but adverse effects are more prominent May work better in melancholic depression TCAs can worsen many cardiac and other medical conditions	Dry mouth, constipation, urinary retention, blurred vision, orthostatic hypotension, cardiac toxicity, sedation	Lethal in overdose Use cautiously in older adults and those with cardiac disorders, elevated intraocular pressure, urinary retention, hyperthyroidism, seizure disorders, or liver or kidney dysfunction Contraindicated in people taking MAOIs

Continued

DRUG TREATMENT OF PATIENTS WITH MAJOR DEPRESSION—cont'd

GENERIC (TRADE)	ACTION	NOTES	ADVERSE EFFECTS	WARNINGS
Monoamine Oxidase Inhibitors (MAOIs)				
Phenelzine (Nardil) Tranylcypromine (Parnate)	Inhibits the enzyme monoamine oxidase, which normally breaks down neurotransmitters, including serotonin and norepinephrine	Efficacy similar to other antidepressants, but dietary restrictions and potential drug interactions make this drug type less desirable	Insomnia, nausea, agitation, confusion Potential for hypertensive crisis or serotonin syndrome with concurrent use of other antidepressants	Contraindicated in people taking other antidepressants Tyramine-rich food could bring about a hypertensive crisis Many other drug interactions
Moclobemide (Aurorix, Manerix)	Acts on serotonin, norepinephrine, and dopamine	MDD and social anxiety	Nausea and dizziness	Contraindicated if known hypersensitivity to moclobemide

Sources: Canadian Pharmacists Association & Canadian Pharmaceutical Association. (2016). *Compendium of pharmaceuticals and specialties: Canada's trusted drug reference.* Toronto: Canadian Pharmaceutical Association; and Lehne, R. A. (2013). *Pharmacology for nursing care* (8th ed.). St Louis: Elsevier.

atypical antidepressants have a low lethality risk in suicide attempts, whereas the tricyclic antidepressants (TCAs) have a very high potential for lethality with overdose.

Indications. The SSRIs have a broad base of clinical use. In addition to their use in treating depressive disorders, the SSRIs have been prescribed with success to treat some anxiety disorders—in particular, obsessive-compulsive disorder and panic disorder (see Chapter 12). Fluoxetine has been found to be effective in treating some women who suffer from late luteal phase dysphoric disorder and bulimia nervosa.

Common adverse reactions. Agents that selectively enhance synaptic serotonin within the CNS may induce agitation, anxiety, sleep disturbance, tremor, sexual dysfunction (primarily anorgasmia), or tension headache. The effect of the SSRIs on sexual performance may be the most significant undesirable outcome reported by patients. Autonomic reactions (e.g., dry mouth, sweating, weight change, mild nausea, loose bowel movements) may also be experienced with the SSRIs.

Potential toxic effects. One rare and life-threatening event associated with SSRIs is serotonin syndrome. This syndrome is thought to be related to overactivation of the central serotonin receptors, caused by either too high a dose or interaction with other drugs, including nonprescription medication like St. John's wort. Symptoms include abdominal pain, diarrhea, sweating, fever, tachycardia, elevated blood pressure, altered mental state (delirium), myoclonus (muscle spasms), increased motor activity, irritability, hostility, and mood change. Severe manifestations can induce hyperpyrexia (excessively high fever), cardiovascular shock, or death.

The risk of this syndrome seems to be greatest when an SSRI is administered in combination with a second serotonin-enhancing agent, such as a monoamine oxidase inhibitor (MAOI). A patient should discontinue all SSRIs for 2 to 5 weeks before starting an MAOI. Box 13-2 lists the signs and symptoms of serotonin syndrome and gives emergency treatment guidelines. Patient and Family Teaching: Selective Serotonin Reuptake Inhibitors (SSRIs) is a useful tool for teaching the patient and family about the SSRIs.

BOX 13-2   SEROTONIN SYNDROME: SYMPTOMS AND INTERVENTIONS

Symptoms
- Hyperactivity or restlessness
- Tachycardia → cardiovascular shock
- Fever → hyperpyrexia
- Elevated blood pressure
- Altered mental states (delirium)
- Irrationality, mood swings, hostility
- Seizures → status epilepticus
- Myoclonus, incoordination, tonic rigidity
- Abdominal pain, diarrhea, bloating
- Apnea → death

Interventions
- Remove offending agents
- Initiate symptomatic treatment:
  - Serotonin receptor blockade with cyproheptadine, methysergide, propranolol
  - Cooling blankets, chlorpromazine for hyperthermia
  - Dantrolene, diazepam for muscle rigidity or rigours
  - Anticonvulsants
  - Artificial ventilation
  - Paralysis

Serotonin–norepinephrine reuptake inhibitors. The serotonin–norepinephrine reuptake inhibitors (SNRIs) inhibit the reuptake of both serotonin and norepinephrine. Pharmacological side effects are similar to those of the SSRIs, although the SSRIs may be tolerated better. The SNRIs are indicated for MDD.

Other newer antidepressants. Several other classifications of antidepressants have been introduced and have provided people with depression and prescribers with more options. The name of the classification describes the action of the antidepressants. They are the serotonin antagonist and reuptake inhibitors (SARIs), a norepinephrine–dopamine reuptake inhibitor (NDRI), and a noradrenergic and specific serotonergic antidepressant (NaSSA). Chapter 11 provides more detail about these drug classifications.

PATIENT AND FAMILY TEACHING
Selective Serotonin Reuptake Inhibitors (SSRIs)

- May cause sexual dysfunction or lack of sex drive. Inform nurse or primary care provider if this occurs.
- May cause insomnia, anxiety, and nervousness. Inform nurse or primary care provider if this occurs.
- May interact with other medications. Tell primary care provider about other medications patient is taking (digoxin, warfarin). SSRIs should not be taken within 14 days of the last dose of a monoamine oxidase inhibitor.
- No over-the-counter drug should be taken without first notifying primary care provider.
- Common adverse effects include fatigue, nausea, diarrhea, dry mouth, dizziness, tremor, and sexual dysfunction or lack of sex drive.
- Because of the potential for drowsiness and dizziness, patient should not drive or operate machinery until these adverse effects are ruled out.
- Alcohol should be avoided.
- Liver and renal function tests should be performed and blood counts checked periodically.
- Medication should not be discontinued abruptly. If adverse effects become bothersome, patient should ask primary care provider about changing to a different drug. Abrupt cessation can lead to serotonin withdrawal.
- Any of the following symptoms should be reported to the primary care provider immediately:
  - Increase in depression or suicidal thoughts
  - Rash or hives
  - Rapid heartbeat
  - Sore throat
  - Difficulty urinating
  - Fever, malaise
  - Anorexia and weight loss
  - Unusual bleeding
  - Initiation of hyperactive behaviour
  - Severe headache

Tricyclic antidepressants. The tricyclic antidepressants (TCAs) inhibit the reuptake of norepinephrine and serotonin by the presynaptic neurons in the CNS, increasing the amount of time norepinephrine and serotonin are available to the postsynaptic receptors. This increase in norepinephrine and serotonin in the brain is believed to be responsible for mood elevations.

Indications. The sedative effects of the TCAs are attributed to the blockage of histamine receptors (Lehne, 2013). Patients must take therapeutic doses of TCAs for 10 to 14 days or longer before they begin to work; full effects may not be seen for 4 to 8 weeks, but an effect on some symptoms of depression, such as insomnia and anorexia, may be noted earlier. Choosing a TCA for a patient is based on what has worked for the patient or a family member in the past and the drug's adverse effects for that patient.

A stimulating TCA, such as desipramine (Norpramin), may be best for a patient who is lethargic and fatigued. If a more sedating effect is needed for agitation or restlessness, drugs such as amitriptyline (Elavil) and doxepin (Sinequan) may be more

appropriate choices. Regardless of which TCA is given, the initial dose should always be low and increased gradually.

Common adverse reactions. The chemical structure of the TCAs closely resembles that of antipsychotic medications, and the anticholinergic actions are similar (e.g., dry mouth, blurred vision, tachycardia, constipation, urinary retention, esophageal reflux). These adverse effects are more common and more severe in patients taking antidepressants than in patients taking antipsychotic medications. They usually are not serious and are often transitory, but urinary retention and severe constipation warrant immediate medical attention. Weight gain is also a common complaint among people taking TCAs.

The α-adrenergic blockade of the TCAs can produce postural-orthostatic hypotension and tachycardia. Postural hypotension can lead to dizziness and increase the risk for falls.

Administering the total daily dose of TCA at night is beneficial for two reasons: (1) most TCAs have sedative effects and thereby aid sleep, and (2) the minor adverse effects occur while the individual is sleeping, which increases adherence to drug therapy.

Potential toxic effects. The most serious effects of the TCAs are cardiovascular: dysrhythmias, tachycardia, myocardial infarction, and heart block have been reported. Because the cardiac adverse effects are so serious, TCA use is considered a risk in older adults and patients with cardiac disease. Patients should have a thorough cardiac workup before beginning TCA therapy.

Adverse drug interactions. A few of the more common medications usually not given while TCAs are being used are MAOIs, phenothiazines, barbiturates, disulfiram (Antabuse), oral contraceptives (or other estrogen preparations), anticoagulants, some antihypertensives (clonidine, guanethidine, reserpine), benzodiazepines, and alcohol. A patient who is taking any of these medications along with a TCA should have medical clearance because some of the reactions can be fatal.

Contraindications. People who have recently had a myocardial infarction (or other cardiovascular problems), those with narrow-angle glaucoma or a history of seizures, and women who are pregnant should not be treated with TCAs, except with extreme caution and careful monitoring.

Patient and family teaching. Topics for the nurse to discuss when teaching patients and their families about TCA therapy are presented in Patient and Family Teaching: Tricyclic Antidepressants (TCAs).

Monoamine oxidase inhibitors. The enzyme monoamine oxidase is responsible for inactivating, or breaking down, certain monoamine neurotransmitters in the brain, such as norepinephrine, serotonin, dopamine, and tyramine. When a person ingests an MAOI, these amines do not get inactivated, and there is an increase of neurotransmitters available for synaptic release in the brain. The increase in norepinephrine, serotonin, and dopamine is the desired effect because it results in mood elevation. The increase in tyramine, on the other hand, poses a problem. When the level of tyramine increases, and it is not inactivated by monoamine oxidase, high blood pressure, hypertensive crisis, and eventually cerebrovascular accident can occur. Therefore people taking these drugs must reduce or eliminate their intake of foods and drugs that contain high amounts of tyramine (Box 13-3; Table 13-5).

PATIENT AND FAMILY TEACHING

Tricyclic Antidepressants (TCAs)

- The patient and family should be told that mood elevation may take from 7 to 28 days. Up to 6 to 8 weeks may be required for the full effect to be reached and for major depressive symptoms to subside.
- The family should reinforce this information frequently to the family member with depression, who may have trouble remembering and may respond to ongoing reassurance.
- The patient should be reassured that drowsiness, dizziness, and hypotension usually subside after the first few weeks.
- The patient should be cautioned to be careful when working around machines, driving cars, and crossing streets because of possible altered reflexes, drowsiness, or dizziness.
- Alcohol can block the effects of antidepressants. The patient should be told to refrain from drinking.
- If possible, the patient should take the full dose at bedtime to reduce the experience of adverse effects during the day.
- If the bedtime dose (or the once-a-day dose) is missed, the patient should take the dose within 3 hours; otherwise, the patient should wait until the usual medication time on the next day. The patient should not double the dose.
- Suddenly stopping TCAs can cause nausea, altered heartbeat, nightmares, and cold sweats within 2 to 4 days. The patient should call the primary care provider or take one dose of the TCA until the primary care provider can be contacted.

Because people with depression are often lethargic, confused, and apathetic, adherence to strict dietary limitations may not be realistic. That is why MAOIs, although highly effective, are not often given as a first-line treatment.

Indications. MAOIs are particularly effective for people with atypical depression (characterized by mood reactivity, oversleeping, and overeating), along with panic disorder, social phobia, generalized anxiety disorder, obsessive-compulsive disorder, post-traumatic stress disorder, and bulimia. The MAOIs commonly used in Canada at present are phenelzine (Nardil) and tranylcypromine sulphate (Parnate).

BOX 13-3	DRUGS THAT CAN INTERACT WITH MONOAMINE OXIDASE INHIBITORS (MAOIS)

- Over-the-counter medications for colds, allergies, or congestion (any product containing ephedrine or phenylpropanolamine)
- Tricyclic antidepressants (imipramine, amitriptyline)
- Narcotics
- Antihypertensives (methyldopa, spironolactone)
- Amine precursors (levodopa, L-tryptophan)
- Sedatives (alcohol, barbiturates, benzodiazepines)
- General anesthetics
- Stimulants (amphetamines, cocaine)

TABLE 13-5	FOODS THAT CAN INTERACT WITH MONOAMINE OXIDASE INHIBITORS (MAOIS)

Foods That Contain Tyramine

CATEGORY	UNSAFE FOODS (HIGH TYRAMINE CONTENT)	SAFE FOODS (LITTLE OR NO TYRAMINE)
Vegetables	Avocados, especially if over-ripe; fermented bean curd; fermented soybean; soybean paste	Most vegetables
Fruits	Figs, especially if over-ripe; bananas, in large amounts	Most fruits
Meats	Meats that are fermented, smoked, or otherwise aged; spoiled meats; liver, unless very fresh	Meats that are known to be fresh (exercise caution in restaurants; meats may not be fresh)
Sausages	Fermented varieties; bologna, pepperoni, salami, others	Nonfermented varieties
Fish	Dried or cured fish; fish that is fermented, smoked, or otherwise aged; spoiled fish	Fish that is known to be fresh; vacuum-packed fish, if eaten promptly or refrigerated only briefly after opening
Milk, milk products	Practically all cheeses	Milk, yogurt, cottage cheese, cream cheese
Foods with yeast	Yeast extract (e.g., Marmite, Bovril)	Baked goods that contain yeast
Beer, wine	Some imported beers, Chianti wines	Major domestic brands of beer; most wines
Other foods	Protein dietary supplements; soups (may contain protein extract); shrimp paste; soy sauce	

Foods That Contain Other Vasopressors

FOOD	COMMENTS
Chocolate	Contains phenylethylamine, a pressor agent; large amounts can cause a reaction.
Fava beans	Contain dopamine, a pressor agent; reactions are most likely with over-ripe beans.
Ginseng	Headache, tremulousness, and mania-like reactions have occurred.
Caffeinated beverages	Caffeine is a weak pressor agent; large amounts may cause a reaction.

Source: Lehne, R. A. (2013). *Pharmacology for nursing care* (8th ed.). St Louis: Elsevier.

TABLE 13-6	ADVERSE REACTIONS TO AND TOXIC EFFECTS OF MONOAMINE OXIDASE INHIBITORS (MAOIs)

ADVERSE REACTIONS	COMMENTS
Hypotension Insomnia Changes in cardiac rhythm Anorgasmia or sexual impotence Urinary hesitancy or constipation Weight gain	Hypotension is a normal adverse effect of MAOIs. Orthostatic blood pressures should be taken—first lying down, then sitting or standing after 1 to 2 minutes. Hypotension may be a dangerous adverse effect, especially in older adults who may fall and sustain injuries as a result of dizziness from the blood pressure drop.
TOXIC EFFECTS	**COMMENTS**
Hypertensive crisis: • Severe headache • Tachycardia, palpitations • Hypertension • Nausea and vomiting	Patient should go to local emergency department immediately—blood pressure should be checked. One of the following may be given to lower blood pressure: • 5 mg intravenous phentolamine (Rogitine) • Sublingual nifedipine to promote vasodilation Patients may be prescribed a 10-mg nifedipine capsule to carry in case of emergency.

Source: Data from Canadian Pharmacists Association & Canadian Pharmaceutical Association. (2016). *Compendium of pharmaceuticals and specialties: Canada's trusted drug reference.* Toronto: Canadian Pharmaceutical Association; and Lehne, R. A. (2013). *Pharmacology for nursing care* (8th ed.). St Louis: Elsevier.

Common adverse reactions. Some common and troublesome long-term adverse effects of the MAOIs are orthostatic hypotension, weight gain, edema, change in cardiac rate and rhythm, constipation, urinary hesitancy, sexual dysfunction, vertigo, overactivity, muscle twitching, hypomanic and manic behaviour, insomnia, weakness, and fatigue.

Potential toxic effects. The most serious reaction to the MAOIs is an increase in blood pressure, with the possible development of intracranial hemorrhage, hyperpyrexia, convulsions, coma, and death. Therefore routine monitoring of blood pressure, especially during the first 6 weeks of treatment, is necessary.

Because many drugs, foods, and beverages can cause an increase in blood pressure in patients taking MAOIs, hypertensive crisis is a constant concern. The hypertensive crisis usually occurs within 15 to 90 minutes of ingestion of the contraindicated substance. Early symptoms include irritability, anxiety, flushing, sweating, and a severe headache. The patient then becomes anxious, restless, and develops a fever. Eventually the fever becomes severe, seizures ensue, and coma or death is possible.

When a hypertensive crisis is suspected, immediate medical attention is crucial. If ingestion is recent, gastric lavage and charcoal may be helpful. Pyrexia is treated with hypothermic blankets or ice packs. Fluid therapy is essential, particularly with hyperthermia. A short-acting antihypertensive agent such as nitroprusside, nitroglycerine, or phentolamine may be used. Intravenous benzodiazepines are useful for agitation and seizure control.

Table 13-6 identifies common adverse effects and toxic effects of the MAOIs, and Patient and Family Teaching: Monoamine Oxidase Inhibitors (MAOIs) can be used as an MAOI teaching guide for patients and their families.

Contraindications. The use of MAOIs may be contraindicated with each of the following:
- Cerebrovascular disease
- Hypertension and congestive heart failure
- Liver disease

PATIENT AND FAMILY TEACHING

Monoamine Oxidase Inhibitors (MAOIs)

- Educate and provide details to the patient and family to avoid certain foods and all medications (especially cold remedies) unless prescribed by and discussed with the patient's primary care provider (see Table 13-5 and Box 13-3 for specific food and drug restrictions).
- Give the patient a wallet card describing the MAOI regimen.
- Instruct the patient to avoid Chinese restaurants (sherry, brewer's yeast, and other contraindicated products may be used).
- Advise the patient to go to the emergency department immediately if he or she has a severe headache.
- Ideally, blood pressure should be monitored during the first 6 weeks of treatment (for both hypotensive and hypertensive effects).
- After the MAOI is stopped, instruct the patient that dietary and drug restrictions should be maintained for 14 days.

- Consumption of foods containing tyramine, tryptophan, and dopamine (see Table 13-5)
- Use of certain medications (see Box 13-3)
- Recurrent or severe headaches
- Surgery in the previous 10 to 14 days
- Age younger than 16 years

Use of antidepressants by pregnant women. The risk of depression in pregnant women may be as high as 20% (Olivier, Akerud, & Promomaa, 2015). There is evidence that depression has a negative effect on birth outcomes. Pre-eclampsia, diabetes, and hypertension have all been associated with maternal depression. Low birth weight, preterm birth, and small size for gestational age have been noted effects in infants born to depressed mothers. We know that antidepressants cross the placenta. Treatment of severe depression, particularly with suicidal ideation, must weigh out the risks versus the benefits.

Use of antidepressants by children and adolescents. In 2005, Health Canada issued a Black Box Warning for all antidepressants, alerting the public to the increased risk for suicidal thinking or suicide attempts in children or adolescents under the age of 18 who are taking antidepressants. Following the Black Box Warning, the number of prescriptions written for SSRIs for children and young adults decreased, but the rates of suicide in those age groups actually increased (Friedman, 2014). Dudley and colleagues concluded that the risk for suicide is greater in children and adolescents with depression who do not take antidepressants. To minimize the risk for suicide in people taking antidepressants, close monitoring by health care providers and patient and caregiver education are essential. Chapter 22 has a more detailed discussion of suicide risk factors and warning signs.

Use of antidepressants by older adults. Polypharmacy and the normal process of aging contribute to concerns about prescribing antidepressants for older adults. SSRIs are a first-line treatment for older adults, but they have the potential for aggravated adverse effects. Starting doses are recommended to be half the lowest adult dose, with dose adjustments occurring no more frequently than every 7 days.

TCAs and MAOIs have adverse-effect profiles that are more dangerous for older adults, specifically cardiotoxicity with TCAs and hypotension with both classes. Any medication with an adverse effect of hypotension or sedation in older adults increases the risk for falls. Older adults should be cautioned against abrupt discontinuation of antidepressants because of the possibility of discontinuation syndrome, which causes anxiety, dysphoria, flulike symptoms, dizziness, excessive sweating, and insomnia.

BIOLOGICAL INTERVENTIONS

Electroconvulsive Therapy

Electroconvulsive therapy (ECT) is a procedure in which electrical currents are passed through the brain, intentionally triggering a brief seizure. ECT seems to cause changes in brain chemistry that can quickly reverse symptoms of certain mental illnesses. It often works when other treatments are unsuccessful. However, despite being a highly effective somatic (physical) treatment for psychiatric disorders, ECT has a bad reputation. This may be due to media portrayals of patients being restrained on a gurney while having a full-blown seizure induced. Given the current sophistication of anesthetic and paralytic agents, ECT is actually not dramatic at all.

Indications

ECT is the most effective acute treatment for depression (Welch, 2016). Psychotic illnesses are the second most common indication for ECT. For drug-resistant patients with psychosis, a combination of ECT and antipsychotic medication has resulted in sustained improvement about 80% of the time. Depression associated with bipolar disorder remits in about 50% of the cases after ECT.

While medication is generally the first line of treatment, ECT may be a primary treatment in the following cases:

- When a patient is experiencing intense suicidal ideation, and there is a need for a rapid, definitive response

- When a patient is severely malnourished, exhausted, and dehydrated due to lengthy depression (after rehydration)
- If previous medication trials have failed
- If the patient chooses
- When there is marked agitation, marked vegetative symptoms, or catatonia
- For major depression with psychotic features
- In pregnant women
- For people with rapid cycling mood swings (four or more in 1 year)

ECT is not effective, however, in patients with dysthymia, atypical depression, personality disorders, drug dependence, or depression secondary to situational or social difficulties.

Risk Factors

Using ECT requires clinicians to weigh the risk of using this method versus the risk of suicide, quality of life, and potential complications. Several conditions pose risks and require careful assessment and management. For example, because the heart can be stressed at the onset of the seizure and for up to 10 minutes after, careful assessment and management of hypertension, congestive heart failure, cardiac arrhythmias, and other cardiac conditions is warranted (Welch, 2016). ECT also stresses the brain as a result of increased cerebral oxygen, blood flow, and intracranial pressure. Conditions such as brain tumours and subdural hematomas may increase the risk of using ECT. Providers of care and patients need to weigh the risk of continued disability or potential suicide from depression against ECT treatment risks.

Procedure

The usual course of ECT for a patient with depression is two or three treatments per week to a total of six to twelve treatments. The procedure is explained to the patient, and informed consent is obtained from the patient or the patient's substitute decision maker. The patient is usually given a general anesthetic to induce sleep and a muscle-paralyzing agent to prevent muscle distress and fractures. These medications have revolutionized the comfort and safety of ECT.

Patients should have a pre-ECT assessment, including a chest X-ray, electrocardiogram, urinalysis, complete blood count, blood urea nitrogen, and electrolyte panel. Benzodiazepines should be discontinued, as they will interfere with the seizure process.

An electroencephalogram (EEG) monitors brain waves, and an electrocardiogram (ECG) monitors cardiac responses. Brief seizures (30 to 60-plus seconds) are deliberately induced by an electrical current (as brief as 1 second) transmitted through electrodes attached to one or both sides of the head (Figure 13-5). To ensure that patients experience a seizure over the entire brain, a blood pressure cuff may be inflated on the lower arm or leg before administration of the paralytic agent. In that way, the convulsion can be visualized in the unparalyzed extremity.

Adverse Reactions

Patients wake about 15 minutes after the procedure. The patient is often confused and disoriented for several hours. The nurse and family may need to orient the patient frequently during the

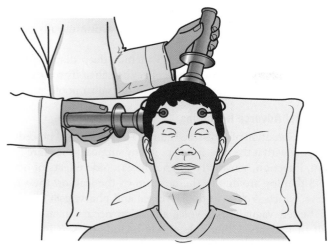

FIGURE 13-5 Electroconvulsive therapy. Source: Illustration from National Institute of Mental Health.

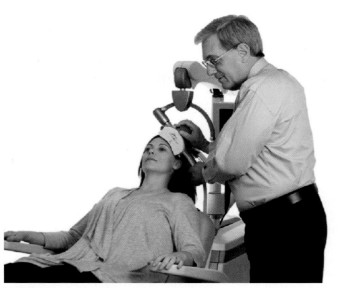

FIGURE 13-6 Transcranial magnetic stimulation. Source: Photo courtesy Neuronetics.

course of treatment. Most people experience what is called retrograde amnesia, which is a loss of memory of events leading up to and including the treatment itself.

Transcranial Magnetic Stimulation

Transcranial magnetic stimulation (TMS) is a noninvasive treatment modality that uses magnetic resonance imaging (MRI)–strength magnetic pulses to stimulate focal areas of the cerebral cortex (Figure 13-6).

Indications

In 2002, Canada approved the use of TMS for patients who have been unresponsive to at least one antidepressant. Researchers suggest that TMS be used to enhance cognitive function in healthy, nondepressed individuals (Clark & Parasuraman, 2013).

Risk Factors

The only absolute contraindication to this procedure is the presence of metal in the area of stimulation. Cochlear implants, brain stimulators, or medication pumps are examples of metals that could interfere with the procedures (Camprodon, Kaur, Rauch, et al., 2016).

Procedure

Outpatient treatment with TMS takes about 30 minutes and is typically ordered for 5 days a week for 4 to 6 weeks. Patients are awake and alert during the procedure. An electromagnet is placed on the patient's scalp, and short, magnetic pulses pass into the prefrontal cortex of the brain (see Figure 13-5). These pulses are similar to those used by MRI scanners but are more focused. The pulses cause electrical charges to flow and induce neurons to fire or become active. During TMS, patients feel a slight tapping or knocking in the head, contraction of the scalp, and tightening of the jaw.

Potential Adverse Reactions

After the procedure, patients may experience a headache and lightheadedness. No neurological deficits or memory problems have been noted. Seizures are a rare complication of TMS. Most of the common side effects of TMS are mild and include scalp tingling and discomfort at the administration site.

Nerve Stimulation

The use of **vagus nerve stimulation (VNS)** originated as a treatment for epilepsy. VNS is approved in Canada for treatment-resistant depression (TRD). Clinicians noted that while VNS decreased seizures, it also appeared to improve mood in a population that normally experiences increased rates of depression. The theory behind VNS relates to the action of the vagus nerve, the longest cranial nerve, which extends from the brainstem to organs in the neck, chest, and abdomen. Researchers believe that electrical stimulation of the vagus nerve results in boosting the level of neurotransmitters, thereby improving mood and also improving the action of antidepressants.

Indications

Nearly a decade after VNS was approved for use in Europe, in 2001 Health Canada granted approval for VNS use for TRD. The cost of the stimulation unit is between $15 000 and $25 000, which is generally not covered by provincial health plans. The efficacy of VNS in treating depression is still being established. Other potential applications of VNS include anxiety, obesity, and pain.

Procedure

The surgery to implant VNS is typically an outpatient procedure. A pacemaker-like device is implanted surgically into the left chest wall. The device is connected to a thin, flexible wire that is threaded upward and wrapped around the vagus nerve on the left side of the neck (Figure 13-7). After surgery, an infrared magnetic wand is held against the chest while a personal computer or personal digital assistant is used to program the frequency

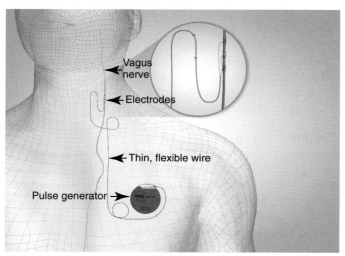

FIGURE 13-7 Vagus nerve stimulation. Source: Image courtesy Cyberonics, Inc.

of pulses. Pulses are usually delivered for 30 seconds, every 5 minutes, 24 hours a day. Antidepressant action usually occurs in several weeks.

Nonsurgical methods of VNS include deep diaphragmatic breathing, "om" chanting, and collecting saliva in your mouth and then submerging your tongue in the saliva pool.

Potential Adverse Reactions

The implantation of VNS (see Figure 13-7) is a surgical procedure, carrying with it the risks inherent in any surgical procedure (e.g., pain, infection, sensitivity to anesthesia). Side effects of active VNS therapy are due to the position of the lead on the vagus nerve, which is close to the laryngeal and pharyngeal branches of the left vagus nerve. Voice alteration occurs in more than half of patients. Other side effects include neck pain, cough, paresthesia, and dyspnea, which tend to decrease with time. The device can be temporarily turned off at any time by placing a special magnet over the implant. This may be especially helpful when engaging in public speaking or heavy exercise.

⚙ INTEGRATIVE THERAPY

Complementary, Alternative, and Integrative Approaches

There are a vast array of complementary, alternative, and integrative approaches in the treatment of depression, including the use of dietary supplements, acupuncture, aromatherapy, meditation, light therapy, homeopathy, and yoga. Herbal products and supplements for depression have become a multimillion-dollar industry; however, the long-term effects of these products is not yet clear. The approaches briefly discussed here are light therapy, use of St. John's wort, and exercise.

Light Therapy

Light therapy has been researched for nearly 20 years and is accepted as a first-line treatment for seasonal affective disorder (SAD). In the *DSM-5* (American Psychiatric Association, 2013), SAD is considered a subtype of major depressive disorder and listed as "with seasonal pattern." People with SAD often live in regions in which there are marked seasonal differences in the amount of daylight.

Light therapy's effectiveness is thought to be the influence of light on melatonin. Melatonin is secreted by the pineal gland and is necessary for maintaining and shifting biological rhythms. Exposure to light suppresses the nocturnal secretion of melatonin, which seems to have a therapeutic effect on people with SAD.

Ideal treatment consists of 30 to 45 minutes of exposure daily to a 10 000-lux light source. Morning exposure is best. However, success has been reported when exposure occurs at other times of the day or in divided doses. Anecdotal reports suggest that increasing the available light by adding additional light sources may also help to elevate mood. For those affected by SAD, light therapy has been found to be as effective in reducing depressive symptoms as medications. Negative side effects include headache and jitteriness.

St. John's Wort

St. John's wort (*Hypericum perforatum*) is a flower that can be processed into tea or tablets. This herb may increase the amount of serotonin, norepinephrine, and dopamine in the brain, resulting in antidepressant effects. Studies of St. John's wort used in the treatment of depression provide mixed evaluations. It has generally been found to be as effective as antidepressants in the treatment of mild to moderate depression, but usefulness in severe depression has not been established (Carpenter, 2011). Because St. John's wort is not regulated in Canada, concentrations of the active ingredients may vary from preparation to preparation, an inconsistency that may account for some variation in research results. St. John's wort has the potential for adverse reactions when taken with other medications, and safety has not been established for use during pregnancy or use in children. For example, when taken with prescribed antidepressants, there is an increased risk of patients experiencing serotonin syndrome.

Exercise

Exercise has biological, social, and psychological effects on symptoms of depression. Research shows that exercise increases the availability of serotonin in the brain. It has also been demonstrated to dampen the activity of the hypothalamic-pituitary-adrenal axis, which is believed to be overly active in depression. People with depression who exercise regularly report feeling an elevated mood and greater happiness, and they become more socially involved. Additional benefits of exercise are that it is more easily accessed, less expensive, and results in fewer side effects than antidepressants.

Sources: Carpenter, D. (2011). St. John's wort and S-adenosyl Methionine as "natural" alternatives to conventional antidepressants in the era of the suicidality boxed warning: What is the evidence for clinically relevant benefit? *Alternative Medicine Health Review, 16*(1), 17–39.

Advanced-Practice Interventions

Nurses and nurse practitioners are qualified to provide counselling, social skills training, and group therapy (Canadian Nurses Association, 2008; Registered Psychiatric Nurses of Canada, 2008). In some provinces, nurse practitioners who have met appropriate educational standards may also be certified to prescribe medication to treat depression.

Psychological Interventions

Psychotherapy. Cognitive behavioural therapy (CBT), interpersonal therapy (IPT), time-limited focused psychotherapy, and behavioural therapy all are considered especially effective in the treatment of mild to moderate depression. However, only CBT and IPT were shown to demonstrate superiority in the maintenance phase. CBT helps people change their negative thought patterns and behaviours, whereas IPT focuses on working through personal relationships that may contribute to depression.

Group therapy. Group therapy is a widespread modality for the treatment of depression; it increases the number of people who can receive treatment at a decreased cost per individual. Another advantage is that groups offer patients an opportunity to socialize and share common feelings and concerns, which decreases feelings of isolation, hopelessness, helplessness, and alienation. Therapy groups also provide a controlled environment in which patients can explore their patterns of interaction and response to others, which may contribute to or exacerbate their depression.

Future of Treatment

Many Canadians continue to have their quality of life negatively affected by depression. As a result, their sense of meaning, fulfillment, and relational connections are affected. To reduce these sequelae, earlier detection, earlier intervention, prevention of progression, achievement of remission, and further integration of neuroscience and behavioural science in the treatment of depression are needed. Priority areas for further development and research are:

- Improving screening for high-risk ages and groups, including:
  - Individuals in late adolescence and early adulthood
  - Women in reproductive years
  - Adults and older adults with medical problems (e.g., pain)
  - People with a family history of depression
- Increasing education, particularly about the link between physical symptoms and depression
- Integrating psychopharmacological treatment augmented with psychological and other nonpharmacological therapies
- Inclusion of more self-care strategies, such as:
  - Promotion of sleep hygiene
  - Increase in exercise
  - Better overall health care

EVALUATION

Short-term indicators and outcome criteria are frequently evaluated during the course of treatment for depression. For example, if the patient with depression came into the unit with suicidal thoughts, the nurse evaluates whether suicidal thoughts are still present, the patient is able to state alternatives to suicidal impulses in the future, the patient is able to explore thoughts and feelings that precede suicidal impulses, and so forth. Outcomes relating to thought processes, self-esteem, and social interactions are frequently formulated, because these areas are often problematic in people with depression.

Physical needs warrant nursing or medical attention. If a patient has lost weight because of anorexia, is the appetite returning? If the patient was constipated, are the bowels now functioning normally? If the patient was suffering from insomnia, is he or she now sleeping 6 to 8 hours per night? If indicators have not been met, an analysis of the data, nursing diagnoses, goals, and planned nursing interventions is made. The care plan is reassessed and reformulated as necessary.

CASE STUDY AND NURSING CARE PLAN 13-1

Depression

Ms. Glessner is a 35-year-old executive secretary. She has been divorced for 3 years and has two sons, 11 and 13 years of age. She is brought into the emergency department (ED) by her neighbour. She has some slashes on her wrists and is bleeding. The neighbour states that both of Ms. Glessner's sons are visiting their father for the summer. Ms. Glessner has become more and more despondent since terminating a 2-year relationship with a married man 4 weeks previously. According to the neighbour, for 3 years after her divorce, Ms. Glessner talked constantly about not being pretty or good enough and doubted that anyone could really love her. The neighbour states that Ms. Glessner has been withdrawn for at least 3 years. After the relationship with her boyfriend ended, she became even more withdrawn and sullen. Ms. Glessner is about 10 kilograms overweight, and her neighbour states that Ms. Glessner often stays awake late into the night, drinking by herself and watching television. She sleeps through most of the day on the weekends.

After receiving treatment in the ED, Ms. Glessner is seen by a psychiatrist. The initial diagnosis is persistent depressive disorder with suicidal ideation. A decision is made to hospitalize her briefly for suicide observation and evaluation for appropriate treatment.

The nurse, Ms. Ward, admits Ms. Glessner to the unit from the ED.

Nurse: *"Hello, Ms. Glessner. I'm Marcia Ward. I'll be your primary nurse."*

Ms. Glessner: *"Yeah, I don't need a nurse, a doctor, or anyone else. I just want to get away from this pain."*

Nurse: *"You want to get away from your pain?"*

Ms. Glessner: *"I just said that, didn't I? Oh, what's the use? No one understands."*

Nurse: *"I would like to understand, Ms. Glessner."*

Ms. Glessner: *"Look at me. I'm fat ... ugly ... and no good to anyone. No one wants me."*

Nurse: *"Who doesn't want you?"*

Continued

CASE STUDY AND NURSING CARE PLAN 13-1—cont'd

Depression

Ms. Glessner: "My husband didn't want me, and now Jerry has left me to go back to his wife."

Nurse: "You think because Jerry went back to his wife that no one else could care for you?"

Ms. Glessner: "Well, he doesn't anyway."

Nurse: "Because he doesn't care, you believe that no one else cares about you?"

Ms. Glessner: "Yes ...."

Nurse: "Who do you care about?"

Ms. Glessner: "No one ... except my sons. I do love my sons, even though I don't often show it."

Nurse: "Tell me more about your sons."

Ms. Ward continues to speak with Ms. Glessner. Ms. Glessner talks about her sons with some affect and apparent affection; however, she continues to state that she does not think of herself as worthwhile.

ASSESSMENT

Self-Assessment

Ms. Ward is aware that when patients have depression, they can be negative, think life is hopeless, and be hostile toward those who want to help. When Ms. Ward was new to the unit, she withdrew from patients with depression and sought out patients who appeared more hopeful and appreciative of her efforts. The unit coordinator was very supportive of Ms. Ward when she was first on the unit. Ms. Ward, along with other staff, was sent to clinical education sessions on working with patients with depression and was encouraged to speak up in staff meetings about the feelings that many of these patients evoked in her. As a primary nurse, she was assigned a variety of patients. She found that as time went on, with the support of her peers and the opportunity to speak up at staff meetings, she was able to take what patients said less personally and not feel so responsible when patients did not respond as fast as she would like.

After 2 years, she had had the experience of seeing many patients who seemed hopeless and despondent on admission respond well to nursing and medical interventions and go on to lead full and satisfying lives. This also made it easier for Ms. Ward to understand that even though the patient with depression may think life is hopeless and may believe there is nothing in life to live for, change is always possible.

Objective Data	Subjective Data
Slashed her wrists	"No one wants me."
Recently broke up with boyfriend	"I just want to get rid of this pain."
Has thought poorly of herself for 3 years, since divorce	"I'm fat ... ugly ... and no good to anyone."
Has two sons she cares about	"I do love my sons, even though I don't often show it."
Is 10 kilograms overweight	
Stays awake late at night, drinking by herself	
Has been withdrawn since divorce	

DIAGNOSIS

The nurse evaluates Ms. Glessner's strengths and weaknesses and decides to concentrate on two initial nursing diagnoses that seem to have the highest priority:

1. *Risk for suicide* related to separation from 2-year relationship, as evidenced by actual suicide attempt

Supporting Data
- Slashed her wrists
- Recently broke up with boyfriend
- Drinks at night by herself
- Withdrawn for 3 years since divorce

2. *Situational low self-esteem* related to divorce and recent termination of love relationship, as evidenced by derogatory statements about self

Supporting Data
- "No one wants me."
- "I'm fat ... ugly ... and no good to anyone."
- "I do love my sons, even though I don't often show it."

OUTCOMES IDENTIFICATION

Patient refrains from attempting suicide.

PLANNING

Because Ms. Glessner is discharged after 48 hours, the issue of disturbance in self-esteem continues to be addressed in her therapy after discharge. Ms. Ward later reviews the goals for her work with Ms. Glessner in the community.

CASE STUDY AND NURSING CARE PLAN 13-1—cont'd

Depression

IMPLEMENTATION

Ms. Glessner's plan of care is personalized as follows:

Short-Term Goal	Intervention	Rationale	Evaluation
1. Patient expresses at least one reason to live, apparent by the second day of hospitalization.	1a. Observe patient every 15 minutes while she is suicidal. 1b. Remove all dangerous objects from patient. 1c. Obtain a "no self-harm" contract with patient for a specific period of time, to be renegotiated (Note: some provinces no longer use contracting). 1d. Spend regularly scheduled periods of time with patient throughout the day. 1e. Assist patient in evaluating both positive and negative aspects of her life. 1f. Encourage appropriate expression of angry feelings. 1g. Accept patient's negativism.	1a, b. Patient safety is ensured. The risk for impulsive self-harmful behaviour is minimized. 1c. Contract may help patient gain a sense of control and a feeling of responsibility. 1d. This interaction reinforces that the patient is worthwhile and builds her experience in relating better to the nurse on a one-to-one basis. 1e. A person with depression is often unable to acknowledge any positive aspects of life unless they are pointed out by others. 1f. Providing for expression of pent-up hostility in a safe environment can reinforce more adaptive methods of releasing tension and may minimize need to act out self-directed anger. 1g. Acceptance enhances feelings of self-worth.	**GOAL MET** By the end of the second day, Ms. Glessner states that she really did not want to die; she just couldn't stand the loneliness in her life. She states that she loves her sons and would never want to hurt them.
2. Patient will identify two outside supports she can call on if she feels suicidal in the future.	2a. Explore usual coping behaviours. 2b. Assist patient in identifying members of her support system. 2c. Suggest a number of community-based support groups she might wish to discuss or visit (e.g., hotlines, support groups, women's groups). 2d. Assist patient in identifying realistic alternatives she is willing to use.	2a. Behaviours that need reinforcing and new coping skills that need to be introduced can be identified. 2b. Strengths and weaknesses in her available support systems can be evaluated. 2c. Patient needs to be aware of community supports to use them. 2d. Unless patient agrees with any plan, she will be unable or unwilling to follow through in a crisis.	**GOAL MET** By discharge, Ms. Glessner states that she is definitely going to try cognitive behavioural therapy. She also discusses joining a women's support group that meets once a week in a neighbouring town.

EVALUATION

During the course of her work with Ms. Ward, Ms. Glessner decides to go to some meetings of Parents Without Partners. She states that she is looking forward to getting back to work and feels much more hopeful about her life. She has also lost 1.5 kilograms while attending Weight Watchers. She states, "I need to get back into the world." Although Ms. Glessner still has negative thoughts about herself, she admits to feeling more hopeful and better about herself, and she has learned important tools to deal with her negative thoughts.

KEY POINTS TO REMEMBER

- There are a number of subtypes of depression and depressive clinical phenomena. The two primary depressive disorders are major depressive disorder (MDD) and persistent depressive disorder (dysthymia).

- The symptoms of major depression are usually severe enough to interfere with a person's social or occupational functioning. A person with MDD may or may not have psychotic symptoms, and the symptoms usually exhibited during an episode of major depression are different from the characteristics of the normal personality prior to the onset of MDD.

- The symptoms of persistent depressive disorder are often chronic (lasting at least 2 years) and are considered mild to moderate. Usually a person's social or occupational functioning is not greatly impaired. The symptoms in persistent depressive disorder are often congruent with the person's usual pattern of functioning.

- Many theories exist about the cause of depression. The most accepted is biological (genetic and biochemical) factors; however, cognitive theory, learned helplessness theory, and the diathesis–stress theory help explain triggers to depression and maintenance of depressive thoughts and feelings.

- Nursing assessment includes the evaluation of affect, thought processes (especially suicidal thoughts), mood, feelings, physical behaviour, communication, and religious beliefs and spirituality. The nurse also must be aware of the symptoms that may mask depression.

- Nursing diagnoses can be numerous. Individuals with depression are always evaluated for risk for suicide. Some other common nursing diagnoses are *Disturbed thought processes, Chronic low self-esteem, Imbalanced nutrition, Constipation, Disturbed sleep pattern, Ineffective coping,* and *Interrupted family processes.*

- Working with people who have depression can evoke intense feelings of hopelessness and frustration in health care workers. Nurses must clarify expectations of themselves and their patients and sort personal feelings from those communicated by the patient via empathy. Peer supervision and individual supervision by an experienced nurse clinician, psychiatric social worker, or psychologist are useful in increasing therapeutic potential.

- Interventions for patients who have depression involve several approaches. Basic-level interventions include using specific principles of communication, planning activities of daily living, administering or participating in psychopharmacological therapy, maintaining a therapeutic environment, and teaching patients about the biochemical aspects of depression.

- Advanced-practice interventions may include several short-term psychotherapies that are effective in the treatment of depression, including IPT, CBT, skills training (assertiveness and social skills), and some forms of group therapy.

- Depression is often overlooked in children, adolescents, and older adults because symptoms of depression are often mistaken for signs of normal development.

- Children and adolescents with disruptive mood dysregulation disorder had previously been diagnosed with bipolar disorder. Usually people with this disorder grow up and are diagnosed with major depressive disorder or an anxiety disorder.

- Planning and interventions for patients with depression are based on the recovery model, which involves a therapeutic alliance with health care providers in order to achieve outcomes based on individual patient needs and values.

- Evaluation is ongoing throughout the nursing process, and patients' outcomes are compared with the stated outcome criteria and short-term and intermediate indicators. The care plan is revised when indicators are not being met.

CRITICAL THINKING

1. You are spending time with Mr. Plotsky, who is undergoing a workup for depression. He hardly makes eye contact, slouches in his seat, and wears a blank but sad expression. Mr. Plotsky has had numerous bouts of major depression in the past and says to you, "This will be my last depression. I will never go through this again."

   a. Since safety is the first concern, what are the appropriate questions to ask Mr. Plotsky at this time?

   b. In terms of behaviours, thought processes, activities of daily living, and ability to function at work and home, give examples of the kinds of signs and symptoms you might find when assessing a patient with depression.

   c. Mr. Plotsky tells you that he has been on every medication there is, but none has worked. He asks you about the herb St. John's wort. What should you tell him about its effectiveness for severe depression, interactions with other antidepressants, and regulatory status?

   d. What might be some somatic options for a person who is resistant to antidepressant medications?

   e. Mr. Plotsky asks what causes depression. In simple terms, how might you respond to his query?

   f. Mr. Plotsky tells you that he has never tried therapy because he thinks it is for weaklings. What information could you give him about various therapeutic modalities that have proven effective for other patients with depression?

2. You are working with Ms. Fok, a 28-year-old with MDD on long-term antidepressant therapy. She asks you about the possibility of pregnancy while taking her SSRIs.

   a. What are some of the things Ms. Fok might want to consider about taking antidepressants if she plans to get pregnant?

   b. If she decides to stop taking her antidepressants, what are some things she might do to help manage her depression?

3. You are working with Mrs. Burton, who has recently been diagnosed with chronic heart failure. In caring for Mrs. Burton, what are two key areas of assessment?

4. What are some of the key areas to consider when working with an older person considering ECT for depression?

CHAPTER REVIEW

1. The nurse is caring for a patient who exhibits disorganized thinking and delusions. The patient repeatedly states, "I hear voices of aliens trying to contact me." The nurse should recognize this presentation as which type of major depressive disorder (MDD)?
   a. Catatonic
   b. Atypical
   c. Melancholic
   d. Psychotic

2. Which patient statement indicates learned helplessness?
   a. "I am a horrible person."
   b. "Everyone in the world is just out to get me."
   c. "It's all my fault that my husband left me for another woman."
   d. "I hate myself."

3. The nurse is planning care for a patient with depression who will be discharged to home soon. What aspect of teaching should be the priority on the nurse's discharge plan of care?
   a. Pharmacological teaching
   b. Safety risk
   c. Awareness of symptoms of increasing depression
   d. The need for interpersonal contact

4. The nurse is reviewing orders given for a patient with depression. Which order should the nurse question?
   a. A low starting dose of a tricyclic antidepressant
   b. An SSRI given initially with an MAOI
   c. Electroconvulsive therapy to treat suicidal thoughts
   d. Elavil to address the patient's agitation

5. Which of the following are considered vegetative signs of depression?
   a. Hallucinations and delusions
   b. Expressions of guilt and worthlessness
   c. Feelings of helplessness and hopelessness
   d. Changes in physiological functioning such as appetite and sleep disturbances

6. Which assessment question asked by the nurse demonstrates an understanding of comorbid mental health conditions associated with major depressive disorder? Select all that apply.
   a. "Do rules apply to you?"
   b. "What do you do to manage anxiety?"
   c. "Do you have a history of disordered eating?"
   d. "Do you think that you drink too much?"
   e. "Have you ever been arrested for committing a crime?"

7. Which chronic medical condition is a common trigger for major depressive disorder?
   a. Pain
   b. Hypertension
   c. Hypothyroidism
   d. Crohn's disease

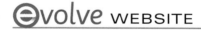 **WEBSITE**

Post-Test interactive review

Visit the Evolve website for Chapter Review Answers and Rationales, Critical Thinking Answer Guidelines, and additional resources related to the content in this chapter: http://evolve.elsevier.com/Canada/Varcarolis/psychiatric/

REFERENCES

American Psychiatric Association. (2013). *Diagnostic and statistical manual of mental disorders* (5th ed.). Arlington, VA: Author.

Beck, A. T., & Rush, A. J. (1995). Cognitive therapy. In H. I. Kaplan & B. J. Sadock (Eds.), *Comprehensive textbook of psychiatry/VI.* (Vol. 2, pp. 1847–1856). Baltimore: Williams & Wilkins.

Camprodon, J. A., Kaur, N., Rauch, S. L., et al. (2016). Neurotherapeutics. In T. Stern, M. Fava, T. E. Wilens, et al. (Eds.), *Massachusetts General Hospital handbook of general hospital psychiatry.* (2nd ed.). Philadelphia: Elsevier.

Canadian Nurses Association. (2008). *Advanced nursing practice: A national framework*. Ottawa: Author.

Carpenter, D. (2011). St. John's wort and S-adenosyl Methionine as "natural" alternatives to conventional antidepressants in the era of the suicidality boxed warning: What is the evidence for clinically relevant benefit? *Alternative Medicine Health Review, 16*(1), 17–39.

Clark, V. P., & Parasuraman, R. (2013). Neuroenhancement: Enhancing brain and mind in health and disease. *Neuroimage, 85,* 889–894.

de Roten, Y., Ambresin, G., Herrera, F., et al. (2017). Efficacy of adjunctive brief psychodynamic psychotherapy to usual inpatient treatment of depression: Results of a randomized controlled trial. *Journal of Affective Disorders, 209*(2017), 105–113. doi:10.1016/j.jad.2016.11.013.

Flaster, M., Sharma, A., & Rao, M. (2013). Poststroke depression. *Topics in Stroke Rehabilitation, 20*(2), 139–150.

Friedman, R. A. (2014). Antidepressants' black-box warning 10 years later. *New England Journal of Medicine, 371,* 1666–1668.

Gillespie, C. F., & Nemeroff, C. B. (2007). Corticotropin-releasing factor and the psychobiology of early-life stress. *Current Directions in Psychological Science, 16,* 85–89. doi:10.1111/j.1467-8721.2007.00481.x.

Krishnadas, R., & Cavanagh, J. (2012). Depression: An inflammatory illness? *Journal of Neurology, Neurosurgery, and Psychiatry, 83*(5), 495–502.

Lehne, R. A. (2013). *Pharmacology for nursing care* (8th ed.). St Louis: Elsevier.

Maughan, B., Collishaw, S., & Stringaris, A. (2013). Depression in childhood and adolescence. *Journal of the Canadian Academy of Child and Adolescent Psychiatry, 22*(1), 35–40. Retrieved from http://www.cacap-acpea.org/en/cacap/Journal_p828.html.

McInnis, M. G., Riba, M., & Greden, J. F. (2014). Depressive disorders. In R. E. Hales, S. C. Yudofsky, & L. W. Roberts (Eds.), *Textbook of psychiatry.* Washington, DC: American Psychiatric Publishing.

Miller, G. E., & Cole, S. W. (2012). Clustering of depression and inflammation in adolescents previously exposed to childhood adversity. *Biological Psychiatry, 72*(1), 34–40.

Moorhead, S., Johnson, M., Maas, M., et al. (2012). *Nursing outcomes classification (NOC)* (5th ed.). St. Louis: Mosby.

National Institute of Mental Health (NIMH). (2012). *Older adults: Depression and suicide facts (fact sheet)*. Retrieved from http://www.nimh.nih.gov/health/publications/older-adults-and-depression/older-adults-and-depression_141998.pdf.

Olivier, J. D. A., Akerud, H., & Promomaa, I. S. (2015). Antenatal depression and antidepressants during pregnancy. *European Journal of Pharmacology, 753*, 257–262.

Paine, D. R., & Sandage, S. J. (2017). Religious involvement and depression: The mediating effect of relational spirituality. *Journal of Religion and Health, 56*(1), 269–283. doi:10.1007/s10943-016-0282-z.

Pearson, C., Janz, T., & Ali, J. (2013). *Mental and substance use disorders in Canada: Health at a glance*. Catalogue no. 82-624-X. Ottawa: Statistics Canada.

Registered Psychiatric Nurses of Canada. (2008). *Guidelines for registered psychiatric nurses in independent practice*. Edmonton: Author.

Ryan, J., & Ancelin, M. (2012). Polymorphisms of estrogen receptors and risk of depression. *Drugs, 72*(13), 1725–1738.

Sadock, B. J., Sadock, V. A., & Ruiz, P. (2015). *Kaplan and Sadock's synopsis of psychiatry* (11th ed.). Philadelphia: Wolters Kluwer.

Seligman, M. E. (1973). Fall into hopelessness. *Psychology Today, 7*(1), 43–48.

Sheikh, J., & Yesavage, J. (1986). Geriatric depression scale (GDS): Recent evidence and development of a shorter version. *Clinical Gerontologist, 5*(1–2), 165–173.

Welch, C. A. (2016). Electroconvulsive therapy. In T. A. Stern, M. Fava, T. E. Wilens, et al. (Eds.), *Comprehensive clinical psychiatry*. (2nd ed.). St. Louis: Elsevier.

CHAPTER 14

Bipolar Disorders

Margaret Jordan Halter
Adapted by Cheryl L. Pollard

KEY TERMS AND CONCEPTS

acute phase
anticonvulsant drugs
bipolar I disorder
bipolar II disorder
clang associations
continuation phase
cyclothymic disorder
euphoric mood

flight of ideas
grandiosity
hypomania
maintenance phase
mania
manic episode
rapid cycling
seclusion protocol

OBJECTIVES

1. Assess a person experiencing mania for (a) mood, (b) behaviour, and (c) thought processes, and be alert to possible dysfunction.
2. Describe the signs and symptoms of bipolar I, bipolar II, and cyclothymic disorder.
3. Distinguish between mania and hypomania.
4. Formulate three nursing diagnoses appropriate for a person with mania, and include supporting data.
5. Explain the rationales behind five methods of communication that may be used with a person experiencing mania.
6. Distinguish the focus of treatment for a person in the acute manic phase from the focus of treatment for a person in the continuation or maintenance phase.
7. Describe common medications used for bipolar disorders.
8. Distinguish between signs of early and severe lithium toxicity.
9. Write a medication care plan specifying five areas of teaching regarding lithium carbonate.
10. Evaluate specific indications for the use of seclusion for a person experiencing mania.
11. Review at least three of the items presented in the patient and family teaching plan (see Patient and Family Teaching: Bipolar Disorder) with a person with bipolar disorder.

⊖volve WEBSITE

Visit the Evolve website for Flashcards, Case Studies, and additional testing resources related to the content in this chapter: http://evolve.elsevier.com/Canada/Varcarolis/psychiatric/

Pre-Test | interactive review

Once commonly known as *manic depression*, bipolar disorder is a chronic, recurrent illness that must be carefully managed throughout a person's life. Bipolar disorder frequently goes unrecognized, and people suffer for years before receiving a proper diagnosis and treatment. Bipolar disorder is marked by shifts in mood, energy, and ability to function. The course of the illness is variable, and symptoms range from mania—an exaggerated euphoria or irritability—to depression (Figure 14-1). Periods of normal functioning may alternate with periods of illness (highs, lows, or a combination of both). However, many individuals continue to experience chronic interpersonal or occupational difficulties even during remission. According to

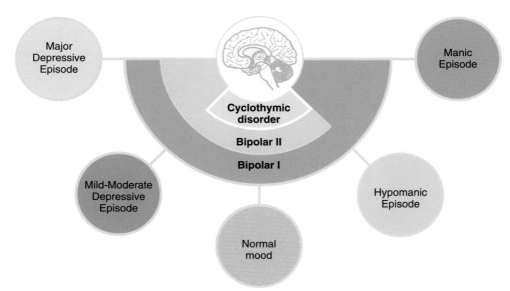

FIGURE 14-1 Continuum of bipolar symptoms.

🌸 HOW A NURSE HELPED ME

Support and Care for My Brother and Me

Life was always different in our house; there were good days and bad days, but there really wasn't a dull day in our house. To my brother and me, Mom was normal—we knew no differently. But to my friends, Mom was strange and "crazy" sometimes. My brother and I often moved around, from relative to relative and from place to place. When I was 17, my mom had another episode and was in hospital once again, and I was left to raise my little brother. Mom was discharged from hospital after 2 months of care—a little longer than usual—but I thought nothing of this as Mom had been in and out of hospital throughout my childhood. Everything was settled for the next couple of months, but I noticed Mom giving away household items as well as buying a lot of new things for the house, this time really quickly. This was a sign, I had learned over the years, that Mom was becoming unwell again. She had bought a new mobile home and airline tickets for an overseas holiday, something we never actually used. Mom had been admitted to hospital again to stabilize, as the nurses always explained to me. This hospital stay was different, as she stayed in for only 2 weeks and was provided with a case manager to follow up with her at home. The case manager was a nurse who was invaluable to Mom's care, but the nurse was also a wealth of help and care to my brother and me. Mom's case manager came over regularly, talked to Mom about her medications and about her signs and symptoms of becoming unwell but,

more importantly, about her ongoing care. The nurse also helped my brother and me understand and watch for signs and symptoms of Mom's bipolar disorder. Mom was stable for a little while, and although she had no money left after the extravagant holiday she'd booked and the new mobile home in our yard, life was more stable, until Mom asked me to join her and the nurse case manager for a chat. I was to find out that Mom had cancer. She'd had it for a while, and the future was not positive. Mom died 2 months after that chat, and life was yet again upside down for my brother and me. It was the nurse who helped us move forward. We all thought that, since Mom had died, there would be no reason for the nurse to visit, but this was not the case. Not only did she make Mom's last days with us comfortable and some of the most stable times we'd had with Mom, but she continued to visit my brother and me, provide support for us both, and help link us with various community supports. The nurse supported my mom but also my brother and me, and without this caring nurse and the continued support after Mom died, my brother and I would not have had the happy memories we have of Mom today. It is the nurse we thank not only for teaching us about bipolar disorder but also for bringing us to an understanding and appreciation of what a good mom we had, even during the rough times, and to the realization that there is support for people who are in the same position as my mom.

the Canadian Mental Health Association's *Fast Facts About Mental Illness* (2011), approximately 1% of Canadians will experience bipolar disorder. The mortality rate among individuals with bipolar disorder is two to three times greater than that of the general population. Suicide accounts for 5% of deaths among women and 10% of deaths among men with bipolar disorder compared with 1% and 2%, respectively, in the general population (Crump, Sundquist, Winkleby, et al., 2013).

CLINICAL PICTURE

The three types of bipolar and related disorders that we discuss in this chapter are bipolar I, bipolar II, and cyclothymic disorder.

Bipolar I Disorder

Bipolar I disorder is marked by severe shifts in mood, energy, and inability to function. Periods of normal functioning may alternate with periods of illness (highs, lows, or a combination of both). Many individuals continue to experience chronic interpersonal or occupational difficulties even during remission.

Individuals with bipolar I disorder have experienced at least one manic episode. Mania is a period of intense mood disturbance with persistent elevation, expansiveness, irritability, and extreme goal-directed activity or energy. These periods last at least 1 week for most of the day, every day. Symptoms of mania are so severe that this state is a psychiatric emergency. Manic episodes usually alternate with depression or a mixed state of anxiety and depression (refer to Chapter 13 for a full discussion of depression).

Initially, individuals experiencing a manic episode feel euphoric and energized, they don't sleep or eat, and they are in perpetual motion. They often take significant risks and engage in hazardous activities. Unfortunately, the person with mania does not recognize the behaviours as being problematic and will usually resist treatment.

As the mania intensifies, individuals may become psychotic and experience hallucinations, delusions, and dramatically disturbed thoughts and behaviour. Hallucinations tend to be auditory, and individuals may begin to hear voices, sometimes the voice of God. They may believe that they are a person of extreme influence and power.

The initial euphoria of mania gives way to agitation and irritability. Utter exhaustion eventually happens, and many people ultimately collapse into depression. Depression and the agitated state of mania is a dangerous combination that can lead to extreme behaviours such as violence or suicide.

People may be at equal risk for developing anxiety as depression after an episode of mania (Olfson, Mojtabai, Merikangas, et al., 2017). They may even experience a major depressive disorder and generalized anxiety disorder simultaneously after a manic event. If clinicians adopted a broader definition of bipolar disorder that includes anxiety as an alternating symptom, we possibly would be able to identify bipolar disorder earlier and develop different treatment approaches. Individuals whose main symptom is anxiety should be assessed for a history of mania before being treated for anxiety (see DSM-5: Diagnostic Criteria for Bipolar I Disorder).

DSM-5
Diagnostic Criteria for Bipolar I Disorder

For a diagnosis of bipolar I disorder, it is necessary to meet the following criteria for a manic episode. The manic episode may have been preceded by and may be followed by hypomanic or major depressive episodes.

Manic Episode

A. A distinct period of abnormally and persistently elevated, expansive, or irritable mood and abnormally and persistently increased goal-directed activity or energy, lasting at least 1 week and present most of the day, nearly every day (or any duration if hospitalization is necessary).

B. During the period of mood disturbance and increased energy or activity, three (or more) of the following symptoms (four if the mood is only irritable) are present to a significant degree and represent a noticeable change from usual behaviour:
   1. Inflated self-esteem or grandiosity.
   2. Decreased need for sleep (e.g., feels rested after only 3 hours of sleep).
   3. More talkative than usual or pressure to keep talking.
   4. Flight of ideas or subjective experience that thoughts are racing.
   5. Distractibility (i.e., attention too easily drawn to unimportant or irrelevant external stimuli), as reported or observed.
   6. Increase in goal-directed activity (either socially, at work or school, or sexually) or psychomotor agitation (i.e., purposeless non–goal-directed activity).
   7. Excessive involvement in activities that have a high potential for painful consequences (e.g., engaging in unrestrained buying sprees, sexual indiscretions, or foolish business investments).

C. The mood disturbance is sufficiently severe to cause marked impairment in social or occupational functioning or to necessitate hospitalization to prevent harm to self or others, or there are psychotic features.

D. The episode is not attributable to the physiological effects of a substance (e.g, a drug of abuse, a medication, other treatment) or to another medical condition.

   Note: A full manic episode that emerges during antidepressant treatment (e.g., medication, electroconvulsive therapy) but persists at a fully syndromal level beyond the physiological effect of that treatment is sufficient evidence for a manic episode and, therefore, a bipolar I diagnosis.

   Note: Criteria A through D constitute a manic episode. At least one lifetime manic episode is required for the diagnosis of bipolar I disorder.

Source: American Psychiatric Association. (2013). *Diagnostic and statistical manual of mental disorders* (5th ed.). Arlington, VA: Author.

Bipolar II Disorder

Individuals with bipolar II disorder have experienced at least one hypomanic episode and at least one major depressive episode. Hypomania refers to a lower-level and less dramatic mania. However, this level of mania still causes significant issues in relationships and occupational functioning. Like mania, hypomania is accompanied by excessive activity and energy for at least 4 days and involves at least three of the behaviours listed under Criterion B in the *Diagnostic and Statistical Manual of Mental Disorders (DSM-5)*. Unlike mania, psychosis is never present with hypomania. Psychotic symptoms may, however, accompany the depressive side of the disorder. Hospitalization is rare. However, the depressive symptoms can be quite profound and may put those who suffer from it at particular risk for suicide.

Among adults, bipolar II disorder is believed to be under-diagnosed and is often mistaken for major depression or personality disorders, when it actually may be the most common form of bipolar disorder. Clinicians may downplay bipolar II and consider it to simply be the milder version of bipolar disorders. However, it is a source of significant morbidity and mortality, particularly due to the occurrence of severe depression. Anyone with major depression should be assessed for symptoms of hypomania because these symptoms are frequently associated with a progression to bipolar disorder.

Cyclothymic Disorder

Cyclothymic disorder has symptoms of hypomania alternating with symptoms of mild to moderate depression for at least 2 years in adults and 1 year in children. Hypomanic and depressive symptoms do not meet the criteria for either bipolar II or major depression, yet the symptoms are disturbing enough to cause social and occupational impairment.

As part of the spectrum of bipolar disorders, cyclothymic disorder may be difficult to distinguish from bipolar II disorder. Individuals with cyclothymic disorder tend to have irritable hypomanic episodes. Children with cyclothymic disorder experience irritability and sleep disturbance.

Some people experience **rapid cycling** and may have at least four changes in mood episodes in a 12-month period. The cycling can also occur within the course of a month or even a 24-hour period. Rapid cycling is associated with more severe symptoms, such as poorer global functioning, high recurrence risk, and resistance to conventional somatic treatments.

Other Bipolar Disorders

Several other bipolar and related disorders are included in the *DSM-5*. They include:

- Substance/Medication-Induced Bipolar and Related Disorder
- Bipolar and Related Disorder Due to Another Medical Condition
- Other Specified Bipolar and Related Disorder
- Unspecified Bipolar and Related Disorder

EPIDEMIOLOGY

The lifetime risk, or the percentage of the population that will ever have a bipolar I or bipolar II disorder, is nearly 4% (Merikangas, Cui, Kattan, et al., 2012). Table 14-1 provides a snapshot of statistics regarding the bipolar disorders in adults and adolescents ages 13 to 18.

Men and women have nearly equal rates of bipolar disorders, yet they respond somewhat differently to their conditions. Men with a bipolar disorder are more likely to have legal problems and commit acts of violence. Women with a bipolar disorder

TABLE 14-1	STATISTICS RELATED TO BIPOLAR I AND II DISORDERS IN ADULTS AND ADOLESCENTS	
	BIPOLAR I	**BIPOLAR II**
Lifetime prevalence: adult	1.0%	1.1%
Lifetime prevalence: adolescent	2.5%	
12-month prevalence: adult	0.6%	0.8%
12-month prevalence: adolescent	2.2%	
Mean age of onset	18 years	20 years

Source: American Psychiatric Association. (2013). *Diagnostic and statistical manual of mental disorders* (5th ed.). Washington, DC: Author.

are more likely to abuse alcohol, commit suicide, and develop thyroid disease.

Women who experience a severe postpartum psychosis within 2 weeks of giving birth have a four times greater chance of subsequent conversion to bipolar disorder (Munk-Olsen, Lauresen, Meltzer-Brody, et al., 2012). Giving birth may act as a trigger for the first symptoms of bipolar disorder. The precipitant may be hormonal changes and sleep deprivation.

Children and Adolescents

The existence of bipolar disorder in nonadults has been the subject of controversy. At the beginning of the twenty-first century, there was an alarming increase in the number of children and adolescents being diagnosed with bipolar disorder. This diagnosis was given to young people who had chronic irritability and anger along with frequent verbal or behavioural outbursts that were an overreaction to the situation. A bipolar diagnosis for this troubled population provided for additional support from the health care and social systems, an answer for bewildered parents, and an established treatment pathway.

However, clinicians and parents alike had concerns over the trend of diagnosing bipolar disorder in children. The most fundamental issue was that these children and adolescents did not usually go on to have bipolar disorder as adults. More commonly, they would eventually be diagnosed with major depression. Unfortunately, a bipolar diagnosis is a lifelong label, one that is stigmatized more than depression. This diagnosis also results in exposure to powerful medications during crucial growth periods. In 2013, the American Psychiatric Association developed a new diagnosis to reverse this troubling diagnostic problem—disruptive mood dysregulation disorder. Chapter 13 discusses this new disorder in more detail.

Bipolar disorder in adolescence, particularly late adolescence, is a serious problem. The prevalence rate in this age group mirrors that of adults (Merikangas, Cui, Kattan, et al., 2012). Researchers estimate that 1 in 5 young people with mania plus depression will attempt suicide. Also, these young people experience nearly 2 months per year of role impairment. This impairment has significant implications for individuals who are positioning themselves for a lifetime and a career, as well as developing relationship patterns.

Cyclothymic Disorder

Cyclothymic disorder usually begins in adolescence or early adulthood. There is a 15% to 50% risk that an individual with this disorder will subsequently develop bipolar I or bipolar II disorder. A major risk factor for developing cyclothymic disorder is having a first-degree relative—parent, sibling, or child—with bipolar I disorder.

COMORBIDITY

Bipolar I Disorder

About 75% of people with bipolar I disorder also experience an anxiety disorder. These individuals may experience panic attacks, social anxiety disorder, and specific phobias.

Other challenging disorders may also complicate the clinical presentation and management of the often dramatic bipolar I disorder. They include attention-deficit/hyperactivity disorder and all of the disruptive, impulse control, or conduct disorders. A substance use disorder is present in more than half of individuals with bipolar I, perhaps in an attempt to self-medicate or as a symptom related to increased risk taking. More than 50% of individuals have an alcohol use disorder, which in turn elevates the risk for suicide.

Further complicating treatment is a higher than normal rate of serious medical conditions. Migraines are more common. Metabolic syndrome, a cluster of problems such as high blood pressure, high blood glucose, excess body fat around the waist, and abnormal cholesterol levels, may lead to premature death due to heart disease, stroke, and diabetes.

Bipolar II Disorder

As with bipolar I, about 75% of individuals with bipolar II disorder have a comorbid anxiety disorder. Typically, the anxiety disorders come about before the hypomania and depressive symptoms. Substance use disorders are also common and affect about 37% of people with bipolar II. Anxiety and eating disorders seem to be associated with the depressive side of bipolar II, while substance use disorder symptoms arise along with hypomanic symptoms. Eating disorders, particularly binge eating disorder, affects about 14% of this population.

Cyclothymic Disorder

As with the bipolar disorders, substance use disorders are common with cyclothymic disorder. This may be due to efforts to self-medicate and subdue the bipolar symptoms. Sleep disorders where people have difficulty going to sleep and staying asleep are often present in this disorder. Attention-deficit/hyperactivity disorder is more common among children with cyclothymic disorder than those with other mental health conditions.

ETIOLOGY

Bipolar disorders are thought to be distinctly different from one another; for example, bipolar I disorder, bipolar II disorder, and cyclothymia have different characteristics. Episodes of depression in bipolar disorders are different from unipolar depression (i.e.,

depression without episodes of mania—see Chapter 13). Depressive episodes in bipolar disorder affect younger people, produce more episodes of illness, and require more frequent hospitalization. They are also characterized by higher rates of divorce and marital conflict.

Theories of the development and onset of bipolar disorders focus on biological, psychological, and environmental factors. Most likely, multiple variables contribute to the occurrence of bipolar disorder. For this reason, a biopsychosocial approach will likely be the most successful approach to treatment.

Biological Factors

Genetic

Bipolar illnesses tend to run in families, and the lifetime risk for individuals with an affected parent is 15% to 30% greater (Fusar-Poli, Howes, Bechdolf, et al., 2012). Recent research suggests that there may be an overlap between rare genetic variations linked to bipolar disorder and those implicated in schizophrenia and autism (Goes, Pierooznia, Parla, et al., 2016).

The concordance rate among identical twins is around 70%. This means that if one twin has the disorder, 70% of the time the other one will, too. Despite the high concordance rate in identical twins, it is uncommon for clinicians to find a positive family history for bipolar disorder in these twins' families (Kerner, 2014). This finding probably means that the disease is polygenic or that a number of genes contribute to its expression.

Some evidence suggests that bipolar disorders are more prevalent in adults who had high intelligence quotients (IQs), and who were particularly verbal, as children (Smith, Anderson, Zammit, et al., 2015). People with bipolar disorders appear to achieve higher levels of education and higher occupational status than individuals with unipolar depression. Also, the proportion of patients with bipolar disorders among creative writers, artists, highly educated men and women, and professionals is higher than in the general population.

Neurobiological

Neurotransmitters (norepinephrine, dopamine, and serotonin) have been studied since the 1960s as causal factors in mania and depression. One simple explanation is that having too few of these chemical messengers will result in depression and having an oversupply will cause mania. However, proportions of neurotransmitters in relation to one another may be more important. Receptor site insensitivity could also be at the root of the problem—even if there is enough of a certain neurotransmitter, it is not going where it needs to go.

Additional research has found that the interrelationships in the neurotransmitter system are complex, and more elaborate theories have been developed since the amine hypotheses were originally proposed. Mood disorders are most likely a result of interactions among various chemicals, including neurotransmitters and hormones.

Brain Structure and Function

Structural neuroimaging techniques (e.g., computed tomography [CT] and magnetic resonance imaging [MRI]) provide still pictures of the scalp, skull, and brain. Structural imaging is useful in viewing bones, tissues, blood vessels, tumours, infection, damage, or bleeding. *Functional* neuroimaging techniques (e.g., positron emission tomography [PET], functional MRI [fMRI], and magnetoencephalography [MEG]) provide measures related to brain activity. Functional imaging reveals activity and chemistry by measuring the rate of blood flow, chemical activity, and electrical impulses in the brain during specific tasks.

With bipolar disorder, functional imaging techniques reveal dysfunction in the prefrontal cortical region, the region associated with executive decision making, personality expression, and social behaviour (Phillips & Swartz, 2014). Dysfunction is also evident in the hippocampus, which is primarily associated with memory, and the amygdala, which is associated with memory, decision making, and emotion. Dysregulation in these areas results in the characteristic emotional lability, heightened reward sensitivity, and emotional dysregulation of bipolar disorder. These abnormalities may be due to grey matter loss in these areas.

Neuroendocrine

The hypothalamic–pituitary–thyroid–adrenal (HPTA) axis has been the object of significant research in bipolar disorder. In fact, hypothyroidism is one of the most common physical abnormalities associated with bipolar disorder. Typically, the thyroid dysfunction is not dramatic and the problem is often undetected.

In both manic and depressive states, peripheral inflammation is increased. This inflammation tends to decrease between episodes (Maletic & Raison, 2014). These findings are consistent with changes in the HPTA axis, which are known to drive inflammatory activation.

The role of estrogen in bipolar disorder is also under review. Childbirth is known to be associated with the onset of mood and anxiety disorders. Estrogen studies have shown that women with postpartum psychosis have very low levels of estrogen and improve after estrogen replacement therapy (Meinhard, Kessing, & Vinberg, 2014). Selective estrogen receptor modulators (e.g., tamoxifen) have also been shown to produce antimanic effects. Further research in this area is required.

Environmental Factors

Bipolar disorder is a worldwide problem that generally affects all races and ethnic groups equally, but some evidence suggests that bipolar disorders may be more prevalent in upper socio-economic classes. The exact reason for this finding is unclear; however, people with bipolar disorders appear to achieve higher levels of education and higher occupational status than individuals with unipolar depression. The educational levels of individuals with unipolar depressive disorders, on the other hand, appear to be no different from those of individuals with no symptoms of depression within the same socioeconomic class.

Children who have a genetic and biological risk of developing bipolar disorder are most vulnerable when their social determinants of health are compromised. Stressful family life and adverse life events may result in a more severe course of illness in these individuals. Stress is also a common trigger for mania and depression in adults.

Psychological Factors

With the advent of improved neuroimaging techniques and treatment advances, psychological theories are largely dismissed. Mania was once thought to be a defence against underlying anxiety and depression. Mania was also thought to help individuals tolerate loss or tragedy, such as the death of a loved one. Psychodynamic theorists believed that a faulty ego uses mania when it is overwhelmed by pleasurable impulses such as sex or feared impulses such as aggression. An overactive and critical superego being replaced with the euphoria of mania has also been suggested as the cause.

 CONSIDERING CULTURE

Influence of Religion and Supernatural Beliefs in Patients With Bipolar Disorder

Background
Religious and supernatural beliefs influence help-seeking and treatment practices in bipolar disorder, but these are rarely explored by clinicians. This study aimed to understand religiousness, magico-religious beliefs, prevalence of religious and supernatural psychopathology, and treatment practices among patients with bipolar disorder in euthymic state.

Methodology
A total of 185 patients with bipolar disorder currently in remission were assessed cross-sectionally for their clinical profile and their current clinical status on the Hamilton Depression Rating Scale (HDRS), Young Mania Rating Scale (YMRS), and Global Assessment of Functioning (GAF). A semistructured instrument for magico-religious beliefs, etiological models, treatment seeking, and treatment practices was administered.

Results
More than a third of patients (37.8%) had psychopathology with either religious or supernatural content, or both, in their lifetime. Almost half of patients (45.4%) believed in a supernatural or religious etiology for their illness. Among the specific causes, planetary influences (13.5%) and God's will (30.8%) were the most common supernatural and religious cause, respectively. Almost half of patients (44.3%) had first treatment contact with religious or supernatural treatment providers. More than 90% of patients reported a belief in God, yet about 70% reported that their doctors did not ask them sufficient questions to understand their religiosity.

Conclusion
Magico-religious beliefs are common among those with bipolar disorder, and a large number of patients attribute these as etiological factors for their illness. Consequently, they tend to seek treatment from traditional practitioners prior to approaching medical practitioners and may continue treatment with them alongside medical management.

Source: Grover, S., Hazari, N., Aaneja, J., et al. (2016). Influence of religion and supernatural beliefs on clinical manifestation and treatment practices in patients with bipolar disorder. *Nordic Journal of Psychiatry, 70*(6), 442-449. Retrieved from http://www.tandfonline.com/doi/abs/10.3109/08039488.2016.1151930. Copyright © 2016 by Taylor & Francis. Reprinted by Permission of Taylor & Francis.

APPLICATION OF THE NURSING PROCESS

ASSESSMENT

Individuals with bipolar disorder are often misdiagnosed or underdiagnosed. Early diagnosis and proper treatment can help people avoid:

- Suicide attempts
- Alcohol or substance abuse
- Marital or work problems
- Development of medical comorbidity

Figure 14-2 presents the Mood Disorder Questionnaire (MDQ). This diagnostic test, while not definitive, is a helpful initial screening device.

General Assessment

Individuals with bipolar disorder tend to spend more time in a depressed state than in a manic state. For a complete discussion of nursing care for the depressive aspects of bipolar disorder, refer to Chapter 13. In this chapter, we focus on nursing care for individuals experiencing mania.

The characteristics of mania discussed in the following sections are (1) mood, (2) behaviour, (3) thought processes and speech patterns, and (4) cognitive function.

Mood

The euphoric mood associated with mania is unstable. During euphoria, patients may state that they are experiencing an intense feeling of well-being, are "cheerful in a beautiful world," or are becoming "one with God." The overly joyous mood may seem out of proportion to what is going on, and cheerfulness may be inappropriate for the circumstances, considering that patients are full of energy with little or no sleep. Their mood may change quickly to irritation and anger when they are thwarted. The irritability and belligerence may be short-lived, or it may become the prominent feature of the manic phase of bipolar disorder.

People experiencing a manic state may laugh, joke, and talk in a continuous stream, with uninhibited familiarity. They often demonstrate boundless enthusiasm, treat others with confidential friendliness, and incorporate everyone into their plans and activities. They know no strangers, and energy and self-confidence seem boundless.

To people experiencing mania, no aspirations are too high, and no distances are too far—no boundaries exist to curtail them. Often during impulsive, intrusive, and demanding behaviours, they can become easily angered and show a shift in mood at anyone attempting to stop them or set limits.

As the clinical course progresses from hypomania to mania, sociability and euphoria are replaced by a stage of hostility, irritability, and paranoia. The following is a patient's description of the painful transition from hypomania to mania:

> At first when I'm high, it's tremendous … ideas are fast … like shooting stars you follow until brighter ones appear … all shyness disappears, the right words and gestures are suddenly there … uninteresting people, things become intensely interesting. Sensuality is pervasive; the desire to seduce and be seduced is irresistible. Your marrow is infused with unbelievable feelings of ease, power,

well-being, omnipotence, euphoria … you can do anything … but somewhere this changes… . The fast ideas become too fast and there are far too many … overwhelming confusion replaces clarity … you stop keeping up with it—memory goes. Infectious humour ceases to amuse—your friends become frightened … everything now is against the grain … you are irritable, angry, frightened, uncontrollable, and trapped in the blackest caves of the mind—caves you never knew were there. It will never end. Madness carves its own reality. (Jamison, 1995, p. 70)

Behaviour

When people experience hypomania, they have appetites for social engagement, spending, and activity, even indiscriminate sex. The increased activity and a reduced need for sleep prevent proper rest. Although short periods of sleep are possible, some patients may not sleep for several days in a row. This nonstop physical activity and the lack of sleep and food can lead to physical exhaustion and worsening of mania.

When in full-blown mania, a person constantly goes from one activity, place, or project to another. Many projects may be started, but few if any are completed. Inactivity is impossible, even for the shortest period of time. Hyperactivity may range from mild, constant motion to frenetic, wild activity. Flowery and lengthy letters are written, and excessive phone calls are made. Individuals become involved in pleasurable activities that can have painful consequences—for example, spending large sums of money on frivolous items, giving money away indiscriminately, throwing lavish parties, visiting expensive night clubs and restaurants, or making foolish business investments that can leave an individual or family penniless. Sexual indiscretion can dissolve relationships and marriages and lead to sexually transmitted infections. Religious preoccupation is a common symptom of mania.

Individuals experiencing mania may be manipulative, profane, fault finding, and adept at exploiting others' vulnerabilities. They constantly push limits. These behaviours often alienate family, friends, employers, health care providers, and others.

Modes of dress often reflect the person's grandiose yet tenuous grasp of reality. Dress may be described as outlandish, bizarre, colourful, and noticeably inappropriate. Makeup may be garish and overdone. People with mania are highly distractible. Concentration is poor, and individuals with mania go from one activity to another without completing anything. Judgement is poor. Impulsive marriages and divorces can take place.

People often emerge from a manic state startled and confused by the shambles of their lives. The following description conveys one patient's experience:

> Now there are only others' recollections of your behaviour—your bizarre, frenetic, aimless behaviour—at least mania has the grace to dim memories of itself … now it's over, but is it? … Incredible feelings to sort through … Who is being too polite? Who knows what? What did I do? Why? And most hauntingly, will it—when will it—happen again? Medication to take—to resist, to resent, to forget, but always to take. Credit cards revoked … explanations at work … bad cheques and apologies overdue … memory flashes of vague men (what did I do?) … friendships gone, a marriage ruined. (Jamison, 1995, p. 86)

MOOD DISORDER QUESTIONNAIRE

Instructions: Please answer each question as best you can.

	Yes	No
1. Has there ever been a period of time when you were not your usual self and....		
you felt so good or so hyper that other people thought you were not your normal self or you were so hyper that you got into trouble?	○	○
you were so irritable that you shouted at people or started fights or arguments?	○	○
you felt much more self-confident than usual?	○	○
you got much less sleep than usual and found you didn't really miss it?	○	○
you were much more talkative or spoke much faster than usual?	○	○
thoughts raced through your head or you couldn't slow down your mind?	○	○
you were so easily distracted by things around you that you had trouble concentrating or staying on track?	○	○
you had much more energy than usual?	○	○
you were much more active or did many more things than usual?	○	○
you were much more social or outgoing than usual; for example, you telephoned friends in the middle of the night?	○	○
you were much more interested in sex than usual?	○	○
you did things that were unusual for you or that other people might have thought were excessive, foolish, or risky?	○	○
spending money got you or your family into trouble?	○	○
2. If you answered "Yes" to more than one of the above, have several of these ever happened during the same period of time?	○	○

3. How much of a problem did any of these cause you — like being unable to work; having family, money, or legal troubles; or getting into arguments or fights? Please select one response only.

○ No problem   ○ Minor problem   ○ Moderate problem   ○ Serious problem

	Yes	No
4. Have any of your blood relatives (children, siblings, parents, grandparents, aunts, uncles) had manic-depressive illness or bipolar disorder?	○	○
5. Has a health care professional ever told you that you have manic-depressive illness or bipolar disorder?	○	○

Criteria for Results: Answering "Yes" to 7 or more of the events in question 1, answering "Yes" to question 2, and answering "Moderate problem" or "Serious problem" to question 3 is considered a positive screen result for bipolar disorder.

FIGURE 14-2 The Mood Disorder Questionnaire (MDQ). Source: Hirschfeld, R., Williams, J., Spitzer, R., et al. (2000). Development and validation of a screening instrument for bipolar spectrum disorder: The Mood Disorder Questionnaire. *American Journal of Psychiatry, 157*(11), 1873–1875. © 2004 Eli Lilly and Company.

Thought Processes and Speech Patterns

Flight of ideas is a nearly continuous flow of accelerated speech with abrupt changes from topic to topic that are usually based on understandable associations or plays on words. At times, the attentive listener can keep up with the flow of words, even though the direction changes from moment to moment. Speech is rapid, verbose, and circumstantial (including minute and unnecessary details). When the condition is severe, speech may be disorganized and incoherent. The incessant talking often includes joking, puns,

RESEARCH HIGHLIGHT

What Youth With Bipolar Disorder Want When Seeking Health Information Online

Problem

People are increasingly using the Internet to search for health-related information. There was no reported research on how best to help youth with bipolar disorder access online mental health information.

Purpose of Study

The purpose of this study was to examine: (1) how Bipolar Youth Action Project (BYAP) participants currently seek mental health information online, and (2) youth preferences and desires for future developments in the arena of online mental health information provision.

Methods

A multidisciplinary collaborative research team that included an academic researcher, health care providers, and community members was established. The work of the research team was guided by the belief that collaborating with those with direct involvement and knowledge about the issues will result in relevant findings. As a result, significant community input was sought throughout the research proves. Focus groups were conducted to gather answers to the following question: What are the best methods for sharing information on self-management strategies with other youth, their families, and the wider community?

Key Findings

- Stigma was a significant barrier to accessing information online. Participants described fears related to posting information and being judged.
- Platforms with more anonymity allowed the participants to participate in a more "faceless" manner. However, this did not result in less stigma or less distressing content.
- Finding credible, high-quality online content was a significant barrier.

Implications for Nursing Practice

Many individuals access information online prior to seeking support and guidance from a health professional. Creating credible online mental health information is critical. Providing online mental health services is also increasing. Nursing competencies related to information management and technology will play a larger part in our future practice.

Source: Noack, K., Balram Elliott, N., Canas, E., et al. (2016). Credible, centralized, safe, and stigma-free: What youth with bipolar disorder want when seeking health information online. *University of British Columbia Medical Journal, 8*(1), 27–30. Retrieved from https://ubcmj.com/.

and teasing: "How are you doing, kid? No kidding around, I'm going home … home sweet home … home is where the heart is, the heart of the matter is I want out, and that ain't hay … hey, Doc … get me out of this place."

The content of speech is often sexually explicit and ranges from grossly inappropriate to vulgar. Themes in the communication of the individual with mania may revolve around extraordinary sexual prowess, brilliant business ability, or unparalleled artistic talents (e.g., writing, painting, dancing). The person may actually have only average ability in these areas.

Speech is not only profuse but also loud, bellowing, or even screaming. One can hear the force and energy behind the rapid words. As mania escalates, flight of ideas may give way to clang associations. Clang associations are the stringing together of words because of their rhyming sounds, without regard to their meaning: "Cinema I and II, last row. Row, row, row your boat. Don't be a cutthroat. Cut your throat. Get your goat. Go out and vote. And so I wrote."

Grandiosity (inflated self-regard) is apparent in both the ideas expressed and the person's behaviour. People with mania may exaggerate their achievements or importance, state that they know famous people, or believe that they have great powers. They boast of exceptional powers, and status can take delusional proportions during mania. Grandiose persecutory delusions are common. For example, people may think that God is speaking to them or that authorities are out to stop them from saving the world. Sensory perceptions may become altered as the mania escalates, and hallucinations may occur. However, no evidence of delusions or hallucinations is present during hypomania.

Cognitive Function

The onset of bipolar disorder is often preceded by comparatively high cognitive function. However, there is growing evidence that about one-third of patients with bipolar disorder display significant and persistent cognitive problems and difficulties in psychosocial areas. Cognitive deficits in bipolar disorder are milder but similar to those in patients with schizophrenia. Cognitive impairments are greater in bipolar I but are also present in bipolar II.

The potential cognitive dysfunction among many people with bipolar disorder has specific clinical implications:

- Cognitive function affects overall function.
- Cognitive deficits correlate with a greater number of manic episodes, history of psychosis, chronicity of illness, and poor functional outcome.
- Early diagnosis and treatment are crucial to prevent illness progression, cognitive deficits, and poor outcome.
- Medication selection should consider not only the efficacy of the drug in reducing mood symptoms but also the cognitive impact of the drug on the patient.

Self-Assessment

The person experiencing mania (who is often out of control and resists being controlled) can elicit numerous intense emotions in a nurse. The person may use humour, manipulation, power struggles, or demanding behaviour to prevent or minimize the staff's ability to set limits on and control dangerous behaviour. People with mania have the ability to "staff split," or divide the staff into the "good guys" and the "bad guys": "The nurse on the day shift is always late with my medication and never talks with me. You are the only one who seems to care." This divisive tactic may pit one staff member or group against another, undermining a unified front and consistent plan of care. Frequent team meetings to deal with the behaviours of the person and the nurses' responses to these behaviours can help minimize staff splitting and feelings of anger and isolation. Limit setting (e.g., lights out after 2300 hours) is the main theme in treating a person with mania. Consistency among staff is imperative if the limit setting is to be carried out effectively.

The person can become aggressively demanding, which often triggers frustration, worry, and exasperation in health care providers. The behaviour of a person experiencing mania is often aimed at decreasing the effectiveness of staff control, which could be accomplished by staff members getting involved in power plays. For example, the person might taunt the staff by pointing out faults or oversights and drawing negative attention to one or more staff members. Usually this taunting is done in a loud and disruptive manner, which provokes staff to become defensive and thereby escalates the environmental tension and the person's degree of mania.

If you are working with a person experiencing mania, you may find yourself feeling helplessness, confusion, or even anger. Understanding, acknowledging, and sharing these responses and counter-transference reactions will enhance your professional ability to care for the person and perhaps promote your personal development as well. Collaborating with the interprofessional team, accessing the supervision (as a nursing student) of your nursing faculty member, and sharing your experience with peers in postconference may be helpful, perhaps essential.

NURSING DIAGNOSIS

Nursing diagnoses vary among people experiencing mania. A primary consideration for a person in acute mania is the prevention of exhaustion and death from cardiac collapse. Because of the person's poor judgement, excessive and constant motor activity, probable dehydration, and difficulty evaluating reality, *Risk for injury* is a likely and appropriate diagnosis. Table 14-2 lists potential nursing diagnoses for bipolar disorders.

OUTCOMES IDENTIFICATION

Outcome criteria will be based on which of the three phases of the illness the patient is experiencing. The *Nursing Outcomes Classification (NOC)* (Moorhead, Johnson, Maas, et al., 2012) provides useful outcomes for each phase.

Acute Phase

The acute phase occurs during an intense manic, hypomanic or depressive episode. The overall outcome of the acute phase is injury prevention. The person may be hospitalized during this phase. Outcomes in the acute phase reflect both physiological and psychiatric issues. For example, the patient will:

- Be well hydrated
- Maintain stable cardiac status
- Maintain and obtain tissue integrity
- Get sufficient sleep and rest
- Demonstrate thought self-control
- Make no attempt at self-harm

Relevant *NOC* outcomes for this phase include *Hydration, Cardiac pump effectiveness, Tissue integrity: Skin and mucous membranes, Sleep, Distorted thought self-control,* and *Suicide self-restraint.* Refer to Chapter 13 for outcomes that also relate to the depressive phase of bipolar disorders.

Continuation Phase

During this stage the presenting symptoms are being controlled but the individual's mental health is still quite fragile. The continuation phase lasts for 4 to 9 months. Although the overall outcome of this phase is relapse prevention, many other outcomes must be accomplished to achieve relapse prevention. These outcomes include:

- Psychoeducational classes for the patient and family related to:
  - Knowledge of disease process
  - Knowledge of medication
  - Consequences of substance addictions for predicting future relapse
  - Knowledge of early signs and symptoms of relapse
- Support groups or therapy (cognitive behavioural, interpersonal)
- Communication and problem-solving skills training

Relevant *NOC* outcomes for this phase include *Compliance behaviour, Knowledge: Disease process, Social support,* and *Substance addiction consequences.*

📋 ASSESSMENT GUIDELINES

Bipolar Disorder

1. Assess whether the person is a danger to self or others:
   - People experiencing mania can exhaust themselves to the point of death.
   - People experiencing mania may not eat or sleep, often for days at a time.
   - Poor impulse control may result in harm to others or self.
   - Uncontrolled spending may occur.
2. Assess the need for protection from uninhibited behaviours. External control may be needed to protect the person from such things as bankruptcy because people experiencing mania may give away all of their money or possessions.
3. Assess the need for hospitalization to safeguard and stabilize the person.
4. Assess medical status. A thorough medical examination helps to determine whether mania is primary (a mood disorder—bipolar disorder or cyclothymia) or secondary to another condition.
   - Mania may be secondary to a general medical condition.
   - Mania may be substance induced (caused by use or abuse of a drug or substance or by toxin exposure).
5. Assess for any coexisting medical condition or other situation that warrants special intervention (e.g., substance abuse, anxiety disorder, legal or financial crises).
6. Assess the person's and family's understanding of bipolar disorder, knowledge of medications, and knowledge of support groups and organizations that provide information on bipolar disorder.

TABLE 14-2	POTENTIAL NURSING DIAGNOSES FOR BIPOLAR DISORDERS
SIGNS AND SYMPTOMS	**NURSING DIAGNOSES**
Excessive and constant motor activity	*Risk for injury*
Poor judgement	*Risk for self-neglect*
Lack of rest and sleep	
Poor nutritional intake (excessive or relentless mix of above behaviours can lead to cardiac collapse)	
Loud, profane, hostile, combative, aggressive, demanding behaviours	*Risk for other-directed violence*
	Risk for self-directed violence
	Risk for suicide
Intrusive and taunting behaviours	*Ineffective coping*
Inability to control behaviour	*Self-neglect*
Rage reaction	
Manipulative, angry, or hostile verbal and physical behaviours	*Defensive coping*
Impulsive speech and actions	*Ineffective coping*
Property destruction or lashing out at others in a rage reaction	*Ineffective impulse control*
Racing thoughts, grandiosity, poor judgement	*Ineffective coping*
	Ineffective impulse control
Giving away of valuables, neglect of family, impulsive major life changes (divorce, career changes)	*Interrupted family processes*
	Caregiver role strain
Continuous pressured speech, jumping from topic to topic (flight of ideas)	*Impaired verbal communication*
Constant motor activity, going from one person or event to another	*Impaired social interaction*
Annoyance or taunting of others, loud and crass speech	*Risk for ineffective relationships*
Provocative behaviours	
Failure to eat, groom, bathe, or dress self because person is too distracted, agitated, and disorganized	*Imbalanced nutrition: less than body requirements*
	Deficient fluid volume
	Self-care deficit (bathing, dressing, feeding, toileting)
Inability to sleep because patient is too frantic and hyperactive (sleep deprivation can lead to exhaustion and death)	*Disturbed sleep pattern*

Maintenance Phase

The overall outcomes for the maintenance phase continue to focus on prevention of relapse and limitation of the severity and duration of future episodes. Relevant *NOC* outcomes include *Knowledge: Disease process, Compliance behaviour,* and *Family support during treatment.* Additional outcomes include:
- Participation in learning interpersonal strategies related to work, interpersonal, and family problems
- Participation in psychotherapy, group, or other ongoing supportive therapy modality

PLANNING

Planning care for an individual with bipolar disorder is usually geared toward the particular phase of mania the person is in (acute, continuation, or maintenance), as well as any other co-occurring issues identified in the assessment (e.g., risk for suicide, risk for violence to person or property, family crisis, legal crises, substance abuse, risk-taking behaviours).

Acute Phase

During the acute phase, planning focuses on medically stabilizing the person while maintaining safety. Therefore the hospital is usually the safest environment for accomplishing this stabilization (see Case Study and Nursing Care Plan 14-1). Nursing care is geared toward managing medications, decreasing physical activity, increasing food and fluid intake, ensuring at least 4 to 6 hours of sleep per night, alleviating any bowel or bladder problems, and intervening to see that self-care needs are met. Some patients may require seclusion or even electroconvulsive therapy (ECT) to assist with stabilization.

Continuation Phase

During the continuation phase, planning focuses on maintaining adherence to the medication regimen and prevention of relapse. Interventions are planned in accordance with the assessment data regarding the person's interpersonal and stress-reduction skills, cognitive functioning, employment status, substance-related problems, and social support systems. During this time, psychoeducational teaching is necessary for the patient and family. The need for referrals to community programs, groups, and support for any co-occurring disorders or problems (e.g., substance abuse, family problems, legal issues, financial crises) is evaluated.

Evaluation of the need for communication skills training and problem-solving skills training is also an important consideration. People with bipolar disorders often have interpersonal and emotional problems that affect their work, family, and social lives. Residual problems resulting from reckless, violent, withdrawn, or bizarre behaviour that may have occurred during a manic episode often leave lives shattered and family and friends hurt and distant. For some patients, cognitive behavioural therapy (in addition to medication management) is useful to address these issues, although the focus of psychotherapeutic treatment will vary over time for each individual.

Maintenance Phase

During the maintenance phase, planning focuses on preventing relapse and limiting the severity and duration of future episodes. Patients with bipolar disorders require medications over long periods of time or even an entire lifetime. Psychotherapy, support groups, psychoeducational groups, and periodic evaluations help patients maintain their family, social, and occupational lives.

IMPLEMENTATION

Patients with bipolar disorders are often ambivalent about treatment. On average, people wait almost 10 years between the onset of symptoms and receiving treatment (Conus, Macneil, & McGorry, 2014). Patients may minimize the destructive consequences of their behaviours or deny the seriousness of the disease, and some are reluctant to give up the increased energy, euphoria, and heightened sense of self-esteem of hypomania. Unfortunately, nonadherence to the regimen of mood-stabilizing medication is a major cause of relapse, so establishing a therapeutic alliance with the individual with bipolar disorder is crucial. Another reason for the delay of adequate treatment is that individuals often present to health care professionals requesting assistance with their depression, and have not yet had a manic episode.

Acute Phase

Depressive Episodes

Depressive episodes of bipolar disorder have the same symptoms and risks as those of major depression (see Chapter 13 for appropriate interventions during the depressive phase of the illness). Hospitalization may be required if suicidal ideation, psychosis, or catatonia is present. Pharmacological treatment is affected by concerns of bringing on a manic phase. A discussion of medication therapy is included in this chapter.

Manic Episodes

Acute phase. Hospitalization provides safety for a person experiencing acute mania (bipolar I disorder), imposes external controls on destructive behaviours, and provides for medication stabilization. There are unique approaches to communicating with and maintaining the safety of the person during the hospitalization period (Table 14-3). Staff members continuously set limits in a firm, nonthreatening, and neutral manner to prevent further escalation of mania and provide safe boundaries for the person and others.

Continuation phase. The continuation phase is crucial for patients and their families. The outcome for this phase is prevention of relapse, and community resources are chosen based on the needs of the person, the appropriateness of the referral, and the availability of resources. Frequently, a case manager evaluates appropriate follow-up care for patients and their families.

Medication adherence during this phase is perhaps the most important treatment outcome. Often, this follow-up is handled in a community mental health clinic. However, adherence to the medication regimen is also addressed in outpatient clinics and psychiatric home care visits. Patients who are not too excitable and are able to tolerate a certain level of stimuli may attend an outpatient clinic. In addition to medication management,

community mental health clinics offer structure, decrease social isolation, and help patients channel their time and energy. If a person is homebound, community psychiatric home care is the appropriate modality for follow-up care.

Maintenance phase. The goal of the maintenance phase is to prevent recurrence of an episode of bipolar disorder. The community resources cited earlier are helpful, and patients and their families often greatly benefit from mutual support and self-help groups, which are discussed later in this chapter.

Pharmacological Interventions

The recommendations for the management of acute mania remain mostly unchanged for the continuation and maintenance phases. Lithium carbonate, valproic acid (Depakene), and several atypical antipsychotics continue to be first-line treatments for acute mania. Tamoxifen is occasionally used as a third-line augmentation option because of the link to altered estrogen levels. Combining olanzapine (Zyprexa) and carbamazepine (Tegretol) is not recommended, as both affect hepatic CYP1A2 metabolism, thereby decreasing the effectiveness of both drugs. For the management of bipolar depression, lithium, divalproex, lamotrigine (Lamictal), and quetiapine (Seroquel) are used for a monotherapy therapy approach. Olanzapine plus a selective serotonin reuptake inhibitor (SSRI) (except paroxetine), or lithium or valproic acid plus an SSRI or bupropion (Wellbutrin) are used as first-line options when combination therapy is required. (Parikh & Goldstein, 2013).

There may be times when a benzodiazepine antianxiety agent can help reduce agitation or anxiety. Due to the concern of dependency, use of benzodiazepines is usually short term until the mania subsides. The high-potency antianxiety benzodiazepines clonazepam and lorazepam are useful in the treatment of acute mania. They may calm agitation and reduce insomnia, aggression, and panic.

Mood Stabilization

Mood stabilizers refer to classes of drugs used to treat symptoms associated with bipolar disorder. The original intent of the term *mood stabilizers* was to indicate that these drugs were effective in the treatment of both mania and depression. This is not precisely true. While all of the medications in this category are effective in treating mania, not all of them do as well in treating depression.

Lithium Carbonate

Lithium carbonate ($LiCO_3$ or $Li+$) is effective in the treatment of bipolar I acute and recurrent manic and depressive episodes. Onset of action is usually within 10 to 21 days. Because the onset of action is so slow, it is usually supplemented in the early phases of treatment by atypical antipsychotics, anticonvulsants, or antianxiety medications.

The clinical benefits of lithium can be incredible. However, newer drugs have been introduced and approved that carry lower toxicity, have more favourable side effects, and require less frequent laboratory testing. The use of these newer drugs has resulted in a decline in lithium use.

Before lithium is administered, a medical evaluation is performed to assess the person's ability to tolerate the drug. In

TABLE 14-3 INTERVENTIONS FOR THE PATIENT EXPERIENCING ACUTE MANIA

INTERVENTION	RATIONALE
Communication	
Use firm and calm approach: "John, come with me. Please eat this sandwich."	Structure and control are provided for the person who is out of control. Feelings of security can result: "Someone is in control."
Use short and concise explanations or statements.	Short attention span limits comprehension to small bits of information.
Remain neutral; avoid power struggles and value judgements.	Person can use inconsistencies and value judgements as justification for arguing and escalating mania.
Be consistent in approach and expectations.	Consistent limits and expectations minimize potential for person's manipulation of staff.
Have frequent staff meetings to plan consistent approaches and set agreed-on limits.	Consistency of all staff is needed to maintain controls and minimize manipulation by patient.
With other staff, decide on limits, and communicate these with the person in simple, concrete terms with consequences. Example: "John, do not yell at or hit Peter. If you cannot control yourself, we will help you." Or, "The seclusion room will help you feel less out of control and prevent harm to yourself and others."	Clear expectations help the person experience outside controls, as well as understand reasons for medication, seclusion, or restraints (if he or she is not able to control behaviours).
Hear and act on legitimate complaints.	Underlying feelings of helplessness are reduced, and acting-out behaviours are minimized.
Firmly redirect energy into more appropriate and constructive channels.	Distractibility is the nurse's most effective tool with the person experiencing mania.
Structure in a Safe Milieu	
Maintain low level of stimuli in patient's environment (e.g., away from bright lights, loud noises, people).	Escalation of anxiety can be decreased.
Provide structured solitary activities with nurse or aide.	Structure provides security and focus.
Provide frequent high-calorie fluids.	Serious dehydration is prevented.
Provide frequent rest periods.	Exhaustion is prevented.
Redirect violent behaviour.	Physical exercise can decrease tension and provide focus.
When warranted in acute mania, use phenothiazines and seclusion to minimize physical harm.	Exhaustion and death can result from dehydration, lack of sleep, and constant physical activity.
Observe for signs of lithium toxicity.	There is a small margin of safety between therapeutic and toxic doses.
Prevent person from giving away money and possessions. Hold valuables in hospital safe until rational judgement returns.	Person's "generosity" is a manic defence that is consistent with irrational, grandiose thinking.
Physiological Safety: Self-Care Needs	
Nutrition	
Monitor intake, output, and vital signs.	Adequate fluid and caloric intake are ensured; development of dehydration and cardiac collapse are minimized.
Offer frequent, high-calorie, protein drinks and finger foods (e.g., sandwiches, fruit, milkshakes).	Constant fluid and calorie replacement are needed. Person may be too active to sit at meals. Finger foods allow "eating on the run."
Frequently remind person to eat. "Tom, finish your milkshake." "Sally, eat this banana."	The person experiencing mania is unaware of bodily needs and is easily distracted. Needs supervision to eat.
Sleep	
Encourage frequent rest periods during the day.	Lack of sleep can lead to exhaustion and death.
Keep person in areas of low stimulation.	Relaxation is promoted, and manic behaviour is minimized.
At night, provide warm baths, soothing music, and medication when indicated. Avoid giving person caffeine.	Relaxation, rest, and sleep are promoted.
Hygiene	
Supervise choice of clothes; minimize flamboyant and bizarre dress (e.g., garish stripes or plaids and loud, unmatching colours).	The potential is decreased for ridicule, which lowers self-esteem and increases the need for manic defence. The person is helped to maintain dignity.
Give simple, step-by-step reminders for hygiene and dress. "Here is your razor. Here are your toothbrush and toothpaste."	Distractibility and poor concentration are countered through simple, concrete instructions.
Elimination	
Monitor bowel habits; offer fluids and foods that are high in fibre. Evaluate need for laxative. Monitor input and output.	Fecal impaction resulting from dehydration and decreased peristalsis is prevented.

particular, baseline physical and laboratory examinations should include assessment of renal function; determination of thyroid status, including levels of thyroxine and thyroid-stimulating hormone; and evaluation for dementia or neurological disorders, which presage a poor response to lithium. Other clinical and laboratory assessments, including an electrocardiogram, are performed as needed, depending on the individual's physical condition.

Indications. Lithium is particularly effective in reducing:

- Elation, grandiosity, and expansiveness
- Flight of ideas
- Irritability and manipulation
- Anxiety
  To a lesser extent, lithium controls:
- Insomnia
- Psychomotor agitation
- Threatening or assaultive behaviour
- Distractibility
- Hypersexuality
- Paranoia

In the acute manic phase lithium is usually started at 600 to 1200 mg a day in two or three divided doses. It is then increased every few days by 300 mg a day with a maximum dose of 1800 mg a day. Lithium must reach therapeutic levels in the patient's blood to be effective. Reaching this level usually takes 7 to 14 days, or longer for some patients. Elderly patients appear to be more susceptible to adverse effects and may experience a higher incidence of neurotoxicity at lithium concentrations considered therapeutic for younger adults.

During the acute phase of the illness, an antipsychotic or a benzodiazepine can be used to prevent exhaustion, coronary collapse, and death until lithium reaches therapeutic levels. Antipsychotics act promptly to slow speech, inhibit aggression, and decrease psychomotor activity. As lithium becomes effective in reducing manic behaviour, the antipsychotic drugs are usually discontinued.

Margaret Trudeau (former wife of the late prime minister Pierre Trudeau and mother to current prime minister Justin Trudeau) struggled with undiagnosed bipolar disorder for more than 30 years. In 2001, after overcoming the stigma and admitting herself to the Royal Ottawa Mental Health Centre, she was finally diagnosed with bipolar depression. In her book *Changing My Mind*, she describes bipolar disorder as a heavy cross to bear, and one she will carry for the rest of her life. She wrote: "[my] contentment, you should know is not solely drug induced. I take a mild dose of mood stabilizer, and will likely for the rest of my days. Family, friends, meaningful work, exercise, diet, meditation, yoga, nature, gardening, lessons, cooking, music and art all play a role these days in keeping my demons at bay" (Trudeau, 2010, p. 12).

Therapeutic and toxic levels. There is a small window between the therapeutic and toxic levels of lithium. Lithium must reach therapeutic blood levels to be effective. This usually takes 7 to 14 days, or longer for some patients. Blood serum levels should reach 0.6 to 1.2 mEq/L (Sadock, Sadock, & Ruiz, 2015). Lithium levels should not exceed 1.5 mEq/L to avoid serious toxicity. Table 14-4 details expected side effects, signs of toxicity, and interventions for both.

TABLE 14-4   LITHIUM ADVERSE EFFECTS AND SIGNS OF LITHIUM TOXICITY

LEVEL	SIGNS AND SYMPTOMS	INTERVENTIONS
Expected Adverse Effects <0.4–1.2 mEq/L (therapeutic level)	Fine hand tremor, polyuria, mild thirst, mild nausea and general discomfort, weight gain	Symptoms may persist throughout therapy. Symptoms often subside during treatment. Weight gain may be helped with diet, exercise, and nutritional management.
Early Signs of Toxicity <1.5 mEq/L	Nausea, vomiting, diarrhea, thirst, polyuria, lethargy, slurred speech, muscle weakness, and fine hand tremor	Medication should be withheld, blood lithium levels measured, and dosage re-evaluated. Dehydration, if present, should be addressed.
Advanced Signs of Toxicity 1.5–2.0 mEq/L	Coarse hand tremor, persistent gastrointestinal upset, mental confusion, muscle hyperirritability, electroencephalographic changes, incoordination, sedation	Interventions outlined above or below should be used, depending on severity of circumstances.
Severe Toxicity 2.0–2.5 mEq/L	Ataxia, confusion, large output of dilute urine, serious electroencephalographic changes, blurred vision, clonic movements, seizures, stupor, severe hypotension, coma; death is usually secondary to pulmonary complications	Hospitalization is indicated. The drug is stopped, and excretion is hastened. If patient is alert, an emetic is administered.
>2.5 mEq/L	Convulsions, oliguria; death can occur	In addition to the interventions above, hemodialysis may be used in severe cases.

Source: Data from Lehne, R. A. (2013). *Pharmacology for nursing care* (8th ed.). St Louis: Elsevier; and Sadock, B. J., Sadock, V. A., & Ruiz, P. (2015). *Synopsis of psychiatry* (11th ed.). Alphen van den Rijn, Netherlands: Wolters Kluwer.

Lithium levels should be measured at least 5 days after beginning lithium therapy and after any dosage change, until the therapeutic level has been reached. Blood levels are determined every month. After 6 months to a year of stability, it is common to measure blood levels every 3 months. Blood should be drawn in the morning, 10 to 12 hours after the last dose of lithium is taken. For older adult patients, the principle of start low and go slow still applies.

Maintenance therapy. Although lithium is an effective intervention for treating the acute manic phase of bipolar disorder, it is not a cure. Some clinicians suggest that patients with bipolar disorder need to be given lithium for 9 to 12 months, and some patients may need lifelong lithium maintenance to prevent further relapses. Individuals receive lithium for maintenance indefinitely and experience manic and depressive episodes if the drug is discontinued. Many patients respond well to lower dosages during maintenance or prophylactic lithium therapy.

Complete suppression occurs in only 50% of patients or fewer, even with adherence to the maintenance therapy regimen. Therefore the patient and family should be given careful instructions about (1) the purpose and requirements of lithium therapy, (2) its adverse effects, (3) its toxic effects and complications, and (4) situations in which the physician should be contacted. The patient and family should also be advised that suddenly stopping lithium can lead to relapse and recurrence of mania. Health care providers must stress to patients and their families the importance of discontinuing maintenance therapy gradually. Patient and Family Teaching: Lithium Therapy outlines teaching regarding lithium therapy for the patient and family.

People taking lithium need to know that two major long-term risks of lithium therapy are hypothyroidism and impairment of the kidneys' ability to concentrate urine. Therefore a person receiving lithium therapy must have periodic follow-ups to assess thyroid and renal function. Health Canada (2014) has also issued warnings that taking lithium carries a high risk of hypercalcemia and hyperparathyroidism. Symptoms of hypercalcemia and hyperparathyroidism can include fatigue, depression, mental confusion, nausea, vomiting, excessive thirst, appetite loss, abdominal pain, frequent urination, muscle and joint aches, and muscle weakness. In the most serious situations, these conditions lead to coma and death.

Contraindications. Lithium therapy is generally contraindicated in patients with cardiovascular disease, brain damage, renal disease, thyroid disease, or myasthenia gravis. Whenever possible, lithium is not given to women who are pregnant because it may harm the fetus. The fear of becoming pregnant and the wish to become pregnant are both major concerns for many women taking lithium. Lithium use is also contraindicated in mothers who are breastfeeding and in children younger than 12 years of age.

Anticonvulsant Drugs

In the 1980s, researchers hypothesized that mood instability could be viewed much the same as epilepsy and that a chain reaction of sensitivity, or *kindling*, was responsible for the worsening of bipolar symptoms over time (Ostacher & Tilley, 2008). This hypothesis led to the use of anticonvulsant drugs, such as carbamazepine (Tegretol), valproic acid (Depakene), and lamotrigine (Lamictal), as a treatment for mania that has been refractory to lithium therapy. They also proved useful in treating people who need rapid de-escalation and who do not respond to other treatment approaches. Subsequent research did not

---

PATIENT AND FAMILY TEACHING

Lithium Therapy

The patient and the patient's family should be given the following information, be encouraged to ask questions, and be given the material in written form as well.

1. Lithium treats your current emotional problem and also helps prevent relapse. Therefore it is important to continue taking the drug after the current episode is over.
2. Because therapeutic and toxic dosage ranges are so close, it is important to monitor lithium blood levels very closely—more frequently at first and then once every several months after that.
3. Lithium is not addictive.
4. It is important to eat a normal diet, with normal salt and fluid intake (1500–3000 mL or six 350-mL glasses of fluid). Lithium decreases sodium reabsorption in the kidneys, which could lead to a deficiency of sodium. A low sodium intake leads to a relative increase in lithium retention, which could produce toxicity.
5. You should stop taking lithium if you have excessive diarrhea, vomiting, or sweating. All of these symptoms can lead to dehydration. Dehydration can raise lithium levels in the blood to toxic levels. Inform your physician if you have any of these problems.

6. Do not take diuretics (water pills) while you are taking lithium.
7. Lithium is irritating to the lining of your stomach. Take lithium with meals.
8. It is important to have your kidneys and thyroid checked periodically, especially if you are taking lithium over a long period. Talk to your doctor about this follow-up.
9. Do not take any over-the-counter medicines without checking first with your doctor.
10. If you find that you are gaining a lot of weight, you may need to talk this change over with your doctor or dietitian.
11. Many self-help groups are available to provide support for people with bipolar disorder and their families. The local self-help group is (give name and telephone number).
12. You can find out more information by calling (give name and telephone number).
13. Keep a list of adverse effects and toxic effects handy, along with the name and number of a person to contact if these effects occur (see Table 14-4).
14. If lithium is to be discontinued, your dosage will be tapered gradually to minimize the risk of relapse.

support the kindling theory, however, suggesting that symptom improvement for bipolar disorder is based on another mechanism of action of these anticonvulsant drugs and not on their seizure prevention mechanism.

Anticonvulsant drugs are thought to be:
- Superior for continuously cycling patients
- More effective when there is no family history of bipolar disorder
- Effective at dampening affective swings in schizoaffective patients
- Effective at diminishing impulsive and aggressive behaviour in some nonpsychotic patients
- Helpful in cases of alcohol and benzodiazepine withdrawal
- Beneficial in controlling mania (within 2 weeks) and depression (within 3 weeks or longer)

Valproate

Divalproex sodium (Epival). Valproate (available as divalproex sodium [Epival] and valproic acid [Depakene]) has surpassed lithium in treating acute mania. Valproate is also helpful in preventing future manic episodes. Although serious complications are rare, it is important to monitor liver function and platelet count periodically. Divalproex doses can cause drowsiness and dizziness and increase thoughts of suicide; therefore mood, ideations, and behaviour should be monitored on a regular basis. Therapeutic serum levels that range from 50 to 100 mcg/mL and 50 to 125 mcg/mL for mania should be monitored to prevent toxicity and overdose (Vallerand, Sanoski, & Deglin, 2013). Symptoms of central nervous system toxicity can include confusion, fatigue, dizziness, hallucinations, headache, and ataxia.

Carbamazepine. Some patients with treatment-resistant bipolar disorder improve after taking carbamazepine (Tegretol) and lithium, or carbamazepine and an antipsychotic. Carbamazepine seems to work better in patients with rapid cycling and in severely paranoid, angry patients experiencing manias rather than in euphoric, overactive, overly friendly patients experiencing manias. It is thought to also be more effective in dysphoric patients experiencing manias.

Liver enzymes should be monitored at least weekly for the first 8 weeks of treatment because the drug can increase levels of liver enzymes that can speed its own metabolism. In some instances, this can cause bone marrow suppression and liver inflammation. Complete blood counts should also be done periodically since carbamazepine is known to cause leukopenia and aplastic anemia.

Lamotrigine. Lamotrigine (Lamictal) is a first-line treatment for bipolar depression and is approved for acute and maintenance therapy. Lamotrigine is generally well tolerated but has one serious, though rare, dermatological reaction: a potentially life-threatening rash. Patients should be instructed to seek immediate medical attention if a rash appears, although most are likely benign.

Adverse drug reactions (ADRs), as indicated by the Canadian Network for Mood and Anxiety Treatments (CANMAT), that require patient safety monitoring are:
- Both valproic acid and carbamazepine may cause blood dyscrasias, hepatotoxicity, and teratogenicity.

- Carbamazepine has also been linked to hyponatremia and serious dermatological adverse effects.
- Valproic acid has been associated with polycystic ovary syndrome, weight gain, acute pancreatitis, and hyperammonemic encephalopathy.
- The severe ADRs associated with lamotrigine are dermatological, namely Stevens-Johnson syndrome.
- Drug interactions such as lamotrigine–valproic acid and carbamazepine–hormonal contraceptives are also important to be aware of.

Antianxiety Drugs

Diazepam (Valium), clonazepam (Rivotril), and lorazepam (Ativan) are antianxiety (anxiolytic) drugs useful in the treatment of acute mania in some patients who are resistant to other treatments. These drugs are also effective in managing the psychomotor agitation seen in mania. They should be avoided, however, in patients with a history of substance abuse.

Atypical Antipsychotics

Many of the second-generation antipsychotics are approved for acute mania. In addition to showing sedative properties during the early phase of treatment (help with insomnia, anxiety, agitation), the second-generation antipsychotics seem to have mood-stabilizing properties. Most evidence supports the use of olanzapine (Zyprexa) or risperidone (Risperdal).

This classification of drugs may bring about serious side effects. These serious side effects stem from a tendency toward weight gain that may lead to insulin resistance, diabetes, dyslipidemia, and cardiovascular impairment.

The Drug Treatment box provides an overview of drugs used to treat bipolar disorder that are approved by Health Canada and the *Canadian Food and Drugs Act.*

Electroconvulsive Therapy

Electroconvulsive therapy (ECT) is used to subdue severe manic behaviour, especially in patients with treatment-resistant mania and in those with rapid cycling (i.e., those who experience four or more episodes of illness per year).

ECT seems to be far more effective than drug-based therapy for treatment-resistant bipolar depression (Schoeyen, Kessler, Andreassen, et al., 2015). Depressive episodes—particularly those with severe, catatonic, or treatment-resistant depression—are an indication for this treatment.

Milieu Management

Control of hyperactive behaviour during the acute phase almost always includes immediate treatment with an antipsychotic drug. However, when a person is dangerously out of control, use of a seclusion room or restraints may also be required. A seclusion room provides comfort and relief to many patients who are unable to control their own behaviour. Seclusion serves the following purposes:
- Reduces overwhelming environmental stimuli
- Protects a person from injuring himself or herself or others, including staff
- Prevents destruction of personal property or property of others

DRUG TREATMENT OF PATIENTS WITH BIPOLAR DISORDER

GENERIC (TRADE)	HEALTH CANADA–APPROVED	OFF-LABEL USES	CANMAT RECOMMENDATIONS
Lithium carbonate	Acute mania Maintenance Mood stabilizer	Depression	First-line treatment for bipolar depression Recommended for acute mania Treatment and prevention of manic episodes
Anticonvulsants			
Valproic acid (Depakene) Divalproex sodium (Epival)	Acute mania	Depression Maintenance	Recommended for acute mania First-line maintenance treatment for bipolar disorder
Carbamazepine (Tegretol)	Acute mania	Depression Maintenance	Recommended for maintenance treatment of bipolar disorder, mood-stabilizing effect
Lamotrigine (Lamictal)	Maintenance	Depression (can worsen mania)	First-line treatment for bipolar depression Recommended for maintenance treatment of bipolar disorder
Gabapentin (Neurontin) and topiramate (Topamax)		Acute mania Maintenance	Recommended for maintenance treatment of bipolar disorder
Atypical Antipsychotics			
Aripiprazole (Abilify)	Mania Maintenance	Depression	
Olanzapine (Zyprexa)	Mania Maintenance	Depression	Recommended for acute mania
Quetiapine fumarate (Seroquel)	Depression Mania Maintenance		
Risperidone (Risperdal)	Mania	Depression Maintenance	First-line treatment for severe mania
Ziprasidone (Zeldox)	Acute mania Mixed features		Acute mania

Sources: Data from Canadian Network for Mood and Anxiety Treatments (CANMAT). (2009). *Canadian Network for Mood and Anxiety Treatments (CANMAT) and International Society for Bipolar Disorders (ISBD) collaborative update of CANMAT guidelines for the management of patients with bipolar disorder.* Toronto: Author; and Health Canada. (2013). *Drugs and health products.* Retrieved from http://www.hc-sc.gc.ca/dhp-mps/index-eng.php.

INTEGRATIVE THERAPY

Omega-3 Fatty Acids as a Treatment for Bipolar Disorder

A few generations ago, children resisted a nightly dose of cod liver oil that mothers swore by as constipation prevention. While the foul-tasting, evil-smelling liquid undoubtedly helped win that particular battle, cod liver oil may have had other benefits as well. It is rich in omega-3 fatty acids, which have drawn increasing attention as being important in mood regulation. Fish oil is the target of this attention. It contains two omega-3 fatty acids, eicosapentaenoic acid (EPA) and docosahexaenoic acid (DHA), which are important in central nervous system functioning.

The interest in these particular fatty acids developed as research began to suggest that people who live in areas with low seafood consumption, especially of cold water seafood, exhibited higher rates of depression and bipolar disorder. This led researchers to explore the influence of omega-3 fatty acids as protective for bipolar disorder.

In 2012, Sarris and colleagues reviewed published research about omega-3 and its influence on mania and depression. They concluded that there is no evidence to support the use of omega-3 in treating mania. However, they found strong evidence that increasing the use of this fatty acid may improve bipolar depressive symptoms.

Source: Sarris, J., Mischoulon, D., & Schweitzer, I. (2012). Omega-3 for bipolar disorder: Meta-analyses of use in mania and bipolar depression. *Journal of Clinical Psychiatry, 73*(1), 81–86.

Seclusion is warranted when documented data collected by the nursing and medical staff reflect the following points:
- Substantial risk of harm to others or self is clear.
- The person is unable to control his or her actions.
- Problematic behaviour has been sustained (continues or escalates despite other measures).
- Other measures have failed (e.g., setting limits beginning with verbal de-escalation or using chemical restraints).

The use of seclusion or restraints is associated with complex therapeutic, ethical, and legal issues. Most provincial and territorial laws prohibit the use of unnecessary physical restraint or isolation. Barring an emergency, the use of seclusion and restraints requires consent. Therefore most hospitals have well-defined protocols for treatment with seclusion. Seclusion protocol includes a proper reporting procedure, through the appropriate channels, when a person is to be secluded. For example, the use of seclusion and restraint is permitted only on the written order of a physician and must be reviewed and rewritten every 24 hours. The order must include the type of restraint to be used. Seclusion and observation levels and care protocols must be carefully adhered to as per individual hospital or agency policy.

Seclusion protocols also identify specific nursing responsibilities, such as how often the patient's behaviour is to be observed and documented (e.g., every 15 minutes), how often the patient is to be offered food and fluids (e.g., every 30 to 60 minutes), and how often the patient is to be toileted (e.g., every 1 to 2 hours). Medication is often administered to patients in seclusion; therefore vital signs should be measured frequently, as per hospital policy.

Careful and precise documentation is a legal necessity. The nurse documents the following:

- The behaviour leading up to the seclusion or restraint
- The actions taken to provide the least restrictive alternative
- The time the patient was placed in seclusion
- Every 15 minutes, the patient's behaviour, needs, nursing care, and vital signs
- The time and type of medications given and their effects on the patient

When a patient requires seclusion to prevent self-harm or violence toward others, it is ideal for one nurse on each shift to work with the patient on a continuous basis. Communication with a patient in seclusion is concrete and direct but also empathic and limited to brief instructions. Patients need reassurance that seclusion is only a temporary measure and that they will be returned to the unit when their behaviour is more controlled and they demonstrate the ability to safely be around others.

Frequent staff meetings regarding personal feelings are necessary to prevent using seclusion as a form of punishment or leaving a patient in seclusion for long periods of time without proper supervision. Restraints and seclusion are never to be used as punishment or for the convenience of the staff. Refer to Chapter 7 for a more detailed discussion of the legal implications of seclusion and restraints.

Support Groups

Patients with bipolar disorder, as well as their friends and families, benefit from forming mutual support groups. Often these are coordinated by organizations such as the Mood Disorders Society of Canada and the Canadian Mental Health Association.

Health Teaching and Health Promotion

Patients and families need information about bipolar disorder, with particular emphasis on its chronic and highly recurrent nature. In addition, patients and families need to be taught the warning signs and symptoms of impending episodes. For example, changes in sleep patterns are especially important because they usually precede, accompany, or precipitate mania. Even a single night of unexplainable sleep loss can be taken as an early warning of impending mania. Health teaching stresses the importance of establishing regularity in sleep patterns, meals, exercise, and other activities. Patient and Family Teaching: Bipolar Disorder lists health-teaching guidelines for patients with bipolar disorder and their families.

 PATIENT AND FAMILY TEACHING

Bipolar Disorder

1. Patients with bipolar disorder and their families need to know:
   - The chronic and episodic nature of bipolar disorder
   - The fact that bipolar disorder is long term. Treatment will require that one or more mood-stabilizing agents be taken for a long time
   - The expected side effects and toxic effects of the prescribed medication, as well as who to call and where to go in case of an adverse reaction
   - The signs and symptoms of relapse that may "come out of the blue"
   - The role of family members and others in preventing a full relapse
   - The phone numbers of emergency contact people, which should be kept in an easily accessed place
2. The use of alcohol, drugs of abuse, caffeine (particularly in energy drinks), and over-the-counter medications can cause a relapse.
3. Good sleep hygiene is critical to stability. Frequently, the early symptom of a manic episode is lack of sleep. In some cases, mania may be averted by the use of sleep medications.
4. Coping strategies are important for dealing with work, interpersonal, and family problems to lower stress, to enhance a sense of personal control, and to increase community functioning.
5. Group and individual therapy are valuable for gaining insight and skills in relapse prevention, providing social support, increasing coping skills in interpersonal relations, improving adherence to the medication regimen, reducing functional morbidity, and decreasing need for hospitalization.

Most of the medications used to treat bipolar disorder may cause weight gain and other metabolic disturbances such as altered metabolism of lipids and glucose. These alterations increase the risk for diabetes, high blood pressure, dyslipidemia, cardiac problems, or all of these in combination (metabolic syndrome). Not only do these disturbances impair quality of life and lifespan, they are also a major reason for nonadherence. Teaching aimed at weight reduction and management is essential to keep patients physically healthy and emotionally stable.

Recovery concepts are particularly important for patients with bipolar disorder, who often have issues with adherence to treatment. The best method of addressing this problem is to follow a collaborative care model in which responsibilities for treatment adherence are shared. In this model, patients are responsible for making it to appointments and openly communicating information, and the health care provider is responsible for keeping current on treatment methods and listening carefully as patients share perceptions. Through this sharing, treatment adherence becomes a self-managed responsibility.

Psychotherapy

Pharmacotherapy and psychiatric mental health care and management are essential in the treatment of acute manic attacks and during the continuation and maintenance phases of bipolar disorder. Individuals with bipolar disorder must deal with the psychosocial consequences of their past episodes and their vulnerability to experiencing future episodes. They also have to face the burden of long-term treatments that may involve unpleasant adverse effects. Many patients have strained interpersonal relationships, marital and family problems, academic and occupational problems, and legal or other social difficulties. Psychotherapy can help them work through these difficulties, decrease some of the psychic distress, and increase self-esteem. Psychotherapeutic treatments can also help patients improve their functioning between episodes and attempt to decrease the frequency of future episodes.

Often the patients receiving medication and therapy place more value on psychotherapy than clinicians do. Kay Redfield Jamison is an American clinical psychologist and mood disorder researcher who has suffered from bipolar disorder since her early adulthood. She describes her feelings about drug therapy and psychotherapy as follows:

> I cannot imagine leading a normal life without lithium. From startings and stoppings of it, I now know it is an essential part of my sanity. Lithium prevents my seductive but disastrous highs, diminishes my depressions, clears out the weaving of my disordered thinking, slows me, gentles me out, keeps me in my relationships, in my career, out of a hospital, and in psychotherapy. It keeps me alive, too. But psychotherapy heals, it makes some sense of the confusion, it reins in the terrifying thoughts and feelings, it brings back hope and the possibility of learning from it all. Pills cannot, do not, ease one back into reality. They bring you back headlong, careening, and faster than can be endured at times. Psychotherapy is a sanctuary, it is a battleground, and it is where I have come to believe that someday I may be able to contend with all of this. No pill can help me deal with the problem of not wanting to take pills, but no amount of therapy alone can prevent my manias and depressions. I need both. (Jamison, 1995, p. 139).

Advanced-Practice Interventions

Many advanced-practice registered nurses are able to diagnose and prescribe medications for treating bipolar disorder. In addition, they may use psychotherapy to help the patient cope more adaptively to stresses in the environment and decrease the risk of relapse. Specific approaches to psychotherapy include cognitive behavioural therapy, interpersonal and social rhythm therapy, and family-focused therapy.

Cognitive Behavioural Therapy

Cognitive behavioural therapy (CBT) is typically used as an adjunct to pharmacotherapy in many psychiatric disorders. It involves identifying maladaptive thoughts ("I am always going to be a loser") and behaviours ("I might as well drink") that may be barriers to a person's recovery and ongoing mood stability.

CBT focuses on adherence to the medication regimen, early detection and intervention for manic or depressive episodes, stress and lifestyle management, and the treatment of depression and comorbid conditions. Some research demonstrates that patients treated with cognitive therapy are more likely to take their medications as prescribed than are patients who do not participate in therapy, and psychotherapy results in greater adherence to the medication regimen.

Interpersonal and Social Rhythm Therapy

Depression and manic-type states impair a person's ability to interact with others. Even in between episodes, relationships have been so damaged it may seem impossible to correct the problems. The advanced-practice nurses can use a specialized approach, interpersonal and social rhythm therapy. This approach aims to regulate social routines and stabilize interpersonal relationships to improve depression and prevent relapse. Psychoeducation is a major component of this therapy and includes symptom recognition, adherence with medication and sleep routines, stress management, and maintenance of social supports.

Family-Focused Therapy

Family-focused therapy helps improve communication among family members. During depressive and manic episodes, family life can become a challenge or even intolerable. Negative patterns of communicating develop and become part of the fabric of the family. Advanced-practice nurses can help people recognize and reduce negative expressed emotion and stressors that provoke episodes.

EVALUATION

Outcome criteria often dictate the frequency of evaluation of short-term and intermediate indicators. Are the person's vital signs stable? Is he or she well hydrated? Is the person able to control personal behaviour or respond to external controls? Is the person able to sleep for 4 or 5 hours a night or take frequent, short rest periods during the day? Does the family have a clear understanding of the patient's disorder and need for medication? Do the patient and family know which community agencies might help them?

If outcomes or related indicators are not achieved satisfactorily, the preventing factors are analyzed. Were the data incorrect or insufficient? Were nursing diagnoses inappropriate or outcomes unrealistic? Was intervention poorly planned? After the outcomes and care plan are reassessed, the plan is revised, if indicated. Longer-term outcomes include adherence to the medication regimen; resumption of functioning in the community; achievement of stability in family, work, and social relationships and in mood; and improved coping skills for reducing stress.

CASE STUDY AND NURSING CARE PLAN 14-1
Mania

Hannah is brought to the emergency department after being found on the highway shortly after her car broke down. She is dressed in a long red dress, a blue and orange scarf, many long chains, and a pair of yellow shoes. The police report that when they came to her aid, she told them she was "driving to fame and fortune." She appeared overly cheerful and was constantly talking, laughing, and making jokes. At the same time, she paced up and down beside the car, sometimes tweaking the cheek of one of the policemen. She was coy and flirtatious with the police officers, saying at one point, "Boys in blue are fun to do."

When she reached into the car and started drinking from an open bottle of vodka, the police decided that her behaviour and general condition might result in harm to herself or others. When they explained to Hannah that they wanted to take her to the hospital for a general checkup, her jovial mood turned to anger and rage, yet 2 minutes after getting into the police car, she was singing "Jailhouse Rock."

On admission to the emergency department, Hannah is seen by a psychiatrist, and her sister is called. The sister states that Hannah stopped taking her lithium about 5 weeks ago and has been becoming more and more agitated and out of control. She reports that Hannah has not eaten in 2 days, has stayed up all night calling friends and strangers all over the province, and finally fled the house when the sister called an ambulance to take her to the hospital. The psychiatrist contacts Hannah's regular physician, and her previous history and medical management are discussed. It is decided that she should be hospitalized during the acute manic phase and restarted on lithium therapy. It is hoped that medications and a controlled environment will prevent further escalation of the manic state and prevent possible exhaustion and cardiac collapse.

ASSESSMENT

Self-Assessment

Jake has worked as a nurse on the psychiatric unit for 2 years. He has learned to deal with many of the challenging behaviours associated with the manic defence. For example, he no longer takes most of the verbal insults personally, even when the remarks are cutting and hit close to home. He is also better able to recognize and set limits on some of the tactics used by the person experiencing mania to split the staff. The staff on this unit work closely with one another, making the atmosphere positive and supportive; therefore communication is good among staff. Frequent and effective communication is needed to prevent staff splitting, maximize external controls, and maintain consistency in nursing care.

The only aspects of Hannah's behaviour Jake thinks he may have difficulty with are the sexual advances and loud sexual comments she makes toward him. He knows that these behaviours could make him anxious, and his concern is that Hannah might pick up on his anxiety. When he discusses this concern with the senior nurse, they decide that two nurses should provide care for Hannah. A female nurse will spend time with her in her room, and Jake will spend time with her in quiet areas on the unit. It is decided that neither Jake nor any male staff member will be alone with Hannah in her room at any time. Jake will ask for relief if Hannah's sexual remarks and acting-out behaviours make him anxious.

Objective Data	Subjective Data
Little if anything to eat for days	"Driving to fame and fortune."
Little if any sleep for days	"Boys in blue are fun to do."
History of mania	
History of lithium maintenance	
Very loud and distracting to others	
Anger when wishes are denied	
Flight of ideas	
Loud and inappropriate dress	
Sexually suggestive remarks and actions	
Remarks that suggest grandiose thinking	
Poor judgement	

DIAGNOSIS

1. *Risk for injury* related to dehydration and faulty judgement, as evidenced by inability to meet own physiological needs and set limits on own behaviour

Supporting Data
- Has not slept for days
- Has not consumed food or fluids for days

CASE STUDY AND NURSING CARE PLAN 14-1—cont'd

Mania

2. *Defensive coping* related to biochemical changes, as evidenced by change in usual communication patterns

Supporting Data

- Remarks suggest sexual themes
- Remarks suggesting grandiose thinking
- Flight of ideas
- Constantly talking, laughing, and making jokes

OUTCOMES IDENTIFICATION

Physical status will remain stable during manic phase.

PLANNING

The nurse plans interventions that will help de-escalate Hannah's activity to minimize potential physical injury (dehydration, cardiac instability) through the use of medication and provision of a nonstimulating environment.

IMPLEMENTATION

Jake makes the following nursing care plan:

Short-Term Goal	Intervention	Rationale	Evaluation
1. Person will be well hydrated, as evidenced by good skin turgor and normal urinary output and specific gravity, within 24 hours.	1a. Give olanzapine (Zyprexa) intramuscularly immediately and as ordered.	1a. Continuous physical activity and lack of fluids can eventually lead to cardiac collapse and death.	**GOAL MET** After 3 hours, person takes small amounts of fluid (60–120 mL per hour). After 5 hours, patient starts taking 250 mL per hour with a lot of reminding and encouragement. After 24 hours, urine specific gravity is within normal limits.
	1b. Check vital signs frequently (every 1–2 hours).	1b. Cardiac status is monitored.	
	1c. Place person in private or quiet room (whenever possible).	1c. Environmental stimuli are reduced—escalation of mania and distractibility are minimized.	
	1d. Stay with person and divert person away from stimulating situations.	1d. Nurse's presence provides support. Ability to interact with others is temporarily impaired.	
	1e. Offer high-calorie, high-protein drink (250 mL) every hour in quiet area.	1e. Proper hydration is mandatory for maintenance of cardiac status.	
	1f. Frequently remind person to drink: "Take two more sips."	1f. Person's concentration is poor; she is easily distracted.	
	1g. Offer finger food frequently, in quiet area.	1g. Person is unable to sit; snacks she can eat while pacing are more likely to be consumed.	
	1h. Maintain record of intake and output.	1h. Such a record allows staff to make accurate nutritional assessment for person's safety.	
	1i. Weigh person daily.	1i. Monitoring of nutritional status is necessary.	

Continued

CASE STUDY AND NURSING CARE PLAN 14-1—cont'd

Mania

Short-Term Goal	Intervention	Rationale	Evaluation
2. Person will sleep or rest 3 hours during the first night in the hospital with aid of medication and nursing interventions.	2a. Continue to direct person to areas of minimal activity.	2a. Lower levels of stimulation can decrease excitability.	Person is awake most of the first night. Sleeps for 2 hours from 0400 to 0600 hours.
	2b. When possible, try to direct energy into productive and calming activities (e.g., pacing to slow, soft music; slow exercise; drawing alone; writing in quiet area).	2b. Directing patient to paced, nonstimulating activities can help minimize excitability.	Person is able to rest on the second day for short periods and engage in quiet activities for short periods (5–10 minutes).
	2c. Encourage short rest periods throughout the day (e.g., 3–5 minutes every hour) when possible.	2c. Person may be unaware of feelings of fatigue. Can collapse from exhaustion if hyperactivity continues without periods of rest.	
	2d. Drinks such as coffee, tea, and colas should be decaffeinated only.	2d. Caffeine is a central nervous system stimulant that inhibits needed rest or sleep.	
	2e. Provide nursing measures at bedtime that promote sleep (e.g., warm milk, soft music).	2e. Such measures promote nonstimulating and relaxing mood.	
3. Person's blood pressure (BP) and pulse (P) will be within normal limits within 24 hours, with the aid of medication and nursing interventions.	3a. Continue to monitor BP and P frequently throughout the day (every 30 minutes).	3a. Physical condition is presently a great strain on patient's heart.	**GOAL MET** Baseline measures on unit are not obtained because of hyperactive behaviour. Information from family physician states that baseline BP is 130/90 mm Hg and baseline P is 88 beats per minute.
	3b. Keep staff informed, by verbal and written reports, of baseline vital signs and patient progress.	3b. Alerting all staff regarding person's status can increase medical intervention if a change in status occurs.	BP at end of 24 hours is 130/70 mm Hg; P is 80 beats per minute.

EVALUATION

After 2 days, the medical staff feel that Hannah's physical status is stable. Her vital signs are within normal limits, she is consuming sufficient fluids, and her urinary output is normal. Although her hyperactivity persists, it does so to a lesser degree; she is able to get periods of rest during the day and is sleeping 3 to 4 hours during the night.

Hannah's hyperactivity continues to be a challenge to the nurses; however, she is able to participate in some activities that require gross motor movement. These activities are useful in channelling some of her aggressive energy. Shortly after her arrival on the unit, Hannah starts a fight with another patient, but seclusion is avoided because she is able to refrain from further violent episodes as a result of medication and nursing interventions. She can be directed toward solitary activities, which channel some of her energies, at least for short periods.

As the effect of the drugs progresses, Hannah's activity level decreases, and by discharge, she is able to discuss issues of concern with the nurse and make some useful decisions about her future. She is to come for follow-up at the community centre and agrees to join a family psychoeducational group for patients with bipolar disorder and their families, which she will attend with her sister.

KEY POINTS TO REMEMBER

- Bipolar I disorder is characterized by the presence or history of at least one manic episode, whereas bipolar II disorder is characterized by the presence or history of at least one hypomanic episode.
- Cyclothymia is a bipolar-related disorder with symptoms of hypomania and symptoms of mild-moderate depression.
- Genetics play a strong role in the risk for the bipolar disorders.
- Neurotransmitter (norepinephrine, dopamine, serotonin) excess and imbalance are also related to bipolar mood swings, supporting the existence of neurobiological influences. Neuroendocrine and neuroanatomical findings provide strong evidence for biological influences.
- Early detection of bipolar disorder can help diminish comorbid substance abuse, suicide, and decline in social and personal relationships and may help promote more positive outcomes.
- Bipolar disorder often goes unrecognized.
- The nurse assesses the person's level of mood (hypomania, acute mania), behaviour, and thought processes and is alert to cognitive dysfunction.
- Analyzing the objective and subjective data helps the nurse formulate appropriate nursing diagnoses. Some of the nursing diagnoses appropriate for patients with mania are *Risk for violence, Defensive coping, Ineffective coping, Disturbed thought processes,* and *Situational low self-esteem.*
- During the acute phase of mania, physical needs often take priority and demand nursing interventions. Therefore *Deficient fluid volume, Imbalanced nutrition, Imbalanced elimination,* and *Disturbed sleep pattern* are usually addressed in the nursing plan.
- The diagnosis of *Interrupted family processes* is vital. Support groups, psychoeducation, and guidance for the family can greatly affect the person's adherence to the medication regimen.

- Planning involves identifying the specific needs of the patient and family during the three phases of mania (acute, continuation, and maintenance). Can the patient benefit from communication skills training, improvement in coping skills, legal or financial counselling, or further psychoeducation? What community resources does the person need at this time?
- Health care workers, family, and friends often feel angry and frustrated by the person's disruptive behaviours. When these feelings are not examined and shared with others, the therapeutic potential of the staff is reduced, and feelings of confusion and helplessness remain.
- Mood stabilizers are usually the first line of defence for bipolar disorder and include lithium and several anticonvulsants.
- Lithium is approved for treating acute mania and maintenance. Blood levels, kidney function, and thyroid function should be assessed regularly.
- Most anticonvulsant drugs are approved for acute mania. Lamotrigine is approved for maintenance.
- Antipsychotic agents, particularly the second-generation antipsychotics, are used for their sedating and mood-stabilizing properties. Screening for metabolic problems (e.g., diabetes) is essential in this population.
- For some patients, ECT may be an appropriate medical treatment.
- Patient and family teaching takes many forms and is most important in encouraging adherence to the medication regimen and reducing the risk of relapse.
- Evaluation includes examining the effectiveness of the nursing interventions, changing the outcomes as needed, and reassessing the nursing diagnoses. Evaluation is an ongoing process and is part of each of the other steps in the nursing process.

CRITICAL THINKING

1. Jian has been diagnosed with bipolar disorder and has been taking lithium for 4 months. During a clinic visit, he tells you that he does not think he will be taking his lithium anymore because he feels fine and misses his old "intensity." He says he is able to function well at his job and at home with his family and that his wife agrees that he "has this thing licked."
   a. What are Jian's needs in terms of teaching?
   b. What are the needs of his family?
   c. Write a teaching plan for Jian, or use an already constructed plan that includes the following teaching topics with sound rationales:

   (1) Use of alcohol, drugs, caffeine, and over-the-counter medications
   (2) Need for sleep and hygiene
   (3) Types of community resources available
   (4) Signs and symptoms of relapse

2. How would you explain the importance of a normal sleep–wake cycle to a patient with bipolar disorder?
   a. Research has shown that a faulty circadian rhythm may be to blame for sleep disruption in the mania phase of bipolar disorder. Therefore it is important to maintain a normal sleep–wake cycle for mood stabilization because sleep disruptions can trigger mania.

CHAPTER REVIEW

1. Which behaviour exhibited by a person with mania should the nurse choose to address first?
   a. Indiscriminate sexual relations
   b. Excessive spending of money
   c. Declaration of "being at one with the world"
   d. Demonstration of flight of ideas

2. The nurse is caring for a person experiencing mania. Which is the most appropriate nursing intervention?
   a. Provide consistency among staff members when working with the person
   b. Negotiate limits so the person has a voice in the plan of care
   c. Allow only certain staff members to interact with the person
   d. Attempt to control the person's emotions

3. The nurse is planning care for a person experiencing the acute phase of mania. Which is the priority intervention?
   a. Prevent injury
   b. Maintain stable cardiac status
   c. Get the person to demonstrate thought self-control
   d. Ensure that the person gets sufficient sleep and rest

4. What critical information should the nurse provide about the use of lithium?
   a. "You will still have hypersexual tendencies, so be certain to use protection when engaging in intercourse."
   b. "Lithium will help you to feel only the euphoria of mania but not the anxiety."
   c. "It will take 1 to 2 weeks and maybe longer for this medication to start working fully."
   d. "This medication is a cure for bipolar disorder."

5. The nurse has provided education for a person in the continuation phase, after discharge from the hospital. What indicates that the plan of care has been successful? Select all that apply.
   a. Person identifies three signs and symptoms of relapse.
   b. Person states, "My wife doesn't mind if I still drink a little."
   c. Person reports that medication has been helpful but he is ready to stop.
   d. Person states, "I no longer have a disease."

6. Luc's family comes home one evening to find him extremely agitated and they suspect in a full manic episode. The family calls emergency medical services. While one medic is talking with Luc and his family, the other medic is counting something on his desk. What is the medic most likely counting?
   a. Hypodermic needles
   b. Fast food wrappers
   c. Empty soda cans
   d. Energy drink containers

7. Which nursing responses demonstrate accurate information that should be discussed with the female patient diagnosed with bipolar disorder and her support system? Select all that apply.
   a. "Remember that alcohol and caffeine can trigger a relapse of your symptoms."
   b. "Due to the risk of a manic episode, you should not take birth control pills."
   c. "It's critical to let your health care provider know immediately if you aren't sleeping well."
   d. "Is your family prepared to be actively involved in helping you manage this disorder?"
   e. "The physical symptoms tend to come and go, so you need to be able to recognize the early signs."

⊖volve WEBSITE

Post-Test | interactive review

Visit the Evolve website for Chapter Review Answers and Rationales, Critical Thinking Answer Guidelines, and additional resources related to the content in this chapter: http://evolve.elsevier.com/Canada/Varcarolis/psychiatric/

REFERENCES

American Psychiatric Association (2013). *Diagnostic and statistical manual of mental disorders* (5th ed.). Arlington, VA: Author.

Canadian Mental Health Association. (2011). *Fast facts about mental illness.* Retrieved from http://www.cmha.ca/bins/content_page.asp?cid=6-20-23-43.

Conus, P., Macneil, C., & McGorry, P. D. (2014). Public health significance of bipolar disorder: Implications for early intervention and prevention. *Bipolar Disorders*, 16(5), 548–556. doi:10.1111/bdi.12137.

Crump, C., Sundquist, K., Winkleby, M. A., et al. (2013). Comorbidities and mortality in bipolar disorder: A Swedish national cohort study. *JAMA Psychiatry*, 70(9), 931–939. doi:10.1001/jamapsychiatry.2013.1394.

Fusar-Poli, P., Howes, O., Bechdolf, A., et al. (2012). Mapping vulnerability to bipolar disorder: A systematic review and meta-analysis of neuroimaging studies. *Journal of Psychiatry Neuroscience*, 37(3), 170–184.

Goes, F. S., Pierooznia, M., Parla, J. S., et al. (2016). Exome sequencing of familial bipolar disorder. *Journal of the American Medical Association Psychiatry*, 73(6), 590–597. doi:10.1001/jamapsychiatry.2016.0251.

Health Canada. (2014). Health professional and consumer advisories. *Canadian Adverse Reaction Newsletter*, 24(2), 5. Retrieved from http://www.hc-sc.gc.ca/index-eng.php.

Jamison, K. R. (1995). *An unquiet mind.* New York: Knopf.

Kerner, B. (2014). The genetics of bipolar disorder. *Application of Clinical Genetics*, 7, 33–42.

Maletic, V., & Raison, C. (2014). Integrated neurobiology of bipolar disorder. *Frontiers in Psychiatry*, 5, 98. Retrieved from http://www.ncbi.nlm.nih.gov/pmc/articles/PMC4142322/.

Meinhard, N., Kessing, L. V., & Vinberg, M. (2014). The role of estrogen in bipolar disorder: A review. *Nordic Journal of Psychiatry*, 68(2), 81–87. doi:10.3109/08039488.2013.775341.

Merikangas, K., Cui, L., Kattan, G., et al. (2012). Mania with and without depression in a community sample of U.S. adolescents. *Archives of General Psychiatry*, 69(9), 943–951.

Moorhead, S., Johnson, M., Maas, M., et al. (2012). *Nursing outcomes classification (NOC)* (5th ed.). St. Louis: Mosby.

Munk-Olsen, T., Lauresen, T. M., Meltzer-Brody, S., et al. (2012). Psychiatric disorders with postpartum onset: Possible early manifestations of bipolar affective disorders. *Archives of General Psychiatry, 69*(4), 428–434.

Olfson, M., Mojtabai, R., Merikangas, K. R., et al. (2017). Reexamining associations between mania, depression, anxiety and substance use disosrders: Results from a prospective national cohort. *Moleculary Psychoatry, 22*(2), 235–241. doi:10.1038/mp.2016.64.

Ostacher, M. J., & Tilley, C. A. (2008). Anticonvulsants. In T. A. Stern, J. F. Rosenbaum, M. Fava, et al. (Eds.), *Comprehensive clinical psychiatry* (pp. 661–666). Philadelphia: Mosby Elsevier.

Parikh, S. V., & Goldstein, B. (2013). CANMAT 2013 update of guidelines for the management of patients with bipolar disorder. *Mood and Anxiety Disorders Rounds, 2*(1), 1–6. Retrieved from http://www.moodandanxietyrounds.ca/cgi-bin/templates/body/accueil.cfm.

Phillips, M. L., & Swartz, H. A. (2014). A critical appraisal of neuroimaging studies of bipolar disorder: Toward a new conceptualization of underlying neural circuitry and roadmap for future research. *American Journal of Psychiatry, 171*(8), 829–843. doi:10.1176/appi.ajp.2014.13081008.

Sadock, B. J., Sadock, V. A., & Ruiz, P. (2015). *Synopsis of psychiatry* (11th ed.). Alphen van den Rijn, Netherlands: Wolters Kluwer.

Schoeyen, H. K., Kessler, U., Andreassen, O. A., et al. (2015). Treatment resistant bipolar depression: A randomized controlled trial of ECT therapy versus algorithm-based pharmacological treatment. *American Journal of Psychiatry, 172*(1), 41–51.

Smith, D. J., Anderson, J., Zammit, S., et al. (2015). Childhood IQ and risk of bipolar disorder in adulthood: Prospective birth cohort study. *British Journal of Psychiatry Open, 1*, 74–80.

Trudeau, M. (2010). *Changing my mind*. Toronto: HarperCollins Publishers Ltd.

Vallerand, A. H., Sanoski, C. A., & Deglin, J. H. (2013). *Davis's drug guide for nurses*. Philadelphia: F. A. Davis.

Schizophrenia Spectrum and Other Psychotic Disorders

Edward A. Herzog
Adapted by Sonya L. Jakubec

KEY TERMS AND CONCEPTS

abnormal motor behaviour
acute dystonia
affective symptoms
akathisia
anosognosia
anticholinergic-induced delirium
associative looseness
boundary impairment
circumstantiality
cognitive symptoms
command hallucinations
concrete thinking
delusions
depersonalization
derealization
disorganized thinking
echolalia
echopraxia

extrapyramidal side effects (EPSs)
hallucinations
ideas of reference
illusions
negative symptoms
neologisms
neuroleptic malignant syndrome (NMS)
paranoia
positive symptoms
pseudoparkinsonism
psychosis
reality testing
recovery model
stereotyped behaviours
tangentiality
tardive dyskinesia (TD or TDK)
word salad

OBJECTIVES

1. Describe the progression of symptoms, focus of care, and intervention needs for the prepsychotic through maintenance phases of schizophrenia.
2. Discuss at least three of the neurobiological, anatomical, and genetic findings that indicate that schizophrenia is a brain disorder.
3. Differentiate among the positive and negative symptoms of schizophrenia in terms of psychopharmacological treatment and effect on quality of life.
4. Discuss the concept of recovery for people living with schizophrenia.
5. Discuss how to deal with common reactions the nurse may experience while working with a person with schizophrenia.

6. Develop teaching plans for people taking conventional antipsychotic drugs (e.g., haloperidol [Haldol]) and atypical antipsychotic drugs (e.g., risperidone [Risperdal]).
7. Compare and contrast the conventional antipsychotic medications with atypical antipsychotics.
8. Identify nonpharmacological interventions that may be used to address symptoms of schizophrenia.
9. Create a nursing care plan that incorporates evidence-informed interventions for key areas of dysfunction in schizophrenia, including hallucinations, delusions, paranoia, cognitive disorganization, anosognosia, and impaired self-care.
10. Role-play intervening with a person who is hallucinating, delusional, and exhibiting disorganized thinking.

⊖volve WEBSITE

Visit the Evolve website for Flashcards, Case Studies, and additional testing resources related to the content in this chapter: http://evolve.elsevier.com/Canada/Varcarolis/psychiatric/

[Pre-Test   interactive review]

Schizophrenia spectrum and other psychotic disorders are potentially devastating brain disorders that affect a person's thinking, language, emotions, social behaviour, and ability to perceive reality accurately. These disorders are characterized by psychosis, which refers to altered cognition, altered perception, and/or an impaired ability to determine what is or is not real (an ability known as reality testing). While symptoms of psychosis may be experienced in response to a number of physical or mental health disorders, in this chapter we review concepts and care specific to schizophrenia spectrum and other psychotic disorders.

The most severe disorder defined by the presence of psychosis is schizophrenia, which is the major focus of this chapter. It affects 1 in every 100 people (more than 350 000 people in Canada) and is among the most disruptive and disabling of mental disorders. Unfortunately, people with this disorder are often misunderstood and stigmatized not only by the general population but also, often, by the medical community. Negative attitudes toward people can interfere with recovery and impair their quality of life (Gaebel, Rössler, & Sartorius, 2017; Walker, Arnfred, Petersen, et al., 2016). For example, many mistakenly believe that people with schizophrenia are likely to be violent or that offenders are likely to have been psychotic preceding episodes of violence. In fact, the rate of psychosis before violence is low even among high-risk offenders (Skeem, Kennealy, Monahan, et al., 2015). Among those with severe forms of mental illness, such as schizophrenia, incidents of violence against strangers are extremely rare—1 incident of homicide per 14.3 million people per year—and usually occur in combination with

✿ HOW A NURSE HELPED ME

They Listen With Compassion and Dignity: I Know I Am Not Alone

I live with schizoaffective disorder. I am 30 now, and I was diagnosed with a mental illness when I was 15. I experience both the psychotic symptoms often present in schizophrenia and a mood disorder, often in the form of rapid cycling of moods from depression to extreme highs. For the first 5 to 10 years of coping with my mental illness, the hospital was like a revolving door for me. It took me numerous years to find the right medications and therapies.

I have been able to overcome my intense symptoms by finding balance in my chaotic moods and a decrease in my delusional symptoms and paranoia. Nurses like Cynthia and Rhonda help me to find that balance when it is lost. Cynthia, who works in the hospital, is a nurse who goes out of her way to be there for her patients. I first met Cynthia 10 years ago on my first admission. She has had such a positive impact on my life because she believes in me even when I don't trust and believe in myself. She brings cheerfulness to the ward that is scary and full of strangeness when you are admitted. If you are depressed or not feeling well, she is most often able to cheer you up. (That is no matter how bad you feel or how painful your day has been.) She has truly listened to me—when I've been really unwell and hospitalized. At those times I am just so scared. I even wonder about the special meaning in the numbers or letter that could be anywhere—even on the menu ordering my food on the ward! It can freak me out a little, but Cynthia listens and talks me through it. Even if I am not cured in that instant, I am comforted and can carry on. Her

dedication to finding ways to work through even my worst suspicions has never wavered. Cynthia is one of a kind.

Rhonda, the community mental health nurse who I work with as an outpatient, is one of the most dedicated and compassionate nurses I have ever met. She has also had a tremendous influence on my life. She often works after-hours to offer full support to her patients. Sometimes I have called her past 6:00 in the evening, thinking I would leave a message, yet to my surprise she is still there, and she works with me on my schedule and needs. She, too, listens to my fears and worries. She treats me with dignity and respect and I know truly wants me to be successful in the world. I have never felt like I have been looked down upon or judged—even if what I bring up to her must seem totally weird or off track sometimes! One of my fears is that I must look stupid when I am fearful of things, but Rhonda has an open mind and her compassion has supported me through many rough and painful times. Rhonda has always believed in me, and this has helped me on my road to recovery. I look forward to appointments with Rhonda because she always allows me to see life situations from a realistic and positive perspective. She provides me with ongoing encouragement. I have been successful at working at the bank now for 3 years and have managed to keep up my friendships and haven't scared my boyfriend away. I know I owe Rhonda for much of that success. Through it all, I know that I am not alone, and with this help I can figure my way out of even the worst thoughts or worries.

Source: Story inspired by Tammy L. (shared with her permission).

substance use and psychosis (Nielssen & Large, 2010). Violence directed to oneself is a greater likelihood, with high levels of self-harm and suicide attempts reported in individuals with psychosis (Witt, van Dorn, & Fazel, 2013). A cross-sectional study of patients with schizophrenia spectrum disorders revealed that close to 50% of patients reported self-harm. Self-harm in these cases was associated with younger age of onset, female gender, comorbid depressive episode, comorbid alcohol abuse or dependence, current suicidality, awareness of illness, and low adherence to prescribed medication (Mork, Mehlum, Barrett, et al., 2012). Overall, people who experience mental illness are much more likely to be victims of crime, hate, and discrimination than to be the perpetrators of them (Mental Health Commission of Canada, 2017).

Practices that concentrate on building trusting therapeutic relationships are practical ways to counter discrimination and promote recovery in the care of those experiencing psychosis and schizophrenia (Mental Health Commission of Canada, 2016). The *How a Nurse Helped Me* story demonstrates the four elements of the LEAP approach (Amador, 2012), which is based on the belief that trusting relationships are key to healing partnerships:

- Listen—Both nurses listened with compassion and genuineness.
- Empathize—It is clear that both nurses were able to convey that they cared about understanding what Tammy was feeling.
- Agree—Both nurses believed in Tammy, affirmed that she was indeed worried and struggling. They supported her in her goals, never looking down on her or judging her but helping her on her own road to recovery.
- Partner—Clearly, both nurses respected Tammy and worked with her as partners for recovery.

LEAP is described as a technique; however, inherent in that description is the risk of seeing it only technically. The LEAP approach must be underpinned by genuineness and caring. Cynthia and Rhonda invited Tammy into a trusting and therapeutic relationship. They did not apply these components as "techniques"; instead, it appears that the LEAP principles flowed naturally out of genuine caring. As genuine understanding, empathy, and respect for Tammy's point of view was communicated, common ground on which the nurses could partner with Tammy followed. Through this process, the professional opinions and support of her "team" started to matter to Tammy. Without this approach, suspicious and delusional ideas can be challenging to understand and manage. Tammy's story demonstrates how empowering and therapeutic it is to experience being truly listened to, empathized with, and collaborated with in all relationships, and particularly with managing psychosis.

CLINICAL PICTURE

There are five key features associated with psychotic disorders:

1. **Delusions**: Alterations in *thought content* (what a person thinks about). Delusions are false fixed beliefs that cannot be corrected by reasoning or evidence to the contrary. "Unusual" beliefs maintained by one's culture or subculture are not delusions.
2. **Hallucinations**: Perception of a sensory experience for which no external stimulus exists (e.g., hearing a voice when no one is speaking).
3. **Disorganized thinking**: The loosening of associations, manifested as jumbled and illogical speech and impaired reasoning.
4. **Abnormal motor behaviour**: Alterations in behaviour, including bizarre and agitated behaviours (e.g., stilted, rigid demeanour; eccentric dress, grooming, and rituals). Grossly disorganized behaviours may include mutism, stupor, or catatonic excitement.
5. **Negative symptoms**: The absence of something that should be present but is not—for example, the ability to make decisions or to follow through on a plan. Negative symptoms contribute to poor social functioning and social withdrawal.

While this chapter concentrates on assessment and treatment of schizophrenia, other psychotic disorders (e.g., schizophreniform, schizoaffective, brief psychotic disorders) are described in Box 15-1.

Adding to observations made by Emil Kraepelin (1856–1926), Eugen Bleuler (1857–1939) coined the term *schizophrenia*. He first proposed that schizophrenia was not one illness but a heterogeneous group of illnesses with different characteristics and clinical courses. Clinicians in Canada use the criteria of the *Diagnostic and Statistical Manual of Mental Disorders*, fifth edition (American Psychiatric Association, 2013), for the diagnosis of schizophrenia spectrum and other psychotic disorders. All those diagnosed with schizophrenia exhibit at least one psychotic symptom, such as delusions, hallucinations, or disorganized thinking, speech, or behaviour. The person experiences extreme difficulty with or an inability to function in family, social, or occupational realms and frequently neglects basic needs such as nutrition or hygiene. Over a period of 6 months, there may be times when the psychotic symptoms are absent, and in their place the person may experience apathy or depression.

EPIDEMIOLOGY

The lifetime prevalence of schizophrenia is 1% worldwide, with no differences related to race, social status, or culture. It is more common in males (1.4:1) and among persons growing up in urban areas (Haddad, Schäfer, Streit, et al., 2015). Schizophrenia usually develops during the late teens and early twenties. Onset in males is usually between the ages of 15 and 25 years and is associated with poorer functioning and more structural abnormality in the brain. The onset tends to be somewhat later in women (ages 25 to 35 years), who tend to have a better prognosis and experience fewer structural changes in the brain (Dean, Orr, Bernard, et al., 2016). People who later are diagnosed with schizophrenia often experience an earlier prodromal phase during which some milder symptoms of the disorder develop, often months or years before the disorder becomes fully apparent (Miller, 2016). Childhood schizophrenia, although rare, does exist, occurring in 1 out of 40 000 children. Early onset (18 to 25 years) occurs more often in males and is associated with poor functioning before onset, more structural brain abnormality, and increased levels of apathy. Individuals with a later onset (25 to 35 years) are more likely to be female, have less structural brain abnormality, and have better outcomes.

BOX 15-1 PSYCHOTIC DISORDERS OTHER THAN SCHIZOPHRENIA

Schizophreniform Disorder

The features of schizophreniform disorder are similar to schizophrenia, but the total duration of the illness is less than 6 months. This disorder may or may not develop into schizophrenia; people who do not develop schizophrenia have a good prognosis.

Brief Psychotic Disorder

This disorder involves a sudden onset of psychosis or grossly disorganized or catatonic behaviour lasting less than 1 month. It is often precipitated by extreme stressors and is followed by a return to premorbid functioning.

Schizoaffective Disorder

Schizoaffective disorder is a subgroup of psychoses in which affective and schizophrenic symptoms are prominent simultaneously. The symptoms are not due to any substance use or to a medical condition and present with either bipolar or depressive affective symptoms alongside psychosis.

Delusional Disorder

Delusional disorder is characterized by nonbizarre delusions (i.e., situations that could occur in real life, such as being followed, being deceived by a spouse, or having a disease). The person's ability to function is not markedly impaired, nor is behaviour otherwise odd or psychotic. A related disorder, Capgras syndrome, involves a delusion about a significant other (e.g., family member, pet) being replaced by an imposter; this disorder may be a result of psychiatric or organic brain disease (Salvatore, Bhuvaneswar, Tohen, et al., 2014).

Substance- or Medication-Induced Psychotic Disorder

Psychosis may be induced by substances such as drugs of abuse, alcohol, medications, or toxins (Mauri, Volonteri, De Gaspari, et al., 2006).

Psychosis or Catatonia Associated With Another Medical Condition or Another Mental Disorder

Psychoses may also be caused by a medical condition (delirium, neurological or metabolic conditions, hepatic or renal diseases, and many others) as well as by mental illness such as post-traumatic stress disorder (Alsawy, Wood, Taylor, et al., 2015) or depression, particularly with coexisting victimization from sexual violence or bullying (Nam, Hilimire, Schiffman, et al., 2016). Medical conditions and substance abuse must always be ruled out before a diagnosis of schizophrenia or other psychotic disorder can be made.

Sources: Alsawy, S., Wood, L., Taylor, P. J., et al. (2015). Psychotic experiences and PTSD: Exploring associations in a population survey. *Psychological Medicine, 45*(13), 2849. doi:10.1017/S003329171500080X; Mauri, M. C., Volonteri, L. S., De Gaspari, I. F., et al. (2006). Substance abuse in first-episode schizophrenic patients: A retrospective study. *Clinical Practice and Epidemiology in Mental Health, 2*, 1–8. doi:10.1186/1745-0179-2-4; Nam, B., Hilimire, M., Schiffman, J., et al. (2016). Psychotic experiences in the context of depression: The cumulative role of victimization. *Journal of Psychiatric Research, 82*, 136–140. doi:10.1016/j.jpsychires.2016.07.023; Salvatore, P., Bhuvaneswar, C., Tohen, M., et al. (2014). Capgras' syndrome in first-episode psychotic disorders. *Psychopathology, 47*(4), 261. doi:10.1159/000357813.

COMORBIDITY

Substance use disorders (particularly alcohol and marijuana related) occur in nearly 50% of persons with schizophrenia (Thoma & Daum, 2013). When substance abuse occurs in people with schizophrenia, it is associated with treatment nonadherence, relapse, incarceration, homelessness, violence, suicide, and a poorer prognosis (Marquez-Arrico, Benaiges, & Adan, 2015). Nicotine dependence rates in schizophrenia are greater than 60%, contributing to an increased incidence of cardiovascular and respiratory disorders and doubling the risk for cancers (Akbarian & Kundakovic, 2015).

Anxiety, depression, and suicide co-occur frequently in schizophrenia. Anxiety may be a response to symptoms (e.g., hallucinations) or circumstances (e.g., isolation, overstimulation) and may worsen schizophrenia symptoms and prognosis. Almost half of all persons with schizophrenia attempt suicide at some point in their lives, and approximately 10% complete suicide, a rate five times that of the general population (Hor & Taylor, 2010). Physical illnesses overall are more common among people with schizophrenia than in the general population. Even after adjusting for demographics and socioeconomic status, the average life expectancy is 15 to 20 years less than for the general population (Rao, Raney, & Xiong, 2015), indeed the risk of premature death is greater for people with schizophrenia (Smith, Langan, McLean, et al., 2013). These significantly higher death rates reflect a combination of (1) higher risk factors for many chronic diseases and some types of cancer; (2) the iatrogenic effects of some psychiatric medications; (3) higher rates of suicide, accidental, and violent death; and (4) disparities in health care access and use (Correll, Detraux, De Lepeleire, et al., 2015; Thornicroft, 2011). Communication problems or difficulties with informed consent may be part of the issue of health care access (Pelletier, Lesage, Boisvert, et al., 2015). Owing to poverty, stigma, or stereotyping (e.g., emergency department personnel attributing symptoms—for example, chest pain—to symptoms of a mental health disorder), patients may not receive adequate health care. Despite having more contact with family physicians than the general population, persons with psychiatric disorders are less likely to be assessed and treated for conditions such as hypertension or to receive preventive care such as smoking cessation (Pelletier, Lesage, Boisvert, et al., 2015).

Incentives and barriers to engaging people with severe mental illness in lifestyle interventions have not been extensively studied, though there is some evidence that these interventions can be effective (Happell, Platania-Phung, & Scott, 2013). Barriers that are reported in the literature include illness symptoms, treatment effects, lack of support, and negative staff attitudes; incentives include peer and staff support, staff participation, reduction of symptoms, knowledge, and personal attributes (Happell, Platania-Phung, & Scott, 2013).

ETIOLOGY

Schizophrenia is a complicated disorder. In fact, what we call "schizophrenia" actually may be a group of disorders with common but varying features and multiple, overlapping etiologies.

What is known is that brain chemistry, structure, and activity are different in a person with schizophrenia from those in a person who does not have the disorder.

The scientific consensus is that schizophrenia occurs when multiple inherited gene abnormalities combine with nongenetic factors (e.g., viral infections, birth injuries, prenatal malnutrition), altering the structures of the brain, affecting the brain's neurotransmitter systems, injuring the brain directly, or doing all three. This effect is called the *diathesis–stress model of schizophrenia* (Berry & Cirulli, 2016).

Biological Factors
Genetic Factors
Evidence suggests that multiple genes on different chromosomes interact with each other in complex ways to create vulnerability for schizophrenia. About 80% of the risk of schizophrenia comes from genetic and epigenetic factors (factors such as toxins or psychological trauma that affect the expression of genes). More than 100 loci in the human genome are associated with an increased risk for schizophrenia (Castellani, Melka, Gui, et al., 2015). While no one particular gene is identified as causal, schizophrenia is said to be inherited, and compared to the usual 1% risk in the general population, having a first-degree relative with schizophrenia increases the risk to 10%. Further, a variability of expression of schizophrenia has been identified, and it depends on environmental factors; schizoaffective disorder and cluster A personality disorders are more common in relatives of people with schizophrenia. Concordance rates (i.e., how often one twin will have the disorder when the other twin has it) are about 50% for identical twins and about 15% for fraternal twins.

Neurobiological Factors
Dopamine theory. The dopamine theory of schizophrenia is derived from the study of the action of the first antipsychotic drugs, collectively known as *conventional* (or *first-generation*) *antipsychotics* (e.g., haloperidol [Haldol] and chlorpromazine [Largactil]). These drugs block the activity of dopamine D_2 receptors in the brain, limiting the activity of dopamine and reducing some of the symptoms of schizophrenia. However, because the dopamine-blocking agents do not alleviate all symptoms of schizophrenia, it is recognized that other neurochemicals are involved in generating the symptoms of schizophrenia. Amphetamines, cocaine, methylphenidate (Ritalin), and levodopa increase the activity of dopamine in the brain and, in biologically susceptible people, may precipitate schizophrenia's onset. If schizophrenia is already present, these substances may also exacerbate its symptoms. Almost any drug of abuse, particularly marijuana, can increase the risk for schizophrenia in biologically vulnerable individuals (Morgan, Freeman, Powell, et al., 2016).

Other neurochemical hypotheses. A newer class of drugs, collectively known as *atypical* (or *second-generation*) *antipsychotics*, block serotonin as well as dopamine, which suggests that serotonin may play a role in schizophrenia as well. A better understanding of how atypical agents modulate the expression and targeting of 5-hydroxytryptamine 2A (5-HT2A) and its receptors would likely lead to a better understanding of schizophrenia.

Researchers have long been aware that phenylcyclohexyl piperidine (PCP) induces a state closely resembling schizophrenia.

This observation led to interest in the *N*-methyl-D-aspartate (NMDA) receptor complex and the possible role of glutamate in the pathophysiology of schizophrenia.

Glutamate, dopamine, and serotonin act synergistically in neurotransmission, and thus glutamate may also play a role in causing psychosis (Andreou, Söderman, Axelsson, et al., 2015). Neurotransmission by another calming neurotransmitter, gamma-aminobutyric acid (GABA), is also impaired in schizophrenia (Frankle et al., 2015). Acetylcholine, active in the muscarinic system, may play a role in psychosis.

Brain Structure Abnormalities
Disruptions in communication pathways in the brain are thought to be severe in schizophrenia. Therefore it is conceivable that structural abnormalities cause disruption of the brain's functioning. Structural differences may be due to errors in neurodevelopment or errors in the normal pruning of neuronal tissue that happens in late adolescence and early adulthood. Inflammation or neurotoxic effects from factors such as oxidative stress, infection, or autoimmune dysfunction may also alter the brain's structure (Sekar, Bialas, de Rivera, et al., 2016).

Using brain imaging techniques—computed tomography (CT), magnetic resonance imaging (MRI), functional MRI (fMRI), and positron emission tomography (PET)—researchers (Dean, Orr, Bernard, et al., 2016) have demonstrated structural brain abnormalities, including:

- Reduced volume in the right anterior insula (may contribute to negative symptoms)
- Reduced volume and changes in the shape of the hippocampus
- Accelerated age-related decline in cortical thickness
- Grey matter deficits in the dorsolateral prefrontal cortex area, thalamus, and anterior cingulate cortex, as well as in the frontotemporal, thalamocortical, and subcortical-limbic circuits
- Reduced connectivity among various brain regions
- Neuronal overgrowth in some areas, possibly due to inflammation or inadequate neural pruning
- Widespread white matter abnormalities (e.g., in the corpus callosum)

In addition, MRI and CT scans demonstrate lower brain volume and more cerebrospinal fluid in people with schizophrenia. PET scans also show a lowered rate of blood flow and glucose metabolism in the frontal lobes, which govern planning, abstract thinking, social adjustment, and decision making, all of which are affected in schizophrenia. (Figure 11-5 in Chapter 11 shows a PET scan demonstrating reduced brain activity in the frontal lobe of a person with schizophrenia.) Such structural changes may worsen as the disorder continues. Postmortem studies on individuals with schizophrenia reveal a reduced volume of grey matter in the brain, especially in the temporal and frontal lobes; those with the most tissue loss had the worst symptoms (e.g., hallucinations, delusions, bizarre thoughts, depression).

Psychological, Social, and Environmental Factors
A number of psychosocial and environmental stressors, particularly those occurring during vulnerable periods of neurological development, are believed to combine with genetic vulnerabilities

to produce schizophrenia. Reducing such stressors is believed to have the potential to reduce the severity of the disorder or even prevent it (Brown, 2011).

Prenatal Stressors

A history of pregnancy or birth complications is associated with an increased risk for schizophrenia. Prenatal risk factors include viral infection, poor nutrition, hypoxia, and exposure to toxins.

Infection during pregnancy increases the risk for mental illness in the child. Prenatal infections in the mother also increase the risk for infection in the child after birth, and those infections in the children also can make them more vulnerable to mental illness (Blomström, Karlsson, Gardner, et al., 2016). Other factors associated with an increased risk for schizophrenia include a father older than 35 years at the child's conception and a child being born during late winter or early spring (Tandon, Keshavan, & Nasrallah, 2008). Psychological trauma to the mother during pregnancy (e.g., the death of a relative) can also contribute to the development of schizophrenia (Khashan, Abel, McNamee, et al., 2008).

Psychological Stressors

Although there is no evidence that stress alone causes schizophrenia, psychological and physical stress increase cortisol levels, impeding hypothalamic development and causing other changes that may precipitate the illness in vulnerable individuals. Schizophrenia often manifests at times of developmental and social stress, such as beginning university or moving away from one's family. Social, psychological, and physical stressors may also play a significant role in both the severity and course of the disorder and the person's quality of life.

Other risk factors include childhood sexual abuse, exposure to social adversity (e.g., chronic poverty), migration to or growing up in a foreign culture, and exposure to psychological trauma or social defeat (Howes & McCutcheon, 2017). These factors may cause structural changes in the brain via epigenetic changes to the genome. Even psychological trauma in a parent or grandparent may cause epigenetic changes that increase vulnerability, and this increased risk can be passed on to one's descendants. It has also been discovered that elevated dopaminergic function places recent immigrants at risk of developing psychosis (Egerton, Howes, Houle, et al., 2017).

Environmental Stressors

Environmental factors such as toxins, including the solvent tetrachloroethylene (used in dry cleaning and to line water pipes, and sometimes found in drinking water), are also believed to contribute to the development of schizophrenia in vulnerable people (Aschengrau, Weinberg, Janulewicz, et al., 2012). Living in urban areas or high-crime environments is also believed to increase the risk for schizophrenia (Haddad, Schäfer, Streit, et al., 2015).

Environmental factors within broader social environments are also believed to contribute to the development of schizophrenia in vulnerable people. These include exposure to social adversity (e.g., living in chronic poverty) and migration to or growing up in a foreign culture (Egerton, Howes, Houle, et al., 2017).

🌐 CONSIDERING CULTURE

The Stigma of Schizophrenia

Mrs. Chou, a 25-year-old woman, left China for North America 6 months ago to join her husband. In China, she lived with her parents and had learned English. She was shy and looked to her parents, and later to her husband, for guidance and support. Shortly after arrival in her new country, her mother developed pneumonia and died. Mrs. Chou later told her husband that if she had stayed in China, her mother would not have become ill and that evil would now come to their 1-year-old child because Mrs. Chou had not taken proper care of her mother.

Mrs. Chou became increasingly lethargic, staring into space and mumbling to herself. When Mr. Chou asked who she was talking to, she answered, "My mother."

Mr. Chou realized that something was terribly wrong with his wife, yet he was reluctant to ask either relatives or professionals for assistance since mental illness is strongly stigmatized in the Chinese culture. In fact, mental illness may be believed to be a punishment for personal failings.

Mrs. Chou was finally admitted to a psychiatric unit when Mr. Chou noticed she had quit eating and taking care of herself and was certainly unable to care for their child. During her admission assessment, she sat motionless and mute. Mr. Nolan, her primary nurse, noticed that after he checked her pulse, her arm remained in midair until he lowered it for her. Mrs. Chou was unkempt and pale, and her skin turgor was poor.

Mr. Nolan also spoke with Mr. Chou, who was visibly distressed by his wife's condition. He discovered that Mr. Chou blamed himself for his wife's illness because his relocation prevented her from caring for her ailing mother. He agreed with his wife that their mutual failings placed their child at risk of retribution. He conceded that coming to the hospital had been very difficult, owing to embarrassment about both his wife's mental illness and his own belief that he should not burden others with the care of himself and his wife. Mr. Nolan helped Mr. Chou recognize that in North American culture, family members shared caregiving burdens, professional help was more available, and stigmatization was less intense.

Gradually, Mr. Chou's distress lessened as he came to appreciate that he would not have to carry the level of burden he had anticipated. As Mrs. Chou's psychosis abated, both she and Mr. Chou came to ascribe more culpability for the illness to fate, reducing their burden of self-blame. They agreed to meet with a healer, who helped them integrate the beliefs and resources of their original and adopted cultures, further reducing their guilt and distress.

Source: Wong, D. F. K., Tsui, H. K. P., Pearson, V., et al. (2004). Family burdens, Chinese health beliefs, and the mental health of Chinese caregivers in Hong Kong. *Transcultural Psychiatry, 4,* 497–513.

Course of the Disorder

The onset of symptoms or forewarning (prodromal) symptoms may appear a month to a year before the first psychotic break or full-blown manifestations of the illness; such symptoms represent a clear deterioration in previous functioning. The course of the disorder thereafter typically includes recurrent exacerbations separated by periods of reduced or dormant symptoms. Some people will have a single episode of schizophrenia without recurrences or have several episodes and none thereafter. A study of more than 2 000 persons found four patterns of the course of the illness. Although the course of schizophrenia varied, all showed an initial deterioration followed by improvement (Levine, Lurie, Kohn, et al., 2011). Remission and recovery are increasingly common outcomes with early detection, appropriate treatment, and social support (Walker, Arnfred, Petersen, et al., 2016). For many people, however, schizophrenia is a chronic or recurring disorder that, like diabetes or heart disease, is managed but rarely cured.

Frequently, the history of a person with schizophrenia reveals that, prior to the illness, the person was socially awkward, lonely, and perhaps depressed and expressed himself or herself in vague, odd, or unrealistic ways. In this prodromal phase, complaints about anxiety, phobias, obsessions, dissociative features, and compulsions may be noted. As anxiety mounts, indications of a thought disorder become evident. Concentration, memory, and completion of school- or job-related work deteriorate. Intrusive thoughts, "mind wandering," and the need to devote more time to maintaining one's thoughts are reported.

The person may feel that something "strange" or "wrong" is happening. Events are misinterpreted, and mystical or symbolic meanings may be given to ordinary events. For example, the person may think that certain colours have special powers or that a song on the radio is a message from God. Discerning others' emotions becomes more difficult, and other people's actions or words may be mistaken for signs of hostility or evidence of harmful intent (Chung, Kang, Shin, et al., 2008).

Prognosis

For the majority of people, most symptoms can be at least somewhat controlled through medications and psychosocial interventions. With support and effective treatments, many people with schizophrenia experience a good quality of life and success within their families, occupations, and other roles. Associates may not even realize that the person has schizophrenia.

An abrupt onset of symptoms is usually a favourable prognostic sign, and those with good premorbid social, sexual, and occupational functioning have a greater chance for a good remission or a complete recovery (Sandler, Kotov & Bromet, 2011).

In other cases, schizophrenia does not respond fully to available treatments, leaving residual symptoms and causing varying degrees of disability. Some cases require repeated or lengthy inpatient care or institutionalization. Studies have shown that most of the deterioration occurs within the first 2 to 5 years after onset of psychosis, followed by a plateau in impairment and symptoms (Srihari, Shah, & Keshavan, 2012). Factors associated with a less positive prognosis include a slow onset (e.g., more than 2 to 3 years), younger age at onset, longer duration between first symptoms and first treatment, longer periods of untreated illness, and more negative symptoms. A childhood history of withdrawn, reclusive, eccentric, and tense behaviour is also an unfavourable diagnostic sign, as is a preponderance of negative symptoms (Freudenreich, Brown, & Holt, 2016). Reducing the frequency,

intensity, and duration of relapse (when previously controlled symptoms return) is believed to improve the long-term prognosis.

Phases of Schizophrenia

Schizophrenia usually progresses through predictable phases, although the presenting symptoms during a given phase and the length of the phase can vary widely. The phases of schizophrenia are as follows (Chung, Kang, Shin, et al., 2008):

- **Phase I—Acute:** Onset or exacerbation of florid, disruptive symptoms (e.g., hallucinations, delusions, apathy, withdrawal) with resultant loss of functional abilities; increased care or hospitalization may be required.
- **Phase II—Stabilization:** Symptoms are diminishing, and there is movement toward one's previous level of functioning (baseline); day hospitalization or care in a residential crisis centre or a supervised group home may be needed.
- **Phase III—Maintenance:** The person is at or nearing baseline (or premorbid) functioning; symptoms are absent or diminished; level of functioning allows the person to live in the community. Ideally, recovery with few or no residual symptoms has occurred. Most people in this phase live in their own residences. Although this phase has been termed *maintenance*, current literature shows a trend toward reframing it with a greater emphasis on recovery. Some clinicians and people with schizophrenia contend that maintenance and recovery are opposing concepts, "maintenance" being a pessimistic view and "recovery" being more optimistic. In a maintenance model, the goal of treatment is stability, whereas in a recovery model, the goal is to extend improvement beyond stability (Mental Health Commission of Canada, 2016; Walker, Arnfred, Petersen, et al., 2016). This new way of looking at this final phase requires recognition that progress is not a linear process and that recovery-focused therapy may be at odds with stability-focused therapy; that is, the health care providers must be able to tolerate instability such as setbacks and struggles in the recovery process (Symanski-Tondora, Miller, Slade, et al., 2014). Further, recovery may not be understood by all involved in the same way and should not be defined by a dominant cultural viewpoint of "productivity" or "success," which can further marginalize the patient. Rather, the defined purpose and goals of the person living with schizophrenia or experiencing psychosis must be supported in pursuit of recovery (Myers, 2010).

Some clinicians also designate an earlier prodromal (or prepsychotic) phase, in which subtle symptoms or deficits associated with schizophrenia are present; such symptoms may or may not herald the onset of schizophrenia. Detection and treatment programs in most major Canadian cities aim to detect psychosis in the prodromal phase and prevent acute episodes of schizophrenia. Strategies of early intervention include reducing the duration of untreated psychosis (DUP), reducing delay in treatment, and providing interventions adapted for younger people and their families in the early course of the illness (Srihari, Shah, & Keshavan, 2012). A list of Canadian programs can be found on the website of IEPA Early Intervention in Mental Health at https://iepa.org.au.

There is controversy as to whether the benefits of early intervention can be maintained over time. However, a study at the Prevention and Early Intervention Program for Psychoses (PEPP) in London, Ontario, found symptom improvement was not only maintained at the 5-year follow-up but increased for an additional 2 to 5 years (Norman, Manchanda, Malia, et al., 2011). This program provides continuity of care for 5 years, with more intense intervention in the initial 2 years and a gradual, individualized transfer to usual services. When compared to programs that provide only 2 years of treatment, the PEPP approach demonstrates better durability of benefit (Srihari, Shah, & Keshavan, 2012). A large longitudinal study in the United Kingdom found that treatment within an early intervention psychosis service was associated with better health and social outcomes and reduced costs (Tsiachristas, Thomas, Leal, et al., 2016). Family involvement in early intervention has been found to be an important component of treatment, the most functional and adaptive family coping approaches being those that involve planning, seeking social support, positive reinterpretation, acceptance and turning to religion, and rare use of "avoidant" coping strategies (e.g., denial or disengagement, use of alcohol and drugs) (Gerson, Wong, Davidson, et al., 2011). A systematic review of family interventions for psychosis established that such interventions improved patient functioning and reduced the likelihood of relapse. Psychotic symptoms were significantly reduced in the longer term; however, caregiver well-being did not sustain the same benefit over time (Fornells-Ambrojo, Claxton, & Onwumere, 2017).

APPLICATION OF THE NURSING PROCESS

ASSESSMENT

Nursing assessment of people who have or may have a psychotic disorder focuses largely on symptoms, coping, functioning, and safety. Assessment involves interviewing the person and observing behaviour and other outward manifestations of the disorder. It also should include mental status and spiritual, cultural, biological, psychological, social, and environmental elements. Sound therapeutic communication skills, an understanding of the disorder and the ways in which the person may be experiencing the world, and the establishment of trust and a therapeutic nurse–patient relationship all strengthen the assessment (see Chapter 10 for more on communication and the clinical interview). Indeed, as discussed in Chapter 9, the therapeutic relationship is of critical importance. A helping partnership between the nurse and the person with schizophrenia facilitates recovery (Chester, Ehrlich, Warburton, et al., 2016).

One effective approach to developing this trusting relationship for patients with psychosis is the LEAP approach described by Amador (2012) and referenced at the beginning of this chapter. It consists of four steps: (1) listen—try to put yourself in the other person's shoes to gain a clear idea of his or her experience; (2) empathize—seriously consider and empathize with the other person's point of view; (3) agree—find common ground and identify facts you can both agree on; (4) partner—collaborate on accomplishing the agreed-upon goals (Amador, 2012). In this way, trust can be gained and an alliance can be formed.

During the Prepsychotic Phase

Experts believe that detection and treatment of symptoms that may warn of schizophrenia's onset lessen the risk of developing the disorder or decrease the severity of the disorder if it does develop. A delay in diagnosis and treatment allows the psychotic process to become more entrenched; it can also result in relational, work, housing, and school problems (Riecher-Rössler, Gschwandtner, Borgwardt, et al., 2006).

Therefore early assessment plays a key role in improving the prognosis for persons with schizophrenia (Chung, Kang, Shin, et al., 2008). This form of primary prevention involves monitoring those at high risk (e.g., children of parents with schizophrenia) for symptoms such as abnormal social development and cognitive dysfunction. Intervening to reduce stressors (i.e., reduce or avoid exposure to triggers), enhancing social and coping skills (e.g., building resilience), and administering prophylactic antipsychotic medication may also be of benefit (Bechdolf, Phillips, Francey, et al., 2006).

Similarly, in people who have already developed the disorder, minimizing the onset and duration of relapses is believed to improve the prognosis. Research suggests that with each relapse of psychosis, there is an increase in residual dysfunction and deterioration. Recognition and personal tracking of the individual early warning signs of relapse, such as reduced sleep and concentration, are important to prevention of relapse. Limiting stress in work, relationships, and social or environmental domains, as well as enlisting the support of friends or loved ones and increasing the frequency of professional supports for monitoring and intensification of treatment, are essential. For this reason, for some, adherence to a drug regimen of antipsychotics can be more important than the risk of adverse effects because most adverse effects are reversible, whereas the consequences of relapse may not be (Brown & Gray, 2015).

General Assessment

Not all people with schizophrenia have the same symptoms, and some of the symptoms of schizophrenia are also found in other disorders such as schizoaffective disorder, delusional disorder, brief psychotic disorder, postpartum psychosis, and substance-induced psychotic disorder. Figure 15-1 describes the four main symptom groups of schizophrenia:
1. **Positive symptoms**: the presence of something that is not normally present
2. Negative symptoms: the absence of something that should be present but is not
3. **Cognitive symptoms**: abnormalities in how a person thinks
4. **Affective symptoms**: symptoms involving emotions and their expression

Positive Symptoms

The positive symptoms usually appear early in the illness, and their dramatic nature captures our attention and often precipitates hospitalization. They are also the symptoms most laypeople associate with insanity, making schizophrenia the disorder most

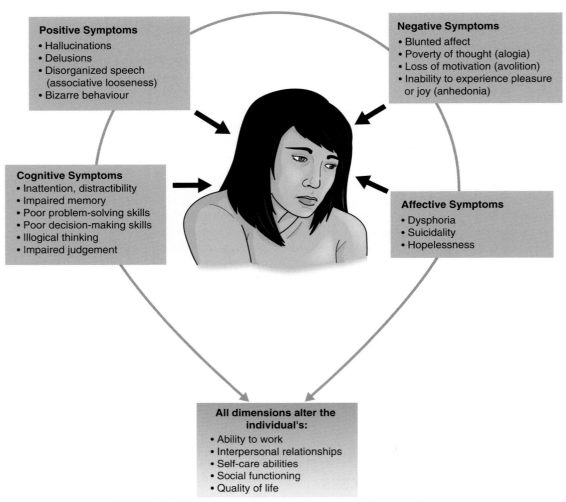

Positive Symptoms
- Hallucinations
- Delusions
- Disorganized speech (associative looseness)
- Bizarre behaviour

Negative Symptoms
- Blunted affect
- Poverty of thought (alogia)
- Loss of motivation (avolition)
- Inability to experience pleasure or joy (anhedonia)

Cognitive Symptoms
- Inattention, distractibility
- Impaired memory
- Poor problem-solving skills
- Poor decision-making skills
- Illogical thinking
- Impaired judgement

Affective Symptoms
- Dysphoria
- Suicidality
- Hopelessness

All dimensions alter the individual's:
- Ability to work
- Interpersonal relationships
- Self-care abilities
- Social functioning
- Quality of life

FIGURE 15-1 The four main symptom groups of schizophrenia.

associated with being "crazy." However, positive psychotic symptoms are perhaps less important prognostically and usually respond to antipsychotic medication. Positive symptoms are associated with:

- Acute onset
- Normal premorbid functioning
- Normal social functioning during remissions
- Normal CT findings
- Normal neuropsychological test results
- Favourable response to antipsychotic medication

The positive symptoms presented here are categorized as alterations in thinking, speech, perception, and behaviour.

Alterations in thinking. All people experience occasional and momentary errors in thinking (e.g., "Why are all these lights turning red when I'm already late? Someone must be trying to slow me down!"), but most can catch and correct the error by using intact **reality testing**—the ability to determine accurately whether an experience is based in reality. People with impaired reality testing, however, maintain the error, which contributes to delusions, or alterations in *thought* content. A person experiencing delusions is convinced that what he or she believes to be real *is* real. Student nurses sometimes try unsuccessfully to argue

a person out of delusions by offering evidence of reality; this approach may irritate the person and slow the development of a therapeutic relationship. Table 15-1 provides definitions and examples of frequent types of delusions.

About 75% of people with schizophrenia experience delusions at some time. The most common delusions are persecutory or grandiose or those involving religious or hypochondriacal ideas. A delusion may be a response to anxiety or may reflect areas of concern for a person; for example, someone with poor self-esteem may believe he is Beethoven or an emissary of God, allowing him to feel more powerful or important. Looking for and addressing such underlying themes or needs can be a key nursing intervention. At times, delusions hold a kernel of truth. One person repeatedly told the staff that the Mafia was out to kill him. Later, staff learned that he had been selling drugs and had not paid his contacts and that gang members *were* trying to find him to hurt or even kill him.

Concrete thinking refers to an impaired ability to think abstractly. The person interprets statements literally. For example, the nurse might ask what brought the person to the hospital, and the person might answer, concretely, "a cab" (rather than explaining that he had attempted suicide). Traditionally,

TABLE 15-1	SUMMARY OF DELUSIONS	
DELUSION	**DEFINITION**	**EXAMPLE**
Thought insertion	Believing that another person, group of people, or external force controls thoughts	Bruce always wears a hat so that aliens don't insert thoughts into his brain.
Thought withdrawal	Believing that others are taking thoughts out of a person's mind	Bernadette covers her windows with foil so the police can't empty her mind.
Thought broadcasting	Believing that one's thoughts are being involuntarily broadcasted to others	Marcel was convinced that everyone could hear what he was thinking at all times.
Ideas of reference	Giving personal significance to trivial events; perceiving events as relating to you when they do not	When Maria noticed staff talking, she believed they were plotting against her.
Ideas of influence	Believing that you have somehow influenced events that are, in fact, out of your control	Jean Pierre is convinced that he caused the flooding in Manitoba.
Persecution	Believing that one is being singled out for harm by others; this belief often takes the form of a plot by people in power	Saied believed that the Royal Canadian Mounted Police were planning to kill him by poisoning his food. Therefore he would eat only food he bought from machines.
Grandeur	Believing that one is a very powerful or important person	Sam believed he was a famous playwright and tennis pro.
Somatic	Believing that the body is changing in an unusual way (e.g., rotting inside)	David told the doctor that his heart had stopped and his insides were rotting away.
Erotomanic	Believing that another person desires you romantically	Although he barely knew her, Millie insisted that Justin would marry her if only his current wife would stop interfering.
Jealousy	Believing that one's mate is unfaithful	Harry wrongly accused his girlfriend of going out with other men. His proof was that she came home from work late twice that week, even though the girlfriend's boss explained that everyone had worked late.

concreteness has been assessed through the patient's interpretation of proverbs. However, this assessment is not accurate if the person is from another culture or is otherwise unfamiliar with the proverb (Haynes & Resnick, 1993). It is preferable to use the *similarities test*, which involves asking the person to explain how two things are similar—for example, an orange and an apple, a chair and a table, or a child and an adult. A description of physical characteristics ("apples and oranges are both round") would be a concrete answer, whereas an abstract answer recognizes ideas such as classifications ("apples and oranges are fruit"). Concreteness reduces one's ability to understand and address abstract concepts such as love or the passage of time or to reality-test delusions or other symptoms. Educational strategies need to take into account a person's ability to think abstractly.

Alterations in speech. Alterations in speech demonstrate difficulties with *thought process* (how a person thinks). *Associations* are the threads that tie one thought logically to another. In associative looseness, these threads are interrupted or illogically connected; thinking becomes haphazard, illogical, and difficult to follow:

Nurse: "Are you going to the picnic today?"

Patient: "I'm not an elephant hunter; no tiger teeth for me."

At times, the nurse may be able to decipher or decode the patient's messages and begin to understand the patient's feelings and needs. Any exchange in which a person feels understood is useful. Therefore the nurse might respond to the patient in this way:

Nurse: "Are you saying that you're afraid to go out with the others today?"

Patient: "Yeah, no tiger getting me today."

Sometimes it is not possible to understand the person's meaning because his or her speech is too fragmented. For example:

Patient: "I sang out for my mother ... for this to hell I went. These little hills hop aboard, share the Christmas mice spread ... the devil will be washed away."

If the nurse does not understand what the patient is saying, it is important that he or she let the patient know this. Clear messages and honesty are a vital part of working effectively in psychiatric mental health nursing. An honest response lets the person know that the nurse does not understand, would like to understand, and can be trusted to be honest.

Other alterations in speech that can make communication challenging are *circumstantiality, tangentiality, neologisms, echolalia, clang association,* and *word salad*:

- Circumstantiality refers to the inclusion of unnecessary and often tedious details in one's conversation (e.g., describing your breakfast when asked how your day is going).
- Tangentiality is a departure from the main topic to talk about less important information; the patient goes off on tangents in a way that takes the conversation off-topic.
- Neologisms are made-up words (or idiosyncratic uses of existing words) that have meaning for the person but a different or nonexistent meaning to others (e.g., "I was going to tell him the *mannerologies* of his hospitality won't do"). This eccentric use of words represents disorganized thinking and interferes with communication.
- Echolalia is the pathological repeating of another's words and is often seen in catatonia.

  Nurse: "Mary, come get your medication."

  Mary: "Come get your medication."

- *Clang association* is the choosing of words based on their sound rather than their meaning, often rhyming and sometimes having a similar beginning sound (e.g., "On the track, have a Big Mac," "Click, clack, clutch, close"). Clanging may also be seen in neurological disorders.
- Word salad is a jumble of words that is meaningless to the listener—and perhaps to the speaker as well—because of an extreme level of disorganization.

Alterations in perception. Alterations in perception are errors in one's view of reality. The most common form of altered perception in psychosis is hallucination, but depersonalization, derealization, and boundary impairment are sometimes experienced as well:

- Depersonalization is a nonspecific feeling that a person has lost his or her identity and that the self is different or unreal. People may feel that body parts do not belong to them or may sense that their body has drastically changed. For example, a person may see her fingers as snakes or her arms as rotting wood.
- Derealization is the false perception that the environment has changed. For example, everything seems bigger or smaller, or familiar surroundings have become somehow strange and unfamiliar. Both depersonalization and derealization can be interpreted as *loss of ego boundaries* (sometimes called *loose ego boundaries*).
- Boundary impairment is an impaired ability to sense where one's self ends and others' selves begin. For example, a person might drink another's beverage, believing that because it is in his vicinity, it is his.
- Hallucinations result from perceiving a sensory experience for which no external stimulus exists (e.g., hearing a voice when no one is speaking). Hallucinations differ from illusions in that illusions are misperceptions or misinterpretations of a real experience; for example, a man sees his coat on a coat rack and believes it is a bear about to attack. He does see something real but misinterprets what it is.

Causes of hallucinations include psychiatric disorders, drug abuse, medications, organic disorders, hyperthermia, toxicity (e.g., digitalis), and other conditions. Hallucinations can involve any of the five body senses. Table 15-2 provides definitions and examples of these types of hallucinations.

Auditory hallucinations are experienced by up to 15% of people without psychotic disorders and 60% of people with schizophrenia at some time during their lives (Hubl, Koenig, Strik, et al., 2004). Voices typically seem to come from outside the person's head, and auditory processing areas of the brain are activated during auditory hallucinations just as they are when a genuine external sound is heard (Hubl, Koenig, Strik, et al., 2004). This abnormal activation may cause hallucinations, but another leading theory is that "voices" are a misperception of one's internally generated conversation (Hoffman & Varanko, 2006). John Nash (n.d.), the world-renowned mathematician portrayed in the 2001 film *A Beautiful Mind*, described the voices he heard during the acute phase of his illness: "I thought of the voices as … something a little different from aliens. I thought of them more like angels. … It's really my subconscious talking, it was really that. … I know that now."

Voices may be of people familiar or unknown, and single or multiple. They may be perceived as supportive and pleasant or derogatory and frightening. Voices commenting on the person's behaviour or conversing with the person are most common. A person who hears voices when no one is present often struggles to understand the experience, sometimes developing related delusions to explain the voices (e.g., the person may believe the voices are from God, the devil, or deceased relatives). People with chronic hallucinations may attempt to cope by drowning them out with loud music or competing with them by talking loudly. Some patients grow to accept the voices, and find ways to cope, including keeping busy with purposeful activities (work or physical recreation), talking about their experiences, and creative writing (Buccheri, Trygstad, Buffum, et al., 2013; Farhall, Greenwood, & Jackson, 2007; Kalhovde, Elstad & Talseth, 2014).

Command hallucinations are "voices" that direct the person to take an action. All hallucinations must be assessed and monitored carefully, because the voices may command the person to hurt self or others. For example, voices might command a person to "jump out the window" or "take a knife and kill my child." Command hallucinations are often terrifying and may herald a psychiatric emergency. In all cases, it is essential to assess what the person hears, the person's ability to recognize the hallucination as real or not real, and the person's ability to resist any commands. A person may falsely deny hallucinations,

TABLE 15-2 SUMMARY OF HALLUCINATIONS

HALLUCINATION	DEFINITION	EXAMPLE
Auditory	Hearing voices or sounds that do not exist in the environment but are misperceptions of inner thoughts or feelings	Juan hit the ambulance attendant when a voice told him the attendant was taking him to a concentration camp.
Visual	Seeing a person, object, animal, colours, or visual patterns that do not exist in the environment	Antoine became very frightened and screamed, "There are rats coming at me!"
Olfactory	Smelling odours that do not exist	Theresa "smells" her insides rotting.
Gustatory	Tasting sensations that do not exist	Simon will not eat his food because he "tastes" the poison they are putting in it.
Tactile	Feeling strange sensations on the skin where no external objects stimulate such feelings; common in delirium tremens	Jack "feels" electrical impulses tingling as they control his mind, and he covers his walls in tinfoil to block them out.

requiring behavioural assessment to support (validate) or refute the person's report. Outward indications of possible hallucinations include turning or tilting the head as if to listen to someone, suddenly stopping current activity as if interrupted, and moving the lips silently.

Visual hallucinations occur less frequently in schizophrenia and are more likely to occur in organic disorders such as acute alcohol withdrawal or dementia. Olfactory, tactile, or gustatory hallucinations are unusual; when present, other physical causes should be investigated (Sadock, Sadock, & Ruiz, 2017).

Alterations in behaviour. Alterations in behaviour include bizarre and agitated behaviours involving such things as stilted, rigid demeanour or eccentric dress, grooming, and rituals. Other behavioural changes seen in schizophrenia include the following:

- Catatonia, a pronounced increase or decrease in the rate and amount of movement. The most common form is stuporous behaviour, in which the person moves little or not at all.
- Psychomotor retardation, a pronounced slowing of movement. It is important to differentiate the slowed movements secondary to schizophrenia from those seen in depression; careful assessment of thought content and thought processes is essential for making this determination.
- Psychomotor agitation, excited behaviour such as running or pacing rapidly, often in response to internal or external stimuli. Psychomotor agitation can pose a risk to others and to the person, who is at risk for exhaustion, collapse, and even death.
- Stereotyped behaviours, repeated motor behaviours that do not presently serve a logical purpose.
- Automatic obedience, the performance by a catatonic person of all simple commands in a robotlike fashion.
- Waxy flexibility, the extended maintenance of posture usually seen in catatonia. For example, the nurse raises the person's arm, and the person retains this position in a statuelike manner.
- Negativism, akin to resistance but may not be intentional. In *active negativism*, the person does the opposite of what he or she is told to do; *passive negativism* is a failure to do what is requested.
- Impaired impulse control, a reduced ability to resist one's impulses. Examples include performing socially inappropriate behaviours such as grabbing another's cigarette, throwing food on the floor, pushing others around, and changing TV channels while others are watching.
- Echopraxia, the mimicking of the movements of another. It is also seen in catatonia.

Negative Symptoms

Negative symptoms develop slowly and are those that most interfere with a person's adjustment and ability to cope. They tend to be persistent and crippling because they render the person inert and unmotivated. Negative symptoms impede one's ability to:

- Initiate and maintain conversations and relationships
- Obtain and maintain a job
- Make decisions and follow through on plans
- Maintain adequate hygiene and grooming

Negative symptoms contribute to poor social functioning and social withdrawal. During the acute phase, they are difficult to assess because positive symptoms (such as delusions and hallucinations) dominate. Selected negative symptoms are outlined in Table 15-3.

In schizophrenia, affect—the external manifestation of feeling or emotion that is manifested in facial expression, tone of voice, and body language—may not always coincide with inner emotions. Affect in schizophrenia can usually be categorized in one of four ways:

- Flat—immobile or blank facial expression
- Blunted—reduced or minimal emotional response
- Inappropriate—emotional response incongruent with the tone or circumstances of the situation (e.g., a man laughs when told that his father has died)
- Bizarre—odd, illogical, emotional state that is grossly inappropriate or unfounded; especially prominent in disorganized schizophrenia and includes grimacing and giggling

Cognitive Symptoms

Cognitive symptoms represent the third symptom group and are evident in most people with schizophrenia. They include difficulty with attention, memory, information processing, cognitive flexibility, and executive functions (e.g., decision making, judgement, planning, problem solving) (Carbon & Correll, 2014). Cognitive symptoms include the following:

- Concrete thinking is an impaired ability to think abstractly, resulting in interpreting or perceiving things in a literal manner. For example, a nurse might ask how the patient found the relaxation class, and the patient answers "by walking down the hall" rather than describing their experience of the class. Interpreting proverbs can be used to assess abstract thought. An abstract interpretation of "The grass is always greener on the other side of the fence" is that it always seems we would

TABLE 15-3	SELECTED NEGATIVE SYMPTOMS OF SCHIZOPHRENIA
NEGATIVE SYMPTOM	**DESCRIPTION**
Affective blunting	A reduction in the expression, range, and intensity of affect (in *flat affect*, no facial expression is present)
Anergia	Lack of energy; passivity or lack of persistence at work or school; may also be a symptom of depression, so needs careful evaluation
Anhedonia	Inability to experience pleasure in activities that usually produce it; result of profound emotional barrenness
Avolition	Reduced motivation; inability to initiate tasks such as social contacts, grooming, and other activities of daily living (ADLs)
Poverty of content of speech	While adequate in amount, speech conveys little information because of vagueness or superficiality
Poverty of speech (alogia)	Reduced amount of speech—responses range from brief to one-word answers

be happier given other circumstances. A concrete interpretation could be "That side gets more sun, so it's greener there." Concreteness reduces one's ability to understand and respond to concepts requiring abstract reasoning, such as love or humour.

Concreteness, especially when combined with an impaired ability to recognize variations in affect or tone of voice, can also make it difficult to recognize social cues such as sarcasm. For example, a patient who had forgotten his wallet asked a store clerk if he could pay later for a bag of chips. When the clerk sarcastically replied, "Oh sure, we let our customers pay whenever they want," the patient took this literally. The patient was distressed when police arrested him for theft despite his protests that he had permission not to pay.

- Impaired memory affects short-term memory and the ability to learn. Repetition and verbal or visual cues may help the patient to learn and recall needed information (e.g., a picture of a toothbrush on the patient's wall as a reminder to brush their teeth).
- Impaired information processing can lead to problems such as delayed responses, misperceptions, or difficulty understanding others. Patients may lose the ability to screen out insignificant stimuli such as background sounds or objects in one's peripheral vision. This can lead to overstimulation.
- Impaired executive functioning includes difficulty with reasoning, setting priorities, comparing options, placing things in logical order or groups, anticipation and planning, and inhibiting undesirable impulses or actions. Impaired executive functioning interferes with problem solving and can contribute to inappropriateness in social situations.

These impairments have a considerable impact on longer term functioning and can leave the person unable to manage personal health care, hold a job, initiate or maintain a support system, or live alone. There are no approved treatments focused on cognitive symptomatology for schizophrenia, but nurses should carefully monitor the areas of cognitive impact and any changes. Some psychosocial treatments, including cognitive behavioural therapy, cognitive remediation, social skills training, and computer-assisted training programs, have shown therapeutic benefits and should be offered in conjunction with antipsychotic treatments (Carbon & Correll, 2014).

Affective Symptoms

Affective symptoms, the fourth symptom group, are common and increase a person's suffering. These involve the experience and expression of emotions. Mood may be unstable, erratic, labile (changing rapidly and easily), or incongruent (not what would be expected for the circumstances).

A serious affective change often seen in schizophrenia is depression. Depression may occur as part of a shared inflammatory reaction affecting the brain or may simply be a reaction to the stress and despair that can come from living with a chronic illness. Assessment for depression is crucial because it may indicate an impending relapse, further impair functioning, and increase risk for substance use disorders. It may also be necessary to assess for a more prolonged and marked affective aspect of the illness, indicating schizoaffective disorder. Most importantly, depression puts people at increased risk for suicide.

This assessment can be done by inquiring into mood and the presence of depressive thoughts or suicidal ideation (see also Chapters 13 and 14).

Self-Assessment

Working with individuals with schizophrenia produces strong emotional reactions in most health care workers. The acutely ill person's intensely anxious, lonely, dependent, and distrustful presentation evokes similarly intense, uncomfortable, and frightening emotions in others. The chronicity, repeated exacerbations, and slow response to treatment that many people experience can lead to feelings of helplessness and powerlessness in staff. Some behaviour (especially violent behaviour) can produce strong emotional responses (called *counter-transference*) such as fear or anger (see Chapter 9).

Ironically, knowledge that schizophrenia is a brain disease may contribute to stigmatizing attitudes and feelings of hopelessness. When public education and nursing practice focus on illness without including personal contact or information about recovery, stigma actually increases or becomes entrenched (Morera, Pratt, & Bucci, 2017). Inpatient nurses, in particular, witness people who are acutely unwell and not able to attend to activities of daily living. It is important for them to build recovery into their inpatient nursing care while such care remains primarily focused on stabilization and symptom relief (Waldemar, Arnfred, Petersen, et al., 2016). The importance of hope in the nursing care of people with schizophrenia and their families is well documented, and being hopeful is an essential characteristic of mental health providers in this field (Koehn & Cutliffe, 2007).

At the same time, it is necessary to be realistic about the length of time it may take for a patient to recover from an acute episode. It can be helpful to remember that the person has essentially had a brain injury; to set realistic, achievable goals; and to acknowledge small steps. Negative symptoms can be particularly slow to resolve. It may also take a long time to gain trust in the therapeutic relationship, so the nurse can expect the orientation phase of the helping relationship to be prolonged.

Without support and the opportunity and willingness to explore feelings with more experienced staff, the nurse may adopt nontherapeutic behaviours—denial, withdrawal, avoidance, and anger, most commonly. These behaviours thwart the patient's progress and undermine the nurse's self-esteem. Comments such as "These patients are hopeless" and "All you can do is babysit these people" are indications of unrecognized or unresolved counter-transference that, if left uncorrected, interfere with both treatment and work satisfaction. Canadian nurse Jan Landeen, cited by Koehn and Cutliffe (2007), found that strategies for increasing hope include getting to know the patient as a person, sharing patient successes, learning about treatments and research, and keeping expectations realistic.

People living with schizophrenia may experience fear, self-stigma, or shame related to their mental illness, leading them to conceal some aspects of their experience. Negativism and alogia (reduced verbalization) can also limit the person's responses. Many people with schizophrenia experience **anosognosia**, an inability to realize that they are ill, which is caused by the illness itself. The resulting lack of insight can make assessment (and treatment) challenging, delaying completion of a full assessment and requiring additional skills on the part of the nurse. Selected techniques that may help you overcome these challenges can be found in Table 15-4.

The Unpleasant Voices Scale has been designed for assessment of the risk of harm related to command hallucinations and can be used in conjunction with the Harm Command Safety Protocol (Gerlock, Buccheri, Buffum, et al., 2010). The items in these assessment tools are found in Figures 15-2 and 15-3.

The Inventory of Voice Experiences, a nursing tool developed in Canada, is another assessment tool for perceptual disturbances

TABLE 15-4 INTERVENTIONS FOR OVERCOMING OBSTACLES TO ASSESSMENT

INTERVENTION	RATIONALE	EXAMPLE
Use empathic comments and observations to prompt the patient to provide information.	Empathy conveys understanding and builds trust and rapport.	*Nurse:* "It must be difficult to find yourself in a psychiatric hospital." *Patient:* "Yes … I'm frightened." "Could you please tell me more about … ?" "Tell me what life has been like for you lately."
Minimize questioning, especially closed-ended questioning. Seek data conversationally, using prompts and open-ended questions.	Extended questioning can increase suspiciousness, and closed-ended questions elicit minimal information. Both become wearing and off-putting.	
Use short, simple sentences and introduce only one idea at a time. Allow time for responses to questions.	Long sentences or rambling questions can confuse a person who has difficulty processing auditory information or is actively hallucinating. Also, a person with alogia requires more time to respond to questions.	*Therapeutic:* "Would you like to join us for a basketball game?" *Nontherapeutic:* "Would you like to join us for a basketball game? Sports can be very good for you, you know, and you seem very lonely, so it would help you a lot. I really hope you will come play a game."
Directly but supportively seek the needed information, explaining the reasons for the assessment. Judiciously use indirect, supportive (therapeutic) confrontation.	Being direct but supportive conveys genuineness, builds rapport, and helps reduce anxiety. Blunt contradiction or premature confrontation increases resistance.	"You seem very sad. Sometimes sad people think about hurting themselves. Have you ever thought about hurting yourself?" "I realize that admitting to hearing voices might be difficult to do. I notice you talking as if to others when no one is there."
Seek other data to support (validate) the person's report (obtain further history from third parties, past medical records, and other treatment providers when possible), preferably with the person's permission.	Patients may be unable or unwilling to provide information fully and reliably. Validating their reports ensures the validity of the assessment.	"Your brother reports that he works at a factory. Is that your understanding?"
Prioritize the data you seek, and avoid seeking nonessential data.	Patients may have limited tolerance for the assessment interview and answer only a limited number of inquiries. Seeking nonessential information does not benefit the person or assessment.	*Patient:* "I hate school! I wish they'd all die!" *Nurse:* (less therapeutic) "Which school do you go to?" *Nurse:* (more therapeutic) "Things would be better if they were dead. …" (Paraphrasing prompts elaboration and confirmation or refutation of the comment.)

1. Please rate your unpleasant "voices" <u>during the past 24 hours</u> by circling one of the following numbers:

0	1	2	3	4	5	6	7	8	9	10
No voices heard	Hardly unpleasant at all									The most unpleasant your voices could be

2. Please rate your unpleasant "voices" <u>over the past week</u> by circling one of the following numbers:

0	1	2	3	4	5	6	7	8	9	10
No voices heard	Hardly unpleasant at all									The most unpleasant your voices could be

3. Do you ever hear pleasant voices? Please circle one   Yes   No

4. Are your voices commanding you to harm yourself?   Yes*   No

5. Do you intend to harm yourself?   Yes*   No

6. Are your voices commanding you to harm someone else?   Yes*   No

7. Do you intend to harm someone else?   Yes*   No

* If you answered "yes", please stay after and speak to one of the group leaders. Thank you.

FIGURE 15-2 Unpleasant Voices Scale. Source: Gerlock, A. A., Buccheri, R., Buffum, M. D., et al. (2010). Responding to command hallucinations to harm self and others: The Unpleasant Voices Scale and Harm Command Safety Protocol. *Journal of Psychosocial Nursing and Mental Health Services, 48*(5), 26–33. doi:10.3928/02793695-20100304-03.

ASSESSMENT GUIDELINES
Schizophrenia and Other Psychotic Disorders

1. Assess for risk to self or others.
2. Assess for suicide risk (see Chapter 22).
3. Assess for command hallucinations (e.g., voices telling the patient to harm self or another). If present, ask the person:
   - Do you recognize the voices?
   - Do you believe the voices are real?
4. Do you plan to follow the command? (A positive response to any of these questions suggests an increased risk that the person will act on the commands.) Assess for ability to ensure self-safety, addressing:
   - Adequacy of food and fluid intake
   - Hygiene and self-care
   - Handling of potentially hazardous activities, such as smoking and cooking
   - Ability to transport self safely
   - Impulse control and judgement
   - Appropriate dress for weather conditions

   Assess whether the person abuses or is dependent on alcohol or drugs. Assess the patient's belief system. Is it fragmented or poorly organized? Is it systematized? Are the beliefs delusional? If yes, then ask:
   - Do you feel that you or your loved ones are being threatened or are in danger?
   - Do you feel the need to act against a person or organization to protect or avenge yourself or your loved ones? (A positive response to either of these questions suggests an increased risk of danger to others.)
5. Assess for the presence and severity of positive and negative symptoms. Complete a mental status examination, noting which symptoms are present, how they affect functioning, and how the patient is managing them.
6. Assess the patient's insight, knowledge of the illness, relationships and support systems, other coping resources, and strengths.
7. Determine if the patient has had a medical workup. Are there any indications of physical medical problems that might mimic psychosis (e.g., digitalis or anticholinergic toxicity, brain trauma, drug intoxication, delirium, fever)?
8. Assess for coexisting disorders:
   - Depression
   - Anxiety
   - Substance abuse or dependency
   - Medical disorders (especially brain trauma, toxicity, delirium, cardiovascular disease, obesity, and diabetes)
9. Assess medications the patient has been prescribed, whether and how the patient is taking the medications, and what factors (e.g., costs, mistrust of staff, adverse effects) are affecting adherence.
10. Assess the family's knowledge of and response to the patient's illness and its symptoms. Are family members overprotective? Hostile? Anxious? Are they familiar with family support groups and respite resources?

that offers increased accuracy of assessment of voices (England, 2007).

DIAGNOSIS

People with schizophrenia have multiple disturbing and disabling symptoms that require a multifaceted approach to care and treatment of both the patient and the family. Table 15-5 lists potential nursing diagnoses for a person with schizophrenia.

OUTCOMES IDENTIFICATION

Desired outcomes vary with the phase of the illness. *Nursing Outcomes Classification (NOC)* (Moorhead, Johnson, Maas, et al., 2013) is a useful guide. Ideally, outcomes should focus on enhancing strengths and minimizing the effects of the patient's deficits and symptoms. Outcomes should be consistent with the recovery model (see Chapter 29), which stresses hope, living a full and productive life, and eventual recovery rather than focusing on controlling symptoms and adapting to disability.

Phase I—Acute

During the acute phase, the overall goal is the person's safety and medical stabilization. Therefore if the person is at risk for violence to self or others, initial outcome criteria address safety issues (e.g., *Person refrains from self-harm*). Another outcome is *Person consistently labels hallucinations as "not real—a symptom of an illness."* Table 15-6 gives selected short-term and intermediate indicators for the outcome *Distorted thought self-control*.

Phase II—Stabilization

Outcome criteria during phase II focus on helping the patient adhere to treatment, become stabilized on medications, and control or cope with symptoms. The outcomes target the negative symptoms and may include ability to succeed in social, vocational, or self-care activities.

Phase III—Maintenance

Outcome criteria for phase III focus on maintaining achievement, preventing relapse, and achieving independence and a satisfactory quality of life.

PLANNING

The planning of appropriate interventions is guided by the phase of the illness and the strengths and needs of the patient. It is influenced by cultural considerations, available resources, and the patient's preferences.

Intent to Harm Self:

When a patient responds *yes* to question 5 on the Unpleasant Voices Scale ("...intent to harm self"), determine whether there is a need for the patient to be assessed for hospitalization. This will be especially important if the patient also indicates the voices are loud and distressing, and the patient does not feel that he or she has much control over the voices (questions on the Characteristics of Auditory Hallucinations Questionnaire—CAHQ; Buccheri et al., 2004).

After class or group, talk privately with the patient and use this script to determine the need for further assessment:

- "You marked here that the voices are commanding you to harm yourself.
  It can be very scary to hear voices telling you to harm yourself."
- "What is (are) the voice(s) commanding you to do to yourself?"
- "Do you plan to carry this out?"
- "Do you have the *means* to carry this out?" (Credible?)
- "Has (have) the voice(s) ever commanded you to do this before?"
- "Have you ever harmed yourself as the voice(s) said to do?"
- "How long ago?"

If the patient indicates that he or she has attempted suicide before (because of the voices), has the means and intent, is distressed, and does not feel much control over the voices, then refer the patient for an evaluation for hospitalization.

- "We (I) would like to get some extra help with this today, and would like you to wait with us (me) until the psychiatrist/crisis team (insert whatever is appropriate for your setting) is able to see you?"

Risk Assessment Checklist*

	YES	NO
Has the means to kill/harm self (credible threat)		
Tried to kill/harm self previously		
Outcome today (who notified):		

* If *yes* to intent to harm self

Continue to monitor for change under these conditions: patient has chronic suicidal command hallucinations, has never acted on them, does not have the means, has no intent, is not distressed, and feels in control.

FIGURE 15-3 Harm Command Safety Protocol. Source: Gerlock, A. A., Buccheri, R., Buffum, M. D., et al. (2010). Responding to command hallucinations to harm self and others: The Unpleasant Voices Scale and Harm Command Safety Protocol. *Journal of Psychosocial Nursing and Mental Health Services, 48*(5), 26–33. doi:10.3928/02793695-20100304-03.

Phase I—Acute

Hospitalization is indicated if the patient is considered a danger to self or others, refuses to eat or drink, or is too disorganized or otherwise impaired to function safely in the community without supervision. The planning process focuses on the best strategies to ensure the person's safety and provide symptom stabilization. In addition, during the patient's hospitalization, this process includes discharge planning.

In discharge planning, the patient and interprofessional treatment team identify aftercare needs for follow-up and support. Discharge planning considers not only external factors, such as the person's living arrangements, economic resources, social supports, and family relationships, but also internal factors, such as resilience and repertoire of coping skills. Because relapse can be devastating to the person's circumstances (resulting in loss of employment, housing, and relationships) and worsen the long-term prognosis, vigorous efforts are made to connect the person and family with (and not simply refer them to) community resources that provide therapeutic programming and social, financial, and other needed support.

Phase II—Stabilization and Phase III—Maintenance

Planning during the stabilization and maintenance phases includes providing individual and family education and skills training (psychosocial education). Relapse prevention skills are vital. Planning identifies interpersonal, coping, health care, and vocational needs and addresses how and where these needs can best be met within the community.

IMPLEMENTATION

Interventions are geared toward the phase of schizophrenia the person is experiencing. For example, during the acute phase, the clinical focus is on crisis intervention, medication for symptom stabilization, and safety. Interventions are often hospital based; however, people in the acute stage are increasingly being treated in the community.

TABLE 15-5   POTENTIAL AREAS THAT WILL REQUIRE NURSING INTERVENTION FOR PEOPLE WITH SCHIZOPHRENIA

SYMPTOM	POTENTIAL AREAS REQUIRING NURSING INTERVENTION
Positive Symptoms	
Hears voices that others do not (*auditory hallucinations*)	*Auditory perceptions*
Hears voices telling him or her to hurt self or others (*command hallucinations*)	*Self-directed violence*
	Other-directed violence
Delusions	*Thought processes*
Shows loose association of ideas (*associative looseness*)	*Thought processes*
Conversation is derailed by unnecessary and tedious details (*circumstantiality*)	*Verbal communication*
Negative Symptoms	
Uncommunicative, withdrawn	*Social isolation*
Expresses feelings of rejection or aloneness (lies in bed all day, positions back to door)	*Social interaction*
	Loneliness
Talks about self as "bad" or "no good"	*Low self-esteem*
Feels guilty because of "bad thoughts"; extremely sensitive to real or perceived slights	*Self-directed violence*
Shows lack of energy (*anergia*)	*Ineffective coping*
Shows lack of motivation (*avolition*), unable to initiate tasks (social contact, grooming, and other aspects of daily living)	*Self-care (bathing, dressing, feeding, toileting)*
	Constipation
Other	
Families and significant others become confused or overwhelmed, lack knowledge about disorder or treatment, feel powerless in coping with the patient	*Family coping*
	Caregiver role strain
	Health literacy
Stops taking medication (because of anosognosia, adverse effects, drugs costs, mistrust of staff), stops going to therapy, is not supported in treatment by significant others	*Decision-making*

TABLE 15-6   *NOC* OUTCOMES RELATED TO DISTORTED THOUGHT SELF-CONTROL

NURSING OUTCOME AND DEFINITION	INTERMEDIATE INDICATORS	SHORT-TERM INDICATORS
Distorted thought self-control: Self-restraint of disruptions in perception, thought processes, and thought content	Maintains affect consistent with mood	Recognizes that hallucinations or delusions are occurring
	Interacts appropriately	Refrains from attending to and responding to hallucinations or delusions
	Perceives environment and the ideas of others accurately	Describes content of hallucinations or delusions
	Exhibits logical thought flow patterns	Reports decrease in hallucinations or delusions
	Exhibits reality-based thinking	Asks for validation of reality
	Exhibits appropriate thought content	

Source: Moorhead, S., Johnson, M., Maas, M. L., et al. (2013). *Nursing outcomes classification (NOC)* (5th ed.). St Louis: Mosby.

Phase I—Acute

Settings

A number of factors affect the choice of treatment setting, including the following:

- Level of care and restrictiveness needed to protect the person from harm to self or others
- Person's need for external structure and support
- Person's ability to cooperate with treatment
- Need for a particular treatment available only in particular settings
- Need for treatment of a coexisting medical condition
- Availability of supportive others who can provide critical information and treatment history to staff and permit stabilization in less restrictive settings

The use of less restrictive and more cost-effective alternatives to hospitalization that work for many people include:

- Partial hospitalization: Patients sleep at home and attend treatment sessions (similar to what they would receive if admitted) during the day or evening.
- Residential crisis centres: Patients who are unable to remain in the community but do not require full in-person services can be admitted (usually for 1 to 14 days) to receive increased supervision, guidance, and medication stabilization.

- Group homes: Patients live in the community with a group of other people, sharing expenses and responsibilities. Staff are present in the house 24 hours a day, 7 days a week to provide supervision and therapeutic activities.
- Day treatment programs: Patients reside in the community and attend structured programming during the day.

These programs may include group and individual therapy, supervised activities, and specialized skill training. It is vital that staff be aware of these and other community resources and make this information available to discharged people and their families, ideally by directly connecting them with these resources. Patients and family members should be given telephone numbers and addresses of local support groups such as their provincial Schizophrenia Society. Northern and rural communities, however, may not have local support groups.

Other community resources include community mental health centres (usually providing medication services, day treatment, access to 24-hour emergency services, psychotherapy, psycho-education, and case management); home health services; supported employment programs, offering services from job training to on-site coaches, who help people learn to succeed in the work environment, often via peer-led services (e.g., drop-in centres, sometimes called "clubhouses," that offer social contact, constructive activities, and sometimes employment opportunities); family educational and skills groups (e.g., Schizophrenia Society of Canada's "Strengthening Families Together" program); and respite care for caregivers.

Interventions

Acute phase interventions include the following:
- Psychiatric, medical, and neurological evaluation
- Psychopharmacological treatment
- Support, psychoeducation, and guidance
- Supervision and limit setting in the milieu

Due to a shortage of inpatient beds, there is pressure to keep the length of hospitalization short. This situation may create an ethical dilemma for treatment teams, as short initial hospital stays have been found to be related to high rates of readmission and shorter intervals between hospitalizations (Canadian Institute for Health Information [CIHI], 2008). Typically, as soon as the acute symptoms are adequately stabilized, the patient is discharged to the community, where appropriate treatment can be continued during the stabilization and maintenance phases. However, in some cases, discharge may be delayed while appropriate housing and supports are sought.

Phase II—Stabilization and Phase III—Maintenance

Effective long-term care of an individual with schizophrenia relies on a three-pronged approach: medication administration and adherence, nursing intervention, and community support. Family psychoeducation, a key role of the nurse, is an essential intervention. All interventions and strategies are geared to the patient's strengths, culture, personal preferences, and needs.

Milieu Management

Effective hospital care provides (1) protection from stressful or disruptive environments and (2) structure. People in the acute phase of schizophrenia show greater improvement in a structured milieu than on an open unit that allows more freedom. A therapeutic milieu is consciously designed to maximize safety, opportunities for learning skills, therapeutic activities, and access to resources. The milieu also provides guidance, supportive peer contact, and opportunities for practising conflict resolution, stress-reduction techniques, and dealing with symptoms.

Activities and Groups

Participation in activities and groups appropriate to the patient's level of functioning may decrease withdrawal, enhance motivation, modify unacceptable behaviours, develop friendships, and increase social competence. Activities such as drawing, reading poetry, and listening to music may be used to focus conversation and promote the recognition and expression of feelings. Self-esteem is enhanced as patients experience successful task completion. Recreational activities such as picnics and outings to stores and restaurants are not simply diversions; they teach constructive leisure skills, increase social comfort, facilitate growth in social concern and interactional skills, and enhance the ability to develop boundaries and set limits on self and others. After discharge, group therapy can provide necessary structure within the patient's community milieu.

Safety

A small percentage of people with schizophrenia, especially during the acute phase, may exhibit a risk for physical violence. Several interrelated risk factors, including demographics (i.e., young, single, male) and social factors (i.e., homelessness, limited education, history of maltreatment or criminality), presence of persecutory delusions or command hallucinations, comorbid antisocial personality pathology, concurrent substance use, inadequate insight, treatment nonadherence, and physiological factors, increase the risk for violence in patients with psychosis. Nonadherence to treatment is a key risk factor predicting violence in patients with psychosis (Lamsma & Harte, 2015). When the potential for violence exists, measures to protect the patient and others become the priority. Interventions include assessing for risk, increasing staff supervision, reducing stimulation (e.g., noise, crowds), addressing paranoia and other contributing symptoms, providing constructive diversion and outlets for physical energy, teaching and practising coping skills, implementing cognitive behavioural approaches (to correct unrealistic expectations or selectively extinguish aggression), de-escalating tension verbally, and, when necessary, using seclusion and chemical (i.e., medi-cation) or physical restraints. The Harm Command Safety Protocol provides guidelines for how to respond when a person indicates intent to harm someone else (Gerlock, Buccheri, Buffum, et al., 2010). Refer to Chapter 24 for more detailed discussions of caring for the aggressive person, seclusion, and restraints.

Counselling and Communication Techniques

Therapeutic communication techniques for patients with schizophrenia aim to lower the person's anxiety, build trust, encourage clear communication, decrease defensiveness, encourage interaction, enhance self-esteem, and reinforce skills such as reality testing and assertiveness. It is important to remember that people with schizophrenia may have memory impairment and require repetition. They may also have limited tolerance for interaction, owing to the stimulation it creates. Therefore shorter (<30 minutes) but more frequent interactions may be more therapeutic. Interventions for paranoia and other selected presentations are discussed later in this chapter.

Hallucinations

When a patient is having a hallucination, the nursing focus is on understanding the person's experiences and responses. Suicidal or homicidal themes or commands necessitate appropriate safety measures. For example, "voices" that tell a patient a particular individual plans to harm him or her may lead to aggressive actions against that person; one-to-one supervision of the patient or transfer of the potential victim to another unit is often essential.

Hallucinations are real to the patient who is experiencing them and may be distracting during nurse–patient interactions. Call the person by name, speak simply but in a louder voice than usual, approach the person in a nonthreatening and nonjudgemental manner, maintain eye contact, and redirect the person's focus to the conversation as needed (Farhall, Greenwood, & Jackson, 2007). Guidelines for Communication: Helping Patients Who Are Experiencing Hallucinations lists other techniques for communicating with patients experiencing hallucinations.

Delusions

Delusions may be the patient's attempts to understand confusion and distorted experiences. They reflect the misperception of one's circumstances, which go uncorrected in schizophrenia due to impaired reality testing. When, as a nurse, you attempt to see the world through the eyes of the patient, it is easier to understand his or her delusional experience. For example:

Patient: "You people are all alike … all in on the RCMP plot to destroy me."

Nurse: "I don't want to hurt you, Tom. Thinking that people are out to destroy you must be very frightening."

In this example, the nurse acknowledges the patient's experience, conveys empathy about the patient's fearfulness, and avoids focusing on the content of the delusion (Royal Canadian Mounted Police and plot to destroy), but labels the patient's feelings so they can be explored, as tolerated. Note that talking about the feelings is helpful, but extended focus on delusional material is not.

It is *never* useful to debate or attempt to dissuade the patient regarding the delusion. Doing so can intensify the patient's retention of irrational beliefs and cause him or her to view you as rejecting or oppositional. However, it *is* helpful to clarify misinterpretations of the environment and gently suggest, as tolerated, a more reality-based perspective. For example:

Patient: "I see the doctor is here; he is out to destroy me."

Nurse: "It is true the doctor wants to see you, but he just wants to talk to you about your treatment. Would you feel more comfortable talking to him in the day room?"

Focusing on specific reality-based activities and events in the environment helps to minimize the focus on delusional thoughts. The more time the patient spends engaged in activities or with

---

GUIDELINES FOR COMMUNICATION

Helping Patients Who Are Experiencing Hallucinations

Nursing Care

1. Watch the patient for hallucinating cues such as eyes tracking an unheard speaker, muttering or talking to self, appearing distracted, suddenly stopping conversing as if interrupted, or intently watching a vacant area of the room.
2. Ask the patient about the content of the hallucinations and how he or she is reacting to it. Assess for command hallucinations and whether the hallucinations are causing fear or distress.
3. Avoid referring to hallucinations as if they are real. Do not ask, "What are the voices saying to you?" Rather, ask, "What are you hearing?"
4. Be alert to signs of anxiety, which may indicate that hallucinations are intensifying or that they are of a command type.
5. Do not negate the patient's experience, but offer your own perceptions and convey empathy. "I don't hear the angry voices that you hear, but that must be very frightening for you."
6. Focus on reality-based "here-and-now" activities such as conversations or simple projects. Tell the patient, "The voice you hear is part of your illness, and it cannot hurt you. Try to listen to me and the others you can see around you."
7. Address any underlying emotion, need, or theme that seems to be indicated by the hallucination, such as fear with menacing voices or guilt with accusing voices.
8. Promote and guide reality testing. If the patient has frightening hallucinations, guide him or her to scan the area to see if others appear frightened; if they are not frightened, encourage the patient to consider that these might be hallucinations.
9. As the patient begins to develop insight, guide him or her to interpret the hallucinations as a symptom of the illness.

Sources: Buccheri, R., Trygstad, L., Buffum, M., et al. (2013). Self-management of unpleasant auditory hallucinations: A tested practice model. *Journal of Psychosocial Nursing and Mental Health Services, 51*(11), 26–34. doi:10.3928/02793695-20130731-02; and Herzog, E. (2014, October 22). *Caring for the hallucinating patient: Non-pharmacological interventions.* Presentation at the 28th annual conference of the American Psychiatric Nurses Association, Indianapolis, IN.

---

people, the more opportunities there are to receive feedback about and become comfortable with reality.

Work with the patient to find out which coping strategies succeed and how the patient can make the best use of them. Guidelines for Communication: People Experiencing Delusions lists techniques for communicating with people experiencing delusions, and Patient and Family Teaching: Coping With Auditory Hallucinations or Delusions presents patient and family teaching topics for coping with hallucinations and delusions.

Associative Looseness

Associative looseness often mirrors the person's abnormal thoughts and reflects poorly organized thinking. An increase in associative looseness often indicates that the person is feeling increased anxiety or is overwhelmed by internal and external stimuli. The person's ramblings may also produce confusion and

GUIDELINES FOR COMMUNICATION
People Experiencing Delusions

- To build trust, be open, honest, and reliable.
- Respond to suspicions in a matter-of-fact, empathic, supportive, and calm manner.
- Ask the person to describe the delusions. Example: "Tell me more about someone trying to hurt you."
- Avoid debating the delusional content, but interject doubt where appropriate. Example: "It seems as though it would be hard for that petite girl to hurt you."
- Focus on the feelings that underlie or flow from the delusions. Example: "You seem to wish you could be more powerful" or "It must feel frightening to think others want to hurt you."
- Once it is understood and addressed, do not dwell further on the delusion. Instead, focus on more reality-based topics. If the person obsesses about delusions, set firm limits on the amount of time you will talk about them, and explain your reason for these limits.
- Observe for events that trigger delusions. If possible, help the person find ways to reduce or manage them.
- Validate a part of the delusion that is real. Example: "Yes, there was a man at the nurses' station, but I did not hear him talk about you."

Source: Data from Farhall, J., Greenwood, K. M., & Jackson, H. J. (2007). Coping with hallucinated voices in schizophrenia: A review of self-initiated strategies and therapeutic interventions. *Clinical Psychology Review, 27*, 476–493. doi:10.1016/j.cpr.2006.12.002.

frustration in the nurse. The following guidelines are useful for intervention with a patient whose speech is confused and disorganized:

- Do *not* pretend you understand the patient's words or meaning when you do not; tell the person you are having difficulty understanding.
- Place the difficulty in understanding on yourself, *not* on the patient. Example: "I'm having trouble following what you are saying," *not* "You're not making any sense."
- Look for recurring topics and themes in the patient's communications, and tie these to events and timelines. Example: "You've mentioned trouble with your brother several times, usually after your family has visited. Tell me about your brother and your visits with him."
- Summarize or paraphrase the patient's communications to role-model more effective ways of making his or her point and to give the person a chance to correct anything you may have misunderstood.
- Reduce stimuli in the vicinity, and speak concisely, clearly, and concretely.
- Tell the person what you *do* understand, and reinforce clear communication and accurate expression of needs, feelings, and thoughts.

Health Teaching and Health Promotion

Education is an essential strategy and includes teaching the patient and family about the illness, including possible causes, medications and medication adverse effects, coping strategies, what to expect, and prevention of relapse. Understanding these things helps the

PATIENT AND FAMILY TEACHING
Coping With Auditory Hallucinations or Delusions

Prevention and Stress Management
- Avoid overly loud or stressful places or activities.
- Avoid negative or critical people and seek out supportive people.
- Learn assertive communication skills so you can tell others "no" if they pressure or upset you.
- When stressed, slow and deepen your breathing. Count slowly from one to four as you inhale, hold the breath, and exhale.
- Gently tense and then relax your muscles, one area of the body at a time, starting at your head (e.g., closing your eyes and then opening them, clenching your teeth and then relaxing your jaw) and working your way down to your hands and feet.
- Discover other ways that help you manage stress (e.g., going for a walk, meditation, taking a hot bath, reading or listening to music, imagining yourself in a less stressful situation [sometimes called a *mental vacation*]).

Distraction
- Listening to music
- Reading (aloud may help more)
- Counting backwards from 100
- Watching television

Interaction
- Observing others—if they do not seem to be hearing or fearing what you are, ignore the voices or thoughts
- Talking with another person

Activity
- Walking
- Cleaning the house
- Having a relaxing bath
- Playing the guitar or singing
- Going to the gym (or any place you enjoy being, where others will be present)

Talking to Yourself
- Telling the voices or thoughts to go away
- Telling yourself that the voices and thoughts are a symptom and not real
- Telling yourself that no matter what you hear, voices can be safely ignored

Social Action
- Talking to a trusted friend or member of the family
- Calling a help line or going to a drop-in centre
- Visiting a favourite place or a comfortable public place

Physical Action
- Taking extra medication when ordered (call your prescriber)
- Going for a walk or doing other exercise
- Using breathing exercises and other relaxation methods

Sources: Buccheri, R., Trygstad, L., Buffum, M., et al. (2013). Self-management of unpleasant auditory hallucinations: A tested practice model. *Journal of Psychosocial Nursing and Mental Health Services, 51*(11), 26–34. doi:10.3928/02793695-20130731-02; and Farhall, J., Greenwood, K. M., & Jackson, H. J. (2007). Coping with hallucinated voices in schizophrenia: A review of self-initiated strategies and therapeutic interventions. *Clinical Psychology Review, 27*, 476–493. doi:10.1016/j.cpr.2006.12.002.

patient and family to recognize the impact of stress, enhances their understanding of the importance of treatment to a good outcome, encourages involvement in (and support of) therapeutic activities, and identifies resources for consultation and ongoing support in dealing with the illness.

PATIENT AND FAMILY TEACHING

Schizophrenia

1. Learn all you can about the illness.
   - Attend psychoeducational and support groups.
   - Join the National Network for Mental Health (http://nnmh.ca/).
   - Contact your provincial Schizophrenia Society.
2. Develop a relapse prevention plan.
   - Know the early warning signs of relapse (e.g., avoiding others, trouble sleeping, troubling thoughts).
   - Know who to call, what to do, and where to go when early signs of relapse appear. Make a list and keep it with you.
   - Relapse is part of the illness, not a sign of failure.
3. Take advantage of all psychoeducational tools.
   - Participate in family, group, and individual therapy.
   - Learn new ways to act and coping skills to help handle family, work, and social stress. Get information from your nurse, case manager, doctor, self-help group, community mental health group, or hospital.
   - Have a plan, on paper, of what to do to cope with stressful times.
   - Recognize that everyone needs a place to address their fears and losses and to learn new ways of coping.
4. Adhere to treatment.
   - People who adhere to treatment that works for them do the best in coping with the disorder.
   - Engaging in struggles over adherence does not help, but tying adherence to the patient's own goals does. ("Staying in treatment will help you keep your job and avoid trouble with the police.")
   - Share concerns about troubling adverse effects or concerns (e.g., sexual problems, weight gain, "feeling funny") with your nurse, case manager, doctor, or social worker; most adverse effects can be helped.
   - Keeping adverse effects a secret or stopping medication can prevent you from having the life you want.
5. Avoid alcohol and drugs; they can act on the brain and cause a relapse.
6. Keep in touch with supportive people—those with shared patient and family experiences and others.
7. Keep healthy—stay in balance.
   - Taking care of one's diet, health, and hygiene helps prevent medical illnesses.
   - Maintain a regular sleep pattern.
   - Keep active (hobbies, friends, groups, sports, job, special interests).
   - Nurture yourself, and practise stress-reduction activities daily.

Further information on facilitating family support is available through the Schizophrenia Society of Canada's third edition of *Strengthening Families Together: Helping Canadians Live with Mental Illness*, http://www.schizophrenia.ca/docs/SFT3_facilitator.pdf, or via the Your Recovery Journey website (Schizophrenia Society of Canada), http://www.your-recovery-journey.ca/.

Including family members in any strategies aimed at reducing psychotic symptoms reduces family anxiety and distress and enables the family to reinforce the staff's efforts. The family plays an important role in the stability of the patient. The patient who returns to a warm, concerned, and supportive environment is less likely to experience relapse. An environment in which people are critical or their involvement in the patient's life is intrusive is associated with relapse and poorer outcomes.

Lack of understanding of the disease and its symptoms can lead others to misinterpret the patient's apathy and lack of drive as laziness, fostering a hostile response by family members, caregivers, or community. Thus public education about the symptoms of schizophrenia can reduce tensions in families, as well as in communities. The most effective education occurs over time and is available when the family is most receptive (Brady, Kangas, & McGill, 2017). Patient and Family Teaching: Schizophrenia offers guidelines for patient and family teaching about schizophrenia.

INTEGRATIVE THERAPY

Mindfulness as an Adjunctive Treatment for Schizophrenia

Mindfulness interventions are gaining popularity as a complementary and integrative practice for people with a number of emotional and psychological concerns. These therapies employ elements of acceptance and compassion in addition to mindfulness. Although these practices are being used with individuals with psychosis, little is known of the effectiveness or value of mindfulness for people experiencing psychosis.

Several RCTs of these interventions have emerged in recent years, and this study sought to systematically review these studies specific to mindfulness interventions for psychosis and schizophrenia.

The review found key benefits of mindfulness therapies included improved insight, medium to larger improvement in mood, trends toward improvement in quality of life, and significant improvements in positive and negative symptoms of schizophrenia. No significant improvement in anxiety was found as a result of the mindfulness therapies. Certain therapies were examined to meet particular needs most effectively; for example, group mindfulness therapy for psychosis was found to improve clinical functioning and enhance mindful response to stressful thoughts. There is also reasonable evidence from one large trial that Internet-based, self-help mindfulness therapy effects moderate reductions in depressive symptoms and symptoms of obsessive-compulsive disorder in outpatients with psychosis.

The review concluded that mindfulness therapies can be safely used with people with psychosis and that they provide a number of therapeutic benefits compared with routine care and, in some cases, other interventions.

Source: Aust, J., & Bradshaw, T. (2017). Mindfulness interventions for psychosis: A systematic review of the literature. *Journal of Psychiatric and Mental Health Nursing, 24*(1), 69–83. doi:10.1111/jpm.12357.

Pharmacological Interventions

Drugs used to treat psychotic disorders, antipsychotics, first became available in the 1950s. Before that time, the available medications provided only sedation, not treatment of the disorder itself. Until the 1960s, people who had even one episode of schizophrenia usually spent months or years in provincial mental health hospitals. Psychotic episodes resulted in great emotional burdens to families and people with schizophrenia. The advent of antipsychotic drugs at last provided symptom control and allowed people to live in the community.

Two groups of antipsychotic drugs exist: conventional antipsychotics (traditional dopamine antagonists [dopamine D_2 receptor antagonists]), also known as *typical* or *first-generation antipsychotics*, and atypical antipsychotics (serotonin–dopamine antagonists [$5\text{-}HT_{2A}$ receptor antagonists]), also known as *second-generation antipsychotics*. A "third generation" of drugs (aripiprazole and brexpiprazole) give hope for enhanced effectiveness and adverse-effect reduction (Howland, 2015). Other drugs, such as anticonvulsants and antiparkinson drugs, are used to augment antipsychotics for patients who do not respond fully. For example, D-serine—an amino acid that enhances NMDA activity—has been shown to increase the effectiveness of selected antipsychotics (Kantrowitz, Malhotra, Cornblatt, et al., 2010).

All antipsychotics are effective for most exacerbations of schizophrenia and for reduction or mitigation of relapse. The conventional antipsychotics affect primarily the positive symptoms of schizophrenia (e.g., hallucinations, delusions, disordered thinking). The atypical antipsychotics can improve negative symptoms (e.g., asociality, blunted affect, lack of motivation) as well.

Antipsychotic agents usually take effect 2 to 6 weeks after the regimen is started. Only about 10% of people with schizophrenia fail to respond to antipsychotic drug therapy; these patients should not continue to take medication that holds only risks and no benefit for them.

Polypharmacy is an issue for patients with severe and persistent symptoms that do not respond easily to a single medication. It is not unusual to find patients being prescribed a combination of antipsychotic medications, sometimes both oral and depot (long-acting injectable) or both typical and atypical. These individuals may also be taking antiparkinson agents and other medications to combat adverse effects. It is important in these cases to have the medication regimen carefully and regularly reviewed by both the physician and a pharmacist and to monitor closely for adverse effects. These patients would be at high risk for anticholinergic toxicity, a potentially life-threatening situation (see Table 15-8).

Antipsychotics are not addictive. However, they should be discontinued gradually to minimize a discontinuation syndrome that can include dizziness, nausea, tremors, insomnia, electric shock–like pains, and anxiety. Antipsychotics are unlikely to be lethal in overdose situations. A lesser-known risk of all antipsychotic medications, due to dopamine blockade or sedation, is impaired swallowing. This may cause drooling and risk of choking (Chen, Chen, Chan, et al., 2015). Also, patients taking antipsychotics are at increased risk for falls due to orthostatic (postural) hypotension, sedation, and gait impairment (Wynaden, Tohotoa, Heslop, et al., 2015).

Additional Medication Administration Issues

Liquid or fast-dissolving forms, available for selected antipsychotics, can make it difficult for a person to "cheek" or "palm" his medicine (hide it in his cheek or palm and later dispose of it).

Some antipsychotics are also available in short-acting injectable form, used primarily for treatment of agitation, behavioural emergencies such as assaultiveness, or when a patient refuses court-mandated oral antipsychotics. Side effects can be intensified and less easily managed when medication is administered directly into the system intramuscularly (IM).

In addition, some medications are available in long-acting injectable (LAI) formulations that need to be administered only every 2 to 4 weeks or, in one case, every 3 months. These may be referred to as "depot" medications. Some require special administration protocols. By requiring less frequent medication administration, adherence is improved and conflict about taking medications is reduced. The downside is lack of dosing flexibility, and patients may feel as if they have less control and are coerced.

Atypical Antipsychotics

Atypical antipsychotics first emerged in the early 1990s with clozapine (Clozaril). Unfortunately, clozapine produces agranulocytosis in 0.8% to 1% of those who take it and also increases the risk for seizures. Clozapine produced dramatic improvement in some patients whose disorder had been resistant to the earlier antipsychotics. Due to the risk for agranulocytosis, however, people taking clozapine must have weekly white blood cell counts for the first 6 months, then frequent monitoring thereafter, to obtain the medication. As a result, clozapine use is declining.

Atypicals are often chosen as first-line antipsychotics because they treat both the positive and the negative symptoms of schizophrenia. Furthermore, they produce minimal to no extrapyramidal side effects (EPSs) or tardive dyskinesia in most people, although these effects may still occur for some patients. Adverse effects tend to be significantly less, resulting in greater adherence to treatment.

Atypical antipsychotics include risperidone (Risperdal), lurasidone (Latuda), olanzapine (Zyprexa), quetiapine (Seroquel), ziprasidone (Zeldox), and aripiprazole (Abilify), the last of which is technically a third-generation drug. These atypicals are free of the potential hematological adverse effects of clozapine and are all first-line agents because of their lower adverse-effect profile.

A subset of the atypicals, or second-generation antipsychotics, is those drugs referred to as third-generation antipsychotics. These drugs are aripiprazole (Abilify), brexpiprazole (Rexulti), and cariprazine (Vraylar). They can be described as dopamine system stabilizers that act by reducing dopamine activity in some brain regions while increasing it in others. Aripiprazole and brexpiprazole act as D_2 partial agonists (meaning that they attach to the D_2 receptor without fully activating it, reducing the effective level of dopamine activity). Cariprazine acts as a partial agonist more on D_3 than D_2 receptors, which may help improve cognitive symptoms.

One significant disadvantage of the atypicals, with the exception of ziprasidone and aripiprazole, is that they have a tendency to cause significant weight gain. Metabolic syndrome—which includes weight gain, dyslipidemia, and altered glucose metabolism—is a significant concern with the administration of most atypicals and increases the risk for diabetes, hypertension, and atherosclerotic heart disease (McDaid & Smyth, 2015). An additional disadvantage of atypicals is cost: they are more expensive than conventional antipsychotics. Table 15-7 lists the classifications, routes, and adverse-effect profiles of the antipsychotic drugs.

Conventional Antipsychotics

Conventional antipsychotics are antagonists at the dopamine D_2 receptor site in both the limbic and the motor centres. This blockage of dopamine D_2 receptor sites in the motor areas causes extrapyramidal side effects (EPSs), which include akathisia, acute dystonias, pseudoparkinsonism, and tardive dyskinesia. Other adverse reactions include anticholinergic effects, orthostasis, photosensitivity, and lowered seizure threshold.

Specific drugs are often chosen for their adverse-effect profiles. For example, chlorpromazine is the most sedating agent and has fewer EPSs than do other antipsychotic agents, but it causes significant hypotension. Haloperidol (Haldol) is less sedating and induces less hypotension but has a high incidence of EPSs. As a result, haloperidol has value for treating hallucinations because of its effectiveness in controlling positive symptoms with minimal hypotension and sedation. People taking these medications may

TABLE 15-7 ANTIPSYCHOTIC DRUGS: CLASSIFICATION, ROUTE, AND ADVERSE-EFFECT PROFILE

GENERIC (BRAND)	ROUTE	EPSS	SEDATION	ORTHOSTATIC HYPOTENSION	ANTICHOLINERGIC	WEIGHT GAIN	DIABETES
Atypical Antipsychotics—Treat Positive and Negative Symptoms							
Aripiprazole (Abilify)	PO	Very low	Low	Low	None	Low	Low
Clozapine (Clozaril)	PO	Very low	High	Moderate	High	High	High
Olanzapine (Zyprexa)	PO, IM	Very low	High	Moderate	High	High	High
Paliperidone (Invega)	PO	Moderate	Low	Low	None	Moderate	*
Quetiapine (Seroquel)	PO	Very low	Moderate	Moderate	None	Moderate	Moderate
Risperidone (Risperdal)	PO, IM	Very low	Low	Low	None	Moderate	Moderate
Ziprasidone (Zeldox)	PO, IM	Moderate	Moderate	Moderate	None	Low	Low
Conventional Antipsychotics—Treat Positive Symptoms							
Low Potency							
Chlorpromazine (generic only)	PO, IM, IV, R	Moderate	High	High	Moderate	Moderate	—
Medium Potency							
Loxapine (Loxapac)	PO	Moderate	Moderate	Low	Low	Low	—
Perphenazine (generic only)	PO	Moderate	Moderate	Low	Low	—	—
High Potency							
Thiothixene (Navane)	PO	High	Low	Moderate	Low	Moderate	—
Fluphenazine (Modecate)	PO, IM	High	Low	Low	Low	—	—
Haloperidol (Haldol)	PO, IM	High	Low	Low	Low	Moderate	—
Pimozide (Orap)	PO	High	Moderate	Low	Moderate	—	—
Conventional Antipsychotics for Which Limited Data Are Available							
Flupentixol (Fluanxol, Fluanxol Depot)	PO, IM	High	Low	Moderate	Low	—	—
Zuclopenthixol (Clopixol, Clopixol Depot, Clopixol Acuphase)	PO IM	—	—	—	May potentiate ACh adverse effects of other drugs	—	—

ACh, Anticholinergic; *EPSs*, extrapyramidal side effects; *IM*, intramuscular; *IV*, intravenous; *PO*, oral; *R*, rectal.
*Data unavailable

Sources: Centre for Addiction and Mental Health. (2012). *Understanding psychiatric medications: Antipsychotics.* Retrieved from https://www.camh.ca/en/education/about/camh_publications/Documents/Flat_PDFs/upm_antipsychotics.pdf; Burchum, J., & Rosenthal, L. (2016). *Lehne's pharmacology for nursing care* (9th ed.). St. Louis: Elsevier; and Freudenreich, O. D., Goff, D. C., & Henderson, D. C. (2016). Antipsychotics. In T. A. Stern, M. Fava, T. E. Wilens, et al. (Eds.), *Massachusetts General Hospital comprehensive clinical psychiatry* (2nd ed., pp. 475–488). Philadelphia: Elsevier.

prefer less sedating drugs, but those who are agitated or excitable may do better with a more sedating medication.

Conventional antipsychotics are becoming less common in the treatment of schizophrenia because of their minimal impact on negative symptoms and their adverse effects. However, conventional antipsychotics are effective against positive symptoms, are much less expensive than atypicals, and come in a depot (long-acting injectable) form, which is given once or twice a month. (*Note:* Risperidone, an atypical antipsychotic, is also available in a depot form [Risperdal Consta].) For people who respond to them and can tolerate their adverse effects, conventional antipsychotics remain an appropriate choice (Rummel-Kluge, Komossa, Corves, et al., 2009), especially when metabolic syndrome or cost is a concern.

The conventional antipsychotics are often divided into low-potency and high-potency drugs on the basis of their anticholinergic (ACh) adverse effects, EPSs, and sedative profiles:

Low potency = high sedation + high ACh + low EPSs

High potency = low sedation + low ACh + high EPSs

Conventional antipsychotics must be used cautiously in people with seizure disorders, as they can lower the seizure threshold. Three of the more common EPSs are acute dystonia (acute sustained contraction of muscles, usually of the head and neck), akathisia (psychomotor restlessness evident as pacing or fidgeting, sometimes pronounced and very distressing to patients), and pseudoparkinsonism (a medication-induced, temporary constellation of symptoms associated with Parkinson's disease: tremor, reduced accessory movements, impaired gait, and stiffening of muscles). Most patients develop tolerance to these EPSs after a few months.

EPSs can usually be minimized by lowering dosages or adding antiparkinson drugs, especially centrally acting anticholinergic drugs such as trihexyphenidyl and benztropine mesylate (Cogentin). Diphenhydramine hydrochloride (Benadryl) is also useful. Lorazepam, a benzodiazepine, may be helpful in reducing akathisia.

Unfortunately, antiparkinson drugs can cause significant ACh adverse effects and worsen the ACh adverse effects of conventional antipsychotics and other anticholinergic medications. These adverse effects include anticholinergic syndrome, which is seen in the peripheral nervous system (tachycardia, hyperthermia, hypertension, dry skin, urinary retention, functional ileus) and central nervous system (mydriasis, hallucinations, delirium, seizures, and, in some cases, coma) (Wilson, Shannon, & Sheilds, 2017). Other troubling adverse effects of conventional antipsychotics include weight gain, sexual dysfunction, endocrine disturbances (e.g., galactorrhea), drooling, and tardive dyskinesia, discussed below. Weight gain, frequently a problem for women, can be more than 45 kilograms; therefore changing the antipsychotic medication may be necessary. Impotence and sexual dysfunction are occasionally reported (but frequently experienced) by men and may also necessitate a medication change.

Table 15-8 identifies common adverse effects of the conventional antipsychotic medications, their usual times of onset, and related nursing and medical interventions.

Tardive dyskinesia (TD or TDK) is a persistent EPS that usually appears after prolonged treatment and persists even after the medication has been discontinued. TD is evidenced by involuntary tonic muscular contractions that typically involve the tongue, fingers, toes, neck, trunk, or pelvis. This potentially serious EPS is most frequently seen in women and older persons and affects up to 50% of individuals receiving long-term, high-dose therapy. TD varies from mild to moderate and can be disfiguring or incapacitating; a common presentation is a guppylike mouth movement sometimes accompanied by tongue protrusion. Its appearance can contribute to the stigmatization of people with mental illness.

Early symptoms of TD are fasciculations of the tongue (described as looking like a bag of worms) or constant smacking of the lips. These symptoms can progress into uncontrollable biting, chewing, or sucking motions; an open mouth; and lateral movements of the jaw. No reliable treatment exists for TD. The National Institute of Mental Health (NIMH) developed the Abnormal Involuntary Movement Scale (AIMS), a brief test for the detection of TD and other involuntary movements (Figure 15-4). It examines facial, oral, extremity, and trunk movement. Regularly administering the AIMS examination to detect TD as early as possible is a key nursing role.

Potentially Dangerous Responses to Antipsychotics

Nurses need to know about some rare—but serious and potentially fatal—effects of antipsychotic drugs, including neuroleptic malignant syndrome, agranulocytosis, liver impairment, and anticholinergic-induced delirium.

Neuroleptic malignant syndrome (NMS) occurs in about 0.2% to 1% of people who have taken conventional antipsychotics, although it can occur with atypicals as well. Acute reduction in brain dopamine activity plays a role in its development. NMS is a life-threatening medical emergency and is fatal in about 10% of cases. It usually occurs early in therapy but has been reported in people after 20 years of treatment.

NMS is characterized by reduced consciousness, increased muscle tone (muscular rigidity), and autonomic dysfunction—including hyperpyrexia, labile hypertension, tachycardia, tachypnea, diaphoresis, and drooling. Treatment consists of early detection, discontinuation of the antipsychotic, management of fluid balance, temperature reduction, and monitoring for complications. Mild cases of NMS may be treated with benzodiazepines, vitamins E and B_6, or bromocriptine. More severe cases may even be treated with electroconvulsive therapy (ECT) (Agar, 2010). Dantrolene, recommended in much of the literature, carries a Black Box Warning (the most serious medication warning required by the U.S. Food and Drug Administration) for hepatotoxicity in the United States (Agar, 2010) and is not available in Canada.

Agranulocytosis is a serious, potentially fatal, adverse effect. Liver impairment may also occur. Nurses need to be aware of the prodromal signs and symptoms of these adverse effects and teach them to patients and their families (see Table 15-8).

Anticholinergic-induced delirium is a potentially life-threatening adverse effect usually seen in older adults, although it can occur in younger people as well. It is also seen in patients taking

TABLE 15-8 ADVERSE EFFECTS OF CONVENTIONAL ANTIPSYCHOTICS AND RELATED NURSING INTERVENTIONS

ADVERSE EFFECT	NURSING INTERVENTIONS
Dry mouth	Provide frequent sips of water, ice chips, and sugarless candy or gum; if severe, provide moisture spray
Urinary retention and hesitancy	Check voiding
	Try warm towel on abdomen, and consider catheterization if no result
Constipation	Usually short term
	May use stool softener
	Ensure adequate fluid intake
	Increase fibre intake
	Use dietary laxatives (e.g., prune juice)
Blurred vision	Usually abates in 1 to 2 weeks
	May require use of reading or magnifying glasses
	If intolerable, consider consult regarding change in medication
Photosensitivity	Encourage person to wear sunglasses, sunscreen, and sun-blocking clothing
	Limit exposure to sunlight
Dry eyes	Use artificial tears
Inhibition of ejaculation or impotence in men	Consult prescriber: person may need alternative medication
Anticholinergic-induced delirium: dry mucous membranes; reduced or absent peristalsis; mydriasis; nonreactive pupils; hot, dry, red skin; hyperpyrexia without diaphoresis; tachycardia; agitation; unstable vital signs; worsening of psychotic symptoms; delirium; urinary retention; seizure; repetitive motor movements	***Potentially life-threatening medical emergency***
	Consult prescriber immediately
	Hold all medications
	Implement emergency cooling measures as ordered (cooling blanket, alcohol, or ice bath)
	Implement urinary catheterization as needed
	Administer benzodiazepines or other sedation as ordered
	Physostigmine may be ordered
Pseudoparkinsonism: masklike facies, stiff and stooped posture, shuffling gait, drooling, tremor, "pill-rolling" phenomenon	Administer prn antiparkinson agent (e.g., trihexyphenidyl or benztropine)
Onset: 5 hours–30 days	If intolerable, consult prescriber regarding medication change
Acute dystonic reactions: acute contractions of tongue, face, neck, and back (usually tongue and jaw first)	Provide towel or handkerchief to wipe excess saliva
Opisthotonos: tetanic heightening of entire body, head and belly up	Administer antiparkinson agent as above—give IM for more rapid effect and because of swallowing difficulty
Oculogyric crisis: eyes locked upward	Also consider diphenhydramine hydrochloride (Benadryl) 25–50 mg IM or IV
Laryngeal dystonia: could threaten airway (rare)	Relief usually occurs in 5–15 minutes
Cogwheel rigidity: stiffness and clicking in elbow joints felt by the examiner during passive range of motion (early indicator of acute dystonia)	Prevent further dystonias with antiparkinson agent (see Table 15-8)
Onset: 1–5 days	Experience can be frightening, and person may fear choking
	Accompany to quiet area to provide comfort and support
	Assist person to understand the event and avert distortion or mistrust of medications
	Monitor airway
Akathisia: motor inner-driven restlessness (e.g., tapping foot incessantly, rocking forward and backward in chair, shifting weight from side to side)	Consult prescriber regarding possible medication change
Onset: 2 hours–60 days	Give antiparkinson agent
	Tolerance to akathisia does not develop, but akathisia disappears when neuroleptic is discontinued
	Propranolol (Inderal), lorazepam (Ativan), or diazepam (Valium) may be used
	In severe cases, may cause great distress and contribute to suicidality
Tardive dyskinesia (TD):	No known treatment
Face: protruding and rolling tongue, blowing, smacking, licking, spastic facial distortion, smacking movements	Discontinuing the drug rarely relieves symptoms
Limbs:	Possibly 20% of people taking these drugs for >2 years may develop TD
Choreic: rapid, purposeless, and irregular movements	Nurses and doctors should encourage people to be screened for TD at least every 3 months
Athetoid: slow, complex, and serpentine movements	Onset may merit reconsideration of medications
Trunk: neck and shoulder movements, dramatic hip jerks and rocking, twisting pelvic thrusts	Changes in appearance may contribute to stigmatizing response
Onset: Months to years	Teach patient actions to conceal involuntary movements (purposeful muscle contraction overrides involuntary tardive movements)

TABLE 15-8	ADVERSE EFFECTS OF CONVENTIONAL ANTIPSYCHOTICS AND RELATED NURSING INTERVENTIONS—cont'd	

ADVERSE EFFECT	NURSING INTERVENTIONS
Hypotension and postural hypotension	Check blood pressure before giving agent: a systolic pressure of 80 mm Hg when standing is indication not to give the current dose Advise person to rise slowly to prevent dizziness and hold on to railings or furniture while rising to reduce falls Effect usually subsides when drug is stabilized in 1–2 weeks Elastic bandages may prevent pooling If condition is dangerous, consult prescriber regarding medication change, volume expanders, or pressure agents
Tachycardia	Always evaluate patients with existing cardiac problems before antipsychotic drugs are administered Haloperidol (Haldol) is usually the preferred drug because of its low ACh effects
Agranulocytosis (a rare occurrence, but a possibility the nurse should be aware of): symptoms include sore throat, fever, malaise, and mouth sores; any flulike symptoms should be carefully evaluated *Onset:* During the first 12 weeks of therapy, occurs suddenly	***A potentially dangerous blood dyscrasia*** Blood work usually done every week for 6 months, then every 2 months Physician may order blood work to determine presence of leukopenia or agranulocytosis If test results are positive, the drug is discontinued, and reverse isolation may be initiated Mortality is high if the drug is not ceased and if treatment is not initiated Teach person to observe for signs of infection
Cholestatic jaundice: rare, reversible, and usually benign if caught in time; prodromal symptoms are fever, malaise, nausea, and abdominal pain; jaundice appears 1 week later	Consult prescriber regarding possible medication change Bed rest and high-protein, high-carbohydrate diet if ordered Liver function tests should be performed every 6 months
Neuroleptic malignant syndrome (NMS): rare, potentially fatal *Severe extrapyramidal:* severe muscle rigidity, oculogyric crisis, dysphasia, flexor-extensor posturing, cogwheeling *Hyperpyrexia:* elevated temperature (over 39°C or 103°F) *Autonomic dysfunction:* hypertension, tachycardia, diaphoresis, incontinence *Delirium, stupor, coma* *Onset:* Variable, progresses rapidly over 2–3 days *Risk factors:* Concomitant use of psychotropics, older age, female, presence of a mood disorder, and rapid dose titration (increase)	***Acute, life-threatening medical emergency*** Stop neuroleptic Transfer stat to medical unit Bromocriptine can relieve muscle rigidity and reduce fever Cool body to reduce fever (cooling blankets, alcohol, cool water, or ice bath as ordered) Maintain hydration with oral and IV fluids; correct electrolyte imbalance Arrhythmias should be treated Small doses of heparin may decrease possibility of pulmonary emboli Early detection increases patient's chance of survival

Ach, Anticholinergic; *IM,* intramuscular; *IV,* intravenous; *prn,* as needed.
Source: Kemmerer, D. A. (2007). Anticholinergic syndrome. *Journal of Emergency Nursing, 33,* 76–78. doi:10.1016/j.jen.2006.10.013.

multiple antipsychotic drugs. See Table 15-8 for symptoms and treatment of this serious adverse effect.

Adjuncts to Antipsychotic Drug Therapy

Antidepressants are recommended along with antipsychotic agents for the treatment of depression, which is common in schizophrenia. Refer to Chapter 13 for a more detailed discussion of depression and antidepressant drugs.

Antimanic (mood-stabilizing) agents have been helpful in enhancing the effectiveness of antipsychotics. Valproic acid (Epival, Valproate) is used during acute exacerbations of psychosis to hasten response to antipsychotics (Freudenreich, Goff, & Henderson, 2016). Lamotrigine may be given along with clozapine to improve therapeutic effects.

Augmentation with benzodiazepines (e.g., clonazepam) can reduce anxiety and agitation and contribute to improvement in positive and negative symptoms (Wilson, Shannon, & Sheilds, 2017).

When to Change an Antipsychotic Regimen

The following circumstances suggest a need to adjust or change the antipsychotic agent or add supplemental medications (e.g., lithium, carbamazepine, valproate):

- Inadequate improvement in target symptoms despite an adequate trial of the drug
- Persistence of dangerous or intolerable adverse effects

Specific Interventions for Paranoia, Catatonia, and Disorganization

The following sections discuss paranoia, catatonia, and disorganization in psychoses and identify pertinent communication guidelines, self-care needs, and milieu needs.

Paranoia

Any intense and strongly defended irrational suspicion can be regarded as paranoia. Paranoia is evident, at least intermittently, in many people without psychotic disorders but is verified as

ABNORMAL INVOLUNTARY MOVEMENT SCALE (AIMS)

Public Health Service
Alcohol, Drug Abuse, and Mental Health Administration
National Institute of Mental Health

Name: _____
Date: _____
Prescribing Practitioner: _____

Code: 0 = None
1 = Minimal, may be extreme normal
2 = Mild
3 = Moderate
4 = Severe

Instructions: Complete Examination Procedure before making ratings.

Movement ratings: Rate highest severity observed. Rate movements that occur upon activation one *less* than those observed spontaneously. Circle movement as well as code number that applies.		Rater Date	Rater Date	Rater Date	Rater Date
Facial and Oral Movements	**1. Muscles of facial expression** (e.g., movements of forehead, eyebrows, periorbital area, cheeks, including frowning, blinking, smiling, grimacing)	0 1 2 3 4	0 1 2 3 4	0 1 2 3 4	0 1 2 3 4
	2. Lips and perioral area (e.g., puckering, pouting, smacking)	0 1 2 3 4	0 1 2 3 4	0 1 2 3 4	0 1 2 3 4
	3. Jaw (e.g., biting, clenching, chewing, mouth opening, lateral movement)	0 1 2 3 4	0 1 2 3 4	0 1 2 3 4	0 1 2 3 4
	4. Tongue: Rate only increases in movement both in and out of mouth — *not* inability to sustain movement. Darting in and out of mouth.	0 1 2 3 4	0 1 2 3 4	0 1 2 3 4	0 1 2 3 4
Extremity Movements	**5. Upper (arms, wrists, hands, fingers):** Include choreic movements (i.e., rapid, objectively purposeless, irregular, spontaneous) and athetoid movements (i.e., slow, irregular, complex, serpentine). *Do not include tremor* (i.e., repetitive, regular, rhythmic).	0 1 2 3 4	0 1 2 3 4	0 1 2 3 4	0 1 2 3 4
	6. Lower (legs, knees, ankles, toes) (e.g., lateral knee movement, foot tapping, heel dropping, foot squirming, inversion and eversion of foot)	0 1 2 3 4	0 1 2 3 4	0 1 2 3 4	0 1 2 3 4
Trunk Movements	**7. Neck, shoulder, hips** (e.g., rocking, twisting, squirming, pelvic gyrations)	0 1 2 3 4	0 1 2 3 4	0 1 2 3 4	0 1 2 3 4
Global Judgments	**8. Severity of abnormal movements overall**	0 1 2 3 4	0 1 2 3 4	0 1 2 3 4	0 1 2 3 4
	9. Incapacitation due to abnormal movements	0 1 2 3 4	0 1 2 3 4	0 1 2 3 4	0 1 2 3 4
	10. Patient's awareness of abnormal movements: Rate only patient's report. No awareness 0 Aware, no distress 1 Aware, mild distress 2 Aware, moderate distress 3 Aware, severe distress 4	0 1 2 3 4	0 1 2 3 4	0 1 2 3 4	0 1 2 3 4
Dental Status	**11. Current problems with teeth and/or dentures**	No Yes	No Yes	No Yes	No Yes
	12. Are dentures usually worn?	No Yes	No Yes	No Yes	No Yes
	13. Edentia	No Yes	No Yes	No Yes	No Yes
	14. Do movements disappear in sleep?	No Yes	No Yes	No Yes	No Yes

FIGURE 15-4 Abnormal Involuntary Movement Scale (AIMS).

AIMS Examination Procedure
Either before or after completing the Examination Procedure, observe the patient unobtrusively, at rest (e.g., in waiting room).

The chair to be used in this examination should be a hard, firm one without arms.

1. Ask patient to remove shoes and socks.
2. Ask patient whether there is anything in his or her mouth (e.g., gum, candy) and, if there is, to remove it.
3. Ask patient about the *current* condition of his or her teeth. Ask patient if he or she wears dentures. Do teeth or dentures bother the patient *now?*
4. Ask patient whether he or she notices any movements in mouth, face, hands, or feet. If yes, ask to describe and to what extent they *currently* bother patient or interfere with his or her activities.
5. Have patient sit in chair with hands on knees, legs slightly apart, and feet flat on floor. Look at entire body movements while in this position.
6. Ask patient to sit with hands hanging unsupported: if male, between legs; if female and wearing a dress, hanging over knees. Observe hands and other body areas.
7. Ask patient to open mouth. Observe tongue at rest within mouth. Do this twice.
8. Ask patient to protrude tongue. Observe abnormalities of tongue movement. Do this twice.
9. Ask patient to tap thumb, with each finger, as rapidly as possible for 10 to 15 seconds, separately with right hand, then with left hand. Observe each facial and leg movement.
10. Flex and extend patient's left and right arms (one at a time). Note any rigidity.
11. Ask patient to stand up. Observe in profile. Observe all body areas again, hips included.
12. Ask patient to extend both arms outstretched in front with palms down. Observe trunk, legs, and mouth.
13. Have patient walk a few paces, turn, and walk back to chair. Observe hands and gait. Do this twice.

FIGURE 15-4, cont'd

irrational and discarded by the reality-testing process. This process fails in people experiencing paranoia concomitant with psychotic disorders. For them, paranoid ideas cannot be corrected by experiences or modified by facts or reality. *Projection* is the most common defence mechanism used in paranoia: when individuals with paranoia feel angry (or self-critical), they project the feeling onto others and believe that others are angry with (or harshly critical toward) them—as if to say, "I'm not angry—you are!"

Schizophrenia with predominantly paranoid symptoms usually has a later age of onset (late twenties to thirties), develops rapidly in individuals with good premorbid functioning, tends to be intermittent during the first 5 years of the illness, and, in some cases, is associated with a good outcome or complete recovery. People with paranoia are usually frightened and may behave defensively (e.g., a delusion that another person is planning to kill the patient can result in the patient attacking or killing that person first). The paranoia is often a defence against painful feelings of loneliness, despair, helplessness, and fear of abandonment. Useful nursing strategies are outlined in the following sections.

Communication guidelines. Because people with paranoia have difficulty trusting those around them, they are usually guarded, tense, and reserved. To ensure interpersonal distance, they may adopt a superior, aloof, hostile, or sarcastic attitude, disparaging and dwelling on the shortcomings of others to maintain their self-esteem. Although they may shun interpersonal contact, functional impairment other than paranoia may be minimal. These people frequently misinterpret the intent or actions of others, perceiving oversights as personal rejection. They also may personalize unrelated events (**ideas of reference**, or *referentiality*). For example, a patient might see a nurse

talking to the psychiatrist and believe that the two are talking about her.

During care, a patient suffering from paranoia may make offensive yet accurate criticisms of staff and of unit policies. It is important that responses focus on reducing the patient's anxiety and fear and not be defensive reactions or rejections of the patient. Staff conferences and clinical supervision help maintain objectivity and a therapeutic perspective about the patient's motivation and behaviour, increasing professional effectiveness.

Self-care needs. People with paranoia usually have stronger ego resources than do individuals in whom other symptoms predominate; this is particularly evident in occupational functioning and capacity for independent living. Grooming, dress, and self-care may not be problems and may, in fact, be meticulous. Nutrition, however, may be affected by a delusion, such as that the food is poisoned. Providing foods in commercially sealed packaging—for example, peanut butter and crackers or nutritional drinks in cartons—can improve nutrition. If people worry that others will harm them when they are asleep, they may be fearful of going to sleep—a problem that impairs restorative rest and warrants nursing intervention.

Milieu needs. A person with paranoia may become physically aggressive in response to his or her paranoid hallucinations or delusions. The person projects hostile drives onto others and then acts on these drives. Homosexual urges are projected onto others as well, and fear of sexual advances from others may stimulate aggression. An environment that provides a sense of security and safety minimizes anxiety and environmental distortions. Activities that distract the patient from ruminating on paranoid themes also decrease anxiety.

Case Study and Nursing Care Plan 15-1 discusses a person with paranoia.

Catatonia: Withdrawn Phase

The essential feature of catatonia is abnormal levels of motor behaviour, either extreme motor agitation or extreme motor retardation. Other associated behaviours include posturing, waxy flexibility (described below), stereotyped behaviour, muteness, extreme negativism or automatic obedience, echolalia, and echopraxia (discussed earlier in this chapter). The onset of catatonia is usually abrupt, and the prognosis favourable. With pharmacotherapy and improved individual management, severe catatonic symptoms are rarely seen today. Useful nursing strategies for intervening in catatonia are discussed in the following sections.

Communication guidelines. People with catatonia can be so withdrawn they appear stuporous or comatose. They can be mute and may remain so for hours, days, or even weeks or months if untreated. Although such patients may not appear to pay attention to events going on around them, they are acutely aware of the environment and may accurately remember events at a later date. Developing skill and confidence in working with withdrawn patients takes practice. The person's inability or refusal to cooperate or participate in activities challenges staff to work to remain objective and avert frustration and anger.

Self-care needs. In extreme withdrawal, a person may need to be hand- or tube-fed to maintain adequate nutritional status. Aspiration is a risk. Normal control over bladder and bowel functions may be interrupted, so the assessment and management of urinary or bowel retention or incontinence is essential. When physical movements are minimal or absent, range-of-motion exercises can reduce muscular atrophy, calcium depletion, and contractures. Dressing and grooming usually require direct assistance.

Milieu needs. The catatonic person's appearance may range from decreased spontaneous movement to complete stupor. Waxy flexibility is often seen; for example, if the patient raises arms over the head, he or she may maintain that position for hours or longer. Caution is advised because, even after holding a single posture for long periods, the patient may suddenly and without provocation show brief outbursts of gross motor activity in response to inner hallucinations, delusions, and changes in neurotransmitter levels.

Catatonia: Excited Phase

Communication guidelines. During the excited stage of catatonia, the patient is in a state of greatly increased motor activity. He or she may talk or shout continually and incoherently, requiring the nurse's communication to be clear, direct, and loud (enough to focus the patient's attention on the nurse) and to reflect concern for the safety of the patient and others.

Self-care needs. A person who is constantly and intensely hyperactive can become completely exhausted and even die if medical attention is not available. Patients with coexisting medical conditions (e.g., congestive heart failure) are most at risk. Intramuscular administration of a sedating antipsychotic is often required to reduce psychomotor agitation to a safer level. During heightened physical activity, the patient requires stimulation reduction and additional fluids, calories, and rest. It is not unusual for the agitated person to be destructive or aggressive to others

in response to hallucinations or delusions or inner distress. Many of the concerns and interventions are the same as those for mania. See Chapter 14 for more information about bipolar disorders.

Disorganization

Disorganization represents the most regressed and socially impaired form of schizophrenia. A person with disorganization may have marked associative looseness, grossly inappropriate affect, bizarre mannerisms, and incoherence of speech and may display extreme social withdrawal. Delusions and hallucinations are fragmentary and poorly organized. Behaviour may be considered odd, and a giggling or grimacing response to internal stimuli is common.

Disorganization has an earlier age of onset (early to middle teens), often develops insidiously, is associated with poor premorbid functioning and a significant family history of psychiatric disorders, and carries a poor prognosis. Often these people reside in long-term care facilities and can live safely in the community only in a structured, well-supervised setting or with intensive follow-up such as a PACT (Program for Assertive Community Treatment) service. Families of patients living at home need significant community support, respite care, and access to day hospital services. Unfortunately, a good portion of these people experience housing instability, which further adds to stressors that contribute to psychosis and difficulties with access to mental health services as well as adherence to anti-psychotic prescription (Rezansoff, Moniruzzaman, Fazel, et al., 2016). See the Case Study and Nursing Care Plan for Disorganized Thinking on the Evolve website.

Communication guidelines. People with disorganization experience persistent and severe perceptual and communication problems. Communication should be concise, clear, and concrete. Tasks should be broken into discrete tasks that are performed one at a time. Repeated refocusing may be needed to keep the patient on topic or to allow task completion. This repetition can be frustrating to the nurse and others, requiring special effort to identify and correct counter-transference and nontherapeutic responses.

Self-care needs. In people with disorganization, grooming is neglected; hair is often dirty and matted, and clothes are unclean and often inappropriate for the weather (presenting a risk to self). Cognition, memory, and executive function are grossly impaired, and the person is frequently too disorganized to carry out simple activities of daily living (ADLs). Areas of nursing focus include encouraging optimal levels of functioning, preventing further regression, and offering alternatives for inappropriate behaviours whenever possible. Significant direct assistance for ADLs is also needed.

Milieu needs. People with disorganization need assistance to conform their behaviour to social expectations. Nurses should provide for the patient's privacy needs. Peer education about the disorder may reduce peer frustration and acting out.

Advanced-Practice Interventions

Services that may be provided by advanced-practice nurses and nurse therapists include psychotherapy, cognitive behavioural

VIGNETTE

Martin, a 36-year-old man, is accompanied to the mental health centre by his mother. Ms. Lam, Martin's nurse, obtains background information from his mother. According to her, he had been in a long-term care facility for treatment of schizophrenia for 3 months and, after his discharge, had been doing well at home until recently. His only employment history was 5 months as a janitor after high school graduation. His mother states that, as a teenager, Martin was an excellent athlete and received average grades. At age 17, he had his first psychotic break, when he took various street drugs. His behaviour became markedly bizarre (e.g., eating cat food and swallowing a rubber-soled heel, which precipitated an emergency laparotomy).

Ms. Lam meets with Martin. He is unshaven and dishevelled. He is wearing a headband that holds Popsicle sticks and paper scraps. He chain-smokes, paces, and frequently changes position. He reports that he is Alice from Alice in the Underground and that people from space hurt him with needles. His speech is marked by associative looseness and occasional blocking, and he often stops in the middle of a phrase and giggles to himself.

He starts to giggle, and Ms. Lam asks what he is thinking about. He states, "You interrupted me." He then begins to shake his head while repeating in a singsong voice, "Shake them tigers ... shake them tigers. ..." He denies suicidal or homicidal ideation. Ms. Lam notes that Martin has great difficulty accurately perceiving what is going on around him. He exhibits regressed social behaviours (e.g., eating with his hands and picking his nose in public). He has no apparent insight into his problems, telling Ms. Lam that his biggest problem is the people in space.

therapy (CBT), group therapy, medication administration, social skills training, cognitive remediation, and family therapy. Family therapy is one of the most important interventions the advanced-practice nurse or nurse therapist can implement for the patient with schizophrenia.

Family Therapy

Family therapy is a service usually delivered by health care providers with specific education in this area, including advanced-practice nurses, nurse therapists, master's-prepared social workers, and registered marriage and family therapists. The field of family therapy was actually originally developed as a treatment for schizophrenia. Families of people with schizophrenia, particularly direct caregivers, often endure considerable hardships while coping with the psychotic and residual symptoms of the illness. The patient and family may become isolated from other relatives, communities, and support systems. In fact, until the 1970s (and sometimes even today), families were often blamed for causing schizophrenia in the affected family member.

Family education and family therapy improve the quality of life for the person with schizophrenia and reduce the relapse rate for many.

Programs that provide support, education, coping skills training, and social network development are extremely effective. This psychoeducational approach brings educational and behavioural approaches into family treatment and does not blame families but, rather, recognizes them as secondary victims of a biological

 RESEARCH HIGHLIGHT

Family Psychoeducation Interventions for Psychosis and Schizophrenia

Problem

Family psychoeducation seeks to engage family members as more sophisticated partners, complementing interventions by clinicians with specialized interactions and coping skills that counter the neurological deficits inherent to the disorder.

Although the scientific evidence is increasingly strong that the major psychotic disorders are based in genetic, neurochemical, inflammatory, and/or neurodevelopmental defects involving brain function and structure, there is also abundant evidence that the first onset, progression, and relapse of psychotic or severe mood symptoms are the result of psychosocial stress. Family psychoeducation is a structured method for incorporating a patient's family members, other caregivers, and friends into acute and ongoing treatment and rehabilitation. Based on a family–patient–professional partnership, the approach differs from family therapy, as the family is not the object of therapy but rather the collaborative implementer of therapy. The most common models are essentially cognitive behavioral therapy with consistent inclusion of family members as collaborators.

Purpose of Study

This study sought to understand particular mechanisms of efficacy of family psychoeducation.

Methods

This study method was a comprehensive scientific, theoretical, and clinical review of the evidence spanning four decades.

Key Findings

Family psychoeducation has proved to be one of the most consistently effective treatments available. Reports on outcome studies now number more than 100, while meta-analyses put relapse rate reduction at 50% to 60% over treatment as usual. The most recent application in first episode and prodromal psychosis, combined with other evidence-based interventions, is yielding some of the most promising results yet achieved—substantial return of functioning and avoidance of psychosis altogether. Patients who experience frequent hospitalizations or prolonged unemployment benefit substantially and often dramatically, as do families who are especially exasperated or confused about the illness or even hostile toward the patient.

Implications for Nursing Practice

Family psychoeducation has been deemed an evidence-based practice and has been included in various treatment guidelines for schizophrenia and other serious mental illnesses. Family intervention is particularly beneficial in the early years of the course of a mental illness, when improvements can have a dramatic and long-term effect and while family members are still involved and open to participation, change in attitude, and interaction with the patient.

Source: McFarlane, W. R. (2016). Family interventions for schizophrenia and the psychoses: A review. *Family Process, 55*(3), 460–482. doi:10.1111/famp.12235.

illness. In family therapy sessions, fears, faulty communication patterns, and distortions are identified; problem-solving skills are taught; healthier alternatives to conflict are explored; and guilt and anxiety can be lessened.

EVALUATION

Evaluation is especially important in planning care for people who have psychotic disorders. Outcome expectations that are unrealistic discourage the patient and staff alike. It is critical for staff to remember that change is a process that occurs over time. For a person with schizophrenia, progress may occur erratically, and gains may be difficult to discern in the short term.

Chronically ill people must be reassessed regularly so that new data can be considered and treatment adjusted when needed. Questions to be asked include the following:

- Is the patient not progressing because a more important need is not being met?
- Is the staff making the best use of the patient's strengths and interests to promote treatment and achieve desired outcomes?
- Are other possible interventions being overlooked?
- Are new or better interventions available?
- How is the patient responding to existing or recently changed medications or other treatments?
- Is the patient becoming discouraged, anxious, or depressed?
- Is the patient participating in treatment? Are adverse effects controlled or troubling?
- Is functioning improving or regressing?
- What is the patient's quality of life, and is it improving?
- Is the family involved, supportive, and knowledgeable regarding the patient's disorder and treatment?

Active staff involvement and interest in the patient's progress communicate concern and caring, help the patient to maximize progress, promote participation in treatment, and reduce staff feelings of helplessness and burnout. Input from the patient can offer valuable information about why a certain desired outcome has not occurred.

CASE STUDY AND NURSING CARE PLAN 15-1

Paranoia in Schizophrenia

Tom, a 34-year-old man, is an inpatient at a Veterans Affairs Canada hospital. He has been separated from his wife and four children for 3 years. His records state that he has been in and out of hospitals for 13 years. Tom is a former master seaman who first "heard voices" at the age of 21 while he was serving as a peacekeeper in Afghanistan. He subsequently received a medical discharge.

The hospitalization was precipitated by an exacerbation of auditory hallucinations. "I thought people were following me. I hear voices, usually a woman's voice, and she's tormenting me. People say that it happens because I don't take my medications. The medications make me tired, and I can't have sex." Tom also uses marijuana, which he knows increases his paranoia. "It makes me feel good, and not much else does." Tom finished 11 years of school but did not graduate. He says he has no close friends. He spent 5 years in prison for manslaughter and was abusing alcohol and drugs when the crime occurred. Drug abuse has also been a contributing factor to Tom's psychiatric hospitalizations.

Jodie is Tom's nurse. Tom is dressed in a T-shirt and jeans, his hygiene is good, and he is well nourished. He reports that "the voices get worse at night, and I can't sleep." Jodie notes in Tom's medical record that he has had two episodes of suicidal ideation, during which the voices were telling him to jump "off rooftops" and "in front of trains." During the first interview, Tom rarely makes eye contact and speaks in a low monotone. At times, he glances about the room as if distracted, mumbles to himself, and appears upset.

Nurse: "Tom, my name is Jodie. I will be your nurse today and every day that I am here. If it is okay with you, we will meet every day for 30 minutes at 10 in the morning. We can talk about areas of concern to you."

Tom: "Well, don't believe what they say about me. I want to start. ... Are you married?"

Nurse: "This time is for you to talk about your concerns."

Tom: "Oh ..." (Looks furtively around the room, then lowers his eyes) "I think someone is trying to kill me. ..."

Nurse: "You seem to be focusing on something other than our conversation."

Tom: "The voices tell me things ... I can't say ..."

Nurse: "It seems like the voices are upsetting to you. I can't hear them. What kinds of things are they saying?"

Tom: "The voices tell me bad things."

Jodie stays with Tom and encourages him to communicate with her. As Tom focuses more on the conversation, his anxiety appears to lessen. His thoughts become more connected, he is able to concentrate more, and he mumbles to himself less.

ASSESSMENT

Self-Assessment

On the first day of admission, Tom assaults another male patient, stating that the other person accused him of being a homosexual and touched him on the buttocks. After assessing the incident, the staff agrees that Tom's provocation came more from his own projections (Tom's sexual attraction to the other person) than from anything the other person did or said.

Tom's difficulty with impulse control frightens Jodie. She has concerns regarding Tom's ability to curb his impulses and the possibility of Tom's striking out at her, especially when Tom is hallucinating and highly delusional. Jodie mentions her concerns to the nursing coordinator, who suggests that Jodie meet with Tom in the day room until he demonstrates more control and less suspicion of others. After 5 days, Tom is less excitable, and the sessions are moved to a room reserved for private interviews. Jodie also speaks with a senior staff nurse regarding her fears. By talking to the senior nurse and understanding more clearly her own fear, Jodie is able to manage her fear and identify interventions to help Tom regain a better sense of control.

CASE STUDY AND NURSING CARE PLAN 15-1—cont'd

Paranoia in Schizophrenia

Objective Data	Subjective Data
Speaks in low monotone	"I hear voices."
Makes poor eye contact	"I think someone is trying to kill me. ..."
Weight appropriate for height	"I don't take my medications. [They] make me tired, and I
Clean, bathed, clothes match	can't have sex."
Impaired reality testing	"The voices get worse at night and I can't sleep."
Has a history of drug abuse (marijuana), which appears to contribute	"[Marijuana] makes me feel good, and not much else does."
to relapses	Voices have told him to jump "off rooftops" and "in front of
Has no close friends, separated from wife and children	trains."
Was first hospitalized at age 21 and has not worked since that time	
Has had suicidal impulses twice, both associated with command	
hallucinations	
Was imprisoned for 5 years for violence (manslaughter) and	
assaulted a peer in the hospital	
Thoughts scattered when anxious	

DIAGNOSIS

1. *Disturbed thought processes* related to alteration in neurological function, as evidenced by persecutory hallucinations and paranoia

Supporting Data

- Voices have told him to jump "off rooftops" and "in front of trains."
- "I think someone is trying to kill me."
- Abuses marijuana (although it increases paranoia) because "it makes me feel good."

2. *Nonadherence to medication regimen* related to adverse effects of therapy, as evidenced by verbalization of nonadherence and persistence of symptoms

Supporting Data

- Failure to take prescribed medications because "they make me tired, and I can't have sex."
- Chronic history of relapse of symptoms

OUTCOMES IDENTIFICATION

1. Tom consistently refrains from acting on his "voices" and suspicions.
2. Tom consistently adheres to treatment regimen.

PLANNING

The nurse plans interventions that will (1) help Tom deal with his disturbing thoughts and (2) minimize drug abuse and adverse effects of medication to increase adherence and decrease the potential for relapse and violence.

IMPLEMENTATION

1. Nursing diagnosis: *Disturbed thought processes*
   Outcome: Tom consistently refrains from acting on his "voices" and suspicions when they occur.

Short-Term Goal	Intervention	Rationale	Evaluation
1. By the end of the first week, Tom will recognize the presence of hallucinations and identify one or more contributing factors, as evidenced by telling his nurse when they occur and what preceded them.	1a. Meet with Tom each day for 30 minutes to establish trust and rapport. 1b. Explore those times when voices are most threatening and disturbing, noting the circumstances that precede them. 1c. Provide noncompetitive activities that focus on the here and now.	1a. Short, consistent meetings help decrease anxiety and establish trust. 1b. Identifying events that increase anxiety and trigger "voices" and then learning to manage triggers, hallucinations can be reduced. 1c. Increased time spent in reality-based activities decreases focus on hallucinations.	**GOAL MET** By the end of the first week, Tom tells the nurse when he is experiencing hallucinations.

Continued

CASE STUDY AND NURSING CARE PLAN 15-1—cont'd

Paranoia in Schizophrenia

Short-Term Goal	Intervention	Rationale	Evaluation
2. By the end of the first week, Tom will recognize hallucinations as "not real" and ascribe them to his illness.	2a. Explore content of hallucinations with Tom. 2b. Educate Tom about the nature of hallucinations and ways to determine if "voices" are real.	2a. Exploring hallucinations identifies suicidal or aggressive themes or command hallucinations. 2b. Education improves Tom's reality testing and helps him begin to attribute his experiences to schizophrenia.	**GOAL MET** Tom identifies that the voices tell him he is a loser and he needs to be careful "because someone is after me." He identifies that the voices are worse at nighttime. He notes that others do not seem to hear what he hears and also states that smoking marijuana produces very threatening voices.
3. By discharge, Tom will consistently report a decrease in hallucinations.	3. Explore with Tom possible actions that can minimize anxiety and reduce hallucinations, such as whistling or reading aloud.	3. Such activities offer alternatives while anxiety level is relatively low.	**OAL MET** Tom states that he is hearing voices less often, and they are less threatening to him. Tom identifies that if he whistles or sings, he stays calm and can control the voices.

2. Nursing diagnosis: *Nonadherence to medication regimen*
Outcome: Tom consistently adheres to medication regimen.

Short-Term Goal	Intervention	Rationale	Evaluation
1. By the end of week 1, Tom will discuss his concerns about medication with staff.	1a. Evaluate medication response and adverse-effect issues. 1b. Initiate medication change to olanzapine (Zyprexa). Administer a large dose at bedtime to increase sleep and a small dose during the day to decrease fatigue. 1c. Educate Tom regarding adverse effects—how long they last and what actions can be taken.	1a. Such evaluation identifies drugs and dosages that have increased therapeutic value and decreased adverse effects. 1b. Olanzapine causes no known sexual difficulties. 1c. This knowledge can give an increased sense of control over symptoms.	**GOAL MET** Tom identifies the reasons for stopping his medication. He agrees to try olanzapine because he trusts staff's assurances that the adverse effects will be reduced. Tom states that he sleeps better at night but is still tired during the day.
2. By the end of week 2, Tom will describe two ways to reduce or cope with adverse effects and two ways the medications help him meet his goals (e.g., avoiding jail, reducing fear).	2. Connect Tom with the local Schizophrenia Society support group.	2. Being part of a group provides peer support and a chance to hear from others (further along in recovery) how medications can be helpful and adverse effects can be managed. The peer group can also offer suggestions for dealing with his loneliness and other problems.	**GOAL MET** Week 1: Tom attends meeting. Week 2: He speaks in the group about "not feeling good." Several group members say they understand and try to help him figure out why he is not feeling good. Peers tell him how taking medication has helped them feel better.

EVALUATION

By discharge, Tom expresses hope that the medications will help him feel better and avoid problems like jail. He has a better understanding of his medications and what to do for adverse effects. He knows that marijuana increases his symptoms and explains that when he gets lonely, he now has ideas of things other than drugs he can do to "feel good." Tom continues with the support group and outpatient counselling, stating that his reason for doing so is "because Jodie really cared about me"; her caring made him want to get better and led him to trust what staff told him. He reports sleeping much better and says that he has more energy during the day.

KEY POINTS TO REMEMBER

- Schizophrenia is a biological disorder of the brain. It is not one disorder but a group of disorders with overlapping symptoms and treatments.
- Recovery is increasingly possible with early identification, new treatments, and adequate social supports.
- The primary differences among subtypes involve the spectrum of symptoms that dominate their severity, the impairment in affect and cognition, and the impact on social and other areas of functioning.
- Psychotic symptoms are often more pronounced and obvious than are symptoms found in other disorders, making psychosis and schizophrenia more likely to be apparent to others and increasing the risk of stigmatization.
- Neurochemical (catecholamines and serotonin), genetic, and neuroanatomical findings help explain the symptoms of schizophrenia. However, no one theory accounts fully for the complexities of schizophrenia.
- There are four categories of symptoms of schizophrenia: positive, negative, cognitive, and affective. Symptoms vary considerably among people and fluctuate over time.
- The positive symptoms of schizophrenia (e.g., hallucinations, delusions, associative looseness) are more pronounced and respond best to antipsychotic drug therapy.
- The negative symptoms of schizophrenia (e.g., social withdrawal and dysfunction, lack of motivation, reduced affect) respond less well to antipsychotic therapy and tend to be more debilitating.
- The degree of cognitive impairment (cognitive symptom) warrants careful assessment and active intervention to increase the patient's ability to adapt, function, and maximize his or her quality of life.

- Coexisting depression (affective symptom) must be identified and treated to reduce the potential for suicide, substance abuse, nonadherence, and relapse.
- Some applicable nursing diagnoses include *Disturbed sensory perception*, *Disturbed thought processes*, *Impaired communication*, *Ineffective coping*, *Risk for self-directed or other-directed violence*, and *Impaired family coping*.
- Outcomes are chosen based on the type and phase of schizophrenia and the person's individual needs, strengths, and level of functioning. Short-term and intermediate indicators are also developed to better track the incremental progress typical of schizophrenia.
- Interventions for people with schizophrenia include trust building, therapeutic communication techniques, support, assistance with self-care, promotion of independence, stress management, promotion of socialization, psychoeducation to promote understanding and adaptation, milieu management, ognitive behavioural interventions, cognitive enhancement or remediation techniques, and medication administration.
- Because antipsychotic medications are essential in the care of people with schizophrenia, the nurse must understand the properties, adverse and toxic effects, and dosages of conventional and atypical antipsychotics and other medications used to treat schizophrenia. The nurse helps the patient and family understand and appreciate the importance of medication to recovery.
- Schizophrenia can produce counter-transference responses in staff; clinical supervision and self-assessment help the nurse remain objective and therapeutic.
- Hope is closely tied to recovery; it is essential for nurses to hold hope for people with schizophrenia.

CRITICAL THINKING

1. Jasmine, a 24-year-old woman, is hospitalized after an abrupt onset of psychosis and is diagnosed with paranoid schizophrenia. Jasmine is recently divorced and works as a legal secretary. Her work had become erratic, and her suspiciousness was attracting negative responses. Jasmine is being discharged in 2 days to her mother's care until she is able to resume her job. Jasmine's mother is overwhelmed and asks the nurse how she is going to cope: "I can hardly say anything to Jasmine without her getting upset. She is still mad at me because I called 911 and had her admitted. She says there is nothing wrong with her, and I'm worried she'll stop her medication once she is home. What am I going to do?"

    a. Explain Jasmine's behaviour and symptoms to a classmate as you would to Jasmine's mother.

    b. How would you respond to the mother's immediate concerns?

    c. What are some of the priority concerns the nurse should address before discharge?

    d. Identify interventions that are based on the concepts of the recovery model.

    e. What are some community resources that can help support this family? Describe how each could be helpful to this family.

    f. What do you think of the prognosis for Jasmine? Support your position with data regarding Jasmine's diagnosis and the treatment you have planned.

CHAPTER REVIEW

1. Which characteristic in an adolescent female is sometimes associated with the prodromal phase of schizophrenia?
   a. Always afraid another student will steal her belongings
   b. An unusual interest in numbers and specific topics
   c. Demonstrates no interest in athletics or organized sports
   d. Appears more comfortable among males

2. Which nursing intervention is particularly well chosen for addressing a population at high risk for developing schizophrenia?
   a. Screening a group of males between the ages of 15 and 25 for early symptoms
   b. Forming a support group for females ages 25 to 35 who are diagnosed with substance use issues
   c. Providing a group for patients between the ages of 45 and 55 with information on coping skills that have proven to be effective
   d. Educating the parents of a group of developmentally delayed 5- to 6-year-olds on the importance of early intervention

3. To provide effective care for the patient diagnosed with schizophrenia, the nurse should frequently assess for which associated conditions? Select all that apply.
   a. Alcohol use disorder
   b. Major depressive disorder
   c. Stomach cancer
   d. Polydipsia
   e. Metabolic syndrome

4. A female patient diagnosed with schizophrenia has been prescribed a first-generation antipsychotic medication. What information should the nurse provide to the patient regarding her signs and symptoms?
   a. Her memory problems will likely decrease.
   b. Depressive episodes should be less severe.
   c. She will probably enjoy social interactions more.
   d. She should experience a reduction in hallucinations.

5. Which characteristic presents the greatest risk for injury to others by the patient diagnosed with schizophrenia?
   a. Depersonalization
   b. Pressured speech
   c. Negative symptoms
   d. Paranoia

6. Gilbert, age 19, is described by his parents as a "moody child" with an onset of odd behaviour at about age 14, which caused Gilbert to suffer academically and socially. Gilbert has lost the ability to complete household chores, is reluctant to leave the house, and is obsessed with the locks on the windows and doors. Due to Gilbert's early and slow onset of what is now recognized as schizophrenia, his prognosis is considered:
   a. Favourable with medication
   b. In the relapse stage
   c. Improvable with psychosocial interventions
   d. To have a less positive outcome

7. Which therapeutic communication statement might a psychiatric mental health registered nurse use when a patient's nursing diagnosis is *Altered thought processes*?
   a. "It must be difficult to hear voices like that, though I cannot hear them."
   b. "Stop listening to the voices, they are NOT real."
   c. "You say you hear voices; what are they telling you?"
   d. "Just tell the voices to leave you alone for now."

8. When patients diagnosed with schizophrenia suffer from anosognosia, they often refuse medication, believing that:
   a. Medications provided are ineffective.
   b. Nurses are trying to control their minds.
   c. The medications will make them sick.
   d. They are not actually ill.

9. Kyle, a patient with schizophrenia, began to take the first-generation antipsychotic haloperidol (Haldol) last week. One day you find him sitting very stiffly and not moving. He is diaphoretic, and when you ask if he is okay he seems unable to respond verbally. His vital signs are BP 170/100, P 110, T 40.1°C/104.2°F. What is the priority nursing intervention?
   a. Hold his medication and contact his prescriber.
   b. Wipe him with a washcloth wet with cold water or alcohol.
   c. Administer a medication such as benztropine IM to correct this dystonic reaction.
   d. Reassure him that although there is no treatment for his tardive dyskinesia, it will pass.
   e. Hold his medication for now and consult his prescriber when he comes to the unit later today.

10. Tomas is a 21-year-old male with a recent diagnosis of schizophrenia. Tomas's nurse recognizes that self-medicating with excessive alcohol is common in this disease and can co-occur along with:
    a. Generally good health despite the mental illness
    b. An aversion to drinking fluids
    c. Anxiety and depression
    d. The ability to express his needs

⊖volve WEBSITE

Post-Test interactive review

Visit the Evolve website for Chapter Review Answers and Rationales, Critical Thinking Answer Guidelines, and additional resources related to the content in this chapter: http://evolve.elsevier.com/Canada/Varcarolis/psychiatric/

REFERENCES

Agar, L. (2010). Recognizing neuroleptic malignant syndrome in the emergency department: A case study. *Perspectives in Psychiatric Care, 46*(2), 143–151. doi:10.1111/j.1744-6163.2010.00250.x.

Akbarian, S., & Kundakovic, M. (2015). CHRNA7 and CHRFAM7A: Psychosis and smoking? Blame the neighbors. *The American Journal of Psychiatry, 172*(11), 1054.

Amador, X. (2012). *I'm not sick, I don't need help!: How to help someone with mental illness accept treatment* (10th anniversary ed.). New York: Vida Press.

American Psychiatric Association (2013). *Diagnostic and statistical manual of mental disorders* (5th ed.). Washington, DC: Author.

Andreou, D., Söderman, E., Axelsson, T., et al. (2015). Cerebrospinal fluid monoamine metabolite concentrations as intermediate phenotypes between glutamate-related genes and psychosis. *Psychiatry Research, 229*(1–2), 497–504. doi.org/10.1016/j.psychres.2015.06.023.

Aschengrau, A., Weinberg, J., Janulewicz, P., et al. (2012). Occurrence of mental illness following prenatal and early childhood exposure to tetrachloroethylene (PCE)-contaminated drinking water: A retrospective cohort study. *Environmental Health: A Global Access Science Source, 11*(1), 1–12.

Bechdolf, A., Phillips, L. J., Francey, S. M., et al. (2006). Recent approaches to psychological interventions for people at risk of psychosis. *European Archive of Psychiatry and Clinical Neuroscience, 256*, 159–173. doi:10.1007/s00406-006-0623-0.

Berry, A., & Cirulli, F. (2016). Toward a diathesis-stress model of schizophrenia in a neurodevelopmental perspective. In V. Mikhail & J. L. Waddington (Eds.), *Handbook of Behavioral Neuroscience* (pp. 209–224). St. Louis: Elsevier.

Blomström, A., Karlsson, H., Gardner, R., et al. (2016). Associations between maternal infection during pregnancy, childhood infections, and the risk of subsequent psychotic disorder—A Swedish cohort study of nearly 2 million individuals. *Schizophrenia Bulletin, 42*(1), 125–133. doi:10.1093/schbul/sbv112.

Brady, P., Kangas, M., & McGill, K. (2017). "Family matters": A systematic review of the evidence for family psychoeducation for major depressive disorder. *Journal of Marital and Family Therapy, 43*(2), 245–263. doi:10.1111/jmft.12204.

Brown, A. S. (2011). The environment and susceptibility to schizophrenia. *Progress in Neurobiology, 93*(1), 23–58. doi:10.1016/j.pneurobio.2010.09.003.

Brown, E., & Gray, R. (2015). Tackling medication non-adherence in severe mental illness: Where are we going wrong? *Journal of Psychiatric and Mental Health Nursing, 22*(3), 192–198. doi:10.1111/jpm.12186.

Buccheri, R. K., Trygstad, L. N., Buffum, M. D., et al. (2013). Self-management of unpleasant auditory hallucinations: A tested practice model. *Journal of Psychosocial Nursing and Mental Health Services, 51*(11), 26. doi:10.3928/02793695-20130731-02.

Canadian Institute for Health Information (CIHI). (2008). *Hospital length of stay and readmission for individuals diagnosed with schizophrenia: Are they related?* Retrieved from https://secure.cihi.ca/estore/productSeries.htm?pc=PCC410.

Carbon, M., & Correll, C. U. (2014). Thinking and acting beyond the positive: The role of the cognitive and negative symptoms in schizophrenia. *CNS Spectrums, 19*(Suppl. 1), 38–53. doi:10.1017/S1092852914000601.

Castellani, C., Melka, M., Gui, J., et al. (2015). Integration of DNA sequence and DNA methylation changes in monozygotic twin pairs discordant for schizophrenia. *Schizophrenia Research, 169*(1–3), 433–440. doi:10.1016/j.schres.2015.09.021.

Chen, C.-F., Chen, Y.-F., Chan, C.-H., et al. (2015). Common factors associated with choking in psychiatric patients. *The Journal of Nursing Research, 23*(2), 94–99. doi:10.1097/jnr.0000000000000060.

Chester, P., Ehrlich, C., Warburton, L., et al. (2016). What is the work of recovery oriented practice? A systematic literature review. *International Journal of Mental Health Nursing, 25*(4), 270–285. doi:10.1111/inm.12241.

Chung, Y. S., Kang, D., Shin, N. Y., et al. (2008). Deficit of theory of mind in individuals at ultra-high risk for schizophrenia. *Schizophrenia Research, 99*, 111–118.

Correll, C. U., Detraux, J., De Lepeleire, J., et al. (2015). Effects of antipsychotics, antidepressants and mood stabilizers on risk for physical diseases in people with schizophrenia, depression and bipolar disorder. *World Psychiatry, 14*(2), 119–136.

Dean, D., Orr, J., Bernard, J., et al. (2016). Hippocampal shape abnormalities predict symptom progression in neuroleptic-free youth at ultrahigh risk for psychosis. *Schizophrenia Bulletin, 42*(1), 161–169. doi:10.1093/schbul/sbv086.

Egerton, A., Howes, O. D., Houle, S., et al. (2017). Elevated striatal dopamine function in immigrants and their children: A risk mechanism for psychosis. *Schizophrenia Bulletin,* doi:10.1093/schbul/sbw181.

England, M. (2007). Accuracy of nurses' perceptions of voice hearing and psychiatric symptoms. *Journal of Advanced Nursing, 58*(2), 130–139. doi:10.1111/j.1365-2648.2006.04162.x.

Farhall, J., Greenwood, K. M., & Jackson, H. J. (2007). Coping with hallucinated voices: A review of self-initiated strategies and therapeutic interventions. *Clinical Psychology Review, 27*, 476–493. doi:10.1016/j.cpr.2006.12.002.

Fornells-Ambrojo, M., Claxton, M., & Onwumere, J. (2017). Do family interventions improve outcomes in early psychosis? A systematic review and meta-analysis. *Frontiers in Psychology, 8*, 371. doi:10.3389/fpsyg.2017.00371.

Frankle, W. G., Cho, R. Y., Prasad, K. M., et al. (2015). In vivo measurement of GABA transmission in healthy subjects and schizophrenia patients. *American Journal of Psychiatry, 172*, 1148–1159.

Freudenreich, O. D., Brown, H. E., & Holt, D. J. (2016). Psychosis and schizophrenia. In T. A. Stern, M. Fava, T. E. Wilens, et al. (Eds.), *Massachusetts General Hospital comprehensive clinical psychiatry* (2nd ed., chapter 28). Philadelphia: Elsevier.

Freudenreich, O. D., Goff, D. C., & Henderson, D. C. (2016). Antipsychotics. In T. A. Stern, M. Fava, T. E. Wilens, et al. (Eds.), *Massachusetts General Hospital comprehensive clinical psychiatry* (2nd ed., pp. 475–488). Philadelphia: Elsevier.

Gaebel, W., Rössler, W., & Sartorius, N. (2017). *The stigma of mental illness: End of the story?* Cham, Switzerland: Springer.

Gerlock, A. A., Buccheri, R., Buffum, M. D., et al. (2010). Responding to command hallucinations to harm self and others: The Unpleasant Voices Scale and Harm Command Safety Protocol. *Journal of Psychosocial Nursing and Mental Health Services, 48*(5), 26–33. doi:10.3928/02793695-20100304-03.

Gerson, R., Wong, C., Davidson, L., et al. (2011). Self-reported coping strategies in families of patients in early stages of psychotic disorder: An exploratory study: Coping by families in early psychosis. *Early Intervention in Psychiatry, 5*(1), 76–80. doi:10.1111/j.1751-7893.2010.00251.x.

Haddad, L., Schäfer, A., Streit, F., et al. (2015). Brain structure correlates of urban upbringing, an environmental risk factor. *Schizophrenia Bulletin, 41*(1), 115–122. doi:10.1093/schbul/sbu072.

Happell, B., Platania-Phung, C., & Scott, D. (2013). Mental health nurse incentive program: Facilitating physical health care for people with mental illness? *International Journal of Mental Health Nursing, 22*(5), 399–408. doi:10.1111/inm.12006.

Haynes, R. M., & Resnick, P. J. (1993). Proverb familiarity and the mental status exam. *Bulletin of the Menninger Clinic, 57*(4), 523–529.

Hoffman, R. E., & Varanko, M. (2006). Seeing voices: Fused visual/auditory verbal hallucinations reported by three persons with schizophrenia-spectrum disorder. *Acta Psychiatrica Scandinavica, 114*, 290–293.

Hor, K., & Taylor, M. (2010). Suicide and schizophrenia: A systematic review of rates and risk factors. *Journal of Psychopharmacology (Oxford, England), 24*(Suppl. 4), 81.

Howes, O. D., & McCutcheon, R. (2017). Inflammation and the neural diathesis–stress hypothesis of schizophrenia: A reconceptualization. *Translational Psychiatry [Electronic Resource], 7*(2), e1024. doi:10.1038/tp.2016.278.

Howland, R. H. (2015). Brexpiprazole: Another multipurpose antipsychotic drug? *Journal of Psychosocial Nursing and Mental Health Services, 53*(4), 23–25. doi:10.3928/02793695-20150323-01.

Hubl, D., Koenig, T., Strik, W., et al. (2004). Pathways that make voices: White matter changes in auditory hallucinations. *Archives of General Psychiatry, 61*(7), 658–668.

Kalhovde, A. M., Elstad, I., & Talseth, A. (2014). "Sometimes I walk and walk, hoping to get some peace": Dealing with hearing voices and sounds nobody else hears. *International Journal of Qualitative Studies on Health and Well-being, 9*(1), 23069. doi:10.3402/qhw.v9.23069.

Kantrowitz, J. T., Malhotra, A. K., Cornblatt, B., et al. (2010). High dose D-serine in the treatment of schizophrenia. *Schizophrenia Research, 121*(1), 125–130. doi:10.1016/j.schres.2010.05.012.

Khashan, A. S., Abel, K. M., McNamee, R., et al. (2008). Higher risk of offspring schizophrenia following antenatal maternal exposure to severe adverse life events. *Archives of General Psychiatry, 65*(2), 146–152.

Koehn, C. V., & Cutliffe, J. R. (2007). Hope and interpersonal psychiatric/mental health nursing: A systematic review of the literature: Part one. *Journal of Psychiatric and Mental Health Nursing, 14*, 134–140. doi:10.1111/j.1365-2850.2007.01054.x.

Lamsma, J., & Harte, J. M. (2015). Violence in psychosis: Conceptualizing its causal relationship with risk factors. *Aggression and Violent Behavior, 24*, 75–82. doi:10.1016/j.avb.2015.05.003.

Levine, S. Z., Lurie, I., Kohn, R., et al. (2011). Trajectories of the course of schizophrenia: From progressive deterioration to amelioration over three decades. *Schizophrenia Research, 126*, 184–191. doi:10.1016/j.schres.2010.10.026.

Marquez-Arrico, J., Benaiges, I., & Adan, A. (2015). Strategies to cope with treatment in substance use disorder male patients with and without schizophrenia. *Psychiatry Research, 228*(3), 752–759. doi.org/10.1016/j.psychres.2015.05.028.

McDaid, T. M., & Smyth, S. (2015). Metabolic abnormalities among people diagnosed with schizophrenia: A literature review and implications for mental health nurses. *Journal of Psychiatric and Mental Health Nursing, 22*(3), 157–170. doi:10.1111/jpm.12185.

Mental Health Commission of Canada. (2016). *Guidelines for recovery-oriented practice: Hope, dignity, inclusion.* Retrieved from http://www.mentalhealthcommission.ca/sites/default/files/2016-07/MHCC_Recovery_Guidelines_2016_ENG.PDF.

Mental Health Commission of Canada. (2017). *Stigma and discrimination.* Retrieved from http://www.mentalhealthcommission.ca/English/focus-areas/stigma-and-discrimination.

Miller, B. (2016). Neuroinflammation marker may foretell psychosis. *Psychiatric Times.* Retrieved from http://www.psychiatrictimes.com/schizophrenia/neuroinflammation-marker-may-foretell-psychosis.

Moorhead, S., Johnson, M., Maas, M. L., et al. (2013). *Nursing outcomes classification (NOC)* (5th ed.). St Louis: Mosby.

Morera, T., Pratt, D., & Bucci, S. (2017). Staff views about psychosocial aspects of recovery in psychosis: A systematic review. *Psychology and Psychotherapy, 90*(1), 1–24. doi:10.1111/papt.12092.

Morgan, C., Freeman, T., Powell, J., et al. (2016). AKT1 genotype moderates the acute psychotomimetic effects of naturalistically smoked cannabis in young cannabis smokers. *Translational Psychiatry, 6*, e738. doi:10.1038/tp.2015.219.

Mork, E., Mehlum, L., Barrett, E. A., et al. (2012). Self-harm in patients with schizophrenia spectrum disorders. *Archives of Suicide Research, 16*(2), 111–123. doi:10.1080/13811118.2012.667328.

Myers, N. L. (2010). Culture, stress and recovery from schizophrenia: Lessons from the field for global mental health. *Culture, Medicine and Psychiatry, 34*(3), 500–528. doi:10.1007/s11013-010-9186-7.

Nash, J. (n. d.) *John Nash quotes.* Retrieved from http://thinkexist.com/quotes/john_nash/.

Nielssen, O., & Large, M. (2010). Rates of homicide during the first episode of psychosis and a systematic review and meta-analysis. *Schizophrenia Bulletin, 36*(4), 702–712. doi:10.1093/schbul/sbn144.

Norman, R. M., Manchanda, R., Malia, A. K., et al. (2011). Symptom and functional outcomes for a 5-year early intervention program for psychoses. *Schizophrenia Research, 129*(2–3), 111–115. doi:10.1016/j.schres.2011.04.006.

Pelletier, J., Lesage, A., Boisvert, C., et al. (2015). Feasibility and acceptability of patient partnership to improve access to primary care for the physical health of patients with severe mental illnesses: An interactive guide. *International Journal for Equity in Health, 14*, 78. doi:10.1186/s12939-015-0200-0.

Rao, S., Raney, L., & Xiong, G. (2015). Reducing medical comorbidity and mortality in severe mental illness: Collaboration with primary and preventive care could improve outcomes. *Current Psychiatry, 14*(7), 14–20.

Rezansoff, S. N., Moniruzzaman, A., Fazel, S., et al. (2016). Adherence to antipsychotic medication among homeless adults in Vancouver, Canada: A 15-year retrospective cohort study. *Social Psychiatry and Psychiatric Epidemiology, 51*(12), 1623–1632. doi:10.1007/s00127-016-1259.

Riecher-Rössler, A., Gschwandtner, U., Borgwardt, S., et al. (2006). Early detection and treatment of schizophrenia: How early? *Acta Psychiatrica Scandinavica, 113*, 73–80. doi:10.1111/j.1600-0447.2005.00722.x.

Rummel-Kluge, C., Komossa, K., Corves, C., et al. (2009). A meta-analysis of head-to-head comparisons of second-generation antipsychotics in the treatment of schizophrenia. *The American Journal of Psychiatry, 166*(2), 152–163. doi:10.1176/appi.ajp.2008.08030368.

Sadock, B. J., Sadock, V. A., & Ruiz, P. (2017). *Concise textbook of clinical psychiatry* (4th ed.). Philadelphia: Lippincott Williams & Wilkins.

Sandler, J., Kotov, R., & Bromet, E. (2011). Predictors of trajectories of illness course over 10 years in schizophrenia. *Comprehensive Psychiatry, 52*(6), e14. doi:10.1016/j.comppsych.2011.04.044.

Sekar, A., Bialas, A., de Rivera, H., et al. (2016). Schizophrenia risk from complex variation of complement component 4. *Nature, 530*(7589), 177–183. doi:10.1038/nature16549.

Skeem, J., Kennealy, P., Monahan, J., et al. (2015). Psychosis uncommonly and inconsistently precedes violence among high-risk individuals. *Clinical Psychological Science,* doi:10.1177/2167702615575879.

Smith, D. J., Langan, J., McLean, G., et al. (2013). Schizophrenia is associated with excess multiple physical-health comorbidities but low levels of recorded cardiovascular disease in primary care: Cross-sectional study. *BMJ Open, 3*(4), e002808. doi:10.1136/bmjopen-2013-002808.

Srihari, V. H., Shah, J., & Keshavan, M. S. (2012). Is early intervention for psychosis feasible and effective? *The Psychiatric Clinics of North America, 35*(3), 613–631. doi:10.1016/j.psc.2012.06.004.

Symanski-Tondora, J. L., Miller, R., Slade, M., et al. (2014). *Partnering for recovery in mental health: A practical guide to person-centered planning* (2nd ed.). Chichester, UK: Wiley-Blackwell.

Tandon, R., Keshavan, M. S., & Nasrallah, H. A. (2008). Schizophrenia, "Just the facts": What we know in 2008. *Schizophrenia Research, 100*(1), 4–19. doi:10.1016/j.schres.2008.01.022.

Thoma, P., & Daum, I. (2013). Comorbid substance use disorder in schizophrenia: A selective overview of neurobiological and cognitive underpinnings. *Psychiatry and Clinical Neurosciences, 67*(6), 367–383. doi:10.1111/pcn.12072.

Thornicroft, G. (2011). Physical health disparities and mental illness: The scandal of premature mortality. *The British Journal of Psychiatry: The Journal of Mental Science, 199*(6), 441–442. doi:10.1192/bjp.bp.111.092718.

Tsiachristas, A., Thomas, T., Leal, J., et al. (2016). Economic impact of early intervention in psychosis services: Results from a longitudinal retrospective controlled study in England. *BMJ Open, 6*(10), e012611. doi:10.1136/bmjopen-2016-012611.

Waldemar, A. K., Arnfred, S. M., Petersen, L., et al. (2016). Recovery-oriented practice in mental health inpatient settings: A literature review. *Psychiatric Services, 67*(6), 596–602. doi:10.1176/appi.ps.201400469.

Walker, A. K., Arnfred, S. M., Petersen, L., et al. (2016). Recovery-oriented practice in mental health inpatient settings: A literature review. *Psychiatric Services, 67*(6), 596–602. doi:10.1176/appi.ps.201400469.

Wilson, B. A., Shannon, M. T., & Sheilds, K. (2017). *Pearson nurse's drug guide 2017.* Upper Saddle River, NJ: Pearson/Prentice Hall.

Witt, K., van Dorn, R., & Fazel, S. (2013). Risk factors for violence in psychosis: Systematic review and meta-regression analysis of 110 studies. *PLoS ONE, 8*(2), e55942.

Wynaden, D., Tohotoa, J., Heslop, K., et al. (2015). Recognizing falls risk in older adult mental health patients and acknowledging the difference from the general older adult population. *Collegian (Royal College of Nursing, Australia), 23*(1), 97–102. http://dx.doi.org/10.1016/j.colegn.2014.12.002.

16

Eating and Feeding Disorders

Carissa R. Enright
Adapted by Sonya L. Jakubec

OBJECTIVES

1. Discuss four theories of eating disorders.
2. Compare and contrast the signs and symptoms (clinical picture) of anorexia nervosa and bulimia nervosa.
3. Identify three life-threatening conditions, stated in terms of nursing diagnoses, for a patient with an eating disorder.
4. Identify three realistic outcome criteria for (a) a patient with anorexia nervosa and (b) a patient with bulimia nervosa.

5. Describe therapeutic interventions appropriate for anorexia nervosa and bulimia nervosa in the acute phase and long-term phase of treatment.
6. Explain the basic premise of cognitive behavioural therapy in the treatment of eating disorders.
7. Differentiate between the long-term prognoses of anorexia nervosa, bulimia nervosa, and binge eating disorder.

⊖volve WEBSITE

Visit the Evolve website for Flashcards, Case Studies, and additional testing resources related to the content in this chapter: http://evolve.elsevier.com/Canada/Varcarolis/psychiatric/

Pre-Test   interactive review

Of all the psychiatric disorders, eating disorders may be the most perplexing. The eating and sharing of food is usually pleasurable and culturally important. It is difficult for many of us to understand how people could starve themselves or induce vomiting and seem to have little regard for how it affects them physically and socially. Cases of anorexia nervosa are documented in ancient writings; however, bulimia and binge eating necessitate an abundance of food and therefore may be more modern-age eating disorders. Many theories of the etiology of these disorders have been postulated, but to date the reasons behind the behaviour are still a mystery that drives research. In this chapter, we focus on the three main types of eating disorders—anorexia nervosa, bulimia nervosa, and binge eating disorder—and introduce feeding disorders (American Psychiatric Association, 2013) with a brief description.

CLINICAL PICTURE

There is not one eating disorder but rather several subtypes, predominantly identified as anorexia nervosa, bulimia nervosa, binge eating disorder, and eating disorder not otherwise specified (NOS). All types of disordered eating have both cognitive and behavioural components (Miller, Vaillancourt, & Hanna, 2009).

Individuals with anorexia nervosa refuse to maintain a minimally normal weight for their height and express an intense fear of gaining weight. The term *anorexia* is a misnomer because it literally means a loss of appetite, which is not specifically the case. Rather, in anorexia nervosa the clinical condition is a behavioural restriction of food intake or, for others, involves binge eating and purging.

HOW A NURSE HELPED ME

A Patient's Challenges

When I was 10 years old, I began overeating. It was at that time that my best friend moved away; I had other friends, but they were not the same. I am not exactly sure why, but eating helped me relax. The food demanded nothing of me—it did not judge me; it did not need me to do anything; it allowed me just to be.

Fortunately, as soon as I finished university, I had no problem finding my first teaching job. It was in a town approximately 300 kilometres away. Moving away was hard for me, but that was where the work was. I was still eating when I felt stressed, and I certainly felt stressed with the new job, in a new town, and with no friends. I was also starting to feel depressed. It was at that point that I went to the local community mental health centre for help. I knew I was smart, as I was successful at school and university, but this was one area I just couldn't seem to get a handle on. I met with a nurse who asked me a number of questions related to my mood, thoughts, feelings, and energy. The nurse helped me change my relationship with food by helping me understand how my thoughts and experiences affected how much I ate. She taught me how to use a journal to record my thoughts and experiences. It helped me identify my thoughts and feelings about food, eating, and not eating. I always hated counting calories and was worried that I would have to do that; to my surprise, we talked about my daily intake of food in relationship to the nutrients my body needed. I was counting food groups and portion sizes, but not calories. Another trick she taught me to manage my stress-related food consumption was to plan ahead for the times and places where I would be eating. This really helped because, when I felt stress, I knew just when I would be eating again, so I did not panic and binge-eat. The nurse did not judge me or criticize me because I was overweight; she listened and took me seriously.

Anorexia nervosa is a chronic illness that waxes and wanes. The 1-year relapse rate approaches 50%, and long-term studies show that up to 40% of patients continue to meet some criteria for anorexia nervosa after 4 years (Harrington, Jimerson, Haxton, et al., 2015). Recovery is evaluated as a stage in the process rather than a fixed event. Factors that influence the stage of recovery include percentage of ideal body weight that has been achieved, the extent to which self-worth is defined by shape and weight, and the amount of disruption existing in the patient's personal life.

Individuals with bulimia nervosa engage in repeated episodes of binge eating followed by compensatory behaviours, such as self-induced vomiting; misuse of laxatives, diuretics, or other medications; fasting; or excessive exercise. This disorder is characterized by a significant disturbance in the perception of body shape and weight.

Individuals with binge eating disorder engage in repeated episodes of binge eating, after which they experience significant distress; they do not regularly use compensatory behaviours, such as those seen in patients with bulimia nervosa. Many individuals have combinations of eating disorder symptoms that are not sufficient for a specific diagnosis of anorexia nervosa, bulimia nervosa, or binge eating disorder; these individuals are therefore diagnosed as having an eating disorder not otherwise specified, or NOS. While distinct, there are a number of both cognitive and behavioural similarities among eating problems, the defining characteristics of which are highlighted in Box 16-1.

Other problems related to eating are identified as feeding disorders, where the patient experiences an inability to or difficulty in eating or drinking sufficient quantities to maintain optimal nutritional status. These disorders have a typical onset in childhood and continue into adulthood. They include avoidant/restrictive food intake disorder, pica, and rumination disorder.

Avoidant/Restrictive Food Intake Disorder

Up to 40% of all toddlers will experience mealtime difficulties that resolve spontaneously with or without caregiver support and education. About 5% to 20% of children without other disorders may have feeding disorders. Prematurity, failure to thrive, autism, and genetic syndromes result in ranges of 40% to 80% with feeding disorders (Romano, 2015). There are no

---

BOX 16-1   CHARACTERISTICS OF EATING PROBLEMS

ANOREXIA NERVOSA	BULIMIA NERVOSA	BINGE EATING

• Intense fear of weight gain
• Distorted body image
• Restricted calories with significantly low body mass index (BMI)
• Subtypes:
  • Restricting (no consistent bulimic features)
  • Binge eating/purging type (primarily restriction, some bulimic behaviours)
	• Recurrent episodes of uncontrollable binging
	• Inappropriate compensatory behaviours: vomiting, laxatives, diuretics, or exercise
	• Self-image largely influenced by body image and external validation
		• Recurrent episodes of uncontrollable binging without compensatory behaviours
		• Binging episodes induce guilt, depression, embarrassment, or disgust and are often preceded by emotional distress with poor coping

unifying etiologies for food refusal. Lack of interest in eating or food may result in weight loss, growth retardation, and nutritional deficiency. It most commonly begins in infancy or early childhood and may continue into adulthood. Anxiety and family anxiety are risk factors.

The primary treatment modality is some form of behavioural modification to increase regular food consumption. Families caring for a child with a feeding disorder often need support and education in specific behavioural techniques, but family therapy is not usually necessary. Treating anxiety and depressive symptoms may be helpful in some cases.

Pica

Pica is the persistent eating of substances such as dirt, chalk, yarn, glue, or paint that have no nutritional value. In institutionalized children, the rate of this disorder may be as high as 26%. Pica usually begins in early childhood and lasts for a few months. Eating nonfood items may interfere with eating nutritional items. Eating nonfood items can also be dangerous. Paint may contain lead and result in brain damage. Objects that cannot be digested, such as stones, can result in intestinal blockage. Sharp objects such as paper clips can result in intestinal damage or laceration. Bacteria from dirt or other soiled objects can result in serious infection. Tooth decay may result from stomach acids. Monitoring the child's eating behaviour is obviously an essential aspect of treating this problem. Behavioural interventions such as rewarding appropriate eating are helpful.

Rumination Disorder

Rumination disorder is characterized by undigested food being returned to the mouth. It is then rechewed, reswallowed, or spit out. It may be diagnosed after 1 month of symptoms. Rumination symptoms can occur at any age, and the onset in infants is between 3 and 12 months. Intellectual development disorder is associated with rumination. Neglect is a predisposing factor to the development of this disorder. The symptoms frequently remit spontaneously but may become habitual and result in severe malnutrition and even death.

Interventions include repositioning infants and small children during feeding. Improving the interaction between caregiver and child and making mealtimes a pleasant experience often reduce rumination. Distracting the child when the behaviour starts is also helpful. Family therapy may be required.

EPIDEMIOLOGY

It is extremely difficult to determine the specific number of people afflicted with eating disorders, as fewer than half seek health care for their illness. Many people with disordered eating patterns do not meet full *Diagnostic and Statistical Manual of Mental Disorders (DSM-5)* criteria and are not included in the statistics gathered in epidemiological reports. Data provided to the Standing Committee on the Status of Women and included in its report *Eating Disorders Among Girls and Women in Canada* (Government of Canada, 2014) suggest that as many as 600 000 to 900 000 Canadians meet the diagnostic criteria for an eating disorder at any given time.

Female sex, younger age, sexual and physical abuse, participation in esthetic or weight-oriented sports, and heritability are found to be most consistently associated with higher eating disorder prevalence and incidence (Mitchison & Hay, 2014). Most eating disorders begin in the early teens to mid-twenties, commonly following puberty, although bulimia generally occurs in later adolescence. Anorexia nervosa may start early (between ages 7 and 12), but bulimia nervosa is rarely seen in children younger than 12 years. For women, the lifetime incidence of anorexia nervosa is 0.9%, and the lifetime incidence for men is 0.24% (Rosenvinge & Petterson, 2015). The 12-month prevalence of bulimia nervosa among young women is 1% to 1.5%. The lifetime incidence of bulimia nervosa for women is 2.3%, and the lifetime incidence for men is 0.5% (Rosenvinge & Petterson, 2015). Bulimia commonly begins in later adolescence, when the prevalence peaks up to young adulthood. Onset of bulimia nervosa is rare in children younger than 12 and adults older than 40.

Binge eating disorder is the most common eating disorder. For women, the lifetime incidence of binge eating disorder is 3.6%, and the lifetime incidence for men is 2.1% (Rosenvinge & Petterson, 2015). Gender differences have been examined, with men being more likely to report overeating; women being more likely to endorse loss of control while eating; and women being significantly more likely than men to report body checking and avoidance, binge eating, fasting, and vomiting (Striegel-Moore, Rosselli, Perrin, et al., 2009). The presence of binge eating disorder is higher in overweight populations (3%) than in the general population (2%). All racial and ethnic groups seem to be represented fairly equally.

Eating disorders among middle-aged women seems to be common, with a greater number of diagnoses of binge eating disorder and eating disorder NOS as compared to the "classical" diagnoses of anorexia and bulimia nervosa. Middle-aged women, even with very broadly defined, subthreshold eating disorders, demonstrated distress and impairment comparable to that of women with full-scale eating disorders (Mangweth-Matzek, Hoek, Rupp, et al., 2014). Eating disturbances appear to be underassessed and underdiagnosed among older men (those ages 40 to 75), though extreme dietary and exercise behaviours, more common in this population, represent an under-recognized form of purging behaviour (Mangweth-Matzek, Kummer, & Pope, 2016).

Patterns of eating disorders, and implications for psychiatric mental health nursing practice, are also prevalent among university and elite sports athletes, as well as among dance and theatre performers. A substantial amount of evidence suggests that collegiate and elite athletes involved in weight-sensitive sports are at particular risk of developing eating disorders (Bar, Cassin, & Dionne, 2016; Thompson & Sherman, 2010), as are those involved in aesthetic performance work (Arcelus, Witcomb, & Mitchell, 2014).

Although culture and ethnicity, socioeconomic status, education, and urbanicity did not appear to have strong associations with eating disorder epidemiology (Mitchison & Hay, 2014), trends are emerging regarding the changing landscape of culture and eating disorders, indicating a stabilization of the incidence of anorexia nervosa and possibly lower incidence rates of bulimia nervosa in White North American and Northern European groups; increasing rates of eating disorders in Asia and the Middle Eastern/ North African region; and increasing rates of binge eating and bulimia nervosa in Hispanic and Black American minority groups in North America (Pike, Hoek, & Dunne, 2014). Boisvert and Harrell (2012), in a Canadian epidemiological study focused on culture and ethnicity, found that younger women, particularly those with higher body shame, higher body mass index (BMI), and lower spirituality, reported more eating disorder symptomatology. Hispanic and Asian women had higher body shame and lower BMI compared to White women. In another Albertan study, Boisvert and Harrell (2009) observed strong differences in age and ethnicity for eating disorders. Hispanic women reported higher body shame than White women. Hispanic women also reported more bulimic behaviour than White, Indigenous, and Asian women. White women reported lower body satisfaction than Asian and Indigenous women. Indigenous women reported the highest body satisfaction. Bulimic behaviour was lowest in older women (65+ years) compared with other age groups. Body satisfaction was greatest in older women (65+ years).

There is some concern that adolescents who go on "extreme diets" that either restrict calories or prohibit certain food groups are at risk for developing an eating disorder, but it does not appear that caloric restriction as a method to reduce body weight in individuals who are overweight is in itself responsible for this risk (Williamson, Martin, Anton, et al., 2008).

Although patients with eating disorders are at risk for medical complications that may result in death, the major cause of death among those affected by eating disorders is suicide. Adolescents diagnosed with anorexia nervosa or bulimia nervosa have a suicide rate that is more than six times greater than the norm for their age group. Overall, among all ages, people with bulimia nervosa make more suicide attempts, and there is a higher incidence of completion in those with anorexia nervosa (Kostro, Lerman, & Attia, 2014).

Self-injurious behaviours are also frequent in people with eating disorders, with higher rates among those whose disorders include binge and purge behaviours and an overall lifetime prevalence of 27.3% in patients with eating disorders (Cucchi, Ryan, Konstantakopoulos, et al., 2016). Self-injurious behaviours, which may or may not include suicidal intent, are especially high among adolescents with eating disorders. Overexercising—often considered a self-injurious behaviour among individuals with eating disorders—may also pose additional risk beyond the physical consequence of the activity itself, contributing to a higher risk for suicide (Kostro, Lerman & Attia, 2014). These alarming rates highlight the need for ongoing safety assessment and evaluation for suicidal ideation and self-injurious behaviours in persons with eating disorders and for routinely taking a family psychiatric history for all patients.

The relevance of specific risk factors that address critical and social or feminist lenses (e.g., weight concerns and dieting, internalization of thinness, negative body image) has not been thoroughly examined or tested yet (Piran, 2010). This complex and emerging epidemiological landscape underscores the public mental health significance of all types of eating disorders.

RESEARCH HIGHLIGHT

Prevention of Eating Disorders

Problem

Body dissatisfaction, prevalent among university students, is considered to be a risk factor for eating pathology, emphasizing the need for prevention programs.

Purpose of Study

To date, most research studies examining the effectiveness of interventions for eating disorders do not mention any stakeholder involvement. The purpose of this study is to pilot, in collaboration with health promotion staff and peer health educators, a prevention program designed to promote positive body image among university students.

Methods

A pre–post design without a control group was used to collect preliminary information about the program. Thirty-seven undergraduate students (6 males; 25 females; mean age 22.6 years) from three Canadian universities were selected from a pool of students enrolled in a peer health education program facilitated by the university-based health promotion staff. Three paper and pencil instruments were used: a survey to collect demographics, the Sociocultural Attitudes Towards Appearance Questionnaire (SATAQ) to measure the degree of internalization of sociocultural stereotypes of weight and appearance, and the Body Satisfaction Scale to assess body satisfaction. The prevention program focused on media literacy, self-esteem enhancement strategies, stress-management skills, and ways to recognize healthy versus unhealthy relationships. Open-ended questions were developed to elicit participants' feedback about the program content and process.

Key Findings

Participants reported significant improvements in body satisfaction and reductions in the internalization of media stereotypes between the baseline and post-program period.

Participants provided positive feedback about the program and the face-to-face format.

Staff also provided positive feedback and expressed interest in incorporating strategies into their routine peer mentoring training activities.

Implications for Nursing Practice

Nurses are often responsible for developing health promotion resources. Knowing how to design sustainable health promotion programs capable of reaching out to students before they develop symptoms of eating disorders is invaluable.

Source: McVey, G. L., Kirsh, G., Maker, D., et al. (2010). Promoting positive body image among university students: A collaborative pilot study. *Body Image, 7,* 200–204. doi:10.1016/j.bodyim.2010.02.005.

COMORBIDITY

Depression and anxiety are common comorbid conditions in people with all types of eating disorders. The estimated lifetime prevalence of mood disorders in anorexia nervosa ranges from 31% to 89% and in bulimia nervosa ranges from 24% to 90%. The fact that depressive symptoms accompany any type of starvation makes determining an exact prevalence difficult (Godart, Perdereau, Rein, et al., 2007).

The incidence of obsessive-compulsive disorder (OCD) has been reported to be as high as 25% in patients with anorexia nervosa. The OCD symptoms centre on food preoccupation and may be manifested in collecting cookbooks, preparing elaborate meals for others, and hoarding food. Anxiety disorders, particularly social phobia, are also common. In addition, significant associations have been found between risk for an eating disorder and alcohol dependence, as well as the lifetime abuse of and dependence on illicit drugs (Piran & Gadalla, 2006).

People with eating disorders who are also living with depression, a substance use disorder, or difficulty with impulse control are at greater risk for relapse. There is some evidence that the younger the person is when anorexic symptoms begin, the better the chance for positive outcomes is (Berkman, Lohr, & Bulik, 2007).

Personality disorders may occur in 42% to 75% of people with eating disorders. There is a high rate of avoidant personality disorders with all eating disorders. Avoidance fits the clinical picture of being overly concerned with acceptance and approval and fearing criticism or rejection. Patients with anorexia nervosa are more likely to have a Cluster C personality disorder (avoidant, dependent, obsessive-compulsive, or passive-aggressive) (Berkman, Lohr, & Bulik, 2007). Obsessive-compulsive and dependent personality disorders are also common in patients with bulimia. Borderline personality disorder is common in patients with binge eating disorder. See Chapter 19 for more information on personality disorders.

There have been several significant conclusions in the research literature examining the relationship between trauma and eating disorders. Associated traumas now include not only childhood sexual abuse but also other forms of abuse and neglect and are more common in eating disorders involving bingeing and purging behaviours. Also, the research findings have been extended to boys and men with eating disorders (Brewerton, 2007).

ETIOLOGY

The eating disorders—anorexia nervosa, bulimia nervosa, binge eating disorder, and eating disorder NOS—are actually entities or syndromes and are not considered to be discrete diseases. Experts tend to agree that there is no single cause of eating disorders. Eating disorders typically develop from a complex interaction of psychological risk factors, sociocultural influences, and biological or genetic predispositions (Mitchell & Wonderlich, 2014). A number of theories attempt to explain eating disorders.

Biological Factors
Genetic
There is a strong genetic link for eating disorders. A review of relevant studies has suggested that the heritability of anorexia nervosa is 60% (Bienvenu, Davydow, & Kendler, 2011). A genetic vulnerability may lead to poor affect and impulse control or to an underlying neurotransmitter dysfunction, but researchers have not discovered any single causative gene to date. It is likely that a gene–environment interaction may predispose a person

to having symptoms of eating disorders and even confer a risk for developing full-blown eating disorders (Campbell, Mill, Uher, et al., 2011).

Neurobiological
Research demonstrates that altered brain serotonin function contributes to dysregulation of appetite, mood, and impulse control in the eating disorders. Patients with eating disorders consistently exhibit personality traits of perfectionism, obsessive-compulsiveness, and dysphoric mood, all of which are modulated through serotonin pathways in the brain. Because these traits appear to begin in childhood—before the onset of actual eating disorder symptoms—and persist into recovery, experts believe that they contribute to a vulnerability to disordered eating (Kaye, Wierenga, Bailer, et al., 2013).

Tryptophan, an amino acid essential to serotonin synthesis, is available only through diet. A normal diet boosts serotonin in the brain and regulates mood. Temporary drops in dietary tryptophan may actually relieve symptoms of anxiety and dysphoria and provide a reward for caloric restriction. Restricting food intake in this way becomes powerfully reinforcing because it provides a temporary respite from dysphoric mood, setting up a feedback loop that further establishes the disordered eating behaviour (Kaye, 2007). The dietary need for tryptophan may account for the fact that antidepressants that boost serotonin do not improve mood symptoms until after an underweight patient has been restored to 90% of optimal weight.

Newer brain imaging capabilities allow for better understanding of the etiological factors of anorexia nervosa (Frank, 2015). There is a consistent finding that patients with eating disorders who are acutely ill and those who have recovered show differences in the frontal, cingulated, temporal, or parietal regions of the brain, or in a combination of these regions, in comparison to controls. Relative to other psychiatric disorders, however, there are few brain scanning studies of the eating disorders, so conclusions are tentative. This is, however, a promising area of research that may contribute to the diagnosis and treatment of this difficult disease. Studies so far suggest that there is a difference in the reward and executive function parts of the brains of people with anorexia (Kaye, Wierenga, Bailer, et al., 2013).

Psychological Factors
Because anorexia nervosa was observed primarily in girls approaching puberty, early psychoanalytic theories linked the symptoms to an unconscious aversion to sexuality. By maintaining a childlike body, the patient avoids the anxiety associated with developing into a mature sexual being. Throughout the 1900s, many authors examined the family dynamics of these patients and concluded that a failure to separate from parents and a rebellion against the maternal bond explained the disordered eating behaviours (Le Grange, Lock, Loeb, et al., 2010). Further work by Bruch (1978) explored the symptoms as a defence against overwhelming feelings of ineffectiveness and powerlessness. Even with further insight into the intrapsychic origin of the behaviour, the process of psychoanalysis—with the goal of making unconscious processes conscious—failed to effect a cure for these syndromes (Caparrotta & Ghaffari, 2006).

Family theorists maintain that eating disorders are a problem of the whole family, and often the symptoms in the child serve to take the attention away from a distressed marriage. Families with a child who has anorexia are often described as enmeshed and perfectionistic; the child feels smothered by protectiveness and at the same time abandoned. The literature gives empirical support for family therapy methods in the treatment of children and adolescents with eating disorders (Haworth-Hoeppner, 2017).

Currently, cognitive behavioural theorists suggest that eating disorders are based on learned behaviour that has positive reinforcement. For example, a mildly overweight 14-year-old has the flu and loses a little weight. She returns to school, and her friends say, "Wow, you look great," and when people say, "Wow, you look really skinny," she still hears, "Wow, you look great." Now she purposefully strives to lose weight. Her behaviour is powerfully reinforced by these comments despite the fact that her health is at risk. Emotional disregulation has been found to be associated with the cognitive (rather than the behavioural) symptoms of those with all types of eating disorders (Pisetsky, Haynos, Lavender, et al., 2017).

Psychological trauma appears to be strongly associated with eating disorders of all types. There is an increased prevalence of sexual trauma for individuals with eating disorders. Recent evidence suggests that sexual trauma precedes and contributes to the development of eating disorders, however further research is needed to assess the potential causal role that sexual trauma may play in the etiology of eating disorders (Madowitz, Matheson, & Liang, 2015).

Environmental Factors

The Western cultural ideal that equates feminine beauty with tall, thin models has received much attention in the media as an etiology for eating disorders. Studies have shown that culture influences the development of self-concept and satisfaction with body size. Further, culture and political support of corporate agencies shape the food regulation and marketing industries. In this context, a 2016 Senate report revealed that almost two thirds of Canadian adults are now considered either overweight or obese. Canada ranks fifth among 40 countries for obesity prevalence, measured at 25.4% of adults (Organisation for Economic Co-operation and Development [OECD], 2015). Obesity rates among children are also dangerously high, with nearly 13% of children between the ages of 5 and 17 being obese and another 20% being overweight. These numbers reflect at least a twofold increase in the proportion of obese adults and a threefold increase in the proportion of obese children since 1980, a trend that is alarming, has a number of health and social implications, and has prompted a concerted effort to address the complex issues at a social level of intervention (Canadian Senate, 2016).

Record numbers of men and women are on diets to reduce body weight, but no study has been able to explain why only an estimated 0.3% to 3% of the population develops an eating disorder. Although a causal link between cultural norms or the social ideal of thinness portrayed in the media and eating disorders has not been proven (Doris, Shekriladze, Javakhishvili, et al., 2015), all patients with eating disorders have low self-esteem

CONSIDERING CULTURE

The Concept of Weight

Although cultural beliefs about physical beauty do not cause eating disorders, they influence self-esteem and set the standard of beauty for men and women. An unhealthy cultural ideal therefore can pose health risks if not addressed.

For centuries, body weight was an indicator of wealth and the availability of food, so the ideal was to achieve a large body. Considering the more recent media focus on the effect of the Western fashion industry and its use of unnaturally thin models, it is of interest that many other cultures still have the more traditional standards that equate obesity with beauty. For example, the Saharawi of Morocco are a nomadic people who see those who are thin as ill. Young Saharawi women, as they reach marriageable age, seek to rapidly increase their weight. To accomplish this, they eat large amounts of traditional foods, restrict their activity, and even take drugs such as corticosteroids to increase appetite and promote weight gain. Of the 249 women interviewed by Rguibi and Belahsen (2006), 225 were unsatisfied with their current weight. The group had a mean body mass index (BMI) of 29.6, with a range from 17.3 to 41.4. Only eight women wished to lose weight; the rest sought to become heavier. The authors suggest that a change in the cultural norm of beauty will be necessary to prevent the known health risks of obesity in that population.

Culturally competent care planning is made very difficult when the cultural ideal is unhealthy. In seeking to change behaviour, the nurse must acknowledge the cultural norm as important to the individual and, at the same time, provide adequate education about the risks and health consequences of the norm and help patients find a solution that respects their culture but promotes health.

Source: Rguibi, M., & Belahsen, R. (2006). Fattening practices among Moroccan Saharawi women. *Eastern Mediterranean Health Journal, 12*(5), 619–624.

that is negatively affected by their inability to conform to an impossible cultural standard of beauty (Malson & Burns, 2009).

Disordered forms of eating behaviour have emerged in the broader society and transnationally, in settings and cultures where eating disorders were not previously identified. Cultural transitions in response to societal changes, as well as the necessity to adapt to changing cultural norms, has been found to produce distress that manifests in some as disordered eating (Nasser, 2009).

ANOREXIA NERVOSA

APPLICATION OF THE NURSING PROCESS

Assessment

Anorexia nervosa and bulimia nervosa are two separate syndromes that present two clinical pictures on assessment. Box 16-2 lists several thoughts and behaviours associated with anorexia nervosa, and Table 16-1 identifies clinical signs and symptoms of anorexia nervosa found on assessment, together with their causes.

Eating disorders are serious and, in extreme cases, can lead to death. Box 16-3 identifies a number of medical complications

BOX 16-2   THOUGHTS AND BEHAVIOURS ASSOCIATED WITH ANOREXIA NERVOSA

- Terror of gaining weight
- Preoccupation with food
- View of self as fat even when emaciated
- Peculiar handling of food:
  - Cutting food into small bits
  - Pushing pieces of food around plate
- Possible development of rigorous exercise regimen
- Possible self-induced vomiting, use of laxatives and diuretics
- Cognition so disturbed that individual judges self-worth by his or her weight

TABLE 16-1   POSSIBLE SIGNS AND SYMPTOMS OF ANOREXIA NERVOSA

CLINICAL PRESENTATION	CAUSE
Low weight	Caloric restriction, excessive exercising
Amenorrhea	Low weight
Yellow skin	Hypercarotenemia
Lanugo	Starvation
Cold extremities	Starvation
Peripheral edema	Hypoalbuminemia and refeeding
Muscle weakening	Starvation, electrolyte imbalance
Constipation	Starvation
Abnormal laboratory values (low triiodothyronine, thyroxine levels)	Starvation
Abnormal computed tomography (CT) scans, electroencephalography (EEG) changes	Starvation
Cardiovascular abnormalities (hypotension, bradycardia, heart failure)	Starvation, dehydration Electrolyte imbalance
Impaired renal function	Dehydration
Hypokalemia (low potassium)	Starvation
Anemic pancytopenia	Starvation
Decreased bone density	Estrogen deficiency, low calcium intake

BOX 16-3   MEDICAL COMPLICATIONS OF ANOREXIA NERVOSA

- Bradycardia
- Orthostatic changes in pulse or blood pressure
- Cardiac arrhythmias
- Prolonged QT interval and ST-T wave abnormalities
- Peripheral neuropathy
- Acrocyanosis
- Symptomatic hypotension
- Leukopenia
- Lymphocytosis
- Carotenemia (elevated carotene levels in blood), which produces skin with yellow pallor
- Hypokalemic alkalosis (with self-induced vomiting or use of laxatives and diuretics)
- Elevated serum bicarbonate levels, hypochloremia, and hypokalemia
- Electrolyte imbalances, which lead to fatigue, weakness, and lethargy
- Osteoporosis, indicated by decrease in bone density
- Fatty degeneration of liver, indicated by elevation of serum enzyme levels
- Elevated cholesterol levels
- Amenorrhea
- Abnormal thyroid functioning
- Hematuria
- Proteinuria

Source: Data from Mitchell, J. E. & Wonderlich, S. A. (2014). Feeding and eating disorders. In R. E. Hales, S. C. Yudofsky, & L. Weiss Roberts (Eds.), *Textbook of psychiatry* (6th ed., pp. 557–587). Washington, DC: American Psychiatric Publishing.

BOX 16-4   CRITERIA FOR HOSPITAL ADMISSION OF PATIENTS WITH EATING DISORDERS

Physical Criteria
- Weight loss, <85% below ideal
- Rapid decline in weight with food refusal even if not <85% below ideal
- Inability to gain weight with outpatient treatment
- Temperature <36°C or <97°F
- Heart rate <40 beats per minute
- Systolic blood pressure <90/60 mm Hg
- Severe dehydration
- Hypokalemia (serum potassium <3 mEq/L) or other electrolyte imbalance
- Glucose <60 mg/dL; poorly controlled diabetes
- Hepatic, renal, or cardiovascular organ compromise requiring acute treatment

Psychiatric Criteria
- Risk for suicide
- Failure to comply with treatment contract
- Severe depression or other psychiatric disorder that would require hospitalization
- Family crisis or dysfunction

Source: American Psychiatric Association (APA). (2006). *Practice guideline for the treatment of patients with eating disorders* (3rd ed.). Washington, DC: Author.

that can occur in individuals with anorexia nervosa and the laboratory findings that may result. Because the eating behaviours in these conditions are so extreme, hospitalization may become necessary. Box 16-4 identifies physical and psychiatric criteria for hospitalization of an individual with an eating disorder.

Fundamental to the care of individuals with eating disorders is establishing and maintaining a therapeutic alliance. Developing this partnership will take both time and diplomacy on the part of the nurse. In treating patients who have been sexually abused or who have otherwise been victims of boundary violations, it is critical that the nurse and other health care workers respect the impact of the patient's history of trauma and associated complex eating disorder (Backholm, Isomaa, & Birgegård, 2013). Establishing therapeutic boundaries and practising with a trauma-informed care approach will facilitate the helping relationship and enhance outcomes (see Unit 5 for more on trauma interventions).

General Assessment

Individuals with the binge–purge type of anorexia nervosa may present with severe electrolyte imbalance (as a result of purging) and enter the health care system through admission to an intensive care unit. The patient with anorexia will be severely underweight and may have growth of fine, downy hair (lanugo) on the face and back. The patient will also have mottled, cool skin on the extremities and low blood pressure, pulse, and temperature readings, consistent with a malnourished, dehydrated state (see Table 16-1).

As with any comprehensive psychiatric nursing assessment, a complete evaluation of biopsychosocial function is mandatory. The areas to be covered include the patient's:

- Perception of the problem
- Eating habits
- History of dieting
- Methods used to achieve weight control (restricting, purging, exercising)
- Value attached to a specific shape and weight
- Interpersonal and social functioning
- Mental status and physiological parameters

INTEGRATIVE THERAPY

Ma Huang

In an attempt to lose weight and fight hunger, many patients with eating disorders turn to weight-loss products that contain herbs, such as ma huang, the Chinese name for the *Ephedra sinica* plant. Health Canada has issued several health advisories warning consumers not to use unauthorized products that contain ephedrine or ephedra in combination with caffeine or other stimulants due to the risk of serious adverse effects. Canadian retailers have also been reminded not to sell unauthorized products containing these ingredients; however, they may still be contained in natural products sold over the Internet. In a small study of patients with eating disorders, 42% of patients who actually experienced adverse effects while using ephedra products decided to continue taking the herb.

Source: Steffen, K. J., Roerig, J. L., Mitchell, J. E., et al. (2006). A survey of herbal and alternative medication use among participants with eating-disorder symptoms. *International Journal of Eating Disorders, 39*, 741–746. doi:10.1002/eat.20233.

Self-Assessment

When caring for the patient with anorexia, you may find it difficult to appreciate the compelling force of the illness, incorrectly believing that weight restriction, bingeing, and purging are self-imposed. If we see such self-destructive behaviours as a lifestyle or personal choice, it is only natural to blame the patient for any consequent health problems. The common personality traits of these patients—perfectionism, obsessive thoughts and actions relating to food, intense feelings of shame, people pleasing,

and the need to have complete control over their therapy—pose additional challenges.

In your efforts to motivate patients and take advantage of their decision to seek help and be healthier, take care not to allow encouragement to cross the line into authoritarianism and the assumption of a parental role. A patient's terror at gaining weight and her or his resistance to clinical interventions may engender significant frustration in the nurse struggling to build a therapeutic relationship and be empathic. Guard against any tendency to be coercive in your approach, and be aware that one of the primary goals of treatment—weight gain—is the very thing the patient fears. When patients appear to be resistant to change, it is helpful to acknowledge the constant struggle that so characterizes the treatment.

ASSESSMENT GUIDELINES

Anorexia Nervosa

Determine whether:
- The patient has a medical or psychiatric condition that warrants hospitalization (see Box 16-4)
- A thorough physical examination with appropriate blood work has been done
- Other medical conditions have been ruled out
- The patient is amenable to receiving or adherent to appropriate therapeutic modalities
- The family and patient need further teaching or information regarding the patient's treatment plan
- The patient and family want to participate in a support group and have been given a referral

DIAGNOSIS

Imbalanced nutrition: less than body requirements is usually the most appropriate initial nursing diagnosis for individuals with anorexia (Herdman & Kamitsuru, 2014). This diagnosis generates further nursing diagnoses—for example, *Decreased cardiac output, Risk for injury* (electrolyte imbalance), and *Risk for imbalanced fluid volume* (which would take first priority when problems are addressed). Other nursing diagnoses include *Anxiety, Chronic low self-esteem, Disturbed body image, Deficient knowledge, Ineffective coping, Powerlessness,* and *Hopelessness.*

OUTCOMES IDENTIFICATION

To evaluate the effectiveness of treatment, outcome criteria are established. Relevant categories of the *Nursing Outcomes Classification (NOC)* (Moorhead, Johnson, Maas, et al., 2013) include *Weight gain behaviour, Weight maintenance behaviour, Anxiety self-control, Nutritional status: nutrient intake,* and *Self-esteem.* Refer to Table 16-2 for examples of short-term *NOC* indicators for the patient with anorexia nervosa.

PLANNING

Planning is affected by the acuity of the patient's situation. When a patient with anorexia is experiencing extreme electrolyte

TABLE 16-2	*NOC* OUTCOMES RELATED TO ANOREXIA NERVOSA

NURSING OUTCOME AND DEFINITION	SHORT-TERM INDICATORS
Nutritional status: nutrient intake: Nutrient intake to meet metabolic needs	Caloric intake Protein intake Fat intake Carbohydrate intake
Weight gain behaviour: Personal actions to gain weight following voluntary or involuntary significant weight loss	Selects a healthy target weight Commits to a healthy eating plan Monitors exercise for caloric requirements Sets achievable weight gain goals
Anxiety self-control: Personal action to eliminate or reduce feelings of apprehension, tension, or uneasiness from an unidentifiable source.	Monitors intensity of anxiety Plans coping strategies for stressful situations Uses effective coping strategies
Self-esteem: Personal judgement of self-worth	Verbalization of self-acceptance Description of self Acceptance of compliments from others Feelings about self-worth

Source: Data from Moorhead, S., Johnson, M., Maas, M. L., et al. (2013). *Nursing outcomes classification (NOC)* (5th ed.). St Louis: Mosby.

imbalance or weighs less than 85% of his or her ideal body weight, the plan is to provide immediate medical stabilization, most likely in an inpatient unit. A person's ideal body weight is based chiefly on height but is modified by factors such as gender, age, build, and degree of muscular development. With the initiation of therapeutic nutrition, malnourished patients may need treatment on a medical unit, owing to *refeeding syndrome*, a potentially catastrophic treatment complication involving a metabolic alteration in serum electrolytes, vitamin deficiencies, and sodium retention (Myatt, 2014).

Once a patient is medically stable, the plan addresses the psychological issues underlying the eating disorder, usually on an outpatient basis. The nature of the treatment is determined by the intensity of the symptoms—which may vary over time—and the experienced disruption in the patient's life.

Discharge planning (living arrangements, school, work, finances, follow-up care) is a critical component of treatment. Often family members also benefit from counselling.

IMPLEMENTATION

Acute Care

Typically, a patient with an eating disorder is admitted to the inpatient psychiatric facility when in a crisis state. The health care team's initial focus, then, depends on the results of a comprehensive assessment that addresses the physical, cognitive, psychological, and social components as well as general mental status baseline. Any acute psychiatric symptoms, such as suicidal ideation, are addressed immediately. The nurse is challenged to establish trust and monitor the patient's eating pattern. Norris

and colleagues (2013) conducted a survey of intensive eating disorder programs specifically for adolescents across Canada, ultimately surveying 11 programs with a 90-item survey that addressed program characteristics and components, governance, staffing, referrals, assessments, therapeutic modalities in place, nutritional practices, and treatment protocols. They discovered a wide diversity of programming available but also the lack of a unified approach or protocols to intensive eating disorder treatment in youth.

Psychosocial Interventions

After addressing any acute symptoms, the patient with anorexia begins a weight-restoration program that allows for incremental weight gain. Based on the patient's height, a treatment goal is set at 90% of ideal body weight, the weight at which most women are able to menstruate.

As patients begin to eat again, they ideally participate in milieu therapy, in which the cognitive distortions (errors in thinking) that perpetuate the illness are consistently addressed by all members of the interprofessional team. Box 16-5 identifies some types of cognitive distortions characteristic of people with eating disorders. Focus should be on the eating behaviour and underlying feelings of anxiety, dysphoria, low self-esteem, and lack of control. When possible, the distortions in body image are avoided because attempts to change this perception are often misinterpreted, as shown in the following vignette.

VIGNETTE

Alicia, a 17-year-old cheerleader, did not come to treatment for weight loss until she fainted at a football game. She insisted that she only needed to "get more energy, not get fat." When the nurse pointed out that Alicia's ribs were clearly visible and that her backbone looked like a skeleton's, Alicia grinned and said, "Thank you."

Pharmacological Interventions

Research has not yet demonstrated that medications are effective as the first course of treatment of anorexia nervosa (Frank & Shott, 2016). Further studies are needed to determine if there is a medication that is effective to treat the core symptoms of the disorder. Despite the lack of rigorous scientific studies, the selective serotonin reuptake inhibitor (SSRI) fluoxetine (Prozac) has been found clinically useful in reducing obsessive-compulsive behaviour after the patient has reached a maintenance weight. Conventional antipsychotics such as chlorpromazine (Thorazine) may be helpful for delusional or overactive patients (Mitchell & Wonderlich, 2014). Atypical antipsychotic agents such as olanzapine (Zyprexa) are helpful in improving mood and decreasing obsessional behaviours and resistance to weight gain (Attia & Walsh, 2007).

Health Teaching and Health Promotion

Self-care activities are an important part of the treatment plan. These activities include learning more constructive coping skills, improving social skills, and developing problem-solving

BOX 16-5   COGNITIVE DISTORTIONS

Overgeneralization
A single event affects unrelated situations.
• "He didn't ask me out. It must be because I'm fat."

All-or-Nothing Thinking
Reasoning is absolute and extreme, in mutually exclusive terms of black or white, good or bad.
• "If I allow myself to gain weight, I'll blow up like a balloon."

Catastrophizing
The consequences of an event are magnified.
• "If I gain weight, my weekend will be ruined."

Personalization
Events are overinterpreted as having personal significance.
• "I know everybody is watching me eat."

Emotional Reasoning
Subjective emotions determine reality.
• "When I'm thin, I feel powerful."

Source: Adapted from Bowers, W. A. (2001). Basic principles for applying cognitive-behavioural therapy to anorexia nervosa. *Psychiatric Clinics of North America, 24,* 293–303. doi:10.1016/S0193-953X(05)70225-2.

and decision-making skills. These skills become the focus of therapy sessions. The following vignette illustrates the need for supportive education.

VIGNETTE

A nursing assessment of a small group of three young women and one young man in a nutrition group finds that all of the participants are very knowledgeable about the caloric value of common foods; as a group, they all avoid any "fatty" foods. The topic of fat-soluble vitamins and the consequences of vitamin deficiencies on the body introduced new information to all of the participants, and one of the young women started to cry, saying, "I had no idea I was doing that to my body." This show of emotion promoted a supportive interaction among the other group members as they shared their own stories of symptoms they could now identify as vitamin deficits.

Milieu Management

Patients admitted to an inpatient unit designed to treat eating disorders participate in a combination of therapeutic modalities provided by an interprofessional team. These modalities are designed to normalize eating patterns and begin to address the medical, family, and social issues raised by the illness.

The milieu of an eating-disorder unit is purposefully organized to assist the patient in establishing more adaptive behavioural patterns, including normalization of eating. The highly structured milieu includes precise mealtimes, adherence to the selected menu, observations during and after meals, and regularly scheduled weigh-ins.

Close monitoring of patients includes monitoring all trips to the bathroom after eating to prevent self-induced vomiting. Often

patient privileges are linked to weight gain and treatment-plan adherence. The following vignette demonstrates monitoring the bathroom as a therapeutic intervention.

VIGNETTE

A 20-year-old woman who primarily restricts her eating but resorts to purging when forced to eat by her family became visibly distressed after eating all of her therapeutic meal. Although her treatment plan was to join other patients in group therapy, the patient requested permission to go to the bathroom alone because she had "embarrassing gas" she did not want overheard. The nurse negotiated to stand away from the bathroom door if the patient agreed not to flush the toilet until the nurse was able to inspect the contents. However, the patient flushed the toilet before inspection. The breaking of the agreement with the nurse was discussed by the treatment team and determined to be an indication that this patient was not able to adhere to her prescribed treatment without additional structure. The treatment team established a new expectation that until the patient had gained 1 kilogram, she was to wait 30 minutes after every meal before she was allowed supervised bathroom breaks.

Advanced-Practice Interventions

Anorexia nervosa is a chronic illness. The 1-year relapse rate approaches 50%, and long-term studies show that up to 20% of patients continue to meet full criteria for anorexia nervosa after several years (Attia & Walsh, 2007). Recovery is evaluated as a stage in the process rather than as a fixed event. Factors that influence the stage of recovery include percentage of ideal body weight that has been achieved, the extent to which self-worth is defined by shape and weight, and the amount of disruption existing in the patient's personal life.

The patient will require long-term treatment that might include periodic, brief hospital stays, admission to a partial hospitalization program, outpatient services, and pharmacological interventions.

Agras and Robinson (2008) reviewed the progress of treatment for eating disorders over the past 40 years. Table 16-3 outlines their findings.

Psychotherapy

The goals of psychotherapy treatment are weight restoration with normalization of eating habits and initiation of the treatment of psychological, interpersonal, and social issues that affect each individual patient. Assisting the patient with a daily meal plan, reviewing a journal of meals and dietary intake maintained by the patient, and providing for weekly weigh-ins (ideally two to three times a week) are essential if the patient is to reach a medically stable weight.

Families frequently report feeling powerless in the face of behaviour that is mystifying. For instance, patients are often unable to experience compliments as supportive and therefore are unable to internalize the support. They often seek attention from others but feel shamed when they receive it. Patients express that they want their families to care for and about them but are unable to recognize expressions of care. When others do respond with love and support, patients do not perceive this as positive. The following vignette demonstrates this phenomenon.

TABLE 16-3	THE STATE OF TREATMENT FOR EATING DISORDERS, 2008	
DISORDER	**EVIDENCE-INFORMED TREATMENTS AVAILABLE (ONE OR MORE LARGE-SCALE CONTROLLED TRIALS)**	**ONE OR MORE CONTROLLED TRIALS**
Anorexia nervosa	None	Moderate number of controlled trials, although sample size and drop-out rates in adults present problems; family therapy for adolescents appears promising
Bulimia nervosa	Cognitive behavioural therapy (CBT); antidepressant medication (fluoxetine is approved by the U.S. Food and Drug Administration); interpersonal therapy	Brief CBT-based therapies appear promising
Binge eating	CBT; antidepressant medication (sibutramine and topiramate reduce both binge eating and weight); interpersonal therapy	Antidepressants appear promising, with the added advantage of weight loss; brief CBT-based therapies appear promising

Source: Adapted from Agras, W. S., & Robinson, A. H. (2008). Forty years of progress in the treatment of the eating disorders. *Nordic Journal of Psychiatry, 62*(47), 19–24. doi:10.1080/08039480802315632.

VIGNETTE

In a multifamily group on an inpatient unit, Pearl (who last saw her daughter before she had gained 18 kilograms) is asked by the group leader how she regards her daughter, Lily. Pearl replies, "She looks healthy." Lily responds with an angry, sullen look. She ultimately verbalizes that she interprets comments about her "healthy" appearance as "You look fat." The group leader points out that it is interesting that Lily equates "healthy" with "fat." In the multifamily group, there is a commonly expressed view that the illness "is not about weight" but that thinness confers a feeling of being special and that being at a normal weight (i.e., healthy) means this special status is lost.

Often family members and significant others seek ways to communicate clearly with the patient with anorexia but find that they are frequently misunderstood and that overtures of concern are misinterpreted. Consequently, families experience the tension of saying or doing the wrong thing and then feeling responsible if a setback occurs. Psychiatric mental health nurses have an important role in assisting families and significant others to develop strategies for improved communication and to search for ways to be comfortably supportive to the patient. Box 16-6 lists strategies for families trying to cope with a family member who has an eating disorder.

EVALUATION

The process of evaluation is built into the outcomes specified by *NOC*. Evaluation is ongoing, and short-term indicators are revised as necessary to achieve the treatment outcomes established. The indicators provide a daily guide for evaluating success and must be continually re-evaluated for their appropriateness. Case Study and Nursing Care Plan 16-1 presents a patient with anorexia nervosa.

BULIMIA NERVOSA

Bulimia first entered the *DSM* as a diagnosis in the third edition in 1980 but without purging or inappropriate compensatory behaviours as criteria. The diagnosis became bulimia nervosa

BOX 16-6 COPING WITH A FAMILY MEMBER WHO HAS AN EATING DISORDER

- Be patient. Eating disorders can be a long-term illness. Recovery takes time.
- Encourage the person to seek professional help. If the family member is truly endangering his or her life, be insistent.
- Seek outside help for yourself. Find a family or friend support group, a counsellor, or other professional who has experience in helping families.
- Recognize that when addressing the problem with the person you suspect has an eating disorder (especially if it is for the first time), the reaction may be one of denial or perhaps even hostility.
- Don't lay blame. This only reinforces the person's feelings of failure.
- Try to ensure that you don't allow the person's problems to interfere with your routine functioning.
- Let the person know that he or she is important to the family, but not more so than any other family member.
- Do not dwell on food-related discussions. Encourage the person to get involved with nonfood-related activities.
- Avoid commenting on the person's weight or appearance—your comments may not be taken in the proper context.
- People with eating disorders must feel control over their daily routine. This can be very frustrating for those around the individual, but the situation often only becomes worse when it is perceived that someone is trying to take that control away.
- Be aware that low self-esteem is often a problem for those with eating disorders. Be careful not to make comparisons to other members of the family or to others within their peer group. Recognize the person for who he or she is.
- Learn about eating disorders. Understanding is a key to coping.

Source: Adapted from Woodside, D. B., & Shekter-Wolfson, L. (1988/2003). *Families and eating disorders. Know the facts.* Retrieved from http://www.nedic.ca/knowthefacts/documents/Familiesandeatingdisorders.pdf.

with the addition of the preceding criteria in 1987. In the *DSM-IV-TR*, it was further subcategorized as purging or non-purging type (Wilfley, Bishop, Wilson, et al., 2007).

APPLICATION OF THE NURSING PROCESS

ASSESSMENT

General Assessment

Initially, patients with bulimia nervosa do not appear to be physically or emotionally ill. They are often at or slightly above or below ideal body weight. However, as the assessment continues and the nurse makes further observations, the physical and emotional problems of the patient become apparent. On inspection, the patient demonstrates enlargement of the parotid glands, with dental erosion and caries if the patient has been inducing vomiting. Box 16-7 identifies a number of medical complications that can occur and the laboratory findings that may result in individuals with bulimia nervosa. The disclosed history may reveal great difficulties with both impulsivity and compulsivity. Family relationships are frequently chaotic and reflect a lack of nurturing. Patients' lives reflect instability and troublesome interpersonal relationships as well. It is not uncommon for patients to have a history of impulsive stealing of items such as food, clothing, or jewellery (Mitchell & Wonderlich, 2014).

> **VIGNETTE**
>
> During the initial assessment, the nurse wonders if Brittany is actually in need of hospitalization on the eating-disorders unit. The nurse is struck by how well the patient appears, seeming healthy, well dressed, and articulate. As Brittany continues to relate her history, she tells of restricting her food intake all day until early evening, when she buys her food and begins to binge as she is shopping. She arrives home and immediately induces vomiting. For the remainder of the evening and into the early morning hours, she "zones out" while watching television and binge eating. Periodically, she goes to the bathroom to vomit. She does this about 15 times during the evening. The nurse admitting Brittany to the unit reminds her of the goals of the hospitalization, including interrupting the binge–purge cycle and normalizing eating. The nurse further explains to Brittany that she has the support of the eating-disorder treatment team and the milieu of the unit to assist her toward recovery.

Box 16-8 lists several thoughts and behaviours associated with bulimia nervosa, and Table 16-4 identifies possible signs and symptoms found on assessment and their causes.

Self-Assessment

In working with someone with bulimia, be aware that the patient is sensitive to the perceptions of others regarding this illness and may feel significant shame and loss of control. In building a therapeutic alliance, try to empathize with the patient's feelings of low self-esteem, unworthiness, and dysphoria. If you believe that the patient is not being honest (e.g., active bingeing or purging goes unreported) or is being manipulative, acknowledge such obstacles and the frustration they provoke, and construct alternative ways to view the patient's thinking and behaviour. An accepting, nonjudgemental approach, along with a comprehensive understanding of the subjective experience of the patient with bulimia, will help to build trust.

BOX 16-7	MEDICAL COMPLICATIONS OF BULIMIA NERVOSA

- Sinus bradycardia
- Orthostatic changes in pulse or blood pressure
- Cardiac arrhythmias
- Cardiac arrest from electrolyte disturbances or ipecac intoxication
- Cardiac murmur, mitral valve prolapse
- Electrolyte imbalances
- Elevated serum bicarbonate levels (although can be low, indicating a metabolic acidosis)
- Hypochloremia
- Hypokalemia
- Dehydration, which results in volume depletion, leading to stimulation of aldosterone production, which in turn stimulates further potassium excretion from kidneys; thus there can be both an indirect renal loss of potassium and a direct loss through self-induced vomiting
- Severe attrition and erosion of teeth, producing irritating sensitivity and exposing the pulp of the teeth
- Loss of dental arch
- Diminished chewing ability
- Parotid gland enlargement associated with elevated serum amylase levels
- Esophageal tears caused by self-induced vomiting
- Severe abdominal pain indicative of gastric dilation
- Russell's sign (callus on knuckles from self-induced vomiting)

Source: Data from Mitchell, J. E. & Wonderlich, S. A. (2014). Feeding and eating disorders. In R. E. Hales, S. C. Yudofsky, & L. Weiss Roberts (Eds.), *Textbook of psychiatry* (6th ed., pp. 557–587). Washington, DC: American Psychiatric Publishing.

BOX 16-8	THOUGHTS AND BEHAVIOURS ASSOCIATED WITH BULIMIA NERVOSA

- Binge eating behaviours
- Often self-induced vomiting (or laxative or diuretic use) after bingeing
- History of anorexia nervosa in one fourth to one third of individuals
- Depressive signs and symptoms
- Problems with:
  - Interpersonal relationships
  - Self-concept
  - Impulsive behaviours
- Increased levels of anxiety and compulsivity
- Possible chemical dependency
- Possible impulsive stealing

ASSESSMENT GUIDELINES

Bulimia Nervosa

1. Medical stabilization is the first priority. Problems resulting from purging are disruptions in electrolyte and fluid balance and cardiac function. Therefore a thorough physical examination is vital, including pertinent laboratory testing:
   - Electrolyte levels
   - Glucose level
   - Thyroid function tests
   - Complete blood count
   - Electrocardiography (ECG)
2. Psychiatric evaluation is advised because treatment of psychiatric comorbidity is important to outcome.

RESEARCH HIGHLIGHT

Screening Eating Disorders

Problem
People with eating disorders request services from primary care providers. The best way to assess the presence of an eating disorder in a primary care setting, however, is not known.

Purpose of Study
This study set out to compare the performance of two short eating-disorder screening tools (the SCOFF [sick, control, one stone, fat, food] Questionnaire and the Eating Disorder Screen for Primary Care [ESP]) in a primary care setting.

Methods
The 233 participants included primary-care-clinic patients and university students. The patients were approached in the clinic waiting room, and the university students were recruited using posters and announcements made in classes. Each participant completed both questionnaires.

Key Findings
It was determined that, for both the primary care patients and the university students, the ESP was a more useful tool than the SCOFF Questionnaire for helping clinicians determine the necessity of a more detailed assessment for a possible eating disorder. The ESP asked the following questions:
1. Are you satisfied with your eating patterns?
2. Do you ever eat in secret?
3. Does your weight affect the way you feel about yourself?
4. Have any members of your family suffered with an eating disorder?
5. Do you currently suffer with or have you ever suffered in the past with an eating disorder?

Implications for Nursing Practice
Using the five ESP questions can be an effective and quick method for screening people for eating disorders. If the patient identifies three or more abnormal responses, a more detailed assessment should be considered.

Source: Cotton, M-A., Ball, C., & Robinson, P. (2003). Four simple questions can help screen for eating disorders. *Journal of General Internal Medicine, 18*, 53–56. doi:10.1046/j.1525-1497.2003.20374.x.

TABLE 16-4	POSSIBLE SIGNS AND SYMPTOMS OF BULIMIA NERVOSA
CLINICAL PRESENTATION	**CAUSE**
Normal to slightly low weight	Excessive caloric intake with purging, excessive exercising
Dental caries, tooth erosion	Vomiting (hydrochloric acid reflux over enamel)
Parotid swelling	Increased serum amylase levels
Gastric dilation, rupture	Binge eating
Calluses, scars on hand (Russell's sign)	Self-induced vomiting
Peripheral edema	Rebound fluid, especially if diuretic used
Muscle weakening	Electrolyte imbalance
Abnormal laboratory values (electrolyte imbalance, hypokalemia, hyponatremia)	Purging: vomiting, laxative and/or diuretic use
Cardiovascular abnormalities (cardiomyopathy, electrocardiography [ECG] changes)	Electrolyte imbalance—*can lead to death*
Cardiac failure (cardiomyopathy)	Ipecac intoxication

DIAGNOSIS

The assessment of the patient with bulimia nervosa yields nursing diagnoses that result from the disordered eating and weight-control behaviours. Problems resulting from purging are a first priority because electrolyte and fluid balance and cardiac function are affected. Common nursing diagnoses include *Decreased cardiac output*, *Powerlessness*, *Chronic low self-esteem*, *Anxiety*, and *Ineffective coping* (substance abuse, impulsive responses to problems).

OUTCOMES IDENTIFICATION

Relevant *NOC* outcomes include *Vital signs*, *Electrolyte and acid/base balance*, *Weight maintenance behaviour*, *Self-esteem*, *Hope*, and *Coping*. Table 16-5 lists selected short-term indicators for patients with bulimia nervosa.

PLANNING

The criteria for inpatient admission of a patient with bulimia nervosa are included in Box 16-4. Like the patient with anorexia

VIGNETTE
Kelsie weighs 85% of her ideal body weight. She has a history of diuretic abuse, and she becomes very edematous when she stops their use and enters treatment. The nurse informs Kelsie that the edema is related to the use of diuretics and thus is transient and will resolve after Kelsie begins to eat normally and discontinues the diuretics. Kelsie cannot tolerate the weight gain and the accompanying edema that occurs when she stops taking diuretics. She restarts the diuretics, perpetuating the cycle of fluid retention and the risk for kidney damage. The nurse empathizes with Kelsie's inability to tolerate the feelings of anxiety and dread she experiences because of her markedly swollen extremities.

TABLE 16-5 *NOC* OUTCOMES RELATED TO BULIMIA NERVOSA

NURSING OUTCOME AND DEFINITION	SHORT-TERM INDICATORS
Vital signs: Extent to which temperature, pulse, respiration, and blood pressure are within normal range	Body temperature Apical heart rate Apical heart rhythm Respiratory rate Systolic blood pressure
Impulse self-control: Self-restraint of compulsive or impulsive behaviours	Identifies harmful impulsive behaviours Identifies feelings that lead to impulsive actions Identifies consequences of impulsive actions Controls impulses
Weight maintenance behaviour: Personal actions to maintain optimum body weight	Maintains recommended eating pattern Retains ingested foods Maintains fluid balance Plans for situations that affect food and fluid intake Expresses realistic body image
Hope: Optimism that is personally satisfying and life supporting	Expresses faith Expresses will to live Expresses optimism Sets goals

Source: Data from Moorhead, S., Johnson, M., Maas, M. L., et al. (2013). *Nursing outcomes classification (NOC)* (5th ed.). St Louis: Mosby.

nervosa, the patient with bulimia may be treated for life-threatening complications such as gastric rupture (rare), electrolyte imbalance, and cardiac dysrhythmias. Planning will also include appropriate referrals for continuing outpatient treatment.

IMPLEMENTATION

Acute Care

A patient who is medically compromised as a result of bulimia nervosa is referred to an inpatient eating-disorder unit for comprehensive treatment of the illness. The cognitive behavioural model of treatment is highly effective and frequently serves as the cornerstone of the therapeutic approach. Inpatient units designed to treat eating disorders are specially structured to interrupt the cycle of binge eating and purging and to normalize eating habits. Therapy is begun to examine the underlying conflicts and distorted perceptions of shape and weight that sustain the illness. The patient is also evaluated for treatment of comorbid disorders, such as major depression and substance abuse. In Canada, the addictions and mental health systems have traditionally functioned as two separate systems, each with its own range of services and particular approaches to treatment and support; however, current best practice supports collaboration in concurrent disorder programs in Canada (refer to Chapter 18 for more information). In addition to specialty or general treatment, there are several centres and programs for those experiencing all types of eating disorders. The National Eating Disorder Information Centre (NEDIC) provides a service provider directory of more than 700 treatment centres (both residential and outpatient-based) and service providers in every province and most cities across Canada. The directory is available at http://nedic.ca/providers/search.

Milieu Management

The highly structured milieu of an inpatient eating-disorder unit has as its primary goals the interruption of the binge–purge cycle and the prevention of disordered eating behaviours. Observation during and after meals (to prevent purging), normalization of eating patterns, and maintenance of appropriate exercise are integral elements of such a unit. The interprofessional team uses a comprehensive treatment approach to address the emotional and behavioural problems that arise when the patient is no longer binge eating or purging. Like the interruption of other obsessive-compulsive behaviours, preventing the binge–purge pattern allows underlying anxiety to surface and be examined.

Pharmacological Interventions

Antidepressant medication together with cognitive behavioural psychotherapy has been shown to bring about improvement in bulimic symptoms. Limited research suggests that the SSRIs and tricyclic antidepressants help reduce binge eating and vomiting over short terms. Fluoxetine (Prozac) treatment may help prevent relapse. Bupropion (Wellbutrin) may be effective, but due to an increased risk for seizures, it is contraindicated in patients who purge (Williams & Goodie, 2007).

Counselling

Compared with the patient with anorexia, the patient with bulimia nervosa often more readily establishes a therapeutic alliance with the nurse, because the eating-disordered behaviours are seen as a problem. The therapeutic alliance allows the nurse, along with other members of the interprofessional team, to provide counselling that gives useful feedback regarding the patient's distorted beliefs.

Health Teaching and Health Promotion

Health teaching focuses on not only the eating disorder but also meal planning, use of relaxation techniques, maintenance of a healthy diet and exercise, coping skills, the physical and emotional effects of bingeing and purging, and the impact of cognitive distortions.

Once patients reach therapeutic goals, it is recommended that they seek long-term care to solidify those goals and address the attitudes, perceptions, and psychodynamic issues that maintain the eating disorder and attend the illness.

Advanced-Practice Interventions
Psychotherapy

Cognitive behavioural therapy is the most effective treatment for bulimia nervosa. Restructuring faulty perceptions and helping individuals to develop accepting attitudes toward themselves and their bodies is a primary focus of therapy. When patients do not engage in bulimic behaviours, issues of self-worth and interpersonal functioning become more prominent.

VIGNETTE

Nadia, a 23-year-old patient with a 6-year history of bulimia nervosa, struggles with issues of self-esteem. She expresses much guilt about "letting her father down" in the past by drinking alcohol excessively and binge eating and purging. She is determined that this time she is not going to fail at treatment. After her initial success in stopping the disordered behaviours, she says defiantly, "I'm doing this for me." Nadia usually experiences her behaviour as either pleasing or disappointing to others, but she begins to realize that her feeling of self-worth is very much dependent on how others see her and that she needs to develop a better sense of herself.

Box 16-9 presents relevant *Nursing Interventions Classification (NIC)* interventions for the management of eating disorders.

EVALUATION

Evaluation of treatment effectiveness is ongoing and built into the *NOC* categories. Outcomes are revised as necessary to reach the desired outcomes. Case Study and Nursing Care Plan 16-2 presents a patient with bulimia nervosa.

BINGE EATING DISORDER

Binge eating disorder is characterized by recurring episodes of eating significantly more food than most in a relatively short

---

BOX 16-9   *NIC* **INTERVENTIONS FOR EATING-DISORDERS MANAGEMENT**

Definition: Prevention and treatment of severe diet restriction and overexercising or bingeing and purging of food and fluids.

Activities:

- Develop a supportive relationship with patient.
- Collaborate with other members of health care team to develop treatment plan; involve patient and significant others as appropriate.
- Confer with team and patient to set a target weight if patient is not within a recommended weight range for age and body frame.
- Establish the amount of daily weight gain that is desired.
- Confer with dietitian to determine daily caloric intake necessary to attain or maintain target weight.
- Teach and reinforce concepts of good nutrition with patient (and significant others as appropriate).
- Encourage patient to discuss food preferences with dietitian.
- Monitor physiological parameters (vital signs, electrolyte levels) as needed.
- Weigh on a routine basis (e.g., at same time of day and after voiding).
- Monitor intake and output of fluids, as appropriate.
- Monitor daily caloric intake.
- Encourage patient self-monitoring of daily food intake and weight gain or maintenance as appropriate.
- Establish expectations for appropriate eating behaviours, intake of food and fluids, and amount of physical activity.
- Use behavioural contracting with patient to elicit desired weight gain or maintenance behaviours.
- Restrict food availability to scheduled, pre-served meals and snacks.
- Observe patient during and after meals and snacks to ensure that adequate intake is achieved and maintained.
- Accompany patient to bathroom during designated observation times following meals and snacks.
- Limit time spent in bathroom during periods when not under direct supervision.
- Monitor patient for behaviours related to eating, weight loss, and weight gain.

- Use behaviour modification techniques to promote behaviours that contribute to weight gain and limit weight-loss behaviours as appropriate.
- Provide reinforcement for weight gain and behaviours that promote weight gain.
- Provide support (e.g., relaxation therapy, desensitization exercises, opportunities to talk about feelings) as patient integrates new eating behaviours, changing body image, and lifestyle changes.
- Encourage patient use of daily logs to record feelings and circumstances surrounding urge to purge, vomit, or overexercise.
- Limit physical activity as needed to promote weight gain.
- Provide a supervised exercise program when appropriate.
- Allow opportunity to make limited choices about eating and exercise as weight gain progresses in desirable manner.
- Assist patient (and significant others as appropriate) to examine and resolve personal issues that may contribute to the eating disorder.
- Assist patient to develop a self-esteem that is compatible with a healthy body weight.
- Confer with the health care team on a routine basis about patient's progress.
- Initiate maintenance phase of treatment when patient has achieved target weight and has consistently shown desired eating behaviours for designated period of time.
- Monitor patient weight on a routine basis.
- Determine acceptable range of weight variation in relation to target range.
- Place responsibility for choices about eating and physical activity with patient as appropriate.
- Provide support and guidance as needed.
- Assist patient to evaluate the appropriateness and consequences of choices about eating and physical activity.
- Reinstitute weight-gain protocol if patient is unable to remain within target weight range.
- Institute a treatment program and follow-up care (medical, counselling) for home management.

Source: Bulechek, G. M., Butcher, H. K., Dochterman, J. M., et al. (2013). *Nursing interventions classification (NIC)* (6th ed., p. 155). St. Louis: Mosby.

period of time accompanied by feelings of guilt or distress. Overeating is frequently noted as a symptom of an affective disorder (e.g., atypical depression). Depression has been associated with binge eating disorder in a number of studies (Araujo, Santos, & Nardi, 2010). Social anxiety (Sawaoka, Barnes, Blomquist, et al., 2012) and family history of anxiety (Blomquist & Grilo, 2015) also have strong associations with the disorder, and thus assessment practices are concerned with clearly determining the points for relevant intervention.

Because of its efficacy with bulimia, the use of SSRIs at or near the high end of the dosage range have been studied to treat binge eating disorder and seem to help in the short term; however, patients regained significant weight after discontinuance of medication. Other medications that are under investigation include the tricyclic antidepressants, antiepileptic agents, and appetite suppressants (Williams & Goodie, 2007).

Cognitive behavioural therapy and interpersonal therapy have been determined to be effective in eliminating binge eating; however, on average, these therapies do not produce clinically significant weight loss (Wilson, Wilfley, Agras, et al., 2010). Dialectical behavioural therapy has been found to be effective in reducing binge eating for those patients seeking weight-loss services (Mushquash & McMahan, 2015).

Binge eating is one of the most common forms of eating disorders documented in individuals who are being considered for bariatric surgery. Approximately 6 000 bariatric surgeries were performed in Canadian hospitals in 2013 (Canadian Institute for Health Information, 2014). Binge eating after bariatric surgery has been associated with poor weight outcomes, however (Kalarchian & Marcus, 2015). Preoperative and postoperative cognitive behavioural therapy, dialectical behavioural therapy, and acceptance and commitment therapy all show promise in reducing binge eating, although their direct impact on longer-term weight loss is unknown (Kalarchian & Marcus, 2015). Many advanced-practice nurses are qualified to provide these therapies. Box 16-10 outlines the recommended preoperative and postoperative standards of care for bariatric surgery.

BOX 16-10 PREOPERATIVE AND POSTOPERATIVE STANDARDS OF CARE FOR BARIATRIC SURGERY

Preoperative Period

Patients:

- Should have a full understanding of the postoperative dietary requirements, the necessary postsurgical supports, and the importance of stress-management strategies
- Should be screened for severe psychiatric comorbidities
- Must have a minimum 12-month period of recovery from any eating disorder, substance abuse, manic episode, psychosis, psychiatric hospitalization, suicide attempt, or trauma-related issue before having bariatric surgery
- Should receive counselling or education to assist with lifestyle changes

Postoperative Period

Patients:

- Will receive close follow-up and support from members of an interprofessional team (surgery, medicine, psychiatry or psychology, nutrition and exercise science) monthly for the first 6 months, then every 2 months for the remainder of the first year after surgery

---

CASE STUDY AND NURSING CARE PLAN 16-1

Anorexia Nervosa

Ella, a 20-year-old woman, is brought to the inpatient eating-disorder unit of a local hospital by two older brothers, who are supporting her on either side. She is profoundly weak, holding her head up with her hands.

ASSESSMENT

Self-Assessment

Nurse Puneet is assigned to care for Ella. Although a young nurse, Puneet has spent the past 3 years working on the eating-disorders unit. When she first began, she had difficulty overidentifying with patients. Ella has struggled with bulimia, but with treatment she has done well. She seeks guidance from her nursing supervisor and the interprofessional team, which have helped her to maintain appropriate boundaries while creating a therapeutic alliance with patients.

Objective Data	Subjective Data
Height: 157 cm	Denies being underweight: "I need treatment because I get fatigued so easily."
Weight: 26.3 kg—50% of ideal body weight	"I check my legs every night. I'm so afraid of getting fat. I hate it if my legs touch each other."
Blood pressure: 74/50 mm Hg	"I don't like to start anything until I know I can do it perfectly the first time. I wouldn't want anyone to see me make a mistake."
Pulse: 54 beats per minute	Depressed mood
Anemic—hemoglobin: 90 g/L (9 g/dL)	
Cachectic appearance, pale, with fine lanugo	
Sad facial expression	
Bruising on inside of each knee from sleeping on her side with knees touching	

Continued

CASE STUDY AND NURSING CARE PLAN 16-1—cont'd

Anorexia Nervosa

DIAGNOSIS

1. *Imbalanced nutrition: less than body requirements* related to restriction of caloric intake secondary to extreme fear of weight gain
2. *Chronic low self-esteem* related to perception that others are always judging her

OUTCOMES IDENTIFICATION

Patient will reach 75% of ideal weight (41.7 kg) by discharge.

PLANNING

The initial plan is to address Ella's unstable physiological state.

IMPLEMENTATION

Ellas's care plan is personalized as follows:

Short-Term Goal	Intervention	Rationale	Evaluation
1. Patient will gain a minimum of 1 kg and a maximum of 1.5 kg weekly through inpatient stay.	1a. Acknowledge the emotional and physical difficulty patient is experiencing. Use patient's extreme fatigue to engage cooperation in the treatment plan.	1a. A first priority is to establish a therapeutic alliance.	**WEEK 1** Patient increases caloric intake with liquid supplement only. Patient unable to eat solid food. Patient does not gain weight. Patient remains hypotensive, bradycardic, anemic (hemoglobin [Hgb] = 90 g/L [9 g/dL]).
	1b. Weigh patient daily for the first week, then three times a week. Patient should be weighed in bra and panties only. There should be no oral intake, including a drink of water, before the early morning weigh-in.	1b. These measures ensure that weight is accurate.	**WEEK 2** Patient gains 1 kg drinking liquid supplement—minimal solid food. Patient remains hypotensive, bradycardic (Hgb = 100 g/L [10 g/dL]).
	1c. Do not negotiate weight with patient or reweigh. Patient may choose not to look at the scale or request that she not be told the weight.	1c. Patient may try to control and sabotage treatment.	**WEEK 3** Patient gains 0.5 kg drinking liquid supplement. Patient selects meal plan but is unable to eat most solid foods. Patient's blood pressure (BP) = 84/60 mm Hg; pulse = 68 beats per minute, regular; Hgb = 110 g/L (11 g/dL).
	1d. Measure vital signs three times a day (tid) until stable, then daily. Repeat electrocardiography (ECG) and laboratory tests until stable.	1d. As patient begins to increase in weight, cardiovascular status improves to within normal range, and monitoring is less frequent.	**WEEKS 4–6** Patient gains an average of 1 kg/week. Patient samples more solid foods selected from meal plan. Patient's BP = 90/60 mm Hg; pulse = 68 beats per minute, regular; Hgb = 115 g/L (11.5 g/dL).
	1e. Provide a pleasant, calm atmosphere at mealtimes. Patient should be told the specific times and duration (usually a half-hour) of meals.	1e. Mealtimes become episodes of high anxiety, and knowledge of regulations decreases tension in the milieu, particularly when patient has given up so much control by entering treatment.	

CASE STUDY AND NURSING CARE PLAN 16-1—cont'd

Anorexia Nervosa

Short-Term Goal	Intervention	Rationale	Evaluation
	1f. Administer liquid supplement as ordered.	1f. Patient may be unable to eat solid food at first.	**WEEK 7** Patient weighs 32.2 kg (almost 60% of ideal body weight); calories are mostly from liquid supplement.
	1g. Observe patient during meals to prevent hiding or throwing away of food and for at least 1 hour after meals and snacks to prevent purging. 1h. Encourage patient to try to eat some solid food. Preparation of patient's meals should be guided by likes and dislikes list because patient is unable to make own selections to complete menu.	1g, h. The compelling force of the illness is such that behaviours related to hiding or discarding food are difficult to stop. A power struggle between staff and patient may emerge, in which patient appears to comply but defies the rules (appearing to eat but throwing away food).	Patient selects balanced meals, eating more varied solid food: turkey, carrots, lettuce, fruit. Patient's Hgb = 125 g/L (12.5 g/dL); normal range of BP and pulse are maintained. Patient continues to increase participation in social aspects of eating. **WEEKS 8–12** Patient gains an average of 1 kg/week and weighs 37.1 kg (approx. 68% of ideal body weight).
	1i. Be empathic with patient's struggle to give up control of her eating and her weight as she is expected to make minimum weight gain on a regular basis. Permit patient to verbalize feelings at these times.	1i. Patient is expected to gain at least 0.25 kg on a specific schedule, usually three times a week (Monday, Wednesday, Friday).	Patient is eating more varied solid food, but most caloric intake is still from liquid supplement. Patient maintains normal vital signs and Hgb levels. Patient maintains social interaction during mealtimes and snacks.
	1j. Monitor patient's weight gain. A weight gain of 1 kg/week to 1.5 kg/week is medically acceptable.	1j. Weight gain of more than 2.25 kg in 1 week may result in pulmonary edema.	**WEEKS 13–16** Patient has reached medically stable weight at the end of 16th week—41.7 kg (approx. 75% of ideal body weight).
	1k. Provide teaching regarding healthy eating as the basis of a healthy lifestyle.	1k. Healthy aspects of eating (e.g., increased energy, rather than gaining weight) are reinforced.	Patient continues to eat more solid food with relatively less liquid supplement. Patient is not able to participate in planned exercise program until she reaches 85% of ideal body weight.
	1l. Use a cognitive behavioural approach to address patient's expressed fears regarding weight gain. Identify and examine dysfunctional thoughts; identify and examine values and beliefs that sustain these thoughts.	1l. Confronting irrational thoughts and beliefs is crucial to changing eating behaviours.	
	1m. As patient approaches her target weight, there should be encouragement to make her own choices for menu selection.	1m. Patient can assume more control of her meals, which is empowering for the patient with anorexia.	
	1n. Emphasize social nature of eating. Encourage conversation that does not have the theme of food during mealtimes.	1n. Eating as a social activity, shared with others and with participation in conversation, serves as both a distraction from obsessional preoccupations and a pleasurable event.	

Continued

CASE STUDY AND NURSING CARE PLAN 16-1—cont'd

Anorexia Nervosa

Short-Term Goal	Intervention	Rationale	Evaluation
	1o. Focus on the patient's strengths, including her good work in normalizing her weight and eating habits.	1o. Patient who is beginning to normalize weight and eating behaviours has achieved a major accomplishment, of which she should be proud. Noneating activities are explored as a source of gratification.	
	1p. Provide for a planned exercise program when patient reaches target weight.	1p. Patient experiences a strong drive to exercise; this measure accommodates this drive by planning a reasonable amount.	
	1q. Encourage patient to apply all the knowledge, skills, and gains made from the various individual, family, and group therapy sessions.	1q. Patient has been receiving intensive therapy and education, which have provided tools and techniques that are useful in maintaining healthy behaviours.	

EVALUATION

By the end of the sixteenth week, Ella has achieved a stable weight of 41.7 kilograms. This weight is approaching congruency with Ella's height, frame, and age. Her vital signs and hemoglobin levels are consistently normal. She is participating in therapy and consistently communicating satisfaction with her body appearance.

CASE STUDY AND NURSING CARE PLAN 16-2

Bulimia Nervosa

Reena is a 30-year-old university graduate who reports that she is an aspiring actress working currently as a "temp" for an insurance agency. She is being admitted to a partial hospitalization program designed for patients with eating disorders. Reena has bulimia nervosa.

ASSESSMENT

Self-Assessment

Matthew, a seasoned nurse in the area of eating disorders, is assigned to care for Reena. Matthew enjoys working with patients with bulimia because he believes that he can help patients move toward health. When he first encounters Reena, he experiences an immediate negative response that surprises him. He speaks to his supervisor about these feelings and raises the question of whether he is the appropriate nurse to care for Reena. As he and the supervisor discuss his feelings, Matthew is able to recognize that Reena reminds him of a girlfriend he had many years earlier. The relationship ended badly. Matthew experiences an emotional release with this realization and believes that he will be able to separate his earlier negative experience from his work with Reena.

Objective Data	Subjective Data
Height: 165 cm	"I can't stand to be fat."
Weight: 57.6 kg—95% of ideal body weight	"I'm ashamed that I can't control my bingeing and vomiting—I know
Blood pressure: 120/80 mm Hg sitting; 90/60 mm Hg standing	it's not good."
Pulse: 70 beats/min sitting; 96 beats/min standing	
Potassium level of 2.7 mmol/L (normal range, 3.3 to 5.5 mmol/L)	
ECG: abnormal—consistent with hypokalemia	
Erosion of enamel, enlarged parotid glands, consistent with a history of binge eating and purging	

CASE STUDY AND NURSING CARE PLAN 16-2—cont'd

Bulimia Nervosa

DIAGNOSIS

1. *Risk for injury* related to low potassium and other physical changes secondary to binge eating and purging
2. *Powerlessness* related to inability to control bingeing and vomiting cycles

OUTCOMES IDENTIFICATION

Reena will demonstrate an ability to regulate eating patterns, resulting in consistently normal electrolyte balance.

PLANNING

Reena is admitted to a partial hospitalization program designed for patients with eating disorders. She attends the program 3 or 4 days a week and participates in individual and group therapy. She will continue to work as a "temp" for an insurance agency.

IMPLEMENTATION

Reena's care plan is personalized as follows:

Short-Term Goal	Intervention	Rationale	Evaluation
1. Patient will identify signs and symptoms of low potassium level (K⁺), and K⁺ level will remain within normal limits throughout hospitalization.	1a. Educate patient regarding the ill effects of self-induced vomiting, low K⁺ level, dental erosion.	1a. Health teaching is crucial to treatment. The patient needs to be reminded of the benefits of normalization of eating behaviour.	**WEEK 1** Patient begins to select balanced meals. Patient demonstrates knowledge of untoward effects of vomiting and K⁺ deficiency. Patient begins to demonstrate understanding of repetitive nature of binge–purge cycle.
	1b. Educate patient about binge–purge cycle and its self-perpetuating nature.	1.b c. The compulsive nature of the binge–purge cycle is maintained by the sequence of intake restriction, hunger, bingeing, purging accompanied by feelings of guilt, and then repetition of the cycle over and over.	**WEEK 2** Patient begins to challenge irrational thoughts and beliefs. Patient continues to plan nutritionally balanced meals, including dinner at home. Patient begins to sample "forbidden foods" and discuss thoughts and attitudes about same.
	1c. Teach patient that fasting sets one up to binge eat.		
	1d. Explore ideas about trigger foods.	1d. Patient needs to understand beliefs about trigger foods to challenge irrational thoughts.	**WEEK 3** Patient discusses triggers to binge and resultant behaviour. Patient continues to challenge irrational thoughts and beliefs in individual and group sessions. Patient plans meals, including "forbidden foods."
	1e. Challenge irrational thoughts and beliefs about "forbidden" foods.	1e. Challenge forces patient to examine own thinking and beliefs.	
	1f. Teach patient to plan and eat regularly scheduled, balanced meals.	1f. This teaching helps to ensure success in maintaining abstinence from binge–purge activity.	**WEEK 4** Patient reports no binge–purge behaviours at day program or outside. Patient demonstrates understanding of repetitive nature of binge–purge cycle. Patient continues to challenge irrational thoughts and beliefs.

EVALUATION

At the end of 4 weeks, Reena reports no binge–purge cycles, and her potassium level remains consistently within normal limits. She is beginning to plan meals and challenge irrational thoughts and beliefs.

KEY POINTS TO REMEMBER

- A number of theoretical models help explain the origins of eating disorders.
- Neurobiological theories identify an association among eating disorders, depression, and neuroendocrine abnormalities.
- Psychological theories explore issues of control related to eating disorders.
- Genetic theories postulate the existence of vulnerabilities that may predispose people toward eating disorders.
- Sociocultural models look at our present societal ideal of being thin.
- Men with eating disorders share many of the characteristics of women with eating disorders.
- The suicide rate of patients with eating disorders is much higher than predicted rates in similar age groups.
- Anorexia nervosa is a potentially life-threatening eating disorder that includes severe underweight; low blood pressure, pulse, and temperature; dehydration; low serum potassium level; and dysrhythmias.
- Anorexia may be treated in an inpatient treatment setting in which milieu therapy, psychotherapy (cognitive), development of self-care skills, and psychobiological interventions can be implemented.
- Long-term treatment is provided on an outpatient basis and aims to help patients maintain healthy weight. It includes treatment modalities such as individual therapy, family therapy, group therapy, psychopharmacology, and nutrition counselling.
- Patients with bulimia nervosa are typically within the normal weight range, but some may be slightly below or above ideal body weight.
- Assessment of the patient with bulimia may show enlargement of the parotid glands and dental erosion and caries if the patient has induced vomiting.
- Acute care may be necessary when life-threatening complications such as gastric rupture (rare), electrolyte imbalance, and cardiac dysrhythmias are present.
- The goal of interventions is to interrupt the binge–purge cycle.
- Psychotherapy and self-care skill training are included in the treatment plan.
- Long-term treatment focuses on therapy aimed at addressing any coexisting depression, substance abuse, or personality disorders that are causing the patient distress and interfering with the quality of life. Self-worth and interpersonal functioning eventually become issues that are useful for the patient to target.
- People with binge eating disorder report a history of major depression significantly more often than people who do not binge eat.
- Effective treatment for obese patients with binge eating disorder integrates modification of the disordered eating, improvement of depressive symptoms, and achievement of an appropriate weight.

CRITICAL THINKING

1. Logan, a 19-year-old male model, has experienced a rapid decrease in weight over the past 4 months after his agent told him he would have to lose some weight or lose a coveted account. Logan is 188 centimetres tall and weighs 60 kilograms, down from his usual 80 kilograms. He is brought to the emergency department with a pulse of 40 beats per minute and severe arrhythmias. His laboratory workup reveals severe hypokalemia. He has become extremely depressed, saying, "I'm too fat! I don't want anything to eat—if I gain weight, my life will be ruined. There is nothing to live for if I can't model." Logan's parents are startled and confused, and his best friend is worried and feels powerless to help: "I tell Logan he needs to eat or he will die. I tell him he is a skeleton, but he refuses to listen to me. I don't know what to do."

   a. Which physical and psychiatric criteria suggest that Logan should be hospitalized immediately?

   b. What are five questions that could be asked to help determine if further assessment is needed regarding the possibility of an eating disorder?

   c. What are some of the questions you would eventually ask Logan when evaluating his biopsychosocial functioning?

   d. What are your feelings toward someone with anorexia? Can you make a distinction between your thoughts and feelings toward women with anorexia and toward men with anorexia?

   e. What are some things you could do for Logan's parents and friend in terms of offering them information, support, and referrals? Identify specific referrals.

   f. Explain the kinds of interventions or restrictions that may be used while Logan is hospitalized.

   g. How would you describe partial hospitalization programs when asked if Logan will have to be hospitalized for an extended period?

   h. What are some of Logan's cognitive distortions that would be a target for therapy?

   i. Identify at least five criteria that, if met, would indicate that Logan was improving.

2. You and Ambreen have been close friends since nursing school and are now working on the same surgical unit. Ambreen told you that in the past she has made several suicide attempts. Today, you come upon her bingeing off-unit, and she looks embarrassed and uncomfortable when she sees you. On several occasions, you notice that she spends time in the bathroom, and you hear sounds of retching. In response to your concern, she admits that she has been bingeing and purging for several years but that she is now getting out of control and feels profoundly depressed.

   a. Although Ambreen does not show any physical signs of bulimia nervosa, what would you look for when assessing an individual with bulimia?

   b. What kinds of emergencies could result from bingeing and purging?

   c. What would be the most useful type of psychotherapy for Ambreen initially, and what issues would need to be addressed?

   d. What kinds of new skills does a person with bulimia need to learn to lessen the compulsion to binge and purge?

   e. What would be some signs that Ambreen is recovering?

3. The high school principal shares with you that several students (male and female) have disclosed to faculty that they have an eating disorder. The principal is concerned about the health of all of the students in the school and asks you to hold a general information session.

   a. What type of health promotion material will be helpful?

   b. How could you deliver this information to the students?

CHAPTER REVIEW

1. Which female patient should the nurse recognize as having the highest risk to have or develop bulimia nervosa? The one who:

   a. Grew up in an underserved area

   b. Lives in a society influenced by Eastern cultural beliefs

   c. Is 20 years old

   d. Is Asian Canadian

2. The nurse is caring for a 16-year-old female patient with anorexia nervosa. What should the initial nursing intervention be upon the patient's admission to the unit?

   a. Build a therapeutic relationship.

   b. Increase the patient's caloric consumption.

   c. Involve the patient in group therapy to build a support group.

   d. Self-assess to decrease tendencies toward authoritarianism.

3. The nurse is caring for a patient with bulimia. Which nursing intervention is appropriate?

   a. Monitor patient on bathroom trips after eating.

   b. Allow patient extensive private time with family members.

   c. Provide meals whenever the patient requests them.

   d. Encourage patient to select foods that she or he likes.

4. The nurse is admitting a patient who weighs 45 kilograms, is 167 centimetres tall, and is below ideal body weight. The patient's blood pressure is 130/80 mm Hg, pulse is 72 beats per minute, potassium is 2.5 mmol/L, and ECG is abnormal. Her teeth enamel is eroded, her hands are visibly shaking, and her parotid gland is enlarged. The patient states, "I am really worked up about coming to this unit." What is the priority nursing diagnosis?

   a. *Powerlessness*

   b. *Risk for injury*

   c. *Imbalanced nutrition: Less than body requirements*

   d. *Anxiety*

5. The nurse is planning care for a patient with an eating disorder. What outcomes are appropriate? Select all that apply.

   a. The patient will experience a decrease in depression.

   b. The patient will identify four methods to control anxiety.

   c. The patient will collect different kinds of cookbooks.

   d. The patient will identify two people to contact if suicidal thoughts occur.

6. What patient statement acknowledges the characteristic behavior associated with a diagnosis of pica?

   a. "Nothing could make me drink milk."

   b. "I'm ashamed of it, but I eat my hair."

   c. "I haven't eaten a green vegetable since I was 3 years old."

   d. "I regurgitate and rechew my food after almost every meal."

⊖volve WEBSITE

Visit the Evolve website for Chapter Review Answers and Rationales, Critical Thinking Answer Guidelines, and additional resources related to the content in this chapter: http://evolve.elsevier.com/Canada/Varcarolis/psychiatric/

REFERENCES

Agras, W. S., & Robinson, A. H. (2008). Forty years of progress in the treatment of the eating disorders. *Nordic Journal of Psychiatry, 62*(47), 19–24. doi:10.1080/08039480802315632.

American Psychiatric Association (APA). (2013). *DSM-5 table of contents.* Retrieved from http://www.psychiatry.org/dsm5.

Araujo, D. M. R., Santos, G. F., & Nardi, A. E. (2010). Binge eating disorder and depression: A systematic review. *World Journal of Biological Psychiatry, 11*(2 Pt. 2), 199–207. doi:10.3109/15622970802563171.

Arcelus, J., Witcomb, G. L., & Mitchell, A. (2014). Prevalence of eating disorders amongst dancers: A systemic review and meta-analysis: Eating disorders and dance. *European Eating Disorders Review, 22*(2), 92–101. doi:10.1002/erv.2271.

Attia, E., & Walsh, B. T. (2007). Anorexia nervosa. *American Journal of Psychiatry, 164*(12), 1805–1810.

Backholm, K., Isomaa, R., & Birgegård, A. (2013). The prevalence and impact of trauma history in eating disorder patients. *European Journal of Psychotraumatology, 4*(1), 22482–22488. doi:10.3402/ejpt.v4i0.22482.

Bar, R. J., Cassin, S. E., & Dionne, M. M. (2016). Eating disorder prevention initiatives for athletes: A review. *European Journal of Sport Science, 16*(3), 325–335. doi:10.1080/17461391.2015.1013995.

Berkman, N. D., Lohr, K. N., & Bulik, C. M. (2007). Outcomes of eating disorders: A systematic review of the literature. *International Journal of Eating Disorders, 40*, 293–309. doi:10.1002/eat.20369.

Bienvenu, O. J., Davydow, D. S., & Kendler, K. S. (2011). Psychiatric "diseases" versus behavioral disorders and degree of genetic influence. *Psychological Medicine, 41*(1), 33–40.

Blomquist, K. K., & Grilo, C. M. (2015). Family histories of anxiety in overweight men and women with binge eating disorder: A preliminary investigation. *Comprehensive Psychiatry, 62*, 161–169. doi:10.1016/j.comppsych.2015.07.007.

Boisvert, J. A., & Harrell, W. A. (2009). Ethnic and age differences in eating disorder symptomatology among Albertan women. *Canadian Journal of Behavioural Science. Revue Canadienne Des Sciences Du Comportement, 41*(3), 143–150. doi:10.1037/a0014689.

Boisvert, J. A., & Harrell, W. A. (2012). The impact of spirituality on eating disorder symptomatology in ethnically diverse Canadian women. *International Journal of Social Psychiatry, 59*(8), 729–738. doi:10.1177/0020764012453816.

Brewerton, T. D. (2007). Eating disorders, trauma, and comorbidity: Focus on PTSD. *Eating Disorders: The Journal of Treatment & Prevention, 15*(4), 285–304. doi:10.1080/10640260701454311.

Bruch, H. (1978). *The golden cage: The enigma of anorexia nervosa.* Cambridge, MA: Harvard University Press.

Campbell, I. C., Mill, J., Uher, R., et al. (2011). Eating disorders, gene-environment interactions and epigenetics. *Neuroscience and Biobehavioral Reviews, 35*(3), 784–793.

Canadian Institute for Health Information. (2014). *Report: Bariatric surgery in Canada.* Retrieved from https://secure.cihi.ca/free_products/Bariatric_Surgery_in_Canada_EN.pdf.

Canadian Senate. (2016). *Report of the Standing Senate Committee on Social Affairs, Science and Technology: Obesity in Canada: A whole-of-society approach for a healthier Canada.* Retrieved from https://sencanada.ca/content/sen/committee/421/SOCI/Reports/2016-02-25_Revised_report_Obesity_in_Canada_e.pdf.

Caparrotta, L., & Ghaffari, K. (2006). A historical overview of the psychodynamic contributions to the understanding of eating disorders. *Psychoanalytic Psychotherapy, 20*(3), 175–196.

Cucchi, A., Ryan, D., Konstantakopoulos, G., et al. (2016). Lifetime prevalence of non-suicidal self-injury in patients with eating disorders: A systematic review and meta-analysis. *Psychological Medicine, 46*(7), 1345. doi:10.1017/S0033291716000027.

Doris, E., Shekriladze, I., Javakhishvili, N., et al. (2015). Is cultural change associated with eating disorders? A systematic review of the literature. *Eating and Weight Disorders: EWD, 20*(2), 149–160. doi:10.1007/s40519-015-0189-9.

Frank, G. K. W. (2015). Advances from neuroimaging studies in eating disorders. *CNS Spectrums, 20*(4), 391–400. doi:10.1017/S1092852915000012.

Frank, G. K. W., & Shott, M. E. (2016). The role of psychotropic medications in the management of anorexia nervosa: Rationale, evidence and future prospects. *CNS Drugs, 30*(5), 419–442. doi:10.1007/s40263-016-0335-6.

Godart, N. T., Perdereau, F., Rein, Z., et al. (2007). Comorbidity studies of eating disorders and mood disorders. Critical review of the literature. *Journal of Affective Disorders, 97*, 37–49. doi:10.1016/j.jad.2006.06.023.

Government of Canada. (2014). *Eating disorders among girls and women in Canada: Report of the Standing Committee on the Status of Women.* Retrieved from https://nedic.ca/sites/default/files//Status%20of%20Women%20Report%20Eating%20Disorders.pdf.

Harrington, B. C., Jimerson, M., Haxton, C., et al. (2015). Initial evaluation, diagnosis, and treatment of anorexia nervosa and bulimia nervosa. *American Family Physician, 91*(1), 46–52.

Haworth-Hoeppner, S. (2017). *Family, culture, and self in the development of eating disorders.* New York: Routledge.

Herdman, T. H., & Kamitsuru, S. (Eds.), (2014). *NANDA international nursing diagnoses: Definitions and classification* (pp. 2015–2017). Oxford, UK: Wiley-Blackwell.

Kalarchian, M. A., & Marcus, M. D. (2015). Psychosocial interventions pre and post bariatric surgery. *European Eating Disorders Review, 23*(6), 457–462. doi:10.1002/erv.2392.

Kaye, W. (2007). Neurobiology of anorexia and bulimia nervosa. *Physiology & Behavior, 94*, 112–135. doi:10.1016/j.physbeh.2007.11.037.

Kaye, W. H., Wierenga, C. E., Bailer, U. F., et al. (2013). Nothing tastes as good as skinny feels: The neurobiology of anorexia nervosa. *Trends in Neuroscience, 36*(2), 110–120. doi:10.1016/j.tins.2013.01.003.

Kostro, K., Lerman, J. B., & Attia, E. (2014). The current status of suicide and self-injury in eating disorders: A narrative review. *Journal of Eating Disorders, 2*(1), 19. doi:10.1186/s40337-014-0019-x.

Le Grange, D., Lock, J., Loeb, K., et al. (2010). Academy for eating disorders position paper: The role of the family in eating disorders. *International Journal of Eating Disorders, 43*(1), 1–5. doi:10.1002/eat.20751.

Madowitz, J., Matheson, B. E., & Liang, J. (2015). The relationship between eating disorders and sexual trauma. *Eating and Weight Disorders: Studies on Anorexia, Bulimia and Obesity, 20*(3), 281–293. doi:10.1007/s40519-015-0195-y.

Malson, H., & Burns, M. (2009). *Critical feminist approaches to eating disorders.* New York: Routledge.

Mangweth-Matzek, B., Hoek, H. W., Rupp, C. I., et al. (2014). Prevalence of eating disorders in middle-aged women: Eating disorders in middle-age. *International Journal of Eating Disorders, 47*(3), 320–324. doi:10.1002/eat.22232.

Mangweth-Matzek, B., Kummer, K. K., & Pope, H. G. (2016). Eating disorder symptoms in middle-aged and older men. *International Journal of Eating Disorders, 49*(10), 953–957. doi:10.1002/eat.22550.

Miller, J. L., Vaillancourt, T., & Hanna, S. E. (2009). The measurement of "eating-disorder-thoughts" and "eating-disorder-behaviors": Implications for assessment and detection of eating disorders in epidemiological studies. *Eating Behaviors, 10*(2), 89–96. doi:10.1016/j.eatbeh.2009.02.002.

Mitchell, J. E., & Wonderlich, S. A. (2014). Feeding and eating disorders. In R. E. Hales, S. C. Yudofsky, & L. Weiss Roberts (Eds.), *Textbook of psychiatry* (6th ed., pp. 557–587). Washington, DC: American Psychiatric Publishing.

Mitchison, D., & Hay, P. J. (2014). The epidemiology of eating disorders: Genetic, environmental, and societal factors. *Clinical Epidemiology, 6*, 89–97. doi:10.2147/CLEP.S40841.

Moorhead, S., Johnson, M., Maas, M. L., et al. (2013). *Nursing outcomes classification (NOC)* (5th ed.). St Louis: Mosby.

Mushquash, A. R., & McMahan, M. (2015). Dialectical behavior therapy skills training reduces binge eating among patients seeking weight-management services: Preliminary evidence. *Eating and Weight Disorders: Studies on Anorexia, Bulimia and Obesity, 20*(3), 415–418. doi:10.1007/s40519-015-0177-0.

Myatt, R. (2014). An overview of cardiac risk in patients with chronic eating disorders. *British Journal of Cardiac Nursing, 9*(6), 287–291.

Nasser, M. (2009). Eating disorders across cultures. *Psychiatry, 8*(9), 347–350. doi:10.1016/j.mppsy.2009.06.009.

Norris, M., Strike, M., Pinhas, L., et al. (2013). The Canadian eating disorder program survey: Exploring intensive treatment programs for youth with eating disorders. *Journal of the Canadian Academy of Child and Adolescent Psychiatry/Journal de l'Académie Canadienne de Psychiatrie de l'Enfant et de l'Adolescent, 22*(4), 310.

Organisation for Economic Co-operation and Development (OECD). (2015). *OECD data: Health: Overweight or obese population.* Retrieved from https://data.oecd.org/healthrisk/overweight-or-obese-population.htm.

Pike, K. M., Hoek, H. W., & Dunne, P. E. (2014). Cultural trends and eating disorders. *Current Opinion in Psychiatry, 27*(6), 436.

Piran, N. (2010). A feminist perspective on risk factor research and on the prevention of eating disorders. *Eating Disorders, 18*(3), 183–198. doi:10.1080/10640261003719435.

Piran, N., & Gadalla, T. (2006). Eating disorders and substance abuse in Canadian women: A national study. *Addiction (Abingdon, England), 102,* 105–113. doi:10.1111/j.1360-0443.2006.01633.x.

Pisetsky, E. M., Haynos, A. F., Lavender, J. M., et al. (2017). Associations between emotion regulation difficulties, eating disorder symptoms, non-suicidal self-injury, and suicide attempts in a heterogeneous eating disorder sample. *Comprehensive Psychiatry, 73,* 143–150. doi:10.1016/j.comppsych.2016.11.012.

Romano, C. (2015). Current findings in pediatric non organic feeding disorders: The gastroenterologist point of view. *Italian Journal of Pediatrics, 41*(Suppl. 2), A61. doi:10.1186/1824-7288-41-S2-A61.

Rosenvinge, J., & Petterson, G. (2015). Epidemiology of eating disorders part II: An update with a special reference to the DSM-5. *Advances in Eating Disorders, 3*(2), 198–220. doi:10.1080/21662630.2014.940549.

Sawaoka, T., Barnes, R. D., Blomquist, K. K., et al. (2012). Social anxiety and self-consciousness in binge eating disorder: Associations with eating disorder psychopathology. *Comprehensive Psychiatry, 53*(6), 740–745. doi:10.1016/j.comppsych.2011.10.003.

Striegel-Moore, R. H., Rosselli, F., Perrin, N., et al. (2009). Gender difference in the prevalence of eating disorder symptoms. *The International Journal of Eating Disorders, 42*(5), 471–474. doi:10.1002/eat.20625.

Thompson, R. A., & Sherman, R. T. (2010). *Eating disorders in sport.* New York: Routledge.

Wilfley, D. E., Bishop, M. E., Wilson, G. T., et al. (2007). Classification of eating disorders: Toward *DSM-V. International Journal of Eating Disorders, 40,* S123–S129. doi:10.1002/eat.20436.

Williams, P. M., & Goodie, J. (2007). Identifying and treating eating disorders. *Family Practice Recertification, 29*(8), 16–23.

Williamson, D. A., Martin, C. K., Anton, S. D., et al. (2008). Is caloric restriction associated with development of eating-disorder symptoms? Results from the CALERIE trial. *Health Psychology, 27*(1), S32–S42. doi:10.1037/0278-6133.27.1.S32.

Wilson, G. T., Wilfley, D. E., Agras, W. S., et al. (2010). Psychological treatments of binge eating disorder. *Archives of General Psychiatry, 67*(1), 94–101. doi:10.1001/archgenpsychiatry.2009.170.

17

Neurocognitive Disorders

Jane Stein-Parbury
Adapted by Cheryl L. Pollard

KEY TERMS AND CONCEPTS

agnosia
Alzheimer's disease (AD)
aphasia
apraxia
catastrophic reactions
confabulation
delirium

dementia
major neurocognitive disorders
mild neurocognitive disorders
neurocognitive disorders
perseveration
pseudodementia
sundowning

OBJECTIVES

1. Compare and contrast the clinical picture of delirium with that of dementia and brain injury.
2. Discuss three critical needs of a person with delirium, stated in terms of nursing diagnoses.
3. Identify three outcomes for patients with delirium.
4. Summarize the essential nursing interventions for a patient with delirium.
5. Recognize the signs and symptoms occurring in the stages of Alzheimer's disease.
6. Give an example of the following symptoms assessed during the progression of Alzheimer's disease: (a) amnesia, (b) apraxia, (c) agnosia, and (d) aphasia.
7. Formulate three nursing diagnoses suitable for a patient with Alzheimer's disease, and define two outcomes for each.
8. Formulate a teaching plan for a caregiver of a patient with Alzheimer's disease, including interventions for communication, health maintenance, and a safe environment.
9. Compose a list of appropriate referrals in the community—including a support group, hotline for information, and respite services—for people with dementia and their caregivers.

⊖volve WEBSITE

Visit the Evolve website for Flashcards, Case Studies, and additional testing resources related to the content in this chapter: http://evolve.elsevier.com/Canada/Varcarolis/psychiatric/

Pre-Test interactive review

The clarity and purpose of an individual's personal journey through life depend on the ability to reflect on its meaning. Cognition, therefore, is a fundamental human feature that distinguishes living from existing. This mental capacity has a distinctive, personalized impact on the individual's physical, psychological, social, and spiritual conduct of life. For example,

the ability to remember the connections between related actions and how to initiate them depends on cognitive processing. Moreover, this cognitive processing has a direct relationship to activities of daily living.

Cognitive functioning involves a variety of domains. Attention and orientation are basic lower-level cognitive domains.

Higher-level cognitive domains are more complex and include the ability to do the following:

- Plan and problem-solve (executive functioning)
- Learn and retain information in long-term memory
- Use language
- Visually perceive the environment
- Interpret social cues (social cognition)

Although primarily an intellectual and perceptual process, cognition is closely integrated with an individual's emotional and spiritual values. Neurocognitive disorders result from changes in the brain and are marked by disturbances in orientation, memory, intellect, judgement, and affect. These disorders may be described as ranging from *minor* to *major* in terms of the level of impairment.

HOW A NURSE HELPED ME

What Happened to the Person I Married?

My husband and I have been married for more than 45 years. Over the past couple of years, he has become more irritable and difficult to live with. In the past, he was always very particular about his appearance and was very kind to everyone. Now, he rarely showers or bathes, almost never brushes his teeth, and wears his dirty clothes for several days. His kindness has been replaced by irritability and sarcasm. We have always had a physical relationship, but now he says sexually explicit comments that are rude and offensive. His comments are sometimes about children—he was never like that. He has also begun to masturbate in public.

I was very upset with these changes in behaviour. Our doctor said that he had a form of dementia that makes his impulses hard to control. Knowing this did not make it easier for me to cope, however. Fortunately, there was a mental health outreach nurse in our area. She came to see my husband and me. She helped me understand my husband's illness and provided me with information on dementia and the impulsive behaviours that are associated with different kinds of dementias. We also discussed how I could set boundaries for myself and understand that my husband's behaviours were not something I had caused. She informed me that my husband's behaviours would change as his dementia got worse. The nurse also helped me figure out what I was going to tell my daughters, who were upset that I did not want the grandchildren staying overnight anymore. We practised role-playing the discussion that I needed to have with my children. This helped build my confidence, knowing that I understood what was happening with my husband's dementia and that I was able to explain it to my kids.

The three main neurocognitive classifications are delirium, mild neurocognitive disorders, and major neurocognitive

disorders. The first syndrome, delirium, tends to be short term and reversible. Mild neurocognitive disorders may or may not progress to being major. Major neurocognitive disorders are commonly referred to as dementia, which is progressive and irreversible. In both mild and major neurocognitive disorders, there is a decline in cognitive functioning from a previous level, although they differ in how much they interfere with independence in everyday activities (American Psychiatric Association [APA], 2013).

The labyrinth of current knowledge about cognitive disorders requires compassionate understanding of the patient and family. Nursing interventions are focused on attending to the needs, desires, and choices of the individual with a cognitive disorder and his or her family. The goals of the interventions are to protect welfare, preserve functional status, and promote well-being for cognitively impaired patients regardless of the reason for the impairment.

This chapter addresses the broad categories of delirium and major neurocognitive disorders, by far the most common conditions nurses encounter. It also introduces psychiatric symptoms of people with brain injuries and compares them with those of people with delirium and major neurocognitive disorders. Table 17-1 offers some guidelines for distinguishing among delirium, major neurocognitive disorders, depression, and brain injury (these last two may have similar symptoms and may co-occur in older adults).

DELIRIUM

CLINICAL PICTURE

Delirium is an acute cognitive disturbance characterized as a syndrome composed of a constellation of symptoms rather than a disorder. The cardinal symptoms of delirium are an inability to direct, focus, sustain, and shift attention; an abrupt onset with clinical features that fluctuate with periods of lucidity; and disorganized thinking and poor executive functioning. Other characteristics include disorientation (often to time and place, but rarely to person), anxiety, agitation, poor memory, and delusional thinking. When hallucinations are present they are usually visual. DSM-5: Diagnostic Criteria for Delirium identifies the diagnostic criteria for delirium.

Delirium is a medical emergency, and immediate attention should be given to prevent irreversible and serious damage (Caplan, Cassem, Murray, et al., 2016). Delirium is associated with increased morbidity and mortality and can have lasting long-term consequences, such as permanent cognitive decline (Inouye, Westendorp, & Saczynski, 2014). In hospitalized patients, delirium is associated with longer hospital stays and increased complications (Anand & MacLullich, 2013). In patients with pre-existing cognitive impairment—for example, major neurocognitive disorder—delirium accelerates cognitive decline. There is also an association with depression postdelirium, and evidence indicates that younger patients who have been delirious while in hospital may develop symptoms resembling those of post-traumatic stress disorder (Bulic, Bennett, & Shehabi, 2015).

TABLE 17-1 COMPARISON OF DELIRIUM, MAJOR NEUROCOGNITIVE DISORDERS, DEPRESSION, AND BRAIN INJURY

	DELIRIUM	MAJOR NEUROCOGNITIVE DISORDERS	DEPRESSION	BRAIN INJURY
Onset	Sudden, over hours to days	Slowly, over months	May have been gradual, with exacerbation during crisis or stress	Usually sudden; symptoms increase as damage becomes more pervasive
Cause or contributing factors	Hypoglycemia, fever, dehydration, hypotension; infection, other conditions that disrupt body's homeostasis; adverse drug reaction; head injury; change in environment (e.g., hospitalization); pain; emotional stress	Alzheimer's disease, vascular disease, human immunodeficiency virus (HIV) infection, neurological disease, chronic alcoholism, head trauma	Lifelong history, losses, loneliness, crises, declining health, medical conditions	Traumatic injury (external physical force) or acquired injury (conditions other than degenerative, such as stroke, anoxia, hypoxia, tumour, toxin)
Cognition	Impaired memory, judgement, calculations, attention span; can fluctuate through the day	Impaired memory, judgement, calculations, attention span, abstract thinking; agnosia	Difficulty concentrating, forgetfulness, inattention	May have difficulty thinking and learning; poor judgement; easily distractible; disoriented, confused, or amnesic depending on injury
Level of consciousness	Altered	Not altered	Not altered	Variable alterations depending on injury
Activity level	Can be increased or reduced; restlessness, which may worsen in evening (sundowning); sleep–wake cycle may be reversed	Not altered; behaviours may worsen in evening (sundowning)	Usually decreased; lethargy, fatigue, lack of motivation; may sleep poorly and awaken in early morning	Depending on injury, may have sleep disturbances, swallowing or appetite changes, weakness or paralysis, balance or coordination difficulties
Emotional state	Rapid swings; can be fearful, anxious, suspicious, aggressive; may have hallucinations, delusions, or both	Flat; delusions	Extreme sadness, apathy, irritability, anxiety, paranoid ideation	Anxiety, depression, agitation, hyper-reactivity, disinhibition, impulsivity, labile mood depending on injury
Speech and language	Rapid, inappropriate, incoherent, rambling	Incoherent, slow (sometimes due to effort to find the right word), inappropriate, rambling, repetitious	Slow, flat, low	Depending on the injury, may experience difficulties with expressive speech, word finding, comprehension
Prognosis	Reversible with proper and timely treatment	Not reversible; progressive	Reversible with proper and timely treatment	Varies depending on the location and the extent of brain damaged

DSM-5

Diagnostic Criteria for Delirium

A. A disturbance in attention (i.e., reduced ability to direct, focus, sustain and shift attention) and awareness (reduced orientation to the environment).

B. The disturbance develops over a short period time (usually hours to a few days), represents a change from baseline attention and awareness, and tends to fluctuate in severity during the course of a day.

C. An additional disturbance in cognition (e.g., memory deficit, disorientation, language, visuospatial ability, or perception).

D. The disturbances in Criteria A and C are not better explained by another preexisting, established, or evolving neurocognitive disorder and do not occur in the context of a severely reduced level of arousal such as coma.

E. There is evidence from the history, physical examination, or laboratory findings that the disturbance is a direct physiological consequence of another medical condition, substance intoxication or withdrawal (i.e., due to a drug of abuse or to a medication), or exposure to a toxin, or is due to multiple etiologies.

Specify whether:

Substance Intoxication Delirium: This diagnosis should be made instead of substance intoxication when the symptoms in Criteria A and C predominate in the clinical picture and when they are sufficiently severe to warrant clinical attention.

Source: American Psychiatric Association. (2013). *Diagnostic and statistical manual of mental disorders* (5th ed.). Washington, DC: Author.

BOX 17-1 COMMON CAUSES OF DELIRIUM

Postoperative States, Drug Intoxications, and Withdrawals
- Anticholinergics, benzodiazepines, alcohol, anxiolytics, opioids, and central nervous system stimulants (e.g., cocaine, crack cocaine)

Infections
- Systemic: pneumonia, typhoid fever, malaria, urinary tract infection, and septicemia
- Intracranial: meningitis and encephalitis

Metabolic Disorders
- Dehydration
- Hypoxia (pulmonary disease, heart disease, and anemia)
- Hypoglycemia
- Sodium, potassium, calcium, magnesium, and acid–base imbalances
- Hepatic encephalopathy or uremic encephalopathy
- Thiamine (vitamin B_1) deficiency (Wernicke's encephalopathy)
- Endocrine disorders (e.g., thyroid or parathyroid)
- Hypothermia or hyperthermia
- Diabetic acidosis

Drugs
- Digitalis, steroids, lithium, levodopa, anticholinergics, benzodiazepines, central nervous system depressants, tricyclic antidepressants
- Central anticholinergic syndrome due to use of multiple drugs with anticholinergic adverse effects

Neurological Diseases
- Seizures
- Head trauma
- Hypertensive encephalopathy

Tumour
- Primary cerebral

Psychosocial Stressors
- Relocation or other sudden changes
- Sensory deprivation or overload
- Sleep deprivation
- Immobilization
- Pain

EPIDEMIOLOGY

Delirium is a common complication of hospitalization, especially in older patients. The reported incidence of delirium in all hospitalized patients is up to 22% in general medical patients, between 11% and 35% in surgical patients, and up to 80% in patients in intensive care units (ICUs) (van Munster & de Rooij, 2014). In patients over 65 years of age, delirium occurs in up to 50% (Inouye, Westendorp, & Saczynski, 2014). The high degree of variability in the reported incidence of delirium is most likely due to its under-recognition (see Research Highlight box).

COMORBIDITY AND ETIOLOGY

Delirium is always secondary to another physiological condition and is often a transient disorder. If the underlying condition is corrected, complete recovery from delirium should also occur. Delirium can be an indicator of increased frailty and vulnerability, not just an exclusively transient and fully reversible condition associated only with acute causes (Clegg, Young, & Siddiqi, 2012). The common acute causes of delirium are nervous system disease, systemic disease (such as cardiac failure) (Box 17-1), and intoxication or withdrawal from a chemical substance (see Chapter 18).

The key to helping patients avoid the consequences of delirium is recognizing and investigating potential causes as soon as possible. Early recognition and diagnosis is challenging for clinicians due to lack of knowledge about cognitive impairment and its clinical assessment and failure to interpret the signs and symptoms. The best evidence for the prevention and management of delirium in hospitalized patients is having clinical protocols for minimizing modifiable risk factors. Early detection of delirium may be improved by consultation with geriatric specialists (Reston & Schoelles, 2013).

APPLICATION OF THE NURSING PROCESS

ASSESSMENT

While symptoms of delirium must be managed, the goal of treatment is to determine the underlying cause and rectify it when possible. Clinicians who suspect delirium should conduct a thorough examination, including mental and neurological status examinations, as well as a physical examination. Blood tests and a urinalysis should also be done. If possible, additional information should be obtained from a person who knows the patient, such as a family member or friend. The patient's medication regimen should be reviewed carefully for drug interactions or toxicity profiles.

General Assessment

There are four cardinal features of delirium that clinicians focus on when using the Confusion Assessment Method (CAM):
1. Acute onset and fluctuating course
2. Inattention
3. Disorganized thinking
4. Disturbance of consciousness

Suspect the presence of delirium when a person's ability to focus, sustain, or shift attention becomes abruptly impaired and his or her awareness of the environment is reduced. Conversation is made more difficult because the person may be easily distracted by irrelevant stimuli. Questions must be repeated because the individual's attention wanders, and the person might easily get off track and need to be refocused. The person may also have difficulty with orientation—first to time, then to place, and last to person. For example, a man with delirium may think that the year is 1972, that the hospital is home, and that the nurse is his wife. Orientation to person is usually intact to the extent that the person is aware of his or her own identity.

Factors That Contribute to Under-Recognition of Delirium

Problem

Delirium is the most frequent complication of hospitalization in older adults. Not only is this problem costly, but delirium is also associated with morbidity and mortality. Timely recognition is essential to offset these negative outcomes.

Purpose of Study

The purpose of the study was to identify factors associated with the recognition of delirium among registered nurses.

Methods

Researchers conducted a literature search for quantitative studies regarding nurses recognizing delirium.

Key Findings

Seven major factors related to poor recognition of delirium by nurses were identified. The factors included:

- Fluctuating nature of delirium
- Lack of delirium education
- Insufficient use of assessment tools
- Poor understanding of delirium
- Perception of delirium as burdensome
- Poor differentiation between dementia and delirium

Implications for Nursing Practice

As a future nurse, you will be in a prime position to notice delirium. Any time a patient experiences an acute onset of confusion, you should consider delirium. Nurses need to be aware of the nature of delirium, especially how it differs from dementia. Standardized assessment scales can improve your ability to detect delirium.

Source: El Hussein, M., Hirst, S., & Salyers, V. (2014). Factors that contribute to under-recognition of delirium by registered nurses in acute care settings: A scoping review of the literature to explain this phenomenon. *Journal of Clinical Nursing, 24,* 906–915. doi: 10.1111/jocn.12693.

A person with delirium may also appear withdrawn, agitated, or psychotic. Fluctuating levels of consciousness are unpredictable. Disorientation and confusion are usually markedly worse at night and during the early morning. In fact, some patients may be confused or delirious only at night and may remain lucid during the day. The phenomenon in which symptoms become more pronounced in the evening is called sundowning (also known as *sundown syndrome*). Sundowning often begins in the late afternoon as the evening approaches. This symptom-exacerbation pattern may occur in people who have either delirium or dementia.

As nurses, our frequent interaction with those in hospital places us in a prime position to prevent, detect, and treat the effects of delirium. Nursing assessment includes observation and evaluation of (1) cognitive and perceptual disturbances, (2) physical needs, and (3) moods and physical behaviours.

Cognitive and Perceptual Disturbances

Patients experiencing delirium may be difficult to engage in conversation because they are easily distracted, display marked attention deficits, and exhibit memory impairment. In mild delirium, memory deficits are noted only on careful questioning. In more severe delirium, memory problems usually take the form of obvious difficulty in processing and remembering recent events. For example, the person might ask when a son is coming to visit, even though the son left only an hour earlier.

Another helpful tool clinicians can use to determine the presence of a component of dementia is the Montreal Cognitive Assessment (MoCA). The MoCA assesses short-term memory, visuospatial abilities, executive functioning, attention, concentration, working memory, language, and orientation to time and place (Nasreddine, Phillips, Bedirian, et al., 2005). The MoCA can be completed by an experienced clinician in approximately 10 minutes.

Perceptual disturbances are also common. *Perception* is the processing of information about one's internal and external environments. Various misinterpretations of reality may take the form of illusions. For example, a person may mistake folds in the bedclothes for white rats or the cord of a window blind for a snake. Or, misinterpretations may take the form of hallucinations. For example, individuals experiencing delirium may become terrified when they "see" giant spiders crawling over the bedclothes or "feel" bugs crawling on or under their skin.

The individual with delirium generally is aware that something is very wrong. Statements like "My thoughts are all jumbled" may signal cognitive problems. When perceptual disturbances are present, the emotional response is often one of fear and anxiety, which may be manifested by psychomotor agitation.

Physical Needs

A person with delirium becomes disoriented and may try to "go home." Alternatively, a person may think that he or she *is* home and jump out of a window in an attempt to get away from "invaders." Wandering, pulling out intravenous lines and Foley catheters, and falling out of bed are common dangers that require nursing vigilance.

An individual experiencing delirium has difficulty processing stimuli in the environment, and confusion magnifies the inability to recognize reality. The physical environment should be made as simple and clear as possible. Objects such as clocks and calendars can maximize orientation to time. Glasses, hearing aids, and adequate lighting without glare can maximize the person's ability to interpret more accurately what is going on in the environment. The nurse should interact with the patient whenever the patient is awake. Short periods of social interaction help to reduce anxiety and misperceptions.

Self-care deficits, injury, or hyperactivity or hypoactivity may lead to skin breakdown and possible infection. Often this condition is compounded by poor nutrition, forced bed rest, and possible incontinence. These situations require nursing assessment and intervention.

Autonomic signs, such as tachycardia, sweating, flushed face, dilated pupils, and elevated blood pressure, are often present in delirium. These changes must be monitored and documented carefully and may require immediate medical attention, as they may be an indication that the underlying physiological condition is worsening.

Changes in the sleep–wake cycle should be assessed and documented. In some cases, a complete reversal of the night–day, sleep–wake cycle can occur. The patient's level of consciousness may range from lethargy to stupor or from semicoma to hypervigilance. In hypervigilance, patients are extraordinarily alert, and their eyes constantly scan the room; they may have difficulty falling asleep or may be actively disoriented and agitated throughout the night.

You should always suspect medications as a potential cause of delirium. This is especially true when there is polypharmacy or use of psychoactive agents. To recognize drug reactions or anticipate potential interactions before delirium actually occurs, it is important to assess all medications, both prescription and over the counter, and other substances (i.e., street drugs, alcohol, herbal or natural therapies) the patient is taking.

Moods and Physical Behaviours

The individual's moods and physical behaviours may change dramatically within a short period. A person with delirium may display motor restlessness (agitation), or he or she may be "quietly delirious" and appear calm and settled. When there is agitation, delirium is considered hyperactive; when there is no agitation, delirium is considered hypoactive. Moods may swing back and forth between fear, anger, anxiety, euphoria, depression, and apathy. A person may strike out from fear or anger or may cry, call for help, curse, moan, and tear off clothing one minute and become apathetic or laugh uncontrollably the next. In short, behaviour and emotions are erratic and fluctuating. The following vignette illustrates the fear and confusion a patient may experience during and after an episode of delirium.

VIGNETTE

Peter Wright, age 43, survived numerous life-threatening complications after open-heart surgery to replace his mitral valve. He spent 3 weeks in an ICU and then moved to a general medical unit.

Peter became suspicious about his bed being moved. "Why are you taking me to another country?" He expressed concern that his organs would be removed and donated for transplan-tation. He began to yell for his wife. Peter knew that the very people who had saved his life were now out to get him.

When he was sure nobody was looking, he climbed out of bed and attempted to leave the unit. The nurses responded by calling security personnel to escort him back to bed. Once he was safely in bed, the nurses applied mechanical restraints and sedated him.

Peter's confusion disappeared the next day. While he realized how distorted his thinking had been during the episode, the anxiety and fear he experienced remained with him for months after discharge from the hospital.

What are some more helpful interventions the nurses could have used? What could the nurses have done differently? What would you have done?

Self-Assessment

Because the behaviours exhibited by the patient with delirium can be directly attributed to temporary medical conditions, intense personal reactions in staff are less likely to arise. In fact, intense, conflicting emotions are less likely to occur in nurses working with a patient with delirium than in nurses working with a patient with dementia, which is discussed later in this chapter. Nonetheless, interacting with these patients can be frustrating for health care providers, especially given the fluctuating nature of the clinical picture.

📋 ASSESSMENT GUIDELINES
Delirium

1. Assess for acute onset and fluctuating levels of consciousness, which are key in delirium.
2. Assess the person's ability to attend to the immediate environment, including responses to nursing care.
3. Establish the person's normal level of consciousness and cognition by interviewing family members or other caregivers.
4. Assess for past cognitive impairment—especially an existing dementia diagnosis—and other risk factors.
5. Identify disturbances in physiological status, especially infection, hypoxia, and pain.
6. Identify any physiological abnormalities documented in the patient's record.
7. Assess vital signs, level of consciousness, and neurological signs.
8. Assess potential for injury, especially in relation to potential for falls and wandering.
9. Maintain comfort measures, especially in relation to pain, cold, or positioning.
10. Monitor situational factors that worsen or improve symptoms.
11. Assess for availability of immediate medical interventions to help prevent irreversible brain damage.
12. Remain nonjudgemental. Confer with other staff readily when questions arise.

DIAGNOSIS

Safety needs play a substantial role in nursing care. Patients with delirium often perceive the environment in a distorted way, and objects are often misperceived (due to illusions or hallucinations). People and objects may be misinterpreted as threatening or harmful, and patients often act on these misinterpretations. For example, if feeling threatened or thinking that common medical equipment is harmful, the patient may pull off an oxygen mask, pull out an intravenous or nasogastric tube, or try to flee. In such a case, the person demonstrates a *Risk for injury* related to confusion as evidenced by sensory deficits or perceptual deficits.

Hallucinations, distractibility, illusions, disorientation, agitation, restlessness, and misperception are major aspects of the clinical picture. When some of these symptoms are present, *Acute confusion* related to delirium is an appropriate nursing diagnosis.

If fever and dehydration are present, fluid and electrolyte balance will need to be managed. If the underlying cause of the patient's delirium results in fever, decreased skin turgor, decreased urinary output or fluid intake, and dry skin or mucous membranes, then the nursing diagnosis of *Deficient fluid volume* is appropriate. Fluid volume deficit may be related to fever, electrolyte imbalance, reduced intake, or infection.

In cases of delirium, restful sleep is not achieved, day or night; the patient may be less responsive during the day and may become disruptively wakeful during the night. *Insomnia* or *Sleep deprivation* related to impaired cerebral oxygenation or disruption in consciousness is a likely diagnosis.

Engaging in communication with a delirious patient is difficult. An example of a nursing diagnosis addressing this problem is *Impaired verbal communication* related to cerebral hypoxia or decreased cerebral blood flow as evidenced by confusion or clouding of consciousness.

Fear is one of the most common of all nursing diagnoses and may be related to illusions, delusions, or hallucinations, as evidenced by verbal and nonverbal expressions of fearfulness. Other nursing concerns include *Self-care deficit, Disturbed thought processes*, and *Impaired social interaction*. Table 17-2 identifies nursing diagnoses for any confused patient with delirium or dementia.

OUTCOMES IDENTIFICATION

The overall outcome is that the delirious patient will return to the premorbid level of functioning. Table 17-3 includes outcomes for acute confusion from the *Nursing Outcomes Classification (NOC)* (Moorhead, Johnson, Maas, et al., 2012). However, for many of the diagnoses we would use for the person experiencing delirium, *NOC* is not specific enough. Although the person can demonstrate a wide variety of needs, *Risk for injury* is always present. Appropriate outcomes are:

- During periods of lucidity, patient will be oriented to time, place, and person with the aid of nursing interventions, such as the provision of clocks, calendars, maps, and other types of orienting information.
- Patient will remain free from falls and injury while confused, with the aid of nursing safety measures while in the hospital.

Because level of consciousness can change throughout the day, the patient needs to be checked frequently for orientation.

PLANNING

Planning nursing care for a patient who is experiencing delirium involves special attention to the safety and security of the environment. You should address the following questions:

- Does the person have the necessary visual and auditory aids?
- Are family members available to stay with the patient?
- Does the environment provide visual cues as to time of day and season of the year?
- Has the person experienced continuity of care providers?

TABLE 17-2	POTENTIAL NURSING DIAGNOSES FOR THE CONFUSED PATIENT
SYMPTOMS	**NURSING DIAGNOSES**
Wanders, has unsteady gait, acts out fear from hallucinations or illusions, forgets things (leaves stove on, doors open)	*Risk for injury*
Awake and disoriented during the night (*sundowning*), frightened at night	*Disturbed sleep pattern*
	Fear
	Acute confusion
Unable to take care of basic needs	*Self-care deficit* (bathing/hygiene, dressing, feeding, toileting)
	Ineffective coping
	Functional urinary incontinence
	Imbalanced nutrition: less than body requirements
	Risk for deficient fluid volume
Sees frightening things that are not there (*hallucinations*), mistakes everyday objects for something sinister and frightening (*illusions*), may become paranoid and think that others are doing things to confuse him or her (*delusions*)	*Anxiety*
	Disturbed sensory perception
	Impaired environmental interpretation syndrome
	Disturbed thought processes
Does not recognize familiar people or places, has difficulty with short- or long-term memory or both, is forgetful and confused	*Impaired memory*
	Impaired environmental interpretation syndrome
	Acute or chronic confusion
Has difficulty with communication, cannot find words, has difficulty recognizing objects or people, is incoherent	*Impaired verbal communication*
	Impaired social interaction
Devastated over losing place in life as known (during lucid moments), fearful and overwhelmed by what is happening to him or her	*Spiritual distress*
	Hopelessness
	Situational low self-esteem
	Grieving
Family and loved ones overburdened and overwhelmed, unable to care for patient's needs	*Disabled family coping*
	Interrupted family processes
	Impaired home maintenance
	Caregiver role strain

TABLE 17-3   *NOC* OUTCOMES RELATED TO ACUTE CONFUSION

Acute confusion: Abrupt onset of reversible disturbance of consciousness, attention, cognition, and perception that develops over a short period of time.

NURSING OUTCOME AND DEFINITION	INTERMEDIATE INDICATORS	SHORT-TERM INDICATORS
Cognitive orientation: Ability to identify person, place, and time accurately	Identifies correct day Identifies correct month Identifies correct year Identifies correct season Identifies current place Identifies significant current events	Identifies self Identifies significant other
Neurological status and level of consciousness: Arousal, orientation, and attention to the environment	Oriented cognitively Communicates appropriately for situation Attends to environmental stimuli	Opens eyes to external stimuli Obeys commands Makes motor responses to noxious stimuli

Source: Moorhead, S., Johnson, M., Maas, M., et al. (2012). *Nursing outcomes classification (NOC)* (5th ed.). St. Louis: Mosby.

BOX 17-2   *NIC* INTERVENTIONS FOR DELIRIUM MANAGEMENT

Definition of *delirium management:* Provision of a safe and therapeutic environment for the patient who is experiencing an acute state of confusion.

Activities:

- Identify etiological factors causing delirium.
- Initiate therapies to reduce or eliminate factors causing delirium.
- Monitor neurological status on an ongoing basis.
- Provide unconditional positive regard.
- Verbally acknowledge patient's fears and feelings.
- Provide optimistic but realistic reassurance.
- Allow patient to maintain rituals that limit anxiety.
- Provide patient with information about what is happening and what can be expected to occur in the future.
- Avoid demands for abstract thinking if patient can think only in concrete terms.
- Limit need for decision making if frustrating or confusing to patient.
- Administer prn (as needed) medications for anxiety or agitation.
- Encourage visitation by significant others, as appropriate.
- Recognize and accept patient's perceptions or interpretation of reality (hallucinations or delusions).
- State your perception in a calm, reassuring, and nonargumentative manner.
- Respond to the theme or feeling tone, rather than the content, of the hallucination or delusion.
- When possible, remove stimuli that create misperception in a particular patient (e.g., pictures on the wall or television).
- Maintain a well-lit environment that reduces sharp contrasts and shadows.
- Assist with needs related to nutrition, elimination, hydration, and personal hygiene.
- Maintain a hazard-free environment.
- Place identification bracelet on patient.
- Provide appropriate level of supervision and surveillance to monitor patient and allow for therapeutic actions, as needed.
- Use physical restraints, as needed.
- Avoid frustrating patient by quizzing with orientation questions that cannot be answered.
- Reorient patient to person, place, and time, as needed.
- Provide a consistent physical environment and daily routine.
- Provide caregivers who are familiar to the patient.
- Use environmental cues (e.g., signs, pictures, clocks, calendars, colour coding of environment) to stimulate memory, reorient, and promote appropriate behaviour.
- Provide a low-stimulation environment for patients disoriented by overstimulation.
- Encourage use of aids that increase sensory input (e.g., glasses, hearing aids, dentures).
- Approach patient slowly and from the front.
- Address patient by name when initiating interaction.
- Reorient patient to health care provider with each contact.
- Communicate with simple, direct, descriptive statements.
- Prepare patient for upcoming changes in usual routine and environment before their occurrence.
- Provide new information slowly and in small doses, with frequent rest periods.
- Focus interpersonal interactions on what is familiar and meaningful to patient.

Source: Bulechek, G. M., Butcher, H. K., & Dochterman, J. M. (2013). *Nursing interventions classification (NIC)* (6th ed.). Toronto: Elsevier.

IMPLEMENTATION

The priorities of treatment are to keep the patient safe while attempting to identify the cause. If the underlying disorder is corrected, complete recovery is possible. If, however, the underlying disorder is not corrected and persists, irreversible neuronal damage can occur. Nursing concerns therefore centre on the following:

- Preventing physical harm due to confusion, aggression, or electrolyte and fluid imbalance

- Performing a comprehensive nursing assessment to aid in identifying the cause
- Assisting with proper health management to eradicate the underlying cause
- Using supportive measures to relieve distress

The *Nursing Interventions Classification (NIC)* (Bulechek, Butcher, & Dochterman, 2013) can be used as a guide to develop interventions for a person experiencing delirium (Box 17-2). Medical management of delirium involves treating the underlying organic causes. If the underlying cause of delirium is not treated, permanent brain damage may ensue. In addition, thoughtful use of antipsychotic or antianxiety agents may also aid in controlling behavioural symptoms.

A patient in acute delirium should never be left alone. Because most hospitals and health facilities are unable to provide one-to-one supervision of the patient, family members can be encouraged to stay with the patient.

EVALUATION

Long-term outcome criteria for a person experiencing delirium include the following:
- Patient will remain safe.
- Patient will be oriented to time, place, and person by discharge.
- Underlying cause will be treated and ameliorated.

MILD AND MAJOR NEUROCOGNITIVE DISORDERS

Dementia is a broad term used to describe progressive deterioration of cognitive functioning and global impairment of intellect. It is a term that does not refer to specific disease but rather to a collection of symptoms. The *Diagnostic and Statistical Manual of Mental Disorders*, fifth edition (*DSM-5*) (APA, 2013), incorporates dementia into the diagnostic categories of mild and major neurocognitive disorders. These disorders are characterized by cognitive impairments that signal a decline from previous functioning.

When mild, the impairments do not interfere with essential activities of daily living although the person may need to make extra efforts. While such impairments may be progressive, a

 DSM-5

Diagnostic Criteria for Mild Neurocognitive Disorder

A. Evidence of modest cognitive decline from previous level of performance in one or more cognitive domains (complex attention, executive function, learning and memory, language, perceptual-motor, or social cognition) based on:
1. Concern of the individual, a knowledgeable informant, or clinician that there has been a mild decline in cognitive function; and
2. A modest impairment in cognitive performance, preferably documented by standardized neuropsychological testing or, in its absence, another quantified clinical assessment.

B. The cognitive deficits do not interfere with capacity for independence in everyday activities (i.e., complex instrumental activities of daily living such as paying bills or accommodation may be required).

C. The cognitive deficits do not occur exclusively in the context of delirium.

D. The cognitive deficits are not better explained by another mental disorder (e.g., major depressive disorder, schizophrenia).

Source: American Psychiatric Association. (2013). *Diagnostic and statistical manual of mental disorders* (5th ed.). Washington, DC: Author.

mild cognitive impairment does not necessarily mean that it will progress to a major neurocognitive disorder (Alzheimer's Association, 2014). DSM-5: Diagnostic Criteria for Mild Neurocognitive Disorder lists diagnostic criteria for mild neurocognitive disorders.

When progressive, these disorders become major neurocognitive disorders because they interfere with daily functioning and independence. While often characterized by memory deficits, neurocognitive disorders affect other areas of cognitive functioning, for example, problem solving (executive functioning) and complex attention. DSM-5: Diagnostic Criteria for Major Neurocognitive Disorder describes the diagnostic criteria for major neurocognitive disorders.

 DSM-5

Diagnostic Criteria for Major Neurocognitive Disorder

A. Evidence of significant cognitive decline from previous level of performance in one or more cognitive domains (complex attention, executive function, learning and memory, language, perceptual-motor, or social cognition) based on:
1. Concern of the individual, a knowledgeable informant, or clinician that there has been significant decline in cognitive function; and
2. A substantial impairment in cognitive performance, preferably documented by standardized neuropsychological testing or, in its absence, another quantified clinical assessment.

B. The cognitive deficits interfere with independence in everyday activities (i.e., at a mini-mum, requiring assistance with complex instrumental activities of daily living such as paying bills or managing medications).

C. The cognitive deficits do not occur exclusively in the context of delirium.

D. The cognitive deficits are not better explained by another mental disorder (e.g., major depressive disorder, schizophrenia).

Source: American Psychiatric Association. (2013). *Diagnostic and statistical manual of mental disorders* (5th ed.). Washington, DC: Author.

Mild and major neurocognitive disorder criteria are general. Specific disorders such as Alzheimer's disease are listed in Table 17-4.

While the underlying etiology varies in neurocognitive disorders, nursing care is based on their behavioural manifestations. Therefore approaches to care are not necessarily different for various etiologies. It is for this reason that the remainder of this chapter focuses on the most frequently occurring major neurocognitive disorder, Alzheimer's disease.

CLINICAL PICTURE

Dementia is the general term used to describe a decline in cognitive functioning that interferes with daily living. **Alzheimer's disease (AD)**, the most common cause of dementia in older adults, is a progressive degenerative neurocognitive disorder marked by impaired memory and thinking skills. It accounts for 60% to

TABLE 17-4   TYPES OF NEUROCOGNITIVE DISORDERS

TYPE OF DEMENTIA	SYMPTOMS
Alzheimer's disease	Early: Difficulty with recent memory, impaired learning, apathy, and depression Moderate to severe: Visual/spatial and language deficits, psychotic features, agitation, and wandering Late: Gait disturbance; poor judgement; disorientation; confusion; incontinence; and difficulty speaking, swallowing, and walking
Frontotemporal dementia	Impaired social cognition, disinhibition, apathy, compulsive behaviour, poor comprehension, and language difficulties
Dementia with Lewy bodies	Fluctuating cognition, early changes in attention and executive function, sleep disturbance, visual hallucinations, muscle rigidity, and other parkinsonian features
Vascular dementia	One or more documented cerebrovascular events. Impaired judgement; poor decision making, planning, and organizing (executive functions); and personality and mood changes
Traumatic brain injury	Trauma to the head with loss of consciousness, post-traumatic amnesia, disorientation and confusion, and/or neurological signs
Substance/medication-induced dementia	Symptoms of neurocognitive impairment persist beyond the usual duration of intoxication and acute withdrawal. Substances include alcohol, inhalants, sedative, hypnotic, or antianxiety agents.
HIV infection	A documented infection with HIV. Impaired executive function, slowing of processing, problems with attention, difficulty learning new information, aphasia. Symptoms dependent on area of brain affected by HIV pathogenic processes.
Prion	Insidious onset and rapid progression of impairment. Motor features such as myoclonus or ataxia. Memory and coordination behaviour changes, rapidly fatal
Parkinson's disease	Progression of Parkinson's disease results in dementia with symptoms similar to dementia with Lewy bodies or Alzheimer's disease; apathetic, depressed, or anxious mood; and sleep disorder.
Huntington's disease	Abnormal involuntary movements, severe decline in thinking and reasoning, mood changes such as irritability and depression, due to genetic defect

TABLE 17-5   MEMORY DEFICIT: NORMAL AGING VERSUS MAJOR NEUROCOGNITIVE DISORDER

PARAMETER	NORMAL AGING	MAJOR NEUROCOGNITIVE DISORDER
Area of impairment	Difficulty in word finding, but no aphasia, dyspraxia, agnosia	Aphasia, dyspraxia, agnosia often found
Extent of impairment	Slowing	Minor to major deceleration
	Cautiousness	Variable cautiousness
	Reduced ability to solve new problems	Minor to major problem-solving impairment
	Mildly impaired memory	Minor to major intellectual impairment
	Mild decline in fluid intelligence	Minor to major decline in fluid intelligence
Rate of impairment	Slow change over many years	More rapid though still gradual changes

80% of all dementias (Alzheimer's Association, 2014). It is a devastating disease that not only affects the person who has it but also places an enormous burden on the families and caregivers of those affected. Nurses practising in any setting will care for patients with AD and must be prepared to respond.

It is important to distinguish between normal forgetfulness and the memory deficit of AD and other dementias. Severe memory loss is *not* a normal part of aging. Slight forgetfulness is a common phenomenon of the aging process (age-associated memory loss), but memory loss that interferes with one's activities of daily living is not. Table 17-5 outlines memory changes in normal aging and memory changes seen in dementia.

Many people who live to a very old age never experience significant memory loss or any other symptom of dementia. Most of us know of people in their eighties and nineties who lead active lives with their intellect intact. Pablo Picasso, Duke Ellington, Ansel Adams, and George Burns are just a few examples of people who were still active in their careers when they died, and all were older than 75 years of age (Picasso was 91; George Burns was 100). The slow, minor cognitive changes associated with aging should not impede social or occupational functioning.

Although dementia often begins with a worsening of ability to remember new information, it is marked by progressive deterioration in intellectual functioning, memory, and the ability to solve problems and learn new skills; a decline in the ability to perform activities of daily living; and a progressive deterioration of personality accompanied by impairment in judgement. A person's declining intellect often leads to emotional changes such as mood lability, depression, and aggressive acting out, as well as to neurological changes that produce hallucinations and delusions.

There are several types of dementias, including dementia of the Alzheimer's type, vascular dementia, Lewy body disease, Pick's disease, alcohol-related dementias (including Korsakoff syndrome), Creutzfeldt-Jakob disease, and the dementias associated with Parkinson's disease, Huntington's disease, acquired immune deficiency syndrome (AIDS), and traumatic and acquired brain injury.

Progression of Alzheimer's Disease

Alzheimer's disease is classified according to the stage of the degenerative process. Table 17-6 outlines the three stages. These

CONSIDERING CULTURE

Cross-Cultural Differences in Dementia

A timely diagnosis provides an opportunity to discuss care options before the person with dementia becomes too cognitively impaired to make decisions. Such an investigation may also result in identifying underlying treatable conditions.

Cultural barriers may result in delays in diagnosis, treatment, and care for dementia. Indi-viduals from racial and ethnic minorities have longer treatment delays and higher levels of cognitive impairment, behavioural issues, and psychological problems when compared with their non-Hispanic White counterparts. There are a variety of reasons for these delays:

- Low levels of acculturation (i.e., adopting of values and customs of a culture)
- Cultural beliefs about memory loss and dementia (i.e., memory loss is normal with age)
- Lack of accurate knowledge about dementia
- Language barriers
- Religious and spiritual beliefs such as possession by evil spirits
- Cultural shame and stigma (e.g., the person's behaviour reflects on the entire family)
- Social isolation and poor education
- Financial limitations (i.e., health insurance)

It is difficult for anyone to care for a family member with dementia. Adding the problems listed here makes a bad situation even worse. Health care workers, especially nurses, can pro-vide education in the context of cultural awareness to reduce treatment delays.

Source: Sayegh, P., & Knight, B. G. (2013). Cross-cultural differences in dementia: The Sociocultural Health Belief Model. *International Psychogeriatrics, 25*(4), 517–530. doi: 10.1017/S104161021200213X.

stages can be used as a guide to understand the progressive deterioration seen in those diagnosed with Alzheimer's disease. The three stages are mild, moderate, and severe. The first stage roughly corresponds to the *DSM-5* criteria for mild neurocognitive disorders. The second and third stages relate to the *DSM-5* criteria for major neurocognitive disorder.

The loss of intellectual ability is insidious. The person with mild Alzheimer's disease loses energy, drive, and initiative and has difficulty learning new things. Because personality and social behaviour remain intact, others tend to minimize and under-estimate the loss of the individual's abilities. The individual may continue to work, but the extent of the dementia becomes evident in new or demanding situations. Depression may occur early in the disease but usually resolves over time.

More severe symptoms appear as Alzheimer's disease pro-gresses. The person experiences agnosia, which is the inability to identify familiar objects or people, even a spouse. Apraxia is a common symptom whereby a person needs repeated instructions and directions to perform the simplest tasks: "Here is the washcloth. Pick up the soap. Now, put water on the face cloth, and rub the face cloth with soap."

Often the individual cannot remember the location of the toilet or is unaware of the process of urinating and defecating,

TABLE 17-6   STAGES OF ALZHEIMER'S DISEASE

STAGE	HALLMARKS
Mild Alzheimer's disease (early stage)	The person and their loved ones notice memory lapses. The person may still be able to function independently but will experience: • Difficulties retrieving correct words or names, previously known • Trouble remembering names when introduced to new people • Greater difficulty performing tasks in social or work settings • Forgetting material that one has just read • Losing or misplacing a valuable object • Trouble with planning or organizing
Moderate Alzheimer's disease (middle stage)	The person confuses words, gets frustrated or angry, or acts in unexpected ways such as refusing to bathe. Symptoms become noticeable to others and the person may: • Forget events or own personal history • Become moody or withdrawn, especially in socially or mentally challenging situations • Be unable to recall his or her own address or telephone number or the high school or university from which he or she graduated • Become confused about where he or she is or what day it is • Need help choosing proper clothing for the season or the occasion • Have trouble controlling bladder and bowels • Change sleep patterns, such as sleeping during the day and becoming restless at night • Be at risk of wandering and becoming lost • Become suspicious and delusional or compulsive, for example, repetitive behaviour such as hand-wringing or tissue shredding
Severe Alzheimer's disease (late stage)	The person loses the ability to respond to his or her environment, to carry on a conversation, and, eventually, to control movement. The person may still say words or phrases, but communicating pain becomes difficult. Personality changes may take place and individuals need extensive help with daily activities. The person may: • Require full-time, around-the-clock assistance with daily personal care • Lose awareness of recent experiences and of his or her surroundings • Require high levels of assistance with daily activities and personal care • Experience changes in physical abilities, including the ability to walk, sit, and, eventually, swallow • Have increasing difficulty communicating • Become vulnerable to infections, especially pneumonia

Source: Adapted from Alzheimer's Association. (2016). *Stages of Alzheimer's.* Retrieved from http://www.alz.org/alzheimers_disease_stages_of_alzheimers.asp?type=alzFooter.

Mrs. White, 78 years old, a retired teacher, has always enjoyed an active life and good health other than an underactive thyroid, which has been successfully controlled. Remarkably, her only hospitalizations were for the births of her two children, now grown and married. She is a vibrant person who takes pride in her appearance and in her beautiful home. She is beginning to forget things that she previously has taken for granted, but jokes about her failing memory as "senior moments."

Recently, her daughter found Mrs. White quite distressed as she attempted to make her famous specialty, lasagna. The ingredients were strewn all over the kitchen, and Mrs. White was frantically searching for a recipe. Her daughter was surprised because neither of them had ever used a written recipe. Her daughter managed to help Mrs. White with step-by-step instructions in the construction of the lasagna. Her daughter was worried about her mother's failing memory, fearing that it was more than usual aging. She tried to broach the subject with her dad, a loving and loyal companion to Mrs. White. His reply was simply, "I don't know what you're talking about."

The situation reached a crisis point when her daughter discovered that Mrs. White was no longer taking her thyroid medication. Since Mrs. White had taken medication for her thyroid for 30 years and could not remember to do so now, this signalled a progression in her condition.

It was painful, but her husband, too, began to realize that Mrs. White was not functioning. Her once-clean house was in a state of disarray. She could no longer coordinate her clothing and usually wore the same outfit for a number of days. Often her clothes were dirty, and her makeup was applied in a disorganized manner.

VIGNETTE

Mrs. White would stare at both the paper and the television, attempting to understand but unable to retain any information. She was often restless during the day, going from one random activity to another, often rearranging her favourite knickknacks in her curio cupboard. She would attempt to wash clothes but forget to put laundry detergent in the machine. She would empty half-filled drinking glasses into the gas range top. If these mistakes were pointed out, she would become angry, stating, "I have always done it this way."

Eating became difficult, as she did not seem to recognize food on her plate, and she was unable to use a knife and fork to cut her food. Sometimes she would pick up a spoon and ask what it was. Her weight began to decrease.

Although Mrs. White always slept well throughout her adult life, she began to wander at night, often waking her husband to ask questions. She would go to the kitchen and empty the cupboards. She would enter her wardrobe and rearrange her clothing, often leaving articles of clothing lying on the floor.

When she set kitchen paper towels on fire on the gas range, her husband and family realized that she could no longer function safely at home. Her husband was unable to leave her alone even for short periods of time, as she would be become extremely distressed, almost to the point of panic. She and her husband moved into an assisted-living facility.

resulting in incontinence. It is usually at this point that total care is necessary. For the family, this burden can be emotionally, financially, and physically devastating. For the individual with Alzheimer's disease, the world is very frightening and nothing makes sense. In response, agitation, paranoia, and delusions are common.

EPIDEMIOLOGY

- Globally, it is estimated that 46.8 million people have dementia (a figure greater than the entire population of Canada) and that the number of people with dementia will double every 20 years to 115.4 million by 2050 (Prince, Wimo, Guerchet, et al., 2015).
- More than 500 000 Canadians are currently living with dementia. Of these, 71 000 are under the age of 65.
- Among Canadians over the age of 65, 1 in 11 has dementia.
- Women comprise 72% of all Canadians living with the Alzheimer's subtype of neurocognitive disorder.
- The Alzheimer's subtype of neurocognitive disorder attacks indiscriminately, striking men and women, people of various ethnicities, rich and poor, and individuals with varying degrees of intelligence.
- Although Alzheimer's disease can occur at a younger age (early onset), most of those with the disease are 65 years of age or older (late onset).

ETIOLOGY

Although the cause of AD is unknown, most experts agree that, like other chronic and progressive conditions, it is a result of multiple factors—genetics, lifestyle, and environment. However, the greatest risk factor is advancing age (Alzheimer's Association, 2014; Lehne, 2013).

Biological Factors

Neurobiological

In the brains of people with Alzheimer's disease, there are signs of neuronal degeneration that begins in the hippocampus, the part of the brain responsible for recent memory. The degeneration then spreads into the cerebral cortex, the part of the brain responsible for problem solving and higher-order cognitive functioning.

There are two processes that contribute to cell death. The first is the accumulation of the protein amyloid outside the neurons, which interferes with synapses. The second is an accumulation of the protein tau inside the neurons, which forms tangles that block the flow of nutrients. Interestingly, some people who have these brain changes do not go on to develop Alzheimer's disease (Alzheimer's Association, 2014).

Genetic

There is an increased risk for AD among those people with an immediate family member who has or had dementia. There are three known genetic mutations that guarantee that a person will develop Alzheimer's disease, although these account for less than 1% of all cases. These mutations lead to the devastating early-onset form of Alzheimer's disease, which occurs before the age of 65 and as young as 30 years (Alzheimer's Association, 2014).

A susceptibility gene has been identified for late-onset Alzheimer's disease as well. It is a gene that makes the protein apolipoprotein E (APOE), which supports lipid transport and injury repair in the brain. Individuals carrying the ε4 allele are at increased risk for Alzheimer's disease compared with those carrying the most common ε3 allele, whereas carrying the ε2 allele decreases risk (Liu, Kanekiyo, Xu, et al., 2013).

Head Injury and Traumatic Brain Injury

Brain injury and trauma are associated with a greater risk for developing AD and other dementias. People who suffer repeated head trauma, such as boxers and football players, may be at greater risk. There is also a suggestion of a greater risk for those who suffer brain injury and carry the gene *APOE4* (Alzheimer's Association, 2014).

Cardiovascular Disease

The health of the brain is closely linked to overall heart health, and there is evidence that people with cardiovascular disease are at greater risk for AD. Likewise, lifestyle factors associated with cardiovascular disease, such as inactivity, high cholesterol, diabetes, and obesity, are considered risk factors for AD (Alzheimer's Association, 2014).

Environmental Factors

There is some evidence that brain health is affected by modifiable factors, such as remaining mentally and socially active and consuming a healthy diet. The research regarding environmental factors is limited by few studies and a low number of participants (Alzheimer's Association, 2014).

APPLICATION OF THE NURSING PROCESS

ASSESSMENT

General Assessment

Alzheimer's disease is commonly characterized by progressive deterioration of cognitive functioning. Initial deterioration may be so subtle and insidious that others may not notice. In the early stages of the disease, the affected person may be able to compensate for loss of memory, sometimes even hide it. This hiding is actually a form of denial, which is an unconscious protective defence against the terrifying reality of losing one's place in the world. Family members may also unconsciously deny that anything is wrong as a defence against the painful awareness that a loved one is deteriorating. As time goes on, symptoms become more obvious, and other defence mechanisms become evident, including (1) denial, (2) confabulation (the creation of stories or answers in place of actual memories, in an attempt to maintain self-esteem; it is not the same as lying because it is done unconsciously), (3) perseveration (the repetition of phrases or behaviour), and (4) avoidance of questions. The following exchange between a nurse and a patient who has remained in a hospital bed all weekend provides an example of confabulation:

Nurse: Good morning, Ms. Jones. How was your weekend?
Patient: Wonderful. I discussed politics with the prime minister, and he took me out to dinner.
or
Patient: I spent the weekend with my daughter and her family. Symptoms observed in AD include the following:

- Amnesia or memory impairment. Initially, the person has difficulty remembering recent events. Gradually, deterioration progresses to include both recent and remote memory.
- Aphasia (loss of language ability), which progresses with the disease. Initially, the person has difficulty finding the correct word, then is reduced to a few words, and finally is reduced to babbling or mutism.
- Apraxia, which is the loss of purposeful movement in the absence of motor or sensory impairment. The person is unable to perform once-familiar and purposeful tasks. For example, in apraxia of gait, the person loses the ability to walk. In apraxia of dressing, the person is unable to put clothes on properly (may put arms in trousers or put a jacket on upside down).
- Agnosia, which is the loss of the sensory ability to recognize objects. For example, the person may lose the ability to recognize familiar sounds (auditory agnosia), such as the ring of the telephone, a car horn, or the doorbell. Loss of this ability extends to the inability to recognize familiar objects (visual or tactile agnosia), such as a glass, magazine, pencil, or toothbrush. Eventually, people are unable to recognize loved ones or even parts of their own bodies.
- Disturbances in executive functioning (planning, organizing, abstract thinking). The degeneration of neurons in the brain results in the wasting away of the brain's working components. These cells contain memories, receive sights and sounds, cause hormones to secrete, produce emotions, and command muscles into motion.

A person with AD loses a personal history, a place in the world, and the ability to recognize the environment and, eventually, loved ones. Alzheimer's disease robs family and friends, husbands and wives, and sons and daughters of valuable human relatedness and companionship, which results in a profound sense of grief. It robs society of productive and active participants. Because of these devastating effects, mental health care professionals and social agencies, the medical and nursing professions, and researchers are challenged to look for possible causes and treatments.

Diagnostic Tests

A wide range of problems may be mistaken for dementia or AD. For example, in older adults, depression and dementia may have similar symptoms. It is important that nurses and other health care providers be able to assess some of the important differences among depression, neurocognitive disorder, and delirium (review Table 17-1).

Other disorders that often mimic dementia include drug toxicity, metabolic disorders, infections, and nutritional deficiencies. A disorder that mimics dementia is sometimes referred to as a pseudodementia. Making a diagnosis of Alzheimer's disease requires ruling out all other pathophysiological conditions

BOX 17-3	BASIC MEDICAL WORKUP FOR DEMENTIA

- Chest and skull radiographic studies
- Electroencephalography
- Electrocardiography
- Urinalysis
- Sequential multiple analyzer 12-test serum profile
- Thyroid function tests
- Folate level
- Venereal Disease Research Laboratory (VDRL) and human immunodeficiency virus (HIV) tests
- Serum creatinine assay
- Electrolyte assessment
- Vitamin B_{12} level
- Liver function tests
- Vision and hearing evaluation
- Neuroimaging (when diagnostic issues are not clear)

through careful assessment, including medical and family history, as well as through physical and laboratory tests, many of which are identified in Box 17-3.

Brain imaging with computed tomography (CT), positron emission tomography (PET), and other developing scanning technologies have diagnostic capabilities because they reveal brain atrophy and rule out other conditions such as neoplasms. The use of mental status questionnaires, such as the Mini–Mental State Examination and various other tests to identify deterioration in mental status and brain damage, is an important part of the assessment.

In addition to performing a thorough physical and neurological examination, it is important to obtain a complete medical and psychiatric history, a description of recent symptoms, a review of medications used, and a nutritional evaluation. The observations and history provided by family members are invaluable to the assessment process.

As mentioned, depression in the older adult is the disorder most frequently confused with dementia. Medical and nursing personnel should be cautioned, however, that dementia and depression or dementia and delirium can coexist. In fact, studies indicate that many people diagnosed with Alzheimer's dementia also meet the *DSM-5* criteria for a depressive disorder.

Self-Assessment

Working with cognitively impaired people in any setting places a tremendous amount of responsibility on caregivers. The behavioural problems that people with dementia may display can cause stress for professionals and family caregivers alike.

Nurses working in facilities designed for people who are cognitively impaired (e.g., assisted-living, supported-living, long-term care, and extended care facilities) need special education and skills. Education must include information about the process of the disease and effective interventions, as well as knowledge regarding antipsychotic drugs. Support and educational opportunities should be readily available, not just to nurses but also to nursing aides, who are often directly responsible for administering basic care.

Because stress is common among those working with patients with cognitive impairments, staff need to be proactive in minimizing its effects through the use of the following strategies:

- Having a clear understanding of the disease so that expectations for the person are realistic
- Establishing realistic outcomes (perhaps as minor as *Patient feeds self with spoon*) for the person and recognizing when they are achieved, remembering that even the smallest achievement can be a significant accomplishment for the impaired individual
- Maintaining good self-care and protecting ourselves from the negative effects of stress by obtaining adequate sleep and rest, eating a nutritious diet, exercising, engaging in relaxing activities, and addressing our own emotional and spiritual needs.

ASSESSMENT GUIDELINES
Neurocognitive Disorders

1. Evaluate the person's current level of cognitive and daily functioning.
2. Identify any threats to the person's safety and security and arrange for their reduction.
3. Evaluate the safety of the person's home environment (e.g., with regard to wandering, eating inedible objects, falling, engaging in provocative behaviours toward others).
4. Review the medications (including herbs and complementary agents) the person is currently taking.
5. Interview family to gain a complete picture of the person's background and personality.
6. Explore how well the family is prepared for and informed about the progress of dementia, depending on cause (if known).
7. Discuss with the family members how they are coping with the requirements of caregiving and what their main issues are at this time.
8. Review the resources available to the family. Ask family members to describe the help they receive from other family members, friends, and community resources. Determine if caregivers are aware of community support groups and resources.
9. Identify the needs of the family for teaching and guidance—for example, how to manage catastrophic reactions (over-reactions to a seemingly normal, nonthreatening situation commonly experienced in AD), lability of mood, aggressive behaviours, and sundowning.

DIAGNOSIS

One of the most important areas of concern identified by both staff and families is safety. Many people with AD wander and may be lost for hours or days. Wandering, along with behaviours such as rummaging, may be perceived as purposeful to the person with AD. Wandering may result from changes in the physical environment, fear caused by hallucinations or delusions, or lack of exercise.

Seizures are common in the later stages of this disease. Injuries from falls and accidents can occur during any stage as confusion and disorientation progress. The potential for burns exists if the person is a smoker or is unattended when using the stove. Prescription drugs can be taken incorrectly, or bottles of noxious fluids can be mistakenly ingested, resulting in a medical crisis. Therefore *Risk for injury* is always present.

As the person's ability to recognize or name objects decreases, *Impaired verbal communication* becomes a problem. As memory diminishes and disorientation increases, *Impaired environmental interpretation syndrome*, *Impaired memory*, and *Confusion* occur.

Additional family issues may emerge. Perhaps some of the most crucial aspects of caregiving are support, education, and referrals for the family. The family loses an integral part of its unit, as well as the love, function, support, companionship, and warmth that this person once provided. *Caregiver role strain* is always present, and planning with the family and arranging community supports are vital parts of appropriate care. *Anticipatory grieving* is also an important phenomenon to assess and may be a significant target for intervention. Helping the family grieve can make the task ahead somewhat clearer and at times less painful. Review Table 17-2 for potential nursing diagnoses for confused patients.

OUTCOMES IDENTIFICATION

Families who have a member with dementia face an exhaustive list of issues that need to be addressed. Table 17-7 provides a checklist that may help nurses and families to identify areas for intervention. Self-care needs, impaired environmental interpretation, chronic confusion, ineffective individual coping, and caregiver role strain are just a few of the areas nurses and other health care providers will need to target (Box 17-4).

PLANNING

Planning care for a person with a major cognitive disorder care is geared toward the person's immediate needs. Refer to Table 17-7 for help in identifying potential areas of care. The Functional Dementia Scale (Figure 17-1) can be used by nurses and families to plan strategies for addressing immediate needs and to track progression of the dementia. The Cognitive Performance Scale, derived from the interRAI assessments, which reflect memory,

TABLE 17-7	PROBLEMS THAT MAY AFFECT PEOPLE WITH MAJOR NEUROCOGNITIVE DISORDERS AND THEIR FAMILIES		
PROBLEM	**EXAMPLES**	**PROBLEM**	**EXAMPLES**
Memory impairment	Forgets appointments, visits, etc.	Uncontrolled behaviour	Restlessness day or night
	Forgets to change clothes, wash, go to the toilet		Vulgar table or toilet habits
	Forgets to eat, take medications		Undressing
	Loses things		Sexual disinhibition
Disorientation	Time: mixes night and day, mixes days of appointments, wears summer clothes in winter, forgets age		Shoplifting
		Incontinence	Urine
			Feces
	Place: loses way around house		Urination or defecation in the wrong place
	Person: has difficulty recognizing visitors, family, spouse	Emotional reactions	Catastrophic reactions
			Demands for attention
Need for physical help	Dressing		Depression
	Washing, bathing		Distress and anxiety
	Toileting		Frustration and anger
	Eating		Embarrassment and withdrawal
	Performing housework		Lack of emotional control
	Maintaining mobility	Other reactions	Suspiciousness
Risks in the home	Falls		Hoarding and hiding
	Fire from cigarettes, cooking, heating	Mistaken beliefs	Still at work
	Flooding		Parents or spouse still alive
	Admission of strangers to home		Hallucinations
	Wandering out	Decision making	Indecisive
Risks outside the home	Competence, judgement, and risks at work		Easily influenced
	Driving, road sense		Refuses help
	Getting lost		Makes unwise decisions
Apathy	Little conversation	Burden on family	Disruption of social life
	Lack of interest		Distress, guilt, rejection
	Poor self-care		Family discord
Poor communication	Aphasia		
Repetitiveness	Repetition of questions or stories		
	Repetition of actions		

BOX 17-4   *NOC* OUTCOMES RELATED TO NEUROCOGNITIVE DISORDERS*

Injury
- Person will remain safe in the hospital or at home.
- With the aid of an identification bracelet and neighbourhood or hospital alert, the person will be returned within 1 hour of wandering.
- With the aid of interventions, person will remain burn free.
- With the aid of guidance and environmental manipulation, person will not hurt himself or herself if a fall occurs.
- Person will ingest only correct doses of prescribed medications and appropriate food and fluids.

Communication
- Person will communicate needs.
- Person will state needs in alternative modes when he or she is aphasic (e.g., will signal correct word on hearing it or will refer to picture or label).
- Person will wear prescribed glasses or hearing aid each day.

Agitation Level
- Person will have rest periods if pacing and restless.
- Person will cooperate with caregiving activities.
- Person will experience minimal frustrating experiences.
- Person will express frustrations in an appropriate manner.

Caregiver Role Strain
- Family members will have the opportunity to express "unacceptable" feelings in a supportive environment.

- Family members will have access to professional counselling.
- Family members will name two organizations within their geographical area that can offer emotional support and help with legal and financial burdens.
- Family members will participate in ill member's plan of care, with encouragement from staff.
- Family members will state that they have outside help that allows them to take personal time for themselves each week or month.

Impaired Environmental Interpretation: Chronic Confusion
- Person will acknowledge the reality of an object or a sound that was misinterpreted (illusion), after it is pointed out.
- Person will state that he or she feels safe after experiencing delusions or illusions.
- Person will remain nonaggressive when experiencing paranoid ideation.

Self-Care Needs
- Person will participate in self-care at optimal level.
- Person will be able to follow step-by-step instructions for dressing, bathing, and grooming.
- Person will put on own clothes appropriately, with aid of fastening tape (Velcro) and nursing supervision.
- Person's skin will remain intact and free from signs of pressure.

*Partial list.
Source: From Moorhead, S., Johnson, M., Maas, M. L., et al. (2012). *Nursing outcomes classification (NOC)* (4th ed.). St. Louis: Mosby.

FUNCTIONAL DEMENTIA SCALE

Circle one rating for each item:
1. None or little of the time
2. Some of the time
3. Good part of the time
4. Most or all of the time

Client: _____
Observer: _____
Position or relation to patient: _____
Facility: _____
Date: _____

1	2	3	4	1. Has difficulty in completing simple tasks on own (e.g., dressing, bathing, doing arithmetic).
1	2	3	4	2. Spends time either sitting or in apparently purposeless activity.
1	2	3	4	3. Wanders at night or needs to be restrained to prevent wandering.
1	2	3	4	4. Hears things that are not there.
1	2	3	4	5. Requires supervision or assistance in eating.
1	2	3	4	6. Loses things.
1	2	3	4	7. Appearance is disorderly if left to own devices.
1	2	3	4	8. Moans.
1	2	3	4	9. Cannot control bowel function.
1	2	3	4	10. Threatens to harm others.
1	2	3	4	11. Cannot control bladder function.
1	2	3	4	12. Needs to be watched so doesn't injure self (e.g., by careless smoking, leaving the stove on, falling).
1	2	3	4	13. Destructive of materials around him/her (e.g., breaks furniture, throws food trays, tears up magazines).
1	2	3	4	14. Shouts or yells.
1	2	3	4	15. Accuses others of doing bodily harm or stealing his or her possessions — when you are sure the accusations are not true.
1	2	3	4	16. Is unaware of limitations imposed by illness.
1	2	3	4	17. Becomes confused and does not know where he or she is.
1	2	3	4	18. Has trouble remembering.
1	2	3	4	19. Has sudden changes of mood (e.g., gets upset, angered, or cries easily).
1	2	3	4	20. If left alone, wanders aimlessly during the day or needs to be restrained to prevent wandering.

FIGURE 17-1 Functional Dementia Scale. Source: Moore, J. T., Bobula, J. A., Short, T. B., et al. (1983). A functional dementia scale. *Journal of Family Practice, 16*(3), 499–503.

decision-making skills, communication, and eating, can also be used as a tool to track the progression of dementia (Canadian Institute for Health Information, 2013).

Identifying a patient's level of functioning and assessing caregivers' needs help health care providers to focus planning and identify appropriate community resources. Does the patient or family need the following?

- Transportation services
- Supervision and care when primary caregiver is out of the home
- Referrals to adult day programs
- Information on support groups within the community
- Meals on Wheels
- Information on respite and residential services
- Telephone numbers for helplines
- Home health aides
- Home care services
- Additional psychopharmaceuticals to manage distressing or harmful behaviours

IMPLEMENTATION

Caring for a person with dementia requires a great deal of patience, creativity, and maturity. The needs of such a person can be enormous for nursing staff and for families who care for their loved ones in the home. As the disease progresses, so do the needs of the person and the demands on the caregivers, staff, and family. The attitude of unconditional positive regard is the nurse's single most effective tool in caring for people with dementia. Positive regard induces patients to cooperate, reduces catastrophic outbreaks, and increases family members' satisfaction with the care provided. Box 17-5 lists *NIC* interventions related to the management of neurocognitive disorders.

A considerable number of individuals with dementia have secondary behavioural disturbances, including depression, hallucinations, delusions, agitation, insomnia, and wandering. Because these symptoms impair the person's ability to function, increase the need for supervision, and influence the need for institutionalization, the control of these symptoms is a priority in managing AD. Helping the individual achieve the highest possible level of independence and function is the foundation of care.

However, intervention with family members is also critical. The effects of losing a family member to dementia—that is, watching the deterioration of a person who has had an important role within the family unit and who is loved and is a vital part of his or her family's history—can be devastating. The following interventions are useful: counselling, health teaching, community supports, family support, and pharmacological interventions and integrative therapies.

Counselling and Communication Techniques

How one chooses to communicate with a person with dementia affects that person's ability to maintain self-esteem and his or her ability to participate in care. People with dementia often find it difficult to express themselves. Potential reasons for this difficulty are listed below.

- Cannot find the right words
- Invent new words to describe things
- Frequently lose their train of thought
- Rely on nonverbal gestures

Guidelines for Communication: People With Dementia provides special guidelines for nurses, family members, and other caregivers to use in communicating with a cognitively impaired person.

Health Teaching and Health Promotion

Educating families who have a cognitively impaired member is one of the most important health-teaching duties nurses encounter. Families who are caring for a member in the home need to know about strategies for communicating and for structuring self-care activities (see Patient and Family Teaching: Guidelines for Self-Care for Individuals With Cognitive Impairment).

Most important, families need to know where to get help. Help includes professional counselling and education regarding the process and progression of the disease. Families especially need to know about and be referred to community-based groups that can help shoulder this burden (e.g., adult support programs, senior citizen groups, organizations providing home visits and respite care, family support groups). A list with definitions of some of the types of services available in the person's community, as well as the names and telephone numbers of the providers of these services, should be given to the family.

Referral to Community Supports

The Alzheimer Society of Canada is a national umbrella agency that provides various forms of assistance to people with the disease and their families. The society offers educational resources on Alzheimer's disease and related dementias, guidelines for providing quality care, ethical guidelines to help people address sensitive issues, and information and referrals for support programs and services, some of which may help prevent total emotional and physical fatigue in caregivers. In partnership with the Royal Canadian Mounted Police, the Alzheimer Society of Canada also has developed the Safely Home registry, a national registry to help find lost Alzheimer's patients and assist them in returning home (Alzheimer Society of Canada, 2011). More information about this registry can be found on the Alzheimer Society of Canada's website: http://www.alzheimer.ca/en. The support programs and services available from the Alzheimer Society vary from community to community; examples of services it provides are found in Table 17-8.

Although many families manage the care of their loved one until death, other families eventually find that they can no longer deal with the labile and aggressive behaviour, incontinence, wandering, unsafe habits, or disruptive nocturnal activity. Family members need to know where and how to place their loved one for care if such a move becomes necessary. Families need information, support, and legal and financial guidance at this time. When the nurse is unable to provide the relevant information, proper referrals by the social worker are needed. Information regarding advance directives, durable power of attorney, and guardianship should be included in the communication with the family. Patient and Family Teaching: Guidelines for Care at

BOX 17-5   *NIC* INTERVENTIONS FOR NEUROCOGNITIVE MANAGEMENT

Definition of *neurocognitive management:* Provision of a modified environment for the patient who is experiencing a chronic confusional state.

Activities:

- Include family members in planning, providing, and evaluating care, to the extent desired by the patient and family.
- Identify usual patterns of behaviour for such activities as sleep, medication use, elimination, food intake, and self-care.
- Determine physical, social, and psychological history of patient, usual habits, and routines.
- Determine type and extent of cognitive deficit(s), using standardized assessment tool.
- Monitor cognitive functioning, using standardized assessment tool.
- Determine behavioural expectations appropriate for patient's cognitive status.
- Provide a low-stimulation environment (e.g., quiet, soothing music; nonvivid and simple decor with familiar patterns; performance expectations that do not exceed cognitive processing ability; dining in small groups).
- Provide adequate but nonglare lighting.
- Identify and remove potential dangers for patient in environment.
- Place identification bracelet on patient.
- Provide a consistent physical environment and daily routine.
- Prepare for interaction with eye contact and touch, as appropriate.
- Introduce self when initiating contact.
- Address patient distinctly by name when initiating interaction, and speak slowly.
- Give one simple direction at a time.
- Speak in a clear, low, warm, respectful tone of voice.
- Use distraction, rather than confrontation, to manage behaviour.
- Provide unconditional positive regard.
- Avoid touch and proximity if they cause stress or anxiety.
- Provide caregivers who are familiar to the patient (e.g., avoid frequent rotations of staff assignments).
- Avoid unfamiliar situations when possible (e.g., room changes and appointments without familiar people present).
- Provide rest periods to prevent fatigue and reduce stress.
- Monitor nutrition and weight.
- Provide space for safe pacing and wandering.

- Avoid frustrating patient by quizzing with orientation questions that cannot be answered.
- Provide cues—such as current events, seasons, location, and names—to assist orientation.
- Seat patient at a small table in groups of three to five for meals, as appropriate.
- Allow patient to eat alone if appropriate.
- Provide finger foods to maintain nutrition for patient who will not sit and eat.
- Provide patient with a general orientation to the season of the year by using appropriate cues (e.g., holiday decorations; seasonal decorations and activities; access to contained, outdoor area).
- Decrease noise levels by avoiding paging systems and call lights that ring or buzz.
- Select television or radio programs based on cognitive processing abilities and interests.
- Select one-to-one and group activities geared to patient's cognitive abilities and interests.
- Label familiar photos with names of the individuals in the photos.
- Select artwork for patient's rooms featuring landscapes, scenery, or other familiar images.
- Ask family members and friends to see patient one or two at a time, if needed, to reduce stimulation.
- Discuss with family members and friends how best to interact with patient.
- Assist family to understand that it may be impossible for patient to learn new material.
- Limit number of choices patient has to make so as not to cause anxiety.
- Provide boundaries, such as red or yellow tape on the floor when low-stimulus units are not available.
- Place patient's name in large block letters in room and on clothing, as needed.
- Use symbols, rather than written signs, to assist patient in locating room, bathroom, or other area.
- Monitor carefully for physiological causes of increased confusion that may be acute and reversible.
- Remove or cover mirrors if patient is frightened or agitated by them.
- Discuss home safety issues and interventions.

Source: Bulechek, G. M., Butcher, H. K., Dochterman, J. M., et al. (2012). *Nursing interventions classification (NIC)* (6th ed.). St. Louis: Mosby.

TABLE 17-8   TYPES OF SERVICES THAT MAY BE AVAILABLE TO PEOPLE WITH DEMENTIA

TYPE OF SERVICE	SERVICES PROVIDED
Family/caregiver	Caregivers have a right to: 　　Easy access to services 　　Respite care 　　Full involvement in decision making 　　Assessment of the needs of both the caregiver and the person with dementia 　　Information and referral
Community services	Case management: coordination of community resources and follow-up Adult support programs: provide activities, socialization, and supervision in an outpatient setting Physician services Protective services: prevent, eliminate, or remedy effects of abuse or neglect Recreational services Transportation Mental health services Legal services

Continued

TABLE 17-8	TYPES OF SERVICES THAT MAY BE AVAILABLE TO PEOPLE WITH DEMENTIA—cont'd
TYPE OF SERVICE	**SERVICES PROVIDED**
Home care	Meals on Wheels
	Home health aide services
	Homemaker services
	Respite services
	Occupational therapy
	Paid companion or sitter services
	Physiotherapy
	Skilled nursing care
	Personal care services: assistance in basic self-care activities
	Social work services
	Telephone reassurance: regular telephone calls to individuals who are isolated and homebound*
	Personal emergency response systems: telephone-based systems to alert others that a person who is alone is in need of emergency assistance*

*Vital for those living alone.

GUIDELINES FOR COMMUNICATION

People With Dementia

Intervention	Rationale
Always identify yourself and call the person by name at each meeting.	The person's short-term memory is impaired—requires frequent orientation to time and environment.
Speak slowly.	The person needs time to process information.
Use short, simple words and phrases.	The person may not be able to understand complex statements or abstract ideas.
Maintain face-to-face contact.	Verbal and nonverbal clues are maximized.
Be near the person when talking, one or two arm-lengths away.	This distance can help the person focus on the speaker while maintaining personal space.
Focus on one piece of information at a time.	The person's attention span is poor, and he or she is easily distracted—bite-sized information helps the person focus. Too much data can be overwhelming and can increase anxiety.
Talk with the person about familiar and meaningful things.	Self-expression is promoted, and reality is reinforced.
Encourage reminiscing about happy times in life.	Remembering accomplishments and shared joys helps distract the person from deficit and gives meaning to existence.
When the person is delusional, acknowledge the person's feelings and reinforce reality. Do not argue or refute delusions.	Acknowledging feelings helps the person feel understood. Pointing out realities may help the person focus on realities. Arguing can enhance adherence to false beliefs.
If the person gets into an argument with another person, stop the argument and temporarily separate those involved. After a short while (5 minutes), explain to each person matter-of-factly why you had to intervene.	Escalation to physical acting out is prevented. The person's right to know is respected. Explaining in an adult manner helps maintain self-esteem.
When the person becomes verbally aggressive, acknowledge the person's feelings, and shift the topic to more familiar ground (e.g., "I know this is upsetting for you, because you always cared for others. Tell me about your children.")	Confusion and disorientation easily increase anxiety. Acknowledging feelings makes the person feel more understood and less alone. Topics the person has mastery over can remind him or her of areas of competent functioning and can increase self-esteem.
Have the person wear prescription glasses or hearing aid(s).	Environmental awareness, orientation, and comprehension are increased, which in turn increase awareness of personal needs and the presence of others.
Keep the person's room well lit.	Environmental clues are maximized.
Have clocks, calendars, and personal items (e.g., family pictures, meaningful books) in clear view of the person while he or she is in bed.	These objects assist in maintaining personal identity.
Reinforce the person's pictures, nonverbal gestures, Xs on calendars, and other methods used to anchor the person in reality.	When aphasia starts to hinder communication, alternative methods of communication need to be instituted.

Source: Data from Bulechek, G. M., Butcher, H. K., Dochterman, J. M., et al. (2012). *Nursing interventions classification (NIC)* (6th ed.). St. Louis: Mosby.

PATIENT AND FAMILY TEACHING

Guidelines for Self-Care for Individuals With Cognitive Impairment

Intervention	Rationale
Dressing and Bathing	
Always have the person perform all tasks within his or her present capacity.	Maintains the person's self-esteem and uses muscle groups
	Impedes staff burnout
	Minimizes further regression
Always have the person wear own clothes, even if in the hospital.	Helps maintain the person's identity and dignity
Use clothing with elastic, and substitute fastening tape (Velcro) for buttons and zippers.	Minimizes the person's confusion
	Eases independence of functioning
Label clothing items with the person's name and name of item.	Helps identify the person if he or she wanders
	Gives the person additional clues when aphasia or agnosia occurs
Give step-by-step instructions whenever necessary (e.g., "Take this blouse. Put in one arm … now the other arm. Pull it together in front. Now …")	Uses the person's ability to focus on small pieces of information more easily
	Allows the person to perform at optimal level
Make sure that water in faucets is not too hot.	Ensures safety for person who is lacking judgement or is unaware of many safety hazards
If the person is resistant to performing self-care, come back later and ask again.	Respects that the person's moods may be labile—the person often complies after a short interval
Nutrition	
Monitor food and fluid intake.	Helps to prevent anorexia or refusal to eat because of confusion
Offer finger food that the person can take away from the dinner table.	Increases intake throughout the day—the person may eat only small amounts at meals
Weigh the person regularly (once a week).	Monitors fluid and nutritional status
During periods of hyperorality, watch that the person does not eat nonfood items (e.g., ceramic fruit or food-shaped soaps).	Ensures safety of the person who puts everything into mouth or who is unable to differentiate inedible objects made in the shape and colour of food
Bowel and Bladder Function	
Begin bowel and bladder program early; start with bladder control.	Helps prevent incontinence by establishing same time of day for bowel movements and toileting—in early morning, after meals and snacks, and before bedtime
Evaluate use of disposable incontinence products.	Prevents embarrassment
Label bathroom door, as well as doors to other rooms.	Maximizes independent toileting by offering additional environmental clues
Sleep	
Because the person may awaken, be frightened, or cry out at night, keep area well lit.	Reinforces orientation
	Minimizes possible illusions
Maintain a calm atmosphere during the day.	Encourages a calming night's sleep
Order nonbarbiturates (e.g., chloral hydrate) if necessary.	Avoids paradoxical reaction of agitation, often caused by barbiturates
If medications are indicated, consider neuroleptics with sedative properties, which may be the most helpful (e.g., haloperidol [Haldol]).	Helps clear thinking
	Sedates
Avoid the use of restraints.	Avoids inciting fear in the person, who may fight against restraints until exhausted to a dangerous degree

Home provides useful guidelines for families for structuring a safe environment and planning appropriate activities.

Pharmacological Interventions

There is currently no cure for Alzheimer's disease. There are, however, four drugs approved by Health Canada that slow the progression of the illness. Although these medications are used widely and have been shown to have statistically significant effects when compared with placebos, they produce only a clinically marginal improvement on cognition and functioning. The benefits of these medications wane after 1 to 2 years, so patients should weigh the potential side effects against the potential benefits. Refer to Figure 17-2 for a brief summary of the neurobiology of Alzheimer's and the effects of medication on the brain.

Cholinesterase Inhibitors

Because a deficiency of acetylcholine has been linked to Alzheimer's disease, medications aimed at preventing its breakdown have been developed. Drugs in this classification work by preventing an enzyme called acetylcholinesterase or, more simply, cholinesterase from break-ing down acetylcholine in the brain. As a result, an increased concentration of acetylcholine leads to temporary improvement of some symptoms of Alzheimer's disease.

There is little evidence that giving cholinesterase inhibitors to individuals who have the mild version of neurocognitive disorders slows the progression to dementia (Buckley & Salpeter, 2015). The cholinesterase inhibitors produce small, but short-lived, improvements in cognitive functioning. There is minimal benefit after 1 year, and risk for side effects doubles in people over 85 years of age.

PATIENT AND FAMILY TEACHING

Guidelines for Care at Home

Intervention	Rationale
Safe Environment	
Gradually restrict use of the car.	Ensures safety as the person's judgement becomes impaired
Remove throw rugs and other objects in person's path.	Minimizes tripping and falling
Minimize sensory stimulation.	Decreases sensory overload, which can increase anxiety and confusion
If the person becomes verbally upset, listen briefly, give support, and then change the topic.	Aims to prevent escalation of anger
	Distracts person to more productive topics and activities
Label all rooms and drawers. Label often-used objects (e.g., hairbrushes, toothbrushes).	May keep the person from wandering into other people's rooms
	Increases environmental clues to familiar objects
Install safety bars in bathroom.	Prevents falls
Supervise the person when he or she smokes.	Minimizes danger of burns
If the person has history of seizures, keep padded tongue blades at beside. Educate family on how to deal with seizures.	Ensures safety—seizure activity is common in advanced Alzheimer's disease
Wandering	
If the person wanders during the night, put his or her mattress on the floor.	Prevents falls when the person is confused.
Have the person wear medical alert bracelet that cannot be removed (with name, address, and telephone number).	Ensures easy identification by police, neighbours, or hospital personnel
Provide police department with recent pictures.	
Alert local police and neighbours about wanderer.	May reduce time necessary to return the person to home or hospital
If the person is in hospital, have him or her wear brightly coloured vest with name, unit, and phone number printed on back.	Makes the person easily identifiable
Put complex locks on door.	Reduces opportunity to wander
Place locks at top of door.	Ensures safety—in moderate and late Alzheimer's-type dementia, ability to look up and reach upward is lost
Encourage physical activity during the day.	May decrease wandering at night
Explore the feasibility of installing sensor devices.	Provides warning if the person wanders
Useful Activities	
Provide picture magazines and children's books when the person's reading ability diminishes.	Allows continuation of usual activities that the person can still enjoy
	Provides focus
Provide simple activities that allow exercise of large muscles.	Provides socialization (e.g., exercise groups, dance groups, walking groups)
	Increases circulation and maintains muscle tone
Encourage group activities that are familiar and simple to perform.	Increases socialization (e.g., activities such as group singing, dancing, reminiscing, working with clay and paint)
	Minimizes feelings of alienation

Tacrine (Cognex), the first approved cholinesterase inhibitor, was used to treat mild to moderate symptoms of Alzheimer's disease. Unfortunately, tacrine was associated with a high frequency of side effects, including gastrointestinal effects, elevated liver transaminase levels, and liver toxicity. As a result, it is rarely prescribed today (Alzheimer's Association, 2015).

The most commonly prescribed cholinesterase inhibitor is donepezil (Aricept). Indications for donepezil include mild, moderate, and severe Alzheimer's disease. It also appears to improve cognitive functions without the potentially serious liver toxicity attributed to tacrine. Some individuals may experience diarrhea and nausea while taking the drug. These side effects are dose related, so a decreased dose helps minimize them.

Rivastigmine (Exelon) is another cholinesterase inhibitor used in the mild to moderate stages of Alzheimer's disease. The most common side effects are nausea, vomiting, loss of appetite, and weight loss. In most cases, these side effects are temporary. Patients should always take rivastigmine with food to reduce gastrointestinal side effects. The Exelon transdermal patch is applied once a day and has no food requirement. It is useful for people who have trouble swallowing pills. Patients and families should be cautioned to always remove the old patch before applying the new one to prevent serious side effects.

Despite slight variations in the mode of action of the cholinesterase inhibitors, there is no evidence of any differences between them with regards to effectiveness. All of the cholinesterase inhibitors have the potential to cause nausea, diarrhea, and vomiting, depending on the dosage level. Bradycardia and syncope have been associated with this class of drugs. They should be used with caution when patients are taking nonsteroidal anti-inflammatory drugs (NSAIDs).

N-Methyl-D-Aspartate (NMDA) Receptor Antagonist

Memantine (Namenda) is typically added after trying the cholinesterase inhibitors. It regulates the activity of glutamate, a neurotransmitter that plays a role in information processing, storage, and retrieval. Memantine blocks NMDA receptors to protect against excessive neuronal stimulation by glutamate. It is approved for use in moderate to severe dementia, but not mild dementia.

▶ Neurobiology of Alzheimer's and the Effects of Medication on the Brain

Two essential neurotransmitters implicated in Alzheimer's disease are acetylcholine and glutamate.

Acetylcholine: is involved with learning, memory, and mood. As Alzheimer's disease progresses. the brain produces less and less acetylcholine. What little acetylcholine is left is rapidly destroyed by the enzyme acetylcholinesterase.

Cholinesterase: inhibitors keep the acetylcholinesterase enzyme from breaking down acetylcholine, thereby increasing both the level and the duration of action of the neurotransmitter acetylcholine.

Glutamate: is involved with cell signalling, learning, and memory. Glutamate binds to cells at the N-methyl-D-aspartate (NMDA) receptor and allows calcium to enter the cell. In Alzheimer's disease, excess glutamate from damaged cells leads to chronic overexposure to calcium.

NMDA: antagonists help reduce excess calcium by blocking some NMDA receptors.

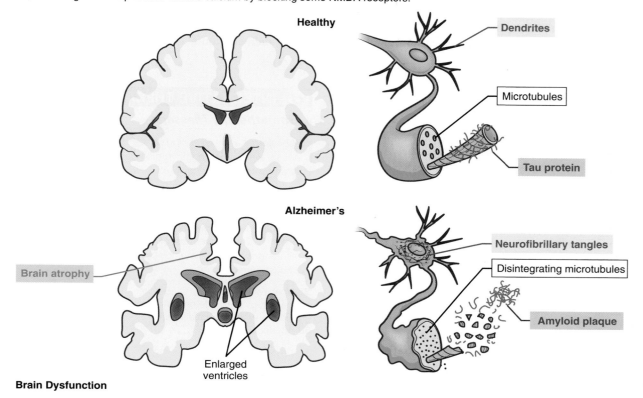

Brain Dysfunction

Amyloid plaques are sticky clumps found between nerve cells that may either cause or be the result of the disease. The clumps block communication at synapses that are normally protected by tau proteins and healthy microtubules. They may also activate immune system cells that trigger inflammation and devour disabled cells.

Neurofibrillary tangles are abnormal collections of protein threads inside nerve cells. They are composed mainly of a protein called tau. Tangles disrupt the transport of food molecules, cell parts, and other key elements. This disruption results in cell death.

Brain atrophy is the cerebral cortex shrivelling up, damaging areas involved in thinking, planning, and remembering. The hippocampus, an area of the cortex that is essential for memory, experiences severe shrinkage. Ventricles, the fluid-filled spaces within the brain, grow larger.

FDA-Approved Drugs for the Treatment of Alzheimer's Disease

Drug Name	Brand Name	Classification	Approved For
galantamine	Razadyne	Cholinesterase inhibitor	Mild to moderate
donepezil	Aricept	Cholinesterase inhibitor	All stages
rivastigmine	Exelon	Cholinesterase inhibitor	All stages
memantine	Namenda	Namenda, an NMDA antagonist, helps reduce excess calcium by blocking some NMDA receptors	Moderate to severe
donepezil and memantine	Namzaric	Cholinesterase inhibitor and NMDA receptor antagonist combination	Moderate to severe

FIGURE 17-2

Refer to Chapter 11 for a more detailed discussion of psychotropic medications.

Medications for Behavioural Symptoms

Other medications are often useful in managing the behavioural symptoms of individuals with cognitive impairment, but these need to be used with extreme caution. The rule of thumb is "start low and go slow." Another is to use the smallest dose for the shortest duration possible and discontinue if the medications are not effective. In addition, because people with cognitive impairment are at high risk for developing delirium, always add medications with caution.

Most people with cognitive impairment will experience behavioural symptoms that reduce their quality of life, are distressing to them and their caregivers, and may lead to placement in a residential care facility. Some of the troubling behaviours are psychotic symptoms (hallucinations, paranoia), severe mood swings (depression is common), wandering, anxiety, agitation, and verbal or physical aggression (combativeness). Not only are these behaviours distressing, but they may also lead to injuries from falls, infections, and incontinence.

Psychotropic medications may be prescribed. Drug classifications that are used off-label include antidepressants, antipsychotics, antianxiety agents, and anticonvulsants. Of these, antipsychotics have been used most often. These medications are associated with risk for mortality, mostly from cardiovascular and infectious causes. As a result, all antipsychotics, both first and second generation, are no longer approved for dementia-related psychosis.

Of clinical relevance to nurses is evidence that suggests that personalized nursing care, in which the idiosyncratic needs of the person are recognized and met, is effective as a nonpharmacological treatment for many symptoms associated with dementia (Ayalon, Gunn, Feliciano, et al., 2006). With this evidence in mind, nurses should try to decipher patients' needs as expressed in their behaviour since people with dementia do not always communicate their needs verbally.

The Future of Drug Therapy

Additional research is ongoing, with focuses on:

- The development of other cholinesterase inhibitors
- The use of cholesterol-lowering agents
- The use of anti-inflammatory agents as a preventive measure
- The use of neurotrophic agents with the potential to regenerate brain cells
- The use of diabetic treatments that might decrease blood vessel inflammation in the brain

Additional information about current clinical studies can be found on the Alzheimer Society of Canada website: http://www.alzheimer.ca.

Integrative Therapy

Aromatherapy, the use of essential oils from fragrant plants such as lavender, peppermint, and sweet marjoram, has been used with people with dementia to promote relaxation and sleep, provide pain relief, and improve mood. At present, there is limited evidence of the effectiveness of aromatherapy in people with dementia. A recent systematic review (Forrester, Maayan, Orrell, et al., 2014) of seven controlled trials demonstrated that there are inconsistent effects of aromatherapy on quality of life, agitation, and behavioural challenges in people with dementia.

⚙ INTEGRATIVE THERAPY

Aromatherapy Massage

Behavioural and psychological symptoms are common in individuals with neurocognitive disorders. Along with the cognitive deficits, agitated behaviours and depressive mood are major causes of caregiver burden. Due to the risks associated with psychotropic medication in this population, clinicians have been reducing or eliminating their use. Therefore nonpharmacological strategies are being recommended to help reduce these symptoms. The effectiveness of nonpharmacological strategies is resulting in broader multidisciplinary teams that include more wholistic practitioners.

Source: Yang, Y., Wang, C., & Wang, J. (2016). Effects of aromatherapy massage on agitation and depressive mood in individuals with dementia. *Journal of Gerontological Nursing, 42*(9), 38–46. doi:10.3928/00989134-20160615-03.

EVALUATION

Outcome criteria for a person with cognitive impairments need to be measurable, within the capabilities of the individual, and evaluated frequently. As the person's condition continues to deteriorate, outcomes must be altered to reflect the person's diminished functioning. Frequent evaluation and reformulation of outcome criteria and short-term indicators also help reduce staff and family frustration and minimize the person with dementia's anxiety by ensuring that tasks are not more complicated than the person can accomplish.

The overall outcomes for treatment are to promote the person's optimal level of functioning and to delay further regression whenever possible. Working closely with family members and providing them with the names of available resources and support sources may help increase the quality of life for both the family and the patient with AD (see Case Study and Nursing Care Plan 17-1).

CASE STUDY AND NURSING CARE PLAN 17-1

Cognitive Impairment

During the past 4 years, Mr. Ludwig has demonstrated rapidly progressive memory impairment, disorientation, and deterioration in his ability to function, related to Alzheimer's disease. He is a 67-year-old man who retired at age 62 to spend some of his remaining "youth" with his wife and to travel, garden, visit family, and finally get to do the things they always wanted to do. At age 63, he was diagnosed with Alzheimer's disease.

Mr. Ludwig has been taken care of at home by his wife and his daughter, Kelly. Kelly is divorced and has returned home with her two young daughters.

The family members find themselves close to physical and mental exhaustion. Mr. Ludwig is becoming increasingly incontinent as he cannot consistently find the bathroom. He wanders away from home, despite close supervision. The police and neighbours bring him back home an average of four times a week. Once, he was lost for 5 days after he had somehow boarded a bus for Vancouver, 1000 kilometres from home. He was robbed and beaten before being found by the police and returned home.

He frequently wanders into his granddaughters' rooms at night while they are sleeping and tries to get into bed with them. Too young to understand that their grandfather is lonely and confused, they fear that he is going to hurt them. Four times in the past 2 weeks, he has fallen while getting out of bed at night, thinking he is in a sleeping bag, camping out in the mountains. After a conflicted and painful 2 months, the family places him in a care facility for people with Alzheimer's disease.

Mrs. Ludwig tells the admitting nurse, Mr. Behar, that her husband wanders almost all the time and that he has difficulty finding the right words for things (aphasia) and becomes frustrated and angry when that happens. Sometimes he does not seem to recognize the family (agnosia). Once, he thought that Kelly was a thief breaking into the house and attacked her with a broom handle. The telling of this story causes Kelly to break down into heavy sobs: "What's happened to my father? He was so kind and gentle. Oh, God ... I've lost my father."

Mrs. Ludwig tells Mr. Behar that her husband can sometimes participate in dressing himself; at other times, he needs total assistance. At this point, Mrs. Ludwig begins to cry uncontrollably, saying, "I can't bear to part with him, but I can't do it anymore. I feel as if I've betrayed him."

Mr. Behar then focuses his attention on Mrs. Ludwig and her experience. He states, "This is a difficult decision for you." Mr. Behar suggests that Mrs. Ludwig talk to other families who have a cognitively impaired member. "It might help you to know that you are not alone, and having contact with others to share your grief can be healing." One of the organizations he suggests is the Alzheimer Society of Canada, a well-known group that provides support and information to caregivers.

ASSESSMENT

Self-Assessment

Mr. Behar has worked on his particular unit for 4 years. It is a unit designed especially for cognitively impaired individuals, which makes nursing care of these patients easier than on a regular unit. He applied for this position shortly after his own father died of complications secondary to Alzheimer's disease. Mr. Behar refers to the process of living and dying with this disease as horrifying; his goal is to help other people go through it with caring, dignity, and the highest level of functioning possible.

Caring for Mr. Ludwig and his family is becoming especially personal. Mr. Behar is struck by the similarity between this family's situation and his own. Mr. Ludwig is about the same age his father had been, looks similar to him, and has many of his mannerisms. Mrs. Ludwig and her daughter Kelly seem to be responding in much the same way his family did. He finds that he is having stronger than usual counter-transference feelings with this family and even became teary when Mrs. Ludwig did.

The evening after he met the Ludwigs, Mr. Behar went home utterly exhausted and continued to think about them and his own father. He shared these feelings with his wife, and the two of them spent some time talking about his father and all they had been through together, good and bad. In the end, Mr. Behar sat back, breathed a long, deep sigh of relief, and thanked his wife for being there for him. He told her that he supposed he will never really get over the death of his father, but he is getting better every day.

When Mr. Behar returned to work, he nearly walked right into Mr. Ludwig, who was standing at the doorway wearing two shirts, a pair of pyjama bottoms, and a baseball cap. "Are you the man who's taking me to pick up my car?" he asks. Mr. Behar smiles and says, "It looks like you have quite a day planned. Let's start with a cup of coffee," and redirects him to the day hall.

Objective Data	Subjective Data
Patient:	"I can't bear to part with him."
• Wanders away from home about four times a week	"I feel as if I've betrayed him."
• Was lost for 5 days and was robbed and beaten	"I've lost my father."
• Is often incontinent when he cannot find the bathroom	
• Has difficulty finding words	
• Has difficulty identifying members of the family at times	
• Has difficulty dressing himself at times	
• Falls out of bed at night	
• Has memory impairment	
• Is disoriented much of the time	
• Gets into bed with granddaughters at night when wandering	
Family is undergoing intense feelings of loss and guilt	

Continued

CASE STUDY AND NURSING CARE PLAN 17-1—cont'd
Cognitive Impairment

DIAGNOSIS

1. *Risk for injury* related to confusion, as evidenced by wandering
Supporting Data
- Wanders away from home about four times a week
- Wanders despite supervision
- Falls out of bed at night
- Gets into other people's beds
- Wanders at night

2. *Functional urinary incontinence* related to disturbed cognition, as evidenced by inability to find the toilet
Supporting Data
- Incontinent when he cannot find the bathroom

3. *Self-care deficit* (self-dressing) related to impaired cognitive functioning, as evidenced by impaired ability to put on and take off clothing
Supporting Data
- Sometimes he is able to dress with help of wife
- At other times he is too confused to dress self at all

4. *Anticipatory grieving* related to loss and deterioration of family member
Supporting Data
- "I can't bear to part with him."
- "I feel as if I've betrayed him."
- "I've lost my father."
- Family undergoing intense feelings of loss and guilt

OUTCOMES IDENTIFICATION

Although Mr. Ludwig has many unmet needs that require nursing interventions, Mr. Behar decides to focus on the four initial nursing diagnoses. As other problems arise, they will be addressed.

Nursing Diagnosis	Long-Term Goals	Short-Term Goals
1. *Risk for injury* related to confusion, as evidenced by wandering	1. Resident will remain safe in nursing home.	1a. Throughout nursing home stay, resident will not fall out of bed.
		1b. Throughout nursing home stay, resident will wander only in protected area.
		1c. Resident will be returned within 2 hours if he succeeds in escaping from the unit.
2. *Functional urinary incontinence* related to disturbed cognition, as evidenced by inability to find the toilet	2. Resident will experience less incontinence (fewer episodes) by fourth week of hospitalization.	2a. By the end of 4 weeks, resident will participate in unit orientation to find toilet.
		2b. By the end of 4 weeks, resident will find the toilet most of the time.
3. *Self-care deficit* (self-dressing) related to impaired cognitive functioning, as evidenced by impaired ability to put on and take off clothing	3. Resident will participate in dressing himself 80% of the time.	3a. By the end of 4 weeks, resident will follow step-by-step instructions for dressing most of the time.
		3b. By the end of 4 weeks, resident will dress in own clothes with aid of fastening tape.
4. *Anticipatory grieving* related to loss and deterioration of family member	4. In 3 months' time, all family members will state that they feel they have more support and are able to talk about their grieving.	4a. After 3 months, family members will state that they have opportunity to express "unacceptable" feelings in supportive environment.
		4b. After 3 months, family members will state that they have found support from others who have a family member with Alzheimer's disease.

PLANNING

Mr. Behar plans care to ensure Mr. Ludwig's safety, provide for the maintenance of his hygiene needs and incontinence, and assist Mrs. Ludwig as she deals with her husband's deterioration.

CASE STUDY AND NURSING CARE PLAN 17-1—cont'd

Cognitive Impairment

IMPLEMENTATION

Using the concepts of *NIC*, Mr. Behar's plan of care (nursing diagnosis: *Risk for injury* related to confusion, as evidenced by wandering) was personalized as follows:

Short-Term Outcome	Intervention	Rationale	Evaluation
1. Throughout stay in nursing home, resident will not fall out of bed.	1a. Spend time with resident on admission.	1a. Time spent with resident lowers anxiety and provides orientation to time and place. Resident's confusion is increased by change.	**GOAL MET** Mattress on floor prevents falls out of bed.
	1b. Label resident's room in big, colourful letters.	1b. Labels offer clues in new surroundings.	
	1c. Remove mattress from bed and place on floor.	1c. Placing the mattress on the floor prevents falls out of bed.	
	1d. Keep room well lit at all times.	1d. Lighting provides important environmental clues and helps lower possibility of illusions.	
	1e. Show resident clock and calendar in room.	1e. These items foster orientation to time.	
	1f. Keep window shade up.	1f. This visibility allows day–night variations.	
2. Throughout nursing home stay, resident will wander only in protected area.	2a. At night, take resident to large, protected, well-lit room.	2a. Resident is able to wander safely in protected environment.	**GOAL MET** Resident continues to wander at night but, with supervision, keeps out of other residents' rooms most of the time. By fourth week, resident starts to nap on couch in large room after snacks during the night.
	2b. Alert physician to check resident for cardiac decompensation.	2b. Physical check addresses possible underlying cause of nocturnal wakefulness and wandering.	
	2c. Offer snacks when resident is up—milk, decaffeinated tea, sandwich.	2c. Snacks help replace fluid and caloric expenditure.	
	2d. Allow soft music on radio.	2d. Music helps induce relaxation.	
	2e. Spend short, frequent intervals with resident.	2e. Time with others decreases resident's feelings of isolation and increases orientation.	
	2f. Take resident to bathroom after snacks.	2f. Bathroom visits after eating help prevent incontinence.	
	2g. During day, offer activities that include use of large muscle groups.	2g. For some residents, using large muscle groups helps decrease wandering.	
3. Resident will be returned within 2 hours if he succeeds in escaping from the unit.	3a. Order MedicAlert bracelet for resident (with name, unit, hospital, and phone number).	3a. If resident gets out of hospital, he can be identified.	**GOAL MET** By fourth week, resident wanders off unit only once; is found in lobby and returned by security guard within 45 minutes.
	3b. Place brightly coloured vest on resident with name, unit, and phone number taped on back.	3b. If resident wanders in hospital, he can be identified and returned.	
	3c. Check resident's whereabouts periodically during the day and especially at night.	3c. Regular checks help monitor resident's activities.	

EVALUATION

Although Mr. Ludwig continues to display wandering behaviours, his wandering is contained to safe areas of the unit, except for one instance when he wanders to the lobby. However, then he is stopped by security and safely returned to the unit within 45 minutes. He has not fallen out of bed. Nursing interventions such as placing his mattress on the floor and ensuring adequate lighting increase his safety while at the same time acknowledge that he continues to exhibit wandering behaviours.

KEY POINTS TO REMEMBER

- *Neurocognitive disorder* is a term that refers to disorders resulting from changes in the brain and marked by disturbances in orientation, memory, intellect, judgement, and affect.
- Delirium and neurocognitive disorders are most frequently seen by health care workers.
- Delirium is marked by acute onset, disturbance in consciousness, and symptoms of disorientation and confusion that fluctuate by the minute, hour, or time of day.
- Delirium is always secondary to an underlying condition; therefore it is transient and may last from hours to days once the underlying cause is treated. If the cause is not treated, permanent damage to neurons can result.
- Signs and symptoms change according to the three stages of Alzheimer's disease: mild, moderate, and severe.

- Behavioural manifestations of Alzheimer's disease include confabulation, perseveration, aphasia, apraxia, agnosia, hyperorality, and sundowning.
- No known cause or cure exists for Alzheimer's disease, although a number of drugs that increase the brain's supply of acetylcholine (a nerve-communication chemical) or regulate glutamate are helpful in slowing the progress of the disease.
- People with Alzheimer's disease have many unmet needs and present numerous management challenges to both their families and health care workers.
- Specific nursing interventions for cognitively impaired individuals can increase communication, safety, and self-care and are described in the chapter. The need for family teaching and support is crucial.

CRITICAL THINKING

1. Mrs. Kendel is an 82-year-old woman who has Alzheimer's disease. She lives with her husband, who has been trying to care for her in their home. Mrs. Kendel is having trouble dressing. She has put her blouse on backwards and sometimes puts her bra on over her blouse. She often forgets where things are. She makes an effort to cook but has recently attempted to "put out" the electric burners of the stove with pitchers of water. Once in a while, she cannot find the bathroom in time, often mistaking a closet for it. At times, she cries because she is aware that she is losing her sense of place in the world. She and her husband have always been close, loving companions, and he wants to keep her at home for as long as possible.
   a. Assist Mr. Kendel by writing out a list of suggestions that he can try at home that might help with (a) communication,

   (b) activities of daily living, and (c) maintenance of a safe home environment.
   b. Identify at least three interventions that are appropriate to this situation for each of the problems Mrs. Kendel is having.
   c. Identify resources available for maintaining Mrs. Kendel in her home for as long as possible. Provide the name of a self-help group that you would urge Mr. Kendel to join.
2. Share with your class or clinical group the name and function of at least three community agencies in your area that could be an appropriate referral for a family with a member with dementia. (For one, you can contact the Alzheimer Society of Canada: http://www.alzheimer.ca).

CHAPTER REVIEW

1. A 73-year-old woman with pneumonia becomes agitated after being admitted to the intensive care unit through the emergency department. She continually tries to leave her bed despite being too weak to walk. Her vital signs are erratic, and her thinking seems disorganized. During her first 24 hours in ICU, the patient varies from somnolent to agitated, and from laughing to angry. Her daughter reports that the patient "was never like this at home." What is the most likely explanation for the situation?
   a. Pneumonia has worsened the patient's early-stage dementia.
   b. The patient is experiencing delirium secondary to the pneumonia.
   c. The patient is sundowning due to the decreased stimulation of the intensive care unit.
   d. The patient does not want to be in the hospital and is angry that staff will not let her leave.

2. Interventions appropriate for a hospitalized patient experiencing delirium include which of the following? Select all that apply.
   a. Immediately placing the patient in restraints if she begins to hallucinate or act in an irrational or unsafe manner
   b. Ensuring that a clock and a sign indicating the day and date is displayed where the patient can see it easily
   c. Being prepared for possible hostile responses to efforts to take vital signs or provide direct physical care
   d. Preventing sensory deprivation by placing the patient near the nurses' station and leaving the television and multiple lights turned on 24 hours per day
   e. Speaking with the patient frequently for short periods for reassurance, assisting the patient in remaining oriented, and ensuring the patient's safety
   f. Anticipating that the patient may try to leave if agitated, and providing a secure environment with direct observation to prevent wandering
   g. Promoting normalized sleep patterns by encouraging the patient to remain awake during the day and facilitating rest at night

3. Which statement about dementia is accurate?
   a. The majority of people over age 85 are affected by dementia.
   b. Disorientation is the dominant and most disruptive symptom of dementia.
   c. People with dementia tend to be distressed by it and complain about its symptoms.
   d. Hypertension, diminished activity levels, and head injury increase the risk for dementia.

4. Mrs. Smythe dies at the age of 82. In the 2 months following her death, her husband, age 84 and in good health, has begun to pay less attention to his hygiene and seems less aware of his surroundings. He complains of difficulty concentrating and sleeping and reports that he lacks energy. His family sometimes has to remind and encourage him to shower, take his medications, and eat, all of which he then does. Which response is most appropriate?
   a. Arrange for an appointment with a therapist for evaluation and treatment of suspected depression.
   b. Reorient Mr. Smythe by pointing out the day and date each time you interact with him.
   c. Meet with family and support persons to help them accept, anticipate, and prepare for the progression of his stage 2 dementia.

   d. Avoid touch and proximity, which are likely to be uncomfortable for Mr. Smythe and may provoke aggression when he is disoriented.

5. Which of the following interventions would be beneficial for those caring for a loved one with Alzheimer's disease? Select all that apply.
   a. Guide the family to restrict the patient's driving as soon as signs of forgetfulness are exhibited.
   b. Recommend switching to hospital-type gowns to facilitate bathing, dressing, and other physical care of the patient.
   c. Discourage wandering by installing complex locks or locks placed at the tops of doors, where the patient cannot readily reach them.
   d. For situations in which the patient becomes upset, teach loved ones to listen briefly, provide support, and then change the topic.
   e. Encourage caregivers to care for themselves, as well as the patient, via use of support resources such as adult day care or respite care.
   f. If the patient is prone to wander away, encourage family to notify police and neighbours of the patient's condition, wandering behaviour, and description.

evolve WEBSITE

Post-Test interactive review

Visit the Evolve website for Chapter Review Answers and Rationales, Critical Thinking Answer Guidelines, and additional resources related to the content in this chapter: http://evolve.elsevier.com/ Canada/Varcarolis/psychiatric/

REFERENCES

Alzheimer Society of Canada. (2011). *About Safely Home registry.* Retrieved from http://www.safelyhome.ca/en/safelyhome/aboutsafelyhome.asp.

Alzheimer's Association. (2014). Alzheimer's Association report: 2014 Alzheimer's disease facts and figures. *Alzheimer's and Dementia, 10,* e47–e92.

Alzheimer's Association. (2015). *FDA-approved treatments for Alzheimer's.* Retrieved from http://www.alz.org/dementia/downloads/topicsheet_treatments.pdf.

American Psychiatric Association (APA) (2013). *Diagnostic and statistical manual of mental disorders* (5th ed.). Washington, DC: Author.

Anand, A., & MacLullich, A. M. J. (2013). Delirium in hospitalized older adults. *Medicine, 41*(1), 39–42.

Ayalon, L., Gunn, A. M., Feliciano, L., et al. (2006). Effectiveness of nonpharmacological interventions for the management of neuropsychiatric symptoms in patients with dementia. *Archives of Internal Medicine, 166*(20), 2182–2188.

Buckley, J. S., & Salpeter, S. R. (2015). A risk–benefit assessment of dementia medications: Systematic review of the evidence. *Drugs and Aging, 32,* 453–467.

Bulechek, G. M., Butcher, H. K., & Dochterman, J. M. (2013). *Nursing interventions classification (NIC)* (6th ed.). Toronto: Elsevier.

Bulic, D., Bennett, M., & Shehabi, M. (2015). Delirium in the intensive care unit and long-term cognitive and psychosocial functioning: Literature review. *The Australian Journal of Advanced Nursing, 33*(1), 44–52. Retrieved from http://www.ajan.com.au/.

Canadian Institute for Health Information. (2010). *Caring for seniors with Alzheimer's disease and other forms of dementia: Describing outcome scales (RAI-HC).* Ottawa: Author.

Canadian Institute for Health Information. (2013). *Caring for seniors with Alzheimer's disease and other forms of dementia.* Ottawa: Author.

Caplan, J. P., Cassem, N. H., Murray, G. B., et al. (2016). Delirium. In T. A. Stern, M. Fava, T. E. Wilkens, et al. (Eds.), *Massachusetts General Hospital comprehensive clinical psychiatry* (pp. 173–183). St. Louis: Elsevier.

Clegg, A., Young, J., & Siddiqi, N. (2012). Delirium in cardiac patients: A clinical review. *British Journal of Cardiac Nursing, 7*(3), 111–115. Retrieved from http://www.cardiac-nursing.co.uk.

Forrester, L. T., Maayan, N., Orrell, M., et al. (2014). Aromatherapy for dementia. *The Cochrane Database of Systematic Reviews,* (2), CD003150, doi:10.1002/14651858.CD003150.pub2.

Inouye, S. K., Westendorp, R. G. J., & Saczynski, J. S. (2014). Delirium in elderly people. *Lancet, 383,* 911–922.

Lehne, R. A. (2013). *Pharmacology for nursing care* (8th ed.). St. Louis: Elsevier.

Liu, C., Kanekiyo, T., Xu, H., et al. (2013). Apolipoprotein E and Alzheimer disease: Risk, mechanisms, and therapy. *Nature Reviews. Neurology, 9*(2), 106–118. doi:10.1038/nrneurol.2012.263.

Moorhead, S., Johnson, M., Maas, M., et al. (2012). *Nursing outcomes classification (NOC)* (5th ed.). St. Louis: Mosby.

Nasreddine, Z., Phillips, N., Bedirian, V., et al. (2005). The Montreal Cognitive Assessment (MoCA): A brief screening tool for mild cognitive impairment. *Journal of the American Geriatrics Society, 53*(4), 695–699. Retrieved from http://onlinelibrary.wiley.com/journal/10.1111/ (ISSN)1532-5415.

Prince, M., Wimo, A., Guerchet, M., et al. (2015). *World Alzheimer report 2015: The global impact on dementia: An analysis of prevalence, in cadence, cost and trends.* London, UK: Alzheimer's Disease International.

Reston, J. T., & Schoelles, K. M. (2013). In-facility delirium prevention programs as a patient safety strategy: A systematic review. *Annals of Internal Medicine, 158,* 375–380.

van Munster, B. C., & de Rooij, S. E. (2014). Delirium: A synthesis of current knowledge. *Clinical Medicine, 14*(2), 192–195.

18

Psychoactive Substance Use and Treatment

Rick Csiernik

KEY TERMS AND CONCEPTS

addiction
alcohol poisoning
alcohol withdrawal
alcohol withdrawal delirium
Alcoholics Anonymous (AA)
blood alcohol level (BAL)
Cannabis sativa
collaboration
compulsive behaviour
concurrent disorder
consultation
contemplation
hallucinogen
harm reduction
inhalants
integrated use

integration
maintenance/adaption
misuse
motivational interviewing
mutual aid
neurotransmitter
opioid
physical dependency
precontemplation
preparation
psychological dependency
relapse prevention
tolerance
transtheoretical model of change
withdrawal

OBJECTIVES

1. Compare and contrast the terms *substance use, abuse, dependence*, and *addiction*.
2. Understand the significance of tolerance and withdrawal and their contribution to the process of physical dependency in creating an addiction.
3. Distinguish between addiction and a compulsive behaviour.
4. Discuss four components of the assessment process, including assessment of readiness for change, to be used with a person who is experiencing substance abuse.
5. Describe the signs of alcohol withdrawal, alcohol delirium, and alcohol poisoning.
6. Identify two short-term goals for a person who abuses alcohol in terms of (a) withdrawal, (b) active treatment, and (c) health maintenance.
7. Distinguish between the symptoms of opioid intoxication and those of opioid withdrawal.
8. Compare and contrast the signs and symptoms of intoxication, overdose, and withdrawal for cocaine and amphetamines.

9. Recognize signs of substance abuse or impaired practice in colleagues and the appropriate steps to take to assist.
10. Present and discuss the stages of the Transtheoretical Model of Change (TTM).
11. Explore the principles and practices of motivational interviewing as an evidence-informed intervention and an approach to communication for recovery.
12. Recognize the phenomenon of relapse as it affects people who abuse substances during different phases of treatment.
13. Evaluate four indications that a person is successfully recovering from substance abuse.
14. Identify the components of the addiction treatment continuum of care, including the various harm reduction options.
15. Identify different treatment approaches for patients with concurrent disorders.
16. Identify distinct treatment needs of Indigenous peoples.

⊖volve WEBSITE

Visit the Evolve website for Flashcards, Case Studies, and additional testing resources related to the content in this chapter: http://evolve.elsevier.com/Canada/Varcarolis/psychiatric/

Pre-Test   interactive review

Canada is a complex multicultural society whose citizens use a variety of psychoactive agents for various biological, psychological, and social purposes: to restore health, reduce pain and anxiety, increase energy, aid weight loss or gain, create a feeling of euphoria, take part in social customs and rituals, induce relaxation or sleep, and create community and intimacy. Most of us both personally and professionally have been affected by the use, misuse, abuse of, and addiction to psychoactive substances. The impact of drugs and also of compulsive behaviours is vast, affecting us not only individually but also on a family level, in the workplace, and as a society. This chapter begins by differentiating between an addiction and a compulsive behaviour and then explores the clinical trajectory and implications of

psychoactive substances, as well as the screening for addiction and the assessment of and nursing care for those experiencing addiction, including nurses themselves.

DISTINGUISHING BETWEEN AN ADDICTION AND A COMPULSIVE BEHAVIOUR

Psychoactive drugs are unique substances that alter the central nervous system (CNS), changing thought, mood, and behaviour. Chronic use leads to **psychological dependency**, which can range from a mild wish to a compelling emotional need for the periodic or continuous use of a drug. Psychological dependence occurs when a drug becomes so important to an individual's thoughts

---

✿ HOW A NURSE HELPED ME

Kari Cared Enough to Take Action

I was introduced to opioids years ago after an injury to my back in a work-related accident. All through my nursing education, I continued to use opioids to control the pain. Eventually, my need for more Dilaudid forced me to see doctors in different cities and towns. I didn't want my family or friends to know; but more importantly I didn't want my employer to know. When my own family doctor suggested going on methadone as a way to control my Dilaudid use and my pain, I willingly agreed. At first, the methadone seemed to be working, but my anxiety and fear about being found out caused nausea and vomiting. One day, I took an ampoule of Gravol 100 mg home from work. I was pleased with the effects; my anxiety abated [as did the nausea and vomiting]. I started carrying two or three ampoules of Gravol 100 mg in my uniform pocket (just in case I needed it at work). Each shift, I would restock my supply of Gravol. I knew how wrong this was, but the feeling of relief I got from the Gravol was profound.

One day, I mentioned this to the nurse at the methadone clinic. I thought by telling her, maybe they would increase my dose or the clinic doctor would prescribe something better.

The nurse, Kari, was kind, nonjudgemental, but very worried about my mixing of these two medications and working under the influence. The next day, Kari asked how much I had used the day before, my plan for stopping, and

solutions I had tried to diminish my anxiety at work. The next day, Kari invited me into her office at the clinic, where we discussed our nursing practice standards and her responsibility for reporting me to the professional nursing association. I think I was angry at first; the clinic is supposed to be confidential; my right to privacy and confidentiality was supposed to be first and foremost!

Then the next day, Kari asked what I had planned to do: was I going to report my using and pilfering of Gravol from my work, or did I want her to? I didn't realize until later how much relief I felt; no more avoiding. It was time to get more help. Thanks to Kari, I booked myself into an inpatient treatment program with the help of my family doctor. I went to my union and my association and told them what was happening. The association suspended my licence, as I knew they would, but because Kari cared enough about my patients—and me—to take action, the association accepted my plan of recovery. I can't begin to imagine my life had that one nurse not taken the initiative to put professional practice into my vision of recovery. My use affected not only myself and my family but my patients and my colleagues. I used to be ashamed and angry about my personal life at work, and my work life at home. Now my recovery is having a positive effect in all aspects of my life and the lives of my patients.

Source: Canadian Nurses Association. (2009). *Position statement: Problematic substance use by nurses.* Ottawa: Author.

and actions that the person believes that she or he cannot manage without the substance. Psychoactive drugs also affect the peripheral nervous system (PNS), creating changes to core biological functioning. Chronic substance use, except to hallucinogens, produces physical dependency, which is a physiological state of cellular adaptation that arises when the CNS and PNS become habituated to a psychoactive agent such that the person physically needs the drug to function or to avoid the physical pain of withdrawal. The use of psychoactive drugs also is affected by the social environment. The classic example of this arose out of the Vietnam War. A visit by an American congressman to Vietnam in 1971 on a fact-finding mission led to urine-screening of all troops to detect use of heroin prior to their redeployment to the United States. In one study, 75% of soldiers, most of whom were drafted and by the age of 21 were combat veterans, tested positive. Upon returning to the United States, only one third continued to use heroin, but of these individuals less than 10% were classified as dependent. Once they were removed from a constant life-threatening situation, there was no longer a need to use the drug. Thus a comprehensive conceptualization of addiction must include three elements: biological, psychological, and social (Figure 18-1) (Csiernik, 2016).

In contrast, compulsive behaviours do not have the biological element but only the psychological and social elements. This is not to diminish the severity of these issues, for they can have substantive impacts on individuals, families, and society, but they simply do not have direct biological risk and thus require distinct treatment approaches, treatment systems, and policies. Examples of compulsive behaviours that are labelled by some as addictive behaviours even in the academic literature are exercising, gaming, gambling, Internet use, pornography viewing, shopping, smartphone use, studying, and work. However, with these compulsive behaviours, there are no biological risks of withdrawal or overdose as would occur with a psychoactive substance. As well, food and sex, which certainly have distinct biological components, have been labelled as addictions by some in the popular and academic literature. The question to ask yourself as you review the remainder of the chapter—given the context of what an addiction entails—is should essential biological processes necessary for our continued survival as individuals, and as a species, be considered an addiction? If the primary addiction treatment protocol remains abstinence, then what are the implications if we label a person as being addicted to food or sex?

THE PROCESS OF ADDICTION DEVELOPMENT

The diagnosis of a substance-related disorder requires knowledge of the class of drug used, patterns of use, the severity of symptoms (mild, moderate, or severe), and the development of tolerance and withdrawal. Figure 18-2 highlights the process of addiction from experimentation to addiction.

No Contact

Prior to a person coming into contact with a psychoactive agent there is no use and thus no risk. In this stage, the individual does not use any psychoactive substances. Just as someone can be predisposed to substance use due to biological (genetic), psychological, or social factors, one's personal disposition or social environment may dissuade the use of certain substances or behaviours. There are many protective factors for not using drugs, including culture, family, other positive social supports, and faith, as well as fear of legal consequences.

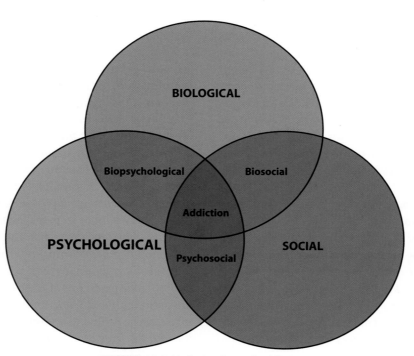

FIGURE 18-1 Holistic view of addiction.

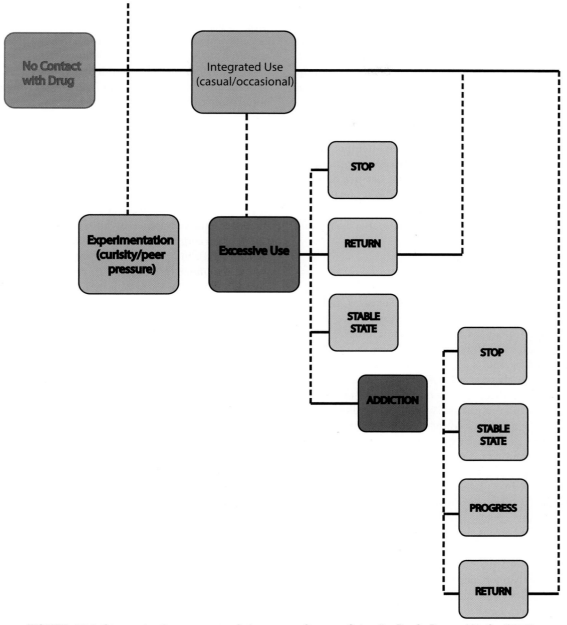

FIGURE 18-2 Stages in the process of drug use. Source: Csiernik, R., & Rowe, W. S. (2017). *Responding to the oppression of addiction.* Toronto: Canadian Scholars Press.

Experimentation

Individuals begin to experiment with drugs for a range of biological, psychological, or social reasons, such as to feel the effects of different substances; to fit in with peers; to reduce the anxiety of intimacy; and to escape from issues of stress, violence, trauma, and oppression.

Integrated Use

Some people may use a substance to enhance an already pleasurable and ongoing experience and therefore consider their use to be a social habit, integrated into their lives and not creating any biological, psychological, or social issues. This can include a glass of wine with dinner or using marijuana before attending a concert. This integrated use of a substance in a socially and culturally accepted manner has few negative consequences.

Excessive Use

The misuse or excessive use of a substance results in problems for users and often for those associated with them. People who misuse drugs may experience lapses in memory; experience conflict in their personal, school, or vocational relationships because of impairment; or engage in acts they would not consider when not under the influence of a psychoactive substance. Treatment intervention becomes appropriate when a person has reached this degree of psychoactive drug consumption.

Addiction

At the stage of addiction, a person has reached the state where they are physically and psychologically dependent. The person has lost the ability to choose to use, and the drug becomes the central organizing principle of the person's life. With regular use of a psychoactive substance, a person develops *tolerance*. Tolerance is a physiological experience that occurs when a person's reaction to a substance decreases with repeated administrations of the same dose. At this point, if the person attempts to stop using the substance, she or he may experience symptoms of withdrawal, which entails cravings for the substance of abuse that are accompanied by decreased physical and emotional health. Withdrawal also produces physiological changes as the blood and tissue concentrations of a drug decrease after heavy and prolonged use of a substance.

EPIDEMIOLOGY

The Canadian Tobacco, Alcohol and Drugs Survey (CTADS) is conducted every 2 years and examines the use of alcohol and illicit drugs among Canadians age 15 years and older. The rate of drug use by youth 15 to 19 years of age remains much higher than that reported by adults 25 years and older: nearly three times higher for cannabis use (22% versus 8%) and nearly five times higher for illicit drugs (5% versus 1%). The overall rate of psychoactive pharmaceutical use was 22% (6.4 million), with youth ages 15 to 19 using at a lower rate than adults 25 years and older (18% to 23%) and with prevalence among females (25%) greater than among males (19%). Of the three categories of pharmaceuticals, opioid pain relievers were the most commonly used in 2013, with 1 in 7 (15%, or 4.3 million) Canadians age 15 years and older reporting their use in the 12 months preceding the survey (Statistics Canada, 2015).

The prevalence of current cigarette smoking in 2015 was 13% (3.9 million smokers), a decrease from 15% (4.2 million smokers) in 2013 and the lowest national smoking rate ever recorded. More males (16%) than females (13%) indicated that they used tobacco products. Daily smokers consumed an average of 13.9 cigarettes per day, lower than the average cigarettes per day smoked in 2012 (15.0). Current smoking among youth ages 15 to 19 years was only 11%, while 15% of Canadians age 25 years and older were current tobacco smokers, with no statistical difference between males and females. CTADS also reported that the prevalence of past-year alcohol use for Canadians was 76%, representing 21.9 million people, with more men than women using this drug. The study also reported that 16% of Canadians age 15 years and older exceeded the quantity of alcohol consumption considered to be a chronic longer-term health risk, and 11% exceeded the quantity considered to be an acute health risk (alcohol poisoning) (Statistics Canada, 2015).

The group most affected by psychoactive drug use is Canada's Indigenous peoples. At the end of the twentieth century, the Royal Commission on Aboriginal Peoples (1996) concluded that alcoholism was the factor creating the greatest problem for Indigenous individuals and communities throughout Canada. Interestingly, Indigenous people's use of alcohol is below the national average, with only 66% of those living on reserves consuming alcohol. However, medical records from Western Canada indicate that Indigenous people, especially men, are admitted to hospitals for problems with substance use more often than other residents within these provinces. The incidence of death due to alcohol use is 43.7 per 100 000 in the Indigenous population of Canada, almost twice the rate in the general population, which is 23.6 per 100 000. This suggests that those who do drink, drink heavily, consuming five or more drinks on one occasion on a regular basis (Khan, 2008). In Indigenous communities, preadolescent youths are two to six times more likely to have already been exposed to alcohol-related problems compared to their non-Indigenous peers (Cotton & Laventure, 2013). Indigenous people who use illicit drugs have a higher incidence and prevalence of human immunodeficiency virus (HIV) when compared to their non-Indigenous drug-using peers (Khan, 2008). Indigenous street youth and female sex workers were also found to have higher HIV prevalence (Duncan, Reading, Borwein, et al., 2011). Also, 1 in 5 Indigenous youth reported having used solvents; of these, 1 in 3 were under the age of 15, with half beginning with sniffing or huffing before the age of 11. Cannabis is also commonly used among both Indigenous adults (27%) and youth (32%) (Aboriginal Healing Foundation, 2007).

COMORBIDITY

Psychiatric Comorbidity

The complex combination of both substance abuse and a mental health condition is referred to as a concurrent disorder. More than 50% of those engaged in treatment for substance use are also struggling with mental illness, and 15% to 20% of those engaged in treatment for mental illness are struggling with addiction. The prevalence of concurrent disorders among those hospitalized for psychiatric concerns in Canada in 2010–2011 was 35.6%. The age group with the greatest percentage of concurrent issues was 25 to 44 year olds (43.0%), followed by 45 to 64 year olds (26.0%), 15 to 24 year olds (22.6%), those 65 years and older (7.0%), and finally 0 to 14 year olds (1.3%). Up to 25% of all Canadians will have an anxiety disorder at some point in their lives, and of these 24% will also have a substance use disorder. The prevalence rate in 2009–2010 of those admitted to a general hospital with anxiety disorder and co-occurring substance use disorder was 4.6%, increasing to 5.5% of those admitted to a psychiatric facility. Major depression will affect 15% to 20% of all Canadians, and among them 27% will also have a substance use disorder. While only a small number of people suffer from bipolar disorders (1% to 2% of the population), of those 56% will also have a substance use disorder. Likewise, only 1% of the population has schizophrenia, yet 47% of these individuals will have a substance use disorder (Canadian Institute for Health Information (CIHI), 2012, 2013; Skinner, O'Grady, Bartha, et al., 2004). Compared with patients who have a single disorder, patients with concurrent disorders often require longer treatment, experience more crises, and progress more gradually in treatment. Among the challenges of meeting the needs of people with concurrent disorders are poorly integrated services that lack attention to cultural or community concerns (Wesley-Esquimaux & Snowball, 2010).

Medical Comorbidity

Alcohol abuse is the most prevalent of the substance abuse disorders. Therefore alcohol-related medical problems are the comorbidities most commonly seen in medical settings. Alcohol can affect all organ systems, in particular the CNS, resulting in disorders such as Wernicke's encephalopathy and Korsakoff's syndrome when there is chronic use. Wernicke's (alcoholic) encephalopathy is an acute and reversible condition, whereas Korsakoff's syndrome is a chronic condition with a recovery rate of only about 20%. The pathophysiological connection between the two problems is a thiamine deficiency, which may be caused by poor nutrition associated with alcohol use or by the malabsorption of nutrients. Wernicke's encephalopathy is characterized by altered gait, vestibular dysfunction, confusion, and several ocular motility abnormalities (horizontal nystagmus, lateral orbital palsy, and gaze palsy). These eye-focused signs are bilateral but not necessarily symmetrical. Sluggish reaction to light and anisocoria (unequal pupil size) are also symptoms. Wernicke's encephalopathy may clear up within a few weeks or may progress into Korsakoff's syndrome, the more severe and chronic version of this problem.

Wernicke's encephalopathy responds rapidly to large doses of intravenous thiamine two to three times daily for 1 to 2 weeks. Treatment of Korsakoff's syndrome is also thiamine for 3 to 12 months. Most patients with Korsakoff's syndrome never fully recover, although cognitive improvement may occur with thiamine and nutritional support.

Chronic alcohol use also produces esophagitis, gastritis, pancreatitis, alcoholic hepatitis, and cirrhosis of the liver and is associated with tuberculosis, cancer, all types of accidents, suicide, and homicide. Alcohol use during pregnancy can have negative consequences for the fetus and result in fetal alcohol spectrum disorder (FASD), which is a lifelong issue affecting cognitive ability.

FASD is a collective term rather than a diagnostic category and includes fetal alcohol syndrome (FAS), alcohol-related neurodevelopmental disorder (ARND), and partial FAS [pFAS]. FASD is the leading cause of developmental disability, affecting 9 out of every 1 000 Canadian infants, although there is a much greater incidence within Indigenous communities. FASD, along with prenatal alcohol exposure (PAE), affects each child differently, though there are commonalities within different diagnostic categories. As alcohol freely moves across the placenta from mother to child, the risks created for the unborn child increase the more a pregnant woman drinks, although at this time no safe level of drinking has been established. Primary disabilities from FASD include impairments in attention, verbal learning, and executive functioning and are the direct result of damage to the brain caused by PAE. It has also been linked to increased risk for childhood leukemia. Secondary disabilities are deficits not evident at birth that arise from primary disabilities and interaction with the environment such as mental health and addiction issues; being in conflict with the law; and education, employment, and family relationship difficulties. Drinking alcohol during pregnancy may lead to cognitive impairment; heart, face,

joint, and limb abnormalities; lower birth weight; and hyperactivity with shorter attention spans, poor self-concept, depression, and aggression. The disabilities created by FASD are not minimized with time and continue to create difficulties and marginalize individuals throughout their adult lives (Burnside & Fuchs, 2013; Latino-Martel, Chan, Druesne-Pecollo, et al., 2010; Rutman & Van Bibber, 2010).

For people who use drugs, the route of drug administration influences the possible comorbid medical complications. Those who use intravenous drugs have a higher incidence of infections and associated problems from infection, including hepatitis and HIV, cellulitis, and sclerosing of veins. Those who use intranasal substances may be prone to sinusitis and perforated nasal septum. Smoking substances increases the likelihood of respiratory problems and saliva or airborne infections if sharing pipes or cigarettes. Table 18-1 lists physical complications associated with various classes of drugs and their routes of administration.

TABLE 18-1	PHYSICAL COMPLICATIONS RELATED TO PSYCHOACTIVE SUBSTANCES BY METHOD OF ADMINISTRATION	
SAMPLE SUBSTANCE	**ROUTE**	**PHYSICAL COMPLICATIONS**
Marijuana	Inhalation	Impaired lung structure
		Micronucleic white blood cells—increased risk for disease due to decreased resistance to infection
		Possible long-term effects on short-term memory
Nicotine	Inhalation	Cancer of the larynx and esophagus
		Cancer of the mouth
		Cardiovascular disease
		Emphysema
		Hypertension
Cocaine hydrochloride	Intranasal (mucous membrane)	Cardiovascular collapse
		Hyperpyrexia
		Perforation of nasal septum
		Respiratory paralysis
Heroin	Intravenous injection	Abscesses—osteomyelitis
		Bacterial endocarditis
		Cardiac arrest
		Dermatitis
		Hepatitis
		Human immunodeficiency virus (HIV)
		Pulmonary emboli
		Renal failure
		Respiratory arrest
		Seizures
		Septicemia
		Tetanus
Caffeine	Oral	Gastroesophageal reflux
		Increased intraocular pressure in unregulated glaucoma
		Increased plasma glucose and lipid levels
		Peptic ulcer
		Tachycardia

ETIOLOGY

Substance use disorders are characterized by use, abuse, and physical and psychological dependence and also by certain patterns of behaviour: (1) loss of control of substance consumption, (2) continued substance use despite associated problems, and (3) cravings and a tendency to relapse after efforts to change behaviour. The reason a person may experience a substance use disorder relates to the intersection of biological, psychological, and social factors.

Biological Factors

During the past two decades, neurobiological studies of addiction have undergone tremendous development and have yielded enormous amounts of valuable information about neuronal response mechanisms and their adaptive changes through an array of techniques ranging from in vitro molecular methods to brain imaging procedures in conscious subjects actively performing a range of behavioural tasks. This research has demonstrated that brain structures do change over time due to exposure to psychoactive drugs until they reach a threshold, at which point the primary symptom of dependence occurs, making it difficult to stop excessive drug use without professional assistance. The brain continually attempts to keep the body at or return the body to a point of balance or homeostasis, and in doing so it will adapt to the prolonged or excessive presence of drugs by making changes in brain cells and neural pathways. When people administer a psychoactive drug, it activates the same reinforcement system in the brain that is normally activated by food, water, and sex, sometimes to a lesser extent but sometimes to a far greater extent. Biological theories have examined the role of the limbic system, particularly the amygdala, the part of the brain responsible for emotions such as fear and anxiety, as being crucial to this process, and the effect of reinforcement of dopamine receptors in the mesolimbic system that originate in the ventral tegmental area (VTA) and terminate in the nucleus accumbens. All of these reinforcers share one physiological effect, and that is increased amounts of dopamine being released in the brain either directly or indirectly through other neurotransmitters being activated. During this process, prominent physical changes occur in areas of the brain that are critical to judgement, decision making, learning and memory, and behavioural control. Neurobiological research focuses on four primary areas:

- Drug actions on intracellular signalling systems that mediate cell responses
- Synaptic plasticity in the course of chronic drug exposure
- The role of dopaminergic and other components of the human reward system
- Genetic factors that will be examined as a distinct theoretical construct (Csiernik, 2016)

Regardless of which neurobiological theory you favour, scientists now know that psychoactive drugs affect specific neurotransmitters and areas of the brain. Neurotransmitters are chemical signalling molecules in the brain that are used to relay, amplify, and modulate signals between neurons and can be grouped into three categories:

- Monoamines, including acetylcholine, norepinephrine, dopamine, histamine, and serotonin
- Peptides and hormones, including endorphins, cortisone, and nitric oxide
- Amino acids, including gamma-aminobutyric acid (GABA) and glutamate (Inaba & Cohen, 2014).

All of the approximately 100 identified neurotransmitters that carry chemical information between cells follow the same chemical transmission pathway. However, they can act in different ways on this pathway. First, a neurotransmitter is released from the sending neuron into the synaptic cleft from a storage vesicle located in the axon terminal. The neurotransmitter then diffuses (travels) across the synaptic cleft. On the receiving neuron, there are specialized receptor areas that are designed to receive one type of neurotransmitter and bind with it. As more and more binding occurs, an electrical signal begins to form in the receiving neuron, and when a sufficient amount of the neurotransmitter is bound, an internal electrical charge is generated and the message is sent forward, following the same pattern of transmission. Once the charge is generated, the neurotransmitter may be broken down by enzymes in the cleft and thus deactivated or actively transported back to its point of origin, the axon terminal of the sending neuron (Figure 18-3).

The chemical structure of many psychoactive drugs is similar to that of neurotransmitters. Similarity in structure allows them to be recognized by neurons and to alter normal brain messaging. This leads to five distinct chemical processes that influence the CNS and change behaviour, which are termed pharmacodynamic interactions:

- Blocking the reuptake of a neurotransmitter back into the axon terminal, allowing more of the neurotransmitter to be available for binding, thus enhancing the message (cocaine)
- Pushing more neurotransmitters out of the storage vesicles into the synaptic cleft, increasing the opportunity for binding and thus enhancing the message (amphetamines)
- Enhancing the binding to the neurotransmitters to further enhance binding to the receptor site to enhance the message (diazepam)

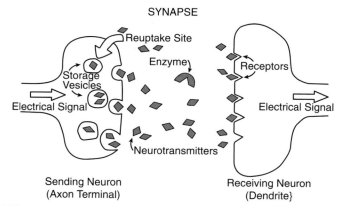

FIGURE 18-3 Chemical transmission between cells. Source: Sproule, B. (2004). *Pharmacology and drug abuse* (2nd ed). Toronto: Centre for Addiction and Mental Health.

- Blocking the enzyme from breaking down the drug in the synaptic cleft, allowing more neurotransmitters to bind to their receptors to enhance the message (monoamine oxidase inhibitors [MAOIs], which are antidepressants, such as phenelzine [Nardil] and tranylcypromine [Parnate])
- Mimicking neurotransmitters and binding directly to receptor sites, but not allowing a message to be transmitted (naloxone).

The main systems that seem to be involved in substance abuse are the endorphin, catecholamine (especially dopamine), serotonin, endocannabinoid, and GABA systems. Cocaine, amphetamines, and lesser stimulants increase levels of nor-epinephrine, serotonin, and dopamine. Opioid drugs act on endorphin receptors with a secondary effect on dopamine. Alcohol and other CNS depressants will act on GABA receptors and, as a result, increase the bioavailability of glutamate, norepi-nephrine, and dopamine. Hallucinogens act to varying degrees on serotonin, whereas marijuana acts on endocannabinoids (Csiernik, 2014).

Psychological Factors

Among the earliest investigations into why people became addicted to substances were learning theories that studied stimuli that give pleasure, relief, or excitement and how reliably and quickly these effects could be produced. Fundamental to this perspective is the belief that people will repeat any behaviour that brings them some kind of pleasure or reward and will discontinue any behaviour that brings them discomfort or punishment. If a drug brings pleasure or relief in a stressful situation, reduces anxiety or fear, or provides status or popularity in an insecure or lonely situation, its use will become a repeated behaviour. Tolerance is also an important process and is associated with habituation. Habituation is seen through reduced responses to a drug either because of prior exposure to the substance or because of the presentation of environmental stimuli that in the past have reliably predicted the presence of the drug. Under specific circumstances, persons who are dependent on opioids have been observed to respond to the mere anticipation of drug effects—to an injection of saline or to an opioid injected while an antagonist is present—as if they had actually administered the drug. Extinction also plays a role and is the process whereby the link between the previously established behaviours of drug seeking and drug using is weakened until a point is reached when the behaviour no longer has any reinforcing benefit or purpose. This is what the treatment process attempts to accomplish in terminating an individual's misuse or abuse of a substance.

Another prominent psychological theory is personality theory. Human personality traits have been grouped into five categories: extraversion, agreeableness, conscientiousness, emotional stability and openness to experience. Of these five, it is the extraversion trait that has been most closely associated with excessive substance use, particularly the attribute of impulsivity. However, the idea of a person having an alcoholic personality had been extremely popular well before the development of the five personality dimensions and contributed to the rise in the popularity of personality tests for those with addiction issues in the mid-twentieth century. The literature generally sides with the view that personality does not predict illness, with research continuing in this area and attempting to determine if those with certain personality characteristics become drug abusers or if drug use creates a specific type of personality.

A third long-established psychological perspective on addiction is based in psychodynamic theory. This view arises from the early work of Freud, although Freud, himself, did not devote much attention to addiction in his extensive writings, despite his own drug dependency to tobacco and cocaine. From this perspective, there are three potential explanations for all mal-adaptive behaviour:
- Seeking sensuous satisfaction
- Conflicts among the components of the self
- Fixation in the infantile past

Freud stated that alcoholism may be due to the inability to successfully resolve issues among the three components of the self: the id or instinctual striving for at times pleasure and at other times pain relief, the superego or conscience, and the ego or coping component of the person. Failure of the ego to resolve issues between conscience and basic instincts can lead to maladaptive coping responses, including use of psychoactive drugs.

A fourth perspective is attachment theory, which focuses on long-term emotional bonds. The core idea of attachment theory is that primary caregivers who are available and responsive to an infant's needs allow the child to develop a sense of security, which some label as love, enabling the child to explore his or her environment in a confident manner, knowing that he or she is protected. Children who are securely attached as infants tend to develop stronger self-esteem and are more sociable and self-reliant as they grow older. They generally becoming independent and have good school performance, which establishes a foundation for successful adulthood interactions. Individuals who are more securely attached in childhood tend to have good self-esteem, positive romantic relationships, and the ability to self-disclose to others. Attachment theory views addiction as an attempt to fill the empty space left by the lack of a secure attachment due to deprivation during childhood, including painful, rejecting, or shaming relationships. Excessive drug use, then, is seen as an individual's attempt to self-repair psychological deficits and fill an emptiness from childhood (Csiernik, 2016).

Sociocultural Factors

Culture is a set of thoughts shared by members of a social unit that include common understandings, patterns of beliefs, and expectations. Cultural guidelines are generally unwritten rules of conduct and direction for acceptable behaviours and actions that reflect the morals, norms, and values of a specific group. Cultural theory begins with this premise in attempting to describe and explain the process of drug use in relation to societal norms. Sociocultural factors express the social relationships, politics, and environments beyond individual psychological environments, and thus sociocultural theories attempt to explain differences in the incidence of substance use in various groups. Sociocultural theorists support the demystification of substance use and the study of drugs within an integrated life model. As early as 1943, Horton asserted that the primary function of alcohol in a culture was to reduce anxiety. Thus substance abuse would be more prevalent in societies in which anxiety abounds and few alternatives to drinking alcohol and using drugs as tension-releasers exist. These societies would also exhibit the highest rates of intoxication. Culture influences alcohol and other socially accepted psychoactive drug use in three distinct ways:

- By the degree to which they operate to bring about acute need for adjustment of inner tensions such as guilt, suppression, aggression, conflict, and sexual tension in their members
- By the attitudes toward drinking that they produce in the members seen in information exchange, including advertising
- By the degree to which the culture provides substitute means of satisfaction beyond substance use in the form of positive alternative lifestyle options

Using alcohol as an example, four prominent cultural patterns of drug use can be observed:

1. Abstinent cultures in which the overall attitude toward drugs, including alcohol, is negative and all alcoholic beverages are forbidden. An example is Saudi Arabia.
2. Ambivalent cultures in which the attitude toward alcohol use is positive in social settings but negative in others. The African nation of Morocco is an example of this cultural pattern. Morocco is a democratic Islamic nation that has a parliament but where the hereditary king's decisions supersede those of parliament. Islam forbids the drinking of alcohol; however, it is widely available throughout the nation.
3. Permissive cultures in which using alcoholic beverages is acceptable, although a negative attitude toward drunkenness remains. An example is Canada.
4. Ultra-permissive cultures in which the attitude is permissive toward both drinking and alcohol-related problems. This last model is most likely to be observed in a culture that is experiencing rapid social change, especially where there is a heavy economic interest in alcohol production and distribution. An example is Russia after the end of communism.

Cultures tend to have lower rates of drug use when the rules governing the use of substances are clear, uniform, and prohibitive and specific social sanctions are associated with use. Lower rates are also more prevalent when members of the culture are exposed to the drug at an early stage and observe adults using it in moderate amounts in settings that discourage the use of the drug as an intoxicant, such as at meals or during religious ceremonies. Sociocultural theories also examine the role of media in the development of drug use, misuse, and addiction. Marketing cues also influence the paths that individuals take both toward becoming addicted and moving away from maladaptive consumption and addiction.

APPLICATION OF THE NURSING PROCESS

ASSESSMENT

Assessment of Substance Use and Substance-Induced Disorders

Assessment of chemical impairment, substance use, abuse, dependence, tolerance, and withdrawal is becoming more complex because of the increase in polydrug abuse, co-occurring psychiatric disorders, and comorbid physical illnesses, including HIV infection, dementia, and encephalopathy. Also, changes in the diagnostic criteria for substance use and substance-induced disorders lead to changes in practice. Depending on the context of the assessment, acute care, intensive care unit, community clinic, or street engaged, different practice guidelines need to be considered. Regardless of the setting, the assessment of safety of the patient and others is always the priority.

Sensitivity to cultural and contextual concerns of patients and families is also important in assessing, interpreting symptoms, making diagnoses, providing clinical care, and designing prevention strategies (see Chapter 8). Steps to follow in assessment include (1) level of acute intoxication, (2) history and past substance use, (3) medical history, (4) psychiatric history, and (5) psychosocial assessment. General nursing assessment can be augmented with specific substance use assessment and addiction screening, family assessment, and assessment of readiness for change in preparation for interventions (Box 18-1).

Assessment of Acute Intoxication and Active and Historical Substance Use

Acute intoxication and history of substance use are important aspects of assessment. Although acute intoxication may or may not be obvious, it is crucial for intoxication to be ascertained to ensure an accurate clinical picture and to prevent possible drug interactions or misdiagnoses. Intracranial hematomas, subdural hematomas, and other conditions can go unnoticed if symptoms of acute alcohol intoxication and withdrawal are not distinguished from the symptoms of a brain injury. Therefore neurological signs such as pupil size, equality, and reaction to light need to be assessed, especially in comatose patients suspected of having traumatic injuries. In addition, questions about alcohol abuse should be asked as part of the assessment of any trauma. **Blood alcohol level (BAL)**, a measurement of the percentage of alcohol in the bloodstream, tested through urinalysis and breath screening devices, can be useful for acute assessment purposes.

Assessment strategies must include collection of data pertaining to both patterns of substance use and psychiatric impairment. Unexplained exacerbations of psychiatric disorders may be due to acute substance abuse or to dependence. Substance abuse can go undetected in patients with depression, anxiety, mania, or suicidal ideation unless a thorough history is taken. Similarly, the understanding and treatment of people with substance use disorders are enhanced by inquiries about symptoms of depression and anxiety.

Once specific data are obtained, it is helpful to know whether the person is abusing or is actively dependent on the substance and the severity of symptoms from mild to severe as assessed by the symptoms present. In addition to an overall assessment interview, any number of more focused rudimentary screening tools may also be used. One measure for assessing alcohol abuse is the Michigan Alcoholism Screening Test (MAST). The MAST, validated for use with many populations, is a 25-point questionnaire designed to provide a rapid and effective screening for lifetime alcohol-related problems and alcoholism (Selzer, 1971; Teitelbaum & Mullen, 2000). Another popular tool is the CAGE

BOX 18-1 KEY AREAS FOR COMPREHENSIVE ASSESSMENT

Client's Goals
- Reasons for seeking care
- Immediate and long-term goals related to health care concerns, including both physical and mental health
- Perceived obstacles to and supports in achieving current goals
- Discussion of the impact of the client's substance use goals on his or her other health care goals
- Client's values and beliefs about the best outcome for himself or herself
- Readiness and stage of change regarding substance use

Demographic and Socioeconomic Information
- Age
- Gender: sexual orientation, gender identity, gender expression
- Cultural and ethnic background
- Education, employment, income
- Housing
- Relationships
- Legal: past or current involvement with the justice system
- Circle-of-care supports: health care providers, family, and other social supports
- Cultural and diversity needs
- Spirituality

Substance Use History
- Substances used by client
- Age of first use of each substance
- Pattern of use, including amount, frequency, duration of use, and historic use looking for issues of tolerance
- Route of substance use: intravenous (IV), intramuscular (IM), subcutaneous (SC), inhalation, via mucous membrane, oral, transdermal
- Withdrawal symptoms associated with substance use
- Tolerance to substances
- Substances of concern, as identified by the client
- Access and use of harm reduction strategies, including safer drug use education and supplies, or supplies as required in each individual case, including but not limited to clean needles
- Triggers of substance use
- Adverse consequences related to use
- Increasing loss of control over use
- Periods of abstinence and factors that supported abstinence
- Past history of seeking help for substance use
- Paradoxical effects to substances

Physical Health History and Medical Conditions
- Diagnosed health conditions past and present
- Medication: past and current, including over-the-counter medications and alternative or complementary medications

- Interventions and procedures
- Experiences with interventions and services
- Chronic pain
- History of seizures
- Dental issues
- Sexually transmitted infections

Potential Infections Resulting From IV Drug Use
- Localized and systemic infections or abscesses
- Cellulitis
- Human immunodeficiency virus (HIV)
- Hepatitis B
- Hepatitis C
- Infective endocarditis
- Osteomyelitis

Mental Health History
- History of mental health problems
- Current mental health concerns
- Current and past interventions for mental health problems, both pharmacological and nonpharmacological
- Experiences with interventions and services for mental health problems
- Trauma: emotional, physical, psychological, and sexual
- History of self-harm
- Suicide attempts or thoughts of suicide
- Feelings of anxiety or depression
- Current ability to cope with emotions
- Resilience and hopefulness

Family History of Substance Use and Mental Health Concerns
- Information about relatives who have or have had issues due to substance use or a substance use disorder, and how they have managed, including use of different medications and therapies and current health status
- Information about relatives who have or have had mental health concerns, and how they have managed, including use of different medications and therapies and current health status

Resilience and Strengths
- Client-identified personal strengths and sources of resilience
- Client-identified needs and supports to enhance resilience and strengths

Sources: American Psychiatric Association (APA). (2006). *Practice guideline for the treatment of patients with substance use disorders* (2nd ed.). Retrieved from http://psychiatryonline.org/pb/assets/raw/sitewide/practice_guidelines/guidelines/substanceuse.pdf; Substance Abuse and Mental Health Services Administration (SAMHSA). (2005). *Substance abuse treatment for persons with co-occurring disorders.* Retrieved from http://www.ncbi.nlm.nih.gov/books/NBK64197/pdf/TOC.pdf; and Registered Nurses' Association of Ontario. (2015). *Engaging clients who use substances* (pp. 35–36). Toronto: Author.

questionnaire (Ewing, 1984). The four questions to be asked in the screening process are remembered by the mnemonic *CAGE*:

1. Have you felt you ought to *Cut* down on your drinking, substance use, or behaviour?
2. Have people *Annoyed* you by criticizing your drinking, substance use, or behaviour?
3. Have you felt *Guilty* about your drinking, substance use, or behaviour?
4. Have you had a drink (or used another substance or behaviour) first thing in the morning to steady your nerves or get yourself going for the day (an *Eye-opener*)?

Each question with an answer of yes scores 1 point, and the higher the score, the greater the problems with the substance or behaviour. A score of 2 or more is considered clinically significant.

If the patient is not able to respond to questions or provide a description of current or historical substance use, the nurse should assess for observable indications of substance abuse, such as dilated or constricted pupils, abnormal vital signs, needle marks, tremors, or alcohol on the breath, and obtain information from family and friends. A patient's clothing and belongings, if he or she is admitted to a health care or addictions services clinic, may also be screened or searched for drug paraphernalia, such as used syringes, crack vials, white powder, razor blades, bent spoons, and pipes.

Signs of Intoxication and Withdrawal

Each class of drugs has its own physiological signs and symptoms of intoxication, which are summarized in the tables for each substance class. Both intoxication and withdrawal may require observation and medical attention or nursing care and can constitute psychiatric emergencies.

 ASSESSMENT GUIDELINES

Acute Chemical Impairment

1. Assess for a severe or major withdrawal syndrome.
2. Assess for an overdose of a drug or alcohol that warrants immediate medical attention.
3. Assess the patient for suicidal thoughts or other self-harming behaviours.
4. Evaluate the patient for any physical complications related to drug abuse.
5. Explore the patient's interests in doing something about his or her drug or alcohol problem.
6. Assess the patient's and family's knowledge of community resources for alcohol and drug treatment.

Central Nervous System Depressants

CNS depressant drugs include alcohol and sedative hypnotics, benzodiazepines, and barbiturates. Symptoms of intoxication, overdose, and withdrawal and possible treatments are presented in Table 18-2.

Withdrawal reactions from alcohol and other CNS depressants are the most problematic and are associated with severe morbidity and mortality, unlike withdrawal from other psychoactive agents (Csiernik, 2014). The syndrome for alcohol withdrawal is the same as that for the entire class of CNS depressant drugs; therefore alcohol is used in this discussion as the prototype. Alcohol withdrawal, if uncomplicated, is typically complete within 5 to 7 days. Symptoms of withdrawal, however, continue for a longer period and are more severe for older than younger patients; as well, psychological craving can last for months and even years.

TABLE 18-2	CENTRAL NERVOUS SYSTEM DEPRESSANTS				
DRUGS	**SIGNS OF INTOXICATION**	**EFFECTS OF OVERDOSE**	**POSSIBLE TREATMENTS FOR OVERDOSE**	**EFFECTS OF WITHDRAWAL**	**POSSIBLE TREATMENTS FOR WITHDRAWAL**
Barbiturates Benzodiazepines Chloral hydrate Glutethimide Meprobamate Alcohol	*Physical:* Slurred speech Incoordination Unsteady gait Drowsiness Decreased blood pressure *Psychological–perceptual:* Disinhibition of sexual or aggressive drives Impaired judgement Impaired social or occupational function Impaired attention or memory Irritability	Cardiovascular or respiratory depression or arrest (mostly with barbiturates) Coma Shock Convulsions Death	Monitor vital signs every 15 minutes. Monitor for respiratory depression. Oxygen, intubation, or mechanical ventilation may be prescribed. If recent ingestion, induced vomiting, gastric lavage, or activated charcoal may be prescribed. Monitor ECG and lab values for shock. Intravenous (IV) fluids may be prescribed. Continue monitoring VS frequently for respiratory complications, cardiac arrest, and possible seizures.	*Cessation of prolonged or heavy use:* Nausea and vomiting Tachycardia Diaphoresis Anxiety or irritability Tremors in hands, fingers, eyelids Marked insomnia Grand mal seizures *After 5–15 years of heavy use:* Delirium	The physician may prescribe a carefully titrated drug in a similar classification so as to minimize symptoms of withdrawal. *Note:* Abrupt withdrawal can lead to death.

ECG, Electrocardiogram; *VS,* vital signs.

Source: Rowe, B., Lang, E. S., Brown, M. D., et al. (2009). *Evidence-based emergency medicine* (Vol. 63). Oxford, UK: Wiley-Blackwell.

Withdrawal may be delayed, however, when another CNS depressant is the main drug of choice or when the patient is withdrawing from a combination of alcohol and other CNS depressants. Multiple drug and alcohol dependencies can result in simultaneous withdrawal syndromes that present a complicated clinical picture among polydrug users and may pose additional problems for safe withdrawal.

Several CNS depressants have become associated with facilitating sexual assaults. These include the benzodiazepine flunitrazepam (Rohypnol, or "roofies) and the solvent gamma-hydroxybutyric acid (GHB) and its congeners. These drugs are odourless, tasteless, and colourless; mix easily with alcoholic drinks; and can render a person unconscious in a matter of minutes due to the pharmacodynamic interaction of two CNS depressants. Perpetrators use these drugs in combination with alcohol because they rapidly produce disinhibition and relaxation of voluntary muscles; they also cause the victim to have lasting anterograde amnesia for events that occur (see also Chapter 26).

Alcohol poisoning. Alcohol poisoning is a state of toxicity that can result when an individual has consumed large amounts of alcohol either quickly or over time. It can produce death from aspiration of emesis or a shutdown of body systems due to severe CNS depression. Signs of alcohol poisoning include an inability to rouse the individual, severe dehydration, cool or clammy skin, respirations less than 10 per minute, cyanosis of the gums or under the fingernails, and emesis while semiconscious or unconscious. Refer to Table 18-2 for important assessment and treatment information regarding alcohol intoxication and poisoning.

Alcohol withdrawal. The early signs of alcohol withdrawal, a physical reaction to the cessation or reduction of alcohol (ethanol) intake, can develop within a few hours of the last intake. Symptoms peak after 24 to 48 hours and then rapidly and dramatically disappear unless the withdrawal progresses to *alcohol withdrawal delirium.* Severity of withdrawal tends to be dose related, with heavier drinkers experiencing more severe symptoms. Withdrawal severity is also related to age, with those over 65 years of age experiencing more severe symptoms. During withdrawal, the patient may appear hyperalert, manifest jerky movements and irritability, startle easily, and experience subjective distress often described as "shaking inside." Grand mal seizures may appear

7 to 48 hours after cessation of alcohol intake, particularly in people with a history of seizures. Careful assessment, including this history and any other risk factors, followed by appropriate medical and nursing interventions can prevent the more serious withdrawal reaction of delirium.

A competent, supportive manner on the part of the nurse can allay anxiety and provide a sense of security. Consistently and frequently orienting the patient to time and place may be necessary. Encouraging family or close friends, one at a time, to remain with the patient in quiet surroundings can also help to increase orientation and minimize confusion and anxiety.

During withdrawal, some patients may experience illusions, which can be both disorientating and terrifying. Illusions are misinterpretations, usually of a threatening nature, of objects in the environment due to excess activation of the CNS by the drug. For example, a person may think that spots on the wallpaper are blood-sucking ants. However, illusions can be clarified to reduce the patient's terror: "See, they are not ants; they are just part of the wallpaper pattern." Some patients withdrawing from alcohol may be argumentative, hostile, or demanding due to the difficult physical experiences but also because of deep-seated anxiety. The nurse can relieve some of these feelings by demonstrating a nonjudgemental attitude, positive affect, and strong support for efforts at recovery. The Clinical Institute Withdrawal Assessment for Alcohol (CIWA-Ar) provides an efficient, objective means of assessing alcohol withdrawal to prevent under- or overtreating patients with benzodiazepines (Table 18-3).

Alcohol intoxication. Alcohol is the only drug for which exact objective measures of intoxication (BAL) currently exist. The relationship between BAL and behaviour in a nontolerant individual is illustrated in Table 18-4. Assessing the patient's behaviour can assist the nurse in (1) ascertaining whether the person accurately reported recent drinking and (2) determining level of intoxication and possible tolerance, as patient behaviours may indicate greater or lesser levels of tolerance. As tolerance develops, a discrepancy is seen between the BAL and expected behaviour: a person with tolerance to alcohol may have a high BAL but minimal signs of impairment. Alternatively, a person who is highly sensitive to alcohol or compromised medically may have a low BAL but demonstrate a high level of intoxication.

TABLE 18-3 CLINICAL INSTITUTE WITHDRAWAL ASSESSMENT FOR ALCOHOL (CIWA-AR)

Nausea/Vomiting		**Tremor**	
Ask "Do you feel sick to your stomach? Have you vomited?"		Arms extended and fingers spread apart.	
No Nausea and No Vomiting	0	No Tremor	0
Mild Nausea and No Vomiting	+1	Not Visible, but can be felt fingertip to fingertip	+1
(Severe Symptoms)	+2	(Severe Symptoms)	+2
(More Severe Symptoms)	+3	(More Severe Symptoms)	+3
Intermittent Nausea with Dry Heaves	+4	Moderate, with Patient's Arms Extended	+4
(Severe Symptoms)	+5	(Severe Symptoms)	+5
(More Severe Symptoms)	+6	(More Severe Symptoms)	+6
Constant Nausea, Frequently Dry Heaves and Vomiting	+7	Severe, even with arms not extended	+7

Continued

TABLE 18-3 CLINICAL INSTITUTE WITHDRAWAL ASSESSMENT FOR ALCOHOL (CIWA-AR)—cont'd

Paroxysmal Sweats

No Sweat Visible	0
Barely perceptible sweating, palms moist	+1
(Severe Symptoms)	+2
(More Severe Symptoms)	+3
Beads of sweat obvious on forehead	+4
(Severe Symptoms)	+5
(More Severe Symptoms)	+6
Drenching Sweats	+7

Anxiety

Ask, "Do you feel nervous?"

No anxiety, at ease	0
Mildly anxious	+1
(Severe Symptoms)	+2
(More Severe Symptoms)	+3
Moderately anxious, or guarded, so anxiety is inferred	+4
(Severe Symptoms)	+5
(More Severe Symptoms)	+6
Equivalent to acute panic states as seen in severe delirium or acute schizophrenic reactions	+7

Agitation

Normal Activity	0
Somewhat more activity than normal activity	+1
(Severe Symptoms)	+2
(More Severe Symptoms)	+3
Moderately fidgety and restless	+4
(Severe Symptoms)	+5
(More Severe Symptoms)	+6
Paces back and forth during most of the interview, or constantly thrashes about	+7

Tactile Disturbances

Ask, "Have you any itching, pins and needles sensations, any burning, any numbness, or do you feel bugs crawling on or under your skin?"

None	0
Very mild itching, pin and needles, burning, or numbness	+1
Mild itching, pin and needles, burning, or numbness	+2
Moderate itching, pin and needles, burning, or numbness	+3
Moderately severe hallucinations	+4
Severe hallucinations	+5
Extremely severe hallucinations	+6
Continuous hallucinations	+7

Auditory Disturbances

Ask, "Are you more aware of sounds around you? Are they harsh? Do they frighten you? Are you hearing anything that is disturbing to you? Are you hearing things you know are not there?"

Not Present	0
Very mild harshness or ability or frighten	+1
Mild harshness or ability or frighten	+2
Moderate harshness or ability or frighten	+3
Moderately severe hallucinations	+4
Severe hallucinations	+5
Extremely severe hallucinations	+6
Continous hallucinations	+7

Visual Disturbances

Ask "Does the light appear to be too bright? Is its color different? Does it hurt your eyes? Are you seeing anything that is disturbing to you? Are you seeing things you know are not there?"

Not Present	0
Very mild sensitivity	+1
Mild sensitivity	+2
Moderate sensitivity	+3
Moderately severe hallucinations	+4
Severe hallucinations	+5
Extremely severe hallucinations	+6
Continous hallucinations	+7

Headache/Fullness in Head

Ask "Does your head feel different? Does it feel like there is a band around your head?" Do not rate for dizziness or lightheadedness. Otherwise, rate severity.

Not Present	0
Very mild	+1
Mild	+2
Moderate	+3
Moderately severe	+4
Severe	+5
Very severe	+6
Extremely severe	+7

Orientation/Clouding of Sensorium

Ask "What day is this? Where are you? Who am I?"

Oriented, can do serial additions	0
Can't do serial additions or is uncertain about date	+1
Disoriented for date by no more than 2 calendar days	+2
Disoriented for date by more than 2 calendar days	+3
Disoriented to place or person	+4

Scoring:

0–9	Absent or minimal withdrawal
10–19	Mild to moderate withdrawal
20+	Severe Withdrawal

Sources: Reoux, J. P., & Miller, K. (2000). Routine hospital alcohol detoxification practice compared to symptom triggered management with an objective withdrawal scale (CIWA-Ar). *The American Journal on Addictions, 9*(2), 135–144; and Sullivan, J. T., Sykora, K., Schneiderman, J., et al. (1989). Assessment of alcohol withdrawal: The revised Clinical Institute Withdrawal Assessment for Alcohol scale (CIWA-Ar). *British Journal of Addiction, 84*(11), 1353–1357.

TABLE 18-4 RELATIONSHIP BETWEEN BLOOD ALCOHOL LEVEL AND EFFECTS IN A NONTOLERANT DRINKER

BLOOD ALCOHOL LEVEL (%)	BLOOD ALCOHOL ACCUMULATION (NUMBER OF DRINKS)	EFFECTS
0.05	1–2	Changes in mood and behaviour; impaired judgement
0.10	5–6	Clumsiness in voluntary motor activity
0.20	10–12	Depressed function of entire motor area of the brain, causing staggering and ataxia; emotional lability
0.30	15–18	Confusion, stupor
0.40	20–24	Coma
0.50	25–30	Death due to respiratory depression

TABLE 18-5 BLOOD ALCOHOL CONTENT (BAC)

FEMALE

LEAN BODY WEIGHT		NUMBER OF DRINKS									
POUNDS	KILOS	1	2	3	4	5	6	7	8	9	10
100	45.4	50	101	152	203	253	304	355	406	456	507
125	56.7	40	80	120	162	202	244	282	324	364	404
150	68.1	34	68	101	135	169	203	237	271	304	338
175	79.4	29	58	87	117	146	175	204	233	262	292
200	90.8	26	50	76	101	126	152	177	203	227	253
225	102.1	22	45	68	91	113	136	159	182	204	227
250	113.4	20	41	61	82	101	122	142	162	182	202

MALE

LEAN BODY WEIGHT		NUMBER OF DRINKS									
POUNDS	KILOS	1	2	3	4	5	6	7	8	9	10
100	45.4	43	87	130	174	217	261	304	348	391	435
125	56.7	34	69	103	139	173	209	242	278	312	346
150	68.1	29	58	87	116	145	174	203	232	261	290
175	79.4	25	50	75	100	125	150	175	200	225	250
200	90.8	22	43	65	87	108	130	152	174	195	217
225	102.1	19	39	58	78	97	117	136	156	175	195
250	113.4	17	35	52	70	87	105	122	139	156	173

Note: milligrams of alcohol in millilitres of blood
rate of elimination 15 millligrams per hour
standard drink 1 beer (12 oz 5% alcohol) = 1 wine (5 oz 12% alcohol) = 1 shot (1.5 oz 40% alcohol)

Source: Csiernik, R. (2014). *Just say know: A counsellor's guide to psychoactive drugs*. Toronto: Canadian Scholars Press.

Alcohol content varies from product to product; nevertheless, a drink is a drink is a drink, with 1.5 ounces of liquor (40% alcohol), a 12-ounce bottle of beer (5% alcohol), and a five-ounce glass of table wine (12% alcohol) all containing the same amount of ethanol. Thus all affect human physiology in a consistent manner as measured by blood alcohol content (BAC), although there are distinct differences between men and women (Table 18-5). Differences in effects from person to person produced by beverage alcohol do not generally result from the type of drink consumed, but rather from the person's size, previous drinking experiences, and rate of consumption. A person's feelings and activities and the presence of other people also play a role in the way the alcohol affects behaviour.

Alcohol withdrawal delirium. Alcohol withdrawal delirium, also referred to as *delirium tremens (DTs)*, is a medical emergency that can result in death in 20% of untreated patients. It is an altered level of consciousness that presents with seizures following acute alcohol withdrawal. Death is usually due to cardiopathy, cirrhosis, or other comorbidities requiring mechanical ventilation (Carlson, Kumar, Wong-Mckinstry, et al., 2012). The state of delirium usually peaks 48 to 72 hours after cessation or reduction of intake, although it can peak later, and lasts 2 to 3 days. Features of alcohol withdrawal delirium include the following:

- Autonomic hyperactivity (tachycardia, diaphoresis, elevated blood pressure)
- Severe disturbance in sensorium (disorientation, clouding of consciousness)
- Perceptual disturbances (visual or tactile hallucinations)
- Fluctuating levels of consciousness (ranging from hyperexcitability to lethargy)
- Delusions
- Anxiety and agitated behaviours
- Fever (38°C to 39°C)
- Insomnia
- Anorexia

If these symptoms are observed, immediate medical attention, including ongoing assessment and supervised treatment, is warranted.

Inhalants. A distinct CNS depressant subgroup is inhalants, which include volatile gases, substances that exist in a gaseous form at body temperature, refrigerants, solvents, general anaesthetics, and propellants. Except for nitrous oxide, more commonly known as laughing gas, and related aliphatic nitrates, all inhalants are hydrocarbons. The misuse of these collective substances has been labelled volatile substance abuse (VSA). As this is typically one of the first drugs misused by adolescents, particularly Indigenous youth, it is a significant public health concern. In addition, long-term exposure to solvents in the workplace has also been linked to a range of health issues in older adults, particularly dementia. It is generally believed that solvents alter CNS functioning through one of three means:

altering the structure of lipid membranes by impairing ion channels, altering enzymes that bind to the brain's membrane, or producing toxic metabolites (Ciechanowski, 2012; McKim & Hancock, 2012).

These substances not only have depressant effects, but also can produce minor hallucinogenic effects on the CNS. As solvents are inhaled, entry into the brain is extremely quick and the onset of effects is virtually immediate, producing feelings of relaxation and warmth within 8 to 15 seconds and with effects generally lasting for several hours. This class of psychoactive drugs has a significant abuse liability. The initial mood-enhancement effect is typically characterized by lightheadedness, exhilaration, fantasy images, and excitation. Negative effects include nausea, increased salivation, sneezing and coughing, loss of coordination, depressed reflexes, and sensitivity to light, along with skin irritation and burns around the mouth and nose. In some users, feelings of invincibility may lead to reckless, dangerous, violent, or erratic behaviour. Physical effects include pallor, thirst, weight loss, nosebleeds, bloodshot eyes, and sores on the nose and mouth (McKim & Hancock, 2012). Chronic use creates a range of medical problems, including damage to the cardiovascular, pulmonary, renal, and hepatic systems as well as to cognitive functioning (Takagi, Lubman, & Yu, 2011). Types of inhalants, signs of intoxication, and adverse effects are outlined in Table 18-6.

Opioids

Opioids are a distinct family of CNS depressants that includes morphine, heroin, codeine, oxycodone, methadone, meperidine, and fentanyl (Box 18-2). An opioid is a derivative or synthetic that affects the CNS and the PNS. Medically, it is used primarily as an analgesic (pain masker). Consistent use causes tolerance

TABLE 18-6 INHALANTS: INTOXICATION, OVERDOSE, AND TREATMENT

DRUGS	INTOXICATION	ADVERSE EFFECTS/OVERDOSE	TREATMENT
Organic solvents (gases or liquids that vaporize at room temperature): Toluene Gasoline Lighter fluid Paint thinner Nail polish remover Benzene Acetone Chloroform Model-airplane glue	Alcohol-like effects: euphoria, impaired judgement, slurred speech, flushing, central nervous system (CNS) depression Visual hallucinations and disorientation	Chronic use is toxic to heart, liver, and kidneys. Toxicity may result in sudden death from anoxia, vagal stimulation, respiratory depression, and dysthymia.	Support affected systems; no antidotes
Volatile nitrites: Room deodorizers Products sold for recreational use	Enhancement of sexual pleasure	Venodilation causes profound systolic blood pressure drop (dizziness, lightheadedness, palpitations, pulsate headache). Toxic dose may result in methemoglobinemia.	Toxicity may be treated with oxygen.
Anaesthetics: Gas—especially nitrous oxide (used in dental procedures and as a propellant for whipped cream) Liquid Local	Giggling, laughter Euphoria	Numbness, weakness, sensory loss, loss of balance. May cause physical dependence. Possible polyneuropathy and myelopathy when use is chronic.	Neuropathy may be treated with vitamin B_{12}.

Sources: Data from Lehne, R. E. (2014). *Pharmacology for nursing care* (9th ed.). Philadelphia: Saunders; and Ruiz, P., Strain, E. C., & Langrod, J. G. (2007). *The substance abuse handbook.* Philadelphia: Lippincott Williams & Wilkins.

BOX 18-2   CANADA'S FENTANYL PUBLIC HEALTH CRISIS

Developed in 1959 for use as a general anesthetic, fentanyl is therapeutically used to provide physical and emotional relief from acute pain, principally for palliative care patients or those with long-term chronic pain who experience breakthrough pain when using other less potent opioids. It has rapid onset and short duration of action; thus it is primarily administered transdermally in a hospital setting to make its use more convenient for those who are severely ill, with each patch designed to slowly release the potent substance over 72 hours.

In 2017, illicit street use of the potent licit synthetic opioid fentanyl became a national public health crisis, with overdose deaths in Canada reaching new levels. A decade before, a less potent licit synthetic opioid oxycontin had likewise become a public health issue, which led to its use being prohibited but without the development of a concurrent treatment strategy for those who had become addicted. In fact, during this time the Harper government appealed all the way to the Supreme Court of Canada in an attempt to shutter the nation's lone supervised injection site; after losing that appeal, the government introduced legislation creating additional barriers to opening any new facility anywhere in Canada.

Historically, whenever a psychoactive substance is prohibited, in its void an alternative arises (Csiernik, 2016). Unfortunately, in this case the prohibition of oxycontin, which was accompanied by its manufacturer, Purdue Pharma, paying a $600 million fine for product misbranding, led to an increase in heroin use. However, heroin is both expensive and illicit, whereas fentanyl, a synthetic drug that is 3 times as potent as uncut heroin and 100 times as potent as morphine, is both far cheaper to manufacture and can be legally produced in nations such as China. Across Canada, the cheaper fentanyl was being mixed with heroin, and at times cocaine, so that less of the expensive drug needed to be used and thus drug dealers could increase their profit margins. Combining the two drugs in street-level labs, however, often creates "hot spots" where more fentanyl is incorporated into the mix and thus the risk of overdose is further increased. Along with fentanyl, another synthetic opioid, even more potent, carfentanil began to be used for this purpose, again increasing the likelihood of each injection leading to an overdose.

TABLE 18-7   OPIOIDS: INTOXICATION, OVERDOSE, AND WITHDRAWAL

DRUGS	EFFECTS OF INTOXICATION	EFFECTS OF OVERDOSE	POSSIBLE TREATMENTS FOR OVERDOSE	EFFECTS OF WITHDRAWAL	POSSIBLE TREATMENTS FOR WITHDRAWAL
Opium (paregoric)	*Physical:*	Possible dilation	Opioid antagonist	Yawning	Methadone tapering*
Heroin	Constricted pupils	of pupils due	(e.g., naloxone	Insomnia	Clonidine–naltrexone
Meperidine (Demerol)	Decreased respiration	to anoxia	[Targin]) to quickly	Irritability	detoxification
Morphine	Drowsiness	Respiratory	reverse CNS	Rhinorrhea	Suboxone substitution*
Codeine	Decreased blood pressure	depression or	depression	Panic	
Methadone (Metadol)	Slurred speech	arrest		Diaphoresis	
Hydromorphone	Psychomotor retardation	Coma		Cramps	
(Dilaudid)	*Psychological–perceptual:*	Shock		Nausea and vomiting	
Fentanyl (Abstral—	Initial euphoria followed	Convulsions		Muscle aches ("bone pain")	
sublingual)	by dysphoria and	Death		Chills	
Fentanyl analogues	impairment of			Fever	
	attention, judgement,			Lacrimation	
	and memory			Diarrhea	

*Methadone tapering is managed very slowly and in careful consultation with the patient with regard to his or her readiness.
Source: Veilleux, J. C., Colvina, P. J., Andersona, J., et al. (2010). A review of opioid dependence treatment: Pharmacological and psychosocial interventions to treat opioid addiction. *Clinical Psychology Review, 30*, 155–166. doi:10.1016/j.cpr.2009.10.006.

and severe, physically painful withdrawal symptoms. Table 18-7 lists signs and symptoms of intoxication, overdose, withdrawal, and possible treatments.

Distinct phases are experienced when injecting an opioid such as heroin. The initial rush that occurs almost immediately is frequently characterized in terms of feelings of sexual arousal and as being superior to sexual intimacy. This initial euphoric phase is characterized physiologically by facial flushing and a deepening of the voice. The second, more prolonged, phase entails a sense of extreme well-being as an intense endorphin reaction is occurring in the brain. This phase can extend for several hours.

The third phase reflects the fact that opioids are CNS depressants and is characterized by a range of responses, from lethargy to virtual unconsciousness. The fourth phase occurs when the heroin is nearly fully metabolized and the person who has used the substance begins to seek additional heroin in order to avoid the painful withdrawal process.

As with alcohol, a protocol has been established to assist with opioid withdrawal. The Clinical Opiate Withdrawal Scale (COWS) was developed for buprenorphine/naloxone induction, though it can also be used in a variety of clinical settings such as assessing acute opioid withdrawal during an opioid detoxification,

TABLE 18-8 CLINICAL OPIATE WITHDRAWAL SCALE (COWS) FOR OPIOID WITHDRAWAL

Resting Pulse Rate (bpm)
Measure pulse rate after patient is sitting or lying down for 1 minute

≤80	0
81–100	+1
101–120	+2
>120	+4

Sweating
Sweating not accounted for by room temperature or patient activity over the last 0.5 hours

No report of chills or flushing	0
Subjective report of chills or flushing	+1
Flushed or observable moistness on face	+2
Beads of sweat on brow or face	+3
Sweat streaming off face	+4

Restlessness Observation During Assessment

Able to sit still	0
Reports difficulty sitting still, but is able to do so	+1
Frequent shifting or extraneous movements of legs/arms	+3
Unable to sit still for more than a few seconds	+5

Pupil Size

Pupils pinned or normal size for room light	0
Pupils possibly larger than normal for room light	+1
Pupils moderately dilated	+2
Pupils so dilated that only the rim of the iris is visible	+5

Bone or Joint Aches
If patient was having pain previously, only the additional component attributed to opiate withdrawal is scored

Not present	0
Mild diffuse discomfort	+1
Patient reports severe diffuse aching of joints/ muscles	+2
Patient is rubbing joints or muscles and is unable to sit still because of discomfort	+4

Runny Nose or Tearing
Not accounted for by cold symptoms or allergies

Not present	0
Nasal stuffiness or unusually moist eyes	+1
Nose running or tearing	+2
Nose constantly running or tears streaming down cheeks	+4

GI Upset
Over last 0.5 hours

No GI symptoms	0
Stomach cramps	+1
Nausea or loose stool	+2
Vomiting or diarrhea	+3
Multiple episodes of vomiting or diarrhea	+5

Tremor Observation of Outstretched Hands

No tremor	0
Tremor can be felt, but not observed	+1
Slight tremor observable	+2
Gross tremor or muscle twitching	+4

Yawning Observation During Assessment

No yawning	0
Yawning once or twice during assessment	+1
Yawning three or more times during assessment	+2
Yawning several times/minute	+4

Anxiety or Irritability

None	0
Patient reports increasing irritability or anxiousness	+1
Patient obviously irritable/anxious	+2
Patient so irritable or anxious that participation in the assessment is difficult	+4

Gooseflesh Skin

Skin is smooth	0
Piloerection of skin can be felt or hairs standing up on arms	+3
Prominent piloerection	+5

Score Interpretation:
- <5 - no active withdrawal
- 5–12 - mild withdrawal
- 13–24 - moderate withdrawal
- 25–36 - moderately severe withdrawal
- >36 - severe withdrawal

GI, Gastrointestinal.
Sources: Tompkins, D. A., Bigelow, G. E., Harrison, J. A., et al. (2009). Concurrent validation of the Clinical Opiate Withdrawal Scale (COWS) and single-item indices against the Clinical Institute Narcotic Assessment (CINA) opioid withdrawal instrument. *Drug and Alcohol Dependence*, *105*(1), 154–159; and Wesson, D. R., & Ling, W. (2003). The Clinical Opiate Withdrawal Scale (COWS). *Journal of Psychoactive Drugs, 35*(2), 253–259.

methadone maintenance, or methadone treatment, as well as during the treatment of chronic pain (Table 18-8).

Central Nervous System Stimulants

This family of drugs includes cocaine hydrochloride as well as crack, amphetamines including crystal meth, caffeine, and nicotine. Central nervous system stimulants are drugs that increase the activity of both the CNS and the PNS. Mood enhancement occurs because of these changes. Upon initial ingestion there is euphoria, followed by excitement and then agitation. Higher doses produce irritability, violent behaviour, spasms, convulsions. and. in infrequent extreme cases, death. More common and

frequent short-term effects include enhanced concentration, increased vigilance, increased blood pressure, increased strength, reduced fatigue, reduced appetite, and feelings of power. While all stimulants increase alertness, as a family they exhibit considerable differences in the nature of their effects and in their relative potencies.

Table 18-9 outlines the physical and psychological effects of intoxication from amphetamines and other psychostimulants, possible life-threatening results of overdose, and emergency measures for both overdose and withdrawal. All stimulants accelerate the normal functioning of the body and affect the CNS and PNS. Upon abrupt discontinuation of drug administration,

TABLE 18-9 CENTRAL NERVOUS SYSTEM STIMULANTS: INTOXICATION, OVERDOSE, AND WITHDRAWAL

DRUGS	EFFECTS OF INTOXICATION	EFFECTS OF OVERDOSE	POSSIBLE TREATMENTS FOR OVERDOSE	EFFECTS OF WITHDRAWAL	POSSIBLE TREATMENTS FOR WITHDRAWAL
Cocaine, crack (short-acting) High obtained by (method) in (time frame): snorted, 2–3 minutes; injected, 15–30 seconds; smoked (for crack), 4–10 seconds Average high lasts 15–30 minutes for cocaine; 5–7 minutes for crack	Physical: Tachycardia Dilated pupils Elevated blood pressure Nausea and vomiting Insomnia Psychological–perceptual: Agitation and aggression Grandiosity Impaired judgement Impaired social and occupational functioning Euphoria	Respiratory distress Ataxia Hyperpyrexia Convulsions Coma Stroke Myocardial infarction Death	Antipsychotics, medical and nursing management for: Fever (ambient cooling) Convulsions (diazepam) Respiratory distress or cardiovascular shock (resuscitation and medical treatment to control hypertension, tachycardia, and respirations) Acidification of urine (ammonium chloride for amphetamine)	Fatigue Depression Agitation Apathy Anxiety Sleepiness Disorientation Lethargy Craving	Supportive measures Diazepam (Valium) or lorazepam (Ativan) may be prescribed for mild to moderate withdrawal symptoms
Amphetamines (long-acting) Dextroamphetamine Methamphetamine/crystal meth	Increased energy Severe effects: State resembling paranoid schizophrenia Paranoia with delusions Psychosis Visual, auditory, and tactile hallucinations Severe to panic levels of anxiety Potential for violence Note: Paranoia and ideas of reference may persist for months afterward	Same as above	Same as above	Same as above	Same as above

Source: Sofuoglu, M., Poling, J., Gonzalez, G., et al. (2006). Cocaine withdrawal symptoms predict medication response in cocaine users. *American Journal of Drug and Alcohol Abuse, 32,* 617–628. doi:10.1080/00952990600920680.

abstinence symptoms observed include fatigue, severe mood depression, lethargy, and irritability; these are commonly referred to as the "crash," which can also include abdominal and muscle cramps, dehydration, and a general apathy. However, unlike with depressants there is generally no risk for fatal withdrawal, although when someone who has ingested a stimulant experiences chest pain, has an irregular pulse, or has a history of heart trouble, the person should immediately be taken to an emergency department.

Cocaine and crack. Cocaine is a naturally occurring stimulant extracted from the leaf of the coca bush, whereas crack is an alkalinized form of coca administrated via inhalation. When smoked, crack takes effect in 6 to 10 seconds, producing a short sense of euphoria, followed by a crash, a period of deep depression as the body works to return to homeostasis, that reinforces the drug-using behaviour. However, as do many psychoactive drugs, cocaine has some recognized medical uses, specifically as an anaesthetic that blocks the conduction of electrical impulses within the nerve cells involved in sensory transmission, primarily pain transmission.

Cocaine works by blocking the reuptake of norepinephrine, dopamine, and serotonin, causing an imbalance of neurotransmitters that, when the drug is metabolized, results in physical

withdrawal symptoms including depression, lethargy, anxiety, insomnia, sweating and chills, and a renewed craving for the drug. Koob and Le Moal (2006) have identified three distinct phases of withdrawal:

1. The first phase, the *crash phase*, can last up to 4 days. Those who use cocaine report depression, anergia, and an acute onset of agitated depression. Craving for the drug peaks during this phase, as do anxiety and paranoia. Inpatient care to prevent access to further doses of the drug is helpful during the first and second phases of withdrawal.

2. During the second phase, the user feels a prolonged sense of dysphoria and anhedonia, a lack of motivation, and intense cravings for the substance of abuse. This phase can last up to 10 weeks. Relapse is most likely during the second phase of withdrawal.

3. The third phase is characterized by intermittent craving and can last indefinitely.

Amphetamines and Methamphetamine

Amphetamines are chemically related to the naturally occurring catecholamine neurotransmitter and work by increasing synaptic levels of dopamine, serotonin (5-HT), and norepinephrine. They

TABLE 18-10	COCAINE– METHAMPHETAMINE COMPARISON	
ACTION	**COCAINE**	**METHAMPHETAMINE**
Length of action		
20–30 minutes	x	
4–6 hours		x
Produces self-esteem	x	x
Increases alertness	x	x
Postpones sleep	x	x
Decreases appetite	x	x
Increases blood pressure	x	x
Produces seizures	x	x
Local anaesthetic	x	
Increases body temperature	x	x
Cardiac arrhythmias	x	x
Elicit paranoid psychosis	x	x
Depression during withdrawal	x	x
High dependency liability	x	x

Source: Csiernik, R. (2014). *Just say know: A counsellor's guide to psychoactive drugs*. Toronto: Canadian Scholars Press.

are used to raise energy levels and reduce appetite and the need for sleep, and provide feelings of clear-headedness and power. Norepinephrine is responsible for methamphetamine's alerting, anorectic, locomotor, and sympathomimetic effects; dopamine also stimulates locomotor effects but in excess can produce psychosis and perception disturbances; and changes to serotonin (5-HT) are responsible for the delusions and psychosis associated with the use of amphetamines. Methamphetamine's effects are similar to those of cocaine, but its onset is slower and the duration is longer (Table 18-10).

Bath Salts (Methylenedioxypyrovalerone and Mephedrone)

Pharmacologically, bath salts are most closely related to khat, a plant that grows and is used widely in the horn of Africa region. Its psychoactive property is derived from the same source, cathinone, though the synthetic version is much more potent. Although cathinone was synthesized by pharmaceutical companies in the late twentieth century, its derivatives did not become broadly used within the drug trade until the beginning of the twenty-first century. It also shares some pharmacological similarity with methylenedioxymethamphetamine (MDMA/ecstasy) but with less hallucinogenic and more stimulant properties closer to the effects of methamphetamine. In a study of the rewarding and reinforcing effects of methylenedioxypyrovalerone (MDPV), rats showed self-administration patterns and escalation of drug intake nearly identical to those seen with methamphetamine (Cameron, Kolanos, Solis, et al., 2013; Cameron, Kolanos, Verkariva, et al., 2013).

This drug can be administered orally, across mucous membranes, or via inhalation or injection. The energizing and often agitating effects occur because of increased levels of dopamine, which also increase a user's heart rate and blood pressure. The surge in dopamine creates feelings of euphoria, increased physical

activity, heightened sexual interest, a lack of hunger and thirst, muscle spasms, sleeplessness, and, when sleep does occur, disrupted dream cycles. Behavioural effects include erratic behaviour, teeth grinding, a lack of recall of how much of the substance has been consumed, panic attacks, anxiety, agitation, severe paranoia, hallucinations, psychosis, self-mutilation, and behaviour that can be aggressive, violent, and and in extreme cases move beyond suicidal ideation to suicidal actions. Overdose is possible due to heart and blood vessel problems because of a lack of any type of regulation of this drug, leading to inconsistency of the psychoactive ingredient between brands. In 2012, the Government of Canada made it illegal to possess, traffic, import, or export methylenedioxypyrovalerone unless authorized by regulation (Antnowicz, Metzger, & Ramanujam, 2011; Ross, Reisfield, Watson, et al., 2012; Wieland, Halter, & Levine, 2012).

Caffeine

Caffeine is the most used psychoactive drug not only in Canada but across the world. It is found in coffee, tea, energy drinks, and soft drinks. Caffeine blocks the actions of adenosine, an inhibitory neurotransmitter, by binding to its receptor and preventing postbinding changes from taking place, which leads to increased firing of dopaminergic neurons, particularly in the nucleus accumbens. Due to its ability to constrict cerebral blood vessels, caffeine is used in combination with other drugs to combat migraine and other cerebrovascular headaches associated with high blood pressure. However, contrary to popular belief, caffeine is not effective in ameliorating headaches due to other causes, and in some cases it may even exacerbate pain. In other medical uses, caffeine is employed to counteract certain symptoms, such as respiratory depression, associated with CNS-depressant poisoning. It is also used:

- As a respiratory stimulant in babies who have had apnea episodes (periods when spontaneous breathing ceases)
- As an emergency bronchodilator in asthmatic children
- As a substitute for methylphenidate for children with attention-deficit/hyperactivity disorder
- As an antifungal agent in the treatment of skin disorders
- As an aid in fertility, because of its ability to enhance sperm mobility
- As a mild stimulant for an assortment of medical problems (Csiernik, 2014)

When taken in moderate amounts, caffeine can produce stimulant effects on the CNS similar to those of small doses of amphetamines. These can include mild mood elevation; feelings of enhanced energy; an increased alertness and reduced performance deficit due to boredom or fatigue; postponement of feelings of fatigue and the need for sleep; and a decrease in hand steadiness, suggesting impaired fine motor performance. Small doses of caffeine can also increase motor activity, alter sleep patterns (including delaying the onset of sleep), diminish sleep time, and reduce the depth of sleep (including altering rapid eye movement [REM] sleep patterns), while also increasing respiration, blood pressure, and metabolism. However, with the increasing use of dietary supplements, caffeine pills, and energy drinks containing far more caffeine than coffee, tea, or cola, there has been an increase in hospitalizations involving the drug and in overdoses leading to death (Banerjee, Ali, Levine, et al., 2014; Campana, Griffin, & Simon, 2014; Eichner, 2014).

Nicotine

Nicotine, in combination with its agent of delivery, tobacco, is the leading cause of premature death from any psychoactive agent in Canada and in the world. Nicotine has a pale-yellow colour and an oily consistency. It turns brown on contact with air, and doses of 60 milligrams can be fatal while amounts as low as 4 milligrams can produce severe illness. Tobacco smoke comprises some 500 compounds, including tar, ammonia, acetaldehyde, acetone, benzene, toluene, benzo(a)pyrene, dimethylnitrosamine, methylethylnitrosamine, naphthalene, carbon monoxide, and carbon dioxide. This drug is thought to affect the brain reward system by increasing dopamine concentrations through interaction with nicotine acetylcholine receptors. Since nicotine is a CNS stimulant, it increases heart rate, pulse rate, and blood pressure; depresses the spinal reflex; reduces muscle tone; decreases skin temperature; increases acid in the stomach; reduces urine formation; precipitates a loss of appetite; increases adrenaline production; and stimulates, then reduces, brain and nervous system activity. In nonsmokers, small doses, even less than one cigarette, may produce an unpleasant reaction that includes coughing, nausea, vomiting, dizziness, abdominal discomfort, weakness, and flushing. Nicotine crosses the placenta, and women who smoke during pregnancy tend to have smaller babies and are more likely to give birth prematurely (Csiernik, 2014).

Marijuana

Marijuana (*Cannabis sativa*) is a member of the hemp family of plants, with one major distinction: it contains delta-9-tetrahydro-cannabinol (THC). This is the psychoactive ingredient found in the resin secreted from the flowering tops and leaves of the female cannabis plant. While this substance has historically been placed within the hallucinogen family of drugs, THC also produces depressant effects and is the only hallucinogen that produces physical dependency; thus it is an addicting agent. Marijuana is generally smoked, but it also can be ingested orally, typically in baked goods. Desired effects include euphoria, detachment, and relaxation. Other effects include talkativeness, slowed perception of time, inappropriate hilarity, heightened sensitivity to external stimuli, and anxiety or paranoia. Long-term use of cannabis can result in lethargy, anhedonia, difficulty concentrating, amotivational syndrome, and memory impairment.

Medical marijuana is used in response to a broad range of issues, including control of chemotherapy-induced nausea, reduction of intraocular pressure in glaucoma, appetite stimulation in acquired immunodeficiency syndrome (AIDS) wasting syndrome, muscle spasms associated with spinal cord injury, and multiple sclerosis, and to decrease seizures caused by some forms of epilepsy. Cannabis can also help alleviate gastrointestinal disorders, depression, anxiety, and tension; can decrease chronic pain; and can aid insomnia (Walsh, Callaway, Belle-Isle, et al., 2013).

Canada plans to legalize recreational use of cannabis in 2018, which will lead to increased use if the pattern follows other jurisdictions. This in turn will likely produce increased health

RESEARCH HIGHLIGHT
Smoking Cessation Support via Mobile Texting

Problem
Most of those killed by tobacco started smoking as teenagers, and smoking contributes to the death of one of every two of those who smoke past 35 years of age. Stopping smoking at an early age conveys greater health benefits.

Purpose of Study
For many people, mobile phones are part of their everyday lives and are always carried with them; therefore a text intervention can take place at any time. The purpose of this study was to assess the effectiveness of a mobile phone–based smoking intervention.

Methods
Participants were recruited through various media, including websites, primary care facilities, and pharmacies. Inclusion criteria were that participants were age 16 or older, had a mobile phone, and were willing to attempt to stop smoking. In the next month, 5 800 participants were randomized into two groups based on age, gender, education, and nicotine addiction score. Individuals in the treatment group received motivational and behavioural text messages, whereas the control group received text messages related only to the importance of participation in the trial. At 6 months post-trial, salivary tests were used to confirm self-reported abstinence.

Key Findings
Text messages via mobile phones doubled smoking cessation rates in the treatment group, but these cessation rates were similar to those seen with other behavioural interventions, such as group, one-to-one, or telephone advice programs. Mobile phones simply provide a new channel for individualized programs to be delivered inexpensively wherever the person is located.

Implications for Nursing Practice
Researchers suggest that the use of mobile text messages should be considered as part of existing cessation programs. The researchers also suggest that using mobile technology may be effective in changing other behavioural risk factors.

Source: Free, C., Knight, R., Robertson, S., et al. (2011). Smoking cessation support delivered via mobile phone text messaging (txt2stop): A single-blind, randomised trial. *The Lancet, 378,* 49–55. doi:10.1016/S0140-6736(11)60701-0

and social issues, including greater rates of impaired driving; child and some adult poisonings, primarily from edibles; increased criminal charges for public intoxication; increased rates of mental health issues such as anxiety and panic attacks, especially among adolescent users; marijuana-associated cyclic vomiting syndrome; and an increase in hospitalizations for burns resulting primarily from flash fires that occur when a user is trying to extract THC and other active marijuana constituents using butane (Monte, Zane, & Heard, 2015).

Hallucinogens

Hallucinogens are distinct psychoactive agents in that they do not primarily produce euphoria, but rather disrupt the CNS and

TABLE 18-11   HALLUCINOGENS: INTOXICATION, OVERDOSE, AND WITHDRAWAL

DRUGS	PHYSICAL EFFECTS OF INTOXICATION	PSYCHOLOGICAL–PERCEPTUAL EFFECTS OF INTOXICATION	EFFECTS OF OVERDOSE	POSSIBLE TREATMENTS FOR OVERDOSE
Lysergic acid diethylamide (LSD) Psilocybin (mushrooms) Mescaline (peyote)	Pupil dilation Tachycardia Diaphoresis Palpitations Tremors Incoordination Elevated temperature, pulse, respiration	Fear of going crazy Paranoid ideas Marked anxiety, depression Synesthesia (e.g., colours are heard, sounds are seen) Depersonalization Hallucinations, although sensorium is clear Grandiosity (e.g., thinking one can fly)	Psychosis Brain damage Death	Keep patient in room with low stimuli—minimal light, sound, activity. Have one person stay with patient. Provide reassurance. Speak slowly and clearly in quiet voice. Diazepam or chloral hydrate may be prescribed for extreme anxiety or tension.
Phencyclidine piperidine (PCP) Ketamine	Vertical or horizontal nystagmus Increased blood pressure, pulse, and temperature Ataxia Muscle rigidity Seizures Blank stare Chronic jerking Agitated, repetitive movements Belligerence, assaultiveness, impulsiveness Impaired judgement, impaired social and occupational functioning	Severe effects: Hallucinations, paranoia Bizarre behaviour (e.g., barking like a dog, grimacing, repetitive chanting speech) Regressive behaviour Violent bizarre behaviours Very labile behaviours	Psychosis Possible hypertensive crisis or cardiovascular accident Respiratory arrest Hyperthermia Seizures	If alert: Put in room with minimal stimuli. Do not attempt to talk down! Speak slowly, clearly, and in a quiet voice. Monitor and be prepared to intervene for: Hyperthermia High blood pressure Respiratory distress Hypertension

Source: Meehan Y. J., Bryant, S. M., & Aks, S. E. (2010). Drugs of abuse: The highs and lows of altered mental states in the emergency department. *Emergency Medicine Clinics of North America, 28,* 663–682. doi:10.1016/j.emc.2010.03.012.

PNS, producing a disconnect between the physical world and the user's perception of the physical world. Effects can include distortion in space and time, hallucinations, delusions both paranoid and grandiose, and synesthesia, which is a blurring and intermingling of the senses, such as smelling a colour or tasting a feeling. Table 18-11 outlines the signs and symptoms of hallucinogen intoxication and overdose.

Hallucinogens, excluding cannabis, are divided into three groups. Indolealkylamines, such as lysergic acid diethylamide (LSD) and psilocybin, have no secondary psychoactive effects; phenylethylamines, such as mescaline, ecstasy, and jimson weed, have structural similarities to amphetamines, producing secondary stimulant effects on the body; and dissociative anaesthetics, psychoactive drugs such as phencyclidine (PCP) and ketamine that are members of the arylcyclohexylamine family, possess depressant properties along with their hallucinatory effects.

A hallucinogen that has received extensive public attention is MDMA (3,4-methylenedioxymethamphetamine), referred to as ecstasy, molly, Adam, yaba, and XTC. Related hallucinogens with stimulant properties include MDA (methylenedioxyamphetamine), the "love drug," and MDE (3,4-methylenedioxyethamphetamine), whose slang name is "Eve." MDMA causes a significant release of the neurochemicals serotonin, dopamine, and norepinephrine. The brain's saturation with these neurotransmitters causes those who use MDMA to exhibit major empathy toward others; reduces inhibitions; elicits introspection; and results in an outpouring of good feelings about others, the current environment, and the world. The release of serotonin also intensely sharpens the senses of those using the substance.

Those using MDMA may be hyperactive and have inexhaustible energy (dancing all night long), dilated pupils with impaired reaction to light, elevated temperature, elevated pulse, elevated blood pressure, diaphoresis, dystonia, bruxism (grinding of the teeth), and other symptoms of stimulant use, such as tachycardia, mydriasis (dilation of the pupils), tremors, arrhythmias, parkinsonism, esophoria (eyes turning inward), serotonin syndrome, and severe hyponatremia. Those using MDMA must drink a large quantity of water during use to prevent dehydration and hyperthermia, which have contributed to occasional deaths. After the effects of MDMA wear off, the person using the substance commonly goes through a period of depression. This affective state is caused by a depletion of serotonin, levels of which do not return to normal within the CNS for at least 3 to 4 days. Two distinct pharmacological processes are most closely associated with this family of drug. The first process is tachyphylaxis, the rapid reduction in the effect produced by the drug, regardless of how much of the drug is consumed. In essence, this is total tolerance that occurs in a short period of time, such that there is no physical withdrawal to the drug. If a drug is taken for a consecutive number of days, after 3 or 4 days, no psychoactive effects of any type are perceived. The secondary effects of hallucinogens such as MDMA or ketamine can still be perceived even when the primary hallucinogenic effect is not. The second process is a flashback, or hallucinogen persisting perceptual disorder (HPPD). These are transitory recurrences of perceptual disturbance that can be caused by a person's earlier hallucinogenic drug use but occur after the fact, when the person is in a drug-free state. Flashbacks can be experienced as pleasant, but most often entail recurrences of frightening images, visual distortions, time expansion, loss of ego boundaries, and intense emotions. However, HPPD is generally talked about more than it is actually experienced (Csiernik, 2014).

HELPING PATIENTS CHANGE

Self-Assessment and Self-Awareness

To offer support and motivation toward recovery, a nurse must begin by examining her or his own attitudes, feelings, and beliefs about addiction and persons with addictions. Such reflection often means that nurses must examine their own substance use and the substance use of others in their lives, a potentially difficult task. A history of substance abuse in a nurse's own family can interfere with the helping relationship and contribute to counter-transference (see Chapter 9). The negative or positive experiences a nurse has had with family members or others with addictions can influence interpersonal interactions with patients and affect treatment outcomes. Therefore attending to personal feelings that arise when working with people experiencing addictions is vital, as are ongoing self-reflection and supervision that encourages reflection on the nurse's responses as well as the patients'. Nurses who do not attend to, and work through, expected negative feelings that arise while providing care may engage in power struggles with patients, resulting in an ineffective therapeutic process, and are more likely to suffer from vicarious trauma (Darnell & Csiernik, 2014).

Psychological Changes

Distinct psychological characteristics are associated with substance abuse, often arising from trauma or oppression, including hopelessness, low self-esteem, anxiety, and depression.

People who abuse substances often feel threatened on many levels in their interactions with nurses in formal hospital and treatment settings. First, they are concerned about being rejected because not all nurses are willing to care for people with addiction issues. In fact, many patients have reported experiences of rejection in past encounters with nursing personnel (Chu & Galang, 2013). Second, people who abuse substances may be anxious about giving up the substance they believe they need to survive; this relates to psychological dependency. Third, people with addictions often are concerned about failing at recovery, as addiction is a chronic, relapsing condition. In fact, relapse is one of the criteria for diagnosing addiction. Most individuals with an addiction have tried recovery at least once before and have since experienced lapse or relapse. As a result, many become discouraged about their chances of ever succeeding. Such feelings of discouragement and a high level of hopelessness can act as barriers to recovery.

Concerns about failure or potential relapse on the path of recovery can threaten the person's sense of security and sense of self, increasing anxiety levels. To protect against these feelings, the person with an addiction may establish self-defensive responses, including defence mechanisms (refer to Chapter 4) such as projection or rationalization, or thought processes such as all-or-none thinking, selective attention, or conflict minimization and avoidance. Typically the person is unable to give up these maladaptive coping styles until more positive and functional skills are learned.

The Transtheoretical Model of Change

Prochaska and DiClemente (1984) revolutionized thinking about addiction treatment with their integrative model of intentional change based on their work with tobacco smokers who stopped without any formal or self-help assistance. They took the idea of motivation and made it into an active counselling skill. Rather than being located exclusively within the patient, they expressed the idea that motivation was an interpersonal, interactional process within which the probability existed for behaviours to lead to positive outcomes. Prochaska and DiClemente identified six specific steps necessary for any type of radical change to occur, which represented a natural process of change that could be adapted by nurses to assist any patient in moving forward (Figure 18-4).

Precontemplation

In the first stage of the model, it is recognized that an individual will be resistant to change and typically has no intention of altering behaviour in the near future; there is typically no or little recognition from the patient's perspective that any type of problem exists. This idea has historically been called denial, and critical to the entire premise of the **transtheoretical model of change** (TTM) is the replacement of the long-standing idea that clients are in denial regarding their addiction with the concept of **precontemplation**. Prochaska and DiClemente (1984) reconceptualized the idea of denial to frame it so that clients are not viewed as willfully deceiving themselves and others and in the process destroying themselves or their families; instead, these individuals are considered to be truly unaware of the impact of their behaviour and the effect it has on those around them. People with substance use disorders are often ambivalent about changing their harmful behaviour regarding alcohol or drug use. They may continue their drug use for a range of reasons, such as being attracted to a particular lifestyle, wanting to be included in a peer group, coping with life's daily stresses, or responding to trauma and oppression in their lives. When the destructive effect of these behaviours becomes obvious, they are then faced with the reality of giving up most of the people, places, and things they have come to enjoy and with which they may strongly identify. Without a clear picture of the future, these individuals may be reluctant to proceed with any change. Thus a considerable effort

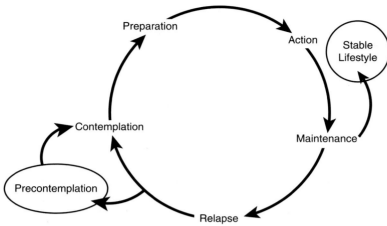

FIGURE 18-4 Transtheoretical model of change. Source: Association of Faculties of Medicine of Canada. (2016). *Primer on population health.* Retrieved from http://phprimer.afmc.ca/Part3-PracticeImprovingHealth/Chapter8IllnessPreventionAndHealthPromotion/Changingbehaviour.

is required by the individual with a substance use disorder, their family members, friends, and helping professionals to become willing to make a commitment to change. Approaches to support the patient at this stage include:

- Validating the lack of readiness
- Encouraging re-evaluation of current behaviour
- Encouraging self-exploration rather than immediate action
- Explaining and personalizing the risk

Contemplation

In the second stage, contemplation, patients become aware that they are stuck in a situation and must decide whether they wish to change or remain where they are. Nurses support patients in gaining understanding of the consequences of their alcohol or drug use but do not force the patient to make a commitment to change. The nurse helps to balance in the patient's mind the delicate equilibrium between the desire to change and the fear of changing and the associated unknown consequences. Nurses need to reflect this ambivalence to help clients be able to move forward to the next stage while recognizing and acknowledging the fear associated with change. Nurses also need to be open to the fact that some patients will drop out at this highly stressful stage, and thus a willingness to work with the patient in the future must be presented when the person is ready and able to move forward again. Supportive approaches include:

- Encouraging evaluation of the pros and cons of behaviour change
- Re-evaluating group image through group activities
- Identifying and promoting new, positive-outcome expectations

Preparation

The third stage, preparation, also known as the determination stage, involves some commitment from the patient that changing the drug-using behaviour is being considered along with anticipation of what this future action may look like. However, the nurse needs to be aware that a significant level of ambivalence

may still exist to the idea and process of actual change. During the preparation phase, probing, reviewing consequences, and self-evaluation are areas of work to perform with the patient, and a specific time frame is established for when the patient agrees to begin changing existing practices and actions, with a maximum target of 1 month. Supportive approaches at this phase include:

- Encouraging the evaluation of the pros and cons of behaviour change
- Identifying and promoting new positive-outcome expectations
- Encouraging realistic, practical, and small initial steps
- Offering referrals to and support of action-oriented programs such as smoking cessation

Action

This is when the work and behavioural change begin, with a heavy emphasis on problem solving and problem-solving skills. However, action also entails changing awareness, emotions, self-image, and thinking. Support of positive decisions and positive reinforcement dominate this stage of moving forward by the patient. Emphasis is on the positive: what patients are doing rather than what they are not (i.e., not using drugs). Supportive approaches include:

- Helping the patient with restructuring cues and triggers and solidifying social support
- Enhancing self-efficacy for dealing with obstacles
- Helping to guard against feelings of loss and frustration, especially if a lapse occurs

Maintenance/Adaption

Stage five, maintenance/adaption focuses on supporting and consolidating the gains made during the action stage and on avoiding lapses or more significant relapse. Social skills training underscores this stage of continued change. This is the skills practice phase of the TTM during which patients are less tempted to lapse and are becoming increasingly confident that they can continue their changed behaviour. Approaches to use include:

- Planning for follow-up support
- Reinforcing internal rewards
- Discussing strategies for coping with triggers and relapse
- Generalizing positive behaviours into more situations

Evaluation/Termination

The final stage of the TTM has the patient move past problem solving with a focus on relapse prevention and dealing with the reality of sobriety. During this phase, clients assess their strengths and areas that may be problematic in the future as they develop a relapse prevention plan that can be undertaken on their own and begin once a lapse occurs. Supportive approaches that are particularly helpful to assist the patient and family include:

- Evaluating triggers for relapse
- Reassessing motivation and barriers to change
- Planning and rehearsing new and stronger coping strategies

Motivational Interviewing

Closely associated with the TTM, and integral to its success, is the idea of motivational interviewing (MI), initially conceptualized by William Miller (1983). MI is a brief, patient-centred, directive method for enhancing change in intrinsic motivation by exploring and resolving patient ambivalence using the ideas of empathy, attribution, cognitive dissonance, and self-efficacy. In MI, motivation is conceptualized not as a personality trait but as an interpersonal process. The model de-emphasizes labelling, replacing confrontation with empathy, and places a much greater emphasis on individual responsibility and internal attribution for change. Cognitive dissonance is created by contrasting the ongoing problem behaviour of a patient with salient awareness of the behaviour's negative consequences. Empathic processes, motivation, and objective assessment feedback are used to channel this dissonance toward a behaviour change, being cognizant of and avoiding the typical patient barriers of low self-esteem, low self-efficacy, and precontemplation. MI is a strength-based counselling style in which the nurse works with the patient rather than doing things for or to the patient. The focus is to look for natural motivating issues within a patient's life or the patient's system. The counsellor needs to anticipate and respond to a patient's genuine hesitation and insecurity to engage in a fundamentally life-altering change in behaviour because simply giving patients advice to change is typically unrewarding and ineffective. MI is nonconfrontational in nature and acknowledges the fact that creating conflict, rather than ambivalence, in the therapeutic relationship is counterproductive and is more likely to create patient resistance than patient change. MI seeks to increase a patient's awareness of his or her problematic behaviour along with unrecognized strengths and opportunities for change. Miller and Rollnick (2002) established eight steps for the MI process: establishing rapport, setting the agenda, assessing readiness to change, sharpening focus, identifying ambivalence, eliciting self-motivating statements, handling resistance, and shifting focus and transition (Box 18-3).

Communication Techniques for Assessment and Interventions

Accurate assessment and effective intervention planning and implementation for colleagues and patients depends on development of a therapeutic relationship (see Chapter 9) and effective communication (see Chapter 10), which can be enhanced by incorporating motivational interviewing and the transtheoretical model of change in a nurse's practice. The nurse's ability to develop a therapeutic relationship with a patient with an addiction can help the patient feel safe enough to start looking at problems with some degree of openness and honesty. The following is a portion of an intake interview with a patient upon admission to a treatment program.

Dialogue	Therapeutic Tool or Comment
Nurse: "Elyse, I get the impression that life must have been very difficult for you lately." **Elyse:** (long pause) "I don't think you would understand."	Validating and empathizing
Nurse: "I guess sometimes it feels as if no one understands, but I would like to try." **Elyse:** "At times I feel I can't go on anymore ... so many losses."	Reflecting and empathizing
Nurse: "Loss is difficult. Elyse, tell me about your losses." **Elyse:** "My brother's sudden death. ... We were so close. ... I depended on him so much."	Encouraging the patient to share her painful feelings
Nurse: "It must have been difficult for you to lose him so suddenly." **Elyse:** (long pause) "No one knows. ... Then Joseph, he left. ..." (Elyse starts to cry)	Empathizing
Nurse: (sitting in silence as Elyse cries, then asking for more information about the feelings expressed) "Tell me about this experience." **Elyse:** "I don't know. ... I just wonder, why does everyone leave me? Oh, I hate them all. ... I wish I had a Valium now."	Encouraging the expression of feelings while feelings are close to the surface
Nurse: "And what does the Valium do to help you?"	Beginning to explore the drug dependence in a gentle, nonthreatening manner

The next example demonstrates the use of therapeutic leverage, making abstinence and sobriety worthwhile for those abusing the substance. It is presented as a dialogue between a nurse and a 17-year-old man whose parents are divorced and whose father

BOX 18-3   THE MOTIVATIONAL INTERVIEWING (MI) PROCESS

1. **Establish rapport.** Chapters 9 and 10 discuss establishing rapport with patients, but in the case of MI, rapport may be fostered by simply asking permission to discuss the patient's behaviour or concern. For example:

   "Do you mind if we spend a few minutes talking about …?"

   "How do you feel about the behaviour (or desired behaviour change)?"

2. **Set the agenda.** Working with the patient to create an agenda helps the nurse and patient to clarify the immediate concerns of interest for the patient and sets the boundaries of the helping relationship. For example:

   "What do you know about …?"

   "Are you interested in learning more about …?"

   "Are you able to come back to the clinic to discuss your plans further?"

3. **Assess readiness to change.** Motivation is not static and can change rapidly from day to day. Patients enter treatment at different levels of motivation or readiness to change, and many are ambivalent about changing, as there are often aspects about the addiction that the patient is still benefiting from in some way. Assessing the patient's readiness to change prepares the nurse to tailor treatment to that stage. Such assessment can be made using a Readiness to Change Ruler, much like a pain scale. This scaling strategy conceptualizes readiness or motivation to change along a continuum and asks patients to use a ruler with a 10-point scale, where 1 equals "definitely not ready to change" and 10 equals "definitely ready to change."

4. **Sharpen the focus.** The nurse can work with the patient to draw a table of costs and benefits of substance use or addiction and also to identify specific facilitators of and barriers to change. For example:

   "Over the past 2 months, you have been talking about stopping using crack, and it seems that just recently you have started to recognize that the fewer good things about using are outweighing the bad things. What is changing for you now that has you leaning toward stopping?"

5. **Identify ambivalence.** While identifying motivators is important, it is also important to address the fluctuation in motivation common in any behaviour change. Uncovering ambivalence and paradox can be achieved through statements that point out the contradictions in the patient's motivations for change. For example:

   "You have been continuing to engage in drinking binges, and yet you say that you want to get your driver's licence back and regain the trust of your parents."

6. **Elicit self-motivating statements.** This approach encourages the patient to state his or her own cognitive recognition of the problem, affective expression of concern, a direct intention toward change, and a sense of optimism. A *cognitive recognition of the problem* may be heard in a statement such as "I guess this is more serious than I thought." While a patient may have heard others express concern many times, self-recognition is a more powerful drive for change. An *affective expression of concern* about the perceived problem, such as "I'm really worried about what is happening to me," anchors the significance of the problem in the patient's own words. A *direct intention to change behaviour*—for example, "I've got to do something about this"—sets out a goal. Last, an expression of *optimism* about one's ability to change reinforces a sense of hope. A nurse may be able to elicit a statement of optimism by asking a patient what he or she can achieve in treatment. A patient may respond with "I know that if I try, I can really do it" or "I have maintained my sobriety for a long period of time before and know it is possible." The nurse can repeat these statements or have the patient write these statements down for future reference.

7. **Handle resistance.** There is a risk involved in recognizing the patient's resistance to change and inviting the patient to argue his or her case, but the nurse, nevertheless, should address resistance head-on and be ready to roll with the counterarguments. The patient may not be able to argue for ongoing change and motivation and may instead retreat to a previous phase of change. In that case, the nurse must be accepting and work with the patient to handle the resistance and the shifting phase of change. Handling resistance requires the nurse to ask questions about readiness and desire for change. The following questions provide examples of addressing the resistance honestly in the interview and reviewing motivation:

   "I know you have been coming to treatment for 2 months, but you are still drinking heavily. Maybe now is not the right time to change?"

   "So, it sounds as though you have a lot going on with trying to balance a career and family, and these priorities are competing with your treatment at this time."

8. **Shift focus and transition.** Through all phases of change, there will be times to illuminate a shift in focus or transition to a new phase of motivation. Making a declaration about such shifts allows the patient to hear your evaluation and to argue for whatever change is developing. One example of shifting focus for motivation is provided by the following long-term outpatient treatment scenario:

   "Your goal to be able to regain visitation of your son, coupled with your girlfriend leaving you because you continued to use crack, makes it easy to understand why you are now committed to not using crack anymore."

Source: Adapted from Sobell, L. C., & Sobell, M. B. (2008). *Motivational interviewing strategies and techniques: Rationales and examples.* Retrieved from http://www.nova.edu/gsc/forms/mi_rationale_techniques.pdf.

abuses him when drinking. He was picked up three times during the preceding 7 months for possession of cocaine.

Dialogue	Therapeutic Tool or Comment
Nurse: "I understand you entered the treatment program yesterday afternoon following your court appearance." **Kang:** "Yeah—it was my dad's idea."	Placing the event in time and sequence; validating the precipitating event
Nurse: "Well, what do you think of the idea?" **Kang:** "I don't like it. I don't need this place. I'm not a junkie—I just use crack … that's all. I can handle it."	Encouraging evaluation (actions first; thoughts; then feelings)
Nurse: "From what I've heard, your involvement with crack has gotten you into trouble." **Kang:** "Yeah, well, I guess I can't deny that … but I still don't think I need this place."	Pointing out realities
Nurse: "Are you saying that you don't think you need a treatment program?" **Kang:** "Well, I don't know. I guess maybe I am a little messed up."	Validating the patient's perception
Nurse: "'Messed up.'" **Kang:** "Yeah."	Restating
Nurse: "What is one thing about you that's messed up?" **Kang:** (silence) "I guess I feel like I don't belong anywhere."	Encouraging the patient to be specific rather than global
Nurse: "Talk more about that."	Clarifying

DIAGNOSIS

Formulation of appropriate nursing diagnoses depends on accurate assessment and screening. Whereas the criteria for medical diagnosis emphasize patterns of use and physical symptoms, nursing diagnoses identify how dependence on substances of abuse interferes with a person's ability to deal with the activities and demands of daily living. Nursing diagnoses for patients with psychoactive substance use disorders are many and varied because of the range of physical and psychological effects of drug abuse or dependence on people using these substances, as well as on their family. Concurrent disorders also need to be addressed. Potential nursing diagnoses for people with substance use disorders are listed in Table 18-12.

OUTCOMES IDENTIFICATION

Nursing Outcomes Classification (NOC) categories (Moorhead, Johnson, Maas, et al., 2012) for outcome criteria for patients

TABLE 18-12   POTENTIAL NURSING DIAGNOSES RELATED TO PSYCHOACTIVE SUBSTANCE USE

SIGNS AND SYMPTOMS	NURSING DIAGNOSES
Vomiting	*Imbalanced nutrition: less than body requirements*
Diarrhea	
Poor nutritional and fluid intake	*Deficient fluid volume*
Audiovisual hallucinations	*Disturbed thought processes*
Impaired judgement	*Disturbed sensory perception*
Memory deficits	
Cognitive impairments related to substance intoxication or withdrawal (e.g., deficits in problem solving, ability to attend to tasks, and grasp ideas)	
Changes in sleep–wake cycle (e.g., interference with stage 4 sleep, inability to sleep, long periods of sleeping related to effects of or withdrawal from substance)	*Disturbed sleep pattern*
Lack of self-care (hygiene, grooming, failure to care for basic health needs)	*Ineffective health maintenance* *Self-care deficit* *Noncompliance to health care regimen*
Feelings of hopelessness, inability to change	*Hopelessness* *Spiritual distress*
Feelings of worthlessness	*Situational low self-esteem*
Feeling that life has no meaning or future	*Chronic low self-esteem* *Risk for self-directed violence* *Risk for suicide*
Family crises and family pain	*Interrupted family processes*
Ineffective parenting	*Impaired parenting*
Emotional neglect of others	*Risk for other-directed violence*
Increased incidence of physical and sexual abuse of others	
Increased self-hate projected to others	
Excessive substance abuse affecting all areas of a person's life: loss of friends, poor job performance, increased illness rates, proneness to accidents and overdoses	*Ineffective coping* *Impaired verbal communication* *Social isolation* *Risk for loneliness* *Anxiety* *Risk for suicide*
Increased health problems related to substance used and route of use, as well as overdose	*Activity intolerance* *Ineffective airway clearance* *Ineffective breathing pattern* *Impaired oral mucous membrane* *Risk for infection* *Decreased cardiac output* *Sexual dysfunction*
Total preoccupation with (and majority of time consumed by) taking and withdrawing from drug	*Delayed growth and development* *Ineffective coping* *Impaired social interaction* *Dysfunctional family processes*

with substance use disorders can be divided into withdrawal, initial and active substance abuse treatment, and health maintenance. When the patient has a concurrent disorder, the nurse will also develop nursing outcomes for that mental health disorder. Specific *NOC* outcomes and examples of patient goals follow.

Withdrawal

Fluid balance: Patient's blood pressure will not be compromised.
Neurological status: Consciousness: Patient will have no seizure activity.
Distorted thought self-control: Patient will consistently describe content of hallucinations.

Initial and Active Substance Abuse Treatment

Risk control: Substance use: Patient will consistently demonstrate a commitment to substance use control strategies.
Risk control: Substance use: Patient will consistently acknowledge personal consequences associated with substance abuse.
Substance addiction consequences: Patient will demonstrate no difficulty supporting self financially.

Health Maintenance

Knowledge: Substance abuse control: Patient will describe actions to prevent and manage relapses in substance use.
Family coping: Family will consistently demonstrate care for the needs of all family members.

PLANNING

Planning care requires attention to the patient's social status, income, ethnic background, faith or religion, gender, age, substance use history, and current condition. Planning must also address the patient's major psychological, social, and medical problems, as well as the substance-using behaviour. Involvement of appropriate family members is also essential whenever possible.

Unfortunately, a person's social status and social relations often deteriorate as a result of addiction. Job demotion or loss of employment, with resultant reduced or nonexistent income, may occur. Meeting basic needs for food, shelter, and clothing is affected. Marriage and other close interpersonal relationships often deteriorate, and the patient is then left alone and isolated. A lack of interpersonal and social supports is a complicating factor in treatment planning for people experiencing addiction. Case Study and Nursing Care Plan 18-2 presents a discussion of a patient with concurrent alcohol dependence and depression.

IMPLEMENTATION

The aim of treatment is self-responsibility and motivation, not compliance with an imposed program. A major challenge is improving treatment effectiveness by matching subtypes of patients to specific types of treatment. Although those experiencing substance-related disorders may share some characteristics and dynamics, significant differences exist with regard to physiological, psychological, and sociocultural processes for all individuals.

Proposing abstinence as a treatment goal is safest for those with more than one substance use disorder. Abstinence is strongly related to good work adjustment, positive health status, comfortable interpersonal relationships, and general social stability. Often the choice of treatment or approach depends on the patient's needs, treatment goals, motivation, and personal circumstances, including family needs and financial resources. Outpatient programs work best for people with substance abuse disorders who are employed and have an active social support system. People who have no support and structure in their day may do better in inpatient or residential programs.

Beyond personal concerns and choice of treatment, neuropsychological deficits have been associated with long-term alcohol abuse and may affect treatment choices or potential benefits. Such deficits have been found in abstract reasoning ability, ability to use feedback in learning new concepts, attention and concentration spans, cognitive flexibility, and subtle memory functions. These cognitive impairments undoubtedly have an impact on the process of treatment for alcohol or other substance abuse.

At all levels of practice, the nurse can play an important role in the intervention process by recognizing the signs of substance abuse in both the patient and the family and by being familiar with the resources available to help with the problem. Approaches to treatment implementation, including substance abuse interventions, motivational interviewing, pharmacological interventions, and advanced-practice interventions, are discussed below, as are implementation strategies at all levels of prevention.

SUBSTANCE ABUSE INTERVENTIONS

Pharmacological Interventions

The predominant biological therapies are intended to support detoxification (management of withdrawal) or to alter drug use (methadone [Metadol], and naltrexone [ReVia]) (Csiernik, 2016).

Detoxification or Alcohol Withdrawal Treatment

Not all people who stop drinking require biological management of withdrawal. The decision to medicate depends on the duration and extent of substance use, the prior history of withdrawal complications, and overall health status. Medication should not be given until the symptoms of withdrawal are observable. Drugs that are useful in treating patients with alcohol withdrawal delirium are listed in Drug Treatment of Patients With Alcohol Withdrawal Delirium.

When the CIWA-Ar reading is abnormal or indicates severe withdrawal, it is likely that the patient is experiencing alcohol withdrawal delirium. In these instances, oral diazepam (Valium) may be useful in the symptomatic relief of acute agitation, tremor, impending or acute delirium tremens, and hallucinosis. Chlordiazepoxide (Librium) may keep your patient out of danger. However, once delirium appears, intravenous lorazepam (Ativan) is used to treat this severe symptom. Seclusion may be necessary. Dehydration, often exacerbated by diaphoresis and fever, can be corrected with oral or intravenous fluids.

DRUG TREATMENT OF PATIENTS WITH ALCOHOL WITHDRAWAL DELIRIUM

DRUG CLASS	SPECIFIC DRUGS	PURPOSE
Benzodiazepines	Chlordiazepoxide (Librax) Diazepam (Valium) (usually not recommended due to its short half-life and frequent dosing schedule) Lorazepam (Ativan)	Decrease withdrawal symptoms, stabilize vital signs, and prevent seizures and delirium tremens
α-adrenergic blockers	Clonidine (Catapres)	Reduce autonomic withdrawal symptoms

Source: Adapted from Lehne, R. E. (2014). *Pharmacology for nursing care* (9th ed.). Philadelphia: Saunders.

Acamprosate. Acamprosate (Campral) was approved by Health Canada in 2008 to treat people who had been alcohol dependent, had stopped drinking, and wished to remain abstinent. In randomized, double-blind, placebo-controlled trials, though without active comparators, acamprosate in conjunction with psychosocial therapy was generally significantly better than placebo plus psychosocial interventions in improving various key outcomes, including the proportion of patients who maintained complete abstinence from alcohol, the average duration of abstinence duration, and the total number of nondrinking days. Acamprosate is believed to effect a reduction in one's intake of alcohol through suppression of excitatory neurotransmission and enhanced inhibitory transmission (Lehne, 2014; Plosker, 2015).

Naltrexone. Naltrexone (ReVia), an agent used in reversing the effects of opioid addiction, is sometimes used in the treatment of alcohol dependency, especially for those with intense cravings and somatic symptoms. Naltrexone works by blocking opioid receptors, thereby interfering with the mechanism of reinforcement and reducing or eliminating the alcohol craving (Vuoristo-Myllys, Lipsanen, Lahti, et al., 2014). Long-acting injectable forms with the brand names Vivitrex or Vivitrol, Naltrel, and Depotrex are being tested and show promise as having relatively stable plasma levels, allowing for more sustained effects (Gordon, Kinlock, Vocci, et al., 2015; Knopf, 2016).

Topiramate. Similar to acamprosate, topiramate (Topamax) is purported to decrease alcohol cravings by inhibiting the release of mesocorticolimbic dopamine, which has been associated with alcohol craving. Currently topiramate is still not approved for use with alcohol-dependent persons, although preliminary findings indicate that it has a beneficial effect in individuals with a typology of craving characterized by drinking obsessions and automaticity of drinking (Guglielmo, Martinotti, Quatrale, et al., 2015).

Pharmacological Treatment of Opioid Addiction

Methadone. Methadone (Metadol) is a synthetic opioid that blocks the craving for and effects of opioids. It has to be taken every day, produces high physical and psychological dependency, and, when stopped, produces withdrawal symptoms that those

in withdrawal have equated to the pain of bone cancer at its peak. Therefore for methadone to be effective, the patient must take a dose at a prescribed level that will prevent withdrawal symptoms, block drug craving, and block any effects of illicit use of short-acting opioids.

Methadone inhibits ascending pain pathways and alters the perception of and response to pain, and although it has morphine-like actions and cross-tolerance, it does not produce euphoria for opioid users when given orally. This has led to its current primary use in substitution therapy for opioid-dependent individuals. However, tolerance and withdrawal do readily occur in methadone users, though their development is much slower than with other opioids. Methadone's side effects include weight gain, constipation, numbness in the extremities, and, for some, hallucinations when they first begin to use the substance.

Buprenorphine. Buprenorphine is a partial μ-opioid receptor agonist and, in combination with the opioid antagonist naloxone in a 4 : 1 ratio, is used as an alternative to methadone in opioid drug substitution. When this combination drug known as Suboxone is taken sublingually, it takes from 2 to 10 minutes to dissolve. Used in this manner, the naloxone exerts no clinically significant effect, leaving only the opioid agonist effects of buprenorphine. However, if a patient attempts to inject Suboxone, the opioid antagonism of naloxone causes the user to go into withdrawal. This nearly immediate physical response greatly reduces the abuse potential of the compound drug. Suboxone users report more clarity of thinking, greater confidence, and lower stigma compared to those using methadone. However, Suboxone, like methadone, produces physical dependency and, as with all opioid substances, can slow and even stop respiration, though it is less likely than methadone to produce an overdose (Orman & Keating, 2009; Tanner, Bordon, Conroy, et al., 2011).

Naltrexone. Naltrexone (ReVia) was originally developed as an opioid antagonist, and as a relatively pure antagonist, it blocks the euphoric effects of opioids well. It has low toxicity and few adverse effects and does not produce dependence, as it is not a psychoactive substance itself. A single dose provides an effective opioid blockade for up to 72 hours. Taking naltrexone three times a week is sufficient to maintain a fairly high level of opioid blockade. For many patients, long-term use results in gradual extinction of cravings.

Clonidine. Clonidine (Catapres) was initially marketed for high blood pressure, but it was also found to be an effective somatic treatment, combined with naltrexone, for some chemical-dependent individuals. Clonidine is a nonopioid suppresser of opioid withdrawal symptoms and as such does not produce physical dependency when used regularly. A Cochrane review found clonidine to be more effective than placebo for the management of withdrawal from heroin or methadone, though methadone is associated with fewer adverse effects than clonidine (Gowing, Farrell, Ali, et al., 2014).

Pharmacological Treatment of Nicotine Addiction

A variety of mechanisms have been introduced to assist individuals to stop smoking, as nicotine produces more lapse and relapse than any other psychoactive agent. One drug substitution approach is a transdermal therapeutic system, or the skin patch.

Looking like a small adhesive bandage, the patch uses a rate-controlling membrane to deliver nicotine via the surface layers of the skin to the bloodstream. A fresh patch is applied once a day to a clean, dry, hair-free area of skin on the upper body or upper arms. For most users, the initial 21 mg/day dosage is used every day for 6 weeks, then is replaced by a 14 mg/day patch for 2 weeks, which in turn is replaced by a 7 mg/day patch for the final 2 weeks of the 10-week treatment program. Clinical studies have indicated greater success with nicotine patches than with placebo control groups, though participants in both groups had members who continued to smoke not only after but also during the trials. The continuation of smoking while using the patches remains a concern with this method of drug substitution, as users can give themselves adverse health effects due to experiencing peak nicotine levels higher than those experienced from smoking alone. Transdermal administration of nicotine doubles long-term tobacco abstinence rates. The nicotine patch is preferred over nicotine gum because compliance with the treatment regimen is better, blood levels are steadier, long-term dependence seldom occurs, and instructions are less complicated. However, this treatment option is also not recommended for use by persons with heart disease, hyperthyroidism, insulin-dependent diabetes, hypertension, or peptic ulcers (Hass, 2011; Tsilajara, Noda, & Saku, 2010).

A controversial new alternative to smoking cigarettes are e-cigarettes, or vaping. Electronic cigarettes contain a battery and an electronic device that produces a vapour when a cartridge containing nicotine and often propylene glycol and some flavouring additive is added. Cartridges can be refilled with different flavours and nicotine concentrations from 0% to 24%. E-cigarettes still contain some carcinogens, including nitrosamines, toxic chemicals such as diethylene glycol, and tobacco-specific components that are harmful to humans. E-cigarettes deliver nicotine to the blood more rapidly than nicotine inhalers but less rapidly than cigarettes. Presently much still needs to be learned about these devices, and their use as an option in nicotine replacement therapy and smoking cessation is undetermined (Callahan-Lyon, 2014).

There are also pharmacological nicotine replacement options, the most prominent being varenicline (Chantix/Champix), a nicotine receptor partial agonist that affects the CNS to reduce cravings and withdrawal symptom by weakly stimulating nicotine receptors. A meta-analysis found varenicline to be twice as effective as the nicotine patch and more than two thirds as likely to assist a person to stop smoking than using nicotine gum (Cahill, Stevens, Perera, et al., 2013). Varenicline nicotine-replacement therapy has proven to be a successful smoking cessation treatment for many individuals, though there remain some lingering concerns, which do not appear to be valid, that it can produce suicidal ideation and action in users (Niaura, 2015).

Implementation at Primary, Secondary, and Tertiary Levels of Prevention

Primary Prevention

Prevention models in health care are classified as primary, secondary, and tertiary. In terms of substance use and addiction prevention, primary approaches are those efforts focused on reducing the demand for a substance or behaviour, as well as stopping the occurrence of alcohol or drug use or abuse. Examples include implementing healthy public policy, offering health education related to addiction, taxing and health-related warning labelling of licit products such as cigarettes and alcohol, and promoting educational campaigns such as addiction and mental health in the workplace.

Secondary Prevention

Secondary prevention seeks to limit further health deterioration and social harm from the use of, abuse of, dependence on, and addiction to substances and behaviours. Examples include programs of early recognition, awareness campaigns, relapse prevention, community support approaches, and strategies for safe prescribing guidelines. Most prominent and most controversial among secondary prevention approaches is harm reduction.

Harm reduction. Harm reduction refers to a range of programs, policies, and interventions designed to reduce or minimize the adverse consequences associated with drug use, such as overdose, infections, and spread of communicable diseases. It is officially one of the four pillars of Canada's drug plan entailing any strategy or behaviour that an individual uses to reduce the potential harm that may exist for him or her. Seven prominent forms of harm reduction programming are reviewed below.

Needle exchange programs. Needle exchange programs allow injection drug users (IDUs) to trade used syringes for new, sterile syringes and related injection equipment, although in recent years many of these fixed and mobile outreach programs have also begun to offer crack pipes and straws for cocaine use. Needle exchange is a harm reduction strategy that arose as a direct result of the bloodborne infections of HIV, hepatitis C virus (HCV), and hepatitis B virus (HBV) that were an unintended outcome of injection drug use. However, this is not only a form of intervention for IDUs but also part of a broader public health model, as funding for these initiatives occurs so as to limit the transfer of these diseases into the general populace.

Methadone treatment and methadone maintenance. Both methadone maintenance (MM) and methadone treatment (MT) consist of an individual drinking a sufficient dose of liquid methadone on a daily basis to eliminate withdrawal symptoms from other opioids. The basic premise of opioid substitution therapy is that a methadone administered daily by mouth is effective in the suppression of withdrawal symptoms and in the reduction of the use of illicit opioids. MM involves determining a correct dose for each individual and providing regular health care and treatment for other addiction issues, while MT programs also entail the provision of counselling and support, mental health services, health promotion, disease prevention and education, along with advocacy and links to community-based supports and services such as housing. As discussed earlier, Suboxone can be used in a similar manner as methadone.

Heroin assisted treatment (HAT). Some individuals do not respond well to methadone or Suboxone, as it may not ease the physical or psychological pain of withdrawal, it may not negate the craving, or an individual may have a negative reaction to the synthetic nature of the drug. Historically, these individuals were forced to endure a painful withdrawal process that would often lead to relapse. This typically led to a return to using street heroin and thus continuing to put themselves at risk for life-threatening health issues, including drug overdoses, blood-borne viral infections, and endocarditis, as well as the violence that accompanies illicit drug transactions. Under a HAT protocol, street heroin users are prescribed pharmaceutical-quality heroin, which is injected in safe, clean specialized medical clinics. In 2005, a randomized controlled trial was funded by the Canadian Institutes of Health Research. The North American Opiate Medication Initiative (NAOMI) was conducted in Vancouver and Montreal to evaluate the feasibility and effectiveness of HAT in Canada. The results of the drug trial found that participants were less likely to use street drugs than those in an MM program and were also less likely to engage in criminal activity, increasing the likelihood of an eventual move toward abstinence (Nosyk, Geller, Guh, et al., 2010).

Supervised injection sites (SISs). Supervised injection sites offer a safe place that drug-dependent individuals can access to inject drugs under the supervision of trained multidisciplinary health and social services staff who can provide education regarding safer injection practices, as well as respond appropriately in the event of an overdose. Typically, needles, syringes, candles, sterile water, paper towels, cotton balls, cookers or spoons, ties, alcohol swabs, filters, ascorbic acid, and bandages are available in the injection areas. SISs allow IDUs to have their privacy, while also offering the comfort of knowing that trained medical staff are available to respond in case of an emergency. SISs do not allow the sharing of drugs or equipment and prohibit assisted injection. This approach has been demonstrated to decrease new HIV and HCV infections and reduce the number of overdose-related deaths while providing access to primary and emergency health care for a traditionally oppressed population.

Controlled drinking. Controlled drinking is an adapted behavioural technique used with persons experiencing low levels of alcohol abuse. Assessment of the client's level of alcohol dependence is necessary to determine if a goal of controlled drinking is feasible. This approach proposes that training in drinking skills is required to teach alcohol misusers to drink in a nonabusive manner as an alternative to abstinence as part of a more broad-based treatment program. The first step in controlled drinking is determining whether a client is a problem drinker or an alcohol-dependent individual. This is accomplished by imposing a 2- to 3-week period of abstinence. If the person can go without drinking, she or he is moved into the next phase. Those who cannot abstain during this baseline period generally do not qualify for a controlled drinking treatment program. In the program itself, clients are provided with a set of goals and rules to help them control their alcohol intake. A common drinking goal of a set number of standard drinks per week is established, with numerous limitations. For a young healthy male approximately 6 feet tall and 180 pounds, the following regimen might be applied:

- No more than two standard drinks per day (one for women)
- No more than one drink per hour
- Sip drinks and avoid carbonated beverages
- Drink only on a full stomach

- Two days per week must be set aside on which no alcohol is consumed
- Limit weekly intake to 14 standard drinks per week (seven for women).

Managed alcohol programs (MAPs). The primary purpose of managed alcohol programs is to offer continuing health and housing services for individuals who have a history of homelessness and alcohol abuse along with chronic health issues and are in many cases deemed to be near the end of their lives. The aim is to provide humane treatment and reduce harm to the clients by eliminating the need to binge drink and to drink nonbeverage alcohol products. Nursing, medical, and rehabilitation care are provided along with a regular, limited amount of alcohol. MAPs' goal is to provide their residents with permanent rather than transient housing, and in this way it falls into the Housing First philosophy. Some MAPs offer private rooms, though the standard is shared accommodation with all programs being staffed 24 hours per day. Care plans are individualized and typically include a recreational component. The overall goal is to improve the quality of life of clients while allowing them to live in a respectful, supportive environment. General strategies for relapse prevention are cognitive and behavioural: recognizing and learning how to avoid or cope with threats to recovery, changing lifestyle, learning how to participate in activities without drugs, and securing help from other people or from social support services.

Relapse prevention and aftercare. Relapse prevention is the process that occurs after formal treatment. The goal is to help prevent individuals who had been addicted from returning to drug use once they have stopped. Relapse to previous psychoactive drug use during recovery is quite common, to the point that the TTM distinguishes between lapse, a brief return or slip, and relapse, a continuing use of the drug after cessation. Relapse prevention aims to help the individual learn from periods of lapse and relapse so that periods of sobriety can be lengthened over time and triggers leading to returning to drug use can be avoided or addressed. Lapses and relapses therefore are not viewed as failures but rather as learning opportunities to assist efforts toward change. Relapse prevention entails supporting the patient post-treatment and monitoring progress so that if an issue does arise, an appropriate referral can be quickly made. Relapse prevention programs also offer patients contacts and a support system after treatment so that an early intervention can be made in the event of a lapse or relapse. The actual length of the follow-up period will vary in terms of how often contact is made and for how long contact is kept, with the most significant restriction being staff resources. A minimally acceptable aftercare program would involve a monthly contact for 1 year, with the provision that the patient can contact the relapse prevention worker whenever needed. Box 18-4 outlines relapse prevention strategies that are of value in a nursing environment. Alcoholics Anonymous and related 12-step groups are a self-help format that also serves as an ongoing relapse prevention support system.

Alcoholics Anonymous (AA) is the prototype for all addiction-related mutual aid self-help programs. Beginning with two members in 1935, it has grown into a global movement premised

BOX 18-4 RELAPSE PREVENTION STRATEGIES

Basics

It is important to keep the program simple at first. Remember that 40% to 50% of patients who abuse substances have mild to moderate cognitive problems while actively using substances. Providing prompts and assistance for the patient's recall may be beneficial. For example:

- Reviewing instructions from health team members
- Encouraging use of a notebook to write down important information, appointments, schedules, and telephone numbers

Skills

Patients may take advantage of cognitive behavioural therapy to increase their coping skills. The patient can identify which important life skills are needed by inquiring about the following:

- Which situations are challenging and stress-producing?
- What situations command new skills or abilities?
- What abilities and skills are currently strong?

Enhancement of Personal Insight

Counselling can help a patient gain insight and control over a variety of psychological concerns. For example:

- What triggers the use or addiction?
- What constitutes a healthy, supportive relationship?
- How can self-esteem, self-worth, and coping be strengthened?
- What does the addiction offer that would be difficult to give up? What would be the loss without the use or addiction? What could replace the loss?

Relapse Prevention Groups

Support membership in a relapse prevention group. These groups help patients work on the following:

- Rehearsing stressful situations using a variety of techniques
- Finding ways to deal with current problems or ones that are likely to arise without the drugs, alcohol, or behavioural addiction
- Providing role models to support change

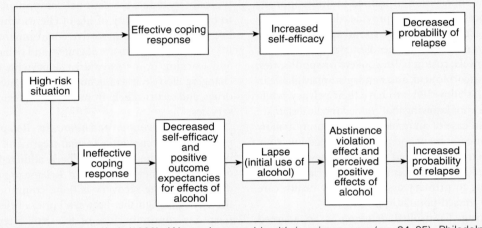

Adapted from Zerbe, K. J. (1999). *Women's mental health in primary care* (pp. 94–95). Philadelphia: Saunders

Source: Adapted from Zerbe, K. J. (1999). *Women's mental health in primary care* (pp. 94–95). Philadelphia: Saunders.

on 12 steps to recovery (Box 18-5). These programs offer properly matched individuals a behavioural, cognitive, and dynamic structure to assist in maintaining their abstinence. Three basic concepts are fundamental to all 12-step programs:

1. Individuals with an addiction are powerless over their addiction, which is no longer conceptualized as a moral failing but rather as a disease, and their lives are unmanageable because of their addiction.
2. Although individuals with an addiction are not responsible for their disease, they are responsible for their recovery.
3. Individuals can no longer blame people, places, and things for their addiction; they must face their problems and their feelings and do so in conjunction with a Higher Power.

Before referring any patient to any mutual aid group, a nurse should attend an open meeting to learn what occurs there and how the fellowship functions in order to facilitate a proper referral. While AA and related groups such as Narcotics Anonymous and Cocaine Anonymous are welcoming resources, they are not a good fit for all patients, and mismatched individuals can be discouraged

from seeking professional treatment if they do not find AA of value to them. However, there are now other options that have arisen in response to the organizational and structural limits of AA that are available both in person and online, including Buddhist Recovery Network (www.buddhistrecovery.org), Millati Islami World Servies (www.millatiislami.org), Moderation Management (www.moderation.org), Rational Recovery (www.rational.org), Secular Organization for Sobriety (www.sossobriety.org), Smart Recovery (www.smartrecovery.org), and Women for Sobriety (www.womenforsobriety.org).

Self-help groups for patient and family or friends. Counselling and support should be encouraged for all family and friends of a person experiencing problems with alcohol, other substance use, or addictions. Al-Anon and Al-ateen are self-help groups that offer support and guidance for adults and teenagers, respectively. Self-help groups assist family members and friends in dealing with many common issues. Their work is based on a combination of educational and operational principles centred on acceptance of the disease model of addiction, including

CASE STUDY 18-1

Bill, a 20-year-old single man, was brought to the emergency department after having been found unconscious in his room at home. He was accompanied by his mother, with whom he shares a small apartment. When his mother was not able to rouse him, she dialled 911 for an ambulance. A syringe and some white powder were found next to Bill.

On admission, Bill had laboured breathing, and his pupils were constricted. Vital signs were taken; his blood pressure was 60/40 mm Hg, and his pulse was 132 beats per minute. Bill's situation was determined to be life threatening. Although extremely distressed, Bill's mother was able to report to the staff that Bill had a substance abuse problem and had been injecting heroin for 6 months before recently entering a methadone maintenance program 1 year ago. It was decided at this point to administer an opioid antagonist, and naloxone was given intramuscularly. Bill's breathing improved, and he was able to respond to verbal stimuli. Bill's mother later told staff that Bill had not been attending his methadone maintenance program for the past week. At the staff's urging, she called the program, and an outreach worker, Sylvain, arranged to talk to her and Bill at the hospital. Bill made an appointment to follow up with Sylvain at the methadone clinic on the following Monday. Sylvain recognized that Bill's future would ultimately depend on Bill's own actions but that he could offer some motivation and guide Bill's insight.

On Monday, Sylvain spoke with Bill about his situation, what changes he wanted for himself, his drug use, some of the factors that led him to lapse, and what Bill thought he might need in order to get back into recovery. Bill stated, "I know I can do it if I can concentrate on health and life. If I lose that concentration, it just is old habit to use again. I can see how I slipped off track." Their interaction included the following exchange:

Dialogue	Therapeutic Tool or Comment
Sylvain: "I was in the emergency department Friday afternoon when you were brought in by ambulance."	Placing the event in time and sequence, validating the precipitating event
Bill: "Were you? I guess a lot of people thought it was over for me."	
Sylvain: "It certainly looked quite serious."	Emphasizing the reality—prevents minimizing the situation
Bill: "Yeah. I should never have left the program. I was doing better, and I just didn't think I needed it anymore."	
Sylvain: "You said you were doing well."	Reflecting
Bill: "Yeah. I had a job, and I was beginning to save some money. Wow! I can't believe I blew this whole thing."	
Sylvain: "I don't know that you really did, it was just one slip and you already seem motivated to keep trying. Your counsellor in the program phoned your doctor this morning to find out how you were doing."	Pointing out reality
Bill: "Do you think they'll take me back?"	
Sylvain: "Why don't we talk some more, and after we finish, I'll speak with the other staff about your situation. If you would like to get back into the program, you can call your counsellor, and we'll support your decision."	Gathering information Supporting decision making

Sylvain and Bill agreed to continue to meet regularly, and while it took several months, Bill stopped using heroin; switched to using Suboxone, as he found the side effects less harsh; and was able to find employment in construction. Bill appears motivated, as he has moved into a methadone treatment program that uses motivational interviewing and is now regularly attending a weekly relapse prevention group. Bill reports that being clear headed and not having to always think about getting and using the drug is worth the time and concentration.

---

pragmatic methods for avoiding enabling behaviours. However, they are not a replacement for, but rather an adjunct to, family counselling, especially in situations where the patient is not ready yet to commit to changing but where the family needs support.

Tertiary Prevention

Tertiary prevention is concerned with limiting and reducing complications and dysfunction related to the experience of addiction. Effective care, treatment, and rehabilitation programs and services are characteristic of tertiary prevention approaches. Specialized addiction detoxification programs, recovery programs, and concurrent disorder programs are examples of tertiary-level services.

Assessment and referral. Once an individual has been identified as having a substance abuse problem, the depth and breadth of the situation needs to be determined. Assessment and referral agencies provide services that use specific instruments and processes to determine the major issues as well as the strengths and supports of the person with a substance issue. These agencies develop individualized plans for assistance, which may entail referral to other organizations for more intensive or residential treatment. A standardized assessment procedure can take anywhere from 2 to 3 hours to complete, typically including a history of the use of alcohol and other drugs, including age of onset, duration, patterns, consequences of use, use of alcohol and drugs by family members, and types of and responses to previous treatment initiatives. It is also recommended that assessments determine a client's physical health, environmental supports (including partner and family), accommodation, employment (if employed), school status (if attending school), leisure activities, legal problems, sexual orientation, gender identification, and any history of sexual or other physical abuse or trauma. It is

BOX 18-5 THE 12-STEPS OF ALCOHOLICS ANONYMOUS

1. We admitted we were powerless over alcohol—that our lives had become unmanageable.
2. Came to believe that a Power greater than ourselves could restore us to sanity.
3. Made a decision to turn our will and our lives over to the care of God as we understood Him.
4. Made a searching and fearless moral inventory of ourselves.
5. Admitted to God, to ourselves, and to another human being the exact nature of our wrongs.
6. Were entirely ready to have God remove all these defects of character.
7. Humbly asked Him to remove our shortcomings.
8. Made a list of all persons we had harmed and became willing to make amends to them all.
9. Made direct amends to such people wherever possible, except when to do so would injure them or others.
10. Continued to take personal inventory and when we were wrong, promptly admitted it.
11. Sought through prayer and meditation to improve our conscious contact with God as we understood Him, praying only for knowledge of His will for us and the power to carry that out.
12. Having had a spiritual awakening as the result of these steps, we tried to carry this message to alcoholics and to practise these principles in all our affairs.

BOX 18-6 REIS TYPOLOGY

MI HIGH SEVERITY, SUD HIGH SEVERITY	MI LOW SEVERITY, SUD HIGH SEVERITY
Serious and persistent mental illness with substance dependence Service: Integrated care	Psychiatrically complicated substance dependence Service: Collaboration
MI HIGH SEVERITY, SUD LOW SEVERITY	**MI LOW SEVERITY, SUD LOW SEVERITY**
Serious and persistent mental illness with substance abuse Service: Collaboration	Mild psychopathology with substance abuse Service: Consultation

MI, Mental illness; *SUD*, substance use disorder.

also essential to initially assess the level and intensity of withdrawal management and stabilization services required. This systematic process must also identify the client's strengths and take into consideration what the client actually wants.

Withdrawal management services: daytox and detox. Withdrawal management or detoxification services are often a first step in the treatment process. This entails total abstinence from not only the drug of misuse but also often all other drugs, including, in some facilities, tobacco. The detoxification process should be of sufficient length to allow all of the psychoactive drugs to be eliminated by the body. A client's safety is the first priority of all withdrawal management staff, though once an individual becomes more stable, staff also typically offer social and environmental support during the stay, including referrals to mutual aid groups.

Community-based (outpatient) treatment. This is treatment provided on a nonresidential basis, usually in regularly scheduled sessions of 1 to 2 hours per week but sometimes two times per week. Treatment may entail individual and/or group sessions to explore all aspects of the person's substance abuse and related problems. Sessions offer information and strategies to assist each individual in her or his recovery process. This is the least intense and intrusive treatment intervention option, primarily offered by nonmedical, community-based counselling agencies. Appropriate matches for this service include clients who:

- Are free of any significant medical problem
- Are self-motivated

- Have a support system in place, including family, friends, or work
- Live within easy access to the facility
- Have not yet had their personal or work life extensively affected by their substance use

Day treatment. This is a more intensive, structured nonresidential treatment, typically provided 5 days per week or alternatively 4 or 5 evenings per week for 3 to 4 hours per session. Treatment involves group activities ranging from formal group treatment sessions, to education groups, to recreational activities. As clients are at home on weekends, evenings, and days, the home environment must be stable, with support from family and friends. This treatment option allows the social aspect of addiction to be acknowledged and addressed early in the treatment process. Day treatment is appropriate for individuals who are able to maintain social competence despite their dependency.

Concurrent disorder programs. Another specialized form of community-based counselling entails work done by agencies whose clients have both an addiction and a mental health issue. Services offered by institutional and community-based psychologists, psychiatrists, social workers, and nurses have long been a part of the extended continuum of care, but traditionally these helping professionals dealt with either the mental health issue or the addiction issue alone, rarely the two together. Concurrent disorder programs move beyond working only with the addiction issue and provide counselling that also addresses issues such as depression, loneliness, suicidal ideation and attempts, paranoia, and violent behaviours. Whether these behaviours are primary or secondary to the use of psychoactive agents is no longer an issue; rather, the mental health problems are categorized as coexisting with the drug misuse or abuse, and vice versa, and thus intervention focuses on both. The Reis Typology (Box 18-6) is used to determine the best service for a client with concurrent disorder (Minkoff, 2005; Skinner, 2005).

Consultation refers to a process that involves informal links between mental health and addiction service personnel, along with additional human services as may be needed for the client. Rather than separate services, the plan is coordinated and facilitated through consultation and acceptance of the role of each service. This may involve parallel or sequential plans. Parallel service is the simultaneous treatment existing or acting together at the same time, whereas sequential service occurs when one treatment follows the other treatment through a referral to another agency or a specialized unit.

Collaboration refers to formal links between mental health and addiction service personnel who work together to develop and implement a recovery plan. This may involve sequential or parallel planning with the client.

Integration refers to the provision of addiction and mental health services in a single treatment setting to meet the often multiple and high needs of the client. In an integrated service, mental health and substance abuse treatments are brought together by the same clinicians in the same program, to ensure that the individual receives a consistent explanation of illness or problems and a coherent prescription for treatment rather than a contradictory set of messages from different providers.

Short-term residential treatment. These programs run for 18 to 28 days, can be sex specific or co-ed, and offer a wide variety of services, including medical evaluation, assessment of the extent of the drug dependency, detoxification in some facilities, individual and group counselling, drug education, spiritual guidance, family involvement, vocational guidance, and even employer involvement. The centres provide a safe, relatively stress-free environment in which the person can recover from the physical and emotional effects of prolonged substance abuse. Planning for rehabilitation upon return to the natural environment is also typically part of the process. Education on the effects of drugs varies between programs, but usually includes the short- and long-term effects of drug use physiologically, socially, spiritually, and psychologically. Often attendance at a 12-step group is either recommended or mandated, even in programs not premised on the philosophy of Alcoholics Anonymous.

Recovery homes. For many struggling with ongoing issues in their recovery, the ability to avoid a relapse is often jeopardized by untenable housing or unsupportive living environments. Recovery residences, also called social model recovery or sober living houses, are designed to provide safe and supportive housing to help individuals initiate and sustain recovery primarily through peer-to-peer interactions guided by staff who themselves have recovery histories. They are gender-specific, residential programs in which the goal is to provide a safe, supportive, therapeutic program of addiction education and life skills counselling. They provide an array of services to individuals with addiction problems within a structured environment either before or after the person has attended a withdrawal management program or has received more intensive treatment through the auspices of a short-term residential program.

Alternative living environment. For many persons with a substance abuse problem, the environment they live in is counterproductive to their successful treatment and recovery. These persons have unstable home lives or no support from family and friends who themselves are not regular substance users. Others come into treatment having no real home, having no role models for healthy living, or needing to relearn or learn socialization skills. Alternative living environments or therapeutic communities provide a protective living environment for people whose substance abuse is not an isolated problem but a major disruption of their entire life. These programs help in setting limits and defining behaviour while satisfying daily needs and desires in a quasi-home setting. Relationships that develop provide a basis on which the members can build the learning or relearning of living with others. Real-life issues of daily existence take precedence at these facilities. Many alternative living settings are affiliated with a religious order, the most prominent being the Salvation Army.

Addiction supportive housing (ASH). Addiction supportive housing programs are another component of the treatment continuum that recognizes the importance of safe and sustainable housing in the recovery process. This resource is part of the Housing First initiative and, while still limited, it provides longer support in a therapeutic environment than do short-term residential programs or recovery homes. The goal is to encourage program participants to develop long-term skills that are necessary to maintain one's own residence. By providing housing supports, ideally in conjunction with but not contingent on addiction treatment, service providers can increase the probability that someone who is marginally housed or homeless will follow through with addiction treatment.

Onen'tó:kon Healing Lodge: an Indigenous treatment approach. The Onen'tó:kon Healing Lodge situated in the Mohawk community of Kanehsatake is one of 59 specialized Indigenous treatment programs in Canada. The 6-week residential program takes a cultural perspective on treatment, including talking and healing circles. Not only is the chemical dependency addressed, but the specific issues that the client identifies, such as anger, resentment, grief, abuse, and low self-esteem, are addressed as well. Talking circles are a variant of group therapy where a person speaks about the issues that are causing pain. The other members of the circle provide individual feedback and confront behaviours that are not helpful in the individual's recovery program. However, healing circles are conducted without confrontation unless an individual behaves in a manner that is disruptive.

Individuals may choose to smudge prior to joining the circle. The act of smudging has a deeply spiritual significance for most Indigenous peoples. The smoke from sage is used to cleanse oneself of evil spirits, and the smoke from sweet grass is used to invite positive influences to help the individual engage in the event in a more positive, integrated, spiritual way that respects the Creator, ancestors, and other participants. People use smudging to find calmness from negative feelings by using the medicines of sweet grass, sage, and cedar. Sweet grass braids and sage are available for people who smudge as a way of communicating with the Creator. Sweat lodges are also available for people who want to do a sweat during the week that they complete treatment. A sweat takes place in an enclosure with hot rocks where people can pray to their higher power. The sweat is used as a healing circle, a peaceful and calm place. It is a safe place to let go of issues.

During the fifth week of a person's treatment program at Onen'tó:kon, an "affirmation circle" takes place in one of the talking circles. Each individual is placed in the centre of the circle, and the other circle members whisper words of affirmation in his or her ear, such as "I am so happy that you were born," "I love you," "You are so special," "You are precious to me," and "I am so proud of you." This activity has a profound effect on the client because for some it may be the first time someone has said those positive words to him or her. The treatment program is geared toward helping people rid themselves of negative thinking and negative "self-talk."

At the conclusion of the 6-week residential treatment program there is a graduation ceremony at which individuals obtain certificates of achievement. This is a very important occasion when the participants' loved ones and friends are invited to help in celebrating each person's accomplishment. The graduates usually feel great pride in having completed the treatment program, as for some it is the first time they have completed something that they have started. During the ceremony, graduates participate through drumming, through singing, and in a greeting circle. The leader starts the greeting with the graduates and continues on to the guests and staff members. The circle gives each individual an opportunity to say the words that need saying, face to face, because those in the circle may not cross paths again (Brownbill & Etienne, 2017).

CASE STUDY AND NURSING CARE PLAN 18-2

Alcohol Dependence With Depression

Mr. Steriovski, age 49 years, and his wife arrive in the emergency department one evening, fearful that he has had a stroke. His right hand is limp, he is unable to hyperextend his right wrist, and sensation to the fingertips in the hand is impaired.

Mr. Steriovski looks much older than his stated age; in fact, he looks about 65. His complexion is ruddy and flushed. History taking is difficult. Mr. Steriovski answers only what is asked of him, volunteering no additional information. He states that he took a nap that afternoon, and when he awakened, he noticed the problems with his right arm.

Ms. Winkler, the admitting nurse, begins the assessment. Mr. Steriovski reveals that he has been unemployed for 4 years because the company he worked for went bankrupt. He has been unable to find a new job but has a job interview in 10 days. His wife is now working full time, so the family finances are stable but less than they were used to when he was employed. They have two grown children who no longer live at home. As he relates this information, his lips momentarily start to tremble and his eyes fill with tears.

Mr. Steriovski does not acknowledge any significant medical illness except for high blood pressure, just diagnosed last year. His father has a history of depression, and his mother has a substance abuse issue but has been abstinent for many years. Ms. Winkler shares with him the fact that depression and alcohol dependency run in families. She asks Mr. Steriovski (1) whether he knows this and (2) whether it concerns him with regard to his own drinking. He says that he knows and that he does not want to think about it.

Ms. Winkler speaks separately with Mrs. Steriovski and asks if there is anything she would like to add. Mrs. Steriovski's shoulders slump; she sighs and says, "I have spent the entire day talking to a counsellor at the local treatment centre to see if I can have him properly assessed. He won't admit that he has a problem." Mrs. Steriovski recounts a 6-year history of steadily increasing alcohol use. She says that she could not admit to herself until now that her husband was an excessive drinker. "He tried to hide it, but gradually I knew. I could tell from little changes that he was intoxicated. I couldn't believe it was happening because he had been through the same thing with his mother. I thought I knew him. Actually, I guess I did when he was working. Being unemployed and unable to find a job has really devastated him. And now he's going to job interviews intoxicated."

She describes her feelings, which are like an emotional roller coaster—elated and hopeful when he seems to be doing okay; dejected and desperate when he loses control. Mrs. Steriovski hates going to work for fear of what her husband might do while she is gone. She says she is terrified that one day he will get into a car wreck and kill himself, because he often drives when intoxicated. He tells her not to worry, because the life insurance policy is paid up.

Meanwhile, the physician in the emergency department has examined Mr. Steriovski. The diagnosis is radial nerve palsy. Mr. Steriovski most likely passed out while lying on his arm. Because he was intoxicated, he did not feel the signals that his nerves sent out to warn him to move (numbness, tingling). He was in this position for so long that the resultant cutoff of circulation was sufficient to cause some temporary nerve damage.

Mr. Steriovski's blood alcohol level (BAL) is 0.15%—nearly twice the legal limit (0.08%) for intoxication in Canada. Even though he has a high BAL, Mr. Steriovski is alert and oriented, not slurring his speech or giving any other outward signs of intoxication. The difference between Mr. Steriovski's BAL and his behaviour indicates the development of tolerance, a symptom of physical dependence.

ASSESSMENT

Self-Awareness

Ms. Winkler has developed capacity and skills in working with people who abuse alcohol. She grew up in a home in which alcohol transformed her father from a caring and responsible parent to one who was physically and verbally abusive to his wife and children. He eventually lost his job and left home. Ms. Winkler was determined to be everything he was not and firmly resolved never to drink or use drugs.

As a new nurse, Ms. Winkler became extremely frustrated and angry with patients like Mr. Steriovski and found herself being overly protective of the patient's family. At the end of a particular day on which she had to work with yet another intoxicated patient, she felt drained, depressed, and despondent. It became such a problem that she knew she needed to either leave her job or deal with the dynamics underlying her responses. She began to attend the support group Al-Anon. There, she was able to talk about her feelings with others who had similar backgrounds. Ms. Winkler was also provided with tools for dealing with her feelings and gained a greater understanding of the pathology behind alcohol abuse.

CASE STUDY AND NURSING CARE PLAN 18-2—cont'd

Alcohol Dependence With Depression

As Ms. Winkler approaches her work with the Steriovski family, she does so with new confidence. She feels empathy and understanding for Mrs. Steriovski, but she is able to maintain emotional boundaries and does not feel drained by their interactions. While she still feels a little frustration with Mr. Steriovski, she recognizes these feelings and focuses on him as a person with a serious disorder.

Ms. Winkler organizes her data into objective and subjective components.

Objective Data	Subjective Data
Driving when intoxicated	Precontemplative with regards to alcohol problem
Covert references to death	Precontemplative with regards to depression
Nerve damage from passing out while lying on arm	
Increased alcohol use since becoming unemployed	
Ability to find employment impaired by alcohol use	
Disruption in marital relationship because of alcohol use	
Inability to see effects of his drinking	
Family history of alcoholism and depression	
BAL twice the legal limit of intoxication; has developed tolerance	

DIAGNOSIS

From the data, the nurse formulates the following nursing diagnoses:

1. *Risk for suicide* related to depressed mood

Supporting Data
- Dangerous behaviour: driving when drinking
- Full payment of life insurance policy

2. *Ineffective coping* related to alcohol use

Supporting Data
- Increased alcohol use during stressful period of unemployment
- Impairment in capacity to obtain employment caused by alcohol use
- Disruption in marital relationship because of alcohol use
- Inability to see effect of his drinking on his life functioning

OUTCOMES IDENTIFICATION

1. The patient will refrain from attempting suicide.
2. The patient will report increase in psychological comfort.

PLANNING

The initial plan is to allow Mr. Steriovski to remain in the emergency department until his blood alcohol level drops to 0.0% in order to discuss his goals. Once he is no longer impaired, the nurse will establish realistic outcomes with him. The risk is that his tolerance has become so substantive he can only function when there is some degree of alcohol in his system. Thus Mr. Steriovski's withdrawal needs to be carefully monitored and managed as per the Clinical Institute Withdrawal Assessment for Alcohol (CIWA-Ar) protocol.

IMPLEMENTATION

Mr. Steriovski's plan of care is personalized as follows:

1. **Nursing diagnosis:** *Risk for suicide*
   Outcome: Patient will consistently demonstrate suicide self-restraint.

Short-Term Goal	Intervention	Rationale	Evaluation
1. Patient will seek treatment for depression from a community mental health care provider.	1a. Determine presence and degree of suicidal risk. 1b. Refer patient to mental health care provider for evaluation and treatment.	1a. Risk for suicide is increased in substance-using patients. 1b. Addressing both substance use and mental health treatment needs improves outcomes.	**Goal Met** After 3 weeks, patient attends appointment at Canadian Mental Health Association and has started taking an antidepressant.

Continued

CASE STUDY AND NURSING CARE PLAN 18-2—cont'd

Alcohol Dependence With Depression

2. Nursing diagnosis: *Ineffective coping*
Outcome: Patient will demonstrate mild to no change in health status and social functioning due to substance addiction.

Short-Term Goal	Intervention	Rationale	Evaluation
1. Patient will consistently acknowledge personal consequences associated with alcohol misuse.	1a. Identify with patient those factors (genetics, stress, unemployment) that contribute to chemical dependence. 1b. Assist patient to identify negative effects of chemical dependency.	1a. Emphasis on alcoholism having biological (genetics), psychological (stress), and social (unemployment) aspects lowers guilt and increases self-esteem. 1b. Identifying negative effects helps patient move from precontemplative to preparation and early action stages (TTM).	**Goal Met** Patient understands how his alcohol use is effecting his ability to find employment.
2. Patient will commit to alcohol-use-control strategies.	2a. Determine history of alcohol use. 2b. Patient attends community addiction treatment program to complete assessment.	2a. Determining history identifies high-risk situations. 2b. Alcohol dependence requires outpatient counselling in conjunction with mutual aid involvement.	**Goal Met** After 3 weeks, patient states that he has arranged for an assessment and has been to one AA meeting and one Rational Recovery meeting and is still deciding which best fits his way of thinking about alcohol but that he will continue to attend both until he decides. His wife has joined the family support group offered at the assessment centre

EVALUATION

See individual outcomes and evaluation in the care plan.

Nurses and addiction in the workplace. "Current estimates place rates of substance misuse, abuse, and addiction rates as high as 20% among practicing nurses" (Monroe & Kenaga, 2011, p. 504), although less than 1% in the United States were in actual monitoring programs (Monroe, Kenaga, Dietrich, et al., 2013).

Fear of disciplinary action up to and including job loss prevents nurses either from seeking help for themselves or from reporting a colleague or friend. Supporting the treatment and recovery of a fellow nurse experiencing an addiction can be challenging, but the situation is not uncommon, nor is being supportive impossible. The choices for action are varied, and the only choice that is clearly wrong is doing nothing. Without intervention or treatment, the problems associated with addiction escalate, and the potential for not only self-harm but also patient harm increases.

A nurse experiencing an addiction may often volunteer to work additional shifts to be nearer to the supply of the substance of abuse. The nurse may leave the unit frequently or spend excessive time in the bathroom. When the nurse with an addiction is on duty, more patients may complain that their pain is unrelieved by their opioid analgesic or that they are unable to sleep, despite receiving sedative medications. Increases in inaccurate drug counts and reports of vial breakage may occur.

The Canadian Nurses Association's (2008) code of ethics requires nurses to recognize when their own personal problems might interfere with their effectiveness and to take action. The code of ethics also requires nurses to recognize signs of substance abuse or impaired practice in colleagues and to report such behaviour to the nurse manager. Intervention is the responsibility of the nurse manager and other nursing administrators. However, clear documentation by co-workers (specific dates, times, events, consequences) is crucial. The nurse manager's major concerns are with job performance and patient safety. Once the nurse manager has been informed, the legal and ethical responsibilities for in-house reporting have been met. If the nurse experiencing an addiction remains in the situation and no action is taken by the nurse manager, co-workers must take the information to the next level in the management structure or look to the provincial or territorial regulatory body for consultation and guidance. These measures can prevent harm to patients under the care of the nurse who is abusing substances and can save a colleague's professional career or even life.

Reporting a colleague who has a problem with misuse, abuse, or addiction is not easy, even though it is a professional responsibility. In efforts to avoid conflict or difficult emotions, nurse

BOX 18-7	SIGNS OF WORKPLACE DIVERSION OF DRUGS

- Arriving early, staying late, and coming to work on scheduled days off
- Excessive wasting of drugs
- Regularly signing out large quantities of controlled drugs
- Volunteering often to give medication to other nurses' patients
- Taking frequent bathroom breaks
- Patients reporting unrelieved pain despite adequate prescription of pain medication
- Discrepancies in the documentation of controlled substance administration
- Medications being signed out for patients who have been discharged or transferred or who are off the unit for procedures or tests
- Minimizing the seriousness of the theft, claiming it would be wasted anyway

Source: Maher-Brisen, P. (2007). Addiction: An occupational hazard in nursing. *American Journal of Nursing, 107*, 78–79. doi:10.1097/01. NAJ.0000282302.49183.67.

colleagues may deny or rationalize the problem, thus allowing the nurse who is abusing substances to continue to put herself or himself at risk. The nurse is also at risk for endangering the lives of those in his or her care. In light of the duty of professional responsibility, nurses can ask themselves the difficult questions: if they have ever co-signed controlled substance "wastes" that were not actually witnessed, if they have ever corrected the narcotic count to account for a discrepancy, or if they have ever excused or rationalized behaviour that might be related to substance abuse. Box 18-7 can be used to assess whether there is a specific drug diversion or a potential misuse of drugs for personal gain in the workplace by a nurse colleague.

Fortunately, most large employers have Employee Assistance Programs, confidential counselling initiatives that are available at no cost, as a viable option through which to seek help for a developing substance use issue before or after it becomes a performance and health issue. As well, formal treatment programs for professionals experiencing addictions have been developed in most Canadian provinces. Some provincial and territorial professional nursing associations support nurses who are experiencing substance misuse or addiction and may withhold disciplinary action if treatment is sought. The aims of supportive policy and specific treatment programs for nurses are to protect patients and to keep the nurse in active practice (perhaps with limitations) or return the nurse to practice after suspension and professional help. More severe consequences—restricting or withholding the ability of the nurse to provide direct patient care—are put into place for nurses who show signs of ongoing impairment.

EVALUATION

Favourable treatment outcome is judged by increased lengths of time of abstinence, decreased denial, acceptable occupational functioning, improved family relationships, and—ultimately—ability to sustain healthy relationships and habits. The ability to use existing supports and skills learned in treatment is important

for ongoing recovery. For example, recovery is actively viable if, in response to cues to use the substance, the patient calls his or her sponsor or other recovering people; increases attendance at 12-step meetings, aftercare, or other group meetings; or writes feelings in a log and considers alternative actions. Although continuous monitoring and evaluation increase the chances for prolonged recovery, it must be stated that no single approach has been found to be universally successful in the treatment of those misusing or abusing a psychoactive substance. Research is conclusive, however, that intervention is superior to no treatment.

Given that addiction is a biopsychosocial phenomenon, an integrated approach of several types of helping modalities will be more successful than recourse to any one alone. Two things are certain: that the treatment used must be tailored to meet the specific needs of each individual and that no patient should be forced into a particular type of rehabilitation merely because of the nurse's convenience or prejudicial choice. Critical factors to always consider are:

- The patient choosing to enter treatment with an expectation of being helped to change his or her behaviour, thus having a motivation to change
- The credibility of the technique being used to both the nurse and the patient
- Consistent application of an empirically proven technique
- The ability to create optimism for a successful outcome
- The ability to create a foundation so that change may occur
- The nurse's discretion, flexibility, and emotional support
- The ability of the nurse to create a supportive environment.

Thus, regardless of the approach used by the nurse, it should always be consistently applied and patient-centred such that the focus is on the individual in relation to her or his needs and wants, both perceived and actual. Evidence from decades of research has slowly begun to indicate that the actual intervention used, while important, is far less vital than the process (Smedslund, Berg, Hammerstrøm, et al., 2011). The process includes the nurse–patient relationship, patient expectations, the model used, and extratherapeutic variables (other factors) such as the patient's attributes, the patient's social system and social environment, and the treatment environment (Figure 18-5). The personal attributes of the nurse—her or his background, understanding, and patience—all play significant roles in the success of the treatment, as the better the reported nurse–patient relationship at all stages of treatment is, the better the outcome for the patient and the patient system. As well, rather than the types of treatment, what tends to matter to a greater degree is the nurse's capacity to structure the treatment so that, regardless of the method or model used, if the patient feels heard and supported, the treatment outcome is more likely to be positive for hope; the nurse being a "hope bringer" is a critical part of the rehabilitation process (Koehn, O'Neill, & Sherry, 2012). What the patient expects, believes, and wants to happen determines what actually happens and contributes to the final outcome. Research indicates that what motivates people to change is positive thoughts, not negative ones. The more one focuses on problems, the more stuck people feel. It is hope that causes people to change, not the pain of addiction or the losses it brings them.

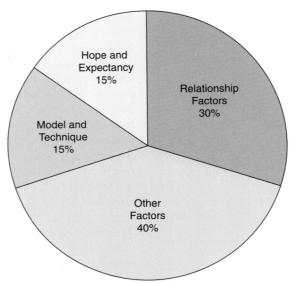

FIGURE 18-5 Contributing factors to positive addiction treatment outcome. Source: Adapted from Hubble, M., Duncan, B., Miller, S., et al. (2010). Introduction. In B. Duncan, S. Miller, B. Wampold, et al. (Eds). *The heart and soul of change: Delivering what works in therapy* (2nd ed., pp. 23–46). Washington, DC: American Psychological Association.

KEY POINTS TO REMEMBER

- Substance use and dependence occur on a continuum, and addiction develops over a period of time and is distinct from compulsive behaviours.
- The cause of substance use disorders is a combination of biological, psychological, and social/environmental factors.
- Assessment of patients with substance use disorders needs to be comprehensive, aimed at identifying common medical and psychiatric comorbidities.
- Patients with concurrent disorders have more severe symptoms, experience more crises, require longer treatment for successful outcomes, and need to be properly assessed and integrated into both treatment systems as per their individual needs.
- Substance use disorders affect the patient's entire family system.
- Assessment of readiness for change is an essential part of the assessment process and can support appropriate treatment strategies.

- Lapse and relapse are expected stages of change from addiction, and treatment needs to include a significant focus on teaching relapse prevention.
- Motivational interviewing, a form of intervention, can lead to appropriate treatment strategies and improved outcomes.
- There is an extensive addiction continuum of care that a nurse should become familiar with, including both professional and mutual aid resources.
- Nurses need to be aware of their own feelings about substance use so they can provide empathy and motivate change for patients.
- Nurses should be vigilant for signs of impairment and addiction in colleagues to ensure patient safety and referral to treatment for the nurse experiencing an addiction.

CRITICAL THINKING

1. The addiction field is a very ambiguous one, filled with myth, belief, half-truths, and ignorance. What are your core beliefs, perception, and knowledge about what addiction is? How has your definition of addiction changed after reading this chapter?
2. Write a paragraph describing reactions you might have to a drug-dependent patient to whom you are assigned.
   a. Would your response be different depending on the substance (alcohol versus heroin, or marijuana versus cocaine)? Give reasons for your answers.
   b. Would your response be different if the substance-dependent person were a professional colleague? How?

3. Aline is a 15-year-old girl who has started using heroin.
   a. When Aline asks you why she needs to take more and more to get "high," how would you explain to her the concept of tolerance?
   b. If she had recently used heroin, what would you find on assessment of physical and psychological–perceptual signs and symptoms?
   c. If she were brought to the emergency department for overdosing on heroin, what would be the emergency care? What might be effective long-term care?

4. Robert is a 45-year-old mechanic. He has a 20-year history of heavy drinking, and he says he wants to quit.
   a. Role-play with a classmate an initial assessment. Identify the kinds of information you would need to have in order to plan holistic care.
   b. Robert decided to stop drinking abruptly. He is now in the emergency department with delirium tremens. What are the dangers for him? What are the appropriate medical interventions?
   c. What are some possible treatment alternatives for Robert when he is safely detoxified? How would you explain to him the usefulness and function of Alcoholics Anonymous? What are some additional treatment options that might be useful to Robert? What are available as referrals for him in your community?

CHAPTER REVIEW

1. Addiction is best explained as
   a. Occuring with games of chance such as roulette or poker
   b. A chronic brain disease
   c. A biopsychosocial phenomenon
   d. The domain of neurobiologists
2. The nurse is caring for a patient with an addictive disorder who is currently drug-free. The patient is experiencing repeated occurrences of vivid, frightening images and thoughts. Which term would the nurse use to document this finding?
   a. Tolerance
   b. Flashbacks
   c. Withdrawal
   d. Physical dependency
3. The condition most concerning for the nurse who is caring for a patient who abuses alcohol would be
   a. Cirrhosis of the liver
   b. Suicidal potential
   c. Wernicke's encephalopathy
   d. Korsakoff's syndrome
4. Which patient response to the question "Have you ever drunk more alcohol or used more drugs than you meant to?" should immediately cause the nurse to assess further?
   a. "No, I have never used drugs or alcohol."
   b. "I have drunk alcohol before but have never let myself get drunk."
   c. "I figured you'd ask me about that."
   d. "Yes, I did that once and will never do it again."
5. Which patient behaviours should the nurse suspect as being related to alcohol withdrawal?
   a. Hyperalert state, jerky movements, easily startled
   b. Tachycardia, diaphoresis, elevated blood pressure
   c. Peripheral vascular collapse, electrolyte imbalance
   d. Paranoid delusions, fever, fluctuating levels of consciousness
6. A patient at your community mental health centre smokes up to a half a pack of cigarettes daily but has tried, with limited success, to cut back over the past 2 weeks. Today he asked the pharmacist about the various products that could aid his attempts to quit smoking in time for him to manage a long overseas flight next month and travel with friends who are allergic to smoke. What phase of change is this patient demonstrating?
   a. Precontemplation
   b. Contemplation
   c. Preparation
   d. Action

Evolve WEBSITE

Post-Test interactive review

Visit the Evolve website for Chapter Review Answers and Rationales, Critical Thinking Answer Guidelines, and additional resources related to the content in this chapter: http://evolve.elsevier.com/Canada/Varcarolis/psychiatric/

REFERENCES

Aboriginal Healing Foundation. (2007). *Addictive behaviours among Aboriginal people in Canada*. Ottawa: Author.

Antnowicz, J., Metzger, A., & Ramanujam, S. (2011). Paranoid psychosis induced by consumption of methylenedioxypyrovalerone: Two cases. *General Hospital Psychiatry, 33*(6), doi:640.e5-640.e6.

Banerjee, P., Ali, Z., Levine, B., et al. (2014). Fatal caffeine intoxication: A series of eight cases from 1999 to 2009. *Journal of Forensic Sciences, 59*(3), 865–868.

Brownbill, K., & Etienne, M. (2017). Understanding the ultimate oppression: Alcohol and drug addiction in Native land. In R. Csiernik & W. Rowe (Eds.), *Responding to the oppression of addiction* (3rd ed.). Toronto: Canadian Scholars Press.

Burnside, L., & Fuchs, D. (2013). Bound by the clock: The experiences of youth with FASD transitioning to adulthood from child welfare care. *First Peoples Child & Family Review, 8*(1), 40–61.

Cahill, K., Stevens, S., Perera, R., et al. (2013). Pharmacological interventions for smoking cessation: An overview and network meta-analysis. *The Cochrane Database of Systematic Reviews*, (5), CD009329.

Callahan-Lyon, C. (2014). Electronic cigarettes: Human health effects. *Tobacco Control, 23*(S2), ii36–ii40.

Cameron, K., Kolanos, R., Solis, E., Jr., et al. (2013). Bath salts components mephedrone and methylenedioxypyrovalerone (MDPV) act synergistically at the human dopamine transporter. *British Journal of Pharmacology, 168*(7), 1750–1757.

Cameron, K., Kolanos, R., Verkariva, R., et al. (2013). Mephedrone and methylenedioxypyrovalerone (MDPV), major constituents of "bath salts," produce opposite effects at the human dopamine transporter. *Psychopharmacology, 227*(3), 493–499.

Campana, C., Griffin, P. L., & Simon, E. L. (2014). Caffeine overdose resulting in severe rhabdomyolysis and acute renal failure. *The American Journal of Emergency Medicine, 32*(1), 111–e3.

Canadian Institute for Health Information (CIHI). (2012). *Hospital mental health services in Canada, 2009–2010.* Ottawa: Author.

Canadian Institute for Health Information (CIHI). (2013). *Hospital mental health services for concurrent mental illness and substance use disorders in Canada: Analysis in brief.* Ottawa: Author.

Canadian Nurses Association. (2008). *Code of ethics for registered nurses.* Ottawa: Author.

Carlson, R. W., Kumar, N. N., Wong-Mckinstry, E., et al. (2012). Alcohol withdrawal syndrome. *Critical Care Clinics, 28*(4), 549–585.

Chu, C., & Galang, A. (2013). Hospital nurses' attitudes toward patients with a history of illicit drug use. *The Canadian Nurse, 109*(6), 29–33.

Ciechanowski, P. (2012). *Exposure assessment report: Risks to toluene exposure and adverse health outcomes.* Retrieved from http://ssrn.com/abstract=2312788 or http://dx.doi.org/10.2139/ssrn.2312788.

Cotton, J., & Laventure, M. (2013). Early initiation to cigarettes, alcohol and other drugs among Innu preadolescents of Quebec. *Canadian Journal of Native Studies, 33*(1), 1–15.

Csiernik, R. (2014). *Just say know: A counsellor's guide to psychoactive drugs.* Toronto: Canadian Scholars Press.

Csiernik, R. (2016). *Substance use and abuse: Everything matters.* Toronto: Canadian Scholars Press.

Darnell, K., & Csiernik, R. (2014). The hazards of being a counsellor for the hazardous workplace. In R. Csiernik (Ed.), *Workplace wellness: Issues and responses.* Toronto: Canadian Scholars Press.

Duncan, K., Reading, C., Borwein, A., et al. (2011). HIV incidence and prevalence among Aboriginal peoples in Canada. *AIDS and Behavior, 15*(1), 214–227.

Eichner, E. R. (2014). Fatal caffeine overdose and other risks from dietary supplements. *Current Sports Medicine Reports, 13*(6), 353–354.

Ewing, J. A. (1984). Detecting alcoholism: The CAGE questionnaire. *Journal of the American Medical Association, 252*, 1905–1907.

Gordon, M. S., Kinlock, T. W., Vocci, F. J., et al. (2015). A phase 4, pilot, open-label study of VIVITROL® (extended-release naltrexone XR-NTX) for prisoners. *Journal of Substance Abuse Treatment, 59*(1), 52–58.

Gowing, L., Farrell, M. F., Ali, R., et al. (2014). Alpha2-adrenergic agonists for the management of opioid withdrawal. *The Cochrane Database of Systematic Reviews,* (3), CD002024, doi:10.1002/14651858.CD002024.pub4.

Guglielmo, R., Martinotti, G., Quatrale, M., et al. (2015). Topiramate in alcohol use disorders: Review and update. *CNS Drugs, 29*(5), 383–395.

Hass, C. (2011). A vaccine against nicotine—New hope or mere hype? *Clinical Correlations.* Retrieved from http://www.clinicalcorrelations.org/?p=3935.

Inaba, D., & Cohen, W. (2014). *Uppers, downers, all arounders.* Medford, OR: CNS Productions.

Khan, S. (2008). Aboriginal mental health: The statistical reality. *Visions, 5*(1), 6–7.

Knopf, A. (2016). Vivitrol: Who's right on the craving question? *Alcoholism & Drug Abuse Weekly, 28*(10), 4–6.

Koehn, C., O'Neill, L., & Sherry, J. (2012). Hope-focused interventions in substance abuse counselling. *International Journal of Mental Health and Addiction, 10*(4), 441–452.

Koob, G. F., & Le Moal, M. (2006). *Neurobiology of addiction.* Oxford, UK: Elsevier.

Latino-Martel, P., Chan, D., Druesne-Pecollo, N., et al. (2010). Maternal alcohol consumption during pregnancy and risk of childhood leukemia: Systematic review and meta-analysis. *Cancer Epidemiology Biomarkers and Prevention, 19*(5), 1238–1260.

Lehne, R. A. (2014). *Pharmacology for nursing care* (9th ed.). Philadelphia: Saunders.

McKim, W., & Hancock, S. (2012). *Drugs and behaviour* (7th ed.). Englewood Cliffs, NJ: Prentice Hall.

Miller, W. R. (1983). Motivational interviewing with problem drinkers. *Behavioural Psychotherapy, 11*, 147–172.

Miller, W. R., & Rollnick, S. (Eds.). (2002). *Motivational interviewing: Preparing people for change* (2nd ed.). New York: Guilford Press.

Minkoff, K. (2005). *Comprehensive continuous integrated system of care: Psychopharmacology practice guidelines for individuals with co-occurring psychiatric and substance use disorders (COD).* Retrieved from http://www.healthcare.uiowa.edu/icmh/documents/changingtheworldarticle.pdf.

Monroe, T., & Kenaga, H. (2011). Don't ask, don't tell: Substance abuse and addiction among nurses. *Journal of Clinical Nursing, 20*, 504–509. doi: 10.1111/j.1365-2702.2010.03518.x.

Monroe, T. B., Kenaga, H., Dietrich, M. S., et al. (2013). The prevalence of employed nurses identified or enrolled in substance use monitoring programs. *Nursing Research, 62*(1), 10–15.

Monte, A. A., Zane, R. D., & Heard, K. J. (2015). The implications of marijuana legalization in Colorado. *Journal of the American Medical Association, 313*(3), 241–242.

Moorhead, S., Johnson, M., Maas, M. L., et al. (2012). *Nursing Outcomes Classification (NOC)* (5th ed.). St. Louis: Mosby.

Niaura, R. (2015). Varenicline and suicide: Reconsidered and reconciled. *Nicotine & Tobacco Research, 18*(1).

Nosyk, B., Geller, J., Guh, D., et al. (2010). The effect of motivational status on treatment outcome in the North American Opiate Medication Initiative (NAOMI) study. *Drug and Alcohol Dependence, 111*(1–2), 161–165.

Orman, J., & Keating, G. (2009). Spotlight on buprenorphine/naloxone in the treatment of opioid dependence. *CNS Drugs, 23*(10), 899–902.

Plosker, G. L. (2015). Acamprosate: A review of its use in alcohol dependence. *Drugs, 75*(11), 1255–1268.

Prochaska, J. O., & DiClemente, C. C. (1984). *The transtheoretical approach: Towards a systematic eclectic framework.* Homewood, IL: Dow Jones Irwin.

Ross, E., Reisfield, G., Watson, M., et al. (2012). Psychoactive "bath salts" intoxication with methylenedioxypyrovalerone. *The American Journal of Medicine, 125*(9), 854–858.

Royal Commission on Aboriginal Peoples. (1996). *Report of the Royal Commission on Aboriginal Peoples.* Ottawa: Indian and Northern Affairs Canada.

Rutman, D., & Van Bibber, M. (2010). Parenting with fetal alcohol spectrum disorder. *International Journal of Mental Health and Addiction, 8*(3), 351–361.

Selzer, M. L. (1971). The Michigan Alcoholism Screening Test (MAST): The quest for a new diagnostic instrument. *American Journal of Psychiatry, 127*, 1653–1658.

Skinner, W. (2005). Introduction. In W. J. Skinner (Ed.), *Treating concurrent disorders: A guide for counsellors* (pp. 1–28). Toronto: Centre for Addiction and Mental Health.

Skinner, W., O'Grady, C. P., Bartha, C., et al. (2004). *Concurrent substance use and mental health disorders: An information guide.* Toronto: Centre for Addiction and Mental Health.

Smedslund, G., Berg, R., Hammerstrøm, K., et al. (2011). Motivational interviewing for substance abuse. *The Cochrane Database of Systematic Reviews,* (5), CD008063, doi:10.1002/14651858.CD008063.pub2.

Statistics Canada. (2015). *Canadian Tobacco, Alcohol and Drugs Survey (CTADS): Summary of results for 2013.* Retrieved from http://healthycanadians.gc.ca/science-research-sciences-recherches/data-donnees/ctads-ectad/summary-sommaire-2013-eng.php.

Takagi, M., Lubman, D., & Yu, M. (2011). Solvent-induced leukoencephalopathy: A disorder of adolescence? *Substance Use and Misuse, 45*(1), 95–98.

Tanner, G., Bordon, N., Conroy, S., et al. (2011). Comparing methadone and suboxone in applied treatment settings: The experiences of maintenance patients in Lanarkshire. *Journal of Substance Abuse, 16*(3), 171–178.

Teitelbaum, L., & Mullen, B. (2000). Validity of the MAST in psychiatric settings: A META-analytic integration. *Journal of Studies on Alcohol, 61*(2), 254–261.

Tsilajara, H., Noda, K., & Saku, K. (2010). A randomized controlled open comparative trial of varenicline vs nicotine patch in adult smokers. *Circulation Journal, 74*(4), 771–778.

Vuoristo-Myllys, S., Lipsanen, J., Lahti, J., et al. (2014). Outcome predictors for problem drinkers treated with combined cognitive behavioral therapy and naltrexone. *The American Journal of Drug and Alcohol Abuse, 40*(2), 103–110.

Walsh, A., Callaway, R., Belle-Isle, L., et al. (2013). Cannabis for therapeutic purposes: Patient characteristics, access, and reasons for use. *International Journal of Drug Policy, 24*(6), 511–516.

Wesley-Esquimaux, C. C., & Snowball, A. (2010). Viewing violence, mental illness and addiction through a wise practices lens. *International Journal of Mental Health and Addiction, 8*, 390–407. doi:10.1007/ s11469-009-9265-6.

Wieland, D., Halter, M., & Levine, C. (2012). Bath salts: They are not what you think. *Journal of Psychosocial Nursing and Mental Health Services, 50*(2), 17–21.

CHAPTER

19

Personality Disorders

Christine A. Tackett, Margaret Jordan Halter, Claudia A. Cihlar
Adapted by Cheryl L. Pollard

KEY TERMS AND CONCEPTS

anger control assistance
callousness
dialectical behaviour therapy (DBT)
diathesis–stress model
emotional dysregulation
emotional lability
impulse-control training
impulsivity

limit setting
persona
personality
personality disorders
personality trait
personality type
splitting
temperament

OBJECTIVES

1. Analyze the interaction of biological determinants and psychosocial stress factors in the etiology of personality disorders.
2. Identify and distinguish among the three clusters of personality disorders.
3. Identify 10 personality disorders.
4. Describe the emotional and clinical needs of nurses and other staff when working with patients who meet criteria for personality disorders.
5. Formulate a nursing diagnosis for each of the personality disorders.
6. Discuss two nursing outcomes for patients with borderline personality disorder.
7. Plan basic nursing care interventions for a patient with impulsive, aggressive, or manipulative behaviours.
8. Identify the role of the advanced-practice nurse when working with patients with personality disorders.

⊖volve WEBSITE

Visit the Evolve website for Flashcards, Case Studies, and additional testing resources related to the content in this chapter: http://evolve.elsevier.com/Canada/Varcarolis/psychiatric/

Pre-Test | interactive review

Often we meet someone and think, "She's quite a strange person" or "What an unusual character he is." When we make evaluations such as these about other people, we are reacting to their personalities. *Personality* comes from the Latin word persona, which means "mask" and may refer to the person as other people see him or her. What is a personality?

Personality is an individual's characteristic patterns of relatively permanent thoughts, feelings, and behaviours that define the quality of experiences and relationships. In mental health nursing there are two key underlying concepts related to an individual's personality. They are personality trait and personality type. A personality trait is a stable characteristic of a person, such as neuoticism, extraversion, openness to experience, agreeableness, and conscientiousness. These can be compared to personality states, which are temporary behaviours and feelings. A personality type is a way to describe a cluster of traits. For example, a person with an authoritarian personality has traits that relate to maintaining orderliness, command, and power. In contrast, a person's character involves defining an individual's integrity.

A personality is considered unhealthy when interpersonal and social relationships and functioning are consistently maladaptive, complicated, or dysphoric. We know that personality can be protective for a person in times of difficulty but may also be a liability if one's personality results in ongoing relationship problems or leads to emotional distress on a regular basis.

Until quite recently, we believed that personalities were fairly fixed entities. More contemporary views challenge this notion. Rather than unchanging patterns of behaviours and thoughts, the rate of personality's change slows over time but does not cease (Newton-Howes, Horwood, & Mulder, 2015). If personality traits evolve continually across the lifespan, we have an opportunity to develop and support more adaptive functioning and social relationships.

CLINICAL PICTURE

Individuals with **personality disorders** display significant challenges in self-identity or self-direction, and they have problems with empathy or intimacy within their relationships. Treating personality disorders is difficult and complex, as people with these disorders have difficulty recognizing or owning the fact that their difficulties are problems of their personality. They may truly believe that the problems originate outside of themselves (Perry, Presniak, & Olson, 2013). People with personality disorders may injure themselves. In Canada in 2009–2010, about 7 in 10 adults hospitalized for self-injury had a mental illness (a diagnosis on the hospital record). Of these admissions, 6% had a personality disorder (Canadian Institute for Health Information, 2011).

Judgements about an individual's personality functioning must take into account the person's ethnic, cultural, and social background. Patients who differ from the majority culture or the culture of the clinician may be at risk for overdiagnosis of a personality disorder. Therefore it is important to obtain additional information from others who are knowledgeable about the particular cultural or ethnic norms before determining the presence of a personality disorder.

According to the American Psychiatric Association (APA, 2013), there are 10 personality disorders. These 10 disorders are

HOW A NURSE HELPED ME

My Reality Check

I was 22 and going through a bitter divorce. I was very angry and felt hopeless. Becoming more depressed, I had thoughts about harming myself and my husband (soon to be ex-husband). I was drinking to help numb my anger. One night, I was drunk and cut my wrists. As I lay bleeding in the bathtub, I phoned my parents to say goodbye. They phoned the ambulance, and I was taken to the hospital and admitted to the "psych" unit. My parents had often told me that I did not make good decisions for myself. I chose the wrong kind of man and the wrong kinds of friends, drank too much, and spent too much. Behind my back, my friends would say that I had a "personality problem." I didn't expect to hear the nurses tell me I had a personality problem, too. I hated being in hospital, but my family felt it was the best thing for me, as they were at their wits' end with me (well, that's what they told me).

I felt I was fairly bright and thought that I would be able to beat the system. I didn't feel I needed any help, and I certainly didn't need to be in hospital. Manipulation was the key: I knew how to sweet-talk to get my way—well, it worked with my family! I went with the routine; I played by the rules, and, yes, I was able to justify my behaviour to the doctor, social worker, and most of the nurses. I behaved the way I did because I had been abandoned. The divorce was my husband's fault, not mine. My parents didn't understand the emotional turmoil I was going through. I had no support. My nurse applied what I felt were strict rules: if I wanted anything, I had to go through her; I couldn't ask the other nurses. This gave me only more reason to try to manipulate my nurse and play the "sweet card." This game, as I referred to it, went on for weeks, but I finally realized she was always one step ahead of me.

My nurse would sit down and talk to me about how I showed patterns of being overly dramatic and displayed erratic behaviour. She gave me some examples of her claim, something I found hard to take, and I became quietly resistive to her "talks." But now, looking back many years later, I see that her description seems fairly close to how I acted. It took me a long time, with two more admissions to hospital (because of self-harming), to understand some of my behaviours. There were other discussions—or as my nurse called them, "therapy"—about my manipulative behaviours. I blamed my parents, my friends, and my ex-husband for my behaviour, and I still do to an extent. But I have learned to control my blaming and emotional behaviours to a degree.

I never said thank you to that particular nurse, who gave me a "reality check," as I didn't think the sessions were in my best interest at the time. But I now realize that the nurse was helping me take control of my life and provided me with various coping skills that I have since applied in my interactions with others. I still have good and bad days, but I know that this particular nurse helped guide me to be stronger and more controlled. I'm now a person who takes responsibility for her behaviours, something I didn't realize she was teaching me through those "therapy" sessions.

grouped into three clusters of similar behaviour patterns and personality traits. These clusters are:

Cluster A: Individuals with these disorders share characteristics of eccentric behaviours, such as social isolation and detachment. They may also display perception distortions, unusual levels of suspiciousness, magical thinking, and cognitive impairment.

- Paranoid personality disorder
- Schizoid personality disorder
- Schizotypal personality disorder

Cluster B: People living with cluster B personality disorders show patterns of responding to life demands with dramatic, emotional, or erratic behaviour. Problems with impulse control, emotion processing and regulation, and interpersonal difficulties characterize this cluster of disorders. Insight into these issues is generally limited. To get their needs met, individuals with cluster B personality disorders may resort to behaviours that are considered desperate or entitled, including acting out, committing antisocial acts, or manipulating people and circumstances.

- Borderline personality disorder
- Narcissistic personality disorder
- Histrionic personality disorder
- Antisocial personality disorder

Cluster C: An individual with these types of personality disorders will demonstrate a consistent patterns of anxious and fearful behaviours, rigid patterns of social shyness, hypersensitivity, need for orderliness, and relationship dependency.

- Avoidant personality disorder
- Dependent personality disorder
- Obsessive-compulsive personality disorder

In this chapter, we begin with an overview of personality disorders, including epidemiology, comorbidity, and risk factors. Afterward, the personality disorders are presented along with prevalence, characteristic pathological responses, nursing care guidelines, and medical treatments. A vignette is provided to illustrate each of these disorders. After reviewing these disorders, application of the nursing process is described.

EPIDEMIOLOGY

In the past decade, the epidemiology of personality disorders has become clearer. Personality disorders are more frequently seen in people receiving extensive medical and psychiatric services (Samuels, 2011). While narcissistic and schizotypal personality disorders are relatively rare, borderline, avoidant, and obsessive-compulsive personality disorders have been established by meta-analyses (which pull together the best and most relevant research) to be common among both community and clinical populations.

While studies vary in their estimates of prevalence depending on their methodologies, the International Classification of Diseases, tenth revision (ICD-10), criteria suggest that personality disorders affect about 10% of the world's population (Samuels, 2011). Culture has a definite influence on the rate of diagnosing personality disorders. For example, an Australian study reports substantially higher prevalence rates than North American studies

do (Samuels, 2011). Differences may reflect the view of personality and behaviour as deviant rather than normal in a particular culture and within certain study methods. Or, it may reflect better diagnosing practices or a system that has more resources to assist people with personality disorders. It is generally agreed that there are insufficient studies to address the role of ethnicity and race on the prevalence of personality disorders (McGilloway, Hall, Lee, et al., 2010).

COMORBIDITY

Personality disorders frequently co-occur with disorders of mood and eating, anxiety, and substance misuse. Personality disorders often amplify emotional dysregulation, a term that describes poorly modulated mood characterized by mood swings. Individuals with emotion regulation problems have ongoing difficulty managing painful emotions in ways that are healthy and effective.

The aging process has some effect on the prevalence of personality disorders. The dramatic, emotional, or erratic cluster B disorders may mute with age as individuals become less impulsive. This dampening may be due to a general tuning down of neurotransmitters (Rosowsky, Abrams, & Zwieg, 2013). Other disorders such as obsessive-compulsive personality disorder or paranoid personality disorder may worsen with age, perhaps due to anxiety regarding declining sensory and cognitive capacity.

Personality traits are amplified during the experience of a crisis and any illness; therefore it is premature and not in the best interest of the individual for a personality disorder to be diagnosed during the active phase of another illness, especially a psychiatric episode or major stressful life event such as grief and loss or trauma.

ETIOLOGY

Personality disorders are the result of complex biological and psychosocial phenomena that are influenced by multifaceted variables involving genetic, neurobiological, neurochemical, and environmental factors.

Biological Factors
Genetics

While genetics are thought to influence the development of personality disorders, individual genes are not believed to be associated with particular personality traits; thus the relationship among genes and traits is a complex one (Taylor, Asmundson, & Jang, 2011).

Several possible hypotheses attempt to account for the personality differences among people in the same family. One may be that a child's temperament can elicit different responses from family members. Individual children may perceive family experiences in unique ways and therefore respond differently from other family members. Children are also affected by forces outside the family that influence personality development. It may be that personality is influenced even by the intrauterine environment, although there are fewer data to support this hypothesis.

Neurobiology and Neurochemistry

Biological influences on personality expression are a promising area of research in understanding these disorders. Influences on the development of personality disorders probably incorporate a complex interaction of genetics, neurobiology, and neurochemistry. The chemical neurotransmitter theory proposes that certain neurotransmitters, including neurohormones, may regulate and influence temperament. Research in brain imaging has also revealed some differences in the size and function of specific structures of the brain in people with some personality disorders (Leichsenring, Leibing, Kruse, et al., 2011).

Psychological Factors

Several psychological theories may help to explain the development of personality disorders. Learning theory emphasizes that children develop maladaptive responses based on modelling of or reinforcement by important people in the child's life. Cognitive theories emphasize the role of beliefs and assumptions in creating emotional and behavioural responses that influence one's experiences within the family environment.

Psychoanalytic theory focuses on the use of primitive defence mechanisms by individuals with personality disorders. Defence mechanisms such as repression, suppression, regression, undoing, and splitting have been identified as dominant (Kernberg, 1985). The role of psychoanalytic theory, while historically relevant and interesting, is not confirmable through evidence-informed research methods.

Environmental Factors

Behavioural genetics research has shown that about half of the variance accounting for personality traits emerges from the environment (Hernandez, Arntz, Gaviria, et al., 2012). These findings suggest that while the family environment is influential on development, there are other environmental factors besides upbringing that shape an individual's personality. One need only think about the individual differences among siblings raised together to illustrate this point.

Childhood neglect and trauma have been established as risk factors for personality disorders (Samuels, 2011). This association has been linked to possible biological mechanisms involving corticotropin-releasing hormone in response to early life stress and emotional reactivity (Lee, Hempel, Tenharmsel, et al., 2012).

System Factors
Diathesis–Stress Model

The diathesis–stress model is a general theory that explains psychopathology using a systems approach. This theory helps us understand how personality disorders emerge from the multifaceted factors of biology and environment (Paris, 2005). *Diathesis* refers to genetic and biological vulnerabilities and includes personality traits and temperament. Temperament is our tendency to respond to challenges in predictable ways. Examples of descriptors of temperament may be *laid back*, referring to a calm temperament, or *uptight*, referring to an anxious temperament. These characteristics remain stable throughout a person's life. In this model, *stress* refers to immediate influences

on personality such as the physical, social, psychological, and emotional environment. *Stress* also includes what happened in the past, such as growing up in one's family with exposure to unique experiences and patterns of interaction. The diathesis–stress model proposes that, under conditions of stress, some people have maladaptive personality development, resulting in the emergence of a personality disorder (Paris, 2005).

There is a two-way directionality among stressors and diatheses. Genetic and biological traits are believed to influence the way an individual responds to the environment while, at the same time, the environment is thought to influence the expression of inherited traits. Many studies have suggested a strong correlation between trauma, neglect, and other dysfunctional family or social patterns of interaction and the development of personality disorders among individuals with particular personality traits and temperament.

The following is a summary of factors that are theorized to influence the development of each disorder (Skodol, Bender, Gunderson, et al., 2014):

- Schizotypal personality disorder (STPD) is a schizophrenia spectrum disorder and is genetically linked, meaning that there is a higher incidence of schizophrenia-related disorders in family members of people with STPD.
- Antisocial personality disorder is genetically linked, and twin studies indicate a predisposition to this disorder. This predisposition is set into motion by a childhood environment of inconsistent parenting, significant abuse, and extreme neglect.
- Borderline personality disorder has traditionally been thought to develop as a result of early abandonment, which results in an unstable view of self and others. This abandonment is made more intense by a biological predisposition, and twin studies identify a heritability of 69%.
- Narcissistic personality disorder may be the result of childhood neglect and criticism. The child does not learn that other people can be a source of comfort and support. As an adult, the individual hides feelings of emptiness with an exterior of invulnerability and self-sufficiency. Little is known about inborn traits or heritability for this disorder.
- Avoidant personality disorder has been linked with parental and peer rejection and criticism. A biological predisposition to anxiety and physiological arousal in social situations has also been suggested. Genetically, this disorder may be part of a continuum of disorders related to social phobia (social anxiety disorder; see Chapter 12).
- Obsessive-compulsive personality disorder may be related to excessive parental criticism, control, and shame. The child responds to this negativity by trying to control his or her environment through perfectionism and orderliness. Heritable traits such as compulsivity, oppositionality, lack of emotional expressiveness, and perfectionism have all been implicated in this disorder.

CLUSTER A PERSONALITY DISORDERS

Paranoid Personality Disorder

Paranoid personality disorder is characterized by a long-standing distrust and suspiciousness of others based on the belief, which is unsupported by evidence, that others want to exploit, harm, or deceive the person. These individuals are hypervigilant, anticipate hostility, and may provoke hostile responses by initiating a counterattack.

The prevalence of paranoid personality disorder has been estimated at about 2% to 4% (APA, 2013). Slightly more men than women are diagnosed with this disorder. Relatives of patients with schizophrenia are more frequently affected with this disorder. A diagnosis of paranoid personality disorder often precedes a schizophrenia diagnosis.

Symptoms may be apparent in childhood or adolescence. Parents may notice that their child does not have friends and experiences social anxiety. Young people with this disorder are frequently teased due to their odd behaviour.

As adults, relationships are difficult due to jealousy, controlling behaviours, and unwillingness to forgive. Projection is the dominant defence mechanism whereby people attribute their own unacknowledged feelings to others. For example, they may accuse their partner of being hypercritical when they themselves are attentively fault finding.

Guidelines for Nursing Care

- Considering the degree of mistrust, promises, appointments, and schedules should be strictly adhered to.
- Being too nice or friendly may be met with suspicion. Instead, give clear and straightforward explanations of tests and procedures beforehand.
- Use simple language and project a neutral but kind affect.
- Limit setting is essential when threatening behaviours are present.

Treatment

Individuals with paranoid personality disorder tend to reject treatment. If they somehow end up in a psychiatric treatment setting, they may appear puzzled and obviously suspicious about why this is happening. Paranoid people are difficult to interview because they are reluctant to share information about themselves for fear that the information will be used against them.

Psychotherapy is the first line of treatment for paranoid personality disorder (Sadock, Sadock, & Ruiz, 2015). Individual therapy focuses on the development of a professional and trusting relationship. Due to their fears, patients may behave in a threatening manner. Therapists should respond by setting limits and dealing with delusional accusations in a realistic manner without humiliating the patients.

Group therapy is threatening to people with paranoid personality disorder. However, the group setting may be useful in improving social skills. Role-playing and group feedback can help reduce suspiciousness. For example, if the patient says, "I think the therapist is singling me out," other groups members may provide a reality check or describe similar feelings in the past.

An antianxiety agent such as diazepam (Valium) may be used to reduce anxiety and agitation (Sadock, Sadock, & Ruiz, 2015). More severe agitation and delusions may be treated with antipsychotic medication such as haloperidol (Haldol) in small doses for brief periods of time to manage the mildly delusional

thinking or severe agitation. The first-generation antipsychotic medication pimozide (Orap) may be useful in reducing paranoid ideation.

VIGNETTE

Ms. Alonzo is a 54-year-old unemployed female who comes to a mental health clinic complaining of depression and pain. She believes that her health maintenance organization has circulated her medical record to all health care providers to prevent her from being treated. She refuses to give any social history and is reluctant to share her telephone number. When the nurse indicates that the psychiatrist does not prescribe pain medications, she smiles bitterly and says, "So they already got to you."

Schizoid Personality Disorder

People with schizoid personality disorder exhibit a lifelong pattern of social withdrawal. They are somewhat expressionless and operate with a restricted range of emotional expression. Others tend to view them as odd or eccentric due to their discomfort with social interaction.

The prevalence rate may be nearly 5% of the population (APA, 2013). Males are more often affected. Symptoms of schizoid personality disorder appear in childhood and adolescence. These young people tend to be loners, do poorly in school, and are the objects of ridicule by their peers for their odd behaviour. There is increased prevalence of the disorder in families with a history of schizophrenia or STPD. Abnormalities in the dopaminergic systems may underlie this problem.

Relationships are particularly affected due to the prominent feature of emotional detachment. People with this disorder do not seek out or enjoy close relationships. Neither approval nor rejection from others seems to have much effect. Friendships, dating, and sexual experiences are rare. If trust is established, the person may divulge numerous imaginary friends and fantasies.

Employment may be jeopardized if interpersonal interaction is necessary. Individuals with this disorder may be able to function well in a solitary occupation such as being a security guard on the night shift. They often endorse feelings of being an observer rather than a participant in life. The patient may describe feelings of depersonalization or detachment from oneself and the world.

Guidelines for Nursing Care

- Nurses should avoid being too "nice" or "friendly."
- Do not try to increase socialization.
- Patients may be open to discussing topics such as coping and anxiety.
- Conduct a thorough assessment to identify symptoms the patient is reluctant to discuss.
- Protect against ridicule from group members due to patient's distinctive interests or ideas.

Treatment

Patients with schizoid personality disorder tend to be introspective (Sadock, Sadock, & Ruiz, 2015). This trait may make them good, if distant, candidates for psychotherapy. As trust develops, these patients may describe a full fantasy life and fears, particularly of dependence. Psychotherapy can help improve sensitivity to others' social cues. Group therapy may also be helpful, even though the patient may frequently be silent. Group therapy provides experience in practising interactions with and receiving feedback from others. Group members may become quite important to the person with schizoid personality disorder and may be the only form of socialization he or she has.

Antidepressants such as bupropion (Wellbutrin) may help increase pleasure in life. Second-generation antipsychotics, such as risperidone (Risperdal) or olanzapine (Zyprexa), are used to improve emotional expressiveness.

> **VIGNETTE**
>
> Mr. Gray, a 30-year-old single male, is a graduate student in mathematics at a large university. He lives alone and has never been married. He works as an assistant in a math classroom in which the professor teaches the course remotely via television. Mr. Gray wears thick glasses, and his clothing is inconspicuous. He rarely smiles and seldom looks directly at the students, even when answering questions. He does get somewhat animated when he writes lengthy solutions to math problems on the blackboard. He is content with his low-paying job and has never been in psychiatric treatment.

Schizotypal Personality Disorder

People with STPD do not blend in with the crowd. Their symptoms are strikingly strange and unusual. Magical thinking, odd beliefs, strange speech patterns, and inappropriate affect are hallmarks of this disorder.

Estimates of the prevalence of STPD vary from 0.6% to 4.6% (APA, 2013). It is more common in men than women. Like the other Cluster A personality disorders, symptoms are evident in young people. People who have first-degree relatives with schizophrenia are at more risk for this disorder. Abnormalities in brain structure, physiology, chemistry, and functioning are similar to schizophrenia. For example, both disorders share reduced cortical volume.

The *Diagnostic and Statistical Manual of Mental Disorders*, fifth edition (*DSM-5*) (APA, 2013), identifies this problem as both a personality disorder and the first of the schizophrenia spectrum disorders. The ICD-10 (World Health Organization, 2016), used throughout the world, classifies schizotypal disorder along with schizophrenia and no longer lists schizotypal disorder as a personality disorder. Chapter 15 discusses the schizophrenia spectrum disorders in greater detail.

Like schizoid personality disorder, individuals with STPD have severe social and interpersonal deficits. They experience extreme anxiety in social situations. Contributions to conversations tend to ramble, with lengthy, unclear, overly detailed, and abstract content. An additional feature of this disorder is paranoia. Individuals with STPD are overly suspicious and anxious. They tend to misinterpret the motivations of others as being out to get them and blame others for their social isolation.

Odd beliefs (e.g., being overly superstitious) or magical thinking (e.g., "He caught a cold because I wished he would") are also common.

Psychotic symptoms seen in people with schizophrenia, such as hallucinations and delusions, may also exist with STPD, but to a lesser degree and only briefly. A major difference between this disorder and schizophrenia is that people with STPD can be made aware of their suspiciousness, magical thinking, and odd beliefs. Schizophrenia is characterized by far stronger delusions.

Guidelines for Nursing Care

- Respect the patient's need for social isolation.
- Nurses should be aware of the patient's suspiciousness and employ appropriate interventions.
- Perform careful assessment as needed to uncover any other medical or psychological symptoms that may need intervention (e.g., suicidal thoughts).
- Be aware that strange beliefs and activities, such as strange religious practices or peculiar thoughts, may be part of the patient's life.

Treatment

The principles of psychotherapy used are similar to those for schizoid personality disorder (Sadock, Sadock, & Ruiz, 2015). However, clinicians should be aware that these patients may also be actively involved in groups such as cults and unusual religious groups and engage in occult activities.

While there is no specific medication for STPD, associated conditions may be treated. People with STPD seem to benefit from low-dose antipsychotic agents for psychotic-like symptoms and day-to-day functioning (Ripoll, Triebwasser, & Siever, 2011). These agents help with such symptoms as ideas of reference or illusions. Depression and anxiety may be treated with antidepressants and antianxiety agents.

> **VIGNETTE**
>
> Raymond is a 55-year-old single male who lives with his mother. He is the youngest of seven children raised in a farming community. Three of his siblings are deaf, and Raymond also has some hearing loss. Raymond started therapy with Wei, an advanced-practice registered nurse (APRN) in psychiatric mental health, after he suffered a career-ending injury, from which he is completely disabled. Wei and Raymond have been working together for several years on quality-of-life issues and depression. Raymond is frequently distressed by his unwavering belief that everyone in his hometown greets him with sexual gestures and believes that he is gay. This belief extends to truck drivers who come through the town; he believes that they talk about his sexuality on their CB radios. These beliefs create great distress and anxiety for him. He occasionally yells at people or gestures back. Wei has been helping Raymond to understand how his perceptions may be faulty and how his hearing loss may contribute to his perceptual difficulties and anxiety. Raymond and Wei have invited his mother into the discussion so she can support him at home.

CLUSTER B PERSONALITY DISORDERS

Borderline Personality Disorder

Borderline personality disorder (BPD) is the most well known and dramatic of the personality disorders. BPD occurs at a rate of about 1.6% in community studies (Skodol, Bender, Morey, et al., 2011). The major features of this disorder are patterns of marked instability in emotion regulation, unstable interpersonal relationships, identity or self-image distortions, and unstable mood. These symptoms result in severe functional impairments, a high mortality rate (approximately 30%), and extensive use of health care services (Madarasz, Manzardo, Mortensen, et al., 2012). People with BPD seek out treatment for depression, anxiety, suicidal and self-harming behaviours, and other impulsive behaviours including substance use. Although hospitalization may decrease self-destructive risk for patients with BPD, it is not regarded as an effective long-term solution. With effective treatment, people with BPD can experience high rates of remission and low rates of relapse (Gunderson, 2011).

Borderline personality disorder is around five times more common in first-degree biological relatives with the same disorder compared with the general population (APA, 2013). This disorder is highly associated with genetic factors such as hypersensitivity, impulsivity, and emotional dysregulation (Gunderson, 2011). A meta-analysis by Amad and colleagues (2014) identified that familial and twin studies support the potential role of genetic vulnerability at approximately 40%.

There is evidence of serotonergic dysfunction that accompanies the borderline trait of impulsivity. It may also contribute to the depression and aggression that commonly accompany this disorder. The serotonin transporter gene *5-HTT* may have shorter alleles, which have been associated with lower levels of serotonin and increased impulsive aggression.

Structural and functional magnetic resonance imaging have revealed abnormalities in the prefrontal cortex and limbic regions. The frontal region is implicated in regulatory control processes, and the limbic region is essential for emotional processing (Krause-Utz, Winter, Niedtfeld, et al., 2014). Limbic hyper-reactivity and diminished control by the frontal brain may explain poor emotion processing, impulsivity, and interpersonal disturbances.

See the Neurobiology of Borderline Personality Disorder feature for more information about the neurobiology of BPD.

Margaret Mahler (1895–1985), a Hungarian-born child psychologist who worked with emotionally disturbed children, developed a framework that is useful in considering BPD. Mahler and colleagues (1975) believed that psychological problems are a result of the disruption of the normal separation-individuation of the child from the mother.

According to Mahler, an infant progresses from complete self-absorption with an inability to separate himself or herself from the mother to a physically and psychologically differentiated toddler. Mahler emphasized the role of the significant other (traditionally the mother) in providing a secure emotional base of support that promotes enough confidence for the child to separate. This support is achieved through a balance of holding (emotionally and physically) a child enough for the child to feel safe, while at the same time fostering and encouraging independence and natural exploration.

Problems may arise in this separation-individuation process. If a toddler leaves his or her mother on the park bench and wanders off to the sandbox, ideally two things should happen. First, the child should be encouraged to go off into the world with smiles and reassurance: "Go on, honey, it's safe to go away a little." Second, the mother needs to be reliably present when the toddler returns, thereby rewarding her efforts. Clearly, parents are not perfect and are sometimes distracted and short tempered. Mahler notes that raising healthy children does not require that parents never make mistakes and that "good enough parenting" will promote successful separation-individuation.

Stages of this process are as follows:

- **Stage 1 (birth to 1 month): Normal autism.** The infant spends most of his or her time sleeping.
- **Stage 2 (1 to 5 months): Symbiosis.** The infant perceives the mother-infant as a single fused entity. Infants gradually distinguish the inner world from the outer world.
- **Stage 3 (5 to 10 months): Differentiation.** The infant recognizes distinctness from the mother. Progressive neurological development and increased alertness draw the infant's attention away from self to the outer world.
- **Stage 4 (11 to 18 months): Practising.** The ability to walk and explore greatly expands the toddler's sense of separateness.
- **Stage 5 (18 to 24 months): Rapprochement.** Toddlers move away from their mothers and come back for emotional refuelling. Periods of helplessness and dependence alternate with the need for independence.
- **Stage 6 (2 to 5 years): Object constancy.** When children comprehend that objects (in this case, the object is the mother) are permanent even when they are not in their presence, the individuation process is complete.

Children who later develop BPD may have had this process disrupted. The rapprochement stage is particularly crucial and coincides with the "terrible twos," which are characterized by darting away and clinging and whining. Some experts suggest that this phase is not a desirable time for extended separation between parent and child.

Consider the previous ideal example of the child who wants to play in the sandbox. If the child wanders off to the sandbox and returns to a caregiver who is emotionally unavailable, perhaps hurt by the attempt at independence, the child feels unsafe to explore. Alternately, if the caregiver has personal issues related to dependency and abandonment, he or she may be threatened by the child's attempts at independence and respond with clinging and halting exploration. The child cannot safely move on to the next stage of development. A fear of abandonment from others, along with a sense of anger, carries over into adulthood.

Pathological Personality Traits Seen in People With BPD

One of the pathological personality traits seen in people with BPD is negative affect. This affect is characterized by **emotional lability**—that is, moods that alternate rapidly from one emotional

Neurobiology of Borderline Personality Disorder

Borderline personality disorder (BPD) is a serious and disabling brain disorder marked by impulsivity and emotional dysregulation.

Serotonin: Altered functioning of serotonin in the brain has been linked to depression, aggression, and difficulty in controlling destructive urges. The serotonin transporter gene *5-HTT* is thought to have shorter alleles in BPD,u which have been associated with lower levels of serotonin and increased impulsive aggression.

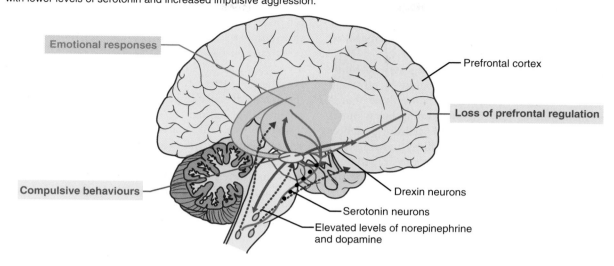

Emotional dysregulation: Emotional responses that are poorly modulated (e.g., angry outbursts, rage, marked fluctuation of mood, self-harm) and that can shift within seconds, minutes, or hours

Brain Imaging (Functional Magnetic Resonance Imaging) Findings
Prefrontal cortex: In times of stress, this part of the brain helps us regulate emotions and refrain from inappropriate actions. The prefrontal cortex helps with reality testing and guides attention and thought. In people with BPD this part of the brain does not respond. Instead, there is an extreme perception and intensity of negative emotions.

Limbic system/amygdala: In BPD, parts of the emotional centre of the brain are overstimulated and take longer to return to normal. Also, **certain neurotransmitters** that act as constraints in normal circumstances may underfunction in BPD, leaving a person in a prolonged fight-or-flight response.

Medications/Therapy to Help Individuals Regulate Their Emotions

Method	What's Involved	What It Does
Medications	Mindfulness, deep breathing, relaxation techniques	Helps brain switch from sympathetic nervous system (arousal) to parasympathetic nervous system (relaxation mode)
Dialectic behavioural therapy (DBT)	Selective serotonin reuptake inhibitors, anticonvulsants, second-generation antipsychotics, lithium	Helps dampen angry, impulsive, labile behaviour

Sources: Dialectical Living. (n.d.). *Emotion dysregulation.* Retrieved from http://www.dialecticalliving.ca/emotion-regulation-disorder-bpd/; Ruocco, A. C., Amirthavasagam, S., Choi-Kain, L. W., et al. (2013). Neural correlates of negative emotionality in borderline personality disorder: An activation-likelihood-estimation meta-analysis. *Biological Psychiatry, 73*(2), 153–160; and Nauert, R. (2015). Brain scans clarify borderline personality disorder. *Psych Central.* Retrieved from http://psychcentral.com/news/2009/09/04/brain-scans-clarify-borderline-personality-disorder/8184.html.

extreme to another. Other characteristics of a negative affect include responding to situations with emotions that are out of proportion to the circumstances, pathological fear of separation, and intense sensitivity to perceived personal rejection. Other disruptive traits common in people with BPD are impulsivity and antagonism. Impulsivity is manifested in acting quickly in response to emotions without considering the consequences. This impulsivity results in damaged relationships and even suicide attempts.

Borderline personality disorder is also characterized by feelings of antagonism, manifested in hostility, anger, and irritability in relationships. Physical violence toward intimate partners and nonintimate partners alike may occur. Rarely, a homicide of family members or others occurs. Violence is also manifested in destructive behaviours such as property damage.

In addition, ineffective and harmful self-soothing habits, such as cutting, promiscuous sexual behaviour, and numbing with substances, are common and may result in unintentional death.

Chronic suicidal ideation is also a common feature of this disorder and influences the likelihood of accidental death. There are high rates of comorbid illnesses such as mood, anxiety, or substance disorders that complicate the treatment and prognosis of BPD. A number of nonpsychiatric diagnoses are also associated with BPD. They include diabetes, high blood pressure, chronic back pain, fibromyalgia, and arthritis, and must be considered when determining treatment approaches.

Splitting, the primary defence or coping style used by people with BPD, is the inability to incorporate positive and negative aspects of oneself or others into a whole image. This kind of dichotomous thinking and coping behaviour is believed to be partly a result of the person's failed experiences with adult personality integration and is likely influenced by exposure to earlier psychological, sexual, or physical trauma. For example, the individual may tend to idealize another person (e.g., friend, lover, health care provider) at the start of a new relationship, hoping that this person will meet all of his or her needs. However, at the first disappointment or frustration, the individual quickly shifts to devaluation, despising the other person.

Guidelines for Nursing Care

- A therapeutic relationship is essential with patients who have BPD because most of them have experienced failed relationships, including therapeutic alliances.
- The therapeutic relationship often follows an initial hesitancy on the part of patient, then an upward curve of idealization by the patient toward the caregiver. This idealization is invariably followed by a devaluation of the staff member when the patient is disappointed by unmet—frequently impossible—expectations.
- Conduct a thorough assessment of current or past physical, sexual, or emotional abuse and level of current risk for harm from self or others.
- Clinical supervision and additional education are helpful and supportive to health care providers.
- Awareness and monitoring of one's own stress responses to patient behaviours facilitate more effective and therapeutic intervention, regardless of the therapeutic approach being used.
- Evaluating treatment effectiveness in this patient population is difficult. Nurses may never know the real results of their interventions.

Treatment

People with BPD are usually admitted to psychiatric treatment programs because of symptoms with comorbid disorders or dangerous behaviour. Emotions such as anxiety, rage, and depression and behaviours such as withdrawal, paranoia, and manipulation are among the most frequent that health care workers must address. When patients blame and attack others, the nurse needs to understand the context of their complaints. These attacks originate from the feeling of being threatened. The more intense the complaints are, the greater the patients' fear of potential harm or loss is. Be aware of manipulative behaviours such as flattery, seductiveness, and instilling guilt.

Case Study and Nursing Care Plan 19-1 presents a patient with BPD.

Realistic outcomes are established for individuals with BPD based on the perspective that personality change occurs with one behavioural solution and one learned skill at a time. This can be expected to take a lot of time and repetition. In the acute care setting, the focus is on the presenting problem, which may be depression or severe anxiety. Health care providers do not expect resolution of chronic behaviour problems during the hospital stay, but rather expect to be met with appropriate therapeutic feedback and incremental steps toward recovery in an outpatient setting.

People with BPD are impulsive and may be suicidal, self-mutilating, aggressive, manipulative, and even psychotic during periods of stress. Provide clear and consistent boundaries and limits. Use straightforward communication. When behavioural problems emerge, calmly review the therapeutic goals.

There are no approved medications for treating BPD. When medications are used, their purposes are to maintain patients' cognitive function, relieve symptoms, and improve quality of life. People with BPD often respond to antidepressants such as selective serotonin reuptake inhibitors (SSRIs), anticonvulsants, and lithium for mood and emotional dysregulation symptoms. Naltrexone, an opioid receptor antagonist, has been found to reduce self-injurious behaviours. Second-generation antipsychotics may control anger and brief psychosis.

When individuals with BPD are admitted to the hospital, partially hospitalized, or in day treatment settings, team management is a significant part of treatment. The primary goal is management of the patient's affect in a group context. Community meetings, coping skills groups, and socializing groups are all helpful for these patients. They have the opportunity to interact with peers and staff to discuss goals and learn problem-solving skills. Dealing with emotional issues that arise in the milieu requires a calm, united approach by the staff to maintain safety and to enhance self-control.

Common problems resulting from staff splitting can be minimized if the unit leaders hold weekly staff meetings in which staff members are allowed to ventilate their feelings about conflicts with patients and each other. This process is often acted out in the treatment milieu and can interrupt the delivery of care. For example, a female patient may briefly idealize her male nurse on the inpatient unit, telling staff and patients alike that she is "the luckiest person because she has the best nurse in the hospital." The rest of the team understands that this comment is an exaggeration. After days of her constant dramatic praise for the nurse and subtle insults to the rest of the staff, some members of the team may start to feel inadequate and resentful of the nurse. They begin to make critical remarks about minor events to prove that the nurse is not perfect. A similar scenario can occur if the person constantly complains about one staff member; some colleagues are then torn between defending and criticizing the targeted staff member. Consistency and a team approach help to ensure the productive use of therapeutic time and structure for the patient. Patient-centred approaches allow the patient to be part of the treatment planning.

Evaluating treatment effectiveness in this patient population is difficult. Freedom from harm to self and others is a tangible and satisfying positive evaluation. Nurses may never know the real results of their intervention, particularly in acute care settings. Even in long-term outpatient treatment, patients with BPD experience too many disruptions to relationships to remain long enough for successful treatment. As noted earlier, however, some motivated patients may be able to learn to change their behaviour, especially if positive experiences are repeated.

VIGNETTE

Shaina is a 38-year-old married woman with one young son. She works full time as a dietitian in a primary care network. Shaina was diagnosed with fibromyalgia 2 years ago and is in treatment at a pain clinic. Most days, she comes home from work fatigued and goes to bed, leaving her son to play by himself after school or with friends until her husband gets home from work. Shaina also has struggled with an eating disorder since she was a teenager. When she feels guilty for ignoring her son's needs, she binges and then purges to relieve her negative emotions. Shaina recognizes that this behaviour helps only temporarily and adds to her fatigue, but she still feels helpless to stop it. When her son asks her to play with him or take him to an activity, she becomes angry with him and then feels angry at herself. Shaina has been referred by the palliative care nurse at the pain clinic to a dialectical behaviour therapy group (discussed later in this chapter) to learn skills to deal with her chronic pain and discover alternative self-soothing strategies for her bingeing and purging behaviours.

Antisocial Personality Disorder

Antisocial personality disorder is a pattern of disregard for, and violation of, the rights of others. People with this disorder may be more commonly referred to as sociopaths. This diagnosis is reserved for adults, but symptoms are evident by the mid-teens. Symptoms tend to peak during the late teenage years and into the mid-twenties. By around 40 years of age, the symptoms may abate and improve even without treatment. The prevalence of antisocial personality disorder is about 1.1% in community studies (Skodol, Bender, Gunderson, et al., 2014). While the disorder is much more common in men (3% versus 1%), women may be underdiagnosed due to the traditional close association of this disorder with males.

Antisocial personality disorder is genetically linked, and twin studies indicate a predisposition to this disorder. Kendler and colleagues (2012) note that there are two main dimensions of genetic risk. One is the trait of aggressive disregard, which refers to violent tendencies without concern for others; the other is the trait of disinhibition, which is a lack of concern for consequences. It is likely that the genetic predisposition for characteristics of antisocial personality disorder such as a lack of empathy may be set into motion by childhood maltreatment. Inconsistent parenting and discipline, significant abuse, and extreme neglect are associated with this disorder. Children reflect parental attitudes and behaviours in the absence of more prosocial influences. Virtually all individuals who eventually develop this disorder have a history of impulse control and conduct problems as children and adolescents.

CONSIDERING CULTURE

Gender Bias in Diagnosing Personality Disorders

There may be a culture-bound gender bias in the diagnosing of personality disorders. Borderline personality disorder (BPD) is an example of such a bias: well-respected diagnostic manuals report a 3:1 gender ratio of females to males for BPD (Sansone & Sansone, 2011). However, Grant and colleagues (2008), in a well-executed epidemiological survey, found BPD to be equally prevalent in men and women. Thus a subtle clinician bias has increased the predominance of BPD diagnosis in women. This bias may have developed because women with BPD undertake more self-harming behaviours, which result in their admission to treatment, whereas men with BPD have more substance abuse and antisocial features, which result in their incarceration. This difference may lead staff working in a psychiatric treatment facility to think that there are more females with BPD. Also, the emotional aspects of BPD may present differently in women and men (Verona, Sprague, & Javdani, 2012), and, as a result, it is important for health care providers to think of this disorder more broadly than as primarily a women's issue.

Sources: Grant, B., Chou, S., Goldstein, R., et al. (2008). Prevalence, correlates, disability, and comorbidity of DSM-IV borderline personality disorder: Results from the wave 2 national epidemiologic survey on alcohol and related conditions. *Journal of Clinical Psychiatry, 69*(4), 533–545. Retrieved from http://www.ncbi.nlm.nih.gov/pubmed/18426259; Sansone, R., & Sansone, L. (2011). Gender patterns in borderline personality disorder. *Innovations in Clinical Neuroscience, 8*(5), 16–20. Retrieved from http://www.ncbi.nlm.nih.gov/pmc/articles/PMC3115767/; and Verona, E., Sprague, J., & Javdani, S. (2012). Gender and factor-level interactions in psychopathy: Implications for self-directed violence risk and borderline personality disorder symptoms. *Personality Disorders, 3*(3), 247–262. doi:10.1037/a0025945.

The main pathological traits that characterize antisocial personality disorder are antagonistic behaviours such as being deceitful and manipulative for personal gain or being hostile if needs are blocked. The disorder is also characterized by disinhibited behaviours such as high level of risk taking, disregard for responsibility, and impulsivity. Criminal misconduct and substance misuse are common in this population.

People with this disorder are mostly concerned with gaining personal power or pleasure, and in relationships they focus on their own gratification to an extreme. They have little to no capacity for intimacy and will exploit others if it benefits them in relationships. One of the most disturbing qualities associated with antisocial personality disorder is a profound lack of empathy, also known as callousness. This **callousness** results in a lack of concern about the feelings of others, the absence of remorse or guilt except when facing punishment, and a disregard for meeting school, family, and other obligations.

These individuals tend to exhibit a shallow, unexpressive, and superficial affect. They may also be adept at portraying themselves as concerned and caring if these attributes help them to manipulate and exploit others. A person with antisocial personality disorder may be able to act witty and charming and be good at flattery and manipulating the emotions of others.

Guidelines for Nursing Care

- Nurses should be aware and monitor their responses to patient behaviours to facilitate effective and therapeutic responses.
- Conduct a thorough assessment of current life stressors, history of violent thoughts and behaviours (including suicidal ideation), and substance use.
- Be aware that distrust, hostility, and a profound inability to connect with others will impair the usual process of developing a therapeutic relationship.
- Evaluating treatment effectiveness in this patient population is difficult. Nurses may never know the real results of their interventions.

Treatment

In the context of antisocial personality disorder, the role of the nurse will be to provide consistency, support, boundaries, and limits. Providing realistic choices (e.g., selection of a particular group activity) may enhance adherence to treatment. People with antisocial personality disorder may be involuntarily admitted to psychiatric units for evaluation. With their freedom limited, they tend to be angry, manipulative, aggressive, and impulsive. Try to prevent or reduce untoward effects of manipulation (flattery, seductiveness, instilling of guilt). Set clear and realistic boundaries and consequences, and ensure that all staff follow these limits. Carefully document behaviours and signs of manipulation. Be aware that antisocial patients can manipulate with feelings of guilt when they are not getting what they want.

The safety of patients and staff is a prime consideration in working with individuals in this population. To promote safety, the entire treatment team should follow a solid treatment plan that emphasizes realistic limits on specific behaviour, consistency in responses, and consequences for actions. Careful documentation of behaviours will aid in providing effective interventions and in promoting teamwork.

Therapeutic communication techniques are valuable tools for working with individuals with antisocial personality disorder. Simply being heard can defuse an emotionally charged situation. For example, the nurse can listen to a patient's emotional complaints about the staff and the hospital without correcting errors, simply noting that the patient truly feels hurt. Showing empathy may also decrease aggressive outbursts if the patient feels that staff members are trying to understand feelings of frustration.

There are no approved medications for treating antisocial personality disorder. Medications are used to treat concurrent comorbid disorders. The advanced-practice psychiatric mental health registered nurse may care for individuals with this type of personality disorder in a variety of inpatient and community settings. Research shows that individuals with this disorder do benefit from therapies to address other mental health conditions. These individuals often require intense and long-term treatment.

Histrionic Personality Disorder

People with histrionic personality disorder are excitable and dramatic yet are often high functioning. They may be referred to in terms of being a "drama queen" or "drama major." Classic

> **VIGNETTE**
>
> Manwell is a 27-year-old divorced cab driver who is referred to the hospital by the court for a mental health evaluation after an assault charge. He told the arresting officer that he has bipolar disorder. He has a history of substance abuse and multiple arrests for disorderly conduct or assault. During his intake interview, he is polite and even flirtatious with the female nurse. He insists that he is not responsible for his behaviour because he is manic. The only symptom he describes is irritability. He points out that he cannot tolerate any psychotropic medications because of the adverse effects. He also notes that he has dropped out of three clinics after several visits because "the staff don't understand me."

characteristics of this population include extraversion, flamboyancy, and colourful personalities. Despite this bold exterior, those with histrionic personality disorder tend to have limited ability to develop meaningful relationships.

Histrionic personality disorder occurs at a rate of nearly 2% in community samples (APA, 2013). In clinical settings, it tends to be diagnosed more frequently in women than in men. Symptoms begin by early adulthood. Inborn character traits such as emotional expressiveness and egocentricity have also been identified as predisposing an individual to this disorder.

This disorder is characterized by emotional attention-seeking behaviours, including self-centredness, low frustration tolerance, and excessive emotionality. The person with histrionic personality disorder is often impulsive and may act flirtatiously or provocatively. Relationships do not last because the partner often feels smothered or reacts to the insensitivity of the histrionic person. The individual with histrionic personality disorder does not have insight into a personal role in breaking up relationships.

In general, individuals with this disorder do not think they need psychiatric help. They may go into treatment for associated problems such as depression, which may be precipitated by losses such as the end of a relationship.

Guidelines for Nursing Care

- Nursing care should reflect an understanding that seductive behaviour is a response to distress.
- Keep communication and interactions professional.
- Patients may exaggerate symptoms and difficulty in functioning.
- Encourage and model the use of concrete and descriptive rather than vague and impressionistic language.
- Assist patients to clarify feelings because they often have difficulty identifying them.
- Teach and role model assertiveness.
- Assess for suicidal ideation. What was intended as a suicide gesture may inadvertently result in death.

Treatment

Individuals with histrionic personality disorder may be out of touch with their feelings (Sadock, Sadock, & Ruiz, 2015). Psychotherapy may promote clarification of inner feelings and appropriate expression. Group therapy may be useful in this population, although distracting symptoms may be disruptive to group functioning.

There are no specific pharmacological treatments available for people with histrionic personality disorder. Medications such as antidepressants can be used for depressive symptoms. Antianxiety agents may be helpful in treating anxiety. Antipsychotics may be used if the patient exhibits derealization or illusions.

VIGNETTE

Ms. Lombard is a 35-year-old twice-divorced female admitted to an inpatient unit after an overdose of asthma medications and antibiotics. She took all of her pills after her primary care provider refused to order a sleeping pill for her. On the first night, she is withdrawn and tearful in her room. By the next morning, she is neatly groomed, even wearing makeup, and is socializing with everyone. She denies thoughts of self-harm. Over the next 2 days, Ms. Lombard monopolizes the community meetings by talking about how unappreciated she is by her family. She seeks special attention from a male evening-shift registered nurse, asking if he can stay late after his shift to sit with her. When he refuses, she demands to be placed back on one-to-one precautions because she feels suicidal again.

Narcissistic Personality Disorder

Narcissistic personality disorder is characterized by feelings of entitlement, an exaggerated belief in one's own importance, and a lack of empathy. In reality, people with this disorder suffer from a weak self-esteem and hypersensitivity to criticism. Narcissistic personality disorder is associated with less impairment in individual functioning and quality of life than the other personality-based disorders.

The prevalence of narcissistic personality disorder ranges from 0% to about 6% in community samples (APA, 2013). It tends to be more common in males than in females. Age of onset is difficult to determine due to the narcissistic traits that are typically found in adolescents. There may be a familial tendency for this disorder, as parents with narcissism may attribute an unrealistic sense of talent, importance, and beauty to their children. These attributions put the children at higher risk for the disorder.

People with narcissistic personality disorder come across as arrogant and as having an inflated view of their self-importance. The individual with this disorder has a need for constant admiration along with a lack of empathy for others, a factor that strains most relationships over time. He or she is very sensitive to rejection and criticism and can be disparaging to others. A sense of personal entitlement paired with a lack of social empathy may result in the exploitation of other people.

Underneath the surface of arrogance, people with narcissistic personality disorder feel intense shame and have a fear of abandonment. In keeping with these descriptions, the main pathological personality trait of narcissism is antagonism, represented by grandiosity and attention-seeking behaviours. Those with narcissistic personality disorder tend to tolerate rejection poorly. As a result, narcissistic individuals may seek help for depression or may seek to be validated by therapists and loved ones for their emotional pain of not being appreciated by others for their efforts or special qualities.

Guidelines for Nursing Care

- Nurses should remain neutral and recognize the source of narcissistic behaviour—shame and fear of abandonment.
- Use the therapeutic nurse–patient relationship as an opportunity to practise engaging in meaningful interaction.
- Avoid engaging in power struggles or becoming defensive in response to the patient's disparaging remarks.
- Role model empathy.

Treatment

Because patients need to confront their problem to make progress, treating people specifically for this disorder is difficult (Sadock, Sadock, & Ruiz, 2015). Because individuals are not likely to seek help for their own problems, they are more likely to be involved in couples or family therapy than in individual treatment. In these family-oriented approaches, narcissistic individuals are likely to deflect suggestions that they contribute to family problems and will instead blame others.

If a person with narcissistic personality disorder somehow seeks treatment, individual cognitive behavioural therapy is helpful in deconstructing faulty thinking. Group therapy can also assist the person in sharing with others, seeing their own qualities in others, and learning empathy.

There are no approved medications for treating narcissistic personality disorder. Medications are used to treat concurrent comorbid disorders.

VIGNETTE

Dr. Abigail McLaughlin is a 40-year-old female attending psychiatrist at a university outpatient centre. She is twice divorced and has no children. Her grooming and makeup are impeccable, and she likes to chat about her expensive shopping habits. She is quite intelligent and is the only doctor on the staff trained in psychoanalysis. In clinical team meetings, she often discusses this fact, repeatedly telling others that psychoanalysis is the best treatment for mental illness. She frequently makes derogatory remarks to psychiatric residents if they suggest alternative treatment approaches for new cases. She is usually late to staff meetings, and when she is not speaking, she yawns and shifts noisily in her seat. She has a reputation for exhibiting angry outbursts at therapists in the hallway over minor mistakes, such as a scheduling error for a patient. She underwent 7 years of psychoanalysis but does not consider it to have been therapy—it "was for training purposes only."

CLUSTER C PERSONALITY DISORDERS

Avoidant Personality Disorder

The main pathological personality traits associated with avoidant personality disorder are low self-esteem related to functioning in social situations, feelings of inferiority compared with peers, and a reluctance to engage in unfamiliar activities involving new people. Some individuals with avoidant personality disorder can function in a protective environment. However, if their support system fails, they can suffer from depression, anxiety, and anger. They are especially sensitive to and preoccupied with rejection, humiliation, and failure. They often avoid new interpersonal relationships or activities due to their fears of criticism or disapproval (APA, 2013).

Avoidant personality disorder occurs in 6.6% of the Canadian population (Langlois, Samokhvalov, Rehm, et al., 2011). It is found equally among men and women. Early symptoms of the disorder are often evident in infants and children. These symptoms include shyness and avoidance that, unlike common shyness, increases during adolescence and early adulthood.

Guidelines for Nursing Care

- Nurses should use a friendly, accepting, reassuring approach and remember that being pushed into social situations can cause extreme and severe anxiety for these patients.
- Convey an attitude of acceptance toward patient fears.
- Provide the patient with exercises to enhance new social skills, but use these with caution because any failure can increase feelings of poor self-worth.
- Assertiveness training can assist the person to learn to express needs.

Treatment

Individual and group therapy is useful in processing anxiety-provoking symptoms and in planning methods to approach and handle anxiety-provoking situations (Sadock, Sadock, & Ruiz, 2015). Psychotherapy focuses on trust and assertiveness training.

Antianxiety agents can be helpful. Beta-adrenergic receptor antagonists (e.g., atenolol) help reduce autonomic nervous system hyperactivity. Antidepressant medications, such as SSRIs like citalopram (Celexa) and serotonin–norepinephrine reuptake inhibitors (SNRIs) like venlafaxine (Effexor), may reduce social anxiety (Ripoll, Triebwasser, & Siever, 2011). Serotonergic agents may help individuals with avoidant personalities feel less sensitive to rejection.

VIGNETTE

Annemarie is a 35-year-old single female who works as a receptionist for a computer repair company. As a child, she had few friends and never participated in extracurricular activities. Annemarie lives alone in her own apartment and has never had an intimate adult relationship. On the job, she rarely talks to co-workers and prefers to work alone. If she has any questions, she asks the supervisor and carefully follows directions. Although she has 7 years of experience and a good work record, she refuses the offer of a promotion because it would require her to interact with customers.

Dependent Personality Disorder

Dependent personality disorder is characterized by a pattern of submissive and clinging behaviour related to an overwhelming need to be cared for. This need results in intense fears of separation.

Dependent personality disorder is fairly rare, with an estimated prevalence rate of about 0.5% (APA, 2013). Dependent personality disorder may be the result of chronic physical illness or punishment for independent behaviour in childhood. The inherited trait of submissiveness may also be a factor.

People with dependent personality disorder have a high need to be taken care of. This need can lead to patterns of submissiveness with fears of separation and abandonment by others. Because they lack confidence in their own ability or judgement, those with dependent personality disorder may manipulate others to assume responsibility for such activities as finances or child rearing. This may create problems by leaving them more vulnerable to exploitation by others because of their passive and submissive nature. Feelings of insecurity about their self-agency and lack of self-confidence may interfere with attempts to become more independent. They may experience intense anxiety when left alone for even brief periods of time (APA, 2013).

Guidelines for Nursing Care

- Nurses can help the patient identify and address current stressors.
- Be aware that strong counter-transference may develop because of the patient's demands for extra time and crisis states.
- The therapeutic nurse–patient relationship can provide a testing ground for increased assertiveness through role modelling and teaching of assertive skills.

Treatment

Psychotherapy is the treatment of choice for dependent personality disorder (Sadock, Sadock, & Ruiz, 2015). Cognitive behavioural therapy can help patients develop more healthy and accurate thinking by examining and challenging automatic thoughts that result in fearful behaviour. This process can help in developing new perspectives and attitudes about the need for other people.

There are no specific medications indicated for this disorder, but symptoms of depression and anxiety may be treated with the appropriate antidepressant and antianxiety agents. Panic attacks can be helped with the tricyclic antidepressant imipramine (Tofranil).

VIGNETTE

Bawaajige is a 32-year-old, married former engineer, and she is mother to two young children, ages 3 years and 11 months. Bawaajige's depression and anxiety have been more severe since she stopped working. She feels inadequate and overwhelmed by her responsibilities, so her mother moved in with the young family at Bawaajige's request. Her therapist, an advanced-practice psychiatric mental health registered nurse, recommended that she receive brief treatment for depression and anxiety at the partial hospitalization program. Bawaajige quickly bonded with the advanced-practice nurse, who is an older woman. She frequently asks her for reassurance that she is doing the right thing by coming to treatment and seeks her out frequently for extra individual sessions. Gradually, as the result of individual and group thereapy, Bawaajige begins to realize that excessive dependence on her mother contributes to long-standing feelings of ineffectiveness, helplessness, and invalidation of her own parenting skills.

Obsessive-Compulsive Personality Disorder

Obsessive-compulsive personality disorder is characterized by limited emotional expression, stubbornness, perseverance, and indecisiveness. Preoccupation with orderliness, perfectionism, and control are the hallmarks of this disorder.

Obsessive-compulsive personality disorder is one of the most prevalent personality disorders. The prevalence rate is about 7.7% (Langlois, Samokhvalov, Rehm, et al., 2011). It is more common in men than in women. Oldest siblings tend to be affected more often than subsequent siblings. Risk factors for this disorder include a background of harsh discipline and having a first-degree relative with this disorder. Obsessive-compulsive personality disorder has been associated with increased relapse rates of depression and an increase in suicidal risks in people with co-occurring depression.

The main pathological personality traits are rigidity and inflexible standards of self and others. People with obsessive-compulsive personality disorder rehearse over and over how they will respond in social situations. They persist in goal seeking long after it is necessary, even if it is self-defeating or relationship defeating. The preoccupation often results in losing the major point of the activity. Projects are often incomplete due to overly strict standards.

There is a difference between obsessive-compulsive disorder and obsessive-compulsive personality disorder. Obsessive-compulsive disorder is characterized by obsessive thoughts and by repetition or adherence to rituals. Those with obsessive-compulsive disorder are aware that these thoughts and actions are unreasonable. Obsessive-compulsive personality disorder is characterized more by an unhealthy focus on perfectionism. Those with obsessive-compulsive personality disorder think that their actions are right and feel comfortable with such self-imposed systems of rules.

People with obsessive-compulsive personality disorder often do feel genuine affection for friends and family, yet leisure activities and friendship are dropped in favour of excessive devotion to work and productivity.

Guidelines for Nursing Care

- Nurses should guard against power struggles with these patients, as their need for control is very high.
- Patients with this disorder have difficulty dealing with unexpected changes.
- Provide structure, yet allow patients extra time to complete habitual behaviour.
- Assist patients to identify ineffective coping and to develop effective coping techniques.

Treatment

Typically, patients seek help for obsessive-compulsive personality disorder, as they are aware of their own suffering. They may also seek treatment for anxiety or depression. The treatment course is often long and complicated. Both group therapy and behavioural therapy can be helpful, so that the person can learn new coping skills for his or her anxiety and see direct benefits for change from feedback within the group.

Clomipramine (Anafranil) may help reduce the obsessions, anxiety, and depression associated with this disorder. Other serotonergic agents such as fluoxetine (Prozac) may also be effective.

VIGNETTE

Robert is a 45-year-old, single, male postal worker in a small town. He lives alone and has never married. He is well groomed and wears a clean, neatly ironed uniform every day. He carefully follows all policies and procedures and is quite resistant whenever there is an update or change. He frequently challenges the supervisor about policy details and has been referred to the regional personnel office countless times for resolution of these conflicts. In staff meetings, he gives excessive circumstantial details and writes extra material on the back of any required report form. When dealing with the public, he sometimes gets into arguments with customers about postal rules or the schedule. Other staff members do not consider him to be a team player because he seldom volunteers to help others. Even if he is asked to help someone, he is quick to criticize his peer's performance. Although he has worked in the same office for 10 years, he has never advanced beyond the front-line position. He is fairly content with his work and has never been in psychiatric treatment.

APPLICATION OF THE NURSING PROCESS

ASSESSMENT

Assessment Tools

The preferred method for determining a diagnosis of personality disorder is the semistructured interview obtained by clinicians. These types of interviews have standard questions and a standard format for asking the questions. These interviews go beyond asking the patient to self-report symptoms because individuals with personality disorders often lack insight into their behaviours and motivations and therefore have difficulty accurately describing themselves. One way to elicit more objective information is to ask the person if family members and colleagues perceive them in a certain way. For example, "You said that you don't think you're emotionally distant. How would your wife describe you?" Cultural norms and expectations also need to be considered when evaluating the presence of a personality disorder. Personality disorders are often assessed through identifying pathology within one or more personality dimensions. The five main dimensions of personalities are (1) extraversion versus introversion, (2) antagonism versus compliance, (3) constraint versus impulsivity, (4) emotional dysregulation versus emotional stability, and (5) unconventionality versus closedness to experience (Simms, Goldberg, Roberts, et al., 2011). See Table 19-1.

Open-ended or subjective interviews, which do not have standard questions or a standard question format, are more likely to result in biased and culturally based decisions about diagnosis (McGilloway, Hall, Lee, et al., 2010). Self-report inventories, such as the well-known Minnesota Multiphasic Personality Inventory (MMPI), are useful because they have built-in validity and reliability scales for the clinician to refer to when interpreting

TABLE 19-1	FIVE DIMENSIONS OF PERSONALITY
PERSONALITY DIMENSIONS	**ATTITUDES AND BEHAVIOURS**
Extraversion versus introversion	Activity, aloofness, assertiveness, detachment, entitlement, excitement seeking, exhibitionism, exploratory excitability, extravagance, gregariousness, histrionic sexualization, intimacy problems, optimism, positive emotionality, restricted expression, schizoid orientation, shyness, sociability, social avoidance, social closeness, social potency, stimulus seeking, warmth, well-being
Antagonism versus compliance	Aggression, agreeableness, alienation, altruism, attachment, callousness, compassion, compliance, conduct problems, dependency, diffidence, empathy, entitlement, helpfulness, insecure attachment, interpersonal disesteem, manipulativeness, mistrust, modesty, narcissism, passive oppositionality, psychopathy, pure-heartedness, rejection, sentimentality, social acceptance, social closeness, straightforwardness, submissiveness, suspiciousness, tender-mindedness, trust
Constraint versus impulsivity	Achievement striving, childishness, competence, compulsivity, conscientiousness, deliberation, disorderliness, dutifulness, eagerness of effort, harm avoidance, impulsivity, irresponsibility, obsessionality, order, perfectionism, propriety, resourcefulness, responsibility, risk taking, self-discipline, traditionalism, workaholism
Emotional dysregulation versus emotional stability	Affective lability, alienation, angry hostility, anticipatory worry, anxiousness, dependency, depressiveness, dysphoria, emotional dysregulation, fear of uncertainty, hostility, hypochondriasis, identity problems, inferiority, introspection, irritability, negative affect, pessimism, self-acceptance, self-consciousness, self-harm, sensitivity, stress reaction, unhappiness, vulnerability, worthlessness
Unconventionality versus closedness to experience	Absorption, dissociation, eccentric perceptions, eccentricity, openness to experience, perceptual cognitive distortion, rigidity, spiritual acceptance, thought disorder, transpersonal identification

Source: Adapted from Simms, L., Goldberg, L., Roberts, J., et al. (2011). Computerized adaptive assessment of personality disorder: Introducing the CAT-PD project. *Journal of Personality Assessment, 93*(4), 380–389. doi:10.1080/00223891.2011.577475. Reprinted by permission of the publisher (Taylor & Francis Ltd, http://www.tandf.co.uk/journals).

test results. Other more focused questionnaires and rating scales can be used to assess several symptoms. These include:

- Feelings of emptiness
- An inclination to engage in risky behaviours such as reckless driving, unsafe sex, substance use, binge eating, gambling, or overspending
- Intense feelings of abandonment that result in paranoia or feeling spaced out
- Idealization of others and becoming close quickly
- A tendency toward anger, sarcasm, and bitterness
- Self-mutilation and self-harm
- Suicidal behaviours, gestures, or threats
- Sudden shifts in self-evaluation that result in changing goals, values, and career focus
- Extreme mood shifts that occur in a matter of hours or days
- Intense, unstable romantic relationships
- Feelings of insecurity
- Rigidity
- Perfectionism

Patient History

Taking a full medical history can help determine if the problem is a psychiatric one, a nonpsychiatric medical one, or both. Nonpsychiatric illness should never be ruled out as the cause for problem behaviour until the data support this conclusion. Important issues in assessing for personality disorders include a history of suicidal or aggressive ideation or actions, current use of medications and illegal substances, ability to handle money, and legal history.

Significant topics about which further details must be obtained include current or past physical, sexual, or emotional abuse and level of current risk for harm from self or others. At times, immediate interventions may be needed to ensure the safety of

the person or others. Information regarding prior use of any medication, including nonprescription substances, is important.

Self-Assessment

Because enduring patterns of interpersonal difficulties are central to the problems faced by people diagnosed with personality disorders, it is understandable that their relationship problems with their caregivers surface in the treatment milieu. Anticipating that people with personality disorders will likely have a disrupted, intense interpersonal experience with caregivers is helpful to the caregivers as they monitor their own personal stress responses. It is important to keep in mind that these dysfunctional behaviours may really represent the person's best efforts to cope because they lack the necessary skills to be effective in their lives.

Finding an approach that works with people in the setting in which they are treated is important. Therapies such as dialectical behaviour therapy and mindfulness-based therapies offer staff evidence-informed interventions, clinical structure, and formalized support for identifying best practices.

DIAGNOSIS

When people with personality disorders are admitted to hospital, it is usually because of symptoms of comorbid disorders, dangerous behaviour, or court-ordered treatment. BPD and antisocial personality disorder both present a challenge for health care providers because the behaviours central to these disorders often cause disruption in psychiatric and medical-surgical settings. Emotions such as anxiety, rage, and depression and behaviours such as withdrawal, paranoia, and manipulation are among the most frequent concerns that health care workers must address. Table 19-2 lists common potential nursing diagnoses related to personality disorders.

RESEARCH HIGHLIGHT

How Do Psychiatric Nurses Respond to Patients With Borderline Personality Disorder?

Problem
People diagnosed with borderline personality disorder (BPD) have problems relating to people in their everyday lives. There is anecdotal evidence that they are also unpopular among mental health nurses.

Purpose of Study
To determine whether mental health nurses respond to people with BPD in problematic ways.

Methods
A systematic integrated literature review of quantitative and qualitative studies was conducted. Forty articles through April 2015 were included. Papers were gathered describing primary research focused on psychiatric nurses' attitudes, behaviour, experience, and knowledge regarding adults with BPD.

Key Findings
- Psychiatric nurses find patients with this diagnosis very challenging to work with.
- Psychiatric nurses report poorer attitudes than other health care professionals toward this population.
- Psychiatric nurses hold poorer attitudes toward patients with BPD than other diagnostic groups.
- Nurses who use a coherent therapeutic framework to guide their practice experience improvement in caregiving.

Implications for Nursing Practice
Mental health nurses have all heard a dismissive, "Oh, she's just a borderline" in response to certain patients. We need a fresh approach to this problem. The authors conclude that developing nurses to lead in the design, implementation, and teaching of coherent therapeutic frameworks will improve the therapeutic relationship.

Source: Dickens, G. L., & Lamont, E. (2016). Mental health nurses' attitudes, behaviour, experience and knowledge regarding adults with a diagnosis of borderline personality disorder: Systematic, integrative literature review. *Journal of Clinical Nursing, 25*(13–14), 1848–1875. doi:10.1111/jocn.13202.

OUTCOMES IDENTIFICATION

Realistic outcomes are established for individuals with personality disorders based on the perspective that personality change occurs with one behavioural solution and one learned skill at a time. This change can be expected to take much time and repetition. In the acute care setting, the focus is on the presenting problem, which may be depression or severe anxiety. During the hospital stay, the chronic behaviour problems of individuals with personality disorders are not expected to be resolved but rather to be met with appropriate therapeutic feedback.

Pertinent categories of nursing outcomes based on the *Nursing Outcomes Classification (NOC)* include aggression self-control, impulse self-control, social interaction skills, personal resiliency, fear level, abusive behaviour self-restraint, and self-mutilation restraint (Moorhead, Johnson, Maas, et al., 2012). Table 19-3 gives

ASSESSMENT GUIDELINES

Personality Disorders

1. Assess for suicidal or homicidal thoughts. If such thoughts are present, the person needs immediate attention.
2. Determine whether the person has a medical disorder or another psychiatric disorder that may be responsible for the symptoms (especially a substance use disorder).
3. View the assessment about personality functioning from within the person's ethnic, cultural, and social background.
4. Ascertain whether the person experienced a recent important loss. Personality disorders are often exacerbated after the loss of significant supporting people or in a disruptive social situation.
5. Evaluate for a change in personality, in middle adulthood or later, that signals the need for a thorough medical workup or assessment for an unrecognized substance use disorder.

TABLE 19-2	POTENTIAL NURSING DIAGNOSES FOR PERSONALITY DISORDERS
SIGNS AND SYMPTOMS	**NURSING DIAGNOSES**
Crisis, high levels of anxiety	*Ineffective coping*
	Anxiety
	Self-mutilation
Anger and aggression; child, elder, or spouse abuse	*Risk for other-directed violence*
	Ineffective coping
	Impaired parenting
	Disabled family coping
Withdrawal	*Social isolation*
Paranoia	*Fear*
	Disturbed sensory perception
	Disturbed thought processes
	Defensive coping
Depression	*Hopelessness*
	Risk for suicide
	Self-mutilation
	Chronic low self-esteem
	Spiritual distress
Difficulty in relationships, manipulation	*Ineffective coping*
	Impaired social interaction
	Defensive coping
	Interrupted family processes
	Risk for loneliness
Failure to keep medical appointments, late arrival for appointments, failure to follow prescribed medical procedure or medication regimen	*Ineffective therapeutic regimen management*
	Nonadherence

examples of other potential nursing outcomes for manipulative, aggressive, and impulsive behaviours.

PLANNING

It is often difficult to create a therapeutic relationship with individuals who have personality disorders because most of them

TABLE 19-3   *NOC* OUTCOMES FOR MANIPULATIVE, AGGRESSIVE, AND IMPULSIVE BEHAVIOURS

NURSING OUTCOME AND DEFINITION	INTERMEDIATE INDICATORS	SHORT-TERM INDICATORS
Social interaction skills: Personal behaviours that promote effective relationships	Uses conflict-resolution methods	Exhibits receptiveness Exhibits sensitivity to others Cooperates with others Uses assertive behaviours as appropriate Uses confrontation as appropriate
Personal resiliency: Positive adaptation and function of an individual following significant adversity or crisis	Uses effective coping strategies	Expresses emotion Seeks emotional support Uses strategies to promote safety Takes responsibility for own actions Uses strategies to avoid violent situations Identifies available community resources Obtains needed support Self-initiates goal-directed behaviour Expresses belief in ability to perform action Expresses that performance will lead to desired outcome
Aggression self-control: Self-restraint of assaultive, combative, or destructive behaviours toward others	Communicates needs appropriately	Identifies when frustrated Identifies when angry Identifies responsibility to maintain control Identifies alternatives to aggression Identifies alternatives to verbal outbursts Vents negative feelings appropriately Refrains from striking or harming others
Impulse self-control: Self-restraint of compulsive or impulsive behaviours	Controls impulses	Identifies harmful impulsive behaviours Identifies feelings that lead to impulsive actions Identifies consequences of impulsive actions to self or others Avoids high-risk environments and situations Seeks help when experiencing impulses

Source: Moorhead, S., Johnson, M., Maas, M., et al. (2012). *Nursing outcomes classification (NOC)* (5th ed.). St. Louis: Mosby.

have experienced failed relationships, including therapeutic alliances. Individuals with BPD or antisocial personality disorder will distrust relationships and demonstrate hostility toward others, thus making the establishment of a therapeutic relationship difficult. People with personality disorders require a sense of control over what is happening to them. Giving them realistic choices (e.g., selection of a particular group activity) may enhance adherence to treatment. It is also important to plan individual patient treatment within the context of their family. Patients, families, and health care providers can access further information on personality disorders from the Internet; two reliable Canadian sites are the Canadian Mental Health Association (www.cmha.ca) and HeretoHelp (www.heretohelp.bc.ca). Refer to Table 19-4 for guidelines for nursing care for the major clusters of personality disorders. Case Study and Nursing Care Plan 19-1 presents a person with BPD.

IMPLEMENTATION

People with BPD are impulsive (e.g., suicidal, self-mutilating), aggressive, manipulative, and even psychotic during periods of stress. Individuals with antisocial personality disorder are often involuntarily admitted and are manipulative, aggressive, and impulsive. Refer to Boxes 19-1, 19-2, and 19-3 for interventions to address these behaviours, based on the *Nursing Interventions*

BOX 19-1   *NIC* INTERVENTIONS FOR MANIPULATIVE BEHAVIOUR LIMIT SETTING

Definition of **limit setting**: Establishing the parameters of desirable and acceptable personal behaviour
  Activities*:
- Discuss concerns about behaviour with person.
- Identify (with input when appropriate) undesirable personal behaviour.
- Discuss with person, when appropriate, what desirable behaviour is in a given situation or setting.
- Establish consequences (with person's input when appropriate) for occurrence or nonoccurrence of desired behaviours.
- Communicate established behavioural expectations and consequences to person in language that is easily understood and nonpunitive.
- Refrain from arguing or bargaining with person about established behavioural expectations and consequences.
- Monitor person for occurrence or nonoccurrence of desired behaviour.
- Modify behavioural expectations and consequences, as needed, to accommodate reasonable changes in person's situation.

*Partial list.
Source: Bulechek, G. M., Butcher, H. K., & Dochterman, J. M. (2013). *Nursing interventions classification (NIC)* (6th ed.). Toronto: Elsevier.

TABLE 19-4   NURSING AND THERAPY GUIDELINES FOR PERSONALITY DISORDER BY CLUSTER

PERSONALITY DISORDER	CHARACTERISTICS	NURSING GUIDELINES	SUGGESTED THERAPIES
Cluster A • Paranoid personality disorder • Schizoid personality disorder • Schizotypal personality disorder	Manifestation of ideas of reference Cognitive and perceptual distortions Social ineptness Anxiety Odd and eccentric behaviours	1. Respect patient's need for social isolation. 2. Be aware of patient's suspiciousness, and employ appropriate interventions. 3. Perform careful diagnostic assessment as needed to uncover any other medical or psychological symptoms that may need intervention (e.g., suicidal thoughts).	Supportive psychotherapy Cognitive and behavioural measures Group therapy to try to improve social skills Low-dose antipsychotics and antidepressants

Cluster B
• Borderline personality disorder
• Narcissistic personality disorder
• Histrionic personality disorder
• Antisocial personality disorder
	Ability to seem normal
	Manipulative
	Exploitive of others
	Disparaging
	Impulsive (suicide, self-mutilation)
	Splitting (adoring then devaluing people)
	Grandiose
	Filled with rage
	Very sensitive to rejection, criticism
	Inability to experience empathy
		1. Try to prevent or reduce untoward effects of manipulation (flattery, seductiveness, instilling of guilt):
		  a. Set clear and realistic limits on specific behaviour.
		  b. Ensure that limits are adhered to by all staff.
		  c. Carefully document signs of manipulation or aggression.
		  d. Document behaviours (give times, dates, circumstances).
		  e. Provide clear boundaries and consequences.
		2. Be aware that patients can instill guilt when they are not getting what they want. Guard against being manipulated through feelings of guilt.
		3. Use clear and straightforward communication.
		4. When behavioural problems emerge, calmly review the therapeutic goals and boundaries of treatment.
		5. Avoid rejecting or rescuing.
		6. Assess for suicidal and self-mutilating behaviours, especially during times of stress.
		7. Remain neutral; avoid engaging in power struggles or becoming defensive in response to the patient's disparaging remarks.
		8. Convey unassuming self-confidence
			Individual psychotherapy
			Dialectical behaviour therapy
			Group therapy
			Pharmacotherapy for anxiety, depression
			Careful use of addictive agents (e.g., benzodiazepines)
			Anticonvulsants may help impulsive behaviour
			Antipsychotics to control anger and brief psychosis

Cluster C • Avoidant personality disorder • Dependent personality disorder • Obsessive-compulsive personality disorder	Excessively anxious in social situations Hypersensitive to negative evaluation Desiring of social interaction Perfectionistic Has need for control Inflexible, rigid Preoccupied with details Highly critical of self and others	1. Being pushed into social situations can cause extreme and severe anxiety. 2. Guard against power struggles with patient. Need for control is very high. 3. A friendly, accepting, reassuring approach is the best way to treat patients. 4. The most common defence mechanisms are intellectualization, rationalization, reaction formation, isolation, and undoing.	Supportive or insightful psychotherapy Group therapy Assertiveness training Antidepressants Antianxiety agents Beta-adrenergic receptor antagonists help reduce autonomic nervous system hyperactivity

BOX 19-2   *NIC* INTERVENTIONS FOR AGGRESSIVE BEHAVIOUR ANGER CONTROL ASSISTANCE

Definition of **anger control assistance**: Facilitation of the expression of anger in an adaptive, nonviolent manner

Activities*:

- Determine appropriate behavioural expectations for expression of anger, given person's level of cognitive and physical functioning.
- Limit access to frustrating situations until person is able to express anger in an adaptive manner.
- Encourage person to seek assistance from nursing staff during periods of increasing tension.
- Monitor potential for inappropriate aggression, and intervene before its expression.
- Prevent physical harm if anger is directed at self or others (e.g., restraint and removal of potential weapons).
- Provide physical outlets for expression of anger or tension (e.g., punching bag, sports, clay, journal writing).
- Provide reassurance to person that nursing staff will intervene to prevent person from losing control.
- Assist person in identifying source of anger.
- Identify function that anger, frustration, and rage serve for person.
- Identify consequences of inappropriate expression of anger.

*Partial list.
Source: Bulechek, G. M., Butcher, H. K., & Dochterman, J. M. (2013). *Nursing interventions classification (NIC)* (6th ed.). Toronto: Elsevier.

BOX 19-3   *NIC* INTERVENTIONS FOR IMPULSIVE BEHAVIOUR IMPULSE-CONTROL TRAINING

Definition of **impulse-control training**: Assisting the person to mediate impulsive behaviour through application of problem-solving strategies to social and interpersonal situations

Activities*:

- Assist person to identify the problem or situation that requires thoughtful action.
- Assist person to identify possible courses of action and their costs and benefits.
- Teach person to cue himself or herself to "stop and think" before acting impulsively.
- Assist person to evaluate the outcome of the chosen course of action.
- Provide positive reinforcement (e.g., praise and rewards) for successful outcomes.
- Encourage person to self-reward for successful outcomes.
- Provide opportunities for person to practise problem solving (role-playing) within the therapeutic environment.
- Encourage person to practise problem solving in social and interpersonal situations outside the therapeutic environment, followed by evaluation of outcome.

*Partial list.
Source: Bulechek, G. M., Butcher, H. K., & Dochterman, J. M. (2013). *Nursing interventions classification (NIC)* (6th ed.). Toronto: Elsevier.

Classification (NIC) (Bulechek, Butcher, & Dochterman, 2013).

Safety and Teamwork

When individuals with personality disorders are receiving treatment from a team of health professionals, milieu management is a significant part of treatment. Most individuals with personality disorders are admitted to hospital because of a risk to themselves or others. Patient and staff safety is a priority.

When patients are actively involved in developing their treatment plans (e.g., being included in daily staff rounds to set goals and evaluate progress), they typically take more responsibility for themselves and the success of implementing the plan. Having limits and being confronted about negative behaviour are better accepted by the person if staff members first employ empathic mirroring (i.e., reflecting back to the person an understanding of the person's distress without a value judgement). For example, the nurse can listen to a person's emotional complaints about the staff and hospital without correcting any errors but simply noting that the person truly feels hurt. Showing empathy may also decrease aggressive outbursts if the person feels that staff members are trying to understand feelings of frustration. Table 19-5 depicts a therapeutic nurse–patient interaction after an antisocial patient initiates a fight with a peer on an inpatient unit.

A final approach that is useful for people with BPD relates to the response to superficial self-destructive behaviours. Acting in accordance with unit policies, the nurse remains neutral and dresses the cutting wound in a matter-of-fact manner. Then the person is instructed to write down the sequence of events leading up to the injury, as well as the consequences, before staff will discuss the event. This cognitive exercise encourages the person to think independently about his or her own behaviour instead of merely ventilating feelings. It facilitates the discussion with staff about alternative actions.

Pharmacological Interventions

There is no direct pharmacological treatment for personality disorders. However, people with personality disorders may be helped by a broad array of psychotropic agents, all geared toward maintaining cognitive function and relieving symptoms. Depending on the chief complaint, antidepressant, anxiolytic, or antipsychotic medication may be ordered for symptom relief and improved quality of life (Ripoll, 2012; Ripoll, Triebwasser, & Siever, 2011), but the treatment efficacy of these medications remains questionable, as they do not specifically treat the underlying personality disorder (Crawford, Kakad, Rendel, et al., 2011). Ripoll (2012) and Ripoll, Triebwasser, and Siever (2011) investigated trends in medication efficacy for the following personality disorders:

- People with STPD seem to benefit from low-dose atypical antipsychotic agents for their psychotic-like symptoms and day-to-day functioning.
- People with antisocial personality disorder respond to mood-stabilizing medications like lithium to help with aggression and impulsivity.
- People with BPD often respond to anticonvulsant mood-stabilizing medications, low-dose antipsychotic

TABLE 19-5 DIALOGUE WITH A PERSON WITH MANIPULATIVE, AGGRESSIVE, AND IMPULSIVE TRAITS

DIALOGUE	THERAPEUTIC TOOL/COMMENT
Nurse: "Borys, I would like to talk with you about what happened this morning." **Borys:** "Okay, shoot."	Be clear as to purpose of interview.
Nurse: "Tell me what started the incident." **Borys:** "Well, as I told you before, I always had to fight to get what I wanted in life. My father and mother abandoned me emotionally when I was a child."	Use open-ended statements. Maintain a nonjudgemental attitude.
Nurse: "Yes, but tell me about this morning." **Borys:** "Okay. I disliked Richard from the first. He has it in for me, I just know it. He doesn't get along with anyone here. Just 2 days ago, he almost had a fight."	Redirect person to present problem or situation.
Nurse: "Borys, what do you mean, Richard has it in for you?" **Borys:** "When I'm talking to one of the nurses, he stares and makes comments under his breath."	Explore situation.
Nurse: "What does he say?" **Borys:** "How I'm 'in' with the nurses. I'm just trying to do what's expected of me here."	Encourage description.
Nurse: "You mean that Richard is envious of your relationship with the nurses?" **Borys:** "Right. He really doesn't want to be here. He doesn't care about all that therapeutic junk."	Validate person's meaning.
Nurse: "You seem to know a lot about how Richard thinks. I wonder how that is." **Borys:** "He reminds me of someone I knew when I was young. His name was Joe. We called him 'Bones.' "	Assist the person to recognize that he or she is assuming to know what others are thinking and that the interpretations may not be based in reality.
Nurse: "Tell me more about Bones." **Borys:** "We called him Bones because he was skinny. He was into drugs and never ate. He was also called Bones because he was selfish. He never shared anything. He never even had a girl that I knew about."	Explore situation further.
Nurse: "So Richard reminds you of someone who is selfish and lonely?" **Borys:** "That's right. I've had three marriages and girlfriends on the side. No one can take them away from me." (angrily) "Just let them try!"	Make interpretation of information. Note increasing anxiety.
Nurse: "What makes you so angry now?" **Borys:** "Richard! I know he wants to be like me, but he can't. I'll hurt him if he makes any more comments about me."	Identify feelings and explore threat or anxiety.
Nurse: "Borys, you will not hurt anyone here on the unit." **Borys:** "I'm sorry, I didn't mean that."	Set limits on, and expectations of, person's behaviour.
Nurse: "It's important that we examine your part in the incident this morning and ways to cope without threats or violence." **Borys:** "Listen, I know I've gotten into trouble because I can't control my temper, but that's because I won't get any respect until I can show them I don't fear them."	Focus on person's responsibility and suggest alternative methods of coping with situation. Person exhibits rationalization.
Nurse: "Who do you mean by 'them'?" **Borys:** "People like Richard."	Clarify pronoun.
Nurse: "You've told me that fighting was a way of survival as a child, but as an adult there are other ways of handling situations that make you angry." **Borys:** "You're right. I've thought about this. Do you think it would help if you gave me some meds to control my anger?"	Show understanding and suggest other means of coping. Person exhibits superficial and concrete thinking—possible manipulation.
Nurse: "I wasn't thinking of medications but of a plan for being aware of your anger and talking it out instead of fighting it out." **Borys:** "I told you before, I have to fight. If I can't fight, I cut myself."	Clarify meaning toward behaviour change. Start to explore alternatives person can use when angry instead of fighting.
Nurse: "Have you thought about the consequences of your fighting or cutting?" **Borys:** "I feel bad afterward. Sometimes I wish it hadn't happened."	Identify results of impulsive behaviour. Person continues to explore.

medications, and omega-3 supplementation for mood and emotion dysregulation symptoms. Naltrexone hydrochloride, an opioid receptor antagonist, has been found to reduce self-injuring behaviours.

- People with avoidant personality disorder seem to respond positively to medications similar to those used for anxiety disorders, such as SSRIs like citalopram (Celexa) and SNRIs such as duloxetine (Cymbalta).

Pharmacological evidence is lacking for the treatment of people with narcissistic and obsessive-compulsive personality disorders.

Case Management

Many people with personality disorders function at a high level, but a significant number need assistance to maintain their independence. Case management is helpful for individuals with personality disorders who are persistently and severely impaired. Many have had multiple hospitalizations, have been unable to maintain work or personal relationships, and are relatively alone in their attempts to care for themselves. In the acute care setting, case management focuses on three goals: to gather pertinent history from current or previous providers; to support reintegration with family or loved ones as appropriate; and to ensure appropriate referrals to outpatient care, including substance disorder treatment, if needed. In the long-term outpatient setting, case-management objectives include reducing hospitalization by providing resources for crisis services and enhancing the social support system.

Advanced-Practice Interventions

The mental health nurse treats individuals with personality disorders in a variety of inpatient and community settings. Research shows that treatment can be effective for many people with personality disorders, especially when a comorbid major mental illness is targeted. See Table 19-4 for a summary of nursing and therapy guidelines for personality disorders.

Advanced-practice nurses are likely to interact with staff members regarding the treatment of individuals with personality disorders as part of their practice and clinical supervision responsibilities. They can assist staff members in a therapeutic alliance. For example, they mentor and teach additional techniques that staff members can use to develop rapport and trust with patients diagnosed with STPD when these patients are experiencing heightened anxiety from being hospitalized. Nurses should understand that the patient's ability to interpret subtle, affective cues is limited and that straightforward communication is necessary (Long, Dolley, & Hollin, 2012).

Psychotherapy

Advanced-practice nurses are highly involved in and are often the clinical leaders in providing individual and group psychotherapy using **dialectical behaviour therapy (DBT)**. DBT is an evidence-informed therapy developed by Dr. Marsha Linehan to treat chronically suicidal people with BPD (Linehan, 1993). DBT is based on a biosocial theory that views the self-harming behaviour as a behaviour used to cope with or eliminate distress brought on by a negatively perceived environmental event, self-generated behaviours, and individual temperaments. There are three primary reasons why individuals use this means of coping: (1) low stress tolerance, (2) deficiencies in emotional regulation, and (3) self-harm is regarded as a reasonable means of problem solving. For example, if an individual is facing an intolerable and inescapable life problem, it would be only reasonable to think about suicide.

DBT combines cognitive and behavioural techniques with mindfulness, which emphasizes being aware of thoughts and actively shaping them. Interventions that are common to DBT and other behaviour therapies include cognitive restructuring, therapist reciprocal vulnerability, skills training, and reinforcement. Unique DBT interventions include the use of emotional regulation and opposite action skills, dialectics, distress tolerance skills, higher degree of therapist self-disclosure, validation as an explicit therapist skill set, and microanalytic chain analysis.

DBT encourages balance and synthesis of acceptance and change. Traditional behavioural treatment modalities focused on change in thoughts, feelings, and behaviours. There was no acknowledgement of why these occur. Patients felt invalidated and criticized and often would drop out of treatment. DBT therapists simultaneously acknowledge the pain and angst of the patient and strategize with the patient on ways of changing—thus there is acceptance and change. The primary philosophical underpinning of dialectical therapies is that in order to understand human suffering, one must understand the system as a whole. The system changes constantly, and each change influences other parts of the system. Patients are treated as a whole person; all aspects of their lives are interrelated and influence their behaviour and those around them.

The goals of DBT are to increase the person's ability to manage distress and improve interpersonal effectiveness. Treatment focuses on behaviour targets, beginning with identification of and interventions for suicidal behaviours and then progressing to a focus on interrupting destructive behaviours (Figure 19-1). Finally, DBT addresses quality-of-life behaviours across a hierarchy of care (Figure 19-2). Optimally, DBT is delivered as a skills training group program combined with individual therapy with a DBT-trained therapist who may be a nurse, social worker, or psychologist.

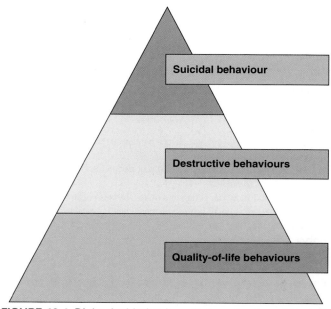

FIGURE 19-1 Dialectical behaviour therapy treatment targets.

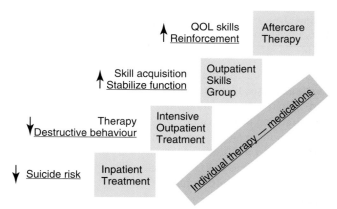

FIGURE 19-2 Dialectical behaviour therapy treatment hierarchy. *QOL*, Quality of life.

EVALUATION

Each therapeutic experience offers an opportunity for the person to observe himself or herself interacting with caregivers who consistently try to teach positive coping skills. Effectiveness can be measured by how successfully the nurse is able to be genuine with the person, maintain a helpful posture, offer substantial instruction, and still care for himself or herself. Specific short-term outcomes may be accomplished, and overall the person can be given the message of hope that quality of life can always be improved.

CASE STUDY AND NURSING CARE PLAN 19-1
Borderline Personality Disorder

Ada is a 24-year-old single administrative assistant who lives alone. She has been seen in the emergency department several times for superficial suicide attempts. She is admitted because she has cut her wrists, ankles, and vagina with glass and has lost a lot of blood. This event is precipitated by her graduation from business college.

Upon admission, she is sweet, serene, and grateful to all the nurses, calling them "angels of mercy." Within a week, she is angry at half of the nurses and demands a new primary nurse, saying that the one she has (to whom she had grown attached) hates her. She has a history of heavy drinking and has managed to sneak alcohol onto the unit. She has been found in bed with a young man. She continually breaks unit rules and then pleads to have this behaviour forgiven and forgotten. When angry, she threatens to cut herself again. When asked why she cut herself, Ada states, "I was tired." She appears restless and tense and frequently asks for antianxiety medication. When asked what she is anxious about, she says, "Uh … I don't know … I feel so empty inside." Ada frequently paces up and down the halls, looking both angry and bored. Her admitting diagnoses include substance abuse disorder and borderline personality disorder.

ASSESSMENT

Self-Assessment

Annie is a recent nurse graduate and Ada's primary nurse. Ada's therapist impresses upon Annie the difficulty that health care workers have in dealing effectively with people with BPD. These patients constantly act out their feelings in self-destructive and maladaptive ways. They usually are not aware of their feelings or what triggered their actions. Most difficult for many health care workers is dealing with the intense feelings and reactions that individuals with BPD can provoke in others. Annie sets up meetings twice a week with Ada's therapist to discuss the quality of the therapeutic relationship with Ada. At the next meeting, common goals and intervention strategies are discussed. This type of staff meeting, sometimes referred to as *supervision*, is a way to facilitate self-reflection for Annie and to help her work more effectively with Ada.

Objective Data	Subjective Data
• Makes frequent, superficial suicide attempts • Requests antianxiety medication frequently • Paces up and down the hall much of the day • Threatens self-mutilation when anxious • Brings alcohol onto the unit • Is found in bed with man	• Initially was attached to her primary nurse; now says her primary nurse "hates" her, and she demands another nurse • Appears restless and tense • Complains of feeling empty inside • Looks angry and bored much of the time

DIAGNOSIS

Annie formulates two initial nursing diagnoses that have the highest priority during this time:

1. *Ineffective coping* related to inadequate psychological resources, as evidenced by self-destructive behaviours
Supporting Data
• After stating that her nurse hates her, Ada sneaks alcohol onto the unit, is found in bed with a man, and demands a new primary nurse.

2. *Self-mutilation* related to borderline personality disorder, as evidenced by suicidal gestures and poor impulse control
Supporting Data
• Is admitted following self-mutilation
• Threatens self-mutilation when anxious
• Threatens self-mutilation on unit

OUTCOMES IDENTIFICATION

1. Person will consistently demonstrate the use of effective coping strategies.
2. Person will refrain from injuring self.

Continued

CASE STUDY AND NURSING CARE PLAN 19-1—cont'd

Borderline Personality Disorder

PLANNING

The initial plan is to maintain personal safety and to encourage verbalization of feelings and impulses instead of action.

IMPLEMENTATION

Annie's plan of care is personalized as follows:

Nursing diagnosis: *Ineffective coping*

Outcome: Ada will consistently demonstrate the use of effective coping strategies.

Short-Term Goal	Intervention	Rationale	Evaluation
Ada will consistently demonstrate a decrease in stress as evidenced by talking about feelings with staff every day and an absence of acting-out behaviours.	1. Encourage verbalization of feelings, perceptions, and fears. 2. Support the use of appropriate defence mechanisms.	1. Discussing and understanding the dynamics of frustration help reduce the frustration by helping the person take positive action. 2. Discussing and understanding the meaning of defences help reduce the potential for acting out.	**Goal Met** Ada was able to experience problems and deal with them appropriately. Acting out was minimal or absent. *Example:* Ada had an appointment for a job interview. She wanted to stay in bed and avoid the interview, but instead she talked with the nurse about her fear of "growing up" and was able to get up and go to the interview.

Nursing diagnosis: *Self-mutilation*

Outcome: Ada will refrain from injuring herself.

Short-Term Goal	Intervention	Rationale	Evaluation
Ada will consistently demonstrate that she will seek help when feeling the urge to injure herself, as evidenced by the absence of self-injurious behaviours and talking to staff about her troubling feelings on a daily basis.	1. Assist the person to identify situations and feelings that may prompt self-harm. 2. Instruct the person in coping strategies. 3. Provide ongoing surveillance of the person and environment.	1. Observing, describing, and analyzing thoughts and feelings reduce the potential for acting them out destructively. 2. Alternative behaviours are offered that can be more satisfying and growth promoting. 3. Times of increased anxiety, frustration, or anger without external controls could increase the probability of the person using self-mutilating behaviours.	**Goal Met** Ada was able to experience troubling thoughts and feelings without self-mutilation. She stated, "I was mad at my therapist today and decided to cut my arms after the session. Instead, I told her I was angry, and together we figured out why."

EVALUATION

See individual outcomes and evaluation in the care plan.

KEY POINTS TO REMEMBER

- All personality disorders share characteristics of inflexibility and difficulties in interpersonal relationships that impair social or occupational functioning.
- Personality disorders are most likely caused by a combination of biological and psychosocial factors.
- People with personality disorders often enter psychiatric treatment because of distress from a comorbid major mental illness.
- Nurses may experience intense emotional reactions to individuals with personality disorders and need to make use of clinical supervision to maintain objectivity.
- Despite the relatively fixed patterns of maladaptive behaviour, some individuals with personality disorders are able to change their behaviours over time as a result of treatment.

CRITICAL THINKING

1. Vasily is undergoing surgery for a broken leg. He is suspicious of the staff and believes that the intravenous (IV) he is receiving for hydration and pre-anaesthesia will be used for harmful purposes. He keeps his eyes closed and refuses to answer or look at his family, who describe him as odd. He has schizotypal personality disorder.
   a. Explain how being friendly and outgoing may be threatening to Vasily.
   b. Explain how being matter-of-fact and neutral and sticking to the facts would be effective with Vasily.
   c. What could be done to give Vasily some control over his situation as a hospitalized person?
   d. How could you best handle Vasily's sarcasm and hostility, so that both you and he would feel most comfortable?
2. Cherie is brought to the emergency department by her brother after slashing her wrist with a razor. She has previously been in the emergency department for drug overdose and has a history of addictions. Cherie can be sarcastic, belittling, and aggressive to those who try to care for her. She has a history of difficulty with interpersonal relationships at her job. When the psychiatric triage nurse comes in to see her, Cherie is initially adoring and compliant, telling him, "You are the best nurse I've ever had, and I truly want to change." However, when he refuses to support her request for diazepam (Valium) and meperidine (Demerol) for "pain," she yells at him: "You are a stupid excuse for a nurse! I want to see the doctor immediately!" Cherie has borderline personality disorder.
   a. What defence mechanisms is Cherie using?
   b. How could the nurse handle this situation while setting limits and demonstrating concern?
   c. How do family members of a person with BPD typically describe their experiences?

CHAPTER REVIEW

1. A person complains that most staff do not like her or care what happens to her, but says that you are special and she can tell that you are a caring person. She talks with you about being unsure of what she wants to do with her life and her "mixed-up feelings" about relationships. When you tell her that you will be on vacation next week, she becomes very angry. Two hours later, she is found using a curling iron to burn her underarms and explains that it "makes the numbness stop." Given this presentation, you would deduce that this person most likely has which personality disorder?
   a. Obsessive-compulsive
   b. Borderline
   c. Antisocial
   d. Schizotypal
2. Which statement about people with personality disorders is most accurate?
   a. Unlike those with mood or psychotic disorders, they are at very low risk for suicide.
   b. They tend not to perceive themselves as having a problem but instead believe that their problems are caused by how others behave toward them.
   c. They are believed to be purely psychological disorders, that is, disorders arising from psychological rather than neurological or other physiological abnormalities.
   d. Their symptoms are not as disabling as most other mental disorders; therefore their care tends to be less challenging and less complicated for staff.
3. A person shows the nurse multiple fresh, serious (but non–life-threatening) self-inflicted cuts on her forearm. Which response would be most therapeutic?
   a. Convey empathy and explore issues that led to the self-injury as you administer first aid to the wounds.
   b. Care for the wounds; then search the person for sharp objects, and place the person on one-to-one observation or in seclusion for her own safety.
   c. Recognizing that the self-injury is, at its heart, a maladaptive attempt to obtain attention, extinguish the behaviour by minimizing the attention paid to it.
   d. Maintain a neutral demeanour while dressing the wounds, and then assign the person to write a list of circumstances that led to the injury before discussing it further.
4. A patient is flirting with a peer and is overheard asking him to intercede with staff so that she will be given privileges to leave the inpatient mental health unit. Later, she offers a back rub to a nurse if that nurse will give her the prn sedation (sedation as needed) early, although it has been ordered for 1000 hours. Which response to such behaviours would be most therapeutic?
   a. Inform the patient that she is being manipulative.
   b. Advise the other nurses that this patient is being manipulative and that they should ignore her when she behaves this way.
   c. Bargain with the patient to determine a reasonable compromise regarding how much of such behaviour is acceptable before the patient crosses the line.
   d. Ignore the behaviour for the time being so that the patient will find it unrewarding and in turn seek other, hopefully more adaptive, ways to meet her needs.
5. A person becomes frustrated and angry when trying to get his MP3 player and headset to function properly and angrily throws it across the room, nearly hitting a peer with it. Which intervention would be the most therapeutic?
   a. Place the person in seclusion for 1 hour to allow him to de-escalate and think about his behaviour.
   b. Point out that the behaviour is unacceptable.
   c. Offer to help him learn about the operation of the MP3 player.
   d. Explore with the person his feelings as he works out how to operate his MP3 player.

⊝volve WEBSITE

Post-Test interactive review

Visit the Evolve website for Chapter Review Answers and Rationales, Critical Thinking Answer Guidelines, and additional resources related to the content in this chapter: *http://evolve.elsevier.com/Canada/Varcarolis/psychiatric/*

REFERENCES

Amad, A., Ramoz, N., Thomas, P., et al. (2014). Genetics of borderline personality disorder: Systematic review and proposal of an integrative model. *Neuroscience and Behavioral Reviews, 40,* 6–19.

American Psychiatric Association (APA) (2013). *Diagnostic and statistical manual of mental disorders* (5th ed.). Arlington, VA: American Psychiatric Publishing.

Bulechek, G. M., Butcher, H. K., & Dochterman, J. M. (2013). *Nursing interventions classification (NIC)* (6th ed.). Toronto: Elsevier.

Canadian Institute for Health Information. (2011). *Health indicators 2011.* Retrieved from https://secure.cihi.ca/free_products/health_indicators_2011_en.pdf.

Crawford, M., Kakad, S., Rendel, C., et al. (2011). Medication prescribed to people with personality disorder: The influence of patient factors and treatment setting. *Acta Psychiatrica Scandinavica, 124*(5), 396–402. doi: 10.1111/j.1600-0447.2011.01728.x.

Gunderson, J. G. (2011). Borderline personality disorder. *The New England Journal of Medicine, 364,* 2037–2042.

Hernandez, A., Arntz, A., Gaviria, A., et al. (2012). Relationships between childhood maltreatment, parenting style, and borderline personality disorder criteria. *Journal of Personality Disorders, 26*(5), 727–736. Retrieved from http://www.ncbi.nlm.nih.gov/pubmed/23013341.

Kendler, K. S., Aggen, S. H., & Patrick, C. J. (2012). A multivariate twin study of the DSM-IV criteria for antisocial personality disorder. *Biological Psychiatry, 71*(3), 247–253.

Kernberg, O. (1985). *Internal world and external reality.* London, UK: Aronson.

Krause-Utz, A., Winter, D., Niedtfeld, I., et al. (2014). The latest neuroimaging findings in borderline personality disorder. *Current Psychiatry Reports, 16*(3), 438. doi:10.1007/s11920-014-0438-z.

Langlois, K. A., Samokhvalov, A. V., Rehm, J., et al. (2011). *Health state descriptions for Canadians: Mental illnesses.* Catalogue no. 82-619-MIE2005002. Ottawa: Statistics Canada.

Lee, R., Hempel, J., Tenharmsel, A., et al. (2012). The neuroendocrinology of childhood trauma in personality disorder. *Psychoneuroendocrinology, 37*(1), 78–86. doi:10.1016/j.psyneuen.2011.05.006.

Leichsenring, F., Leibing, E., Kruse, J., et al. (2011). Borderline personality disorder. *Lancet, 377*(9759), 74–84. doi:10.1016/S0140-6736(10)61422-5.

Linehan, M. M. (1993). *Cognitive behavioral treatment of borderline personality disorder.* New York: Guilford.

Long, C., Dolley, O., & Hollin, C. (2012). Engagement in psychosocial treatment: Its relationship to outcome and care pathway progress for women in medium-secure settings. *Criminal Behaviour & Mental Health, 22*(5), 336–349. doi:10.1002/cbm.1824.

Madarasz, W., Manzardo, A., Mortensen, E., et al. (2012). Forty-five-year mortality rate as a function of the number and type of psychiatric diagnoses found in a large Danish birth cohort. *Canadian Journal of Psychiatry, 57*(8), 505–511. Retrieved from http://www.ncbi.nlm.nih.gov/pubmed/22854033.

Mahler, M. S., Pine, F., & Bergman, A. (1975). *The psychological birth of the human infant.* New York: Basic Books.

McGilloway, A., Hall, R., Lee, T., et al. (2010). A systematic review of personality disorder, race, and ethnicity: Prevalence, aetiology and treatment. *BMC Psychiatry, 10*(33), 1–14. doi:10.1186/1471-244X-10-33.

Moorhead, S., Johnson, M., Maas, M., et al. (2012). *Nursing outcomes classification (NOC)* (5th ed.). St. Louis: Mosby.

Newton-Howes, G., Horwood, J., & Mulder, R. (2015). Personality characteristics in childhood and outcomes in adulthood: Findings from a 30 year longitudinal study. *Australian & New Zealand Journal of Psychiatry, 49*(4), 377–386. doi:10.1177/0004867415569796.

Paris, J. (2005). A current integrative perspective on personality disorders. In J. M. Oldham, A. E. Skodol, & D. S. Bender (Eds.), *Textbook of personality disorders* (pp. 119–128). Washington, DC: American Psychiatric Publishing.

Perry, J., Presniak, M., & Olson, T. (2013). Defense mechanisms in schizotypal, borderline, antisocial, and narcissistic personality disorders. *Psychiatry: Interpersonal & Biological Processes, 76*(1), 32–52. doi:10.1521/psyc.2013.76.1.32.

Ripoll, L. (2012). Clinical psychopharmacology of borderline personality disorder: An update on the available evidence in light of the *Diagnostic and Statistical Manual of Mental Disorders–5. Current Opinion in Psychiatry, 25*(1), 52–58. doi:10.1097/YCO.0b013e32834c3f19.

Ripoll, L., Triebwasser, J., & Siever, L. (2011). Evidence-based pharmacotherapy for personality disorders. *The International Journal of Neuropsychopharmacology / Official Scientific Journal of the Collegium Internationale Neuropsychopharmacologicum (CINP), 14*(9), 1257–1288. doi:10.1017/S1461145711000071.

Rosowsky, I., Abrams, R. C., & Zwieg, R. A. (2013). *Personality disorders in older adults.* New York: Routledge.

Sadock, B. J., Sadock, V. A., & Ruiz, P. (2015). *Kaplan & Sadock's synopsis of psychiatry* (11th ed.). Philadelphia: Wolters Kluwer.

Samuels, J. (2011). Personality disorders: Epidemiology and public health issues. *International Review of Psychiatry, 23*(3), 223–233. doi:10.3109/09540261.2011.588200.

Simms, L., Goldberg, L., Roberts, J., et al. (2011). Computerized adaptive assessment of personality disorder: Introducing the CAT-PD project. *Journal of Personality Assessment, 93*(4), 380–389. doi:10.1080/00223891.2011.577475.

Skodol, A., Bender, D., Morey, L., et al. (2011). Personality disorder types proposed for DSM-5. *Journal of Personality Disorders, 25*(2), 136–169. doi:10.1521/pedi.2011.25.2.136.

Skodol, A. E., Bender, D. S., Gunderson, J. G., et al. (2014). Personality disorders. In R. E. Hales, S. C. Yudofsky, & G. O. Gabbard (Eds.), *Textbook of psychiatry* (6th ed., pp. 851–894). Washington, DC: American Psychiatric Publishing.

Taylor, S., Asmundson, G., & Jang, K. (2011). Etiology of obsessive-compulsive symptoms and obsessive-compulsive personality traits: Common genes, mostly different environments. *Depression & Anxiety, 28*(10), 863–869. doi:10.1002/da.20859.

World Health Organization. (2016). *International classification of diseases and related health problems, 10th revision—Clinical modification.* Retrieved from https://www.cdc.gov/nchs/icd/icd10cm.htm.

Sleep–Wake Disorders

Margaret Jordan Halter, Margaret Trussler
Adapted by Sonya L. Jakubec

KEY TERMS AND CONCEPTS

confusional arousal disorders
dyssomnias
excessive sleepiness (ES)
hypersomnia disorders
insomnia disorders
melatonin
polysomnography
sleep architecture

sleep continuity
sleep deprivation
sleep efficiency
sleep fragmentation
sleep hygiene
sleep latency
sleep restriction
stimulus control

OBJECTIVES

1. Discuss the impact of inadequate sleep on health and well-being.
2. Describe the social and economic impact of sleep disturbance and chronic sleep deprivation.
3. Identify the risks to personal and community safety imposed by sleep disturbance and chronic sleep deprivation.
4. Describe normal sleep physiology, and explain the variations in normal sleep.
5. Differentiate between insomnia and hypersomnia, and identify at least two examples of each.
6. Identify the predisposing, precipitating, and perpetuating factors for patients with insomnia.

7. Identify and describe the use of two assessment tools in the evaluation of patients experiencing sleep disturbance.
8. Develop a teaching plan for a patient with insomnia, incorporating principles of sleep restriction, stimulus control, and cognitive behavioural therapy.
9. Formulate three nursing diagnoses for people experiencing a sleep disturbance.
10. Develop a nursing care plan for the person experiencing sleep disturbance incorporating basic sleep hygiene principles.

℮volve WEBSITE

Visit the Evolve website for Flashcards, Case Studies, and additional testing resources related to the content in this chapter: http://evolve.elsevier.com/Canada/Varcarolis/psychiatric/

Pre-Test   interactive review

Sleep disturbances vary in severity, duration, quality, or timing, all of which can have adverse health consequences. These disturbances are broadly referred to as dyssomnias. Understandably, energy level and cognitive focus can be impaired as a result of dyssomnias, but mood can also be affected. Disturbed sleep certainly worsens the distress and impairment caused by mental illnesses and is also a potential warning sign for additional mental or physical conditions. For instance, disturbed sleep may be a

sign of medical or neurological problems such as Parkinson's disease, heart failure, or osteoarthritis, among other conditions, and can also exacerbate symptoms of post-traumatic stress disorder, which is characterized by night terrors (Brownlow, McLean, Gehrman, et al., 2016).

Sleep and sleep–wake disorders are receiving increased attention in medical, nursing, research, and social science literature. The Canadian Sleep Society was established in 1986 to facilitate research, training, dissemination of health information, and other activities with respect to the basic understanding of sleep and sleep–wake disorders. Over the past 30 years, there has been an exponential growth in our scientific understanding of these disorders. However, despite the investment in sleep-related research and tremendous growth in our understanding of sleep physiology and pathology, application of the findings has been slow.

In this chapter, we briefly review the components of normal sleep, sleep regulation, and functions of sleep and give an overview of the most common sleep disturbances encountered in the clinical environment, with a focus on their relationship to psychiatric illness. Pediatric sleep disorders and treatments are discussed in brief. Finally, in this chapter we discuss the nurse's role in the assessment and management of a patient with a sleep disturbance.

✺ HOW A NURSE HELPED ME

Worrying the Night Away

Kelly, a 30-year-old woman, was referred to the mental health nurse by her family physician for an assessment of her insomnia. Kelly reported a 3-month history of insomnia that had resulted in a progressively harder time falling asleep. Kelly reported that she would toss and turn for 2 to 3 hours before falling asleep. Due to her children's schedules, she was usually up early, so was becoming more fatigued and irritable because of her lack of sleep. Kelly was adamant with her physician that she did not want to take sleeping pills.

The mental health nurse visited Kelly at her home and conducted a complete mental status examination, including formal depression or anxiety inventories and psychosocial, sleep history, and sleep hygiene surveys. Kelly reported no other signs of mental health problems and no acute stressors other than the ongoing challenges of parenting two young children ages 2 and 3. She reported difficulty winding down in the evening and felt that, at bedtime, she was constantly thinking of things she should be getting done. During the winter, she had decreased her exercise and was drinking four or five cups of coffee a day due to her fatigue. The mental health nurse spent the first session with Kelly educating her about sleep hygiene and some cognitive strategies for decreasing worrying at bedtime. Kelly felt she could try decreasing her caffeine intake to two to three cups of coffee before 4 p.m. and wanted to try getting out for a walk each day for 20 minutes. She agreed to try a worry list each day at 3 p.m. rather than at bedtime.

The second session, a week later, focused on Kelly's new bedtime routine practices, which included a warm shower and a book rather than TV and cleaning. She reported surprise at how the "worry time" strategies seemed to be working. At the final follow-up visit 1 month later, Kelly was reporting improved sleep and energy levels.

SLEEP

In a fast-paced society, people subject themselves to schedules that disrupt normal sleep physiology, so sleep is often forfeited. The National Sleep Foundation (2016a) recommends that the average adult get 7 to 9 hours of sleep each night, yet epidemiological surveys suggest that mean sleep duration among Canadian adults has decreased during the past century, with 31% of Canadians reporting ongoing difficulties with sleep, making Canada the third most sleep-deprived country after the UK and Ireland. Sleep has become an expendable commodity. People frequently cut back on sleep to meet other social and professional demands, with compensated work time and travel time being the most potent determinants of total sleep time (Aviva, 2016).

CONSEQUENCES OF SLEEP LOSS

The major consequence of acute or chronic sleep curtailment is **excessive sleepiness (ES)**. ES is a subjective report of difficulty staying awake that is serious enough to affect social and vocational functioning and increase the risk for accident or injury. The terms *excessive sleepiness, excessive daytime sleepiness, hypersomnia,* and *hypersomnolence* are often used interchangeably. While hypersomnia is considered a disease classification, ES is a symptom of a sleep disorder or other disease but not itself a disease per se. While self-imposed sleep restriction is a common cause of ES, disruption of the normal sleep cycle (as seen in those who do shift work and people who use electronic devices late into the night), underlying sleep–wake disorders, medications, alcohol, and many medical disorders are important causes of excessive sleepiness (Ohayon, Dauvilliers, & Reynolds, 2012).

We need only look to our own experiences with acute or total sleep loss to recognize its consequences. After a poor night's sleep, we feel tired, lethargic, and irritable. The effects of chronic sleep deprivation may be less obvious but may have a greater overall impact on health and well-being. The discrepancy between hours of sleep obtained and hours of sleep required for optimal functioning creates a state of **sleep deprivation**, which has widespread implications for health, safety, and quality of life. Poor general health, frequent physical distress, frequent mental distress, limitations in activities of daily living, depressive symptoms, anxiety, pain, poor memory, learning and motor function are all consequences of sleep deprivation (Banks, Dorrian, Mathias, et al., 2017). Specifically, chronic sleep deprivation has been linked to diabetes, obesity, and heart disease, which often relate to endocrine and breathing problems that affect sleep. For instance, the breathing-related sleep disorder sleep apnea is believed to cause and worsen medical disorders such as hypertension, diabetes, obesity, coronary artery disease, congestive heart failure, cardiac arrhythmias, substance use, and anxiety (Khurshid, 2015).

Sleep loss also diminishes safety, resulting in the loss of lives and property. Some of the most devastating environmental and human tragedies of our time can be linked to human error due to sleep loss and fatigue. The grounding of the *Exxon Valdez*, the nuclear meltdown at Chernobyl, and the explosion of the Union

Carbide chemical plant in India are prime examples (Pishka Upender, 2017). The Canadian Council of Motor Transport Administrators reports that fatigue is the key factor in more than 20% of vehicle collisions, resulting in over 300 deaths and 2 000 serious injuries every year. This makes fatigue the highest measurable cause of collisions, after driving drunk and driving aggressively (Government of Canada, 2017). In fact, sleep deprivation can produce psychomotor impairments equivalent to those induced by alcohol consumption at or above the legal limit for drivers. Currently, a blood alcohol concentration (BAC) of 0.08%, or 80 milligrams of alcohol in 100 millilitres of blood, is the legal limit in Canada, with individual provincial and territorial acts existing to respond to those driving with lower BACs (Canada Safety Council, 2013). Interestingly, daytime wakefulness in excess of 17 to 19 hours is known to affect psychomotor ability to the same degree as a BAC of between 0.05% and 0.1% (Gaines, 2016). In this way, driving while fatigued is like driving drunk.

There are relatively few comprehensive data available on the economic burden of sleep disruption. However, considering its prevalence, its impact on overall health and quality of life, and the indirect costs associated with property loss and damage, the economic burden has been estimated to reach several billions of dollars in North America (Gaines, 2016).

Formal training in sleep or sleep–wake disorders within medical and nursing education is limited, and the number of trained clinicians and scientists is insufficient. Awareness among health care providers regarding the prevalence and burden of sleep disruption and the problem of inadequate sleep is lacking, so providers do not routinely screen for sleep disturbance or inquire about overall sleep quality (Ye, Keane, Hutton Johnson, et al., 2013). Consequently, there is inadequate recognition, diagnosis, management, and treatment of sleep disturbance, and clinicians do not gain the health education vital to their own professional success and public health safety (see Research Highlight for an innovative training program for nursing students).

NORMAL SLEEP CYCLE

Sleep is a dynamic neurological process that involves complex interaction between the central nervous system and the environment. Behaviourally, sleep is associated with low or absent motor activity, a reduced response to environmental stimuli, and closed eyes. Neurophysiologically, sleep is categorized according to specific brainwave patterns, eye movements, and general muscle tone. Sleep is measured electrophysiologically through an electroencephalogram (EEG) and consists of two distinct physiological states: non–rapid eye movement (NREM) sleep and rapid eye movement (REM) sleep.

NREM sleep is divided into four stages characterized by progressive or deeper sleep. Stage 1 is a brief transition between wakefulness and sleep and accounts for between 2% and 5% of sleep time. The time it takes to go to sleep is referred to as *sleep latency*. During stage 1 sleep, body temperature declines and muscles relax. Slow, rolling eye movements are common. People lose awareness of their environment but are generally easily aroused. Stage 2 sleep occupies 45% to 55% of total sleep time.

🔍 RESEARCH HIGHLIGHT

Sleep Education for Nursing Students

Problem

Despite the multiple health and mental health comorbidities and significant consequences of sleep problems and sleep disorders, as yet there is no established curriculum for sleep in nursing education. As a result, most nurses start their clinical practice without any instruction or training related to sleep and sleep disorders. The need to educate the future nursing workforce to increase understanding of healthy sleep practices, adverse health consequences of impaired sleep, and common sleep disorders is pressing.

Purpose of Study

The purpose of this study was to develop and test an educational intervention for undergraduate nursing students.

Methods

This study method was a pre-post intervention test developed to accompany a 10-hour sleep education program that included three sequential components: traditional in-classroom teaching, guided online virtual self-learning, and interactive simulation-based discussion. This innovative education program was implemented in a core course offered to senior nursing students, and testing on knowledge of sleep disorders and interventions followed. The effect of the education program on students' knowledge related to sleep and sleep disorders was tested statistically by the paired t-test.

Key Findings

For the sample of 57 students (all females in upper levels of their program), significant improvement was observed in the quiz performance after the education program, compared with the scores at baseline. The self-rated level of knowledge of sleep and sleep disorders was also significantly increased, compared with the level at baseline. Overall, the sleep education program was well received, with great feedback from the participants. Some students suggested starting the sleep education earlier during undergraduate study.

Implications for Nursing Practice

Translating this curriculum into undergraduate nursing programs, the addition of an important component of clinical practice in assessment of and intervention for sleep disorders will lay a foundation for improving the health care of patients and decreasing the health risks for nurses as care providers themselves.

Source: Ye, L., & Smith, A. (2015). Developing and testing a sleep education program for college nursing students. *Journal of Nursing Education, 54*(9), 532. doi:10.3928/01484834-20150814-09.

Heart rate and respiratory rate decline. Arousal from stage 2 sleep requires more intense stimuli than does arousal from stage 1. Stages 3 and 4 are collectively known as slow wave sleep or delta sleep. Stage 3 is relatively short and constitutes only about 3% to 8% of sleep time; stage 4 is longer and represents 10% to 15% of sleep time. Slow wave sleep is characterized by further reduction in heart rate, respiratory rate, blood pressure, and response to external stimuli. The four stages of NREM sleep make up 75% to 80% of total sleep time (Carskadon & Dement, 2017).

REM sleep comprises 20% to 25% of total sleep time and is characterized by reduction and absence of skeletal muscle tone (muscle atonia), bursts of rapid eye movement, myoclonic twitches of the facial and limb muscles, reports of dreaming, and autonomic nervous system variability. The atonia in REM sleep is thought to prevent the acting out of nightmares and dreams (Carskadon & Dement, 2017).

Sleep normally begins with NREM sleep. Continuous EEG recordings of sleep demonstrate an alternating cycling between NREM and REM sleep. Typically, four to six cycles of NREM and REM sleep occur over 90- to 120-minute intervals across the sleep period. There is also a distinct organization to sleep, with NREM sleep predominating during the first half of the sleep period and REM sleep predominating during the second half. The shortest REM period occurs 60 to 90 minutes after sleep onset and lasts only for several minutes. The longest REM period occurs at the end of the sleep period and can last up to an hour. This later REM cycle is why many people remember dreaming upon waking in the morning (Carskadon & Dement, 2017).

The structural organization of NREM and REM sleep is known as **sleep architecture** and is often displayed graphically as a hypnogram, as in Figure 20-1, which depicts the progression of the stages of sleep in a young adult and an older adult. The visual depiction of sleep is helpful in identifying **sleep continuity** (the distribution of sleep and wakefulness across the sleep period) as well as changes in sleep that may occur as a result of aging, illness, or certain medications. Disruption of sleep stages as indicated by excessive amounts of stage 1 sleep, multiple brief arousals, and frequent shifts in sleep staging is known as **sleep fragmentation**.

The function of alterations between NREM and REM sleep is not yet understood, but irregular cycling, absent sleep stages, and sleep fragmentation are associated with many sleep–wake disorders (McGinty & Szymusiak, 2017). For example, in people with depression, the latency to REM sleep—or the period of time to go from a full, wakeful state to REM sleep—is frequently reduced. People with depression also experience a reduction in the percentage of slow wave sleep. Benzodiazepines tend to suppress slow wave sleep, whereas serotonergic drugs suppress REM sleep.

REGULATION OF SLEEP

Although the regulation of sleep and wakefulness is not completely understood, it is believed to be a complex interaction between two processes: one that promotes sleep, known as the *homeostatic*

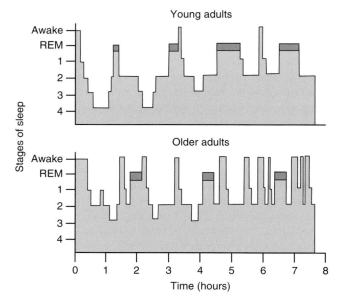

FIGURE 20-1 Hypnogram depicting the progression of the stages of sleep in a young adult and an older adult. A comparison of the two hypnograms illustrates the typical sleep architecture differences found between older and young adults. The hypnogram for the older adult shows more awakenings (shown as the spikes in the graph), less rapid eye movement (REM) sleep (purple rectangles), and delayed sleep latency (length of line on far left of graph) than those of the young adult. Source: Duthie, E. H., Katz, P. R., & Malone, M. (2007). *Practice of geriatrics* (4th ed.). Philadelphia: Saunders.

process or *sleep drive*, and one that promotes wakefulness, known as the *circadian process* or *circadian drive*. The homeostatic process is dependent on the number of hours a person is awake. The longer the period of wakefulness, the stronger the sleep drive. During sleep, the sleep drive gradually dissipates.

Circadian drives are near-24-hour cycles of behaviour and physiology generated and influenced by endogenous and exogenous factors. The exogenous factors are various clues from the environment known as *zeitgebers* (time-givers) that help set our internal clock to a 24-hour cycle. The strongest external cue for wakefulness is light, whereas darkness is a cue for sleep. Other environmental cues include the timing of social events, such as meals, work, or exercise (Czeisler & Buxton, 2017). The endogenous component, known as the *master biological clock*, is located in the suprachiasmatic nucleus (SCN) of the hypothalamus. This clock regulates not only sleep but also a host of other biological and physiological functions within the body. Information about the lighting conditions of the external environment is relayed to the SCN from the retina via the retinohypothalamic tract. The SCN also receives information from the thalamus and the midbrain. These two pathways transmit photic (light-related) and nonphotic information to the circadian clock through an expansive network. They also exert control over endocrine regulation, body temperature, sleep–wake cycles, metabolism, autonomic regulation, psychomotor and cognitive performance, attention, memory, and emotion (Czeisler & Buxton, 2017).

In addition to the circadian and homeostatic processes, several neurotransmitter systems are responsible for sleep and wakefulness. The neurotransmitters responsible for wakefulness are dopamine, norepinephrine, acetylcholine, histamine, glutamate, and hypocretin. Sleep-promoting neurotransmitters include adenosine, gamma-aminobutyric acid (GABA), and serotonin (McGinty & Szymusiak, 2017). Any medication that crosses the blood–brain barrier may affect sleep and wakefulness through the modulation of these neurotransmitters. Many of the medications used in psychiatry manipulate these neurotransmitter systems. For example, amphetamines—which promote wakefulness—increase the release of dopamine and norepinephrine. Caffeine (methylxanthine)—which promotes alertness—functions by blocking adenosine. Prescribers of medications must be aware of the effects of drugs on neurotransmitters that are involved in sleep and wakefulness.

FUNCTIONS OF SLEEP

Despite remarkable advances in the understanding of sleep–wake disorders and the biological and physiological process of sleep, very little is known about the true function of sleep. Most of the information on the function of sleep comes to us from animal models of sleep deprivation and human models of partial sleep deprivation. Based on these models, several theories have been proposed and include brain tissue restoration, body restoration (NREM sleep), energy conservation, memory reinforcement and consolidation (REM sleep), regulation of immune function, metabolism and regulation of certain hormones, and thermoregulation (Arun, Sathiamma, & Bindu, 2014; Siegel, 2017). In brief, the essence of these theories suggest general adaptation and regulation processes. For instance, restorative theory purports that sleep serves to restore what the body loses while awake, giving the body a chance to rejuvenate and repair itself. Energy conservation theory suggests that the main function of sleep is to minimize energy demand and expenditure during the day or night, especially when it is least efficient to search for food (Banks, Dorrian, Mathias, et al., 2017; Siegel, 2017).

SLEEP REQUIREMENTS

Sleep architecture and efficiency may change over time, but there is little change in the amount of sleep required once we reach adulthood. Sleep requirement varies considerably from individual to individual and to some degree is probably genetically mediated. Most adults require 7 to 9 hours, and adolescents require 8 to 10 hours of sleep for optimal functioning (Hirshkowitz, Whiton, Albert, et al., 2015). The amount of sleep required is determined by the amount after which a person feels fully awake and able to sustain normal levels of performance during the period of wakefulness. Considerable variability also exists in children's sleep duration requirements, with toddlers and preschool-aged children requiring 11 to 13 hours, school-aged children 9 to 12 hours, and adolescents 8 to 10 hours of sleep over a 24-hour period (Paruthi, Brooks, D'Ambrosio, et al., 2016).

Many people have a misconception regarding sleep need and tend to allow circumstances to dictate the amount of sleep

CONSIDERING CULTURE

The Role of Sleep in Canadian Culture

Jane is a busy, full-time professional and mother of three teenage girls. It is not unusual for her to leave the house by 6 a.m. and return home at 6:00 or 7:00 in the evening. She is active in the School Parent Committee and Girl Guides and also coaches the girls' soccer team during the spring. Her 86-year-old mother's health is failing, and Jane spends weekends helping her shop and running errands. She estimates that between her "real job" and her "second shift" domestic and community responsibilities, she works 16 to 18 hours a day, 7 days a week. How does she do it? Jane sleeps only 4 or 5 hours a night, some nights less. If she feels tired or fatigued, she reaches for a double latte and is on her way again. Sleep just is not a priority for her.

In Canada, the individual who seems to be able to do it all is held in high regard. Employers have come to expect near-24-hour access to their employees, making sleeplessness a cultural phenomenon. What some individuals describe as insomnia may actually be symptomatic of inadequate sleep opportunity and lack of leisure time to recharge and rejuvenate. Have you ever wondered what toll this may be having on health, functioning, relationships, and quality of life?

Nurses can play a key role in educating patients and the public about the health and societal consequences of inadequate sleep. Helping people strike a healthy balance between work and home may have significant implications for primary prevention.

Sources: Henry, D., McClellen, D., Rosenthal, L., et al. (2008). Is sleep really for sissies? Understanding the role of work in insomnia in the US. *Social Science and Medicine, 66,* 715–726. doi:10.1016/j.socscimed.2007.10.007; and Hurst, M. (2008). Who gets sleep these days? Sleep patterns of Canadians (Statistics Canada, Catalogue no. 11-008-X). *Canadian Social Trends, 85*(Spring), 39–45. Retrieved from http://www.statcan.gc.ca/pub/11-008-x/2008001/article/10553-eng.pdf.

obtained. The most accurate way to determine one's sleep requirement is to establish a routine bedtime and allow oneself to sleep undisturbed without an alarm for several days. This test is usually best accomplished during an extended period of leisure time, such as during a vacation. The average of several nights' undisturbed sleep is a good estimate of total sleep requirement (Epstein, 2007).

SLEEP PATTERNS

Sleep architecture changes over the lifespan. The percentage of each stage of sleep, as well as the overall sleep efficiency, or ratio of sleep duration to time spent in bed, varies according to age. For example, infants sleep 16 to 18 hours a day, enter sleep through REM (not NREM) sleep, and spend up to 50% of sleep time in REM sleep. By age 3, the percentage of REM sleep decreases to 20% to 25% and stays relatively constant throughout old age. The amount of slow wave sleep is maximal in young children and declines with age to almost none, particularly in men. This deficit results in a tendency for middle-of-the-night awakenings and reduced sleep efficiency with age (Bliwise & Scullin, 2017).

SLEEP–WAKE DISORDERS

The causation of sleep–wake disorders is multifactorial, with distinct and often overlapping biological (neurological or neurochemical), psychological, and social origins. Distinct aspects of causation affect specific disorders, and since different causes call for different treatment approaches, the assessment phase of the nursing process must be emphasized.

Sleep testing is often indicated for people complaining of sleep disturbance or ES that impairs social and vocational functioning. Four common diagnostic procedures are used in the evaluation of sleep–wake disorders: polysomnography (PSG), the multiple sleep latency test (MSLT), the maintenance of wakefulness test (MWT), and actigraphy.

The polysomnogram (PSG) is the most common sleep test. It is used to diagnose and evaluate people with sleep disorders related to breathing, nocturnal seizure disorders, and various parasomnias, or unusual sleep patterns that interrupt functioning.

A PSG is a noninvasive, pain-free procedure that usually requires spending a night or two in a sleep facility for what are commonly referred to as sleep studies (National Sleep Foundation, 2016b). During a PSG, a technologist records multiple biological functions during sleep, such as brainwave activity, eye movement, muscle tone, heart rhythm, and breathing, via electrodes and monitors placed on the head, chest, and legs.

After a full night's sleep is recorded, the data are tabulated and presented to a physician for interpretation. Depending on the interpretation and needs, patients may be even given therapy during the course of the study, which could include medication, oxygen, or a device called continuous positive airway pressure (CPAP) therapy.

The MSLT is a daytime nap test used to measure sleepiness objectively in a sleep-conducive setting. One day following a PSG evaluation, the MSLT is routinely performed for patients suspected of having narcolepsy. An MWT evaluates a person's ability to remain awake in a situation conducive to sleep and is used to document adequate alertness in individuals with careers for which sleepiness would pose a risk to public safety (Kirsch, 2012).

As an adjunct to clinical interviews, sleep diaries and, even alongside the overnight sleep studies mentioned here, actigraph devices are also used to measure sleep and track alterations, in particular for those with insomnia or circadian rhythm disorders. These watch-like devices are worn on the wrist and record movements that can be used to estimate sleep parameters with specialized algorithms in computer software programs. Actigraphy has been well validated across age groups and has the advantage of providing objective information on sleep habits in the patient's natural sleep environment (Slater, Botsis, Walsh, et al., 2015).

CLINICAL PICTURE

In the *Diagnostic and Statistical Manual of Mental Disorders*, fifth edition (*DSM-5*), sleep–wake disorders are classified into three major categories: insomnia, hypersomnia, and confusional arousal disorders, with a variety of subtypes for each (Reynolds, Redline, & DSM-V Sleep-Wake Disorders Workgroup and Advisors, 2010).

Additional clusters of sleep–wake disorders include those related to breathing and circadian rhythm. Diagnostic criteria for all include disturbed sleep causing marked distress and impaired daytime functioning. As introduced at the start of this chapter, sleep–wake disorders may be experienced independently or as co-occurring disorders and require clinical attention so as to achieve optimal outcomes for sleep, mental health, and physical health. The most common insomnia, hypersomnia, and confusional arousal disorders, as well as breathing and sensory and movement disorders affecting sleep, are described in more detail in this chapter, with particular attention to diagnostic criteria, care, and interventions for insomnia disorders.

Insomnia Disorders

Insomnia disorders are those sleep disturbances not directly attributable to another medical, psychiatric, or substance abuse disorder. Individuals who experience insomnia complain that they have difficulty with sleep initiation, sleep maintenance, early awakening, or nonrefreshing, nonrestorative sleep. People experiencing insomnia disorders will also have altered daytime functioning associated with the sleep disturbance, such as impaired social or vocational functioning, decreased concentration or memory impairment, somatic complaints, or mood disturbance. A disorder is not manifested by a few nights of poor sleep. To be classified as a disorder, symptoms must be present for three or more nights a week for more than 3 months, with an impairment in functioning.

Insomnia is best understood as a state of constant hyperarousal that involves biological, psychological, and social factors (Institute of Medicine, 2006). In addition to a thorough medical, psychiatric, and substance use history, it is helpful to use Spielman's 3P model of insomnia to comprehensively assess the causes of insomnia, suggest appropriate interventions, and provide rationales for treatment (Sadock, Sadock, & Ruiz, 2017). This model suggests that three factors contribute to the insomnia complaint: predisposing, precipitating, and perpetuating factors.

Predisposing factors are individual factors that create a vulnerability to insomnia. These may include a prior history of poor-quality sleep, a history of depression and anxiety, or a state of hyperarousal. People at risk for insomnia may describe themselves as light sleepers and "night owls." Pediatric insomnia has other precipitating factors that include neurological and other disorders. For example, 25% to 50% of children with attention-deficit/hyperactivity disorder report disturbed sleep patterns, particularly in the form of a sleep onset form of insomnia (Holvoet & Gabriëls, 2013).

Precipitating factors are external events that trigger insomnia. Personal and vocational difficulties, medical and psychiatric disorders (often comorbidly experienced with mood disorders, anxiety, post-traumatic stress disorder, cognitive disorders, and others), grief, and changes in role or identity (as seen with retirement) are examples. *Perpetuating factors* are sleep practices and attributes that maintain the sleep complaint, such as excessive caffeine or alcohol use, spending excessive amounts of time in bed or napping, and worry about the consequences of insomnia (Spielman & Glovinsky, 2004).

BOX 20-1 SLEEP HYGIENE

- Maintain a regular sleep–wake schedule.
- Develop a presleep routine that signals the end of the day.
- Reserve the bedroom for sleep and a place for intimacy.
- Create an environment that is conducive to sleep (taking into consideration light, temperature, and clothing).
- Avoid clock watching.
- Limit caffeinated beverages to one or two a day and none in the evening.
- Avoid heavy meals before bedtime.
- Use alcohol cautiously, and avoid use for several hours before bed.
- Avoid daytime napping.
- Exercise daily but not right before bed.
- Restrict use of light emitting devices

Source: Epstein, L. (2007). *The Harvard Medical School guide to a good night's sleep.* New York: McGraw-Hill.

Successful treatment of insomnia involves an integration of the basic principles of sleep hygiene (conditions and practices that promote continuous and effective sleep) (Box 20-1), behavioural therapies, and, in some instances, the use of hypnotic medication. Treatment is always targeted to the particular subtype, so, in some cases, lifestyle and breathing interventions are indicated (for instance, with sleep apnea disorders). Sedative and hypnotic medication is always used with caution, particularly when the patient has breathing-related insomnia, when addiction may be a concern, or when physical health or illness compromise breathing or central nervous system functioning. Both sedative or anxiolytic medications and over-the-counter sleeping aids have adverse effects; over-the-counter products also demonstrate limited effectiveness. Melatonin, a naturally occurring hormone, is a popular over-the-counter nutraceutical, but few data support its use in the management of insomnia (see Integrative Therapy: Melatonin for Insomnia).

Hypersomnia Disorders

Hypersomnia

Hypersomnia disorders are defined as excessive sleepiness that occurs three or more times per week for 3 or more months despite a main sleep lasting 7 hours or longer. The disorder is evidenced by either prolonged nighttime sleep episodes or daytime sleep episodes that occur almost daily and cause significant distress and social and vocational impairment. Key diagnostic features of hypersomnia disorders are a report of continuous yet not refreshing nor restorative sleep and difficulty waking up, either in the morning or at the end of a nap. Some individuals with these disorders can sleep up to 20 hours a day. Diagnosis is determined by clinical evaluation and a PSG and MSLT. Treatment is through lifestyle modification and stimulant medication.

Narcolepsy

The classic tetrad of narcolepsy includes episodes of irresistible attacks of refreshing sleep, cataplexy (muscle weakness), sleep paralysis (waking in a state of temporary paralysis), and hypnagogic hallucinations (dreaming while awake). While everyone with narcolepsy reports impairing degrees of excessive sleepiness, not everyone experiences cataplexy, sleep paralysis, and hypnagogic hallucinations, making diagnosis sometimes difficult. Diagnosis focuses on narcolepsy with or without cataplexy, so all points of assessment are important. When cataplexy is present, narcolepsy is almost always caused by an immune-mediated destruction of orexin (also referred to as hypocretin) neuropeptides located in the lateral hypothalamus. This condition is not considered a hypersomnia but rather its own category of disorder, and the cataplexy is then typically managed with sodium oxybate and antidepressant drugs.

Narcolepsy is also distinguished from other hypersomnia disorders in that patients generally feel refreshed upon waking. Associated symptoms include disturbed nighttime sleep with multiple middle-of-the-night awakenings and automatic behaviours characterized by memory lapses. Diagnosis is determined by clinical evaluation and a PSG and MSLT. Treatment is through lifestyle modifications and stimulant medication.

Confusional Arousal Disorders

Confusional arousal disorders are recurrent episodes of incomplete awakening from sleep with or without terror or movement, usually occurring during the first third of the major sleep episode and contributing to impaired nighttime and daytime safety or functioning. Varying subtypes exist and include sleepwalking, sleep terrors, nightmare disorder, sleep paralysis, and rapid eye movement behaviour disorder.

Sleepwalking

Also referred to as *somnambulism*, sleepwalking consists of a sequence of complex behaviours that begin in the first third of the night during deep NREM sleep (stages 3 and 4) and usually progress, without full consciousness or later memory, to leaving bed and walking about (activities may include dressing, going to the bathroom, screaming, and even driving). Because of the possibility of accident or injury, somnambulism in adults should be evaluated by a sleep specialist. A PSG is sometimes indicated to rule out the possibility of an underlying disorder of sleep fragmentation. Treatment consists of instructing the person and family regarding safety measures such as installing alarms or locks on windows and doors and gating stairways. Attention to sleep hygiene, limiting alcohol prior to bed, obtaining adequate amounts of sleep, and stress reduction help to prevent episodes.

Sleep Terrors

Sleep terrors are recurrent episodes of abrupt awakening from sleep, usually occurring during the first third of the major sleep episode and beginning with a panicky scream. There is intense fear and signs of autonomic arousal, such as mydriasis, tachycardia, rapid breathing, and sweating, during each episode.

Nightmare Disorder

Characterized by long, frightening dreams from which people awaken scared, nightmares almost always occur during REM sleep, usually after a long REM period late in the night. For some people, nightmare disorder is a lifetime condition; for others, nightmares occur only at times of stress and illness. Diagnosis is determined by clinical evaluation. Recurring nightmares can occur with post-traumatic stress disorder, so a thorough psychiatric exam and psychosocial history is necessary. Treatment is dependent on the frequency and severity of the symptoms, as well as the underlying cause. Treatment can include cognitive behavioural strategies, pharmacotherapy, or both. Many people do well with lifestyle modification measures, attention to sleep hygiene, and stress reduction.

Sleep Paralysis

Sleep paralysis is the sensation of paralysis at sleep onset or upon waking. The patient describes a complete awareness of his or her surroundings but is unable to move. For many people, sleep paralysis causes extreme anxiety and even panic. For a number of people, sleep paralysis events are rare or isolated and do not require any long-term treatment. Reassurance that the sensation is harmless and temporary is helpful. For those individuals with more frequent or severe episodes, further evaluation and treatment by a sleep specialist are warranted. Because sleep paralysis can be seen in people with narcolepsy, screening for narcolepsy is also indicated.

Rapid Eye Movement Behaviour Disorder

Rapid eye movement behaviour disorder (RBD) is characterized by the absence of muscle atonia during sleep. People with this disorder display elaborate motor activity associated with dream mentation. These people are actually acting out their dreams. RBD is most frequently seen in older-adult men but can be the heralding symptom of neurological pathology such as Parkinson's disease. Serotonergic medications (such as selective serotonin reuptake inhibitors [SSRIs] or selective serotonin–norepinephrine reuptake inhibitors [SNRIs]) can induce or exacerbate episodes. Diagnosis is determined by clinical evaluation and a PSG with video recording. Treatment focuses on patient and sleep partner safety. Placing the mattress on the floor is sometimes necessary to prevent injury as a result of falling out of bed. The use of intermediate-acting benzodiazepines can be helpful, especially in cases of severe disruption to the sleep partner and concerns about safety.

Kleine–Levin Syndrome

Kleine–Levin syndrome is characterized by recurrent episodes of excessive sleep (more than 11 hours per day). These episodes of hypersomnia occur at least once a year and are between 2 days and 4 weeks in duration. When awake, during at least one of these episodes, cognition is abnormal, with a feeling of disorientation, unreality, or confusion. During episodes, patients may experience abnormal behaviour such as megaphagia or hypersexuality. Between episodes, the patient experiences normal alertness, cognitive functioning, and behaviours.

Sleep–Wake Disorders Related to Breathing
Obstructive Sleep Apnea Hypopnea Syndrome
The most common disorder of breathing and sleeping is obstructive sleep apnea hypopnea syndrome, which is characterized by repeated episodes of upper airway collapse and obstruction that result in sleep fragmentation. Essentially, patients with obstructive sleep apnea hypopnea syndrome are not able to sleep and breathe at the same time. Typical symptoms include loud, disruptive snoring; witnessed apnea episodes; and excessive daytime sleepiness. Obesity is an important risk factor for obstructive sleep apnea. Diagnosis is determined by clinical evaluation and a PSG. Treatment is with CPAP therapy.

Primary Central Sleep Apnea

Another form of sleep disorder related to breathing, primary central sleep apnea is characterized by experiences of at least one of the following: excessive daytime sleepiness, frequent arousals and awakenings during sleep or insomnia complaints, or awakening short of breath. The PSG will show five or more central apneas per hour of sleep.

Primary Alveolar Hypoventilation

In the case of primary alveolar hypoventilation, PSG monitoring demonstrates episodes of shallow breathing longer than 10 seconds in duration associated with arterial oxygen desaturation and frequent arousals from sleep associated with the breathing disturbances or bradytachycardia. Patients often report excessive daytime sleepiness, frequent arousals and awakenings during sleep, or insomnia complaints.

Circadian Rhythm Sleep Disorder

Circadian rhythm sleep disorder is characterized by a persistent or recurrent pattern-of-sleep disruption. It results from an altered function of the circadian timing system or from a mismatch between the individual's natural circadian sleep–wake cycle and external demands regarding the timing and duration of sleep—for example, as occurs with shift work or jet lag. Diagnosis is determined by clinical evaluation, sleep diaries, and actigraphy. Treatment is with aggressive lifestyle management strategies aimed at adapting to or modifying the required sleep schedule (Abbott, Reid, & Zee, 2015).

Restless Legs Syndrome (Willis-Ekbom Disease)

Restless legs syndrome (RLS) is a sensory and movement disorder characterized by an uncomfortable sensation in the legs (occasionally affecting the arms and trunk) accompanied by an urge to move. Symptoms begin or worsen during periods of inactivity and are relieved or reduced by physical activity such as walking, stretching, or flexing. Symptoms are worse in the evening and at bedtime and can have a significant impact on the individual's ability to fall asleep and stay asleep. Symptoms may be induced or exacerbated by serotonergic agents such as SSRIs or SNRIs (Goldstein, 2011; Pack & Pien, 2011). Diagnosis is determined by clinical evaluation. Many people with RLS also have periodic limb movements during sleep that are observed during a PSG. Treatment is through lifestyle modification and dopamine agonist therapy, such as pramipexole (Mirapex) and ropinirole (Requip) (Reynolds, Redline, & DSM-V Sleep-Wake Disorders Workgroup and Advisors, 2010).

Nahla is a 32-year-old woman who was referred by her primary care provider for a psychiatric evaluation for complaints of anxiety and restlessness. She reported feeling fine during the day, but in the evening, she felt nervous and anxious. The symptoms always started at the same time. As soon as she would settle down for the evening to watch some television, she would begin to have a restless sensation in her legs that would make her jump up and pace back and forth. She described the sensation as having "soda pop fizzing through my veins." Sometimes she would go out for a walk at night even if it was very late in order to "calm down." These episodes began to occur almost nightly, and, as a result, she was having difficulty getting a good night's sleep. She began to dread the approach of nightfall. A full clinical evaluation suggested the diagnosis of RLS, and a course of the dopamine agonist pramipexole was initiated in the evening, resulting in dramatic improvement in her symptoms and total resolution of her sleep complaint.

EPIDEMIOLOGY

Sleep–wake problems are highly prevalent and occur across all age groups, cultures, and genders. It is estimated that 40% of Canadians experience some form of insomnia (Morin, LeBlanc, Belanger, et al., 2011). Further, 5.4 million Canadian adults have been diagnosed with sleep apnea or are at high risk for experiencing obstructive sleep apnea (Evans, Skomro, Driver, et al., 2014). In Canada, 34% of shift workers report sleep onset and maintenance difficulties compared to 25% of daytime workers, and circadian rhythm sleep disorder, a misalignment of the normal sleep–wake pattern, affects 2% to 5% of workers (Boivin & Boudreau, 2014).

COMORBIDITY

Multiple studies suggest that sleeping less than 7 hours per night may have a significant impact on cardiovascular, endocrine, immune, and neurological function (Institute of Medicine, 2006). Short sleep duration has been associated with obesity, cardiovascular disease and hypertension, and impaired glucose tolerance and diabetes (Barone & Menna-Barreto, 2011). Many sleep–wake disorders increase the risk for the development of certain medical conditions. For example, obstructive sleep apnea has been associated with hypertension, diabetes, cardiovascular disease, and stroke (Badran, Yassin, Fox, et al., 2015). A Canadian study by Kling, McLeod, and Koehoorn (2010) showed that sleep problems were associated with increased risk for workplace injury and that women were at higher risk for work injuries related to sleep problems. Individuals with neurological disease, such as Alzheimer's and Parkinson's disease, frequently experience sleep disturbance that worsens with the progression of the illness. Sleep disturbance is a major factor contributing to placement of people with dementia in a long-term care facility.

Most psychiatric disorders are associated with sleep disturbance. Insomnia is the most frequent complaint, but reports of hypersomnia are also common. About 85% of people with a major mood disorder will report some type of a sleep disturbance over the course of the illness. In addition, there is evidence to demonstrate that sleep disruption itself may be a precipitating factor in triggering mood and other psychiatric disorders and increases the risk for relapse, making the identification and management of sleep disturbance in people with affective disorders critical (Herrick & Sateia, 2016; Kaplan, Talbot, Gruber, et al., 2012; Staner, 2010). Of special concern is that depressed people who experience a sleep disturbance demonstrate greater degrees of suicidal ideation (Chellappa & Araujo, 2007). Sleep disturbance is common in people with alcoholism, and insomnia occurs in 36% to 72% of patients in early recovery and persists for months or even years. Sleep disturbance increases the risk for relapse to alcohol abuse. Targeting sleep disturbance during recovery may support continued abstinence (Arnedt, Conroy, & Bower, 2007).

Sleep–Wake Disorders and Mental Illness

People with sleep–wake disorders tend to focus on their sleep problems and may ignore the symptoms of other mental health or physical health disorders. It is not unusual for patients to present to a sleep–wake disorders centre for a sleep evaluation and later be diagnosed with an additional sleep–wake disorder, a psychiatric disorder, or both. For example, a person may be assessed for a breathing-related sleep–wake disorder and also diagnosed with insomnia, or may be diagnosed with comorbid RLS and insomnia. People with major depressive disorder frequently experience insomnia that involves relatively normal sleep onset followed by repeated awakenings during the second half of the night and early-morning waking. They usually then are in a difficult mood in the morning. Many patients point to the sleep disruption as the cause of the mood disturbance and report that if they could just get a good night's sleep, the mood symptoms would improve.

Difficulty with sleep latency is common with all anxiety disorders, and it is not unusual for people with a previously undiagnosed anxiety disorder to present for treatment of an insomnia complaint of lifelong duration. Management of the underlying anxiety diagnosis in conjunction with the insomnia complaint results in the best clinical outcome. Finally, people with schizophrenia have prolonged sleep latencies, sleep fragmentation, and multiple middle-of-the-night awakenings. It is believed that decreased slow wave sleep plays a factor in the cognitive and negative symptoms of schizophrenia (Lee & Douglass, 2010). Poor health habits such as excessive caffeine use, smoking, and inattention to a regular sleep schedule also contribute to sleep complaints. Those who take medications used to treat schizophrenia are at increased risk for weight gain, an adverse effect, and consequently the development of obstructive sleep apnea and should be screened accordingly (Lee & Douglass, 2010).

Hypersomnia is seen in many patients with mental conditions, including mood disorders. Many people report excessive daytime sleepiness in the beginning stages of a mild depressive disorder. A similar complaint is characteristic of the depressed phase of

VIGNETTE

Margret had been living with treatment-resistant schizophrenia for many years. Despite multiple medication trials, she had poor control of her symptoms and was frequently hospitalized. Last year she was started on clozapine (Clozaril); within a few months, she had a dramatic reduction in her command hallucinations and total resolution of paranoid delusions. Her family was thrilled. She was finally working and living in a group home. Over the past few months, however, the group home staff noticed a change in Margret's sleep patterns. She frequently wakes during the night and, in the morning, complains of a headache and a sore throat. When she returns home from work in the afternoon, it is not unusual for her to take a nap for 60 minutes or longer. In addition, the group home staff members express concern that she has gained more than 18 kilograms in the past year and feel that she is out of shape. They have been trying to get her motivated to exercise, but she complains of feeling too tired. While Margret was home on a family visit, her mother noted loud snoring and discussed this detail with the psychiatrist. A PSG was performed and demonstrated a severe degree of obstructive sleep apnea, most likely related to her recent weight gain. Continuous positive airway pressure (CPAP) therapy was initiated, and she was able to return to her baseline level of functioning.

bipolar I disorder. Uncomplicated grief may temporarily be associated with hypersomnia. Personality disorders, dissociative disorders, somatoform disorders, and dissociative fugue are all associated with hypersomnia. Treatment is directed at both the sleep–wake disorder and the psychiatric disorder (Reynolds, Redline, & DSM-V Sleep-Wake Disorders Workgroup and Advisors, 2010).

Sleep and General Health

Many medical conditions are also associated with insomnia. For instance, people with conditions accompanied by pain and

VIGNETTE

Robbie Carson is a student nurse assigned to Mrs. Ventresca in a nursing home. Robbie is in his psychiatric nursing rotation, part of which is spent in a skilled nursing facility taking care of people with dementia. When Robbie receives the report in the morning, he learns that Mrs. Ventresca has been experiencing significant sleep disturbance. She seems to have difficulty falling asleep and frequently wakes up groaning during the night. Robbie notes that Mrs. Ventresca is very confused, as well as agitated. She grimaces whenever she moves. Robbie believes that Mrs. Ventresca is in pain. He checks her history to find that she has had arthritis for many years. He then checks her medication profile and discovers that Mrs. Ventresca is not on any pain medication for her arthritis. He speaks to the charge nurse, who calls the physician. Immediately, the physician orders acetaminophen at bedtime for Mrs. Ventresca. Over the next few days, not only is there a dramatic improvement in Mrs. Ventresca's sleep, but her confusion abates and the agitation disappears.

discomfort, such as arthritis and cardiovascular and pulmonary disease, frequently complain of insomnia. Insomnia is also associated with neoplasms, vascular lesions, infections, and degenerative and traumatic conditions. Chronic fatigue syndrome and hypothyroidism have been associated with hypersomnia. The relationship between chronic medical disorders and sleep disturbance highlights the importance of screening people with medical disorders for sleep complaints. Treatment is directed at both the sleep–wake disorder and the underlying medical condition (Sadock, Sadock, & Ruiz, 2017).

A substance-induced sleep disorder can result from the use or recent discontinuance of a substance or medication. While it is quite obvious that many prescriptions and over-the-counter medications may affect sleep, there is less appreciation for the effects of commonly used substances on sleep. Alcohol, nicotine, and caffeine all have an impact on sleep quantity and quality. Alcohol—despite its great soporific effects—decreases deep sleep (stages 3 and 4) and REM sleep and is responsible for middle-of-the-night awakenings with difficulty returning to sleep. Nicotine is a central nervous system stimulant, increasing heart rate, blood pressure, and respiratory rate. As nicotine levels decline through the night, people wake in response to mild withdrawal symptoms. Caffeine blocks the neurotransmitter adenosine, promoting wakefulness. It increases sleep latency, reduces slow wave sleep, and acts as a diuretic, causing middle-of-the-night awakening for urination (Garcia & Salloum, 2015).

APPLICATION OF THE NURSING PROCESS

Regardless of the clinical environment or the presenting complaint, every patient can benefit from a sleep evaluation. Assessment of the person's sleep allows the nurse to identify short- and long-term health risks associated with sleep–wake disorders and sleep deprivation, provide health teaching and counselling regarding sleep needs, and improve clinical outcomes in those experiencing a sleep disturbance.

ASSESSMENT

General Assessment

Sleep Patterns

People frequently do not report sleep difficulties or discuss their sleep-related concerns with health care providers. They tend to minimize or adapt to the consequences of sleep disturbance. Furthermore, there is a lack of knowledge about the impact that sleep disturbance and sleep deprivation have on overall functioning and health. Many people do not complain of sleep disturbance directly but, rather, complain of associated symptoms such as fatigue, decreased concentration, mood disturbance, or physical ailments.

In assessing the patient with a sleep complaint, you must recognize the 24-hour nature of the sleep disturbance. Sleep disturbance is not confined to the 7 or 8 hours devoted to sleep. Sleep diaries (Figure 20-2) are helpful in identifying sleep patterns and behaviours that may be contributing to the sleep complaint. Assigning the person the homework of completing a sleep diary for 2 weeks will help guide the assessment and direct the plan

Two-week sleep diary

INSTRUCTIONS:
1 Write the date, day of the week, and type of day: Work, School, Day off, or Vacation.
2 Put the letter "C" in the box when you have coffee, cola, or tea. Put "M" when you take any medicine. Put "A" when you drink alcohol. Put "E" when you exercise.
3 Put a line (I) to show when you go to bed. Shade in the box that shows when you think you fell asleep.
4 Shade in all the boxes that show when you are asleep at night or when you take a nap during the day.
5 Leave boxes unshaded to show when you wake up at night and when you are awake during the day.

SAMPLE ENTRY BELOW: On a Monday when I worked, I jogged on my lunch break at 1 PM, had a glass of wine with dinner at 6 PM, fell asleep watching TV from 7 to 8 PM, went to bed at 10:30 PM, fell asleep around midnight, woke up and couldn't get back to sleep at about 4 AM, went back to sleep from 5 to 7 AM, and had coffee and medicine at 7:00 AM.

Today's Date	Day of the Week	Type of Day Work, School, Off, Vacation	Noon	1 PM	2	3	4	5	6 PM	7	8	9	10	11 PM	Midnight	1 AM	2	3	4	5	6 AM	7	8	9	10	11
sample	Mon.	Work		E					A				I									C M					

Week 1

Week 2

FIGURE 20-2 **Two-week sleep diary.** Source: Adapted from American Academy of Sleep Medicine. (n.d.). *Two week sleep diary.* Retrieved from http://yoursleep.aasmnet.org/pdf/sleepdiary.pdf.

of care. The following questions and comments provide direction for the assessment:

- When did you begin having trouble with sleep? Have you had trouble with sleep in the past?
- Describe your pre-bedtime routine. What are the activities you customarily engage in before sleep?
- Describe your sleeping environment. Are there things in your sleep environment that are hampering your sleep (such as noise, light, temperature, overall comfort)?
- Do you use your bedroom for things other than sleep or sexual activity (such as working, eating, or watching television)?
- What time do you go to bed? How long does it take to fall asleep?
- Once asleep, are you disturbed by middle-of-the-night awakening? If so, what wakes you up? Are you able to return to sleep?
- If you are unable to sleep, what do you do?
- What time do you wake up? What time do you get out of bed?
- How much time do you actually think you sleep?
- Do you sleep longer on weekends or days off?
- Do you nap? If so, for how long? Do you feel refreshed after napping?
- Can you identify any stress or problem that may have initially contributed to your sleep difficulties? Is there any particular issue or problem troubling you now?
- How have you dealt with that stress or problem?
- Tell me about your daily habits. I am interested in your diet, exercise, and medications you take. I am interested in whether or not you smoke or drink caffeinated or alcoholic beverages.
- Can you describe for me the thoughts you experience when you are lying in bed unable to get to sleep?
- What changes, if any, have you made to improve your sleep? What were the results?

Identifying Sleep–Wake Disorders

It is helpful to think about sleep–wake disorders according to the predominant symptoms of insomnia, hypersomnia, and arousal disorders. Box 20-2 provides pertinent screening questions for each diagnosis. An affirmative answer to any of these questions demands further investigation and evaluation.

Functioning and Safety

As previously described, sleep disturbance can result in increased risk for accident and injury and impose serious limitations on quality of life. Several screening tools are available to assist the clinician in evaluating sleep quality and the safety risk associated with ES. The Pittsburgh Sleep Quality Index (PSQI) is a subjective measure of sleep quality. A global sum of five or greater indicates poor quality and patterns of sleep (Buysse, Reynolds, Monk, et al., 1989). The Epworth Sleepiness Scale (ESS) is a validated psychometric tool used to measure subject reports of sleepiness and has been validated by objective measures using the MSLT. Scores of less than 10 are considered normal, 10 to 15 is

---

BOX 20-2   PRIMARY SYMPTOMS OF SLEEP–WAKE DISORDERS SCREENING QUESTIONS

Insomnia

- Do you have difficulty falling asleep, difficulty staying asleep, or early-morning awakenings?
- Do you feel not refreshed and not restored in the morning?
- Have you noticed any problems with your energy, mood, concentration, or work quality as a result of your sleep problem?
- Is your desired sleep schedule in conflict with your social and vocational goals? What is your preferred sleep schedule? (*also for circadian rhythm disturbance*)

Hypersomnia

- Have you ever been told that you snore or that it looks as though you stop breathing in your sleep? (*obstructive sleep apnea*)
- Do you have an unpleasant or uncomfortable sensation in your legs (or arms) that prevents you from sleeping or wakes you up from sleep and makes you want to move? (*restless legs syndrome*)
- Do you have episodes of sleepiness you cannot control? (*narcolepsy*)
- Do you ever feel unrested even after an extended sleep period? (*hypersomnia*)

Confusional Arousal Disorders

- Have you ever been told that you have done anything unusual in your sleep, such as walking (*somnambulism*) or talking (*somniloquy*)?
- Have you ever been told that you act out your dreams? (*REM sleep behaviour disorder*)
- Have you ever had an unusual experience associated with sleep, such as the inability to move upon awakening or falling asleep? (*sleep paralysis*)

---

moderately sleepy, and greater than 15 is excessively sleepy. In addition to these screening tools, the following questions provide direction for further assessment:

- Have you had an accident or injury as a result of sleepiness?
- Are you sleepy when you drive a car? What do you do if you are sleepy while driving?
- What kind of work do you do? Do you operate heavy equipment or machinery? How many hours a week do you work? How long is your commute?
- How does your sleep disturbance affect your work performance?
- Do you avoid social obligations as a result of your sleep problems?
- Do you feel as though your sleep disturbance is affecting your physical health? How so?

Sleep Studies

Alongside screening questionnaires and tools such as sleep diaries, and in cases where more complex medical diagnostics are necessary, a patient may participate in diagnostic sleep studies, often using polysomnography or actigraphy (National Sleep Foundation, 2016b), described earlier.

Self-Assessment

Nurses are especially vulnerable to the effects of sleep deprivation and sleep disruption. Rotating shifts and night work result in circadian rhythm disruption that can cause problems with insomnia and excessive sleepiness. Long shifts and overtime hours may lead to a decrease in total available sleep time, and on average, a night-shift worker sleeps for nearly 1.5 to 2 hours less over a 24-hour period than a daytime worker. This lack of sleep accumulates over the course of several working nights and cannot be entirely recovered during the worker's days off. Consequently, this lack of sleep can eventually accumulate over the years and may contribute to the development of certain health problems (Canadian Sleep Society, n.d.; Government of Alberta, 2017). Inadequate sleep time and sleep quality have been shown to impair performance and judgement, both of which may affect personal safety and quality of care. In addition, nurses who work rotating or night shifts may pose an increased risk for accident or injury to self and the community, as night-shift work increases driver drowsiness, degrading driving performance and increasing the risk of near-crash drive events (Lee, Howard, Horrey, et al., 2016).

Nurses need to be able to track their own sleep patterns, recognize the effects of chronic partial sleep deprivation on their performance and functioning, and take measures to ensure that they are well rested and able to provide safe and competent care. Self-evaluation for a possible sleep disorder and for the ability to cope with the rigours of shift work is warranted. Consultation with a sleep professional is indicated if there is significant disruption to sleep, physical and mental health, job performance, job satisfaction, and social functioning.

Paying attention to issues of sleep hygiene, obtaining 7 to 8 hours of sleep within a 24-hour period, limiting overtime hours, and limiting shift work to 8 hours are general recommendations for nurses and others working extended, night, and evening shifts, all of which can alter sleep quality and duration. Going to bed as soon as possible after a night shift will ensure a longer and a deeper sleep. It is advised to plan a fixed duration (e.g., from 9 a.m. till 11 a.m.) that will always be dedicated to sleep, both during working days and days off. This strategy of a regular sleeping period helps stabilize the biological clock and allows a worker to sleep better after a night shift without causing major disruptions during the days off. Avoiding exposure to morning light (i.e., by wearing sunglasses) between finishing work and during bedtime enables less stimulation of the biological clock and improved sleep. Increasing exposure to light in the evening and during the first half of the working night is also beneficial, as is sleeping in the darkest possible environment (Canadian Sleep Society, n.d.).

Sleeping the evening before a night shift is another strategy that supports adaptation to the altered sleep pattern, and could be appropriate as workers age and natural changes in sleep patterns occur, and for anyone starting their first night shift after some time. This strategy can reduce fatigue and stress during the night shift and allows workers to benefit from greater exposure to daylight, especially in winter. It is a strategy that facilitates moving onto a daytime schedule. For this strategy to be effective, the workers must be exposed to morning light; however, during the summer, sunglasses must be worn in the evening. Once again, sleeping in the darkest possible room is necessary (Canadian Sleep Society, n.d.).

DIAGNOSIS

There are four specific North American Nursing Diagnosis Association International (NANDA-I) nursing diagnoses for sleep disturbance (Herdman & Kamitsuru, 2014):

1. *Sleep deprivation*—prolonged periods of time without sleep (sustained natural, periodic suspension of relative consciousness)
2. *Insomnia*—a disruption in amount and quality of sleep that impairs functioning
3. *Readiness for enhanced sleep*—a pattern of natural, periodic suspension of consciousness that provides adequate rest, sustains a desired lifestyle, and can be strengthened
4. *Disturbed sleep pattern*—Time-limited interruptions of sleep amount and quality due to external factor

OUTCOMES IDENTIFICATION

The *Nursing Outcomes Classification (NOC)* (Moorhead, Johnson, Maas, et al., 2013) identifies several appropriate outcomes for the person experiencing sleep disruption, including *Sleep, Rest, Risk control*, and *Personal well-being*. Table 20-1 provides selected intermediate and short-term indicators for these categories.

PLANNING

The majority of people with sleep–wake disorders are treated in the community. The exceptions are cases in which the person has a primary psychiatric disorder or a medical condition that requires hospitalization. Because long-standing sleep problems are associated with a host of occupational, social, interpersonal, psychiatric, and medical conditions, the treatment is multifaceted and frequently requires a team approach under the leadership of a sleep disorder specialist. The role of the nurse is generally to conduct a full assessment, provide support to the patient and family while the appropriate interventions are determined, and teach the patient and family strategies that may improve sleep.

IMPLEMENTATION

Counselling

The nurse's counselling role begins with the assessment of the sleep disorder. The nurse's questions and responses to the patient and family provide support and reassurance that the sleep problems are treatable. For many people, the distress caused by chronic sleep difficulties sets up a conditioned barrier of hopelessness. Through the nurse's counselling approach, this hopelessness is identified and countered with encouragement, positive suggestions, and the belief that the person will be able to manage sleep difficulties.

TABLE 20-1	*NOC* OUTCOMES FOR SLEEP DISTURBANCES	
NURSING OUTCOME AND DEFINITION	**INTERMEDIATE INDICATORS**	**SHORT-TERM INDICATORS**
Sleep: Natural periodic suspension of consciousness during which the body is restored	Sleeps through the night consistently with improvements to sleep pattern and sleep quality	Hours of sleep improve to enable restorative state
		Sleep routine established
		Appropriate and functional wakefulness resumes
Rest: Quantity and pattern of diminished activity for mental and physical rejuvenation	Physically rested	Amount of rest sufficient
	Emotionally rested	Rest pattern supports functioning
	Mentally rested	Rest quality supports functioning
	Energy restored after rest	Rested appearance
Risk control: Personal actions to prevent, eliminate, or reduce modifiable health risks	Acknowledges risk factors	Develops effective risk-control strategies
	Modifies lifestyle to reduce risk factors	Commits to risk-control strategies
Personal well-being: Extent of positive perception of one's health status and life circumstances	Spiritual life is satisfactory	Performance of activities of daily living
	Physical health is satisfactory	Performance of usual roles
	Cognitive functioning is improved	

Source: Data from Moorhead, S., Johnson, M., Maas, M., et al. (2013). *Nursing outcomes classification (NOC)* (5th ed.). St. Louis: Mosby.

Health Teaching and Health Promotion

The nurse's role in health teaching cannot be overemphasized. Most individuals do not think about their sleep. This means that they also do not recognize the importance of a sleep routine or consider factors that influence good sleep. Many patients with sleep problems that can affect their mental health or with mental illnesses that affect sleep can learn sleep-promoting practices, practices they can put into place—for instance, adding a routine or taking away a sleep-impairing routine (such as use of light-emitting devices before bed). In addition, there are many myths regarding what constitutes "good sleep" and what factors contribute to sleep quality (see Box 20-1). Education about sleep testing, sleep–wake disorders, and sleep hygiene can be done verbally or with the use of educational materials such as those available through the Canadian Sleep Society or Canadian Lung Association. The nurse may also be involved in teaching relaxation techniques, such as meditation, guided imagery, progressive muscle relaxation, or controlled breathing exercises. Use of these techniques has been linked to sustained benefits for patients with primary insomnia (Sadock, Sadock, & Ruiz, 2017).

Pharmacological Interventions

Many people use medication to address their sleep problems. Nurses frequently provide education about the benefits of a particular drug, the adverse effects, and the fact that medications are usually prescribed for no more than 2 weeks because tolerance and withdrawal may result (Sadock, Sadock, & Ruiz, 2017). In many settings, the nurse also monitors the effectiveness of the medication.

The Drug Treatment box provides information about hypnotics approved by Health Canada for treatment of insomnia.

Generally, however, long-term use of hypnotic medication is discouraged because nonpharmacological treatments have shown efficacy in reducing insomnia. Many antidepressants and atypical antipsychotics are also used off-label (i.e., without specific approval from Health Canada) in the treatment of sleep–wake disorders because of their sedative properties.

Cognitive Behavioural Therapy for Insomnia

Cognitive behavioural therapy for insomnia (CBT-I) includes educational, behavioural, and cognitive components; it targets factors that perpetuate insomnia over time (Morin, 2004). It is the most researched nonpharmacological intervention for insomnia and is considered to be a first-line treatment option (Mitchell, Gerhman, Perlis, et al., 2012). The counsellor's first objectives are to provide education regarding sleep and sleep needs and help the person to set realistic expectations regarding sleep. Patients should be asked what they believe constitutes healthy sleep, and counsellors should then clarify any misconceptions. Eliciting information about the total number of hours spent sleeping typically has little value. Many people are stuck on a set number of sleep hours rather than on the quality of sleep obtained. Focusing on the number of hours slept rather than the quality of sleep and daytime functioning increases the insomnia experience.

The next approach involves modifying poor sleep habits and establishing a regular sleep–wake schedule. Keeping a sleep diary (see Figure 20-2) for a period of 2 weeks is helpful in establishing overall sleep patterns and determining overall sleep efficiency ([total sleep time divided by total time in bed] × 100). After reviewing sleep diaries, patients are sometimes surprised to discover that their sleep problems are not as bad as previously believed. Sleep restriction, or limiting the total sleep time, creates a temporary, mild state of sleep deprivation and strengthens the sleep homeostatic drive. This technique decreases sleep latency and improves sleep continuity and quality. If, for example, a person's sleep diary indicates that he or she is in bed for 8 hours but sleeping only 6 hours, sleep is restricted to 6 hours, and the bedtime and wake time are adjusted accordingly. The sleep time should not be reduced below 5 hours, regardless of sleep efficiency, and patients should be cautioned about the dangers of driving while undergoing a trial of sleep restriction. Once sleep efficiency is improved, total sleep time is gradually increased by 10- to 20-minute increments.

CBT-I also involves using stimulus control. Based on classical conditioning theory, stimulus control employs five basic principles that decrease the negative associations with the bed or

DRUG TREATMENT OF PATIENTS WITH INSOMNIA

GENERIC (BRAND) NAME	ONSET OF ACTION (MIN.)	DURATION OF ACTION	HEALTH CANADA– APPROVED FOR INSOMNIA	HABIT FORMING
Benzodiazepines				
Flurazepam (Dalmane, Som Pam)	30–60	Long	Yes	Yes, all drugs in this class are Schedule IV
Nitrazepam (Mogadon, Nitrazadon)	30–60	Long	Yes	
Temazepam (Restoril)	45–60	Intermediate	Yes	
Triazolam	15–30	Short	Yes	
Benzodiazepine-Like Drugs				
Zopiclone (Imovane, Rhovane)	60	Intermediate	Yes	Yes, all drugs in this class are Schedule IV
Antidepressant				
Trazodone (Oleptro)	60–120	Long	No	No
Antihistamines				
Diphenhydramine (Benedryl, Nytol)	60–180	Long	Yes	Tolerance to hypnotic effects develops in 1–2 weeks

Source: Adapted from Health Canada. (2009). *Authorized sleep-aid medications in Canada.* Retrieved from http://www.hc-sc.gc.ca/ahc-asc/media/advisories-avis/_2009/2009_161-list-eng.php.

INTEGRATIVE THERAPY

Melatonin for Insomnia

Many people with insomnia turn to over-the-counter solutions. Melatonin is a hormone secreted by the pineal gland in response to information it receives from the suprachiasmatic nucleus regarding light and dark. It is available as a synthetic product at most health food stores and pharmacies. Normally, as night approaches, melatonin is secreted and blood levels rise, producing a sensation of sleepiness. Melatonin levels stay elevated throughout the night but begin to decline in the early morning hours and are essentially undetectable during the day. It would stand to reason, then, that melatonin supplementation would be a safe and effective complementary therapy. Many patients reach for melatonin supplements in some situations to help align the body's circadian rhythms with the outside environment.

Unfortunately, research into the role of melatonin in the management of insomnia has been disappointing, with most data pointing to little to no benefit at all. It does seem, however, that melatonin may be effective in the management of circadian rhythm disorders such as jet lag, shift-work disorder, and advances and delays in the sleep cycle.

Although there have been no documented reports of toxicity or overdose of synthetic melatonin, it is important to tell patients that (1) there is no identified effective dosage range and (2) because melatonin is available over the counter and unregulated by Health Canada, there is no standardization of nutraceutical ingredients. Reported adverse effects include nausea, headache, and orthostatic blood pressure changes. Potential contraindications to melatonin use have included excessive sedation with ingestion, pregnancy or nursing, seizure disorders, and warfarin therapy. More recently, the question of the potential effects of melatonin on glucose tolerance has emerged in the literature.

There is evidence available indicating that melatonin can be effective in the treatment of chronic insomnia in children and, on the whole, is well tolerated. However, there are limited evidence-based guidelines about the dosage and timing of intake for children, which makes the practice concerning. Very little systematic research has been done into the possible impact of melatonin intake on puberty and the endocrine system. Therefore treatment with melatonin in children with attention-deficit/hyperactivity disorder and chronic insomnia is advised to be reserved for only those children with sleep disorders that have a severe impact on daily functioning.

bedroom and strengthen the stimulus for sleep (Morin, 2004). Patients should be instructed to do the following:

1. Go to bed only when sleepy.
2. Use the bed or bedroom only for sleep and intimacy (no television, reading, or other activities in the bedroom).
3. Get out of bed if unable to sleep and engage in a quiet-time activity such as reading or crossword puzzles (no television, work, or computer).
4. Maintain a regular sleep–wake schedule, with getting up at the same time each day being the most important factor.
5. Avoid daytime napping (if napping is necessary to avoid accident or injury, it should be limited to 20 to 30 minutes maximum).

Other objectives of CBT-I are aimed at identifying and correcting maladaptive attitudes and beliefs about sleep that perpetuate insomnia. For example, people frequently amplify the consequences of their insomnia and attribute most daytime experiences to their sleep complaint. They may rationalize maladaptive coping behaviours such as excessive time in bed to "catch up" on lost sleep and may exhibit unrealistic expectations about sleep. The practitioner offers alternative interpretations regarding the sleep complaint to assist the person to think about the insomnia in a different way, empowering the patient to be in control of his or her sleep (Haynes, 2015). Because CBT-I approaches are not immediately effective and may take several weeks of practice before improvement is seen, success is dependent on both a high degree of motivation in the patient and a commitment on the part of the practitioner.

Other nonpharmacological methods for treating insomnia are exercise, tai chi, acupuncture, yoga, and mindfulness. All of these approaches have been researched and demonstrate some evidence of improvement in sleep quality and insomnia, but the quantity and quality of research available is limited (Cheuk, Yeung, Chung, et al., 2012).

Advanced-Practice Interventions

Although psychotherapy offers little value in the treatment of primary insomnia, there is a component of primary insomnia that involves a conditioned response. The initial episode of insomnia is frequently associated with a stressful event or crisis that produces anxiety. This anxiety becomes associated with worry about not being able to get to sleep and leads to preoccupation with getting enough sleep. The more the person tries to sleep, the more elusive sleep becomes, and the greater the person's anxiety. The advanced-practice nurse may be closely involved in the use of cognitive behavioural therapy to manage insomnia.

EVALUATION

Evaluation is based on whether the person experiences improved sleep quality as evidenced by decreased sleep latency, fewer nighttime awakenings, and a shorter time to get back to sleep after waking. This evaluation is accomplished through an individual's report and maintenance of a sleep diary. Just as important as objective changes in the person's sleep pattern is the person's perception of improvement. Objectively, the improvement may be quite modest, but the person may perceive that he or she is no longer controlled by sleep (or the lack of it) but is exerting control over sleep through lifestyle changes and a better sleep routine.

> **VIGNETTE**
>
> Josette Harris is a 52-year-old woman who complains of difficulty falling asleep and staying asleep every night. It is not unusual for Josette to take several hours to fall asleep, and once she does fall asleep, she is able to sleep for only 2 to 3 hours at a time. She tosses and turns and lies in bed "hoping to fall asleep." She estimates that she is sleeping only about 4 or 5 hours a night. Josette reports that this has been going on for at least a year but that it seems to have been getting progressively worse over the past several months. Because she sleeps poorly at night, she has been staying in bed until 9:00 or 10:00 in the morning and has been late for work several times during the past 3 months. She feels tired during her waking hours and has difficulty focusing on the task at hand in her accounting job. To improve her work performance, she has been drinking five or six cups of coffee during the day. Even though she feels tired, she is unable to nap. Family members complain that she is irritable and short tempered with them. Interestingly, she reports that she was able to sleep fairly well while on vacation last month. Josette completes a sleep diary for a 2-week period and undergoes a complete assessment. There seems to be no underlying medical or psychiatric disorder associated with her sleep complaint. She is diagnosed with an insomnia disorder and begins a cognitive behavioural therapy program.

■ KEY POINTS TO REMEMBER

- Sleep disturbance has major implications for overall health, quality of life, and personal and community safety.
- Research into the physiology of normal sleep, as well as sleep–wake disorders, is expanding.
- Most people with a mood disorder will report sleep disturbance; recognition and treatment of sleep disturbance in people with psychiatric disorders improves clinical outcomes.
- Regardless of the clinical environment or the presenting complaint, all patients can benefit from an evaluation of their sleep needs.

- It is helpful to categorize sleep disturbance according to the three major symptom categories of insomnia, hypersomnia, and confusional arousal disorders.
- Primary insomnia can be effectively treated with nonpharmacological interventions such as CBT-I, sleep restriction, stimulus control, and attention to issues of sleep hygiene. Long-term pharmacological management is generally not indicated.

■ CRITICAL THINKING

1. Jabar is a 46-year-old man who complains of waking frequently at night. Consequently, he is tired all day and knows that he has not been functioning as well as he should. Whenever he can manage it, he goes out to his car at lunchtime to take a 60-minute nap because he has fallen asleep at his desk in the past and been given a disciplinary warning. He is drinking two to three cups of coffee in the afternoon so that he does not feel sleepy while driving home.

a. What questions would you ask to determine whether Jabar might have a sleep disorder?

b. What recommendations will you make for him to improve his sleep hygiene?

c. What instructions and education should you give Jabar regarding personal and community safety?

2. Your patient, Vivian, has been using temazepam (Restoril) for several years to treat insomnia. She has been reading that long-term use of hypnotics is not healthy or productive and wants to quit taking them. However, she is focused on needing 9 hours of sleep each night and is extremely worried about what will happen when she quits the temazepam.

a. What instructions would you provide to Vivian regarding stimulus control, sleep restriction, and cognitive restructuring of her sleep complaint?

b. Identify alternative pharmacological therapies.

3. Mrs. Levine is a 72-year-old woman with a history of major depression. She takes fluoxetine (Prozac) 10 mg every day and has experienced significant relief from depression. While listing her medications, she tells you she is using a variety of over-the-counter sleep aids because she has been having some difficulty sleeping recently. These over-the-counter products include diphenhydramine, melatonin, valerian, and something that her neighbour gave her to try.

a. In light of the person's age and history of depression, what are your concerns?

b. What further assessment is required?

c. What specific question would you need to ask concerning her use of Prozac?

d. What instructions and education will you provide?

4. Suzie Au, a 47-year-old business executive and single mother of two teenage sons, has presented to the urban mental health centre complaining that she is "hanging on by my fingernails," that taking care of her business and her boys is taking all of her energy, and that she has suffered from constant insomnia for several years but that it has worsened over the past few months. Her lack of sleep has forced her to give up her social life, including gym workouts. She feels stressed and worries that her ability to cope will soon disappear unless she can improve the quality of her sleep. She has begun to drink four or five cups of coffee per day to keep awake and tries to catch a nap whenever possible.

a. What strategy or tool would enable Suzie to provide an accurate self-appraisal of the characteristics of her sleep?

b. What further assessments would you need to do?

c. What immediate instructions and education will you offer Suzie in regard to her current coping strategies?

d. What short-term goals would be appropriate for Suzie?

CHAPTER REVIEW

1. A person states that he needs only 5 to 6 hours of sleep per night to feel rested. How should the nurse interpret this statement?
   a. The person is not sleeping enough.
   b. The person is sleeping too much.
   c. The person is sleeping according to his own body's needs.
   d. The person is not getting enough REM sleep.

2. The nurse is planning care for a person with primary insomnia. What is an appropriate outcome?
   a. The person will sleep 12 hours nightly.
   b. The person will go to bed and wake up at consistent times daily.
   c. The person will take one nap daily to restore energy.
   d. The person will drink a cup of warm tea before bedtime.

3. The nurse is providing teaching for a person who has been taking a hypnotic medication to sleep. What statement by the nurse is appropriate?
   a. "You can use this medication for as long as you would like."
   b. "It would be better to take an over-the-counter medication instead."
   c. "Melatonin has been shown to be just as effective as hypnotic medications."
   d. "Be certain to follow up with your doctor regularly while you take this medication."

4. Because of the likelihood of underestimated or inaccurate self-assessment of sleep, what tool would be most appropriate for the nurse to use in obtaining an assessment from a patient suspected of having a sleep–wake disorder?
   a. A mini-mental state examination
   b. An anxiety inventory
   c. A sleep diary
   d. A family history assessment

5. Which behaviour would alert the nurse to a circadian rhythm sleep disorder?
   a. Excessive sleepiness for at least 1 month, accompanied by prolonged sleep episodes
   b. Multiple episodes of brief daytime sleeping followed by disturbed nighttime sleep
   c. Persistent patterns of sleep disruption after travelling for business
   d. Repeated episodes of upper airway collapse and obstruction that results in sleep fragmentation

⊖volve WEBSITE

Post-Test   interactive review

Visit the Evolve website for Chapter Review Answers and Rationales, Critical Thinking Answer Guidelines, and additional resources related to the content in this chapter: http://evolve.elsevier.com/ *Canada/Varcarolis/psychiatric/*

REFERENCES

Abbott, S. M., Reid, K. J., & Zee, P. C. (2015). Circadian rhythm sleep-wake disorders. *The Psychiatric Clinics of North America, 38*(4), 805.

Arnedt, J. T., Conroy, D. A., & Bower, K. J. (2007). Treatment options for sleep disturbance during alcohol recovery. *Journal of Addictive Diseases, 26,* 41–54. doi:10.1300/J069v26n04_06.

Arun, S., Sathiamma, S., & Bindu, K. (2014). Current understanding on the neurobiology of sleep and wakefulness. *International Journal of Clinical and Experimental Psychology, 1*(1), 3–9.

Aviva. (2016). *Health Check UK Report: Family health: Habits across the generations.* Retrieved from http://www.aviva.com/media/news/item/ uk-nation-of-sleepless-nights-one-in-four-uk-adults-want-a-better-night s-sleep-17693/.

Badran, M., Yassin, B. A., Fox, N., et al. (2015). Epidemiology of sleep disturbances and cardiovascular consequences. *The Canadian Journal of Cardiology, 31*(7), 873–879. doi:10.1016/j.cjca.2015.03.011.

Banks, S., Dorrian, J., Mathias, B., et al. (2017). Sleep deprivation. In M. Kryger, T. Roth, & W. Dement (Eds.), *Principles and practice of sleep medicine.* (6th ed., pp. 49–55). Philadelphia: Elsevier.

Barone, M. T., & Menna-Barreto, L. (2011). Diabetes and sleep: A complex cause-and-effect relationship. *Diabetes Research and Clinical Practice, 91,* 129–137. doi:10.1016/j.diabres.2010.07.011.

Bliwise, D., & Scullin, M. K. (2017). Normal aging. In M. Kryger, T. Roth, & W. Dement (Eds.), *Principles and practice of sleep medicine.* (6th ed., pp. 25–38). Philadelphia: Elsevier.

Boivin, D. B., & Boudreau, P. (2014). Impacts of shift work on sleep and circadian rhythms. *Pathologie-Biologie, 62*(5), 292. doi:10.1016/j. patbio.2014.08.001.

Brownlow, J. A., McLean, C. P., Gehrman, P. R., et al. (2016). Influence of sleep disturbance on global functioning after posttraumatic stress disorder treatment. *Journal of Traumatic Stress, 29*(6), 515–521. doi:10.1002/ jts.22139.

Buysse, D. J., Reynolds, C. F., III, Monk, T. H., et al. (1989). The Pittsburgh Sleep Quality Index: A new instrument for psychiatric practice and research. *Psychiatry Research, 28,* 193–213. doi:10.1016/0165-1781(89)90047-4.

Canada Safety Council. (2013). *Canada's blood alcohol laws among the strictest in the Western world.* Ottawa: Author. Retrieved from https:// canadasafetycouncil.org/traffic-safety/canada-s-blood-alcohol-laws-among -strictest-western-world.

Canadian Sleep Society. (n.d.). *Strategies for night shift workers.* Retrieved from https://css-scs.ca/resources/brochures/night-shift-workers.

Carskadon, M. A., & Dement, W. C. (2017). Normal human sleep: An overview. In M. Kryger, T. Roth, & W. Dement (Eds.), *Principles and practice of sleep medicine.* (6th ed., pp. 15–24). Philadelphia: Elsevier.

Chellappa, S. L., & Araujo, J. F. (2007). Sleep disorders and suicidal ideation in patients with depressive disorder. *Psychiatry Research, 153,* 131–136. doi:10.1016/j.psychres.2006.05.007.

Cheuk, D. K., Yeung, W. F., Chung, K. F., et al. (2012). Acupuncture for insomnia. *The Cochrane Database of Systematic Reviews,* (9), doi:10.1002/14651858.CD005472.pub3.

Czeisler, C., & Buxton, O. M. (2017). The human circadian timing system and sleep–wake regulation. In M. Kryger, T. Roth, & W. Dement (Eds.), *Principles and practice of sleep medicine.* (6th ed., pp. 362–376). Philadelphia: Saunders.

Epstein, L. (2007). *The Harvard Medical School guide to a good night's sleep.* New York: McGraw-Hill.

Evans, J., Skomro, R., Driver, H., et al. (2014). Sleep laboratory test referrals in Canada: Sleep apnea rapid response survey. *Canadian Respiratory Journal, 21*(1), e4–e10. doi:10.1155/2014/592947.

Gaines, K. K. (2016). Sleepless in America: Burning the candle at both ends? At what cost? *Urologic Nursing, 36*(3), 109. doi:10.7257/1053-816X.2016.36.3.109.

Garcia, A. N., & Salloum, I. M. (2015). Polysomnographic sleep disturbances in nicotine, caffeine, alcohol, cocaine, opioid, and cannabis use: A focused review. *The American Journal on Addictions, 24*(7), 590–598. doi:10.1111/ ajad.12291.

Goldstein, C. A. (2011). Parasomnias. *Disease-A-Month, 57*(7), 364–388.

Government of Alberta. (2017). *Fatigue, extended work hours, and workplace safety.* Retrieved from https://work.alberta.ca/documents/ OHS-bulletin-ERG015.pdf.

Government of Canada. (2017). *Road safety in Canada.* Retrieved from https://www.tc.gc.ca/eng/motorvehiclesafety/tp-tp15145-1201.htm.

Haynes, P. (2015). Application of cognitive behavioral therapies for comorbid insomnia and depression. *Sleep Medicine Clinics, 10*(1), 77.

Herdman, T. H., & Kamitsuru, S. (Eds.), (2014). *NANDA international nursing diagnoses: Definitions and classification, 2015–2017.* Oxford, UK: Wiley-Blackwell.

Herrick, D. D., & Sateia, M. J. (2016). Insomnia and depression: A reciprocal relationship. *Psychiatric Annals, 46*(3), 164. doi:10.3928/00485713-20160121-01.

Hirshkowitz, M., Whiton, K., Albert, S. M., et al. (2015). The National Sleep Foundation's sleep time duration recommendations: Methodology and results summary. *Sleep Health, 1*(1), 40–43.

Holvoet, E., & Gabriëls, L. (2013). Disturbed sleep in children with ADHD: Is there a place for melatonin as a treatment option? *Tijdschrift Voor Psychiatrie, 55*(5), 349.

Institute of Medicine. (2006). *Sleep disorders and sleep deprivation: An unmet public health problem.* Washington, DC: National Academies Press.

Kaplan, K. A., Talbot, L. S., Gruber, J., et al. (2012). Evaluating sleep in bipolar disorder: Comparison between actigraphy, polysomnography, and sleep diary. *Bipolar Disorders, 14*(8), 870–879. doi:10.1111/ bdi.12021.

Khurshid, K. A. (2015). *A review of changes in DSM-5 sleep-wake disorders.* Retrieved from https://psychiatry.ufl.edu/files/2015/10/Psychiatric_Times_ Khurshid.pdf.

Kirsch, D. B. (2012). A neurologist's guide to common subjective and objective sleep assessments. *Neurologic Clinics, 30*(4), 987.

Kling, R. N., McLeod, C. B., & Koehoorn, M. (2010). Sleep problems and workplace injuries in Canada. *Sleep, 33*(5), 611–618.

Lee, E. K., & Douglass, A. B. (2010). Sleep in psychiatric disorders: Where are we now? *The Canadian Journal of Psychiatry, 55*(7), 403–412.

Lee, M. L., Howard, M. E., Horrey, W. J., et al. (2016). High risk of near-crash driving events following night-shift work. *Proceedings of the National Academy of Sciences, 113*(1), 176–181. doi:10.1073/pnas.1510383112.

McGinty, D., & Szymusiak, R. (2017). Neural control of sleep in mammals. In M. Kryger, T. Roth, & W. Dement (Eds.), *Principles and practice of sleep medicine.* (6th ed., pp. 62–77). Philadelphia: Elsevier.

Mitchell, M. D., Gerhman, P., Perlis, M., et al. (2012). Comparative effectiveness of cognitive behavioural therapy for insomnia: A systematic review. *BMC Family Practice, 13*(40), doi:10.1186/1471-2296-13-40.

Moorhead, S., Johnson, M., Maas, M. L., et al. (2013). *Nursing outcomes classification (NOC)* (5th ed.). St. Louis: Mosby.

Morin, C. (2004). Cognitive-behavioural approaches to the treatment of insomnia. *The Journal of Clinical Psychiatry, 65*(Suppl. 16), 33–40.

Morin, C. M., LeBlanc, M., Belanger, L., et al. (2011). Prevalence of insomnia and its treatment in Canada. *Canadian Journal of Psychiatry, 56*(9), 540–548.

National Sleep Foundation. (2016a). *How much sleep do we really need?* Retrieved from https://sleepfoundation.org/how-sleep-works/how-much-sleep-do-we-really-need.

National Sleep Foundation. (2016b). *Sleep studies.* Retrieved from https://sleepfoundation.org/sleep-topics/sleep-studies/page/0/1.

Ohayon, M. M., Dauvilliers, Y., & Reynolds, C. F. (2012). Operational definitions and algorithms for excessive sleepiness in the general population: Implications for DSM-5 nosology. *Archives of General Psychiatry, 69,* 71–79.

Pack, A. I., & Pien, G. W. (2011). Update on sleep and its disorders. *Annual Review of Medicine, 62,* 447–460. doi:10.1146/annure v-med-050409-104056.

Paruthi, S., Brooks, L. J., D'Ambrosio, C., et al. (2016). Recommended amount of sleep for pediatric populations: A consensus statement of the American Academy of Sleep Medicine. *Journal of Clinical Sleep Medicine : JCSM : Official Publication of the American Academy of Sleep Medicine, 12*(6), 785–786.

Pishka Upender, R. P. (2017). Sleep medicine, public policy, public health. In M. Kryger, T. Roth, & W. Dement (Eds.), *Principles and practice of sleep medicine.* (6th ed., pp. 638–645). Philadelphia: Elsevier.

Reynolds, C. F., Redline, S., & DSM-V Sleep-Wake Disorders Workgroup and Advisors. (2010). The DSM-V sleep–wake disorders nosology: An update

and an invitation to the sleep community. *Journal of Clinical Sleep Medicine : JCSM : Official Publication of the American Academy of Sleep Medicine, 6*(1), 9–10.

Sadock, B. J., Sadock, V. A., & Ruiz, P. (2017). *Concise textbook of clinical psychiatry* (4th ed.). Philadelphia: Lippincott Williams & Wilkins.

Siegel, J. M. (2017). Sleep in animals: A state of adaptive inactivity. In M. Kryger, T. Roth, & W. Dement (Eds.), *Principles and practice of sleep medicine.* (6th ed., pp. 103–114). Philadelphia: Elsevier.

Slater, J. A., Botsis, T., Walsh, J., et al. (2015). Assessing sleep using hip and wrist actigraphy. *Sleep and Biological Rhythms, 13*(2), 172–180. doi:10.1111/sbr.12103.

Spielman, A., & Glovinsky, P. (2004). A conceptual framework of insomnia for primary care providers: Predisposing, precipitating, and perpetuating factors. *Sleep Medicine Alert, 9*(1), 1–6.

Staner, L. (2010). Comorbidity of insomnia and depression. *Sleep Medicine Reviews, 14*(1), 35–46. doi:10.1016/j.smrv.2009.09.003.

Ye, L., Keane, K., Hutton Johnson, S., et al. (2013). How do clinicians assess, communicate about, and manage patient sleep in the hospital? *Journal of Nursing Administration, 43,* 342–347.

Trauma Interventions

21. Crisis and Disaster

22. Suicide and Nonsuicidal Self-Injury

23. Anger, Aggression, and Violence

24. Interpersonal Violence: Child, Older Adult, and Intimate Partner Abuse

25. Sexual Assault

Crisis and Disaster

Sonya L. Jakubec

KEY TERMS AND CONCEPTS

adventitious crisis
coping
coping methods
crisis
crisis intervention
critical incident stress debriefing (CISD)
disasters
maturational crisis

mental health emergency
mental health first aid (MHFA)
phases of crisis
primary care
secondary care
situational crisis
tertiary care
trauma

OBJECTIVES

1. Differentiate among the three types of crisis.
2. Delineate six aspects of crisis relevant for nurses involved in crisis intervention.
3. Understand areas of assessment and approaches to assessment during crisis.
4. Discuss four common problems in the nurse–patient relationship encountered by beginning nurses when starting crisis intervention. Discuss resolutions to these problems.
5. Compare and contrast the differences among primary, secondary, and tertiary intervention, including appropriate intervention strategies.
6. Identify modalities of crisis intervention.
7. List at least five resources in the community that could be used as referrals for a patient in crisis.

⊖volve WEBSITE

Visit the Evolve website for Flashcards, Case Studies, and additional testing resources related to the content in this chapter: http://evolve.elsevier.com/Canada/Varcarolis/psychiatric/

Pre-Test   interactive review

In a matter of a few hours, a May 2016 wildfire destroys entire neighbourhoods in Fort McMurray, Alberta, taking the homes of many. A train derailment and resulting explosion in downtown Lac-Mégantic, Quebec, leaves 47 people dead on July 6, 2013. Floods in Calgary and High River, Alberta, in June 2013, and in central Canada in May 2017, leave hundreds homeless and without their livelihoods. A young man is killed by a bullet intended for a neighbourhood drug dealer in a drive-by shooting; the deceased man's family recently emigrated from Sudan, where several other family members had been killed or injured during years of war. A middle-aged woman serves on a jury for a gruesome torture and homicide murder trial, observing numerous grotesque exhibits and hearing emotional, distressing victim impact statements. Thousands of refugees settle into new homes in Canada, only to hear daily of destruction and death in Syria. A 35-year-old automotive manufacturing employee is laid off and, after months of desperately trying to pay his family's bills, finds his family and himself homeless. A young nursing student discovers she is pregnant, and the father of the baby abandons her. A retired executive relocates to her cottage, quickly discovering she lacks hobbies, purpose, and a social network.

What do these situations have in common? Each scenario could be the precipitant of a crisis—leaving individuals, families, or whole communities struggling to cope with the impact of the event. In 2014, more than 12.4 million Canadians age 15 years and older reported having personally experienced a major emergency or disaster within their community in their lifetime (Statistics Canada, 2016).

Everyone experiences crises, which are not in themselves a mental illness but rather are representative of a struggle for equilibrium and adaptation. Crisis and disaster experiences do, however, create vulnerable populations and conditions that require mental health services (Kolski & Jongsma, 2014). Further, crises and disasters highlight vulnerabilities and risks for mental illness and disproportionately affect those who are marginalized (Raphael, 2015). A **crisis** is an acute state of psychological imbalance resulting in poor coping with evidence of distress and functional impairment. The primary cause of a crisis is an intensely felt threat or a stressful event (Registered Nurses' Association of Ontario, 2002). Two necessary conditions for a crisis identified by Yaeger and Roberts (2015) are (1) the individual's perception of the event as the cause of considerable upset, disruption, or both; and (2) the individual's inability to resolve the disruption by previously used coping mechanisms (p. 6).

Crisis both threatens personality organization and presents an opportunity for personal growth and development. Successful crisis resolution results from the development of adaptive coping methods, reflects ego development, and suggests the employment of physiological, psychological, and social resources. Crisis, or rather *coping* with crisis, is an essential component of individual growth and development. **Coping** can be defined as "finding ways to accomplish goals despite obstacles and challenges" (Goldner, Palma, Jenkins, et al., 2016, p. 233). **Coping methods** are the thinking, behavioural, and emotional processes individuals use to support functioning in the face of stressors (Registered Nurses' Association of Ontario, 2006).

Crises are acute and time limited, usually lasting 4 to 6 weeks. They are associated with events that precipitate overwhelming emotions of increased tension, helplessness, and disorganization. As shown in Figure 21-1, resolution from the state of crisis depends on the following three factors:

1. The realistic perception of the event: People vary in the way they absorb, process, and use information from the environment (Aguilera, 1998).

2. Adequate situational supports: Situational supports include nurses, other health care providers, and community members who use *crisis intervention* to assist those in crisis. **Crisis intervention** is a process focused on resolution of the immediate problem through personal, social, and environmental resources. The goals of early intervention are as follows (Registered Nurses' Association of Ontario, 2002, p. 15):

- Stabilization of the situation
- Rapid resolution of the crisis experience
- Prevention of further deterioration or trauma
- Achievement of (at least) pre-crisis level of functioning
- Promotion of effective problem solving and realistic understanding of the experience
- Facilitation of a sense of self-reliance and belief in one's ability to return to independence and apply new coping skills to future challenges

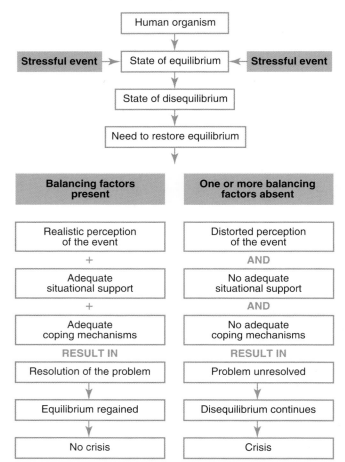

FIGURE 21-1 Paradigm: The effect of balancing factors in a stressful event. Source: Aguilera, D. C. (1998). *Crisis intervention: Theory and methodology* (8th ed.). St. Louis: Mosby.

In general, interventions are responsive to the situation, timing, environment, and resources available. Modalities may include mental health first aid, including early identification and comfort measures; telephone support; home visits or mobile response interventions; reflection and goal setting to promote coping; or even emergency psychiatric services and hospitalization (Goldner, Palma, Jenkins, et al., 2016; Mental Health Commission of Canada, 2017).

3. Adequate coping mechanisms: Coping skills are acquired through a variety of sources, such as cultural responses, modelling behaviours of others, and life opportunities that broaden experience and promote new adaptive coping responses (Aguilera, 1998). Many factors compromise a person's ability to cope with a crisis event—for example, the number of other stressful life events the person is currently coping with, the presence of other unresolved losses, the presence of coexisting psychiatric or medical problems, the presence of excessive fatigue or pain, and the quality and quantity of a person's usual coping skills.

THE DEVELOPMENT OF CRISIS THEORY

An early crisis theorist, Erich Lindemann, studied the grief reactions of relatives of victims who died in the 1942 fire at

Boston's Coconut Grove nightclub. His research formed the foundation of crisis theory and intervention. Lindemann (1944) concluded that while acute grief is a normal reaction to a distressing situation, preventive interventions could eliminate or decrease the serious psychological consequences of the anxiety associated with crisis. He believed that the same interventions helpful in bereavement would prove helpful in crises.

In the 1960s, Gerald Caplan advanced crisis theory and intervention strategies. Since then, clinicians and theorists have further extended our understanding of crisis and interventions. The significant impact of crisis on individual and population health has been well articulated. Mental health first aid training, early intervention, and support crisis intervention are all priorities for strategic action in Canada's evolving national mental health framework for action (Mental Health Commission of Canada, 2017). Donna Aguilera and Janice Mesnick provided a classic framework for nurses related to crisis assessment and intervention, and Aguilera continues to set a standard in the practice of crisis assessment and intervention, including examination of the individual's reactions, education, coping, and problem solving. Albert R. Roberts's seven-stage model of crisis intervention (Figure 21-2) provides another useful model for addressing the suffering experienced in acute situational crises, as well as in acute stress disorder.

More recently, in an effort to establish consensus on mass disaster intervention principles, Hobfoll and colleagues (2007)

identified five essential, empirically supported elements of mass trauma interventions that promote (1) a sense of safety, (2) calming, (3) a sense of self-efficacy and collective efficacy, (4) connectedness, and (5) hope.

The effects of a mass disaster such as the 2015 mass shooting that killed 49 people and wounded 53 others in a terrorist attack/hate crime inside an Orlando, Florida, nightclub; the sexual assault of a young man in a rural town; or the fatal motor vehicle accident of a young Australian tourist en route to a ski hill all represent the need for crisis assessment and intervention at the community level. Regardless of the type of crisis and whether traumatized individuals are victims, families, rescue workers, or witnesses, those with access to crisis assessment and intervention are more likely to feel safe, supported, and able to make sense of their response to the disaster, as compared to those without such access (Hobfoll, Watson, Bell, et al., 2007; Raphael, 2015).

Components of crisis assessment and intervention are derived from established crisis theory and evidence base. An understanding of three areas of crisis theory enables application of the nursing process: (1) types of crisis, (2) phases of crisis, and (3) aspects of crisis that have relevance for nurses.

Types of Crisis

There are three basic types of crisis situation: (1) developmental or maturational crises; (2) situational crises; and (3) disasters, or adventitious crises. Disadvantaged and stigmatized people, such as those with pre-existing mental health problems, substance abuse, or limited external resources, are especially vulnerable to crisis (Raphael, 2015).

Maturational Crisis

A process of maturation occurs across the life cycle. Erik Erikson conceptualized the process by identifying eight stages of ego growth and development (see Table 4-2). Each stage represents a time during which physical, cognitive, instinctual, and sexual changes prompt an internal conflict or crisis, which results in either psychosocial growth or regression. Therefore each developmental stage represents a maturational crisis (i.e., a critical period of increased vulnerability and heightened potential—a turning point).

When a person arrives at a new stage, formerly used coping styles are no longer effective, and new coping mechanisms have yet to be developed. Thus, for a time, the person is without effective defences. This deficit often leads to increased tension and anxiety, which may manifest as variations in the person's normal behaviour. Examples of events that can precipitate a maturational crisis include leaving home during late adolescence, marriage, the birth of a child, retirement, and the death of a parent. Successful resolution of these maturational tasks leads to the development of basic human qualities.

Erikson (1959) believed that the way these crises are resolved at one stage affects the ability to pass through subsequent stages, because each crisis provides the starting point for movement toward the next stage. If a person lacks support systems and adequate role models, successful resolution may be difficult or may not occur. Unresolved problems in the past and inadequate coping mechanisms then adversely affect what is learned in each

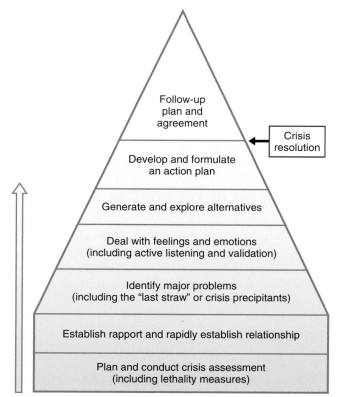

FIGURE 21-2 Roberts's seven-stage model of crisis intervention. Source: Roberts, A. R., & Ottens, A. J. (2005). The seven-stage crisis intervention model: A road map to goal attainment, problem solving, and crisis resolution. *Brief Treatment and Crisis Intervention, 5*, 329–339.

developmental stage. Experiencing severe difficulty during a maturational crisis may disrupt progression through the maturational stages and warrant professional intervention. For example, Steve developed addictive behaviours in early adolescence and therefore may lack adult coping and problem-solving skills when dealing with a situational (financial) crisis as a result of gambling debts at age 25.

Situational Crisis

A situational crisis arises from events that are extraordinary, external rather than internal, and unanticipated (Roberts & Ottens, 2005). Examples of precipitating events to a situational crisis are job loss or change, the death of a loved one, an unplanned pregnancy, financial troubles, relationship breakup, and severe physical or mental illness. Whether these events precipitate a crisis depends on factors such as the degree of support available from caring friends, family members, and others; general emotional and physical status; and the ability to understand and cope with the meaning of the stressful event. As in all crises, the stressful event involves loss or change that threatens a person's self-concept, self-esteem, and sense of security.

Adventitious Crisis

An adventitious crisis results from events not part of everyday life, such as a natural disaster (e.g., flood, fire, earthquake) or a national disaster (e.g., acts of terrorism, war, riots, airplane crashes). Disasters are those events that threaten (physically or psychologically) the well-being of citizens. Adventitious crises may also result from a violent crime (e.g., rape, assault or murder in the workplace or school, bombing in public areas, spousal or child abuse). Experiencing or witnessing such events that threaten an individual's very survival (physical or psychological) is referred to as trauma. An important development in the field of adventitious crisis theory has been the recognition of just how differently people respond to and are affected by disaster. It is known that traumatizing events may overwhelm an individual's usual coping skills and be of such intensity that lasting psychological harm occurs, including the potential for post-traumatic stress disorder (PTSD) (Goldner, Palma, Jenkins, et al., 2016). For more information on PTSD and interventions, see Chapter 12. PTSD is among several post-trauma disorders that also include acute stress disorder, dissociative disorder, and depression.

While certain people may be more vulnerable to crisis than others, the need for intervention for all people who experience crisis cannot be overemphasized. Situational and adventitious crises can challenge the basic assumptions that underlie individuals' world views. Vulnerability to a stressful event, and challenges to one's ability to cope, depend on the newness, intensity, and duration of the stressful event (Yaeger & Roberts, 2015). At times, the newness and shock that render a personal vulnerable to a stressful event can result in numbness that protects the patient from being overwhelmed by the magnitude of the crisis or disaster. The response of numbness from a crisis may be adaptive in the short term; however, if sustained over a longer duration, it may ultimately interrupt daily functioning. In such cases, coping can become exhausted, and further intervention may be required to re-establish balance (Yaeger & Roberts, 2015).

Vulnerability also depends on the number of crises experienced simultaneously. Consider a 51-year-old woman who may be going through a midlife transition (maturational) when her husband dies suddenly of cancer (situational).

Phases of Crisis

Caplan (1964) first identified four distinct phases of crisis:

Phase 1

A person confronted by a conflict or problem that threatens the self-concept responds with increased feelings of anxiety. The increase in anxiety stimulates the use of problem-solving techniques and defence mechanisms in an effort to solve the problem and lower anxiety.

Phase 2

If usual defensive responses fail and the threat persists, anxiety continues to rise and produces feelings of extreme discomfort. Individual functioning becomes disorganized. Trial-and-error solutions, in an effort to restore a normal balance, begin.

Phase 3

If the trial-and-error attempts fail, anxiety can escalate to the severe or panic level, and the person may mobilize automatic relief behaviours, such as withdrawal and flight. Some form of resolution (e.g., compromising needs or redefining the situation to reach an acceptable solution) may be made in this stage.

Phase 4

If the problem remains unresolved and new coping skills are ineffective, an individual may transition to a mental health emergency—a state of overwhelming anxiety that can lead to serious personality disorganization, depression, confusion, and behavioural disturbances. In a mental health emergency, there are urgent issues of safety, potentially because of risk for self-care limitations (e.g., lack of nutrition, exposure to physical risks), self-harm behaviour (e.g., substance abuse, risk for suicide), or violence against others (Goldner, Palma, Jenkins, et al., 2016).

APPLICATION OF THE NURSING PROCESS

Because people typically experience increased stress and anxiety in medical, surgical, and psychiatric hospital settings, as well as in community settings, nurses are often positioned to implement mental health first aid and crisis intervention. Crisis theory defines aspects of crisis that are basic to crisis intervention and relevant to the nursing process (Box 21-1).

ASSESSMENT

General Assessment

As shown in Figure 21-1, a person's equilibrium may be adversely affected by one or more of the following: (1) an unrealistic perception of the precipitating event, (2) inadequate situational supports, and (3) inadequate coping mechanisms (Aguilera, 1998). It is crucial for nurses to assess these factors during a crisis. Data gained from the assessment guide the nurse and the

BOX 21-1 FOUNDATION FOR CRISIS INTERVENTION

- A crisis is self-limiting and usually resolves within 4 to 6 weeks.
- At the resolution of a crisis, the patient will emerge at one of three different functional levels:
  - A higher level of functioning
  - The same level of functioning
  - A lower level of functioning
- The goal of crisis intervention is to return the patient to at least the pre-crisis level of functioning.
- The level of crisis resolution depends on the patient's actions and others' interventions.
- During a crisis, people are often more receptive than usual to outside intervention. With intervention, the patient can learn new approaches to the problem.
- The patient in a crisis situation is assumed to be mentally healthy and to have previously functioned well but is currently in a state of disequilibrium.
- Crisis intervention deals only with the patient's present problem and resolution of the immediate crisis (i.e., the here and now).
- The nurse must take an active, even directive, role in intervention, which is in contrast to conventional therapeutic intervention that stresses a more nondirective role.
- Early intervention increases the potential for a good prognosis.
- The patient is encouraged to set realistic, focused goals and interventions with the nurse.

patient in planning realistic and meaningful goals and interventions.

The steps of the nursing assessment follow:

1. Promote a sense of safety by assessing the patient's potential for suicide or homicide. If the patient is suicidal, homicidal, or unable to take care of personal needs, hospitalization should be considered (Aguilera, 1998). Sample questions to ask include:
   - Do you feel you can keep yourself safe?
   - Have you thought of killing yourself or someone else? If yes, have you thought of how you would do this?

   After establishing that the patient poses no danger to self or others, the nurse assesses three main areas: (1) the patient's perception of the precipitating event, (2) the patient's situational supports, and (3) the patient's personal coping skills.

VIGNETTE

A 25-year-old woman named Caitlin is brought to the emergency department by police after being beaten by her husband. Caitlin is seen by the emergency physician and then interviewed by the emergency department's psychiatric mental health nurse. The nurse calmly introduces herself and tells Caitlin she would like to spend some time with her. The nurse says, "It looks as if things are pretty overwhelming. Is that how you're feeling?" The nurse makes the observation that things must be very bad if Caitlin stays with an abusive husband. Caitlin sits slumped in a chair, her hands in her lap, head hanging down, and tears in her eyes.

---

2. Assess the patient's perception of the precipitating event. The nurse's task is now to assess the individual or family and the problem. The more clearly the problem can be defined, the more likely effective solutions will be identified. Sample questions that may facilitate assessment include:
   - Has anything particularly upsetting happened to you within the past few days or weeks?
   - What was happening in your life before you started to feel this way?
   - What leads you to seek help now?
   - Describe how you are feeling right now.
   - How does this situation affect your life?
   - How do you see this event affecting your future?
   - What would need to be done to resolve this situation?

VIGNETTE

Nurse: "Caitlin, tell me what has happened."
Caitlin: "I can't go home. ... No one cares. No one believes me. I can't go through it again."
Nurse: "Tell me what you can't go through again."
(Caitlin cries, shaking with sobs. The nurse sits quietly for a while and then speaks.)
Nurse: "Tell me what is so troublesome. Let's look at it together."
After a while, Caitlin tells the nurse that her husband, Dan, has been beating her regularly, particularly after drinking. The beatings have progressively become more violent, and Caitlin states, "I'm afraid I'll end up dead."

---

3. Assess the patient's situational supports. Next, the nurse determines resources available to the patient. The following are sample questions:
   - Who do you live with?
   - Who do you talk to when you feel overwhelmed?
   - Who can you trust?
   - Who is available to help you?
   - Do you belong to a spiritual community?
   - Where do you go to school or to other community-based activities?
   - During difficult times in the past, who did you want most to help you?
   - Who is the most helpful?

VIGNETTE

Nurse: "Caitlin, who can you go to? Do you have any other family?"
Caitlin: "No. My family is in another province. Dan and I are pretty much alone."
Nurse: "Do you have anyone you can talk to?"
Caitlin: "I really don't have any friends. Dan's jealousy makes it difficult for me to have friends. He doesn't like anyone who I would want as a friend."
Nurse: "What about co-workers?"
Caitlin: "My co-workers are nice, but I can't tell them things like this. They wouldn't believe me anyway."
The nurse learns that Caitlin feels successful at her job and that work is a refuge from her troubles. Getting good job reviews also has another reward: it is the only time Dan says anything nice about her.

4. Assess the patient's personal coping skills. Finally, the nurse evaluates the patient's anxiety level and identifies his or her established coping patterns. Common coping mechanisms may be overeating, drinking, smoking, withdrawing, seeking out someone to talk to, yelling, fighting, or engaging in other physical activity (Behrman & Reid, 2002). It is important to remember that coping strategies vary widely, that they may be influenced by culture, and that the specific coping strategy, particularly in the early phase of crisis assessment and intervention, is not as critical as whether it enables the person to cope (Substance Abuse and Mental Health Services Administration, 2014). In this way, coping is assessed and addressed through harm reduction and trauma-informed approaches (Canadian Centre on Substance Abuse, 2014). Sample questions to ask include:

- What do you usually do to feel better?
- Did you try it this time? If so, what was different?
- What do you think might happen now?
- What helped you through difficult times in the past?
- What role does your culture play in handling situations like this? (See Considering Culture: How Acknowledging Culture Supports Crisis Resolution.)

VIGNETTE

Nurse: "What do you think would help your situation?"

Caitlin: "I don't want to be in an abusive marriage. I just don't know where to turn."

The nurse tells Caitlin that she wants to work with her to find a solution and that she is concerned for Caitlin's safety and well-being.

Self-Assessment

Nurses' self-awareness when dealing with a patient in crisis is crucial. It is important for them to recognize their own anxiety level and negative feelings to prevent patients from closing off their expression of painful feelings.

There may be times when nurses feel they cannot deal effectively with a patient's situation. When this happens, the nurse should ask a colleague to work with the individual rather than limit the required assessment and intervention in order to avoid troublesome feelings. Asking for support and supervision will help the nurse separate his or her own needs from the patient's and identify ways to address uncomfortable or painful personal issues to care more effectively for patients in crisis.

Essential aspects of the therapeutic relationship include clear verbal and nonverbal communication skills, assertiveness, responsiveness to patient needs, strong problem-solving abilities, attention to diversity and power relations, and genuine empathy for the lived experience of the patient. As examined in Chapters 9 and 10, the therapeutic relationship and communication demands are even more pronounced in crisis situations, in which rapid decisions and more extreme emotions are expected. It is crucial that the nurse engages in ongoing self-reflection and self-awareness and that expert supervision be available as an integral part of crisis intervention nursing.

CONSIDERING CULTURE

How Acknowledging Culture Supports Crisis Resolution

Consider your client, who has lost his job with the closure of the local paper mill and presents in crisis at a rural health centre. Consider also your Indigenous client at the clinic on a reserve who has experienced the stillbirth of her third child and the new-immigrant woman you are assessing in the psychiatric emergency department of a large urban hospital who has attempted suicide following a relationship breakdown. While rapid resolution of the crisis is the goal, there are many reasons a nurse should consider culture during such a crisis intervention. Culture can influence one's interpretation of and the meaning attributed to a disaster or crisis event. Culture can also influence an individual's personal coping or a community's reaction to an event. Despite the significance of culture on the assessment and intervention process, the immediacy of crisis intervention nursing often results in cultural factors and issues of cultural identity being overlooked in favour of efficient assessment and interventions. Ignoring the important role of culture, however, may get in the way of effective and efficient crisis resolution.

Acknowledging the client's personal history and context, as well as the distinct history, context, and cultures of the client and nurse (i.e., occupation, income, age, gender, nationality, physical abilities, language, ethnic heritage, sexual orientation, education), allows for more rapid development of the trust and rapport necessary to communicate both verbally and nonverbally for assessment and intervention. Addressing context and culture in this way assists the nurse to convey acceptance and trust to assist with the immediate problems.

After the symptoms of crisis are stabilized and controlled, knowledge of the client's culture can assist in identifying important resources available for follow-up care, such as family, religious community, or cultural heritage agencies, which can provide continuing support after the symptoms are controlled. In short, culture is crucial to the three balancing factors to a crisis: perception of the event, coping, and support. A nurse's capacity to acknowledge the client's context, history, and culture will enhance crisis intervention and trauma-informed approaches and will support resolution and good patient outcomes. See also Chapter 8.

Sources: British Columbia Provincial Mental Health and Substance Use Planning Council. (2013). *Trauma informed practice guide.* Retrieved from http://bccewh.bc.ca/wp-content/uploads/2012/05/2013_TIP-Guide.pdf; and Muskett, C. (2014). Trauma-informed care in inpatient mental health settings: A review of the literature. *International Journal of Mental Health Nursing, 23*(1), 51–59. doi:10.1111/inm.12012.

Even experienced nurses can become overwhelmed when witnessing severe suffering, catastrophic loss of human life (e.g., acts of war, plane crashes, workplace shootings), or mass destruction of people's homes and belongings (e.g., floods, fires, earthquakes). Mental health care providers may experience psychological distress from working with traumatized populations, a phenomenon called *secondary traumatic stress* or *vicarious traumatization* (Bercier & Maynard, 2015). Particular risk factors for secondary traumatic stress of mental health workers working with victims of trauma include a larger volume of patients in a caseload with trauma counselling needs, personal trauma or abuse history, perceived quality of work support and supervision, and social support outside of the clinical setting (Hensel, Ruiz, Finney, et al., 2015). Supervision and critical incident stress debriefing are strategies that support nurses' ability to cope with overwhelming violent and disastrous situations (Registered Nurses' Association of Ontario, 2002).

ASSESSMENT GUIDELINES
Crisis

1. Identify whether the patient's response to the crisis warrants psychiatric treatment or hospitalization to minimize decompensation (e.g., suicidal or violent behaviour, psychotic thinking).
2. Identify whether the patient is able to identify the precipitating event.
3. Assess the patient's understanding of his or her present situational supports.
4. Identify the patient's usual coping styles, determining coping mechanisms suited to the present situation.
5. Determine any cultural beliefs or spiritual practices that should be responded to in assessing and intervening in this patient's crisis.
6. Assess whether this situation is one in which the patient needs primary (education, environmental manipulation, or new coping skills), secondary (crisis intervention), or tertiary (rehabilitation) interventions.

DIAGNOSIS

The North American Nursing Diagnosis Association International (NANDA-I) provides nursing diagnoses that can be considered for patients experiencing anxiety and anxiety disorders. When a person is in crisis, the nursing diagnosis of *Ineffective coping* is often useful (Herdman & Kamitsuru, 2014). This diagnosis is not to suggest that people in crisis are inadequate or do not have coping abilities, but because anxiety may escalate to moderate or severe levels in times of crisis, the ability to solve problems may be impaired. *Ineffective coping* may be experienced as an inability to meet basic needs, an inability to meet role expectations, an alteration in social participation, the use of inappropriate defence mechanisms, or the impairment of usual patterns of communication. The "related to" component of the diagnosis will vary according to the individual patient. Table 21-1 identifies potential nursing diagnoses for people in crisis and provides signs and symptoms that might be present to support the diagnosis.

In the preceding vignettes, the assessment of Caitlin's perception of the precipitating event, situational supports, and personal coping skills provides the nurse with enough data to formulate two diagnoses and set goals and plan interventions with Caitlin.

VIGNETTE

Caitlin's nurse formulates the following nursing diagnoses:
- *Anxiety (moderate or severe)* related to mental and physical abuse, as evidenced by ineffectual problem solving and feelings of impending doom
- *Compromised family coping* related to the constant threat of violence

TABLE 21-1 POTENTIAL NURSING DIAGNOSES FOR CRISIS INTERVENTION

SIGNS AND SYMPTOMS	NURSING DIAGNOSIS
Inability to meet basic needs, decreased use of social support, inadequate problem solving, inability to attend to information, isolation	*Ineffective coping* *Risk for compromised resilience*
Denial, exaggerated startle response, flashbacks, horror, hypervigilance, intrusive thoughts and dreams, panic attacks, feeling numb, substance abuse, confusion, incoherence	*Post-trauma syndrome* *Rape-trauma syndrome* *Anxiety (moderate, severe, panic)* *Acute confusion* *Sleep deprivation*
Minimizes symptoms, delays seeking care, displays inappropriate affect, makes dismissive comments when speaking of distressing events	*Ineffective denial*
Overwhelmed, depressed, states has nothing in life worthwhile, self-hatred, feelings of being ineffectual, sees limited alternatives, feels strange, perceives a lack of control	*Risk for suicide* *Chronic low self-esteem* *Disturbed personal identity* *Hopelessness* *Powerlessness*
Has difficulty with interpersonal relationships, isolated, has few or no social supports	*Social isolation* *Impaired social interaction*
Changes in family relationships and functioning, difficulty performing family caregiver role	*Interrupted family processes* *Caregiver role strain*

OUTCOMES IDENTIFICATION

Relevant outcomes of the *Nursing Outcomes Classification (NOC)* (Moorhead, Johnson, Maas, et al., 2013) for a person experiencing a crisis include *Coping, Decision making, Role performance,* and *Stress level.* The planning of realistic outcomes is done with the patient and family so as to determine outcomes congruent with the patient's cultural and personal values. Without the patient's involvement, the outcome criteria (i.e., goals at the end of 4 to 8 weeks) may be irrelevant or unacceptable solutions to that patient's crisis. Table 21-2 lists selected *NOC* outcomes with intermediate and short-term indicators for a patient in crisis.

Mental health first aid (MHFA) is the help provided to a person developing a mental health problem or experiencing a mental health crisis. We know that physical first aid is administered to an injured person before medical treatment can be obtained; likewise, MHFA is given until appropriate treatment is found or until the crisis is resolved, and it is often life saving. Many laypeople in communities are receiving this training that, like physical first aid, is found to support early intervention and disease prevention by preserving life when there is a danger or threat to life, to promote recovery and good mental health, and to provide comfort to those experiencing mental health problems. Psychological first aid (World Health Organization, 2011) is another crisis response approach, one that is more specifically focused on unique crisis mental health responses to disasters (Milligan & McGuinness, 2009).

The MHFA approach and the training of people in MHFA represent a growing area of health promotion in Canada (Mental Health Commission of Canada, 2017). Overall, this approach aims to provide skills and knowledge to help people manage developing mental health problems in themselves, family members, friends, or co-workers. It does not attempt to train amateur therapists but, rather, teaches people to (1) recognize the signs and symptoms of mental health problems, (2) provide initial help, and (3) guide a person toward appropriate professional help. Lessons learned about MHFA from Scotland and Australia (see the Research Highlight box), in particular, are being drawn upon for current initiatives by the Mental Health Commission of Canada (2017).

VIGNETTE

The nurse consults a social worker about Caitlin, and the three meet together. All agree that Caitlin should not return to her home. Caitlin and the nurse then establish goals and plan interventions. The goals are as follows:
- Caitlin will return to her pre-crisis state within 2 weeks.
- With the support of the staff, Caitlin will find a safe environment.
- With the support of the staff, Caitlin will have at least two outside supports available within 24 hours.
- Caitlin will receive continued evaluation and support until the immediate crisis is over (6 to 8 weeks).

TABLE 21-2   *NOC* OUTCOMES FOR PATIENT IN CRISIS

NURSING OUTCOME AND DEFINITION	INTERMEDIATE INDICATORS	SHORT-TERM INDICATORS
Coping: Personal actions to manage stressors that tax an individual's resources	Modifies lifestyle as needed Uses effective coping strategies Reports decrease in physical symptoms of stress Reports decrease in negative feelings	Identifies effective coping patterns Identifies ineffective coping patterns Reports decrease in stress Uses personal support system Verbalizes need for assistance
Decision making: Ability to make judgements and choose between two or more alternatives	Chooses among alternatives	Identifies relevant information Identifies alternatives Weighs alternatives
Role performance: Congruence of an individual's role behaviour with role expectations	Able to meet role expectations	Performs family role behaviours Describes role changes with illness or disability Describes role changes with older-adult dependents, new family member, or family member who is leaving home Performs family, parental, intimate, community, work, or friendship role behaviours
Stress level: Severity of manifested physical or mental tension resulting from factors that alter an existing equilibrium	Able to modulate stress level	Reduction in elevated blood pressure Reduction in increased radial pulse rate Reduction in symptoms of upset stomach Reduced level of restlessness Improved sleep Reduction in interruption of thought process Reduced forgetfulness Infrequent cognitive mistakes Improved ability to concentrate on tasks Decrease in emotional outbursts

Source: Based on Moorhead, S., Johnson, M., Maas, M., et al. (2013). *Nursing outcomes classification (NOC)* (5th ed.). St. Louis: Mosby.

RESEARCH HIGHLIGHT

Mental Health First Aid: Lessons From Drought-Affected Rural Australia

Problem
Crisis mental health care in rural communities with few services and resources can be challenging, particularly when a large population may be affected.

Purpose of Study
Mental health first aid (MHFA) training was part of a strategy to improve capacity among farming communities for early intervention for mental health problems. This strategy was viewed as particularly important in those regions affected by drought and wildfire and often lacking in professional mental health systems.

Methods
A survey of 99 participants from 12 New South Wales towns was administered before and after delivery of MHFA training, emphasizing the role of front-line workers from agriculture-related services.

Key Findings
Participants' abilities to identify high-prevalence disorders and promote evidence-informed interventions for both high- and low-prevalence disorders and their confidence in providing appropriate help and referrals all increased following MHFA training.

Implications for Nursing Practice
The conclusion from the study was that MHFA training is an effective part of a strategy to improve early intervention in rural communities by using local networks to provide mental health support. Nurses play an important role in teaching, training, and health promotion to support MHFA training, particularly in rural or resource-poor communities.

Source: Sartore, G. M., Kelly, B., Stain, H. J., et al. (2008). Improving mental health capacity in rural communities: Mental health first aid delivery in drought-affected rural New South Wales. *Australian Journal of Rural Health, 16*, 313–318. doi:10.1111/j.1440-1584.2008.01005.x.

PLANNING

Nurses are called on to plan and intervene in a variety of crisis intervention modalities, such as disaster nursing, mobile crisis units, group work, MHFA training, health education and crisis prevention, victim outreach programs, and crisis lines or telephone outreach. The nurse may be involved in planning interventions for individuals (e.g., cases of physical abuse), groups (e.g., students after a classmate's suicide or shooting), or communities (e.g., disaster nursing after fires, shootings, or airplane crashes). Data from the answers to the following questions guide the nurse in determining immediate actions (Aguilera, 1998):

- How much has this crisis affected the patient's life? Can the patient still go to work? Attend school? Care for family members?
- How is the state of disequilibrium affecting significant people in the patient's life (e.g., wife, husband, children, other family members, boss, boyfriend, girlfriend)?

IMPLEMENTATION

Crisis intervention is a function of the basic-level nurse and has two initial goals:
1. Patient safety. External controls may be applied for protection of the patient in crisis if the patient is suicidal or homicidal.
2. Anxiety reduction. Anxiety-reduction techniques are used so that inner resources can be mobilized.

During the initial interview, the patient in crisis first needs to gain a feeling of safety. Solutions to the crisis may be offered so that the patient is aware of various options. Feelings of support and hope will temporarily diminish anxiety. The nurse needs to play an active role by indicating that help is available, conveyed by the competent use of crisis intervention skills and genuine interest and support. The availability of help is not conveyed by the use of false reassurances and platitudes, such as "Everything will be all right." Crisis intervention requires a creative and flexible approach through the use of traditional and nontraditional therapeutic methods. The nurse may act as educator, advisor, and role model, always keeping in mind that it is the patient who solves the problem, not the nurse. At times, highly directive interventions will be required to assist in problem solving, ensure safety, prioritize actions, and provide new information. Alongside this active and directive role, the following are important assumptions when working with a patient in crisis:
- The patient is in charge of his or her own life.
- The patient is able to make decisions.
- The crisis counselling relationship is one between partners.

The nurse helps the patient refocus to gain new perspectives on the situation, drawing on supportive interventions. In this way, the nurse validates the patient experience and supports the patient during the process of finding constructive ways to solve or cope with the problem. It is important for nurses to be mindful of the fact that coping will look different for all patients and how difficult it is for the patient to change behaviours. Table 21-3 offers guidelines for nursing interventions and corresponding rationales.

> **VIGNETTE**
> After talking with the nurse and the social worker, Caitlin seems open to going to a safe house for battered women. She also agrees to talk to a counsellor at a mental health centre. The nurse sets up an appointment at which she, Caitlin, and the counsellor will meet. The nurse will continue to see Caitlin twice a week.

Counselling
Primary Care

Psychotherapeutic crisis interventions are directed toward three levels of care: (1) primary, (2) secondary, and (3) tertiary. Primary care promotes mental health and reduces mental illness to decrease the incidence of crisis. On this level, the nurse can:
1. Work with a patient to recognize potential problems by evaluating the patient's experience of stressful life events

TABLE 21-3   GUIDELINES FOR CRISIS INTERVENTION

INTERVENTION	RATIONALE
Assess for suicidal or homicidal thoughts or plans.	Safety is always the first consideration.
Take initial steps to make patient feel safe and less anxious.	A person who feels safe and less anxious is able to more effectively problem-solve solutions with the nurse.
Listen carefully (e.g., make eye contact, give frequent feedback to verify and convey understanding, summarize what patient says).	A person who believes someone is really listening is more likely to believe that someone cares about his or her situation and that help may be available. This belief offers hope.
Crisis intervention calls for directive and creative approaches. Initially, the nurse may make phone calls to arrange babysitters, schedule a visiting nurse, find shelter, or contact a social worker.	A person who is confused, frightened, or overwhelmed may be temporarily unable to perform usual tasks.
Identify needed social supports (with patient's input) and mobilize the priority.	A person's need for shelter, help with care for children or older-adult dependents, medical workup, emergency medical attention, hospitalization, food, safe housing, and self-help groups is determined.
Identify needed coping skills (e.g., problem solving, relaxation, assertiveness, job training, newborn care, self-esteem building).	Increasing coping skills and learning new ones can help with current crisis and help minimize future crises.
Involve patient in identifying realistic, acceptable interventions.	The person's involvement in planning increases his or her sense of control, self-esteem, and compliance with the plan.
Plan regular follow-up (e.g., phone calls, clinic visits, home visits) to assess patient's progress.	Plan is evaluated to see what works and what does not.

2. Teach the patient specific coping skills, such as decision making, problem solving, assertiveness skills, meditation, and relaxation skills

3. Assist the patient in evaluating the timing or reduction of life changes to decrease the negative effects of stress as much as possible

The third intervention may involve working with a patient or client, such as a government or a health services department, to plan environmental changes, make important interpersonal decisions, and rethink changes in occupational roles. The Public Health Agency of Canada plays an important role in mass disaster planning and prevention—for instance, with H1N1 pandemic flu planning and G8 meetings on disaster planning in Kananaskis and Toronto—and has recorded many lessons learned for future disaster planning (Public Health Agency of Canada, 2015).

Secondary Care

Secondary care includes intervention during an acute crisis to prevent prolonged anxiety from diminishing personal effectiveness and personality organization. The nurse's primary focus is to ensure the safety of the patient. After safety issues are dealt with, the nurse works with the patient to assess the patient's problem, support systems, and coping styles. Desired goals are explored, and interventions are planned. This level of care lessens the time a patient is mentally disabled during a crisis. Secondary care occurs in hospital units, emergency departments, clinics, and mental health centres, usually during daytime hours. Psychological first aid programs are another approach to secondary care, aimed at helping survivors of disasters gain skills to manage distress

and cope with postdisaster stress and adversity (Vernberg, Steinberg, Jacobs, et al., 2008; World Health Organization, 2011).

Tertiary Care

Tertiary care provides support for those who have experienced a severe crisis and are now recovering from a disabling mental state. Social and community facilities that offer tertiary intervention include rehabilitation centres, sheltered workshops, day hospitals, and outpatient clinics. Primary goals are to facilitate optimal levels of functioning and prevent further emotional disruptions. People with severe and persistent mental problems are often extremely susceptible to crisis, and community facilities provide the structured environment that can help prevent problem situations. Box 21-2 lists *Nursing Interventions Classification (NIC)* (Bulechek, Butcher, Dochterman, et al., 2013) interventions for responding to a crisis.

Critical incident stress debriefing. A critical incident stress debriefing (CISD) is a group-level crisis intervention carried out very soon after a traumatic event. Individuals involved in or witnessing the event (e.g., those in a school, workplace, or emergency responder group) are brought together in a safe and confidential environment to talk about what happened, discuss feelings and behavioural responses, and obtain health education about the crisis process for early intervention purposes. Generally, the discussion is guided by a professional or trained peer. There is evidence promoting CISD as an important strategy to prevent PTSD, one that should be implemented as part of a broad approach to crisis intervention that includes formal assessment and referrals for individual and family counselling and a range of other supports (Goldner, Palma, Jenkins, et al., 2016).

BOX 21-2 CRISIS INTERVENTION

Definition of crisis intervention: Use of short-term counselling and other interventions to help the patient cope with a crisis and resume pre-crisis state of functioning modalities. Interventions may include:

- Crisis lines—telephone support provided by trained volunteers (for first aid and support) or professionals (for assessment, triage, and referral)
- Mobile crisis outreach—outreach crisis response services often provided by collaborative teams, including police or other first responders
- Urgent or walk-in crisis care—services through which people can present their crisis needs to professionals for assessment, intervention, and referral
- Psychiatric emergency care—services such as emergency mental health care in hospital triage; assessment; crisis counselling; emergency medical treatment, often for brief-stay admissions

Activities:

- Provide an atmosphere of support.
- Avoid giving false reassurances.
- Provide a safe haven.
- Determine whether the patient presents a safety risk to self or others.
- Initiate necessary precautions to safeguard the patient or others at risk for physical harm.
- Encourage expression of feelings in a nondestructive manner.

- Assist in identification of the precipitants and dynamics of the crisis.
- Encourage patient to focus on one implication at a time.
- Assist in identification of personal strengths and abilities that can be used in resolving the crisis.
- Assist in identification of past and present coping skills and their effectiveness.
- Assist in development of new coping and problem-solving skills, as needed.
- Assist in identification of available support systems.
- Link the patient and family with community resources, as needed.
- Provide guidance about how to develop and maintain support systems.
- Introduce the patient to people (or groups) who have successfully undergone the same experience.
- Assist in identification of alternative courses of action to resolve the crisis.
- Assist in evaluation of the possible consequences of the various courses of action.
- Assist the patient to decide on a particular course of action.
- Assist in formulating a time frame for implementation of the chosen course of action.
- Evaluate with the patient whether the crisis has been resolved by the chosen course of action.
- Plan with the patient how adaptive coping skills can be used to deal with crises in the future.

Sources: Adapted from British Columbia Ministry of Health. (2002). *Best practices in mental health: Crisis response and emergency services.* Retrieved from http://www.health.gov.bc.ca/library/publications/year/2000/MHABestPractices/bp_crisis_response.pdf; and Bulechek, G. M., Butcher, H. K., Dochterman, J. M., et al. (2013). *Nursing interventions classification (NIC)* (6th ed.). St. Louis: Mosby.

> **VIGNETTE**
>
> The nurse performs secondary crisis intervention and meets with Caitlin twice weekly for 4 weeks. At first, Caitlin is motivated to work with the social worker and the nurse to find another permanent place to live. The nurse suggests Caitlin see a counsellor in the outpatient clinic after the crisis is over so that she can talk about some of her pain. Caitlin becomes ambivalent and is already thinking she will return to her husband.

EVALUATION

Guided by nursing best practice guidelines, the nurse might consider asking the following in the evaluation of interventions (Registered Nurses' Association of Ontario, 2002, p. 28):

- Did the patient carry out the crisis plan, and what was the outcome?
- Does the patient have a plan to work toward meeting, through alternative actions, his or her goals?
- Does the patient require additional or alternative links to community resources and supports?

NOC includes a built-in measurement for each outcome and for the indicators that support the outcome. Each indicator is measured on a five-point Likert scale, which helps the nurse evaluate the effectiveness of the crisis intervention. This evaluation is usually performed 4 to 8 weeks after the initial interview,

although it can be done earlier (e.g., by the end of the visit, the anxiety level has decreased from 1 = severe to 3 = moderate). If the intervention has been successful, the patient's level of anxiety and ability to function should be at pre-crisis levels. A patient may wish to follow up on additional areas of concern and get referrals to other agencies for more long-term work. Crisis intervention frequently serves to prepare a patient for further treatment.

> **VIGNETTE**
>
> Caitlin returns to her husband 5 weeks after the battering episode. She has convinced herself that he has changed his behaviour, even though he has not sought any help to control his anger.
>
> Caitlin continues to see the nurse, as planned; however, Caitlin is aloof and distant. After 6 weeks, Caitlin and the nurse decide that the crisis is over. The nurse evaluates Caitlin as being in a moderate amount of emotional pain, but Caitlin feels she is doing well. The nurse's assessment indicates that Caitlin has other serious issues (e.g., low self-esteem, childhood abuse), and the nurse strongly suggests that she could benefit from further counselling. The decision, however, belongs to Caitlin, who says she is satisfied with the way things are and again states that if she has any future problems, she will return to the women's shelter counsellor.

HOW A NURSE HELPED ME

Helping the Team Debrief From Not One Event but Accumulated Tragedies

As a member of our local critical incident stress management (CISM) committee representing our provincial parks managers, I was most intrigued by a recent debriefing. The participants included community members, ambulance staff, emergency physicians, nurses, and many of my co-workers with provincial and national parks who witnessed and supported the victims of a tragic incident last September. In that incident, two teenagers were fatally injured in a mountaineering accident witnessed by park guides and other young people. Ginette, the community mental health nurse who is the leader of our CISM committee, facilitated the team process. It was intriguing because this process has changed my work with my parks colleagues—and changed me.

Even though I knew about crisis response and the need for debriefing, I had started to wear a shield as a manager. These incidents occurred all too often and became things we just didn't talk about in our office. Sure, we talked about safety and strategy for prevention and education for mountaineers, but we never talked about the luggage we were carrying from these events. But it didn't stop these events—especially this event—from making me angry and sad. Truly, if I heard "they died doing what they loved" one more time, I was going to explode!

You see, during a crisis, our adrenaline pumps to help us provide the best response we can deliver, but then having to deliver horrible news to a family that their children have been severely injured and that they must get to the hospital, and must be prepared for the worst, is most certainly not an easy task for any of us. I had to do that twice on that day last September. The adrenaline only gets you so far!

But, in the debriefing last September, Ginette, guided us to think about many questions—even unanswerable ones. How exactly could we remain mentally healthy? How can we go on without the answers? Ginette was so calm, and just by raising these questions, she made me realize I had those questions all the time, but I just kept putting the luggage of our crisis work further back into the closet of my mind. I know now that we need to talk it out. We have to express feelings, or at least listen to the experiences of others. I needed to start listening—in a regular and real way—with my co-workers. The questions about what happened on scene in the park, and what happened in the hospital, must be discussed. Knowing the answers to the assumptions we naturally make may allow us to connect the dots to make more sense of an incident. I believe now that those questions are answered, or at least acknowledged, and we can start to move through the grieving period ourselves. I believe that the other incidents that have been stuffed into the luggage have also been let out. Ginette has been a great role model. I have learned new ways to respond better to the next incidents that will inevitably happen in our park … and to respond better to the whole team. I know I am a better manager because of how Ginette helped me. I have managed my anger by talking about even the unanswerable questions—instead of putting all my questions and feelings back in the luggage!

RESEARCH HIGHLIGHT

Crisis-Service Needs for Urban and Rural Areas—One Size Does Not Fit All

Problem

Law enforcement officers are often faced with difficult decisions about how to best respond to individuals experiencing a psychiatric crisis. The Crisis Intervention Team (CIT) program fosters collaborative ties between law enforcement, the mental health treatment system, consumers, and consumer advocates. The CIT model was originally developed as an urban model for police officers responding to calls about persons experiencing a mental illness crisis. Little is known of the practical challenges of adapting this model in rural settings.

Purpose of Study

This study attempts to better understand the unique challenges of implementing the CIT model in a rural community and undertakes an exploration of the barriers and challenges that community stakeholders in rural areas may face in implementing CIT programs.

Methods

A qualitative analysis of data gathered through observations and focus groups of service providers.

Key Findings

The study revealed that there were both external and internal barriers to developing CIT programs in their respective communities. Some of these barriers were a consequence of working in small communities and working within small police departments. Participants actively overcame these barriers through the realization that CIT programs were needed in their community, through collaborative efforts across disciplines, and through the involvement of mental health advocacy groups.

Implications for Nursing Practice

These results indicate that CIT programs can be successfully implemented in rural communities.

Source: Skubby, D., Bonfine, N., Novisky, M., et al. (2013). Crisis intervention team (CIT) programs in rural communities: A focus group study. *Community Mental Health Journal, 49*(6), 756–764. doi:10.1007/s10597-012-9517-y.

CASE STUDY AND NURSING CARE PLAN 21-1

Crisis

Gurpreet Sidhu, the psychiatric clinical nurse specialist, is called to the neurological unit. She is told that Alexzy, a 43-year-old man with Guillain-Barré syndrome, is demonstrating challenging behaviours, and the staff has requested a consult. The disease has caused severe muscle weakness to the point that Alexzy is essentially paralyzed; however, he is able to breathe on his own.

The nurse manager says that Alexzy is hostile and sexually abusive, and his abusive language, demeaning attitude, and angry outbursts are having an adverse effect on the unit as a whole. The staff nurses state that they feel ineffective and angry and have tried to be patient and understanding; however, Alexzy's difficult behaviours have persisted. The situation has affected the morale of the staff and, the nurses believe, the quality of their care.

Alexzy, a new Canadian from Eastern Europe, was employed as a taxicab driver. Six months before his hospital admission, he had given up drinking after years of episodic alcohol abuse. His fiancée visits him every day. He needs a great deal of assistance with every aspect of his activities of daily living: he has to be turned and repositioned every 2 hours and is fed through a gastrostomy tube.

ASSESSMENT

Gurpreet gathers data from Alexzy, the nursing staff, and Alexzy's fiancée.

Perception of the Precipitating Event

During the initial interview, Alexzy speaks to Gurpreet angrily, using profanity and making lewd sexual suggestions. He also expresses anger about needing a nurse to "scratch my head and help me blow my nose." He cannot figure out how his illness suddenly developed. He says the doctors told him that it was too early to know for sure if he would recover completely but that the prognosis was good.

Support System

Gurpreet speaks with Alexzy's fiancée. Alexzy's relationships with his fiancée, within his Eastern European cultural group, and with his taxi company co-workers are strong. Neither Alexzy nor his fiancée has much knowledge of supportive agencies.

Personal Coping Skills

Alexzy comes from a strongly male-dominated subculture, in which the man is expected to be a strong leader. His independence and power to affect the direction of his life are central to his perception of being acceptable as a man.

Alexzy feels powerless, out of control, and enraged. He is handling his anxiety by displacing these feelings onto the environment—namely, the staff and his fiancée. This redirection of anger temporarily lowers his anxiety and distracts him from painful feelings. When he intimidates others, he feels temporarily in control and experiences an illusion of power. He uses displacement to relieve his painful levels of anxiety.

Alexzy's unconscious use of displacement is maladaptive and does not resolve the issues causing his distress. His anxiety continues to escalate. Furthermore, his behaviour leads others to avoid him, further increasing his sense of isolation and helplessness.

Self-Assessment

Gurpreet meets with the staff twice. The staff members discuss feelings of helplessness and lack of control stemming from their feelings of rejection by Alexzy. They talk of their anger about Alexzy's demeaning behaviour and frustration about the situation. Gurpreet points out to the staff that Alexzy's feelings of helplessness, lack of control, and anger at his situation are the same feelings the staff are experiencing. His displacement of his feelings of helplessness and frustration by intimidating the staff gives Alexzy a brief feeling of control. It also distracts him from his own feelings of helplessness.

The nurses become more understanding of the motivation for the behaviour Alexzy employs to cope with moderate to severe levels of anxiety. The staff begins to focus more on the patient and less on personal reactions, and decides on two approaches to try as a group. First, they will not take Alexzy's behaviour personally. Second, Alexzy's displaced feelings will be refocused back to him.

On the basis of her assessment, Gurpreet identifies three main problem areas of importance and formulates the nursing diagnoses.

DIAGNOSIS

1. *Ineffective coping* related to inadequate coping methods, as evidenced by inappropriate use of defence mechanisms (displacement)

Supporting Data
- Anger directed toward staff and fiancée
- Profanity and crude sexual remarks aimed at staff
- Isolation related to staff withdrawal
- Continued escalation of anxiety
2. *Powerlessness* related to lack of control over his health care environment, as evidenced by frustration over inability to perform previously uncomplicated tasks

Continued

CASE STUDY AND NURSING CARE PLAN 21-1—cont'd

Crisis

Supporting Data
- Anger over nurses having to "scratch my head and help me blow my nose"
- Minimal awareness of available supports in larger community
- *Ineffective coping* related to exhaustion of staff's supportive capacity toward patient, as evidenced by staff withdrawal and limited personal communication with patient

Supporting Data
- Staff feels ineffective.
- Morale of staff is poor.
- Nurses believe that the quality of their care has been adversely affected.

OUTCOMES IDENTIFICATION

Gurpreet speaks to Alexzy and tells him she would like to spend 15 minutes with him every morning to talk about his concerns. She suggests that he might be able to handle his feelings in alternative ways and notes that they can also explore community resources. Alexzy gruffly agrees, saying, "You can visit me if it will make you feel better." They make arrangements to meet each morning at 0730 hours.

The following outcomes are set:

Nursing Diagnosis	Short-Term Goal
1. *Ineffective coping* related to inadequate coping methods, as evidenced by inappropriate use of defence mechanisms (displacement)	1. Alexzy will be able to name and discuss at least two feelings about his illness and lack of mobility by the end of the week.
2. *Powerlessness* related to lack of control over health care environment, as evidenced by frustration over inability to perform previously uncomplicated tasks	2. Alexzy will be able to name two community organizations that can offer him information and support by the end of 2 weeks.
3. *Ineffective coping* related to exhaustion of staff's supportive capacity toward patient, as evidenced by staff withdrawal and limited personal communication with patient	3. Staff and nurse consultant will discuss reactions and alternative nursing responses to Alexzy's behaviour twice within the next 7 days.

PLANNING

Gurpreet creates a nursing care plan and shares it with the staff.

Nursing diagnosis: *Ineffective coping* related to inadequate coping methods, as evidenced by inappropriate use of defence mechanisms (displacement)

Outcome: By discharge, Alexzy will state that he feels more comfortable discussing difficult feelings.

Short-Term Goal	Intervention	Rationale	Evaluation
1. By the end of the week, Alexzy will be able to name and discuss at least two feelings about his illness and lack of mobility.	1a. Nurse will meet with patient daily for 15 minutes at 0730 hours.	1a. Night is usually the most frightening for patient; in early morning, feelings are closer to surface.	**Goal Met** Within 7 days, Alexzy speaks to nurse more openly about feelings.
	1b. When patient lashes out, nurse will remain calm.	1b. Patient perceives that nurse is in control of her feelings. This belief can reassure patient and increase patient's sense of security.	
	1c. Nurse will consistently redirect and refocus anger from environment back to patient (e.g., "It must be difficult to be in this situation").	1c. Refocusing feelings offers patient opportunity to cope effectively with his anxiety and decreases need to act out.	
	1d. Nurse will come on time each day and stay for allotted time.	1d. Consistency sets stage for trust and reinforces that patient's anger will not drive nurse away.	

Nursing diagnosis: *Powerlessness* related to lack of control over health care environment, as evidenced by frustration over inability to perform previously uncomplicated tasks

Outcome: By discharge, Alexzy will contact at least one community support source.

CASE STUDY AND NURSING CARE PLAN 21-1—cont'd

Crisis

Short-Term Goal	Intervention	Rationale	Evaluation
2. By the end of 2 weeks, Alexzy will name and discuss at least two community organizations that can offer information and support.	2a. Nurse will spend time with patient and fiancée. Role and use of specific agencies will be discussed. 2b. Nurse will introduce one agency at a time. 2c. Nurse will not push patient to contact any of the agencies.	2a. Both patient and fiancée will have opportunity to ask questions of nurse. 2b. Gradual introduction allows time for information to sink in and minimizes feeling of being pressured or overwhelmed. 2c. Patient is able to make own decisions once he has appropriate information.	**Goal Met** By the end of 10 days, Alexzy and his fiancée can name two community resources they are interested in. At the end of 6 weeks, Alexzy has contacted the Guillain-Barré Society.

IMPLEMENTATION

Gurpreet goes into Alexzy's room at 0730 hours the following morning and sits by his bedside. At first, Alexzy's comments are hostile.

Dialogue	Therapeutic Tool or Comment
Nurse: "Alexzy, I'm here as we discussed. I'll be spending 15 minutes with you every morning. We could use this time to talk about some of your concerns."	Nurse offers herself as a resource, gives information, and clarifies her role and patient expectations. Night is Alexzy's most difficult time. In the early morning, he will be the most vulnerable and open for therapeutic intervention and support.
Alexzy: "Listen, sweetheart, my only concern is how to get a little sexual relief, get it?"	
Nurse: "Being hospitalized and partially paralyzed can be overwhelming for anyone. Perhaps you wish you could find some relief from your situation."	Nurse focuses on the process "need for relief," not the sexual content, and encourages discussion of feelings. Sexual issues often challenge new nurses, and discussing their feelings and appropriate interventions with an experienced professional is important for their growth and the quality of the care they give.
Alexzy: "What do you know, Ms. Know-it-all? I can't even scratch my nose without getting one of those fools to do it for me … and half the time those bitches aren't even around."	
Nurse: "It must be difficult to have to ask people to do everything for you."	Nurse restates what the patient says in terms of his feelings and continues to refocus away from the environment back to the patient.
Alexzy: "Yeah. … The other night a fly kept landing on my face. I had to shout for 5 minutes before one of those bitches came in, just to take the fly out of the room."	
Nurse: "Having to rely on others for everything can be a terrifying experience for anyone. It sounds extremely frustrating for you."	Nurse acknowledges that frustration and anger would be a natural response for anyone in this situation. This response encourages the patient to talk about these feelings instead of acting them out.
Alexzy: "Yeah. … It's a bitch … like a living hell."	

Gurpreet continues to spend time with Alexzy. He gradually talks more about his feelings and shows less hostility toward the staff. As he begins to feel more in control, he becomes less defensive about others caring for him. After 2 weeks, Gurpreet decreases her visits to twice a week. Alexzy is beginning to experience gross motor movements but is not walking yet. He still displaces much of his frustration and lack of control onto the environment, but he is better able to acknowledge the reality of his situation. He can also identify and briefly talk about his feelings.

Dialogue	Therapeutic Tool or Comment
Nurse: "What's happening? Your face looks tense this morning, Alexzy."	Nurse observes the patient's clenched fists, rigid posture, and tense facial expression.
Alexzy: "I had to wait 10 minutes for a bedpan last night."	
Nurse: "And you're angry about that."	Nurse verbalizes the implied.
Alexzy: "Well, there were only 2 nurses on duty for 30 people, and the nursing assistant was on his break. … You can't expect them to be everywhere, but still …"	
Nurse: "It may be hard to accept that people can't be there all the time for you."	Nurse validates the difficulty of accepting situations one does not like when one is powerless to make changes.
Alexzy: "Well … that's the way it is in this place."	

Continued

CASE STUDY AND NURSING CARE PLAN 21-1—cont'd

Crisis

EVALUATION

After 6 weeks, Alexzy is able to get around with assistance, and his ability to perform his activities of daily living is increasing. Although Alexzy still feels angry and overwhelmed at times, he is able to identify more of his feelings and acts them out less often, and he is able to talk to his fiancée about his feelings and lashes out at her less often. He is looking forward to going home, and his boss is holding his old job for him.

Alexzy makes arrangements for a meeting with the Guillain-Barré Society, and he is thinking about Alcoholics Anonymous but believes that he can handle this problem himself.

Staff members feel more comfortable and competent in their relationships with Alexzy. The goals have been met. Alexzy and Gurpreet agree that the crisis is over and terminate their visits. Alexzy is given the number of the crisis line and encouraged to call if he has questions or feels the need to talk.

KEY POINTS TO REMEMBER

- A crisis is not a pathological state but a struggle for emotional balance.
- Crises offer opportunities for emotional growth but can also lead to personality disorganization.
- There are three types of crisis: maturational, situational, and adventitious.
- Crises are usually resolved within 4 to 6 weeks.
- Assessment involves reviewing the balancing factors of the patient's perception of the problem, usual coping mechanisms, and situational supports.
- Social support and intervention can promote successful resolution.
- Resolution of a crisis takes three forms: a patient emerges at a higher level, at the pre-crisis level, or at a lower level of functioning.
- Crisis therapists take an active and directive approach with the patient in crisis.
- The patient is an active participant in setting goals and planning possible solutions.
- Crisis intervention is usually aimed at the mentally healthy patient who generally is functioning well but is temporarily overwhelmed and unable to function.
- The steps in crisis intervention are consistent with the steps of the nursing process.
- Specific qualities in the nurse that can facilitate effective intervention are a caring attitude, flexibility in planning care, an ability to listen, and an active, directive approach.
- The basic goals of crisis intervention are to reduce the individual's anxiety level and to support the effort to return the patient to his or her pre-crisis level of functioning.
- Crisis intervention therapy is short term—from 1 to 6 weeks—and focuses on the present problem only.
- Modalities of crisis intervention depend on the situation and services available at the time and locale (e.g., mental health first aid, which may be provided by professionals or community members; crisis lines; mobile response teams; urgent care clinics; in-hospital emergency psychiatric care, including medical and other interventions).
- The goals of mental health first aid are much like those of physical first aid: to assist in early intervention, health promotion, protection from harm, and application of comfort until other measures are obtained.
- A critical incident stress debriefing is a group approach that helps groups of people who have been exposed to a crisis situation.

CRITICAL THINKING

1. List the three important areas of crisis assessment once safety concerns have been identified. Give examples of two questions in each area that need to be answered before planning can take place.
2. Carley, a 21-year-old nursing student, tells her clinical instructor that her father (age 50 years) has just lost his job. Her father has been drinking heavily for years, and Carley is having difficulty coping. Because of her father's alcoholism and the increased stress in her family, Carley wants to leave school. Her mother has multiple sclerosis and thinks that Carley should quit school to take care of her.
   a. How many different types of crisis are going on in this family? Discuss each crisis from the viewpoint of each individual family member.
   b. If you were providing crisis counselling for this family, what areas would you assess? What kinds of questions would you ask to evaluate each member's individual needs and the needs of the family as a unit (perception of events, social supports, coping styles)?
   c. Formulate some tentative goals you might set in conjunction with the family.
   d. Identify specific referral agencies in your area that would be helpful if members of this family were willing to expand their use of outside resources and stabilize the situation.
   e. How would you set up follow-up visits for this family? Would you see the family members together, alone, or in combination during the crisis period (4 to 6 weeks)? How would you decide whether follow-up counselling was indicated?

3. Why is it important for nurses to promote mental health first aid (MHFA) training in rural or resource-poor communities?

4. What are some of the unique characteristics of rural versus urban settings and the distinct facilitators and barriers each setting poses for crisis workers and services?

CHAPTER REVIEW

1. Jack had a psychotic episode when he was 15 years old. He did not respond well to treatments available at the time and continued to have a significant number of residual symptoms. At the age of 42, he began taking olanzapine (Zyprexa), which significantly reduced his remaining symptoms, allowing him to leave his group home and live independently for the first time. However, once his mental health became more stable and he was living in his own apartment, he was unsure of what to do with his time, how to go about getting a job, and how to meet his sexual and companionship needs appropriately. What type of crisis situation is represented by this case?
   a. Maturational crisis
   b. Situational crisis
   c. Adventitious crisis
   d. Phase 4 crisis

2. Rashid witnessed a car suddenly careen out of control and onto the sidewalk where he and his best friend were walking. Rashid's friend pushed him out of the way at the last second but was struck and killed instantly. Rashid was treated for minor injuries and released but was referred for mental health evaluation because he was very distraught over the death of his friend. Which response should be used first during your assessment of Rashid?
   a. "Tell me about what happened that day."
   b. "What would you like to accomplish during your treatment?"
   c. "Do you think you are coping well with this very tragic event?"
   d. "Tell me what has been going through your mind since the accident."

3. Rashid confides that he feels so guilty that his friend died while pushing him to safety that he has found himself having overwhelming impulses to kill himself by crashing his car, which he almost did yesterday. Which intervention would be most therapeutic?
   a. Admit Rashid to an inpatient mental health unit to ensure his safety until his condition can improve.

   b. Work with Rashid's family to ensure that he does not have access to a car, and set up emergency counselling sessions.
   c. Persuade Rashid to agree to remain safe pending counselling, as admitting him would only further traumatize him.
   d. Consult with a psychiatrist or prescribing physician so that Rashid can be started immediately on antianxiety and antidepressant medications.

4. Justine Lee, a mother of two teenagers and a nurse with 15 years of experience in the crisis centre, fails to show up for work several days in a row not long after providing crisis intervention to area high school students following a shooting at their school. Co-workers complain that she is not taking her share of crisis calls. As Justine's manager, you attempt to address the issue, but she responds irritably and denies that anything is wrong. Justine most likely:
   a. Is becoming burned out on crisis work
   b. Is experiencing vicarious traumatization
   c. Has developed a hidden substance abuse problem
   d. Has lost her objectivity, owing to having children of her own

5. Suzanne experiences a crisis after witnessing the brutal assault of her friend during a robbery in their office tower parkade. Which outcome is the most appropriate for Suzanne?
   a. Suzanne reports greater satisfaction with her life within 2 months.
   b. Suzanne attends all treatment sessions specified in her treatment plan.
   c. Within 3 weeks, Suzanne reports that she no longer feels distressed.
   d. Suzanne returns to her pre-crisis level of functioning within 2 weeks.

℮volve WEBSITE

Post-Test   interactive review

Visit the Evolve website for Chapter Review Answers and Rationales, Critical Thinking Answer Guidelines, and additional resources related to the content in this chapter: http://evolve.elsevier.com/Canada/Varcarolis/psychiatric/

REFERENCES

Aguilera, D. C. (1998). *Crisis intervention: Theory and methodology* (8th ed.). St. Louis: Mosby.

Behrman, G., & Reid, W. J. (2002). Post-trauma intervention: Basic tasks. *Brief Treatment and Crisis Intervention, 2*, 39–48. doi:10.1093/brief-treatment/2.1.39.

Bercier, M. L., & Maynard, B. R. (2015). Interventions for secondary traumatic stress with mental health workers: A systematic review. *Research on Social Work Practice, 25*(1), 81–89. doi:10.1177/1049731513517142.

Bulechek, G. M., Butcher, H. K., Dochterman, J. M., et al. (2013). *Nursing interventions classification (NIC)* (6th ed.). St. Louis: Mosby.

Canadian Centre on Substance Abuse. (2014). *Trauma-informed care toolkit.* Retrieved from http://www.ccsa.ca/Resource%20Library/CCSA-Trauma-informed-Care-Toolkit-2014-en.pdf.

Caplan, G. (1964). *Symptoms of preventive psychiatry.* New York: Basic Books.

Erikson, E. H. (1959). *Identity and the life cycle.* New York: International Universities Press.

Goldner, E. M., Palma, J., Jenkins, E., et al. (2016). *A concise introduction to mental health in Canada* (2nd ed.). Toronto: Canadian Scholars Press.

Hensel, J. M., Ruiz, C., Finney, C., et al. (2015). Meta-analysis of risk factors for secondary traumatic stress in therapeutic work with trauma victims. *Journal of Traumatic Stress, 28*(2), 83–91. doi:10.1002/jts.21998.

Herdman, T. H., & Kamitsuru, S. (Eds.), (2014). *NANDA international nursing diagnoses: Definitions and classification, 2015–2017.* Oxford, UK: Wiley-Blackwell.

Hobfoll, S., Watson, P., Bell, C., et al. (2007). Five essential elements of immediate and mid-term mass trauma intervention: Empirical evidence. *Psychiatry, 70*(4), 283–315.

Kolski, T. D., & Jongsma, A. E. (2014). *The crisis counseling and traumatic events treatment planner, with DSM-5 updates* (2nd ed.). Hoboken, NJ: Wiley.

Lindemann, E. (1944). Symptomatology and management of acute grief. *American Journal of Psychiatry, 101*(9), 141–148.

Mental Health Commission of Canada (2017). *Advancing the mental health strategy for Canada: A framework for action.* Ottawa: Author. Retrieved from http://www.mentalhealthcommission.ca/English/framework-action-2017-2022.

Milligan, G., & McGuinness, T. M. (2009). Mental health needs in a post-disaster environment. *Journal of Psychosocial Nursing and Mental Health Services, 47*(9), 23–30. doi:10.3928/02793695-20090731-01.

Moorhead, S., Johnson, M., Maas, M. L., et al. (2013). *Nursing outcomes classification (NOC)* (5th ed.). St. Louis: Mosby.

Public Health Agency of Canada. (2015). *Emergency response services.* Retrieved from http://www.phac-aspc.gc.ca/emergency-urgence/index-eng.php.

Raphael, B. (2015). Disaster, hope, help, reality. *Epidemiology and Psychiatric Sciences, 24*(6), 500–503. doi:10.1017/S204579601500075X.

Registered Nurses' Association of Ontario (2002). *Crisis intervention.* Toronto: Author.

Registered Nurses' Association of Ontario (2006). *Crisis intervention.* Toronto: Author.

Roberts, A. R., & Ottens, A. J. (2005). The seven-stage crisis intervention model: A road map to goal attainment, problem solving, and crisis resolution. *Brief Treatment and Crisis Intervention, 5,* 329–339.

Statistics Canada. (2016). *Canadians' experiences with emergencies and disasters, 2014.* Retrieved from http://www.statcan.gc.ca/pub/85-002-x/2016001/article/14469-eng.htm.

Substance Abuse and Mental Health Services Administration (2014). *Trauma informed care in behavioral health services.* Rockville, MD: Author. Treatment Improvement Protocol (TIP) Series 57. HHS Publication No. (SMA) 13-4801.

Vernberg, E. M., Steinberg, A. M., Jacobs, A. K., et al. (2008). Innovations in disaster mental health: Psychological first aid. *Professional Psychology, Research and Practice, 39*(4), 381–388. doi:10.1037/a0012663.

World Health Organization. (2011). *Psychological first aid: Guide for field workers.* Retrieved from http://www.who.int/mental_health/publications/guide_field_workers/en/.

Yaeger, K. R., & Roberts, A. R. (2015). *Crisis intervention handbook: Assessment, treatment, and research* (4th ed.). New York: Oxford.

Suicide and Nonsuicidal Self-Injury

Sonya L. Jakubec

KEY TERMS AND CONCEPTS

cluster suicide
death by suicide
euthanasia
lethality
medically assisted death
nonsuicidal self-injury
postvention
primary intervention

SAD PERSONS scale
secondary intervention
suicidal behaviour
suicidal ideation
suicide
survivors of suicide
tertiary intervention

OBJECTIVES

1. Describe the profile of suicide in Canada, noting psychosocial and cultural factors that affect risk.
2. Identify three common precipitating events.
3. Describe risk factors and warning signs for suicide, including coexisting psychiatric disorders.
4. Name the most frequent coexisting psychiatric disorders.
5. Use the SAD PERSONS scale to assess suicide risk.
6. Describe three expected reactions a nurse may have when beginning work with suicidal patients.
7. Give examples of primary, secondary, and tertiary (postvention) interventions.
8. Describe basic-level interventions that take place in the hospital or community.
9. Identify key elements of suicide precautions and environmental safety factors in the hospital.
10. Distinguish suicide from nonsuicidal self-injury
11. Identify appropriate interventions for nonsuicidal self-injury in the clinical setting.

⊖volve WEBSITE

Visit the Evolve website for Flashcards, Case Studies, and additional testing resources related to the content in this chapter: http://evolve.elsevier.com/Canada/Varcarolis/psychiatric/

Pre-Test | interactive review

Sadly, it is the rare individual who has yet to encounter, directly or indirectly, the significant public health problem that is suicide. Approximately every 40 seconds, a human life ends as a result of suicide (World Health Organization, 2014). Nursing students and practising nurses at all levels encounter individuals suffering from the pain and hopelessness that all too frequently culminate in some type of suicidal behaviour. These individuals can be identified in inpatient settings, in outpatient treatment settings, and in the community. Studies have shown that 83% of people who die by suicide had received inpatient or outpatient health services in the year before their death (Ahmedani, Simon, Stewart, et al., 2014), with 45% consulting a primary care physician within a month before death (Turecki & Brent, 2016). This highlights the important role clinicians have in identifying risks and preventing these suicides. All too often, however, the focus of concern is concentrated on individuals who are at immediate risk (Hogan

& Grumet, 2016). It is critical for nursing and primary health care providers to be advocates for this devastating problem and to mobilize the community to reduce factors that may contribute to suicide. Nurses at the primary, secondary, and tertiary levels of intervention can play a crucial role in the care of these patients, their families, and the survivors of suicide (family and friends of a person who has died by suicide). This chapter presents the facts about suicide and discusses approaches for assessment and care of suicidal patients and their loved ones.

This chapter uses definitions that represent current thinking in reference to suicide and suicidal behaviours. The terms suicide or death by suicide are used to describe the act of taking one's own life. The term suicidal behaviour is used to describe potentially self-injurious actions with a nonfatal outcome for which there is evidence that a person intended to kill himself or herself (Turecki & Brent, 2016). Examples of suicidal behaviours include self-harm, suicidal ideation, desire to hasten death, risky behaviour, and suicide threats. Suicidal behaviour may or may not result in injury. Nonsuicidal self-injury is discussed in brief at the end of the chapter and is characterized by self-harming behaviour with no intent to die.

Several terms used in association with suicide add to the stigma and alienation experienced both by people with suicidal ideation (referred to as self-stigma) and by survivors of suicide (Boyd, Adler, Otilingam, et al., 2014). Terms such as *committed suicide, failed suicide,* and *successful suicide* are avoided. Words like *commit* and *attempt* evoke connotations of criminality, which are inappropriate and potentially stigmatizing to suicidal individuals and those touched by suicide. Certainly, the notions of failure and success in this regard are equally disrespectful and distort what could never be considered a success. Some suicide prevention activists use the term *completed suicide*; however, professionalized jargon is rarely helpful in this context, and the term *complete* expresses a connotation of incompleteness for those who nonfatally attempt suicide. For those surviving, there is nothing that feels "complete" amid the many unanswered questions and loss of hopes and dreams for and with their loved one. For these reasons, the neutral and factual expression "died by suicide" is preferred (Beaton, Forster, & Maple, 2012). Changing the language that we use to describe suicide and suicidal behaviours is a first step in addressing the ways in which nurses can sensitively and empathically begin working with individuals who are suicidal.

EPIDEMIOLOGY

According to Statistics Canada (2016), 4 000 deaths by suicide were recorded in 2015, or 12 suicides for every 100 000 people. These numbers are thought to be understated, with the actual number of suicide deaths much higher. On their own, these numbers represent a considerable loss. Four thousand people is the equivalent of losing a small town from our national map every year. It is like twelve 747 jets crashing and killing everyone on board every year. It is more than double the annual number of traffic fatalities and nearly 10 times the annual number of homicides. These are unnecessary, preventable losses—the loss of life of the person who dies plus the grief of all the people touched by that person.

In Canada, 10 people die by suicide every day, and suicide is the ninth leading cause of death. For every 1 suicide death, there are 5 self-inflicted injury hospitalizations, 25 to 30 suicide attempts, and 7 to 10 people profoundly affected by suicide loss. Suicide and mental illness are deeply connected, and 90% of the 4 000 individuals who die by suicide each year were living with a mental health problem or illness (Government of Canada, 2016). The statistics are concerning across the lifespan. The highest rates of suicide were among those ages 50 to 54, with considerable increases from previous years in that age group and among individuals ages 55 to 59 and 60 to 64. The annual number of suicides in the 15- to 19- and 20- to 24-year-old groups actually decreased in 2013. However, suicide was still the leading cause of death for people ages 15 to 34 (Statistics Canada, 2016).

It is also important to consider that the number of suicides may actually be double or triple the reported statistics due to under-reporting in general (Rocket, 2010). Purposefully aiming a car at a bridge abutment and crashing may look like an accident. But, in fact, many reported accidents, homicides, and deaths ruled as "undetermined" are actually suicides.

Studies of suicide in the Canadian Armed Forces between 1995 and 2015 have demonstrated that suicide rates did not significantly increase over time, after age standardization. Suicide rates among the Armed Forces were also not statistically higher than those in the general Canadian population. History of deployment continued to be a possible risk factor for suicide in the Armed Forces, and deployment-related trauma (especially that related to the mission in Afghanistan) and resulting mental disorders are likely related to these associations (National Defense and the Canadian Armed Forces, 2016). Studies have indicated that Canadian veterans can, however, experience a greater incidence of depression, alcohol abuse (Fetzner, Abrams, & Asmundson, 2013), and post-traumatic stress disorder (Zamorski, Rolland-Harris, Jetly, et al., 2015) than those who were not in the military. The *Life After Service Studies,* a joint research venture of Veterans Affairs Canada (VAC), the Department of National Defence/Canadian Forces (DND/CF), and Statistics Canada, continues to examine Canadian veterans' mental health issues as they transition to civilian life (Veterans Affairs, 2016).

Racial and Ethnic Statistics

Indigenous peoples (First Nations, Inuit, and Métis) in Canada are especially vulnerable to death by suicide. For First Nations male youth, the situation is particularly alarming. While there is much variation among communities, overall rates are high, with suicide rates five to seven times higher for First Nations youth than for non-Aboriginal youth and suicide rates among Inuit youth among the highest in the world, at 11 times the national average (Health Canada, 2016). Many of the same risk factors for the general population, such as depression and substance misuse, are related to suicidal behaviour among Indigenous youth. There is also evidence of the predisposing risk factors that affect other young people with elevated rates of suicide, especially early developmental adversity, such as trauma and abuse, including childhood sexual abuse.

In response to this growing crisis, in 2005 Health Canada, the Assembly of First Nations (AFN), and the Inuit Tapiriit Kanatami (ITK) established the First Nations and Inuit Mental Wellness Advisory Committee (MWAC) to develop community-based solutions to mental health issues such as the disproportionate rate of suicide among First Nations youth. One MWAC initiative, the Alianait Inuit-Specific Mental Wellness Task Group, is mandated to explore mental wellness issues in the context of the distinct circumstances and culture of Inuit. Another initiative, the National Aboriginal Youth Suicide Prevention Strategy (NAYSPS) is a multimillion-dollar federal strategy providing funds to support community-based research and capacity building for suicide prevention plans. NAYSPS posits that suicide prevention initiatives should be evidence informed; support for community-based approaches should be provided by publicly funded agencies; support must be culturally appropriate; all levels of prevention must be offered; youth should be involved in the process; varying levels of community readiness must be considered; suicide prevention is the responsibility of all people, communities, agencies, organizations, and governments; and the promotion of life and well-being is as important as suicide prevention.

Risk Factors

Suicide is not a psychiatric disorder per se; rather, self-harm is the manifestation of inner pain, hopelessness, and helplessness suffered by people experiencing suicidal ideation, also known as suicidal thoughts. These thoughts can range from a fleeting idea about one's own death (or about not being here) that does not include the act of killing oneself to a detailed plan, including the final act of killing oneself. In Canada, in 2009–2010, approximately 7 in 10 hospitalizations for self-harm included a mental health illness diagnosis. The percentages of hospitalizations for self-harm attributable to specific psychiatric disorders are listed in Table 22-1.

It is estimated that 90% of people who die by suicide are experiencing depression, another mental health illness, or a substance use disorder, all of which are potentially treatable (Government of Canada, 2016). About 15% of patients who have major depression or bipolar disorder (during the depressed phase) will die by suicide (Brendel, Breezing, Lagomasino, et al., 2016). Loss of relationships, financial difficulty, and impulsivity are contributing factors in this population.

Suicide risk is 50 times higher among patients with schizophrenia than among the general population, especially during the first few years of the illness, and suicide is the leading cause of early death among those with the illness. About 40% of all patients—and 60% of males—with schizophrenia attempt suicide at least once. Up to 10% of these patients die by suicide, usually related to depressive symptoms rather than to command hallucinations or delusions. The more risk factors that are present, the higher is the risk for suicide (Figure 22-1).

Patients with alcohol or substance use disorders also have a higher suicide risk. Comorbidity of substance abuse and depression or antisocial personality disorder is also associated with increased risk. Up to 15% of those with alcohol or substance abuse die by suicide (Sadock, Sadock, & Ruiz, 2017).

Keep in mind that suicide is not necessarily synonymous with a mental health disorder. The act of purposeful self-destruction represented by taking one's own life is usually accompanied by intensely conflicted feelings of pain, hopelessness, guilt, and self-loathing, coupled with the belief that there are no solutions and that things will not improve. Self-harming actions have been associated with the feeling that there is no one to turn to for support (Muehlenkamp, Brausch, Quigley, et al., 2013). People who survive serious suicide attempts often report that it is these feelings that fuelled the sense of isolation and despair. They describe an all-consuming psychic pain that shuts out thoughts of the loved ones and heartache they will leave behind. To understand this phenomenon, imagine the pain of your hand on a hot stove burner. At that moment, you are unlikely to think of anything but putting an immediate end to the pain. Emotional pain can render the individual void of thought and without even enough motivation to leave a suicide note. Antoon Leenars, a Canadian psychologist and researcher who has studied suicide notes extensively, has stated that only between 12% and 37% of people who died by suicide left suicide notes (Canadian Association for Suicide Prevention, 2009).

Besides psychiatric disorders, other risk factors associated with the psychic pain that can trigger suicidal behaviour include victimization by bullying, pathological gambling, incarceration, and nonheterosexuality. The term *bullycide* was coined by Marr and Field (2000) to refer to suicidal behaviour in response to bullying. In a larger survey across Canada it was found that 1 in 5 teens has seriously considered suicide in the last 12 months, with twice as many girls as boys reporting having considered suicide. Of this group, nearly half reported that they did not speak to anyone about suicide (47%) and that they had formulated a plan (46%). Bullying, relationship problems, and body and self-image problems are all related to suicidal thoughts in this group (Kids Help Phone, 2016).

Researchers have also established connections between pathological gambling and suicidal ideation, bipolar disorder, personality disorders, anxiety disorder, major depression, and substance use disorders. It is estimated that more than 200 Canadians experiencing problems related to gambling end up taking their own lives every year (Smith, 2014).

TABLE 22-1	PERCENTAGE OF HOSPITALIZATIONS FOR SELF-HARM ATTRIBUTABLE TO PSYCHIATRIC DISORDERS
DISORDERS	**PERCENTAGE**
Affective illnesses (major depression and bipolar disorder)	23%
Substance-related disorders	12%
Anxiety disorders	11%
Disorders of personality and behaviour	6%
Schizophrenia	3%
Multiple mental health–related diagnoses (coexisting disorders)	14%

Source: Data from Canadian Institute for Health Information. (2013). *Health indicators 2013*. Ottawa: Author. Retrieved from https://secure.cihi.ca/free_products/HI2013_Jan30_EN.pdf.

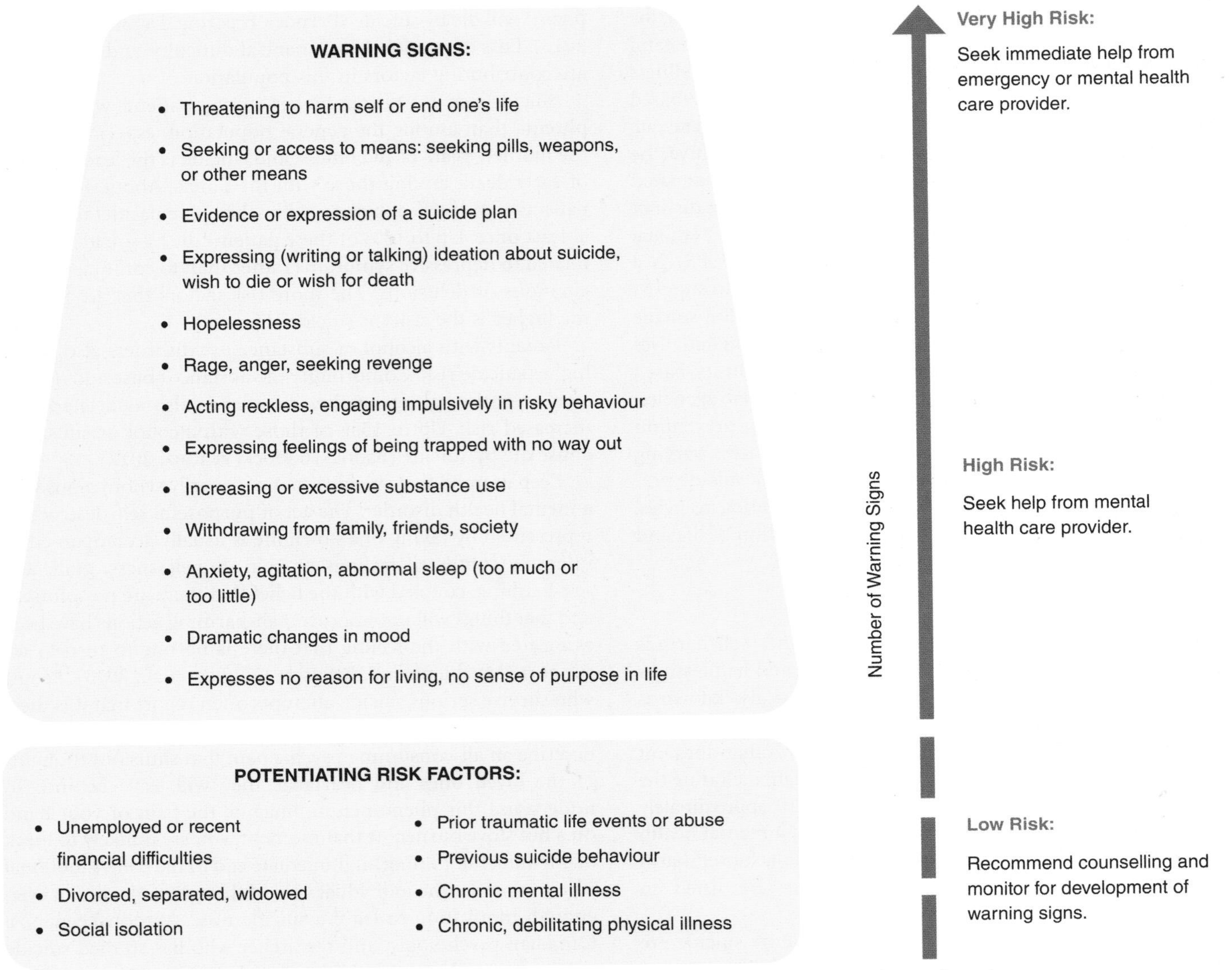

WARNING SIGNS:

- Threatening to harm self or end one's life

- Seeking or access to means: seeking pills, weapons, or other means

- Evidence or expression of a suicide plan

- Expressing (writing or talking) ideation about suicide, wish to die or wish for death

- Hopelessness

- Rage, anger, seeking revenge

- Acting reckless, engaging impulsively in risky behaviour

- Expressing feelings of being trapped with no way out

- Increasing or excessive substance use

- Withdrawing from family, friends, society

- Anxiety, agitation, abnormal sleep (too much or too little)

- Dramatic changes in mood

- Expresses no reason for living, no sense of purpose in life

Very High Risk:

Seek immediate help from emergency or mental health care provider.

Number of Warning Signs

High Risk:

Seek help from mental health care provider.

POTENTIATING RISK FACTORS:

- Unemployed or recent financial difficulties

- Divorced, separated, widowed

- Social isolation

- Prior traumatic life events or abuse

- Previous suicide behaviour

- Chronic mental illness

- Chronic, debilitating physical illness

Low Risk:

Recommend counselling and monitor for development of warning signs.

FIGURE 22-1 Illustration of the accumulation of potentiating risk factors and warning signs on risk for suicide. Source: Perlman, C. M., Neufeld, E., Martin, L., et al. (2011). *Suicide risk assessment inventory: A resource guide for Canadian health care organizations.* Toronto: Ontario Hospital Association and Canadian Patient Safety Institute. Retrieved from http://www.oha.com/KnowledgeCentre/Documents/Final%20-%20Suicide%20Risk%20Assessment%20Guidebook.pdf.

There are 10 suicide deaths each year in federal penitentiaries, a rate seven times higher than in the general population (Office of the Correctional Investigator Canada, 2014).

Researchers have established that suicidal behaviour is significantly higher in nonheterosexual populations. Among youth, those who are lesbian, gay, bisexual, or transgender and those questioning their sexuality are at higher risk for suicide than their heterosexual peers (Ahuja, Webster, Gibson, et al., 2015). Although most mortality data do not include sexual orientation, nonheterosexual youth are believed to experience suicidal ideation and engage in suicidal behaviour to a greater extent than heterosexual adolescents and young adults. The stigma and discrimination associated with their sexual orientation elevate risk and lower protective factors among this group.

Refer to Box 22-1 for a description of significant psychosocial risk and protective factors for suicide and to Box 22-2 for warning signs.

ETIOLOGY

Biological Factors

Researchers continue to study biological factors in order to better understand and screen for suicidal behaviour, although none of the biological markers identified to date are sensitive or precise enough for use in the clinical setting. Failures in neurotransmitter and neuroendocrine systems, such as the serotonergic, noradrenergic, dopaminergic, and hypothalamic–pituitary–adrenal (HPA) systems, have been investigated (Ganz, Braquehais, & Sher, 2010) but have not yet yielded any evidence strong enough to

RESEARCH HIGHLIGHT

Understanding Self-Harm and Suicidal Behaviour

Problem

Suicide is among the top causes of mortality worldwide, especially in adolescents and young adults. Considerable attention has been given to the possible link between peer victimization and self-harm, suicidal ideation, or suicide attempt. Victimization by peers is highly prevalent in adolescence, with rates ranging from 11% to 40%. Surprisingly, however, conflicting results appear in existing research about the association between recent bullying victimization and suicide risk.

Purpose of Study

The purpose of this study was to describe the association between recent bullying victimization and risk for suicide among pediatric emergency department patients.

Methods

Patients presenting to one of three different urban pediatric emergency departments with either medical-surgical or psychiatric chief complaints completed structured interviews as part of a study to develop a suicide risk screening instrument, the Ask Suicide-Screening Questions. Seventeen candidate items and the criterion reference Suicidal Ideation Questionnaire were administered to patients ages 10 to 21 years. Bullying victimization was assessed by a single candidate item ("In the past few weeks, have you been bullied or picked on so much that you felt like you couldn't stand it anymore?").

Key Findings

A total of 524 patients completed the interview (34.4% psychiatric chief complaints; 56.9% female; mean [SD] age, 15.2 [2.6] years). Sixty patients (11.5%) reported recent bullying victimization, and of these, 33 (55.0%) screened positive for suicide risk. After controlling for demographic and clinical variables, including a history of depression and drug use, the odds of screening positive for suicide risk were significantly greater in patients who reported recent bullying victimization. Recent bullying victimization was associated with increased odds of screening positive for elevated suicide risk among pediatric emergency department patients presenting with medical-surgical complaints.

Implications for Nursing Practice

Understanding this important correlate of suicide risk in pediatric emergency department patients may help inform emergency department–based suicide prevention interventions.

Source: Stanley, I. H., Horowitz, L. M., Bridge, J. A., et al. (2016). Bullying and suicide risk among pediatric emergency department patients. *Pediatric Emergency Care, 32*(6), 347.

BOX 22-1 SUICIDE RISK FACTORS AND PROTECTIVE FACTORS

Risk Factors

- Suicidal ideation with intent
- Lethal suicide plan
- History of previous suicide attempt
- Co-occurring psychiatric illness
- Co-occurring medical illness
- History of childhood abuse
- Family history of suicide
- Lack of social support
- Unemployment
- Recent stressful life event (e.g., death, other loss, legal conflict, relationship breakup, conflict)
- Hopelessness
- Helplessness
- Panic attacks
- Feeling of shame or humiliation
- Impulsivity
- Aggressiveness
- Loss of cognitive function (e.g., loss of impulse control)
- Access to firearms and other highly lethal means
- Substance use (without formal disorder)
- Impending incarceration
- Low frustration tolerance
- Sexual orientation and gender identity issues
- Social isolation
- Key demographic risk (widowed, divorced, single, white, elderly, adolescent, young adult, Indigenous, lesbian, gay, bisexual and transgendered).

Protective Factors

Note that, although patients who exhibit protective factors may attempt and die by suicide, multiple protective factors generally contribute to patient resiliency in the face of stress and adversity. Protective factors may be considered in each of the domains of the individual, family, work and community. Important protective factors may include:

- children in the home, except among those with postpartum psychosis
- responsibility to others
- pregnancy
- personal, social, cultural and religious beliefs that discourage suicide and support self-preservation
- life satisfaction
- reality testing ability
- positive coping skills
- positive social support
- positive therapeutic relationship
- attachment to therapy, social or family support
- hope for future
- self-efficacy
- supportive living arrangements
- fear of act of suicide
- fear of social disapproval

Sources: Centre for Addiction and Mental Health. (2015). *Suicide prevention and assessment handbook.* Retrieved from https://www.camh.ca/en/hospital/health_information/a_z_mental_health_and_addiction_information/suicide/Documents/sp_handbook_final_feb_2011.pdf.

BOX 22-2 WARNING SIGNS

The American Association of Suicidology (AAS) uses the mnemonic IS PATH WARM to assist people in recognizing and identifying the warning signs of suicide.

SUICIDE WARNING SIGNS

I	Ideation
S	Substance use
P	Purposelessness
A	Anxiety or agitation
T	Trapped
H	Hopelessness or helplessness
W	Withdrawal
A	Anger
R	Recklessness
M	Mood changes

The presence of any warning sign may signify that someone is thinking about suicide. The presence of more than one warning sign indicates a higher risk for suicide. The presence of one or more warning signs should signal the need to begin a dialogue into a person's circumstances and a follow-up with a more in-depth suicide risk assessment.

Source: American Association of Suicidology. (n.d.). *Know the warning signs.* Retrieved from http://www.suicidology.org/stats-and-tools/suicide-warning-signs.

significantly change clinical practice. For example, evidence suggests a potentially causal association between suicidal behaviour and the serotonin neurotransmission system (Carballo, Akamnonu, & Oquendo, 2008). Further, low cerebrospinal fluid 5-hydroxyindoleacetic acid (5-HIAA, the main serotonin metabolite) is considered a promising biological predictor of suicidal behaviour (Ganz, Braquehais, & Sher, 2010).

Recent studies indicate a combined effect of genetic and epigenetic (external gene altering) factors. Guintivano and colleagues (2014) found that the *SKA2* gene expression was lower in individuals with suicidal ideation. This lowered gene expression along with anxiety and stress could account for about 80% of suicidal behaviours and the progression from suicidal ideation to suicide attempt. These findings are consistent with the diathesis–stress model or the dual-risk hypothesis.

Another consideration is the involvement of protein kinase A (PKA), a crucial enzyme in the adenylyl cyclase signal transduction pathway, which regulates gene transcription, cell survival, and plasticity. When stress affects PKA's synaptic and structural plasticity, an association with suicide has been identified (Dwivedi & Pandey, 2011).

Psychosocial Factors

Sigmund Freud originally theorized that suicide resulted from unacceptable aggression toward another person that is turned inward. Karl Menninger added to Freud's thought by describing three parts of suicidal hostility: the wish to kill, the wish to be killed, and the wish to die (Sadock, Sadock, & Ruiz, 2017). Aaron Beck identified a central emotional factor underlying suicide intent: hopelessness. Certain cognitive styles that contribute to higher risk are rigid all-or-nothing thinking, inability to see different options, and perfectionism (Hewitt, Caelian, Chen,

et al., 2014). Maladaptive perfectionist thinking, in which anything less than perfect is unacceptable, can leave individuals vulnerable to depression and suicide (Kiamanesh, Dieserud, & Haavind, 2015).

Recent theories of suicide have focused on the lethal combination of suicidal fantasies accompanied by loss (e.g., of love, self-esteem, job, freedom due to imminent incarceration), rage or guilt, or identification with a suicide victim (cluster suicide). A cluster suicide, sometimes referred to as a copycat suicide, follows a highly publicized suicide of a public figure, an idol, or a peer in the community. Adolescents are at especially high risk for cluster suicide, owing to their immature prefrontal cortex, the portion of the brain that controls the executive functions involving judgement, frustration tolerance, and impulse control.

Athletes, at both elite and amateur levels, can feel constant pressure to perform. Loss of status in their sport, steroid use, or an injury such as postconcussion syndrome can leave them susceptible to suicidal fantasies. Persistent pain has been found to increase depression in retired professional athletes (Riley, 2016).

Cultural Factors

Cultural factors, including religious beliefs, family values, and attitude toward death, can influence suicide rates. Yet, as Leong and Leach (2008) observed, "Pain is pain…. The suicidal mind is the suicidal mind … whether in any cultural group" (p. 3). Special consideration must be made for populations. Described earlier, the high rate of suicide among Indigenous peoples in Canada is alarming. The numerous risk factors exist in a context of historical and social trauma (see Chapter 8). The National Inuit Suicide Prevention Strategy was established in 2016 to address broader social and cultural conditions in order to prevent suicide among Inuit; it targets six priority areas: (1) creating social equity, (2) creating cultural continuity, (3) nurturing healthy Inuit children from birth, (4) ensuring access to a continuum of mental wellness services for Inuit, (5) healing unresolved trauma and grief, and (6) mobilizing Inuit knowledge for resilience and suicide prevention (Inuit Tapiriit Kanatami, 2016). Of particular importance in both population health promotion strategy and caring for patients who are experiencing the pain of suicidal behaviour is an understanding of the relational concept of cultural safety (refer to the Considering Culture box).

Societal Factors

No discussion about current societal attitudes and trends would be complete without an examination of the way in which suicide is viewed in a general context. In Canada, at this time, although euthanasia is against the law, the federal government has passed legislation that allows eligible Canadian adults to request medical assistance in dying. At the core of the argument supporting medically assisted death are the twin goals of minimizing human suffering and maximizing individual autonomy. Medically assisted death (also referred to as assisted suicide or death with dignity) and euthanasia are different.

Medically assisted death involves providing another with the knowledge or means to intentionally end his or her own life through medicine, for example, when a physician prescribes

Factors: Cultural Safety

Grounded in the principle of safety as a nursing expectation and standard, cultural safety seeks to overcome situations wherein people from one cultural group feel demeaned, disempowered, or "unsafe" as a consequence of the actions of a more dominant group from another culture. From a critical theory perspective, culture is a complex, dynamic, political, historical, and relational process that shifts over time and one that has significantly been influenced by our social, professional, and gendered location (Registered Nurses' Association of Ontario, 2009). Cultural safety is not about ethnocultural differences, customs, and practices. Rather, cultural safety calls us to view our way of providing nursing care through a lens of critical consciousness and to question the inherent power differentials in the health care systems in which we learn and work.

Originating in New Zealand, the concept of cultural safety emerged as indigenous Maori nurse leaders began to link the poor health outcomes of Maori people, in part, to the cultural inappropriateness and insensitivity of health care providers, who were descendents of European settlers, the dominant culture (Syme, Josewiski, & Kendall, 2010). In essence, "cultural safety analyzes power imbalances, institutional discrimination, colonization, and colonial relationships" (National Aboriginal Health Organization, 2009, p. 3). The approach continues to gain international recognition, primarily in relation to indigenous peoples' experiences with mainstream health care, and is particularly relevant in caring for patients with suicidal behaviour in Canada's multicultural context. Health care providers must remember that, although knowledge of practices that may be associated with different cultural groups can be valuable in assessing some suicidal behaviour, this same knowledge can also be construed as stereotyping, labelling, and marginalizing patients.

Sources: National Aboriginal Health Organization. (2009). *Cultural competency and safety in First Nations, Inuit and Métis health care.* Ottawa: Author; Registered Nurses' Association of Ontario. (2009). *Assessment and care of adults at risk for suicidal ideation and behaviour.* Toronto: Author; and Syme, V., Josewiski, V., & Kendall, E. (2010). *Cultural safety: An overview.* Report to the First Nations, Inuit, and Métis Advisory Committee and Mental Health Commission of Canada. Retrieved from http://www.mooddisorderscanada.ca/documents/Publications/CULTURAL%20SAFETY%20AN%20OVERVIEW%20%28draft%20mar%202010%29.pdf.

medication to a patient with advanced terminal illness, who uses the drugs to end his or herself. Regarding medically assisted death, the "General: Consent to Death" section of the *Criminal Code* (1985) is now amended to read that "No medical practitioner or nurse practitioner commits culpable homicide if they provide a person with medical assistance in dying in accordance with section 241.2" (c. C-46, s. 247(1)). This amendment extends also to assistants to the clinical practitioners and to those who provide counsel to those seeking medical assistance in death.

Euthanasia is a deliberate act undertaken by a person with the intention of ending the life of another person in order to relieve that person's suffering and where that act is the cause of death. An example of euthanasia is a physician who administers a lethal dose of medication to a woman suffering from severe dementia with the intention of ending her life in order to relieve the pain and suffering caused by her condition where the medication cause death (Health Law Institute, 2017). Regarding euthanasia, the "General: Consent to Death" section of the *Criminal Code* (1985) states: "No person is entitled to consent to have death inflicted on him, and such consent does not affect the criminal responsibility of any person by whom death may be inflicted on the person by whom consent is given" (c. C-46, s. 14).

The efforts to decriminalize euthanasia and medically assisted death in Canada have been under way for many years and are part of a global trend in this direction. The Netherlands allows for this practice in nonterminal cases of "lasting and unbearable" suffering (Appel, 2007). Belgium authorizes physician-assisted suicide for nonterminal cases when suffering is deemed to be "constant and cannot be alleviated." And no country has laws as liberal as Switzerland, in which assisted suicide has been legal since 1918 and allows nonresidents to terminate their lives without a physician involved in the process (Appel, 2007).

The ethical and moral dilemmas in this evolving trend are clear. Questions continue to be posed about whether chronic and serious mental illness is no different in the depth and breadth of suffering from chronic and serious physical illness (Appel, 2007). Ethicists question whether the "slippery slope" of legally sanctioned suicide will result in abuse of vulnerable groups such as the clinically depressed (Battin, van der Heide, Ganzini, et al., 2007; Finlay & George, 2011). Until more effective treatment or a cure is found, some individuals who obtain little or no benefit from existing psychiatric treatments may choose to end suffering by suicide.

APPLICATION OF THE NURSING PROCESS

The process of suicide risk assessment is comprehensive and requires identifying specific risk factors, taking a psychosocial and medical history, and interacting with the patient during the interview. The nurse usually completes this assessment in conjunction with other clinicians since comparison of data from two interviewers is often a significant element of the evaluation.

Not all patients who show suicidal ideation or who engage in suicidal behaviour truly want to die. Suicidal behaviour can include a variety of behaviours, including self-harm either with or without clear intent to cause bodily harm or death. Any previous suicidal behaviour is a risk factor for suicide—about half of all people who kill themselves have a history of some form of suicidal behaviour. Especially prevalent in the adolescent and young adult populations, self-harm (usually in the form of cutting) is most often done with the intent to either alleviate psychic pain or pierce the psychic numbness these individuals describe (Doyle, Sheridan, & Treacy, 2017). They do not engage in this behaviour as a means of seeking attention and will often go to great lengths to conceal the evidence. Self-harm often carries a lethal risk for death or permanent injury. It is important for nurses to try to understand what is behind the behaviour, as it is often a sign that the individual is trying to communicate his or her pain and despair.

Nonacute suicidal or self-destructive thoughts and feelings can be treated in the outpatient setting. Alternative services available to suicidal patients include crisis intervention, community mental health services, assertive community treatment (ACT), addiction treatment, social services, and legal assistance. While suicide risk assessment is a reasoned and inductive process rather than an intuitive one, there is no one single predictor of suicide and a wide individual variation occurs across all demographics. A central purpose of a suicide assessment is to appreciate the complexity of risk factors that contribute to suicidality in a systematic way (Centre for Addiction and Mental Health, 2015). These types of interventions are also individualized and realistic, both of which are essential aspects of the person-centred recovery model. The Mental Health Commission of Canada (2017) advocates for a mental health system that focuses on recovery and hope, choice, responsibility, dignity, and respect.

ASSESSMENT

The *Suicide Risk Assessment Guide: A Resource for Health Care Organizations* (Perlman, Neufeld, Martin, et al., 2011) is a general guide to help health care organizations with understanding and standardizing the practice of high-quality suicide risk assessment. The guide emphasizes the importance of thorough documentation in assessing suicide. Box 22-3 provides a sample of recommended documentation, summarizing eight important points to include in nursing assessments.

Organizations should also develop standard protocols for the location of documentation regarding suicide risk within the patient's record so that documentation is consistently located and, therefore, easily identified by others within the organization or by those involved in the care of the person.

Verbal and Nonverbal Clues

Almost all people considering suicide send out clues, especially to people they think of as supportive. Nurses and other health care workers often fit into this category. There may be overt or covert verbal clues and nonverbal signals. Examples include:

- Overt statements
  - "I can't take it anymore."
  - "Life isn't worth living anymore."
  - "I wish I were dead."
  - "Everyone would be better off if I died."
- Covert statements
  - "It's okay now. Soon everything will be fine."
  - "Things will never work out."
  - "I won't be a problem much longer."
  - "Nothing feels good to me anymore and probably never will."
  - "How can I give my body to medical science?"

Most often, it is a relief for people contemplating suicide to finally talk to someone about their despair and loneliness. Asking about suicidal thoughts does not "give a person ideas" and is, in fact, a professional responsibility similar to asking about chest pain in cardiac conditions. Talking openly leads to a decrease in isolation and can increase problem-solving alternatives for living. People who contemplate suicide, those who act on their suicidal

---

BOX 22-3 SAMPLE OF RECOMMENDED DOCUMENTATION

1. The overall level of suicide risk
   The level of risk should be clearly documented, along with information to support this assertion, which can include the following:
   - The types of assessment tools used to inform risk assessment
   - Details from clinical interviews and from communication with others (e.g., the person's family and friends, other professionals), including:
     - The circumstances and timing of the event
     - Method chosen for suicide
     - Degree of intent
     - Availability of resources to carry out plan
     - Description of actions taken by the health care provider or family members
     - Consequences of previous suicidal ideation or self-harming behaviours (e.g., Were there any permanent injuries?)
2. Prior history of suicide attempt(s) and self-harming behaviour
   - The prior care or intervention plan that was in place
   - The length of time since previous suicide attempt(s) or self-harming behaviour(s)
   - The rationale for not being admitted to a more intensive environment or discharged to a less restrictive environment, and what safety plans were put into place
   - Details about family concerns and how these were addressed
3. Details about all potentiating risk factors, warning signs, and protective factors
4. The degree of suicide intent
   The degree of intent may include, for example, what the person thought or hoped would happen.
5. The person's feeling and reaction following suicidal behaviour
   Record, for example, whether the person feels a sense of relief or regret at being alive.
6. Evidence of an escalation in potential lethality of self-harm or suicidal behaviours
   Document whether the person has begun to consider, plan, or use increasingly lethal means (e.g., from cutting to hanging, seeking a gun).
7. Similarity of person's current circumstances to those surrounding previous suicide attempt(s) or self-harming behaviour(s)
8. History of self-harm or suicidal behaviour(s) among family or friends or significant loss of family or friends
   This history should include anniversary dates of these events as risk may be elevated at such times.

Source: Centre for Addiction and Mental Health. (2015). *Suicide prevention and assessment handbook*. Toronto: Author. Retrieved from https://www.camh.ca/en/hospital/health_information/a_z _mental_health_and_addiction_information/suicide/Documents/ sp_handbook_final_feb_2011.pdf.

thoughts, and even those who regret the "failure" of their actions are often extremely receptive to talking about their suicide crisis. Specific questions to ask about suicidal ideation include the following (Meerwijk, van Meijel, van den Bout, et al., 2010):

- Have you ever felt that life was not worth living?
- Have you been thinking about death recently?
- Have you been feeling so bad that you have thought about taking your own life?
- Did you ever think about suicide?
- Have you ever tried to end your life?
- Do you have a plan for what you would do to end your own life?
- If so, what is your plan?

Lethality of Suicide Plan

The evaluation of a suicide plan is extremely important in determining the degree of suicidal risk. Five main elements must be considered when evaluating lethality (the degree of suicidal risk) (Toth, Schwartz, & Kurka, 2007):

1. Presence of risk factors for suicide
2. Degree of suicidal ideation
3. Intent to carry out suicide plan
4. Means and availability of resources to carry out selected method of suicide
5. Degree of hope for improvement of psychological state

People who have definite plans for the time, place, and means are at high risk.

People experiencing psychotic episodes are at high risk—regardless of the specificity of details—because their impulse control and judgement are grossly impaired. A person suffering psychosis is particularly vulnerable when depressed or having command hallucinations. Regardless of whether the nurse considers a patient high or low risk, *all* threats of suicide should be taken seriously, and a suicide risk assessment should be completed.

Assessment Tools

Many tools have been developed to aid a health care worker in assessing suicidal potential. Patterson and colleagues (1983) devised an assessment aid with the acronym *SAD PERSONS* to evaluate 10 major risk factors for suicide (Table 22-2). The SAD PERSONS scale is a simple and practical guide for triaging potentially suicidal patients, particularly in an emergency department environment. Ten categories are described in the assessment tool, and the person being evaluated is assigned one point for each applicable characteristic. The total point score for the individual correlates with an action scale that assists health care workers to determine whether hospital admission is advisable. If a patient scores in the 3- to 4-point range, a psychiatric or mental health care provider must conduct a full mental status examination and interview.

The SAD PERSONS tool has its shortcomings. It does not address whether the patient is taking either illicit or prescribed drugs that may have a significant impact on him or her, and it is also dated (from 1983).

Prescription medications such as antidepressants should be evaluated for their contribution to suicide risk. Health Canada

TABLE 22-2	SAD PERSONS SCALE	
S	Sex	1 if male
A	Age	1 if <19 or >45 years
D	Depression	1 if present
P	Previous attempt	1 if present
E	Ethanol use	1 if present
R	Rational thinking loss	1 if psychotic for any reason
S	Social supports lacking	1 if lacking, especially recent loss
O	Organized plan	1 if plan with lethal method
N	No spouse	1 if divorced, widowed, separated, or single male
S	Sickness	1 if severe or chronic

Guidelines for Actions

POINTS	CLINICAL ACTION
0–2	Send home with follow-up
3–4	Closely follow up; consider hospitalization
5–6	Strongly consider hospitalization
7–10	Hospitalize or commit

Source: From Patterson, W. M., Dohn, H. H., Bird, J., et al. (1983). Evaluation of suicidal patients: The SAD PERSONS scale. *Psychosomatics, 24*(4), 343–345, 348–349.

advisories warn against the use of selective serotonin reuptake inhibitor (SSRI) antidepressants in pregnant women and in children and young adults up to age 24 due to their potential to increase the risk for suicide. Health Canada monitors the safety of these and other psychiatric medications and posts ongoing alerts on its website. Some patients taking psychiatric medications develop extreme restlessness and agitation (akathisia) that can make life intolerable and thereby increase the risk for suicide. The impulsivity associated with mania, and the regret that may be felt because of acts committed during a manic state, may also increase suicidal risk factors. Health care practitioners need to be aware that several medications can induce a manic state (e.g., antidepressants, steroids) and ensure that responses to medications are carefully monitored and that screening for suicide potential is completed (Harvard Medical School, 2007).

Self-Assessment

All health care professionals who work with suicidal people need to collaborate with other clinicians. Fear, grief, anger, puzzlement, and condemnation of suicidal feelings or intent are common. If these intense emotional responses are not acknowledged, counter-transference may limit effective intervention. Understanding the suicidal patient, as well as acknowledging, understanding, and accepting the emotions that arise from working with and caring for these patients, is essential.

IMPLEMENTATION

Nursing interventions for suicide take place at three different levels: primary, secondary, and tertiary. Because improving *overall* community mental health can reduce the incidence of suicide more effectively than extensive efforts directed at identifying imminently suicidal individuals, more attention focused on primary interventions that involve community-wide participation

📋 ASSESSMENT GUIDELINES

Suicide

1. Assess risk factors, including history of suicide (in family, friends), degree of hopelessness and helplessness, and lethality of plan.
2. If there is a history of a suicide attempt, assess intent, lethality, and injury.
3. Determine whether the patient's age, medical condition, psychiatric diagnosis, or current medications put the patient at higher risk.
4. Further assessment is necessary if the patient suddenly goes from sad or depressed to happy and peaceful. Often a decision to kill oneself gives a feeling of relief and calm.
5. If the patient is to be managed on an outpatient basis, also assess social supports and helpfulness of significant others.

can improve outcomes at the community level (Canadian Association for Suicide Prevention, 2009).

Primary Intervention

Primary intervention includes activities that provide support, information, and education to prevent suicide (Box 22-4). The foundation of any intervention for suicide or suicidal behaviours is establishing a therapeutic relationship. Understanding and appreciating clients' unique situations and treating individuals with respect and openness are essential. Nurses who remain informed, empathic, and nonjudgemental are well positioned to initiate interventions at both the individual and the community levels. Primary intervention can be practised in a wide variety of community settings, such as schools, homes, churches, hospitals, and work settings. Elementary school children are screened using evidence-informed tools that focus on both risk factors and warning signs (Joe & Bryant, 2007). Several high schools are

---

BOX 22-4   GOALS OF THE NATIONAL STRATEGY FOR SUICIDE PREVENTION

In 2009, the Canadian Association for Suicide Prevention (2009), released the second edition of the *Blueprint for a National Suicide Prevention Strategy* (the first edition having been released in 2004). It was developed out of the belief that many suicidal behaviours are potentially preventable and that it is the collective responsibility of Canadians to work together toward prevention, intervention, and postvention.

Six principles guided the development of the national strategy (Canadian Association for Suicide Prevention, 2009, p. 9):

1. Suicide prevention is everyone's responsibility.
2. Canadians respect our multicultural and diverse society and accept responsibility to support the dignity of human life.
3. Suicide is an interaction of biological, psychological, social and spiritual factors and can be influenced by societal attitudes and conditions.
4. Strategies must be humane, kindly, effective, caring and should be:
   a. Evidence or experience based
   b. Active and informed
   c. Respectful of community and culture-based knowledge
   d. Inclusive of research, surveillance, evaluation, accountability, and reporting
   e. Reflective of evolving knowledge and practices
5. Many suicides are preventable by knowledgeable, caring, compassionate, and committed communities.
6. We must have the courage to confront the stigma of suicide and the patience to address mental health literacy on both a national and local level.

Awareness and Understanding Goals

1. Promote awareness in every part of Canada that suicide and suicide-related behaviour is our problem and is preventable.
2. Develop broad-based support for suicide prevention, intervention, and postvention.
3. Develop and implement a strategy to reduce stigma, to be associated with all suicide prevention, intervention, and bereavement activities.
4. Increase media knowledge regarding suicide.

Prevention, Intervention and Postvention Goals

1. Develop, implement, and sustain community-based suicide prevention, intervention, and postvention programs, respecting diversity and culture at local, regional, and provincial or territorial levels.
2. Reduce the availability and lethality of suicide methods.
3. Increase training for recognition of risk factors, warning signs and at-risk behaviours and for provision of effective intervention and postvention, targeting key gatekeepers, volunteers, and professionals.
4. Develop and promote effective clinical and professional practice (effective strategies, standards of care) to support patients, families, and communities.
5. Improve access and integration with strong linkages between the continuum-of-care components/services/families.
6. Prioritize intervention and service delivery for high-risk groups while respecting local, regional, and provincial or territorial uniqueness.
7. Increase crisis intervention and support.
8. Increase services and support to those bereaved by suicide or who have attempted suicide.
9. Increase the number of primary prevention activities.

Knowledge Development and Transfer

1. Improve and expand surveillance systems.
2. Promote and support the development of effective evaluation tools.
3. Promote and develop suicide-related research.
4. Increase opportunities for reporting.

Funding and Support

1. Increase funding and support for all activities connected with the CASP Blueprint for a Canadian National Suicide Prevention Strategy (2nd edition).
2. Ensure access to appropriate and adequate health, wellness and recovery services for all Canadians in keeping with the *Canada Health Act.*

Source: Canadian Association for Suicide Prevention. (2009). *The CASP national suicide prevention strategy* (2nd ed., pp. 10–16). Winnipeg: Author. Retrieved from http://www.suicideprevention.ca/wp-content/uploads/2009/10/2010strategy-final-september.pdf.

adopting suicide prevention curricula that involve elements of education, peer support and referral, and discussions about risk factors and warning signs (Ciffone, 2007).

The World Health Organization recommends that any suicide prevention strategy contain the following best practices: timely access to mental health care; responsible and nonsensational media reportage; reduction of access to means of suicide; and education, including awareness raising, stigma reduction, gatekeeper training, research, and surveillance (World Health Organization, 2014).

Secondary Intervention

Secondary intervention is treatment of the actual suicidal crisis. It is practised in clinics, hospitals, and jails and on telephone hotlines. Involving the entire community, especially in primary and secondary interventions, is essential to reducing suicides. Often secondary interventions are the determinants of life or death, and nurses with good crisis intervention skills are in a position to use, role model, and teach these skills to others.

Tertiary Intervention

Tertiary intervention (or **postvention**) refers to interventions with the family and friends of a person who has died by suicide. Postvention aims to both reduce the traumatic aftereffects and explore effective means of addressing survivor problems using primary and secondary interventions. Nurses understand grief or loss well and are in a position to refer, consult, and collaborate in the best interests of those left behind, a vital service since the suicide rate increases for those left behind (Jordan & McIntosh, 2011). Survivors of suicide are in immediate need of supportive avenues for coping with such complicated grief.

Milieu Management
Suicide Precautions

In accordance with unit policies and procedures, the patient is observed continuously by nursing staff. Refer to Table 22-3 for a general description of suicide precautions. This intense attention from the nurse provides for safety and allows for constant reassessment of risk. Monitoring flow sheets for suicide precautions are more clinically useful if they include a description of affect as well as behaviour. For example, instead of noting "Patient watching television," the nurse can describe the patient's affect at each observation interval (e.g., hostile, fearful, calm). Flow sheets should also indicate clear accountability for staff starting and ending their periods of observation. In addition to observing the patient, the nurse is responsible for monitoring the environment for safety hazards. Review Box 22-5 for guidelines on how to minimize physical risks in the milieu.

Studies show that acute care of suicidal patients is usually effective. Suicide risk is highest in the first few days of admission and during times of staff rotation, particularly rotation of psychiatric residents. Assessment of suicidal risk must be an ongoing process; assessment should be performed particularly before a change in level of observation or upon sudden improvement or worsening of symptoms.

Counselling

Counselling skills, including interviewing, crisis care, and problem-solving techniques, are used in both inpatient and outpatient settings. The key element is establishing a working alliance to encourage the patient to engage in more realistic problem solving. Helpful staff characteristics include warmth, sensitivity, interest, and consistency. Once patients leave the hospital, the nurse may see them in the clinic, in a partial hospital program, or in home care.

Talking openly and honestly about suicide and the feelings a patient is having is an important part of the process of ongoing assessment and intervention. Encouraging patients to consult with their physician, community mental health worker, or emergency department if they are experiencing suicidal ideation can be a first step in helping to link them with appropriate resources. While the use of "no-suicide contracts" has been a past practice in mental health work, these contracts are now discouraged, as there is limited evidence to support their value.

TABLE 22-3	SUICIDE PRECAUTIONS WITH CONSTANT ONE-TO-ONE OBSERVATION	
STAFF ASSESSMENT	**POSSIBLE PATIENT SYMPTOMS**	**NURSING RESPONSIBILITIES**
Patient with suicidal ideation or delusions of self-mutilation who, according to assessment by unit staff, presents clinical symptoms that suggest a clear intent to follow through with the plan or delusion	• Patient is currently verbalizing a clear intent to harm self. • Patient shows no insight into existing problems. • Patient has poor impulse control. • Patient has already attempted suicide in the recent past by a particularly lethal method (e.g., hanging, gun, carbon monoxide poisoning).	1. Conduct one-to-one nursing observation and interaction 24 hours a day (never let patient out of staff's sight). 2. Maintain arm's length observation at all times. 3. Chart patient's whereabouts and record mood, verbatim statements, and behaviour every 15 to 30 minutes per protocol. 4. Ensure that meal trays contain no glass or metal silverware. 5. When patient is sleeping, patient's hands should always be in view, not under the bedcovers. 6. Carefully observe patient swallow each dose of medication. 7. Respectfully maintain observation even when patient is in the bathroom. 8. The nurse and physician should explain to the patient what they will be doing and why; both document this explanation in the chart.

BOX 22-5 ENVIRONMENTAL GUIDELINES FOR MINIMIZING SUICIDAL BEHAVIOUR ON THE PSYCHIATRIC UNIT

- Conduct frequent environmental tours of all areas of the unit, including patient bathrooms and other private spaces.
- Provide plastic eating utensils.
- Do not assign patient to a private room, and ensure that the door remains open at all times.
- Jump-proof and hang-proof the bathrooms by installing break-away shower rods and recessed shower nozzles.
- Keep electrical cords to a minimal length.
- Install unbreakable glass in windows. Install tamper-proof screens or partitions too small to pass through. Keep all windows locked.
- Lock all utility rooms, kitchens, adjacent stairwells, and offices. All nonclinical staff (e.g., housekeepers, maintenance workers) should receive instructions to keep doors locked.
- Take all potentially harmful gifts (e.g., flowers in glass vases) from visitors before allowing them to see patients.
- Go through personal belongings with patient present, and remove all potentially harmful objects (e.g., belts, shoelaces, metal nail files, tweezers, matches, razors, perfume, shampoo).
- Ensure that visitors do not bring in or leave potentially harmful objects in patient's room (e.g., matches, nail files).
- Search patient for harmful objects (e.g., drugs, weapons, sharp objects, cords) on return from pass.

Health Teaching and Health Promotion

The nurse teaches the patient about psychiatric diagnoses, medications and complementary therapies, and age-related crises. Teaching regarding community resources, coping skills, stress management, and communication skills is also important. When possible, the family or significant others are included to strengthen the patient's support system. A focus on personal strengths and positive thoughts and emotions (e.g., hope) is essential (Harvard Medical School, 2007). Talk therapy, in addition to medications, should be incorporated.

Case Management

Case management is an important aspect of nursing care for the suicidal patient. The patient's perception of being alone without supports often blinds the person to the real support figures who are present. Reconnecting the patient with family and friends is a major focus, whether in the hospital or the community. Aftercare referral may be given and may include information on the following resources: substance treatment centres, crisis hotlines, support groups for patients or families, and recreational activities to enhance socialization and self-esteem. Encouraging the patient to get reacquainted with a previous spiritual support system can also be beneficial.

Pharmacological Interventions

A significant nursing intervention to assist the suicidal patient in regaining self-control is the careful administration of medication. All medications given to high-risk patients are monitored carefully, although lethal overdose is nearly impossible with SSRIs, unlike with the risky tricyclic antidepressants and monoamine oxidase inhibitors. Mouth checks may be used to be sure patients are not saving (hoarding) medications in the hospital; in the community, provision of a limited day supply or family supervision is required.

Antidepressants should be ordered for patients who have depressive or anxiety disorders, with an emphasis on administering an adequate dosage and providing appropriate clinical evaluation when using SSRIs. Close monitoring must occur during the 2- to 3-week postinitiation period, when energy increases can lead to acting on suicidal ideation, and during times of dosage adjustment. Astute nursing care involves careful patient (and family, if appropriate) teaching about the identified benefits and risks of antidepressant therapy.

There is clear evidence that long-term lithium treatment for bipolar disorder and major depression significantly reduces suicide and suicide attempts. Some studies have shown a reduced suicide rate among patients with schizophrenia receiving clozapine. Thus far, no clinical studies have examined the effect of antianxiety treatment on suicide risk.

An alternative somatic treatment for acute suicidal risk is electroconvulsive therapy (ECT). Evidence suggests that ECT decreases acute suicidal ideation. Refer to Chapter 13 for further discussion of ECT.

Postvention for Survivors of Suicide

A discussion of suicidal patients is incomplete without noting the issues surrounding a death by suicide. Surviving family and friends can experience overwhelming guilt and shame, compounded by the difficulty of discussing the frequently taboo subject of suicide (Peters, Murphy, & Jackson, 2013). The usual social supports of neighbours and church are sometimes lacking for these mourners.

Evidence collected in a systematic review that investigated differences in mental health and grief reactions between suicide survivors and other bereaved groups found no significant differences. However, the variables of rejections, shame, stigma, concealing the cause of death, and blaming showed significant difference among those grieving suicide (Sveen & Walby, 2008). See Box 22-6 for suggestions that survivors have made to health care providers who want to be sure to meet the survivors' needs.

Staff members who have cared for a suicide victim are similarly traumatized by suicide. Staff may also experience symptoms of post-traumatic stress disorder, with guilt, shock, anger, shame, and decreased self-esteem. Group support is essential as the treatment team conducts a thorough psychological postmortem assessment. The event is carefully reviewed to identify the potential overlooked clues, faulty judgements, or changes that are needed in employer protocols.

Most facilities have a clear policy about communication with families after suicide. Although some lawyers advise having no contact except through them, others recommend designating a spokesperson who can address the feelings of the family without discussing the details of the patient's care. Referrals should be

BOX 22-6 SURVIVORS' ADVICE TO HEALTH CARE PROVIDERS

- If being a survivor is the main reason treatment has been sought, remember that the survivor, not the deceased, is the patient. Focus on the patient's thoughts and feelings, and do a thorough assessment as you usually would.
- Remember that the most difficult time for survivors is not so much in the immediate aftermath of the suicide; rather, it is in the weeks, months, and years following it. Make frequent efforts to reach out to these individuals, especially on the most difficult anniversary dates. Do not be afraid of talking about the deceased person—in fact, speak of him or her often. While this may seem counterintuitive and may feel uncomfortable, survivors of suicide universally want their loved one to be remembered in this way. Talking reduces the hurt, isolation, and stigma.
- If being a survivor comes out as an incidental finding during an assessment, ask open-ended questions and evaluate how much the loss has been resolved.
- Recommend community resources and survivor support groups, and show empathy about the loss of someone to suicide. Know about local Survivors of Suicide (SOS) support groups in your area, and refer the survivors and their families as soon as possible following the suicide.

Source: Centre for Addiction and Mental Health. (2011). *Hope and healing after suicide. A practical guide for people who have lost someone to suicide in Ontario.* Retrieved from http://knowledgex.camh.net/amhspecialists/resources_families/Documents/hope_and_healing.pdf.

given to family members to try to assist them in dealing with their grief and to address any emotional problems that develop, especially in adolescents. Alberta Health Services (2017) has published *Healing Your Spirit: Surviving After the Suicide of a Loved One*, a practical guidebook for people who have lost someone to suicide. British Columbia (Centre for Applied Research in Mental Health and Addiction, 2007) and Ontario (Centre for Addiction and Mental Health, 2011) have adapted that booklet, tailoring the practical information to their own provincial resources. These booklets are all available online.

As for documentation, all staff members need to ensure that the record is complete and that any late entries are identified. Courts require that the patient be periodically evaluated for suicide risk, that the treatment plan provide for high-level security, and that staff members follow the individual treatment plan. Despite adherence to institution protocols, treatment plans, and the appropriate standards of practice, suicides do occasionally still happen, especially with patients in the community. Human behaviour is simply not predictable.

EVALUATION

Evaluation of a suicidal patient is ongoing. The nurse must be constantly alert to changes in the suicidal person's mood, thinking, and behaviour. The nurse also looks for indications that the patient is communicating thoughts and feelings more readily and that the patient's social network is widening. For example,

it is a positive sign if the person is able to talk about his or her feelings and engage in problem solving with the nurse. Is the patient increasing his or her social activities and expanding his or her interests? The nurse must remember that suicidal behaviour is the result of interpersonal turmoil. If an episode of major depression is the main admitting diagnosis and a serious suicidal gesture resulted from this depression, both problems are initially assessed and treated. When the patient is no longer an acute suicide risk, treating the depression becomes the main focus of care. Essentially, the nurse evaluates each short-term goal and establishes new ones as the patient progresses toward the long-term goal of resolving suicidal ideation.

Once stabilized, the patient may qualify for transfer to an intensive outpatient (IOP) treatment program, which involves continuing treatment after discharge, or a partial hospitalization program (PHP), which allows patients to go home in the evenings to practise new coping skills. Community-based support groups are also available and are both effective and free of charge. Nurses need to be knowledgeable about, and proactive in, referring patients to these support groups.

NONSUICIDAL SELF-INJURY

A problem closely related to suicidal behaviour is nonsuicidal self-injury. Nonsuicidal self-injury is also commonly known as self-injurious behaviour, self-mutilation, parasuicide, deliberate self-harm, self-abuse, and self-inflicted violence (Klonsky, Muehlenkamp, Lewis, et al., 2011). These self-injuries are deliberate and direct attempts to inflict shallow yet painful injuries to the surface of the body without intending to end one's life. The behaviour most commonly consists of cutting, burning, scraping or scratching skin, biting, hitting, skin or hair picking, and interfering with wound healing. Often the self-injurers report multiple methods of self-injury.

For these behaviours to be considered significant, they typically last at least a year and happen repeatedly. The majority of self-injurers do not seek professional help. Even when they are not engaged in the behaviours, those who self-harm tend to be preoccupied with self-injury. Self-injurious actions are most often done with the intent to self-punish, to alleviate psychic pain, or to pierce the psychic numbness these individuals describe, in what is referred to as "antidissociation" (Doyle, Sheridan, & Treacy, 2017, p. 134).

EPIDEMIOLOGY

The lifetime prevalence of nonsuicidal self-injury is difficult to accurately determine due to attempts to conceal the behaviour. However, some have estimated that between 13% and 23% of adolescents engage in the behaviours. It is a global problem, peaking between 20 to 29 years of age with 17% to 35% reporting engaging in the behaviour. There is a decline in the behaviour beyond this age. Estimates are that approximately 6% of the U.S. population has engaged in the behaviour at some time in their lives. Research regarding prevalence by gender is inconclusive. Some studies report that there is less discrepancy between the sexes than there is with suicidal behaviour.

COMORBIDITY

Nonsuicidal self-injury often occurs with other mental health disorders, including depression, anxiety, eating disorders, and substance use disorders. In the past, researchers thought there was a direct relationship between borderline personality disorder and nonsuicidal self-injury. However, Bracken-Minor and McDevitt-Murphy (2014) conducted research and concluded that the emotional regulation and distress tolerance found in individuals with nonsuicidal self-injury was distinctly different than characteristics found in borderline personality disorder.

RISK FACTORS

Biological Factors

Studies related to the physiological mechanism of action in nonsuicidal self-injury are inconclusive; however, researchers continue to investigate the neurobiological mechanisms behind the disorder. Several neurochemical pathways in the brain play a role in the development of these behaviours. Although studies are inconclusive, the neurotransmitter group of monoamines including serotonin, dopamine, and norepinephrine may play a role in the mediation of self-injury, and research is ongoing. As practitioners continue to search for an effective treatment, clinical research will seek to find the neurobiological basis of nonsuicidal self-injury.

Environmental Factors
Cultural

Recent studies have investigated the prevalence of nonsuicidal self-injury behaviours internationally to determine best practices for treatment and whether culturally different approaches to care are relevant. Similar rates of the behaviour occur among adolescents in the United States and among several European countries, with the behaviour stabilizing among youth over the last several years and no significant increases seen internationally. With this stabilization in occurrence rates, researchers have an opportunity to further investigate cultural differences in the behaviour and whether these differences lead to different treatment modalities.

Societal

Self-injurious behaviours such as cutting may be a social phenomenon that is rampant in society. Individuals often learn about the behaviour from a peer who is engaging in nonsuicidal self-injury and begin using the behaviours themselves in an attempt to alleviate personal discomfort. In fact, when an individual who engages in nonsuicidal self-injury is admitted to an inpatient unit, others on the unit begin to engage in the behaviour.

CLINICAL PICTURE

Nonsuicidal self-injury is not an official disorder in the *Diagnostic and Statistical Manual of Mental Disorders (DSM-5)*. It is still under review to determine whether it will become a recognized disorder by the American Psychiatric Association. However, the behaviours associated with the disorder are often seen in both inpatient and outpatient settings. This self-harm differs from suicide attempt in terms of motivation, familial transmission (found only in suicidal behaviour), age of onset (younger in nonsuicidal self-injury), psychopathology, and functional impairment (greater in suicide attempt) (Turecki & Brent, 2016). There is limited research on the effectiveness of nursing care for patients who engage in nonsuicidal self-injury. However, holistic interdisciplinary approaches to care where patients are included in planning their care will likely lead to best outcomes.

ASSESSMENT

A history from the patient regarding the self-injurious behaviour includes types of self-injury, triggers for the behaviour, and frequency of the behaviour (Tofthagen, Talseth, & Fagerström, 2014). In addition, ask the patient what has worked effectively in stopping the behaviours in the past. Appropriate physical assessment to determine the condition of wounds, if present, allows you to plan appropriate interventions.

Self-Assessment

Nurses caring for patients who engage in self-injury report that they are emotionally affected by caring for these patients. Emotions experienced include feeling defeated by relapses, discouragement, and powerlessness (Tofthagen, Talseth, & Fagerström, 2014). In addition, nurses need to be aware that transference may occur through projection of the patient's emotions onto the nurse. Establishing appropriate professional boundaries with the patient is important for self-care, as is collaboration with other clinicians.

DIAGNOSIS

The nursing diagnoses with the highest priorities are *Self-mutilation* and *Risk for self-mutilation*. Patients may be experiencing feelings of anxiety, tension, and self-reproach. Consider any nursing diagnosis that is appropriate for underlying comorbid psychiatric disorders as appropriate (see the chapters in Unit 4 for further information).

OUTCOMES CRITERIA

The relevant *Nursing Outcomes Classification (NOC)* is *Mutilation self-restraint*, which is defined as "personal actions to refrain from intentional self-inflected injury" (Moorhead, Johnson, Maas, et al., 2013, p. 1406). Measurements for this outcome include:

- Refrains from gathering means for self-injury
- Obtains assistance as needed
- Refrains from injuring self
- Uses available support groups
- Uses medication as prescribed
- Uses effective coping strategies

PLANNING

The plan of care for individuals who engage in self-injury includes demonstration of a caring attitude toward the patient, bearing hope for recovery, observing for signs of self-harm, evaluating the need for medication, and providing appropriate interventions for patients' wounds and injuries. Engage patients in their recovery plan, which encompasses a six-step approach to recovery including (1) limit setting for safety, (2) developing self-esteem, (3) discovery of the motive for self-injury and the role it served for the patient, (4) learning that self-injury can be self-controlled, (5) replacing the self-injury with coping skills, and (6) entering a maintenance phase (Gonzales & Bergstrom, 2013).

INTERVENTIONS

Basic nursing interventions for patients with nonsuicidal self-injury include caring for the patient's wounds and injuries, establishing a therapeutic alliance, and teaching coping skills to replace the self-injurious behaviours. A therapeutic relationship will provide support and an alternative to self-injury when anxiety increases.

Advanced-practice psychiatric mental health nurses may work with patients who use self-injury to cope. Psychotherapeutic interventions for this population should facilitate the patient's ability to learn coping strategies. Specific therapies that are used include cognitive behavioural therapy, dialectical behaviour therapy, and problem-solving therapy, which may take place in individual or group therapy. There are no specific medical treatments for self-harm or self-injury. Treating underlying psychiatric disorders using psychopharmacology is an additional role of the advanced-practice nurse.

EVALUATION

Similar to suicidal behaviour, the evaluation of patients with nonsuicidal self-injury behaviours is ongoing. The development of a therapeutic alliance with the patient allows for the patient to trust the care provider. The nurse must continue to evaluate whether the patient is communicating his or her thoughts and feelings accurately and whether the patient's perception is that engagement in the behaviours is declining while being replaced with appropriate coping skills.

KEY POINTS TO REMEMBER

- Suicide is a significant public health problem in Canada.
- Suicide is everyone's business.
- Specific biological, psychosocial, and cultural factors are known to increase the risk for suicide.
- Most suicidal patients can be helped by treatment of a coexisting psychiatric disorder.
- Certain medical conditions and psychiatric diagnoses are associated with increased risk for suicide.
- Suicidal ideation must be taken seriously, even if the person has a history of multiple attempts.
- The nurse can have a real impact on suicide prevention through primary, secondary, and tertiary interventions.
- Nursing care of the suicidal patient is challenging but rewarding: patients' desperate feelings evoke intense reactions in staff, but most people with suicidal ideation respond to treatment and do not complete suicide.
- If a patient dies by suicide, family, friends, and health care workers are traumatized and need support, possibly including referrals for mental health intervention.

CRITICAL THINKING

1. Locate and review the suicide protocol at your hospital unit or community centre. Are there any steps you anticipate having difficulty carrying out? Discuss these difficulties with your peers or clinical group.
2. Knowing that nurses can suffer postsuicide stress and that they need support when those in their care are involved in suicidal behaviour, do you believe that help is available for nurses? What sort of support do you feel would be most helpful to you in this situation? How would you respond to another staff member who expresses guilt over the death by suicide of a patient on your unit?
3. Identify three common and expected emotional reactions that a nurse might have when initially working with people who are suicidal.
   a. How do you think you might react?
   b. What actions could you take to deal with the event and obtain support?
4. In addition to psychiatric mental health nursing practice areas, are there other practice areas in which nursing assessments for self-harm would strengthen client care? How does knowing the reason for a patient self-harming make a difference in planning care?

CHAPTER REVIEW

1. Which assessment statements would be appropriate for a patient who may be suicidal? Select all that apply.
   a. Do you ever think about suicide?
   b. Are you thinking of hurting yourself?
   c. Do you sometimes wish you were dead?
   d. Has it ever seemed like life is not worth living?
   e. If you were to kill yourself, how would you do it?
   f. Does it seem as though others might be better off if you were dead?

2. Jon, 15 years old, asks the community health nurse what the greatest health risk for his age group is. How should the nurse respond?
   a. Suicide
   b. Substance abuse
   c. Eating disorders
   d. Unintentional injuries

3. Ms. Rallyea, 58 years old, is admitted with severe clinical depression and started on antidepressant medications. Her mood has remained low and she has not initiated conversation. On her fifteenth day of hospitalization, she informs the nurse that she is feeling great and energetic. What should the nurse do?
   a. Notify the social worker of the improvement to schedule a discharge planning conference.
   b. Invite Ms. Rallyea to talk and ask her if she is thinking of hurting herself.
   c. Report to the team that the antidepressant medication is effective.
   d. Chart the mood change and share the observation at the team meeting the next day.

4. A nurse has great difficulty distancing herself from the care of a client when she leaves work. What should the nurse do?
   a. Recognize that she is too compassionate.
   b. Request that the client be assigned to another nurse.
   c. Share her concern with the patient.
   d. Confide in a colleague she trusts.

℮volve WEBSITE

Post-Test interactive review

Visit the Evolve website for Chapter Review Answers and Rationales, Critical Thinking Answer Guidelines, and additional resources related to the content in this chapter: http://evolve.elsevier.com/Canada/Varcarolis/psychiatric/

REFERENCES

Ahmedani, B., Simon, G., Stewart, C., et al. (2014). Health care contacts in the year before suicide death. *Journal of General Internal Medicine, 29*(6), 870–877. doi:10.1007/s11606-014-2767-3.

Ahuja, A., Webster, C., Gibson, N., et al. (2015). Bullying and suicide: The mental health crisis of LGBTQ youth and how you can help. *Journal of Gay & Lesbian Mental Health, 19*(2), 125–144. doi:10.1080/19359705.2015.1007417.

Alberta Health Services. (2017). *Healing your spirit: Surviving after the suicide of a loved one.* Retrieved from http://www.albertahealthservices.ca/assets/healthinfo/ipc/hi-ip-pipt-chc-healing-your-spirit-2017.pdf.

Appel, J. M. (2007). A suicide right for the mentally ill? A Swiss case opens a new debate. *Hastings Center Report, 37,* 21–23. doi:10.1353/hcr.2007.0035.

Battin, M., van der Heide, A., Ganzini, L., et al. (2007). Legal physician-assisted dying in Oregon and the Netherlands: Evidence concerning the impact on patients in "vulnerable" groups. *Journal of Medical Ethics, 33,* 591–597. doi:10.1136/jme.2007.022335.

Beaton, S., Forster, P., & Maple, M. (2012). The language of suicide. *The Psychologist, 25,* 731. Retrieved from http://blog.une.edu.au/crnmentalhealth/2012/10/08/the-language-of-suicide/.

Boyd, J. E., Adler, E. P., Otilingam, P. G., et al. (2014). Internalized Stigma of Mental Illness (ISMI) Scale: A multinational review. *Comprehensive Psychiatry, 55,* 221–231.

Bracken-Minor, K., & McDevitt-Murphy, M. (2014). Differences in features of non-suicidal self-injury according to borderline personality disorder screening status. *Archives of Suicide Research, 18,* 88–103.

Brendel, R. W., Breezing, A., Lagomasino, I. T., et al. (2016). The suicidal patient. In T. A. Stern, J. R. Rosenbaum, M. Fava, et al. (Eds.), *Massachusetts General Hospital comprehensive clinical psychiatry* (2nd ed., pp. 589–598). St. Louis: Mosby.

Canadian Association for Suicide Prevention (2009). *The CASP national suicide prevention strategy* (2nd ed.). Winnipeg: Author. Retrieved from http://www.suicideprevention.ca/wp-content/uploads/2009/10/2010strategy-final-september.pdf.

Carballo, J. J., Akamnonu, C. P., & Oquendo, M. A. (2008). Neurobiology of suicidal behavior: An integration of biological and clinical findings. *Archives of Suicide Research, 12,* 93–110. doi:10.1080/13811110701857004.

Centre for Addiction and Mental Health. (2011). *Hope and healing after suicide: A practical guide for people who have lost someone to suicide in Ontario.* Retrieved from http://knowledgex.camh.net/amhspecialists/resources_families/Documents/hope_and_healing.pdf.

Centre for Addiction and Mental Health. (2015). *Suicide prevention and assessment handbook.* Retrieved from https://www.camh.ca/en/hospital/health_information/a_z_mental_health_and_addiction_information/suicide/Documents/sp_handbook_final_feb_2011.pdf.

Centre for Applied Research in Mental Health and Addiction. (2007). *Hope and healing: A practical guide for survivors of suicide.* Retrieved from http://www.comh.ca/publications/resources/pub_hh/HopeandHealing.pdf.

Ciffone, J. C. (2007). Suicide prevention: An analysis and replication of a curriculum-based high school program. *Social Work, 52*(1), 41–49.

Criminal Code, R. S. C. *1985, c. C-46.* (2011). Retrieved from http://laws-lois.justice.gc.ca/eng/acts/C-46/page-103.html#s-241.

Criminal Code, R. S. C. *1985, c. C-46.* (2016). Retrieved from http://laws-lois.justice.gc.ca/eng/AnnualStatutes/2016_3/FullText.html.

Doyle, L., Sheridan, A., & Treacy, M. P. (2017). Motivations for adolescent self-harm and the implications for mental health nurses. *Journal of Psychiatric and Mental Health Nursing, 24*(2–3), 134. doi:10.1111/jpm.12360.

Dwivedi, Y., & Pandey, G. (2011). Elucidating biological risk factors in suicide: Role of protein kinase A. *Progress in Neuro-Psychopharmacology & Biological Psychiatry, 35,* 831–841. doi:10.1016/j.pnpbp.2010.08.025.

Fetzner, M. G., Abrams, M. P., & Asmundson, G. J. G. (2013). Symptoms of posttraumatic stress disorder and depression in relation to alcohol-use and alcohol-related problems among Canadian Forces veterans/Symptômes du trouble de stress post-traumatique et de dépression relatifs à la consommation d'alcool et aux problèmes liés à l'alcool chez les anciens combattants des forces Canadiennes. *Canadian Journal of Psychiatry, 58*(7), 417.

Finlay, I., & George, R. (2011). Legal physician-assisted suicide in Oregon and the Netherlands: Evidence concerning the impact on patients in vulnerable groups—Another perspective on Oregon's data. *Journal of Medical Ethics, 37*, 171–174. doi:10.1136/jme.2010.037044.

Ganz, D., Braquehais, M. D., & Sher, L. (2010). Secondary prevention of suicide. *PLoS Medicine, 7*, 1–4. doi:10.1371/journal.pmed.1000271.

Gonzales, A., & Bergstrom, L. (2013). Adolescent non-suicidal self-injury (NSSI) interventions. *Journal of Child and Adolescent Psychiatric Nursing, 26*, 124–130. doi:10.1111/jcap.12035.

Government of Canada. (2016). *Working together to prevent suicide in Canada: The 2016 progress report on the federal framework for suicide prevention.* Retrieved from http://www.healthycanadians.gc.ca/publications/healthy-living-vie-saine/framework-suicide-progress-report-2016-rapport-d-etape-cadre-suicide/alt/64-03-15-1430-suicideprev-progressreport-eng.pdf.

Guintivano, J., Brown, T., Newcomer, A., et al. (2014). Identification and replication of a combined epigenetic and genetic biomarker predicting suicide and suicidal behaviors. *American Journal of Psychiatry, 171*(12), 1287–1296.

Harvard Medical School. (2007). Antidepressants and suicide. *Harvard Mental Health Letter, 24*(1), 1–4.

Health Canada. (2016). *First Nation and Inuit health: Suicide prevention.* Retrieved from http://www.hc-sc.gc.ca/fniah-spnia/promotion/suicide/index-eng.php.

Health Law Institute. (2017). *End of life law and policy in Canada.* Retrieved from http://eol.law.dal.ca/?page_id=221.

Hewitt, P. L., Caelian, C. F., Chen, C., et al. (2014). Perfectionism, stress, daily hassles, hopelessness, and suicide potential in depressed psychiatric adolescents. *Journal of Psychopathology and Behavioral Assessment, 36*(4), 663–674. doi:10.1007/s10862-014-9427-0.

Hogan, M., & Grumet, J. G. (2016). Suicide prevention: An emerging priority for health care. *Health Affairs, 35*(6), 1084–1090.

Inuit Tapiriit Kanatami. (2016). *National Inuit suicide prevention strategy.* Retrieved from https://www.itk.ca/wp-content/uploads/2016/07/ITK-National-Inuit-Suicide-Prevention-Strategy-2016.pdf.

Joe, S., & Bryant, H. (2007). Evidence-based suicide prevention screening in schools. *Children & Schools, 29*(4), 219–227.

Jordan, J. R., & McIntosh, J. L. (2011). *Grief after suicide: Understanding the consequences and caring for the survivors.* New York: Routledge.

Kiamanesh, P., Dieserud, G., & Haavind, H. (2015). From a cracking façade to a total escape: Maladaptive perfectionism and suicide. *Death Studies, 39*(5), 316–322. doi:10.1080/07481187.2014.946625.

Kids Help Phone. (2016). *Teens Talk 2016: A Kids Help Phone report on the well-being of teens in Canada.* Retrieved from http://org.kidshelpphone.ca/main-data/uploads/2015/09/kids-help-phone-teens-talk-2016.pdf.

Klonsky, E. D., Muehlenkamp, J. J., Lewis, S. P., et al. (2011). *Nonsuicidal self-injury.* Toronto: Hogrefe Publishing.

Leong, F., & Leach, M. (2008). *Suicide among racial and ethnic minority groups: Theory, research and practice.* New York: Routledge.

Marr, N., & Field, T. (2000). *Bullycide: Death at playtime.* Didcot, UK: Success Unlimited.

Meerwijk, E., van Meijel, B., van den Bout, J., et al. (2010). Development and evaluation of a guideline for nursing care of suicidal patients with schizophrenia. *Perspectives in Psychiatric Care, 46*(1), 65–73. doi:10.1111/j.1744-6163.2009.00239.x.

Mental Health Commission of Canada (2017). *Advancing the mental health strategy for Canada: A framework for action.* Ottawa: Author. Retrieved from http://www.mentalhealthcommission.ca/English/framework-action-2017-2022.

Moorhead, S., Johnson, M., Maas, M. L., et al. (2013). *Nursing outcomes classification (NOC)* (5th ed.). St Louis: Mosby.

Muehlenkamp, J., Brausch, A., Quigley, K., et al. (2013). Interpersonal features and functions of nonsuicidal self-injury. *Suicide and Life-Threat Behavior, 43*(1), 67–80. doi:10.1111/j.1943-278X.2012.00128.x.

National Defence and the Canadian Armed Forces. (2016). *2016 Report on Suicide Mortality in the Canadian Armed Forces (1995 to 2015).* Retrieved from http://www.forces.gc.ca/en/about-reports-pubs-health/report-on-suicide-mortality-caf-2016.page.

Office of the Correctional Investigator Canada. (2014). *A three-year review of federal inmate suicides (2011–2014).* Retrieved from http://www.oci-bec.gc.ca/cnt/rpt/pdf/oth-aut/oth-aut20140910-eng.pdf.

Patterson, W. M., Dohn, H. H., Bird, J., et al. (1983). Evaluation of suicidal patients: The SAD PERSONS scale. *Psychosomatics, 24*(4), 343–345, 348–349.

Perlman, C. M., Neufeld, E., Martin, L., et al. (2011). *Suicide risk assessment guide: A resource for Canadian health care organizations.* Toronto: Ontario Hospital Association and Canadian Patient Safety Institute. Available at http://www.oha.com/KnowledgeCentre/Documents/Final%20-%20Suicide%20Risk%20Assessment%20Guidebook.pdf.

Peters, K., Murphy, G., & Jackson, D. (2013). Events prior to completed suicide: Perspectives of family members. *Issues in Mental Health Nursing, 34*(5), 309–316. doi:10.3109/01612840.2012.751639.

Riley, E. T. (2016). Chronic traumatic encephalopathy and professional athletes: Suicides are contagious. *World Neurosurgery, 94*, 576–577. doi:10.1016/j.wneu.2016.04.055.

Rocket, I. (2010). Counting suicides and making suicide count as a public health problem. *Journal of Crisis Intervention and Suicide Prevention, 31*, 227–230. doi:10.1027/0227-5910/a000071.

Sadock, B. J., Sadock, V. A., & Ruiz, P. (2017). *Kaplan and Sadock's concise textbook of clinical psychiatry* (4th ed.). Philadelphia: Lippincott Williams & Wilkins.

Smith, G. (2014). The nature and scope of gambling in Canada. *Addiction (Abingdon, England), 109*(5), 706–710. doi:10.1111/add.12210.

Statistics Canada. (2016). *Table 02-0563—Leading causes of death, total population, by sex, Canada, provinces and territories, annual.* Retrieved from http://www5.statcan.gc.ca/cansim/a47.

Sveen, C., & Walby, F. A. (2008). Suicide survivors' mental health and grief reactions: A systematic review of controlled studies. *Suicide & Life-Threatening Behavior, 38*(1), 13–29. doi:10.1521/suli.2008.38.1.13.

Tofthagen, R., Talseth, A., & Fagerström, L. (2014). Mental health nurses' experiences of caring for patients suffering from self-harm. *Nursing Research and Practice, 2014*, 1–10. doi:10.1155/2014/905741.

Toth, M., Schwartz, R., & Kurka, S. (2007). Strategies for understanding and assessing suicide risk in psychotherapy. *Annals of the American Psychotherapy Association, 10*(4), 18–25. Retrieved from http://www.annalsofpsychotherapy.com/index.php.

Turecki, G., & Brent, D. A. (2016). Suicide and suicidal behaviour. *The Lancet, 387*(10024), 1227–1239. doi:10.1016/S0140-6736(15)00234-2.

Veterans Affairs. (2016). *2013 Life After Service Studies (LASS).* Retrieved from http://www.veterans.gc.ca/eng/news/vac-responds/just-the-facts/life-after-service-studies.

World Health Organization. (2014). *Preventing suicide: a global imperative.* Retrieved from http://www.who.int/mental_health/suicide-prevention/world_report_2014/en/.

Zamorski, M. A., Rolland-Harris, E., Jetly, R., et al. (2015). Military deployments, posttraumatic stress disorder, and suicide risk in Canadian Armed Forces personnel and veterans. *The Canadian Journal of Psychiatry, 60*(4), 200. doi:10.1177/070674371506000407.

23

Anger, Aggression, and Violence

Melodie B. Hull

KEY TERMS AND CONCEPTS

aggression
bullying
de-escalation techniques
locus of control (LOC)

rage
trauma-informed care
violence

OBJECTIVES

1. Compare and contrast three theories that explore the determinants for anger, aggression, and violence.
2. Distinguish between the emotions of anger and rage and the behavioural manifestations of aggression and violence.
3. Identify precipitators to anger, aggression, or violence.
4. Compare and contrast interventions for a patient with healthy coping skills with those for a patient with marginal coping behaviours.
5. Identify four principles of de-escalation with a moderately angry patient.
6. Describe two criteria for the use of seclusion or restraint.

⊖volve WEBSITE

Visit the Evolve website for Flashcards, Case Studies, and additional testing resources related to the content in this chapter: http://evolve.elsevier.com/Canada/Varcarolis/psychiatric/

Pre-Test | interactive review

Anger, aggression, and violence are the subject of daily news headlines. Anger is a normal, natural emotion that occurs on a continuum, stemming from a wide variety of feelings that are sometimes misinterpreted as anger (e.g., jealousy, confusion). Evidence of the scope and prevalence of the problem can been seen in an expanding list of terminology used to describe specific types of aggression. For example, *road rage* is a dangerous aggressive response to anger that is accompanied by cursing, offensive gestures, and cutting off others while driving. Road rage is rampant in high-stress industrialized societies. *Workplace violence* includes lashing out at work. Hospitals are potential sites for this particular type of violence. Violence can also be experienced through engagement with online activities. It often occurs through social media sites. Posts, photos, messages, and so forth that are distributed online and are intended to harm the target are expressions of anger and aggression and result in

psychological violence. One example of online violence is *revenge porn* sites, where suggestive, intimate photos are shared with the intent to demean and punish. In many of these cases, provocative sexual photos are used and the face of the target victim is Photoshopped into the picture. Harsh, hostile, and explicit commentary is written by the perpetrator seeking revenge.

CLINICAL PICTURE

Once the anger response is triggered, it can escalate into overt or passive aggression, even violence. Not everyone responds to anger with aggression and violence. A healthy and appropriate release of anger might lead to talking about the trigger in an effort to reduce its impact or to provide a signal to the person expressing it that an anger-provoking stressor is present. There are also instances when anger is suppressed. For example, victims

BOX 23-1   FEELINGS THAT MAY PRECIPITATE ANGER

- Discounted, ignored, or rejected
- Embarrassed or humiliated
- Frightened
- Guilty
- Hurt
- Inadequate
- Insecure
- Unheard
- Overwhelmed
- Powerlessness: no control of the situation
- Threatened
- Tired
- Vulnerable

of bullying experience the fight or flight response with each bullying incident. However, this response is frequently not acted on by the victim for fear of an escalation of the bullying. In the case of cyberbullying, however, this may not be the case. Research has begun to show that some victims react impulsively and reciprocate the anger and aggression (Pabian & Vandebosch, 2016). This is an example of reactive aggression. In addition, Frey, Higheagle Strong, and Onyewuenyi (2017) have found that when perpetrators believe their dominance is challenged, they perceive this as a threat to goal attainment and therefore feel justified in retaliating, which further escalates bullying behaviours. Thus cyberbullying can be a vicious cycle. Understanding the emotion of anger, its etiology, and its psychological and behavioural manifestations are key to accurate assessment, intervention, and treatment. Box 23-1 provides examples of feelings that may precipitate anger.

Anger is a key diagnostic criteria in intermittent explosive disorder, oppositional defiant disorder, disruptive mood dysregulation disorder, borderline personality disorder, and bipolar disorder (American Psychiatric Association, 2013). Anger is an

VIGNETTE

Solange is a 41-year-old woman with a diagnosis of bipolar disorder. She has a history of eight hospital admissions to acute care psychiatry over the past 20 years. She is experiencing a manic episode, which includes affect dysregulation. She has been admitted as an involuntary patient to the psychiatric unit of a general hospital. Being admitted against her wishes frustrates and angers her. She attempts to intimidate the staff with verbal aggression and threats. She refuses to take her mood-stabilizing medications. She exhibits hyperactivity, racing thoughts, poor judgement, distractibility, pressured speech, and sleep deprivation. She has very low frustration tolerance and reacts spontaneously and impulsively to stressors. Solange feels trapped. She is able to voice her feelings of being overwhelmed and out of control, but she is quite incapable of dealing with these feelings. Nursing interventions require setting clear and consistent limits on her behaviours to promote a low-stimulus environment. Seclusion is ordered when Solange is unable to exhibit self-control of her behaviour.

emotional response that can be released appropriately or inappropriately, suppressed over periods of time, or controlled in its release (emotional regulation). It does not always lead to violence. Anger can be functional when it prompts individuals to remove obstacles and barriers to achieving their goals but is also seen as an enhancer of creativity in, for example, problem solving, conflict resolution, and restructuring environments (Yang & Hung, 2015). For some people, anger is a coping response to embarrassment, jealousy, or fear of rejection or replacement. Personal appraisals of self-worth and self-efficacy also factor into the anger response. Suppressed anger, a learned response from decades of political and societal oppression, is not uncommon for those who have experienced historical trauma, such as that experienced by Indigenous peoples of Canada.

Rage is an uncontrollable, violent state of anger and is quite uncommon. Once the person has begun expressing rage, he or she cannot think clearly or logically, and psychosocial or cognitive behavioural interventions are not possible. Rage must dissipate on its own. Protective strategies are necessary both for the person in a state of rage and for those around him or her.

Aggression is an emotion that results in a verbal or physical attack. *Aggression* is often used interchangeably with the term *violence*. This is not accurate. Aggression is not always inappropriate. Instrumental aggression is sometimes necessary for self-protection. Reactive or hostile aggression is violence. Causality for reactive or hostile aggression is multifactorial. States of high arousal, hyperexcitability, psychosis, and confusion are all possible antecedents to acts of violence. Bullying is also a form of aggression that results from issues of low self-esteem. The goal of bullying is to dominate another person through fear and humiliation, and the desired outcome is achievement of power and prestige (Lantos & Halpern, 2015).

Violence includes the intent to harm. It can be directed at self, others, or objects. The *Criminal Code*, section 265(1) (2011), includes violence under its definition of *assault*: physical or verbal. Violence includes psychological and emotional abuse, damage to property, suicide, and self-harm. Predatory aggression leads to violence as an instrumental means to get needs and wants met. Affective or impulsive, spontaneous murder is also a form of reactive aggression that has led to violence (Shiina, 2015). Violence is almost always an objectionable act. Exceptions include the work of armed forces and police officers.

Sometimes, when individuals have difficulty identifying the actual, specific source of their anger, they may suppress it (Kashdan, Goodman, Mallard, et al., 2015). Although suppressing anger is sometimes necessary based on situations or sociocultural or sociopolitical structures over time, it can be quite maladaptive. An example of this is the oppression of race. "Racial oppression is a traumatic form of interpersonal violence which can lacerate the spirit, scar the soul, and puncture the psyche" (Hardy, 2013, p. 25). In Canada, the oppression of Indigenous peoples has included marginalization, disenfranchisement, discrimination, and loss of culture. Suppression of race (and culture) can result from the cumulative effects of voicelessness and powerlessness over long periods of time (Hardy, 2013). This suppression differs from anger in that it is not connected to an immediate triggering situation, but rather to one that has had a long duration.

Workplace violence, a type of lateral violence, is not uncommon in health care. Nurses are at the highest risk due to the amount of contact they have with patients. However, not all workplace aggression or violence stems from patients, visitors, or family members; 44% of Canadian nurses have experienced hostility from their co-workers, whereas in the general workforce fewer than 30% have had the same experience (Canadian Institute for Health Information [CIHI], 2015).

EPIDEMIOLOGY

As a nurse, you will deal with the effects of violent behaviour. The Public Health Agency of Canada identified physical assault as the third leading cause of injury-specific admission to hospital in those ages 15 to 34 years (Pike, Richmond, Rothman & Macpherson, 2015). In our society, the rise of intentional assault among youth is concerning. Its intention is to inflict serious injury or cause death. The typical perpetrator of an assault is a male between the ages of 14 and 17. However, the CIHI (2015) reports that intentional assaults by young females has increased by 22%.

Violence against nurses in dementia care, acute inpatient psychiatric units, and emergency departments in hospitals remains a concern in Canada (Kim, Young, & Berry, 2017; National Emergency Nurses Association, 2014; Stevenson, Jack, O'Mara, et al., 2015). The National Survey of the Work and Health of Nurses found that nurses were physically assaulted by patients most frequently in geriatric or long-term care (50%), palliative care (47%), psychiatric mental health care (44%), critical care (44%), and the emergency room (42%) (Shields & Wilkins, 2009). Box 23-2 identifies milieu characteristics in the hospital or institutional setting that are conducive to violence.

Dissatisfaction with the organization's practices and policies, workplace constraints, poor communication or collaboration among the team, and incivility can all contribute to workplace stress and violence (Hamblin, Essenmacher, Upfal, et al., 2015). Workplace violence of this type can include bullying, and perhaps some of this type of violence is caused by the defence mechanism of projection when individuals feel powerless and voiceless to implement change. This is not so different from the causes of violence in general. Employers, unions, and policymakers have moved to a zero-tolerance position on all types of workplace violence (Canadian Nurses Association & Canadian Federation of Nurses Unions, 2015), and this includes bullying. Accreditation

Canada (2012) now makes workplace violence prevention a required operational practice (ROP).

Beyond the physical ramifications, being the victim of workplace violence can lead to occupational stress disorder (OSD) or post-traumatic stress disorder (PTSD). Nursing staff are not alone in this. Incidents of violence leading to OSD or PTSD in first responders, health care workers, and military personnel are well documented (Standing Committee on Public Safety and National Security, 2016). The Centers for Disease Control and Prevention (2015) has also determined that social determinants of health, individual personalities, and health status contribute to violence and victimization.

COMORBIDITY

Anger can coexist with multiple psychiatric and nonpsychiatric disorders. There is increasing evidence for the comorbidity of aggression and violence in people with PTSD, particularly within the military and among veterans, who frequently having thoughts of harming self or others (Gonzales, Novaco, Reger, et al., 2016). The same is being found among those with substance use disorders and with neuropsychiatric disorders, including psychosis and dementia (Volicer, Citrome, & Volavka, 2017). Patients with acute, severe mental illnesses who abuse substances are at a significantly greater risk for being a victim of violence than the general public (Pickard & Faze, 2013).

ETIOLOGY

Biological Factors

A biological predisposition to respond to life events with irritability, low frustration tolerance, and anger may be a function of neurological development or neurochemical changes.

Neurological

Any neurological condition affecting areas of the brain that are involved with impulse control and emotion regulation can result in increased violence, severe behavioural disorders, and low levels of frustration tolerance. Certain brain tumours, dementias, and temporal lobe epilepsy are associated with anger and aggression. Temporal lobe dysfunction, violence, and aggression are correlated (Bannon, Salis, & O'Leary, 2015). The brain's temporal lobes share some memory function with the limbic system. Memory of previous insult or assault is important in the cognitive appraisal of a threat and can play a determining role in the expression of anger. When there is damage to the frontal lobes of the brain, particularly lesion in the frontal ventromedial area, the potential for aggression and violence is not uncommon (Brodie, Besag, Ettinger, et al., 2016). Prefrontal cortex damage is also implicated in aggressive behaviour (Bannon, Salis, & O'Leary, 2015), as this structure is needed for anger, aggression, impulse control, judgement, and reasoning.

Epilepsy is also linked to aggression and violence. It is important to note that aggressive behaviour in this disease in general is not symptomatic of it but unrelated, and any such behaviours are more likely symptomatic of co-occurring psychiatric disorders (Brodie, Besag, Ettinger, et al., 2016). Seizure activity should also

BOX 23-2	MILIEU CHARACTERISTICS CONDUCIVE TO VIOLENCE IN THE HOSPITAL OR INSTITUTIONAL SETTING

- Overcrowding
- Staff inexperience
- Provocative or controlling staff
- Poor limit setting
- Arbitrary revocation of privileges
- Language or other communication barriers
- Cultural barriers

be actively explored in the elderly when aggression is a concern (Klein, 2016). Aggression can be the result of undiagnosed partial onset and complex partial seizures that occur in the frontal lobe of the elderly (rather than temporal lobes in younger people). Understanding the true cause of the behaviour is essential to providing the most appropriate treatment.

Neurochemical

Serotonin, dopamine, gamma-aminobutyric acid (GABA), glutamate, and acetylcholine all have an impact on anger and aggression (Crockett, Siegel, Kurth-Nelson, et al., 2015; Fanning & Coccaro, 2016). Studies have shown a relationship between anger, aggression, violence, and low levels of serotonin (de Boer, Olivier, Veening, et al., 2015; Hendricks, Bore, Aslinia, et al., 2013). Dopamine has also been linked to aggressive outbursts. There is some indication that this may be based on whether a reward–avoidance process is engaged when dopamine transmission occurs (Crockett, Siegel, Kurth-Nelson, et al., 2015). For example, increased dompanine can lead to increased reward seeking and inhibit the sociomoral response to not cause harm to another (Crockett, Siegel, Kurth-Nelson, et al., 2015).

Selye's (1976) *general adaptation syndrome* can be applied to the natural anger response. When a response occurs to an anger-provoking stressor, the alarm stage is initiated. Neurotransmitters are released, and the ability to think with reason and good judgement diminishes and is replaced by the self-protective mechanisms of fight or flight. *Fight* is the aggressive response to a threat; its goal is to remove or extinguish the dangerous or noxious stimuli. *Flight* is the flee response. Once a fight or flight response is initiated, the neurochemical processes in the body need time to dissipate. It is not prudent to engage a client who is already in an agitated or hostile state in any manner that may continue the escalation of emotion or lead to further misinterpretation of the situation.

Finally, steroid hormones can influence the ability to cope with or express anger, particularly in pubescent, adolescent, and young adult males who experience surges in testosterone. Research reveals that higher levels of testosterone combined with low levels of cortisol in males are positively associated with impulsivity and aggression (Platje, Popma, Vermeiren, et al., 2015).

Psychological Factors

Development of the perception of emotions plays a crucial role in the psychology of anger. Behaviourists hold that emotions are learned responses to environmental stimuli (Skinner, 1953). When a stimulus is perceived as a threat, this thought leads to the emotional and physiological arousal necessary to take action (Selye, 1976). A perceived assault on areas of personal domain (e.g., values, moral code, self-esteem) can lead to anger (Beck, 1976). For example, bullying has long-term effects on the development of self-esteem, self-efficacy issues, anxiety disorders, and self-harming behaviours (Evans-Lacko, Takizawa, Brimblecombe, et al., 2016).

In 1966, Rotter identified locus of control (LOC) as an inherent factor in our experience and expression of mood (April, Dharani, & Peters, 2012). Today, we might refer to LOC as *personal power*. We all wish to exert or maintain control over our lives. An internal

 RESEARCH HIGHLIGHT

Intimate Partner Violence in the Canadian Armed Forces: Psychological Distress and the Role of Individual Factors Among Military Spouses

Problem

Unique military demands can have a significant impact on family life. Although most Canadian Armed Forces families are able to cope effectively with the stressors of military life, some experience marital conflicts, contributing to spousal violence.

Purpose of Study

The purpose of this study was to examine the impact of physical and emotional violence on the psychological well-being of spouses or partners of Canadian Armed Forces members and the potential protective role of individual factors such as social support seeking and problem-focused coping as well as on mastery and perceived social support.

Methods

Canadian Armed Forces spouses were contacted by mail and asked to complete a survey in either English or French. The survey collected demographic information, experiences of intimate partner violence, psychological distress, coping strategies, and information on the individual's perceived ability to exercise control over his or her life circumstances. The final information gathered in the survey related to perceived social support.

Key Findings

Violence has an important impact on the psychological distress of Canadian Armed Forces spouses. Individuals who experience intimate partner violence generally report experiencing multiple forms of violence (psychological, emotional, physical). In addition, individuals who used only one type of coping (problem-focused or support-seeking coping) generally did not engage with alternative coping strategies.

Implications for Nursing Practice

The psychological effects of violence have a lasting impact on victims. This study highlights the risks related to spousal violence in the military and the psychological consequences of such violence. Nurses working with individuals who are trying to modify their behavioural responses to anger need to recognize that these individuals' spouses may need support and interventions. Therefore, when planning and delivering anger management programs, an essential component relates to enhancing spousal well-being.

Source: Skomorovsky, A. & LeBlanc, M. M. (2017). Intimate partner violence in the Canadian armed forces: Psychological distress and the role of individual factors among military spouses. *Military Medicine, 182*(1/2), e1568. doi:10.7205/MILMED-D-15-00566.

locus of control exists when one has a sense of control over the external world. A person with an external locus of control is more likely to feel powerless and blame others for what occurs. This person sees himself or herself as a victim of life. If our personal power or our control is threatened, we experience trauma, and it is from that trauma that anger, aggression, and violence may originate. A person who believes that he or she has a strong, positive internal locus of control believes that any rewards and successes that occur are the result of self-efficacy. Happiness and satisfaction are based on a positive internal locus of control (April, Dharani, & Peters, 2012). Beisswingert and colleagues (2015) found that, on the contrary, perceived loss of control can provoke anger and lead to an increase in risk-taking behaviours. In other words, response to this loss decreases a person's aversion to risk, self-harm, or harm to others. Nursing interventions often reflect LOC as we strive to empower patients in their own care.

Cognitive therapist Albert Ellis (1973) asserts that our own irrational thinking, as well as our appraisals about how the world should be and how others should behave in relation to us, personally leaves us frustrated, dissatisfied, and angry. A person who believes that he or she should be loved and accepted by absolutely everyone at all times is demonstrating irrational or faulty thinking. Anger, hostile aggression, and violence are not uncommon behaviours used by these individuals to deal with any perceived sense of rejection, devaluing, or disrespect.

Cognitive behaviourists Beck, Emery, and Greenberg (2005) believe that dysfunctional anger is rooted in our predispositions, beliefs, memories, learning, and interpretations of self and others in relation to self. Our personal self-appraisal of efficacy and confidence determines how we deal with all situations, including perceived threats. A patient who is kept waiting in a clinic for long periods of time without explanation may interpret this situation as neglect and a lack of respect. Anger may escalate when the initial appraisal is followed by thoughts such as "They have no right to treat me this way. I am a person, too." For some individuals, escalation can be rapid. In contrast, patients who are less predisposed to anger might interpret the wait as a sign that the clinic is busy. These patients might be frustrated by the situation, but in the absence of anger, they might access and use strategies such as asking how much longer the wait is likely to be, finding distractions in the environment, or rescheduling the appointment. For patients who have been suppressing anger, this situation might be the trigger that suddenly releases pent-up anger, even though the situation has little or nothing to do with the original causes of the anger. Long-term suppression of anger may decrease the ability to deal effectively with new anger-provoking stimuli, and there is some suggestion that chronic anger suppression can potentiate a sudden outburst of built-up anger (Ellis, 1990). This built-up anger is often misdirected when released.

Sociological Factors

Social learning theory asserts that children learn aggression by imitating others and that people repeat behaviour that is rewarded (Bandura, 1973). Based on this theory, children exposed to violence often grow up to be aggressive and violent because that behaviour was originally imitated and subsequently rewarded. Children exposed to television and video-game violence learn that violence is an option for resolving conflict and that those violent acts have no real negative consequences. Bullying can be learned this way—what seems like a funny thing to do is actually hurtful and demeaning. Parents, teachers, peers, and the media can contribute to normalizing and justifying this behaviour when they laugh or ignore it. Based on the social learning theory, when a person's behaviour is neither modelled nor rewarded, its

occurrence will decrease. When norms of behaviour are communicated and modelled consistently for youth, incidents of bullying decrease.

Although all people experience the emotion of anger, it is not expressed in the same way across cultures. Biologically and psychologically based anger responses are inextricably entwined with folkways (group habits that are common to a society or culture) that mediate the actual expression of anger. In a multicultural context, this difference in expression of anger provides a challenge to both nurses and patients. Language difficulties and culturally based acceptance of how anger is and can be expressed can easily confound a person's abilities to experience and deal successfully with an anger-producing situation. In Western cultures, the functionality of anger is acknowledged and accepted. The expression of anger is a way to protect rights, personal freedoms, and self-esteem. Anger is seen as a means to find clarity. In other cultures, the expression of anger would be seen as inappropriate and disrespectful.

The Considering Culture box provides an example of the culture of bullying in schools.

🌐 CONSIDERING CULTURE

The Culture of Bullying in Schools

Bullying is a repetitive behaviour that sustains an imbalance of power. It includes any negative activity intended to bother or harm someone, including verbal actions that are demeaning and intimidating such as teasing, gossiping, insulting, or threatening. It can be done in person, by phone, by letter, or online. The physical actions of bullying include all forms of assault.

Wendy Craig and Heather McCuaig Edge (2010) report on a research study of Canadian school-aged children that found that 22% of students were victims of bullying and 12% were students who bully. The study also found that 41% of these students both bullied others and were victimized. Victims are more likely than those not experiencing bullying to feel unsafe at school, have lower grade point averages (GPAs), and feel sad most days. They may develop anxiety disorders, depression, or suicidal thoughts. Suicide can be and has been the result of incessant bullying.

Psychologically, bullies seem to lack empathy, have poor interpersonal skills, and have no respect for authority. Bullies are more likely to develop enduring aggressive behaviour styles and persistent negative attitudes. Scholastically, they are less focused than other students (Public Safety Canada, 2010). In a health care setting, whether adults or youths, bullies have the potential for aggressive verbal and physical acting out against staff.

Sources: Craig, W., & McCuaig Edge, H. (2010). The health of Canada's young people: A mental health focus. In J. G. Freeman, M. King, W. Pickett, et al. (Eds.), *Canadian report on the 2009/10 Health Behaviour in School-aged Children (HBSC) Study*. Retrieved from http://www.phac-aspc.gc.ca/hp-ps/dca-dea/publications/hbsc-mental-mentale/bullying-intimidation-eng.php; Public Safety Canada. (2010). Bullying prevention: Nature and extent of bullying in Canada. In *Building the evidence—Bullying prevention*. April 200-8BP-01. National Crime Prevention Centre Publications. Retrieved from https://www.publicsafety.gc.ca/cnt/rsrcs/pblctns/bllng-prvntn/bllng-prvntn-eng.pdf.

APPLICATION OF THE NURSING PROCESS

ASSESSMENT

General Assessment

Most reactions to stimuli come from previous experiences; therefore identifying patient triggers to anger and aggression through a comprehensive history is essential. Initial and ongoing assessment of the patient can reveal problems before they escalate to anger and aggression. When patients are experiencing anger, it may manifest as increased demands, irritability, frowning, redness of the face, pacing, twisting of the hands, or clenching and unclenching of the fists. Speech may be increased in rate and volume or may be slowed, pointed, and quiet. Any change in behaviour from what is typical for that patient must be addressed. The Assessment Guidelines box highlights various predictors and precipitators of anger, aggression, or violence.

An older concept of providing care has recently been reintroduced. Trauma-informed care refers to care focused on the patient's past experiences of violence or trauma and the role it currently plays in their lives. When a history of trauma is present, it is important for the nursing team to be aware of this and to avoid any situations that may retraumatize the patient. Consider the following examples:

- A woman who was raped may be retraumatized by being catheterized for a medical procedure years later.
- An Indigenous person who was starved and beaten in a residential school as a small child may be retraumatized by the lights and sounds in the environment when hospitalized, especially at night, or may be triggered when meals are late or reflective of the types of food from that earlier traumatic time.
- A Canadian veteran who was wounded and confined as a prisoner by the enemy years ago may be retraumatized if confined to a hospital bed in traction.

These traumatic histories can impede a patient's ability to self-soothe, resulting in negative coping responses and creating a vulnerability to coercive interventions by staff.

Self-Assessment

Nurses may have their own histories with anger, aggression, and violence, and these experiences can influence their ability to intervene safely and effectively in a similar incident. Nurses should reflect on self-assessment of personal responses to anger and aggression, including choice of words, tone of voice, and nonverbal communication. It is essential to be aware of personal dynamics that may trigger nontherapeutic emotions and reactions with specific patients. Finally, the nurse must assess situational factors (e.g., fatigue, insufficient staff) that may decrease normal competence in the management of complex patient problems. Self-assessment promotes calm responses to patient anger and potential aggression. These responses are further supported by the creation of an environment that encourages staff to express feelings, use humour, and develop a professional support system.

DIAGNOSIS

Some patients have coping skills that are adequate for day-to-day events, but they may be overwhelmed by the stresses of illness or hospitalization. Others may have a maladaptive coping pattern that is marginally effective for them but consists of coping strategies that are unhealthy and may potentiate anger and aggression. When the nursing assessment identifies the potential for anger or aggression, *Ineffective coping* (overwhelmed or maladaptive), *Stress overload*, *Risk for self-directed violence*, and *Risk for other-directed violence* are relevant nursing diagnoses (Kamitsuru & Herdman, 2014).

OUTCOMES IDENTIFICATION

Having clearly defined outcome criteria is important for identifying the behaviours that staff can encourage. These outcomes should be identified in initial planning, prior to intervening.

The *Nursing Outcomes Classification (NOC)* outlines specific outcome criteria for use with angry and aggressive patients (Moorhead, Johnson, Maas, et al., 2012). Table 23-1 lists outcome indicators for aggression self-control.

PLANNING

Planning interventions requires a sound assessment of history, present coping skills, and the patient's willingness and capacity to learn alternative and nonviolent ways of handling angry feelings. In addition, the nurse needs to consider whether:

- The situation calls for:
  - Psychoeducational approaches to teach the patient new skills for handling anger
  - Immediate intervention to prevent overt violence (e.g., de-escalation techniques, restraint or seclusion, medications)
- The environment provides:
  - Privacy for the patient
  - Enough space for patients
  - A healthy balance between structured and quiet time
  - Adequate personnel to safely and effectively deal with potentially violent situations
- Staff skills call for:
  - Education in verbal de-escalation techniques
  - Education about positive and consistent approaches to patients
  - Education for appropriate use of restraints

IMPLEMENTATION

Ideally, intervention begins prior to any sign of escalation of anger. This intervention includes developing a trusting relationship with the patient by having numerous brief, nonthreatening, nondirective interactions to get to know the patient. In certain settings (e.g., crisis units, emergency departments), episodes of patient anger and aggression can be predicted; therefore education and practice of verbal and nonverbal interventions with patients

ASSESSMENT GUIDELINES

Anger, Aggression, or Violence

Assessment for Adaptive Versus Maladaptive Expression of Anger	Assessment for Aggression or Violence
Demographic assessment:	Demographic assessment:
• History of difficulty with anger management	• History of violence is the best predictor of future violence
• History of ineffective coping	• Male gender
• Difficulty expressing or dealing with emotions	• Age 14 to 24 years
• Diagnosis of borderline, histrionic, or antisocial personality disorder	• Low socioeconomic status
• Diagnosis of dementia or brain injury	• Substance abuse
• Puberty and adolescence (mood swings, hormonal surges, peer pressures)	• Inadequate support system
	• Prison time
	• History of limited coping skills increases risk for using violence

Preassaultive Assessment of Mental State

Feelings of …
- Frustration, fear, anxiety, embarrassment, shame, or rejection
- Irritability, hypersensitivity to perceived criticism, or attempts by others to control

Voicing …
- Lack of control over life or situation
- Defiance
- Need for support of anger from others

Behaviours indicative of …
- Hyperactivity, impulsivity, or withdrawal
- Confusion or delusions
- Intoxication or other impairment
- Rumination, sullenness, or pacing

Assaultive Stage—Risk Assessment

Voicing …
- Verbal abuse (profanity, argumentativeness, threats)
- Loud voice; change of pitch; or very soft voice, forcing others to strain to hear
- Negative or hostile response in the context of limit setting by the nurse

Thinking (cognition or decision making) …
- Diminishing ability to recognize the anger
- Diminishing ability or desire to diffuse own anger
- Inability to differentiate between assertiveness and aggressive expressions of anger
- Plan, wish, or intent to harm and capacity or means to do so
- Possession of a weapon or object that may be used as a weapon (fork, knife, rock)

Behaviours …
- Hyperactivity most important predictor of imminent violence (pacing, restlessness)
- Increasing anxiety and tension (clenched jaw or fist, rigid posture, fixed or tense facial expression, mumbling to self, shortness of breath, sweating, and rapid pulse)
- Intense or avoidant eye contact
- Assault (hitting, punching, striking, throwing, intimidating, or threatening)

and staff are essential. Cultural competency is an essential part of staff education.

Psychosocial Interventions

As the nurse determines a patient's emotional state, intervention begins. During this process, the nurse listens to the patient's story and acknowledges his or her needs. Summarizing what the patient has said demonstrates the nurse's empathy, compassion, and acceptance of the patient. Acceptance of the patient does not indicate an acceptance of aggressive or violent behaviour. It is important to clearly and simply state expectations for the patient's behaviour. In some situations, the anger may not be resolved before the risk for violence arises.

TABLE 23-1	SIGNS AND SYMPTOMS, NURSING DIAGNOSES, AND OUTCOMES FOR AGGRESSION	
SIGNS AND SYMPTOMS	**NURSING DIAGNOSES**	**OUTCOMES**
Body language (rigid posture, clenching of fists and jaw, hyperactivity, pacing), history of violence, history of family violence, history of substance use	*Risk for other-directed violence*	Identifies when angry, identifies alternatives to aggression, refrains from verbal outbursts, avoids violating others' personal space, maintains self-control
Impulsivity; suicidal ideation (has plan, ability to carry it out); overt or covert statements regarding killing self; feelings of worthlessness, hopelessness, helplessness	*Risk for self-directed violence*	Expresses feelings, verbalizes suicidal ideas, refrains from suicide attempts, plans for the future
Difficulty with simple tasks, inability to function at previous level, poor problem solving, poor cognitive functioning, verbalizations of inability to cope	*Ineffective coping*	Identifies ineffective and effective coping, uses support system, uses new coping strategies, engages in personal actions to manage stressors effectively
Demonstrates feelings of anger, impatience; reports feelings of pressure, tension, difficulty in functioning, anger, impatience; experiences negative impact from stress; reports problems with decision making	*Stress overload*	Expresses feelings constructively, reports feelings of calmness and acceptance, physical symptoms of stress are reduced or absent, decision making is optimal

Sources: Kamitsuru, S., & Herdman, T. H. (Eds.). (2014). *NANDA international nursing diagnoses: Definitions and classification, 2015–2017.* Oxford, UK: Wiley-Blackwell; and Moorhead, S., Johnson, M., Maas, M. L., et al. (2013). *Nursing outcomes classification (NOC)* (5th ed.). St. Louis: Elsevier.

Approaching an angry patient can be unnerving or frightening. The goal is to facilitate the expression of anger in an adaptive, nonviolent manner.

When approaching the patient, convey a calm, relaxed, open, nonthreatening, and caring demeanour. The ability to maintain a calm exterior while feeling inner distress comes with experience.

Pay attention to the environment. If the patient is in a state of low arousal, choose a quiet place to talk, but one that is visible to other staff. This approach is most beneficial in helping a patient to regain control. If the patient is in a state of moderate arousal, pacing up and down a corridor together while the patient vents can be effective. The use of advanced communication skills to de-escalate the situation can help to dissipate pent-up energy fuelled by the release of neurotransmitters and hormones. This technique is helpful when the patient is unable to use the flight response and may feel trapped. Box 23-3 lists some principles underlying **de-escalation techniques**.

Personal space changes when the body and mind are in a heightened state of arousal. Patients in the preassaultive stage need much more space. Do not crowd the patient in or attempt to touch him or her. Allow the patient enough personal space so that you are not perceived as intrusive but not so much space that the patient cannot speak in a normal voice. Always stay about 30 cm (1 foot) farther than the patient can reach with his or her arms or legs.

An angry patient may invade your space with verbal abuse and profanity. This means of communicating may be the only way the patient can express his or her feelings. As uncomfortable as this kind of communication may make you feel, you cannot take the patient's words personally or respond in kind. During an escalating situation is not the time to forbid the patient to communicate in this way or to end the conversation because of the patient's verbal abusiveness. The patient who is about to lose emotional control should not be abandoned. For the protection of the patient and others, the nurse needs to remain engaged while a preplanned crisis intervention begins to unfold.

BOX 23-3	DE-ESCALATION TECHNIQUES: PRACTICE PRINCIPLES

- Respond as early as possible
- Assess for personal safety
- Maintain calmness for self and patient
- Use a calm, clear tone of voice
- Assess the patient and the situation for stressors and stress indicators
- Maintain the patient's self-esteem and dignity
- Establish what the patient considers to be needed
- Invest time; be goal oriented
- Remain honest
- Maintain a large personal space
- Avoid verbal struggles
- Make the options clear
- Use a nonaggressive posture
- Use genuineness and empathy
- Be assertive, not aggressive

Source: Adapted from Price, O., & Baker, J. (2012). Key components of de-escalation techniques: A thematic synthesis. *International Journal of Mental Health Nursing, 21*(4), 310–319. doi:10.1111/j.1447-0349.2011.00793.x.

As escalation increases, the patient's ability to process stimuli decreases. Keep your voice audible, but at a lower volume than the patient's. Eventually the patient will match it and begin to listen more closely. Ensure that you are speaking at an appropriate level and not whispering. Choose your words carefully, speak in short sentences, be clear and concise, and listen to the patient's response. Use open-ended statements and questions to elicit the patient's thoughts. Avoid punitive, threatening, accusatory, or challenging statements.

Honestly verbalize the patient's options and encourage the individual to assume responsibility for choices made. During the preassaultive stage, you may want to give two options, such as "Do you want to go to your room or to the quiet room for a while?" This approach decreases the sense of powerlessness that often precipitates violence. This type of question is quite appropriate in the preassaultive stage, but not during the assaultive stage. In the preassaultive stage, the patient's lack of clarity in thinking and poor decision making become key elements in the intervention. Therefore open-ended questions create too much confusion. You might say, "Some quiet time in your room might help now" or "The quiet room is free." Again, be sure your voice is calm and confident, with a tone that demonstrates that these statements to the patient are options, not directions.

In the assaultive stage, when aggression is deemed likely, seclusion, restraint, or pharmacological means of de-escalation may be necessary to ensure the safety of patients and staff. These measures should be used only when other interventions have failed. Canadian care facilities are mandated by policies that dictate the use of the least restrictive means to care for patients whenever possible. Nurses are also guided by position statements set out by their regulatory bodies.

Staff Safety

Staff should know who is working with a potentially violent patient, keep an eye on the interaction, and be prepared to intervene if the situation escalates. At that time, other patients should be moved away from the incident, and the environment around the specific patient should be free from any object that could be used as a weapon. On psychiatric units, policies and procedures for working as a team in a critical incident of violence (or potential for violence) are in place. All staff should become familiar with the protocols. Discussing and rehearsing the protocols ensures confidence, safety, security, and trust. Facility policies and workers' compensation boards dictate that dangling earrings, necklaces, and similar jewellery should never be worn on duty.

Considerations for Engaging the Angry or Aggressive Patient

Prior to engaging an angry or aggressive patient, ensure that sufficient staff members are available for support. Avoid confrontation with the patient. If security personnel are called to stand by, keep them in the background until they are needed to assist.

Do not stand directly in front of the patient or in front of a doorway; this position could be interpreted as confrontational. Instead, stand slightly off to the side. Encourage the patient to have a seat. An angry person may sit. An aggressive person will not.

If a patient's behaviour begins to escalate, provide feedback. "You seem to be very upset." Such an observation allows exploration of the patient's feelings and may lead to de-escalation of the situation. If the patient validates what you have said, invite him or her to sit down and talk about it. It is best to use a closed-ended statement here. "Let's sit down and talk about it."

Call a Code White if you believe that the aggression and violence are going to require additional help. In many hospitals, nurses with experience dealing with anger, aggression, and violence and who have completed special training may be designated as *Code White responders*. In British Columbia, this role may fall

to the psychiatric nurse clinician in the emergency department. When a Code White is called, the Code White nurse attends an incident occurring in the facility and is met there by members of a trained Code White team. Upon arrival on the scene, the staff initiating the call defers to the expertise of the Code White nurse, who is supported in the action by the Code White team.

Generally, the first staff member on the scene is the only person who should talk to the patient. That person takes the lead while other staff maintain an unobtrusive presence. They may be directed to call for additional help, prepare a seclusion room, gather restraints, or prepare to give medications.

NOTE: Code White policies and procedures are not in place in all jurisdictions nationally. Also, the procedures may differ across jurisdictions. It is important to check with the employer or institution regarding that institution's policies and procedures.

Pharmacological Interventions

When a patient is showing increased signs of anxiety or agitation, it is appropriate to offer antianxiety or antipsychotic medication to alleviate symptoms. When used in conjunction with psychosocial interventions and de-escalation techniques, these medications may prevent a violent incident. Drug Treatments for Emergency Management of Violent Behaviour identifies medications of choice, routes, and indications. Note: Some medications are given concurrently for optimal therapeutic effect.

It is the nurse's role to assess for appropriateness of prn (as needed) medications. Many patients feel traumatized by the use of intramuscular injections; therefore the decision to use this route of administration needs to be determined by what is in the best interests of the patient and the speed with which effects of the medication are needed. Nurses must provide the patient with information about the medication, the reason it is being given, and potential adverse effects, even if the patient is out of control.

The long-term treatment of anger, aggression, and violence is based on treating the underlying psychiatric disorder. Selective serotonin reuptake inhibitors (SSRIs), lithium, anticonvulsants, benzodiazepines, atypical antipsychotics, and beta blockers are all used successfully for specific patient populations. Anger and aggression related to attention deficit disorder or attention-deficit/hyperactivity disorder may be reduced through the use of psycho-stimulants. Drug Treatments for Long-Term Management of Chronic Aggression provides an overview of the drugs used to treat chronic aggression.

Health Teaching and Health Promotion

A nurse can model appropriate responses and ways to cope with anger, teach a variety of methods to appropriately express anger, and educate patients regarding coping mechanisms, identification of personal triggers, de-escalation techniques, and self-soothing skills to manage emotions. These skills include removing themselves from a situation or taking a personal time out. Working with patients to explore their own psychological and somatic responses to anger or anger-provoking stimuli enhances self-awareness related to personal triggers and facilitates learning about how to intervene and exert self-management skills during these stressful events. Box 23-4 provides an example of

DRUGS TREATMENTS FOR EMERGENCY MANAGEMENT OF VIOLENT BEHAVIOUR

GENERIC (TRADE)	ROUTES	INDICATIONS
Antianxiety Agents (Benzodiazepines)		
Lorazepam (Ativan)	PO, SL, IM, IV	Drug of choice in this class
		Use with caution with hepatic dysfunction
Alprazolam (Xanax)	PO	Paradoxical (opposite response) with personality disorders and older adults
Diazepam (Valium)	PO, IM, IV	Rapid onset of calming and sedating
		Long half-life; use with caution in older adults
Conventional Antipsychotics		
Haloperidol	PO, IM, IV	Favourable adverse-effect profile
		Due to risk for neuroleptic malignant syndrome, keep hydrated, check vital signs, and test for muscle rigidity
Loxapine (Loxapac)	PO, IM, SC	Decreases abnormal excitement in the brain; decreases agitation and aggression
		Incompatible with other medications in a syringe
		Avoid or minimize use with the frail elderly
Chlorpromazine	PO, PR, IM	Very sedating
		Injections can cause pain; watch for hypotension
Atypical Antipsychotics		
Risperidone (Risperdal)	PO, IM	Calms while treating underlying condition
		Watch for hypotension
		Increased risk for stroke in older adults
Olanzapine (Zyprexa, Zyprexa Zydis)	PO, IM, SL	Useful in patients who are unresponsive to haloperidol
		Calms while treating underlying condition
		Avoid when using lorazepam
		Increased risk for stroke in older adults
Zuclopenthixol acetate (Clopixol-Acuphase)	IM	Rapid acting to decrease psychotic symptoms and excitability
		Watch for drowsiness
		Avoid if prior alcohol consumption or substance abuse is suspected
Combinations		
Haloperidol, lorazepam (Ativan), and benztropine	IM	Commonly used in the acute setting
		Men who are young and athletic are at increased risk for dystonia
		Consider akathisia (sensations of inner restlessness that manifest as an inability to sit or remain seated) if agitation increases
Loxapine (Loxapac), lorazepam (Ativan), and benztropine	IM, PO	Consider this combination if patient has difficulty taking haloperidol
		Loxapine must be given PO, whereas lorazepam and benztropine may be given PO or IM

IM, Intramuscular; *IV,* intravenous; *PO,* oral; *PR,* rectal; *SC,* subcutaneous; *SL,* sublingual.
Source: Data adapted from Canadian Pharmacists Association. (2011). *Compendium of pharmaceuticals and specialties: The Canadian drug reference for health professionals.* Ottawa: Author.

confrontational assertion when dealing with angry and aggressive people.

Case Management

A multidisciplinary approach is important for a patient with behavioural issues. Consistency and planning are key to the patient's success. Intervention strategies should be discussed during treatment team meetings and then with the patient, before implementation. A discharge plan outlining follow-up, anger management classes, and counselling is essential.

Milieu Management

Behaviours rarely occur in a vacuum. A thorough, proactive examination of the environment is important when considering the potential for anger and aggression on a unit. It is hard to determine how the stimulation of any unit might affect someone whose anxiety is extremely high or who is delusional or confused.

Patients' ability to cope with their acute illness is confounded by unfamiliar environments full of unfamiliar and often unpredictable fellow patients. Feelings of frustration, fear, anxiety, and confusion can escalate to aggression and acting out. Frequent rounds on the unit are important as part of the ongoing assessment of the milieu.

If an escalating patient has enough self-control, sometimes taking a time out in his or her room is sufficient to enable the person to regain composure. Some inpatient psychiatric units, group homes, residential care facilities, and correctional centres offer a therapeutic quiet room. The room is partially lit and has relaxing music and comfortable furniture that promote feelings

DRUGS TREATMENTS FOR LONG-TERM MANAGEMENT OF CHRONIC AGGRESSION

CLASS	POPULATION	CONSIDERATIONS
Selective serotonin reuptake inhibitors (SSRIs)	Antisocial personality disorder, schizophrenia, dementia, brain injury	Reduces irritability, impulsivity, and aggression Stabilizes mood Use cautiously with bipolar disorder
Lithium	Antisocial personality disorder, prison inmates, intellectual disability, brain injury	TSH levels measured prior to treatment Due to antiaggressive properties, blood levels can be lower than those necessary to treat mania
Anticonvulsants	Prison inmates, antisocial personality disorder, borderline personality disorder, substance use, ADD, brain injury, schizophrenia, and intermittent explosive disorder (IED; rages)	Significantly reduces impulsive aggression Similar doses with bipolar disorder Multiple drug interactions Periodic blood levels Monitor CBC and LFTs
Gabapentin	Anxiety disorder, personality disorders	No interactions with other anticonvulsants
Benzodiazepines	Anxiety disorder	Potential for abuse, dependence, and withdrawal May cause paradoxical aggression
Atypical antipsychotics	Schizophrenia, psychosis, mania, borderline personality disorder, intellectual disability	Clozapine superior to other atypical antipsychotics Fewer adverse effects and greater adherence than conventional antipsychotics Risperidone reduces irritability in autistic disorder
Beta blockers	Schizophrenia, brain injury, dementia, intellectual disability	Propranolol (Inderal) contraindicated with asthma, COPD, and type 1 diabetes Sedation adverse effects may explain antiaggressive effects
Psychostimulants	ADD or ADHD in children and adults	Potential for addiction and abuse

ADD, Attention deficit disorder; *ADHD,* attention-deficit/hyperactivity disorder; *CBC,* complete blood count; *COPD,* chronic obstructive pulmonary disease; *LFTs,* liver function tests; *TSH,* thyroid-stimulating hormone.
Source: Data from Canadian Pharmacists Association. (2011). *Compendium of pharmaceuticals and specialties: The Canadian drug reference for health professionals.* Ottawa: Author.

BOX 23-4   CONFRONTATIONAL ASSERTION

Assertiveness is an essential skill for psychiatric/mental health nurses. It can be particularly helpful when dealing with confrontation. Whether the confrontation that happens with clients or colleagues occurs in the spur of the moment or in a planned meeting, the assertive nurse remembers that mutual respect and open, honest communication are necessary for an effective engagement.

Confrontation includes thoughts and feelings. When someone opposes, challenges or fights the ideas of another, their behaviours or what they perceive as a violation of personal rights, conflict can turn into confrontation. Conflict and confrontation by someone can quickly escalate when anger or fear are also evident in the nurse. Confrontational assertion is used to remove the emotional charge from the situation and deal with the core issues effectively. The assertive nurse will consider and apply the following as appropriate:

Planned Confrontational Assertion (prior to engagement)
- Prepare and rehearse what will be said about the issues, not the people involved
- Employ self-awareness to clarify and manage own emotions
- Prepare for respectful engagement (review assertiveness skills)
- Identify possible effective outcomes and consequences
- Prepare to give and receive feedback professionally
- Plan to meet the person/group in a neutral setting
- Agree to meet at a time when both parties are not acutely angry

Acute/Immediate Confrontational Assertion
- Initiate the interaction
- Remain calm
- Keep tone of voice neutral
- Use short, clear and concise sentences and responses
- Use attentive listening to ascertain the issues
- Reflect the issues back, clearly and concisely
- Seek clarification
- Maintain professional language and deportment
- Identify solutions in collaboration
- State potential consequences of the confrontational behaviour or solutions in a non-threatening manner

Source: Adapted from Gooding, L. (n.d.). *Assertiveness: A key to success.* Retrieved from http://lonestar.edu/blogs/lgooding/files/2009/10/assertiveness-a-key-to-success.pdf.

of security and safety. Patients who identify their own need for a time out in a therapeutic quiet room are able to use it of their own volition. In many institutions, quiet rooms are locked and used as seclusion rooms. The decision to lock the door is based on the patient's risk assessment and the discretion of the multidisciplinary team.

Use of Restraints or Seclusion

Seclusion or restraint is used only if the patient presents a clear danger to self or others. Restraints of any type should be used only when alternatives fail to protect the patient and others from harm. There are three different types of restraints (Brickell, Nicholls, Procyshyn, et al., 2009):

1. Environmental restraint: Seclusion is an example of an environmental restraint. The patient's locomotion is restricted by confinement to a defined area or locked room. The situation is temporary, the patient is alone, and there is no furniture or other amenities in the room.
2. Physical or mechanical restraints: These are techniques or devices used to physically restrict or subdue whole or partial body movements (e.g., transfer belts, four-point restraints, geriatric chairs).
3. Chemical restraints: Chemical restraint is achieved through the use of medications, with the sole intent of managing behaviour.

Additional guidelines for the use of mechanical restraints are given in Box 23-5.

Prior to seclusion, a patient must be assessed for contraindications, including pregnancy, chronic obstructive pulmonary disorder (COPD), head or spinal injury, seizure disorder, abuse, history of surgery or fracture, morbid obesity, and sleep apnea. A patient can be secluded or restrained with an order from a psychiatrist or physician in accordance with a provincial or territorial mental health act.

Staff work as a team when secluding a patient. The team leader briefly describes the rationale for seclusion and directs the team. One nurse prepares the seclusion room while others promote safety and privacy by clearing the area of onlookers. A nurse prepares prn (as needed) or stat (immediate) medication. Options are provided to the patient, including taking a time out, accepting medication orally, or walking with the nursing team into the seclusion room. When these options fail, the staff intervenes to physically restrain the patient and escort him or her into seclusion. The patient may be required to change into pyjamas, and medication may be administered despite patient objections. One by one, team members back out of the room, locking the door behind them. Close or constant observation protocols are initiated per hospital policy. The patient remains in seclusion until assessed as being less at risk for harm to self or others.

Following seclusion of a patient, the treatment team should debrief the incident, and when seclusion is discontinued, the nurse and patient should also debrief. It is important to identify precipitating factors, explore coping resources, and develop a plan of action for a time when another incident is likely to occur. Questions to be answered during the team debriefing may include the following:

BOX 23-5	**ADDITIONAL GUIDELINES FOR USE OF MECHANICAL RESTRAINT OR SECLUSION**

Indications for Use
- To protect the patient from self-harm
- To prevent the patient from assaulting others

Legal Requirements
- Multidisciplinary involvement
- Appropriate health care provider's signature according to provincial and territorial law
- Patient advocate or relative notification
- Restraint or seclusion discontinuation as soon as possible

Documentation Describes
- Patient's behaviour leading to restraint or seclusion
- Nursing interventions used and the patient's responses (including least restrictive measures used prior to restraint or seclusion)
- Evaluation of the interventions used and patient's response

Plan of Care for Restraint Use or Seclusion Implementation
- Ongoing evaluations by nursing staff and appropriate health care providers
- Method of reintegration into the unit milieu
- Evidence of least restrictive measures used prior to restraint or seclusion
- Critical Incident or Unusual Occurrence Report form completed

Clinical Assessments
- Patient's mental state at time of restraint or seclusion (i.e., preassaultive, assaultive, postassaultive)
- Physical examination for medical problems possibly causing behaviour changes
- Need for restraints or seclusion

Observation and Ongoing Assessment
- Staff in constant or close attendance
- Written record completed every 15 minutes
- Range of movement frequently assessed if limbs are restrained
- Vital signs monitored
- Circulation assessed: blood flow observed in hands or feet
- Observation to ensure that restraint is not rubbing or causing friction on skin
- Provision for nutrition, hydration, and elimination

Release Procedure
- Patient able to follow commands and stay in control
- Termination of restraints or seclusion
- Debriefing with patient

- Could we have done anything that would have prevented the violence? If yes, how will we ensure this approach is taken another time?
- Did we respond as a team? Were team members acting according to the policies and procedures of the unit? If not, what could we do another time?

- How do staff members feel about this patient now and about the incident that occurred?

Feelings of fear and anger must be discussed and worked through; otherwise staff may deal with the patient in a punitive and nontherapeutic manner. Employee morale, productivity, use of sick leave time, transfer requests, and absenteeism are all affected by patient violence, especially if a staff member has been injured. Staff members must feel supported by their peers as well as by the organizational policies and procedures established to maintain a safe environment.

- Is there a need for additional staff education regarding how to respond to violent patients?
- How did the actual restraining process go? What could be done differently?
- If injury occurred, has it been reported and cared for?

Incidents that require the use of seclusion or restraints provoke anxiety for the staff and may trigger their stress responses. Skills in nonviolent crisis intervention techniques are critical. Nurses should not be put into positions such as these without this additional training. Many health authorities, care facilities, and health institutions across Canada provide this training at the time of hiring and intermittently during employment.

Reintegration to the unit occurs when the patient is assessed as being able to handle increasing amounts of stimulation. Reintegration should be gradual. If the process proves to be too much for the patient and increased agitation results, the individual is returned to the seclusion room or another quiet area or restraints are reapplied. Prior to release from restraint or seclusion, patients must be able to follow directions and control behaviours. With restraints, a structured reintegration is the best approach. Begin by removing one of the four-point restraints, then another, and so on. Close observation of the patient is essential as the restraints are removed and for several hours afterward. If the patient is unable to manage his or her behaviour, further seclusion or restraint may be necessary.

It is important to remember once again that psychiatric patients are not the only patients who exhibit anger and have the potential for aggression and violence.

Caring for Patients in General Hospital Settings
Patients With High Anxiety Related to Hospitalization

Caring for hospitalized patients who exhibit signs of anxiety begins with listening to the patient's story and helping the patient to identify immediate goals. Mild anxiety can be moderated by the provision of comfort items before they are requested (beverage, deck of cards, access to TV). This kind of response can build rapport and reassure the patient. Anxiety can also be minimized by reducing ambiguity. This strategy includes clear and concrete communication. An interaction providing clarity about what the nurse can and cannot do is most usefully ended by offering something within the nurse's power to provide (i.e., leaving the patient with a "yes").

Interventions for anxiety might also include the use of distractions such as magazines, action comics, and video games. Generally, distractions that are colourful and do not require sustained attention work best, although the choice of distraction varies according to the patient's interests and abilities. When a patient is anxious, frustrated, angry, or fearful, pacing with the patient up and down the corridor can be a helpful strategy. Continue to converse with the patient as you do so.

Patients with a high level of baseline anxiety and limited coping skills are helped when their interactions with the treatment team are predictable. This predictability may include speaking with the physician at a specific time each day and providing consistency in nursing assignments. Individuals from outside the unit, such as a chaplain or a volunteer, may help by giving the patient more attention.

Patients With Healthy Coping Skills Who Are Overwhelmed

A patient loses autonomy and control when hospitalized, which can cause a great deal of related distress. When this stress is combined with the uncertainty of illness, a patient may respond in ways that are not usual for him or her. A careful nursing assessment, with history and information from family members, helps evaluate whether a patient's anger is a usual or unusual way for that patient to manage stress.

Interventions for patients whose usual coping strategies are healthy involve finding ways to re-establish or substitute similar means of dealing with the hospitalization. This problem solving occurs in collaboration with the patient, in interactions that demonstrate that the nurse acknowledges the patient's distress, validates it as understandable under the circumstances, and indicates a willingness to search for solutions. Validation includes making an apology to the patient when appropriate, such as when a promised intervention (e.g., changing a dressing by a certain time) has not been delivered, or sympathizing with the patient about the "horrible food" and assisting him or her to make tastier choices on the menu.

Patients who have become angry may be unable to moderate this emotion enough to problem-solve with their nurses; others may be unable to communicate the source of their anger. Often the nurse—knowing the patient and the context of the anger—can make an accurate guess at what feeling is behind the anger and help name it for the patient. Doing so can lead to a sense of being understood and dissipation of the anger, resulting in a calmer discussion of the event.

Patients With Marginal Coping Skills

Patients whose coping skills were marginal before hospitalization need a different set of interventions from those who have basically healthy ways of coping. They are poorly equipped to use alternatives when initial attempts to cope are unsuccessful or are found to be inappropriate. Such patients frequently manifest anxiety that moves quickly to anger and on to aggression. For some, anger and intimidation are primary coping strategies used to obtain short-term goals of control or mastery. For others, the anger occurs when their limited or primitive attempts at coping are unsuccessful and alternatives are unknown. For these patients, anger and violence are particular risks in inpatient settings.

The potential for violence is especially true for hospitalized patients with chemical dependence, who may be anxious about being cut off from the substance to which they are addicted.

VIGNETTE

Jagwinder, a 21-year-old patient who had been in an automobile accident, was admitted to the medical unit with a pelvic fracture and is bedridden. Since admission, he has yelled at each nurse who walks by his room, using expletives to demand that the nurse enter and attend to his needs.

Intervention: The nurse assigned to the patient for the evening stops in his doorway after he yells at her and assertively states, "Jagwinder, it is inappropriate to yell and swear at the staff. If you would like our attention, please address us courteously." She continues on her way, and Jagwinder is left to process the message. He is unable to offer a retort or to engage the nurse in argument. He is initially angry and profane in response. However, the nurse will not return to him. Should he repeat this behaviour on her next encounter with him, she will repeat her original message, consistently setting limits on his behaviour. She will not engage in conversation with him until he is prepared to act and speak appropriately. At each negative encounter, the patient is left to think about his behaviour.

Response: Jagwinder eventually comes to realize how to get the attention he needs in a more appropriate manner. He gains insight and modifies his behaviour. His anger and frustration triggered by not getting his needs met immediately begin to dissipate. When the nurse meets with him, she engages him in the primary topic of his concern, followed by a debriefing of his inappropriate behaviour. Together they explore how to communicate his needs more effectively, more appropriately, and more assertively. They discuss his anger and frustration with hospitalization and explore his pattern of coping. At each step of the encounter, the nurse applies principles of behavioural therapy to her intervention strategies.

They may have well-founded concerns that any physical pain will be inadequately addressed. Many chemically dependent patients may see the source of their discomfort and anxiety as being outside themselves (i.e., impaired locus of control); relief must therefore also come from an outside source (e.g., the nurse, medication). These patients exhibit frustration intolerance and can be quite verbally aggressive. An understanding of the patient's lived experience with addiction helps the nurse and other staff determine a course of action for dealing with hostile aggression and the potential for violent acting out (see Chapter 18). Most hospitals have a withdrawal protocol that ensures that patients do not go through withdrawal without medication. Medication administration needs to be provided promptly and consistently to communicate to patients that nurses can be trusted. Attention to patients' need for the medication can be very anxiety relieving for those patients with a chemical-dependency problem. Precautionary measures may be in place on the hospital unit to limit certain visitors, to protect the sobriety or withdrawal and maintenance protocols for chemically dependent patients.

Interventions for patients who externalize blame require firm and consistent limit setting on inappropriate behaviours. Anger may be communicated by verbal abuse targeting the staff. If attempts to teach alternative methods of coping and communicating are unsuccessful, three interventions can be used:

1. Leave the room as soon as the verbal abuse begins. Inform the patient that you, the nurse, will return in a specific amount of time (e.g., 20 minutes) when the situation is calmer. A matter-of-fact, neutral demeanour is important because fear, indignation, and arguing are gratifying to many verbally abusive patients. Alternatively, if the nurse is in the middle of a procedure and cannot leave immediately, she or he can break off conversation and eye contact, completing the procedure quickly and matter-of-factly before leaving the room. The nurse avoids chastising, threatening, or responding punitively to the patient.

2. Withdraw attention from the abuse. Withdrawal of attention to verbal or emotional abuse is successful only if a second intervention is also used. This step requires attending positively to, and thus reinforcing, nonabusive communication by the patient. Interventions can include discussing non–illness-related topics, responding to requests, and providing emotional support, particularly when the patient is calm and approachable. This technique is quite effective when used in conjunction with the third one.

3. Schedule routine interactions. Patients who are verbally abusive may respond best to the predictability of routine, such as scheduled contacts with the nurse (every 30 or 60 minutes). Use of such contacts provides nursing attention that is not contingent on the patient's behaviour; therefore it does not reinforce the abuse. Of course, the patient's illness or injury may sometimes require nursing visits for assessment or intervention outside the scheduled contact times. These visits can be carried out in a calm, brief, matter-of-fact manner. For patients with marginal coping skills, once anxiety is moderated, nursing interventions include teaching alternative behaviours and coping strategies.

Implementing appropriate interventions can be difficult when the nurse is feeling threatened. Remaining matter-of-fact with patients who habitually use anger and intimidation can be difficult, as they are often skillful at making personal and pointed statements. It is important to remember that patients do not know their nurses personally and thus have no basis on which to make judgements. Nurses can discuss their feelings and beliefs with other staff members or with the critical incident debriefing team.

Caring for Patients in Inpatient Psychiatric Settings

Patients Who Are Acutely Psychotic

Assault on inpatient psychiatric units is of worldwide concern. On a psychiatric unit, the potential for hostile aggression and violence is most often demonstrated by those who are acutely psychotic, in a manic phase, substance dependent, or being held under the authority of a mental health act.

Caring for Patients With Cognitive Deficits in Long-Term Residential Care Settings

Patients (or residents) with cognitive deficits are particularly at risk for acting aggressively. Such deficits may result from delirium, dementia, or brain injury (see Chapter 17). Traditional approaches to disorientation and to the agitation it can cause rely heavily on reality orientation and medication. Reality orientation consists

VIGNETTE

Ken is a 32-year-old patient with a diagnosis of schizophrenia who has lived in a group home for 10 years. He is well maintained on his medications and attends daily programs and recreation at a local psychosocial clubhouse. He has a delusion that the Canadian Security Intelligence Service (CSIS) is listening in on him because he has some intimate knowledge of nuclear weapons design. When well, he continues to suffer from delusions and auditory hallucinations, but they are less intense and less intrusive, and they do not interfere with his daily living or ability to cope. Currently, Ken is experiencing an exacerbation of his symptoms. He is increasingly paranoid, and this paranoia has led to admission to an acute psychiatric inpatient unit. Ken is yelling at the nurses and accusing them of being part of the conspiracy against him. He believes they will force him to take medications that will erase his knowledge about the secret weapon. He insists that he must remain alert, vigilant, and self-protective.

Intervention: Ken is escalating, and the potential for violence is determined. The staff prepare to intervene. James, a nurse, engages Ken in the hallway. The nurse acknowledges Ken's concerns for his safety. (The use of skillful communication facilitates development of rapport, respect, and trust.) To help Ken settle, James offers him a prn medication or one-to-one time to talk with the staff. He gives the patient time to process the options. James continues to set limits and attempts to de-escalate the situation with Ken. Sensing that the patient is unable to use reason at that moment or regulate his emotions, the nurse signals the care team and they prepare for an intervention of seclusion. James advises Ken and also gives him one more opportunity to take medication to help him settle.

Response: Despite Ken's altered thought content, he is able to understand the potential for being secluded. When the nurse offers him medication to settle, Ken makes some choices. He chooses not to be put in seclusion, commenting that he believes the room is "bugged." He adds that he prefers to take a tablet form of medication rather than liquid or a capsule. The nurse is able to provide a tablet. James has been able to meet the need for safety and security for everyone on the unit through the pre-emptive strategies of listening, setting limits, offering options, and providing space and time for the patient to process the information. These actions also allowed Ken to maintain a sense of control.

VIGNETTE

Mrs. Green, an 81-year-old woman with a diagnosis of Alzheimer's disease, always becomes agitated during her morning care; her caregivers have come to dread this time. Careful observation of antecedents to the episodes of agitation reveals a pattern. Mrs. Green is initially calm when care begins; however, one staff person gives morning care to the patient and her roommate at the same time, moving between the two. Observation of the process reveals that the patient becomes distracted by cues being given to her roommate and often startles when the caregiver returns to her. As this process continues over several minutes, Mrs. Green becomes increasingly distressed and then agitated.

When a change is made to ensure that patient care is provided on an individual basis, Mrs. Green becomes receptive to the nursing care provided.

of providing the correct information to the patient about place, date, and current life circumstances. For many patients, this orientation is comforting because it reminds them of pertinent information and helps them feel in touch with their world. For others, reality orientation does not work. Because of their cognitive disorder, they can no longer "enter into our reality"; they become frightened and more agitated and may become aggressive. Sometimes the patient with a cognitive disorder experiences such severe agitation and aggression that it is referred to as a *catastrophic reaction*. The patient may scream, strike out, or cry because of overwhelming fear. Adopting a calm and unhurried manner is the best approach.

Patients who misperceive their setting or life situation may be calmed by validation therapy. Some disoriented older patients believe that they are young and feel the need to return to important tasks that were a significant part of those earlier years. For example, a woman may insist that she must go home to take care of her babies. Telling the patient that her babies have grown up and there is no home to return to is nontherapeutic and results in increased agitation. It is often more helpful to reflect back to the patient the feelings behind her demand and to show understanding and concern for her worry. During the conversation, the nurse can comment on what appears to be underlying the patient's distress, thereby validating it. For example, when working with Mrs. Green in the vignette, the nurse may note that Mrs. Green misses her children and that she gets lonely at times:

Nurse: "Mrs. Green, you miss your children, and this can be a lonely place."

The nurse shows interest in aspects of the patient's life, thereby establishing herself as a safe, understanding person. Mrs. Green finds more focus and is less overwhelmed by the stimulus occurring in her environment. The patient often becomes calmer and more open to redirection. As patients reminisce in this fashion, they often bring themselves into the present.

Mrs. Green: "Of course, they're all grown and doing well on their own now."

Refer to Chapter 17 for a more detailed discussion of interventions for people with cognitive impairments. Refer to Chapter 28 for a more detailed discussion of the use of validation and reminiscent therapeutic modalities for older adults.

EVALUATION

Evaluation of the nursing care plan (NCP) is essential for patients with a potential for anger, aggression, and violence. Evaluation provides information about the extent to which the interventions have achieved the outcomes. The initial NCP may have included assessment of the environmental stimuli that precede a patient's agitation. Once stimuli are identified, interventions specific to those stimuli are developed. Results of the interventions are evaluated and documented, and the NCP is revised.

KEY POINTS TO REMEMBER

- Angry emotions and aggressive, violent actions are difficult targets for nursing intervention, and self-awareness of personal responses to angry or threatening patients is essential.
- Nurses benefit from an understanding of how to intervene with an angry, aggressive, or violent patient.
- Understanding precipitating factors that can lead to an escalation of aggression facilitates care planning for individuals in a variety of situations.
- The expression of anger can lead to negative physiological changes.
- Psychosocial, cognitive, sociocultural, and biological theories provide explanations for anger and aggression.
- A patient's past aggressive behaviour is the most important indicator of future aggressive episodes.
- A variety of interventions are used to help patients de-escalate and maintain control, depending on their coping abilities, cognitive and mental status, and potential for violence.
- Administration of antipsychotics, mood stabilizers, and antianxiety medications may be indicated.
- Seclusion or restraints may be necessary to ensure safety for the patient and others on the unit.
- Clear protocols for the safe use of seclusion or restraints and for the humane management of care during this time are essential.
- The nurse is expected to have a clear understanding of policies, protocols, and legalities related to anger, aggression, and violence, as well as how to intervene.

CRITICAL THINKING

1. Jennifer admits a 24-year-old man with a diagnosis of mania to an inpatient unit. She notes that the patient is irritable, has trouble sitting during the interview, and has a history of assault.
   a. Identify appropriate responses the nurse can make to the patient.
   b. What interventions should be built into the care plan?
   c. Identify at least three long-term outcomes to consider when planning care.
2. What are the two indicators for the use of seclusion and restraint rather than verbal interventions? Provide a rationale.
3. Enter into a debate on the use of restraint and seclusion with your clinical group or in class. Choose a side and defend it, even if you do not necessarily agree with it. Use these topics:
   a. There are always better alternatives to seclusion and restraint.
   b. Seclusion and restraint are underused—people who have tried to limit their use have gone too far.
   c. Using chemical restraint with medication is preferable to seclusion and restraint.
4. Jordan is a 24-year-old male who is prone to alcohol and drug abuse. He likes to fight and initiate fights. He prides himself on his strength and aggressive personality. When another person looks directly at Jordan for more than just a few seconds, based on research, how is he likely to interpret the person's staring?

CHAPTER REVIEW

1. Which statement about violence and nursing is accurate?
   a. Unless working in psychiatric or mental health settings, nurses are unlikely to experience patient violence.
   b. About 3 in 10 nurses will face an injury due to patient violence during their careers.
   c. Emergency, psychiatric, and step-down units have the highest rates of violence toward staff.
   d. Violence primarily affects inexperienced or unskilled staff who cannot calm their patients.
2. A nurse working with a patient who describes himself as "always angry" should assess the patient for which problems? Select all that apply.
   a. Pain
   b. Dementia
   c. Tachycardia
   d. Hypertension
   e. Traumatic brain injury
3. Which statements by a patient indicate an increased likelihood of violent behaviour? Select all that apply.
   a. "People push me, but they can only push me so far."
   b. "I have a right to feel angry, and right now I am angry."
   c. "You are really stupid. I'd get better nursing care from a monkey."
   d. "A man has to do what a man has to do when somebody crosses him."
   e. "This is frustrating; I wish people would leave me alone. That's what would help me."
4. A nurse, Sarah, responds to loud, angry voices coming from the day room, where she finds that Mr. Christopher is pacing and shouting that he "isn't going to take this (expletive) anymore." Which reaction by Sarah is likely to be helpful in de-escalating the situation with Mr. Christopher?
   a. Acts calm, quiet, and in control.
   b. States, "You are acting inappropriately and must calm yourself now."
   c. Matches the patient's volume level so that he is able to hear over his own shouting.
   d. Stands close to the patient so she can intervene physically, if needed, to protect others.

5. Andrea, a patient, is anxiously waiting her turn to speak with a nurse. The nurse is very busy, however, and asks Andrea if she can wait a few minutes so she can finish her task. The nurse is distracted and forgets her promise temporarily, and 45 minutes pass before the nurse remembers and approaches Andrea. On seeing the nurse, Andrea accuses the nurse of lying and refuses to speak with her. Which response by the nurse is most likely to be therapeutic at this time?

a. "You seem angry that I didn't speak with you when I promised I would."
b. "Look, I'm sorry for being late, but screaming at me is not the best way to handle it."
c. "You are too angry to talk right now. I'll come back in 20 minutes and we can try again."
d. "Why are you angry? I told you that I was busy and would get to you soon as I could."

⊖volve WEBSITE

Post-Test   interactive review

Visit the Evolve website for Chapter Review Answers and Rationales, Critical Thinking Answer Guidelines, and additional resources related to the content in this chapter: http://evolve.elsevier.com/Canada/Varcarolis/psychiatric/

REFERENCES

Accreditation Canada. (2012). *Required organizational practices: Emerging risks, focused improvements.* Ottawa: Author. Retrieved from https://accreditation.ca/sites/default/files/char-2012-en.pdf.

American Psychiatric Association. (2013). *Diagnostic and statistical manual of mental disorders* (5th ed.). Arlington, VA: American Psychiatric Publishing.

April, K. A., Dharani, B., & Peters, K. (2012). Impact of locus of control expectancy on level of well-being. *Review of European Studies, 4*(2), 124–137. doi:10.5539/res.v4n2p124.

Bandura, A. (1973). *Aggression: A social learning analysis.* New York: Prentice Hall.

Bannon, S. M., Salis, K. L., & O'Leary, K. D. (2015). Structural brain abnormalities in aggression and violent behavior. *Aggression and Violent Behavior, 25,* 323–331. doi:10.1016/j.avb.2015.09.016.

Beck, A. (1976). *Cognitive therapy and the emotional disorders.* New York: International Universities Press.

Beck, A., Emery, G., & Greenberg, R. (2005). *Anxiety disorders and phobias* (15th anniversary ed.). New York: Basic Books.

Beisswingert, B. M., Zhang, K., Goetz, T., et al. (2015). The effects of subjective loss of control on risk-taking behavior: The mediating role of anger. *Frontiers in Psychology, 6,* 774. doi:10.3389/fpsyg.2015.00774.

Brickell, T., Nicholls, T., Procyshyn, R., et al. (2009). *Patient safety in mental health.* Edmonton: Canadian Patient Safety Institute and Ontario Hospital Association.

Brodie, M. J., Besag, F., Ettinger, A. B., et al. (2016). Epilepsy, antiepileptic drugs, and aggression: An evidence-based review. *Pharmacological Reviews, 68*(3), 563–602. doi:10.1124/pr.115.012021.

Canadian Institute for Health Information (CIHI). (2015). *Intentional assault among children and youth in Canada.* Retrieved from https://www.cihi.ca/web/resource/en/info_child_assault_en.pdf.

Canadian Nurses Association & Canadian Federation of Nurses Unions. (2015). *Joint position statement: Workplace violence and bullying.* Retrieved from https://www.cna-aiic.ca/en/advocacy/policy-support-tools/cna-position-statements#sthash.GBV4839P.dpuf.

Centers for Disease Control and Prevention. (2015). The social-ecological model: A framework for prevention. *Injury Prevention & Control: Division of Violence Prevention.* Retrieved from http://www.cdc.gov/violenceprevention/overview/social-ecologicalmodel.html.

Criminal Code, R.S.C. 1985, c. C-46. (2011). Section 265. Retrieved from http://laws-lois.justice.gc.ca/eng/acts/C-46/.

Crockett, M., Siegel, J. Z., Kurth-Nelson, Z., et al. (2015). Dissociable effects of serotonin and dopamine on the valuation of harm in moral decision making. *Current Biology, 25*(14), 1852–1859. doi:10.1016/j.cub.2015.05.021.

de Boer, S. F., Olivier, B., Veening, J., et al. (2015). The neurobiology of offensive aggression: Revealing a modular view. *Physiology & Behavior, 146,* 111–127. doi:10.1016/j.physbeh.2015.04.040.

Ellis, A. (1973). *Humanistic psychotherapy: The rational-emotive approach.* New York: McGraw-Hill.

Ellis, A. (1990). *Anger: How to live with and without it.* New York: Citadel Press.

Evans-Lacko, S., Takizawa, R., Brimblecombe, N., et al. (2016). Childhood bullying victimization is associated with use of mental health services over five decades: A longitudinal nationally representative cohort study. *Psychological Medicine, 47*(1), 1–9. doi:10.1017/S0033291716001719.

Fanning, J. R., & Coccaro, E. F. (2016). Neurobiology of impulsive aggression. In P. M. Kleepsies (Ed.), *The Oxford handbook of behavioral emergencies and crises.* New York: Oxford University Press. doi:10.1093/oxfordhb/978-19935277.001.0001.

Frey, K. S., Higheagle Strong, Z., & Onyewuenyi, A. C. (2017). Individual and class norms differentially predict proactive and reactive aggression: A functional analysis. *Journal of Educational Psychology, 109*(2), 178–190. doi:10.1037/edu0000118.

Gonzales, O. I., Novaco, R. W., Reger, M. A., et al. (2016). Anger intensification with combat-related PTSD and depression comorbidity. *Psychological Trauma: Theory, Research, Practice, and Policy, 8*(1), 9–16. doi:10.1037/tra0000042.

Hamblin, L. E., Essenmacher, L., Upfal, M. J., et al. (2015). Catalysts of worker-to-worker violence and incivility in hospitals. *Journal of Clinical Nursing, 24,* 2458–2467. doi:10.1111/jocn.12825.

Hardy, K. V. (2013). Healing the hidden wounds of racial trauma. *Reclaiming Children and Youth, 22*(1), 24–28. Retrieved from http://www.reclaimingjournal.com.

Hendricks, L. H., Bore, S., Aslinia, D., et al. (2013). The effects of anger on the brain and body. *National Forum Journal of Counseling and Addiction, 2*(1).

Kamitsuru, S., & Herdman, T. H. (Eds.). (2014). *NANDA international nursing diagnoses: Definitions and classification, 2015–2017.* Oxford, UK: Wiley-Blackwell.

Kashdan, T. B., Goodman, F. R., Mallard, T. T., et al. (2015). What triggers anger in everyday life? Links to the intensity, control, and regulation of these emotions, and personality traits. *Journal of Personality, 84*(6), 737–749. doi:10.1111/jopy.12214.

Kim, S. C., Young, L., & Berry, B. (2017). Aggressive behaviour risk assessment tool for newly admitted residents of long-term care homes. *Journal of Advanced Nursing, 73*(7), 1747–1756. doi:10.1111/jan.13247.

Klein, R. B. (2016). Aggression and violence in the elderly. In P. M. Kleepsies (Ed.), *The Oxford handbook of behavioral emergencies and crises.* New York.: Oxford University Press. doi:10.1093/oxfordhb/978-19935277.001.0001.

Lantos, J. D., & Halpern, J. (2015). Bullying, social hierarchies, poverty and health outcomes. *Pediatrics, 135*(Suppl. 2), doi:10.1542/peds.2014-3549B.

Moorhead, S., Johnson, M., Maas, M. L., et al. (2012). *Nursing Outcomes Classification (NOC)* (5th ed.). St. Louis: Mosby.

National Emergency Nurses Association. (2014). *Position statement: Violence in the emergency department*. Retrieved from http://nena.ca/w/wp-content/uploads/2015/11/Violence-in-the-ED.pdf.

Pabian, S., & Vandebosch, H. (2016). (Cyber)bullying perpetration as an impulsive, angry reaction following (cyber)bullying victimisation? In M. Walrave, K. Ponnet, E. Vanderhoven, et al. (Eds.), *Youth 2.0: Social media and adolescence: Part III* (pp. 193–209). Cham, Switzerland: Springer International Publishing. doi:10.1007/978-3-319-27893_11.

Pickard, H., & Faze, S. (2013). Substance abuse as a risk factor for violence in mental illness: Some implications for forensic psychiatric practice and clinical ethics. *Current Opinion in Psychiatry, 26*(4), 349–354. doi:10.1097/YCO.0b013e328361e798.

Pike, I., Richmond, S., Rothman, L., et al. (Eds.). (2015). *Canadian injury prevention resource*. Toronto, ON: Parachute, publisher.

Platje, E., Popma, A., Vermeiren, R. R., et al. (2015). Testosterone and cortisol in relation to aggression in a non-clinical sample of boys and girls. *Aggressive Behavior, 41*(5), 478–487. doi:10.1002/ab.21585.

Selye, H. (1976). *The stress of life*. New York: McGraw-Hill.

Shields, M., & Wilkins, K. (2009). Factors related to on-the-job abuse of nurses by patients. *Health Reports, 20*(2). Retrieved from http://www.statcan.gc.ca/pub/82-003-x/2009002/article/10835-eng.pdf.

Shiina, A. (2015). Neurobiological basis of reactive aggression: A review. *International Journal of Forensic Science & Pathology, 3*(3), 94–98. doi:10.19070/2332-287X-1500023.

Skinner, B. (1953). *Science and human behaviour*. New York: Macmillan.

Standing Committee on Public Safety and National Security. (2016). Healthy minds, safe communities: Supporting our public safety officers through a national strategy for operational stress injuries. *Report of the Standing Committee on Public Safety and National Security 2016*. Retrieved from http://www.parl.gc.ca/HousePublications/Publication.aspx?Mode=1&Parl=42&Ses=1&DocId=8457704&Language=E.

Stevenson, K. N., Jack, S. M., O'Mara, L., et al. (2015). Registered nurses' experiences of patient violence on acute care psychiatric inpatient units: An interpretive descriptive study. *BMC Nursing, 14*, 35. doi:10.1186/s12912-015-0079-5.

Volicer, L., Citrome, L., & Volavka, J. (2017). Measurement of agitation and aggression in adult and aged neuropsychiatric patients: Review of definitions and frequently used measurement scales. *CNS Spectrums*, 1–8. doi:10.1017/S1092852917000050.

Yang, J. S., & Hung, H. V. (2015). Emotions as constraining and facilitating factors for creativity: Companionate love and anger. *Creativity and Innovation Management, 24*(2), 217–230. doi:10.1111.caim/12089.

24

Interpersonal Violence: Child, Older Adult, and Intimate Partner Abuse

Margaret Jordan Halter, Judi Sateren
Adapted by Sonya L. Jakubec

KEY TERMS AND CONCEPTS

abuse
aggression
assault
crisis situation
cultural violence
ecological model
emotional violence
financial abuse
interpersonal violence
neglect
perpetrators
physical violence

primary prevention
psychological violence
safety plan
secondary prevention
sexual violence
spiritual (religious) violence
survivor
tertiary prevention
typology of interpersonal violence
verbal abuse
violence
vulnerable person

OBJECTIVES

1. Differentiate anger, aggression, and interpersonal violence.
2. Identify nine types of violence: physical, sexual, psychological, emotional, spiritual, cultural, verbal abuse, financial abuse, and neglect.
3. Discuss the ecological model of violence in terms of etiology of violence (e.g., stresses on the perpetrator, vulnerable person, and environment that could escalate anxiety to the point at which abuse becomes the relief behaviour).
4. Compare and contrast three characteristics of a perpetrator with three characteristics of a vulnerable person.
5. Describe signs of escalating aggression and nursing interventions for de-escalation.

6. Describe four areas to assess when interviewing a person who has experienced violence.
7. Formulate four nursing diagnoses for the survivor of violence, and list supporting data from the assessment.
8. Write out a safety plan with the essential elements for a victim of intimate partner abuse.
9. Compare and contrast primary, secondary, and tertiary levels of intervention, giving two examples of intervention for each level.
10. Discuss three psychotherapeutic modalities that are useful in working with people experiencing violence.

evolve WEBSITE

Visit the Evolve website for Flashcards, Case Studies, and additional testing resources related to the content in this chapter: http://evolve.elsevier.com/Canada/Varcarolis/psychiatric/

Pre-Test   interactive review

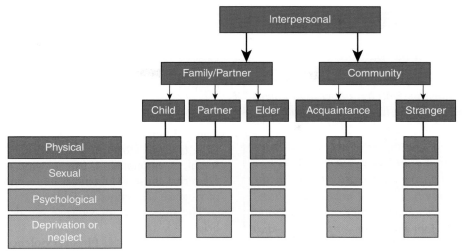

FIGURE 24-1 Typology of interpersonal violence. Source: Krug, E. G., Dahlberg, L. L., Mercy, J. A., et al. (Eds.). (2002). *World report on violence and health.* Geneva: World Health Organization. Retrieved from http://www.who.int/violence_injury_prevention/violence/world_report/en/.

According to the World Health Organization (WHO) (Krug, Dahlberg, Mercy, et al., 2002), interpersonal violence refers to violence between individuals and is subdivided into family and intimate partner violence and community violence. The former category includes child abuse, intimate partner violence, and older adult abuse, whereas the latter is broken down into acquaintance and stranger violence and includes youth violence, assault by strangers, violence related to property crimes, and violence in workplaces and other institutions. Figure 24-1 illustrates this typology of interpersonal violence, identifying four modes of violence that we elaborate on further in this chapter as nine types of violence: physical, sexual, psychological, emotional, spiritual, cultural, verbal abuse, financial abuse, and neglect. Interpersonal violence includes child abuse, intimate partner violence, and older adult abuse and can involve all nine types of violence. Both acquaintance and stranger experiences of violence are described at the community level.

To be effective in working with victims, the nurse needs an understanding of the conditions for violence, the types of violence, and how the types of violence may be experienced. Fundamental to this entire discussion is self-understanding (see the Self-Assessment section later in the chapter).

CLINICAL PICTURE

Violence is defined by the WHO as "the intentional use of physical force or power, threatened or actual, against oneself, another person, or against a group or community, that either results in or has a high likelihood of resulting in injury, death, psychological harm, maldevelopment or deprivation" (WHO, 2017). The essential element of violence is power and control. Violence is used to establish and maintain power and control over another person and often reflects an imbalance of power between the victim and the abuser. In this way, violence may be experienced through expressions of anger, but it is not caused by anger.

Anger can be understood as misunderstood and misaligned emotion that often follows fear, depression, stress, fatigue, or a perceived threat or personal attack. The situation that causes anger (for instance, the perceived threat) is not the problem; rather, the unhealthy response to anger is the problem (see Chapter 23 for more on anger and aggression). In How a Nurse Helped Me, Rachel's reflection on receiving expert nursing care in a health crisis illustrates how understanding anger amid multiple vulnerabilities can make a difference to both patient experiences and health outcomes.

Further clarity is also needed concerning the terms *aggression*, *violence*, *abuse*, and *assault*. These may sometimes be used interchangeably, though there are particular distinctions regarding clinical and legal requirements and practices. For example, abuse is a term used for legal purposes to describe violence perpetrated against children and dependent adults, and the term assault is used to describe the intentional threat or application of force to another person (an assault can be physical or sexual in nature) (*Criminal Code*, 1985).

Understanding anger, aggression, cycles of violence, and interventions at multiple levels (individual, interpersonal, community, and societal) with an ecological perspective on violence enables mental health nurses to support patients experiencing relationship violence and to address prevention.

Aggression is an action or behaviour in response to misaligned anger that results in a verbal or physical attack. Aggression tends to be used synonymously with violence. However, aggression is not always inappropriate and is sometimes necessary for self-protection. On the other hand, violence is always an objectionable act that involves intentional use of force that results in, or has the potential to result in, injury to another person.

Effective nursing intervention becomes more difficult when patient anger becomes personal and is directed at the nurse or nursing student or when aggression interrupts functioning and threatens the safety of individuals or communities. In the clinical setting, nursing interventions should ideally begin before anger

HOW A NURSE HELPED ME

Maybe We Can Trust Each Other a Bit More: Understanding Anger Amid Multiple Vulnerabilities

I have diabetes and ended up with a number of problems with my circulation and then landed in hospital with severe pain in my left foot. Tests showed that the vessels to that foot were blocked. No surgery could fix it, so I just took medications, but that didn't always work out because I was in and out of housing and mostly living in the homeless shelter downtown. That the medication didn't work and my foot slowly blackened—they called it necrotic. When they told me the foot should be amputated—that was the last straw. I just refused. Well, I should say I "lost it"—nothing physical, just yelling—it was all I could do, I was so upset. I know they thought I was a problem on the ward; they ended up calling security to watch me like a prisoner or something. But, really, shouldn't we talk about options or at least try other things first? It is hard enough living downtown and trying to stay away from heroin—now they think I should do that with half a leg? But one of the nurses, Nadija, on the hospital ward spent time with me. She really asked about my day-to-day life and how unbalanced things had become for me over the past years without a stable home, money, or family. I will never forget that she really found out about how I was living in the street community. When she said, "It must be hard when your body is also turning on you," well, that was it exactly. My foot was like my family—not coming back. As soon as I thought about it that way, I could face the facts, though. I was able to think about what this would mean for me, for housing and getting around, and made an appointment with my social worker. Nadija said things would be okay—there would be changes, but there would be some help for me. I don't always trust the help out there, but am willing to try. And I didn't totally lose it in the hospital ward, so maybe we can all trust each other a bit more.

and aggression become a problem. Anxiety is often the precipitant for negative feelings and behaviours. Assessing and responding to this anxiety can have extremely positive returns. Refer to Chapter 12 for interventions to reduce anxiety before it becomes a crisis (with crisis interventions discussed in more detail in Chapter 21).

Violence

Types of Violence

Nine types of violence have been identified: (1) physical, (2) sexual, (3) emotional, (4) psychological, (5) spiritual, (6) cultural, (7) verbal abuse, (8) financial abuse, and (9) neglect. The types of violence are defined in Table 24-1.

The nine types of violence are described in more detail below.

Physical violence. Physical violence may be experienced or perpetrated in a number of ways, including the following:
- Using physical force that results in pain, discomfort, or injury
- Hitting, pinching, hair-pulling, arm-twisting, strangling, burning, stabbing, punching, pushing, slapping, beating, shoving, kicking, choking, biting, force-feeding, or any other rough treatment
- Assault with a weapon or other object
- Threats with a weapon or other object
- Deliberate exposure to severe weather or inappropriate room temperatures
- Murder
- Medication abuse. Inappropriate use of medication, including:
  - Withholding medication
  - Not complying with prescription instructions
  - Overmedication or undermedication
- Restraints abuse:
  - Forcible confinement
  - Excessive, unwarranted, or unnecessary use of physical restraints
  - Forcing a person to remain in bed
  - Unwarranted use of medication to control a person (also called "chemical restraint")

Covert indicators of violence could include minor accidents—especially falls—and a series of minor complaints, such as low energy, fatigue, sleep problems, pain, swollen joints, sore muscles,

TABLE 24-1	TYPES OF VIOLENCE
Physical violence	The infliction of physical pain or bodily harm (e.g., slapping, punching, hitting, choking, pushing, restraining, biting, throwing, burning).
Sexual violence	When a person is forced to unwillingly take part in sexual activity. Sexual violence against adults may be referred to as *rape,* or in legal terms as *sexual assault* (see Chapter 25).
Emotional violence	When someone says, or does something to make a person feel belittled or worthless.
Psychological violence	When someone uses threats and causes fear in an individual to gain control.
Spiritual (or religious) violence	When someone uses an individual's spiritual beliefs to manipulate, dominate, or control that person.
Cultural violence	When an individual is harmed as a result of practices that are part of her or his culture, religion, or tradition.
Verbal abuse	When someone uses language, whether spoken or written, to cause harm to an individual.
Financial abuse	The withholding of financial support or the illegal or improper exploitation of funds or other resources for one's personal gain.
Neglect	When someone has the responsibility to provide care or assistance for an individual but does not.

BOX 24-1	COMMON PRESENTING PROBLEMS OF VICTIMS OF PHYSICAL VIOLENCE

Emergency Department
- Bleeding injuries, especially to head and face
- Internal injuries, concussions, perforated eardrum, abdominal injuries, severe bruising, eye injuries, strangulation marks on neck
- Back injuries
- Broken or fractured jaw, arms, pelvis, ribs, clavicle, legs
- Burns from cigarettes, appliances, scalding liquids, acids
- Psychological trauma, anxiety, attacks of hyperventilation, heart palpitations, severe crying spells, suicidal tendencies
- Miscarriage

Ambulatory Care Settings
- Perforated eardrum, twisted or stiff neck and shoulder muscles, headache
- Depression, stress-related conditions (e.g., insomnia, violent nightmares, anxiety, extreme fatigue, eczema, loss of hair)
- Talk of having "problems" with spouse; describing person as very jealous, impulsive, or an alcohol or drug abuser
- Repeated visits with new complaints
- Bruises of various ages and specific shapes (fingers, belt)

Any Setting
- Signs of stress due to family violence: emotional, behavioural, school, or sleep problems and increase in aggressive behaviour
- Injuries in a pregnant woman
- Recurrent visits for injuries attributed to being "accident prone"

faintness, dizziness, memory loss, difficulty concentrating, ringing in ears, indigestion, and appetite loss (Ford-Gilboe, Varcoe, & Merritt-Gray, 2010). Overt signs of battering include bruises, scars, burns, and other wounds in various stages of healing, particularly around the head, face, chest, arms, abdomen, back, buttocks, and genitalia. Injuries that should arouse the nurse's suspicion are listed in Box 24-1.

If the explanation does not match the injury or if the patient minimizes the seriousness of the injury, abuse may be suspected. Ask directly, but in a nonthreatening manner, if the injury has been caused by someone close to the patient. Observe the nonverbal response, such as hesitation or lack of eye contact, as well as the verbal response. Then ask specific questions such as "When was the last time it happened?" "How often does it happen?" "In what ways are you hurt?" Inconsistent explanations serve as a warning that further investigation is necessary. Vague explanations should alert the nurse to possible abuse ("She fell from a chair"; "The hot water was turned on by mistake"). The key to identification is a high index of suspicion.

Nonspecific bruising in older children is a common sign of abuse. Any bruises on an infant younger than 6 months of age should be considered suspicious. *Shaken baby syndrome*, one of the most serious types of child abuse, is the result of the brain moving in the opposite direction as the baby's head (Mian, Shah, Dalpiaz, et al., 2015). A baby who has been shaken

may present with respiratory problems, bulging fontanels, and central nervous system damage, resulting in seizures, vomiting, and coma.

Sexual violence. Sexual violence may be experienced or perpetrated in a number of ways, including but not limited to the following:
- Touching in a sexual manner without consent (i.e., kissing, grabbing, fondling)
- Forced sexual intercourse
- Forcing a person to perform sexual acts that may be degrading or painful
- Beating sexual parts of the body
- Forcing a person to view pornographic material; forcing participation in pornographic filming
- Using a weapon to force compliance
- Exhibitionism
- Making unwelcome sexual comments or jokes; leering behaviour
- Withholding sexual affection
- Denial of a person's sexuality or privacy (watching)
- Denial of sexual information and education
- Humiliating, criticizing, or trying to control a person's sexuality
- Forced prostitution
- Unfounded allegations of promiscuity or infidelity
- Purposefully exposing the person to human immunodeficiency virus (HIV) or other sexually transmitted infections

There are a variety of emotional and behavioural consequences of sexual violence, including depression, anxiety, suicide, aggression, chronic low self-esteem, and post-traumatic stress disorder (PTSD) (Carter-Snell & Jakubec, 2013). Childhood sexual abuse is a significant factor in the development of depression in many women (Kendler & Aggen, 2014). Girls are at higher risk for sexual abuse, although boys may be less likely to report it, and therefore sexual abuse of boys is less recognized and less treated (Ramsey & Abrams, 2010).

Emotional violence. Emotional violence occurs when someone says or does something to make a person feel belittled. It includes but is not limited to the following:
- Name calling
- Blaming all relationship problems on the person
- Not allowing the person to have contact with family and friends
- Destroying possessions
- Humiliating or making fun of the person
- Recalling a person's past mistakes
- Expressing negative expectations
- Expressing distrust
- Telling a person that she or he is worthless or a burden

Emotional violence may exist on its own or as a result of co-occurring physical, sexual, or psychological violence or other forms of abuse. Emotional abuse has devastating effects on children. Although it is less obvious and more difficult to assess than physical violence, studies have shown that those who were emotionally abused as children show higher rates of anxiety, depression, interpersonal sensitivity, and dissociation (Public Health Agency of Canada, 2016).

Psychological violence. **Psychological violence** occurs when someone uses threats and causes fear in a person to gain control. It includes but is not limited to the following:

- Threatening to harm the person or her or his family if she or he leaves
- Threatening to harm oneself
- Threats of violence
- Threats of abandonment
- Stalking or criminal harassment
- Socially isolating the person
- Not allowing access to a telephone
- Not allowing a competent person to make decisions
- Inappropriately controlling the person's activities
- Treating a person like a child or a servant
- Withholding important information
- Withholding companionship or affection
- Use of undue pressure to:
  - Sign legal documents
  - Not seek legal assistance or advice
  - Move out of the home
  - Make or change a legal will or beneficiary
  - Make or change an advance health care directive
  - Give money or other possessions to relatives or other caregivers
  - Do things the person does not want to do

Spiritual violence. **Spiritual (religious) violence** occurs when someone uses a person's spiritual beliefs to manipulate, dominate, or control the person. Spiritual violence includes but is not limited to the following:

- Not allowing the person to follow her or his preferred spiritual or religious tradition
- Forcing a spiritual or religious path or practice on another person
- Belittling or making fun of a person's spiritual or religious tradition, beliefs, or practices
- Using one's spiritual or religious position, rituals, or practices to manipulate, dominate, or control a person

Cultural violence. **Cultural violence** occurs when a person is harmed as a result of practices that are part of her or his culture, religion, or tradition (Gill, Strange, & Roberts, 2014). It includes but is not limited to the following:

- Committing "honour" or other crimes against women in some parts of the world, where women especially may be physically harmed, shunned, maimed, or killed for:
  - Falling in love with the "wrong" person
  - Seeking divorce
  - Infidelity; committing adultery
  - Being raped
  - Practising witchcraft
  - Being older

Cultural violence may take place in some of the following ways:

- Lynching or stoning
- Banishment
- Abandonment of an older person at hospital by family
- Genital mutilation
- Rape-marriage

- Sexual slavery
- Murder

Verbal abuse. **Verbal abuse** occurs when someone uses language, whether spoken or written, to cause harm to a person. It includes but is not limited to the following:

- Expressing distrust
- Yelling
- Lying
- Name-calling
- Insulting, swearing
- Unreasonably ordering around

Financial abuse. **Financial abuse** occurs when someone controls a person's financial resources without the person's consent or misuses those resources. It includes but is not limited to the following:

- Not allowing the person to participate in educational programs
- Forcing the person to work in a certain job
- Refusing to let the person work outside the home or attend school
- Controlling the person's choice of occupation
- Illegally or improperly using a person's money, assets, or property
- Acts of fraud
- Taking funds from the person without permission for one's own use
- Misusing funds through lies, trickery, or controlling or withholding money
- Not allowing access to bank accounts, savings, or other income
- Requiring excessive detailed justification for all money spent
- Persuading the person to buy a product or give away money
- Selling the house or other possessions without permission
- Forging a signature on pension cheques or legal documents
- Misusing a power of attorney, an enduring power of attorney, or a legal guardianship
- Not paying bills
- Opening mail without permission
- Living in a person's home without paying fairly for expenses
- Destroying personal property

Neglect. **Neglect** is the failure to provide basic needs for a dependant. It can take several forms, including but not limited to the following:

- Failing to meet the needs of a person who is unable to meet those needs alone
- Abandonment in a public setting
- Not remaining with a person who needs help
- Physical neglect; disregarding necessities of daily living, including failing to provide adequate or necessary:
  - Nutrition or fluids
  - Shelter
  - Clean clothes and linens
  - Social companionship
- Failing to turn a bed-ridden person frequently to prevent stiffness and bedsores
- Medical neglect:
  - Ignoring special dietary requirements
  - Not providing needed medications

- Not calling a physician; not reporting or taking action on a medical condition, injury, or problem
- Not being aware of the possible negative effects of medications

Neglected children and older adults often appear undernourished, dirty, and poorly clothed. Neglect is also manifested by inadequate medical care, such as lack of immunizations or untreated medical conditions. Adults who were neglected in childhood are more likely to report current symptoms of anxiety, depression, somatization, paranoia, and hostility than those who were physically abused but did not suffer neglect (Raposo, Mackenzie, Henriksen, et al., 2014; Registered Nurses' Association of Ontario, 2014).

Cycle of Violence

Dr. Donald Dutton studied the relationship of borderline personality characteristics to the characteristics of both chronic and intermittent family abusers. Dutton (2007) identified three borderline personality characteristics: (1) an unstable sense of self with dependency and fear of abandonment, (2) unstable interpersonal relationships with manipulation, and (3) intense and impulsive behaviours, relating to the cycle of violence perpetrators use to control their partners.

The *cycle of violence*, first proposed by Walker (1979), includes three recurring phases of violence. These phases are characterized by periods of intense violence that tend to increase in severity and frequency, alternating with periods of safety, hope, and trust. Phase I of the borderline, or *cyclic*, personality consists of an internal buildup of tensions as a result of the abuser not knowing how to verbalize inner feelings of dysphoria. The abuser converts dysphoria into abuse through the assertion that it is the partner's fault for not being able to soothe the abuser's bad feelings (Dutton, 1998, 2007). The *tension-building stage* is characterized by relatively minor incidents, such as pushing, shoving, and verbal abuse. During this time, the victim often ignores or accepts the abuse for fear that more severe abuse will follow. Abusers then rationalize that their abusive behaviour is acceptable. As the tension escalates, both participants may try to reduce it. The abuser may try to reduce the tension through the use of alcohol or drugs, and the victim may try to reduce the tension by minimizing the importance of the incidents ("I should have had the house neater … dinner ready"). The abuser may become increasingly demanding. The splitting characteristics of borderline personality become evident, as the abuser sees the partner as "all bad"—unloving, unfaithful, and malevolent (Dutton, 1998, 2007). During the *acute battering stage*, the unexpressed rage builds until the abuser with borderline personality releases the built-up tension through brutal beatings. Severe injuries can and do result, driving the victim further away and increasing the abuser's feelings of abandonment. Consequently, the abuser promises anything to get the victim back. The opposite side of splitting here becomes evident, as the abuser describes the victim as "all good" (Dutton, 1998, p. 96). This phase coincides with the *honeymoon stage*, which may be characterized by kindness and loving behaviours. The abuser, at least initially, feels remorseful and apologetic and may bring presents, make promises, and tell the victim how much she or he is loved and needed. The victim usually believes

the promises, feels needed and loved, and drops any legal proceedings or plans to leave that may have been initiated during the acute battering stage.

Unfortunately, without intervention, the cycle will repeat itself. Over time, the periods of calmness and safety become briefer, and the periods of anger and violence increase. With each repetition of the pattern, the victim's self-esteem becomes more and more eroded. The victim either believes that the violence was deserved or accepts the blame for it. This self-blame can lead to feelings of depression, hopelessness, immobilization, and self-deprecation. Figure 24-2 illustrates the cycle of violence.

EPIDEMIOLOGY

Violence within families is among the most important Canadian public health issue and is therefore a significant nursing concern. The abusive behaviours exist within a context in which their purpose is to gain power and control and to induce fear. Abusive behaviour may involve one or more of the types of violence already described and may be inflicted on a child, an intimate partner, an older adult, or other populations. While the true prevalence of child, older adult, and intimate partner abuse is unknown (because of under-reporting and variability in reporting methods, instruments, sites, and reporters), it is clear that abuse is a significant problem.

Child Abuse

In 2016, the Public Health Agency of Canada estimated 85 440 substantiated child abuse investigations that year (14.19 investigations per 1 000 children). Thirty-four percent identified exposure to intimate partner violence as the primary type of abuse, and another 34% identified neglect as the overriding concern, followed by physical abuse (20%), emotional abuse (9%), and sexual abuse (3%). There was some variation by age and sex in the incidence of investigated abuse, with rates being highest for infants. The rate of family-related sexual offences was more than four times higher for girls than for boys, and the rate of physical assault was similar for girls and boys (Statistics Canada, 2017). According to the Criminal Intelligence Service (Public Health Agency of Canada, 2016), 94% of substantiated investigations involved children whose primary caregiver was a biological parent, and 2% involved children whose primary caregiver was a parent's partner or an adoptive parent.

Indigenous children have been identified as a key group to examine because of concerns about their over-representation in the foster care system (Fallon, Chabot, Fluke, et al., 2013). The rate of substantiated child abuse investigations was four times higher in investigations involving Indigenous children than in those involving non-Indigenous children.

Intimate Partner Violence

According to Statistics Canada (2017), in 2015 almost 92 000 people in Canada were victims of intimate partner violence, representing just over a quarter (28%) of all victims of police-reported violent crime. Violence against spouses and dating partners in current and former relationships is referred to as

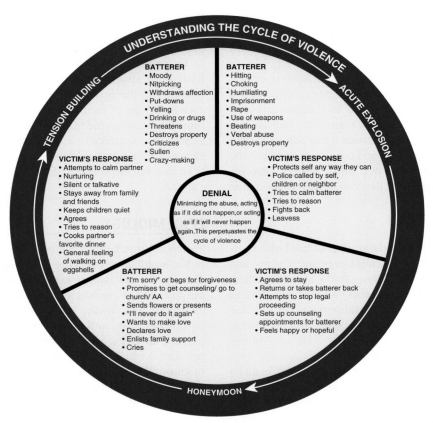

FIGURE 24-2 The cycle of violence. Source: Mayfield, C. (2016). Understanding the cycle of violence. Retrieved from http://dvbleedingheart.com/understanding-the-cycle-of-violence/.

intimate partner violence (IPV) or *domestic violence (DV)*. The definition of spouse includes current or former legally married, separated, divorced, and common-law partners, and the term *dating relationships* includes current or former boyfriends and girlfriends as well as other intimate relationships (i.e., casual sexual relationships or encounters not considered to be boyfriend–girlfriend relationships). In 2015, violence within dating relationships was more common than violence within spousal relationships, according to police-reported data. IPV was more likely to be perpetrated by current or former dating partners (54% of victims) than by current or former married or common-law spouses (44% of victims). These proportions were similar among male and female victims. Four out of five victims of police-reported IPV were women, representing about 72 000 female victims. Similar to the general crime data reported to police (Allen, 2016), rates of IPV were highest in the territories. Nunavut had the highest rate of police-reported IPV in Canada (3 575 per 100 000 population), more than five times that of the highest provincial rate (Statistics Canada, 2017).

The rate of intimate partner physical assault (the most common type of police-reported IPV) increased slightly between 2014 and 2015 (up 2%). Overall, the rate of intimate partner physical assault declined by 8% between 2010 and 2015. The rate of intimate partner sexual assault was 36 times higher among women than men (18 female victims per 100 000 versus 0.5 male victims per 100 000), according to police-reported 2015 data (Statistics Canada, 2017).

Homicides committed by intimate partners decreased 46% between 1995 and 2015. According to police-reported data, between 2005 and 2015, females ages 25 to 29 years were at the highest risk for intimate partner homicide (8.2 per 1 million population). Most (74%) of the 964 intimate partner homicides between 2005 and 2015 were committed by a current or former legally married or common-law spouse.

Older Adult Abuse

A recent large-scale 2015 Canadian survey uncovered that about 7.5% of older adults (approximately 695 248) were abused in the previous year. When neglect was added to psychological, physical, sexual, and financial abuse, this number increased to 8.2%, or 766 247 older Canadian adults. Survey respondents were, for the most part, relatively healthy adults in their sixties and early seventies, and very few were ill or identified as frail. Most common was psychological or emotional abuse, affecting 2.7% of older Canadians daily or almost daily and involving repeated criticism, yelling, or insults. Second most common was financial abuse, affecting 2.6% of older adults. Physical abuse was the third most common form of elder abuse and affected 2.2% of older people. Fewer older Canadians reported that they were sexually assaulted, though 1.6% of survey respondents reported being sexually abused in the past 12 months. Finally, 1.2% of older adults were neglected a few times or more in the last year, typically by being denied assistance with housework and meals (Canadian Medical Association, 2016).

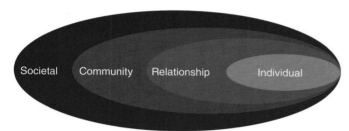

FIGURE 24-3 The ecological model of violence. Source: Krug, E. G., Dahlberg, L. L., Mercy, J. A., et al. (Eds.). (2002). *World report on violence and health.* Geneva: World Health Organization. Retrieved from http://www.who.int/violence_injury_prevention/violence/world _report/en/.

COMORBIDITY

Common long-term psychological and social effects of abuse include depression, suicidal ideation, chronic post-traumatic stress symptoms, dissociation, interpersonal disturbances, substance abuse, and revictimization (Coles, Lee, Taft, et al., 2015). Family violence is common in the childhood histories of juvenile offenders, runaways, violent criminals, prostitutes, and those who in turn are violent toward others. Exposure to abuse has been associated with decrements in children's optimal development in the areas of social behaviour, academic performance, physical health, and mental health (Public Health Agency of Canada, 2016).

Box 24-2 identifies some of the long-term effects of family violence.

ETIOLOGY

In any form, anger, aggression, violence, and abuse profoundly affect individual mental health and well-being. The roots of all forms of violence are founded in the many types of inequality that continue to exist and grow in society, and ecological understanding of causation assists nurses in assessment and planning of interventions at multiple levels. The etiology of anger and aggression also provides a useful framework for mental health nursing practice (refer to Chapter 23).

The Ecological Model of Violence

The WHO adopted an "ecological model" in its *World Report on Violence and Health* to help understand the multilevel, multifaceted nature of violence (Krug, Dahlberg, Mercy, et al., 2002). As an analytical tool, the ecological model (Figure 24-3) recognizes and identifies personal history and characteristics of the victim or perpetrator, other family members, the immediate social context (often referred to as *community factors*), and the larger society. In contrast to simplistic explanations, the ecological model emphasizes that it is a *combination* of factors, acting at different levels, that influences the risk for and resiliency to violence and the potential for recurrence of abuse. The various factors relevant to the different levels of the ecological model are also affected by the context of the settings children interact with—in their home and family environment, at school, in institutions and workplaces, as well as in their community and broader society.

BOX 24-2   LONG-TERM EFFECTS OF FAMILY VIOLENCE

- People involved in family violence are found to have a higher incidence of:
  - Depression
  - Suicidal feelings
  - Self-contempt
  - Inability to trust
  - Inability to develop intimate relationships in later life
- Victims of severe violence are also at higher risk for experiencing recurring symptoms of post-traumatic stress disorder (PTSD):
  - Flashbacks
  - Dissociation—out-of-body experiences
  - Poor self-esteem
  - Compulsive or impulsive behaviours (e.g., substance abuse, excessive spending, gambling, promiscuity)
  - Multiple somatic complaints
- Children who witness violence in their homes are at greater risk for developing behavioural and emotional problems throughout their lives.
- After the age of 5 or 6, children who witness violence at home show an indication of identifying with the aggressor and losing respect for the victim.
- Some mental and behavioural conditions are associated with childhood abuse or witnessing of abuse:
  - Depressive disorders
  - PTSD
  - Somatic complaints
  - Low self-esteem
  - Phobias (agoraphobia, social and specific phobias)
  - Antisocial behaviours
  - Potential for future child or spousal abuse
- Adolescent victims or witnesses of abuse are more likely to have behavioural symptoms, such as:
  - Failing grades
  - Difficulty forming relationships
  - Increased incidence of theft, police arrest, and violent behaviours
  - Seductive or promiscuous behaviours
  - Running away from home

Environmental Factors

Violence and abuse occur across all segments of Canadian society. While some risk factors may be unique to a particular type of violence, the various types of violence more commonly share a number of risk factors. Prevailing cultural norms, poverty, social isolation, and such factors as alcohol abuse, substance abuse, and access to firearms are risk factors for more than one type of violence (Krug, Dahlberg, Mercy, et al., 2002).

The occurrence of abuse requires the following participants and conditions:

- A perpetrator
- Someone who, by age or situation, is vulnerable (e.g., child, woman, older adult, mentally ill or physically challenged person)
- A crisis situation

BOX 24-3 CHARACTERISTICS OF ABUSIVE PARENTS

- A history of abuse, neglect, or emotional deprivation as a child
- Family authoritarianism: a commitment to raising children as they were raised by their own parents
- Low self-esteem, feelings of worthlessness, depression
- Poor coping skills
- Social isolation (may be suspicious of others): few or no friends, little or no involvement in social or community activities
- Involvement in a crisis situation: unemployment, divorce, financial difficulties
- Rigid, unrealistic expectations of child's behaviour
- History of severe mental illness
- Violent temper outbursts
- Looking to child for satisfaction of need for love, support, and reassurance (often unmet because of parenting deficits in family of origin)
- Projecting blame onto the child for parents' "troubles" (e.g., step-parent may project hostility toward new mate onto a child)
- Lack of effective parenting skills
- Inability to seek help from others
- Perception of the child as bad or evil
- History of drug or alcohol abuse
- Feeling of little or no control over life
- Low tolerance for frustration
- Poor impulse control

Perpetrator

Perpetrators, those who initiate violence, often consider their own needs to be more important than anyone else's and look to others to meet their needs. The term *perpetrator* applies to any member of a household who is violent toward another member (e.g., children, siblings, same-sex partners, extended family members). Risk factors for those who may become abusive to their children are summarized in Box 24-3.

Control and power are acted out by perpetrators of abuse in all stages of the cycle of violence. The abuse of power and control is the foundational etiology of relationship violence (Figure 24-4), with additional ecological risk and resiliency factors determining the typology. Because of extreme pathological jealousy, many perpetrators of relationship violence refuse to allow their partners to work outside the home; others demand that their partners work in the same place as they do so they can monitor activities and friendships. Many accompany their partners to and from all activities and forbid them to have personal friends or participate in recreational activities outside the home. Even after imposing such restrictions, perpetrators often accuse their partners of infidelity. Many perpetrators maintain their control and possessiveness by controlling the family finances so tightly that there is barely enough money for daily living. Typically, perpetrators believe in male supremacy—being in charge and being dominant. Messages of male dominance are reinforced via observations of the partner dyad, parent–child interactions, peer group experiences, and the influence of the media (Internet, television, movies, comics, computer games).

Culturally driven violence against women is a growing problem in Canada's immigrant communities (Papp, 2010). However, it is important to recognize that a wide variety of cultural norms in Canadian society dictate the dynamics of relationships between intimate partners and child-rearing practices. Learning about the cultural backgrounds of patients can assist health care providers in identifying risk factors and culturally appropriate interventions.

Vulnerable Person

The **vulnerable person** is an adult or child who, as a result of illness, physical condition, or experiences, is at greater risk than the general population for being harmed. The term **survivor** recognizes the recovery and healing process that follows victimization and does not have the connotation of passivity that *victim* has.

Women. Pregnancy may trigger or increase violence (Taillieu, Brownridge, Tyler, et al., 2016). The Public Health Agency of Canada (2016) reported the prevalence of abuse during pregnancy to be 5.7% to 6.6% based on two major studies done in Saskatoon and Toronto. A past history of abuse is one of the strongest predictors of abuse during pregnancy. Other risk factors include social instability (e.g., young, unmarried, failed to complete high school, unemployed, having an unplanned pregnancy), an unhealthy lifestyle (e.g., unhealthy diet, alcohol use, illicit drug use, emotional problems), and physical and psychological health problems (including prescription drug use). Multiple, cumulative effects of violence toward women in workplaces revealed that lifetime sexual harassment was associated with higher PTSD symptomology, highlighting the importance of including bullying in studying women and relationship violence (MacIntosh, Wuest, Ford-Gilboe, et al., 2015).

Children. The Canadian Incidence Study (Public Health Agency of Canada, 2016) found that, in 46% of substantiated child abuse investigations, at least one child functioning issue was indicated. Academic difficulties were the most frequently reported functioning concern (23%), with 11% involving intellectual or developmental disabilities. The second most common functioning concern was depression, anxiety, or withdrawal (19%). Fifteen percent of cases involved child aggression, whereas 14% involved attachment issues. Eleven percent of investigations involved children experiencing attention-deficit disorder (ADD) or attention-deficit/hyperactivity disorder (ADHD). The increased risk for abuse could be due to the added stress of caring for a child with functioning difficulties as well as to the differences between the parents' expectations of their child and the reality of who the child is. Parental substance abuse is associated with an increase in the risk of exposure to both childhood physical and sexual abuse (Wallström, Persson, & Salzmann-Erikson, 2016). As with relationship violence more broadly, the abuse of power and control and particular risks for child abuse are described in the Duluth model (Figure 24-5).

Older adults. Older adult abuse is recognized as a serious problem in Canada. Risk factors for older adult abuse include cognitive disability (e.g., Alzheimer's disease) or other mental illness, poor physical health, impairment in the activities of daily living (ADLs), dependency on the caregiver, isolation, stressful events, and a history of intergenerational conflict between the

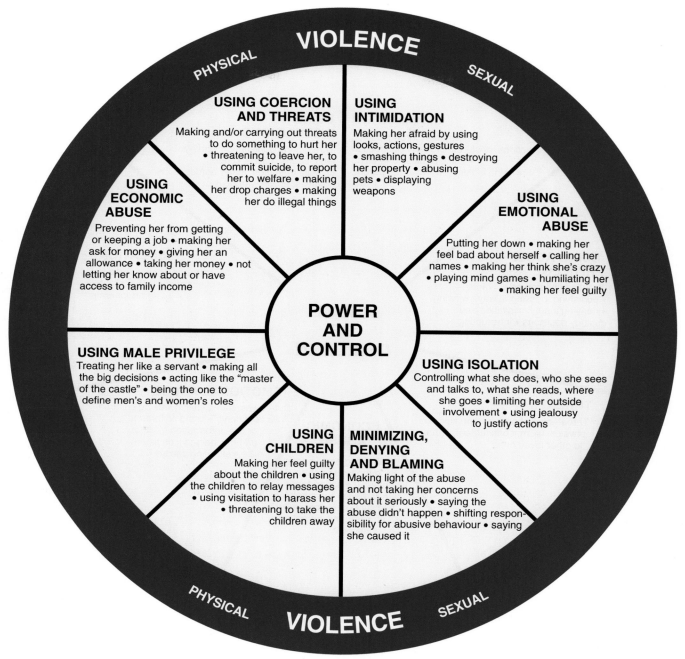

FIGURE 24-4 The Duluth "Power and Control" wheel. Source: Redrawn from Domestic Abuse Intervention Project, 202 East Superior Street, Duluth, MN 55802, Tel. 218-722-2781. Retrieved from http://www.theduluthmodel.org/training/wheels.html.

older adult and the caregiver (Pillemer, Burnes, Riffin, et al., 2016; Podnieks, Rietschlin, & Walsh, 2012).

Crisis Situation

Anyone may be at risk for abuse in a crisis situation—crises of all kinds contribute to an increased risk for interpersonal violence. Refer to Chapter 21 for more on crisis and crisis intervention.

APPLICATION OF THE NURSING PROCESS: INTERPERSONAL VIOLENCE

ASSESSMENT

General Assessment

It has been increasingly recommended that routine universal screening for both perpetrators and victims of violence be

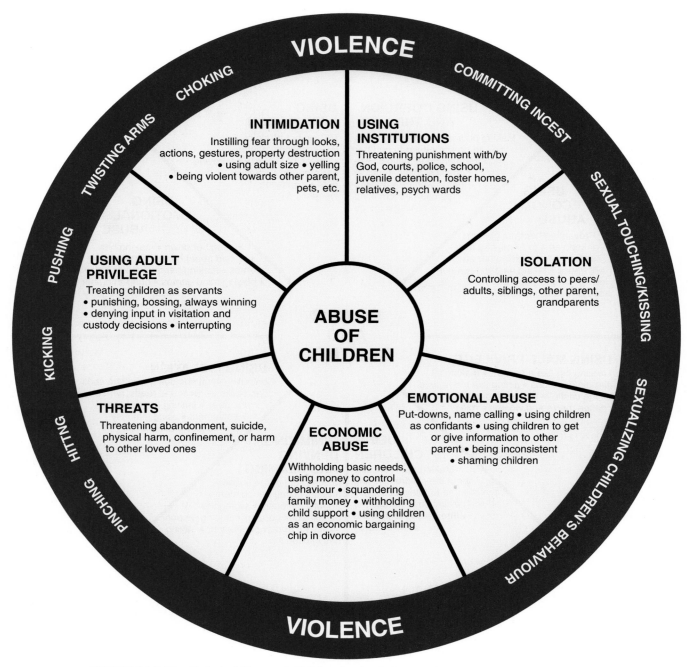

FIGURE 24-5 The Duluth "Abuse of Children" wheel. Source: Redrawn from Domestic Abuse Intervention Project, 202 East Superior Street, Duluth, MN 55802, Tel. 218-722-2781. Retrieved from http://www.theduluthmodel.org/training/wheels.html.

implemented within all manner of health care settings (Registered Nurses' Association of Ontario, 2005; Wathen, Macgregor, Sibbald, et al., 2013). The nurse is often the first point of contact for people experiencing violence and thus is in an ideal position to contribute to prevention, detection, and effective intervention. Organizations need to develop policies that support nursing practice while considering the unique setting where the

screening is to take place, patient needs, and outcomes (Paterno & Draughon, 2016).

Effective programs to assess and intervene with violence target specific populations based on the risk and resiliency factors described as part of the clinical picture. Pregnant women are just one population considered at risk for violence and abuse (see Research Highlight box).

ASSESSMENT GUIDELINES

Interpersonal Violence

During assessment and counselling, maintain an interested and empathetic manner. Assess the following:
- Presenting signs and symptoms of victims of abuse
- Potential indicators of vulnerable parents who might benefit from education and instruction in effective coping techniques
- Physical, sexual, or emotional abuse; neglect; and economic maltreatment of older adults
- Family coping patterns
- Patient's support system
- Drug or alcohol use
- Suicidal or homicidal ideas
- Post-traumatic stress

  If the patient is a child or older adult, identify the protective services in your province or territory that must be notified.

Interview Process and Setting

Important and relevant information about the family situation can be incorporated into a routine health history process. Because many victims of violence do not disclose abuse the first time they are asked about it, nor do they recognize violence as a health issue, screening for violence among women and their families should occur not only on the initial health history but also each time the health history is updated (Registered Nurses' Association of Ontario, 2005). For screening strategies, refer to Woman Abuse: Screening, Identification and Initial Response at http://rnao.ca/bpg/guidelines/woman-abuse-screening-identification-and-initial-response.

Screening tools use specific terminology that describes the *actions* of perpetrators of violence rather than general terminology such as "abuse." Therefore screening questions need to be clear, and examples of abusive behaviour may be needed to help the patient understand what constitutes abusive behaviour. There are validated tools that can be used in screening (e.g., the Abuse Assessment Screen [AAS], the Abuse Assessment Screen—Disability [AAS-D], the Woman Abuse Screening Tool [WAST]), or nurses can develop their own style, keeping in mind these principles (Registered Nurses' Association of Ontario, 2005). The AAS, developed by the Nursing Research Consortium on Violence and Abuse (McFarlane, Hughes, Nosek, et al., 2001), has been used extensively to assist in the routine identification of intimate partner abuse (Figure 24-6). More research does need to be conducted, however, on culturally sensitive screening, as well as on screening for male victims (Arkins, Begley, & Higgins, 2016).

Guiding principles for screening for abuse will assist the nurse in implementing effective interventions. The adapted mnemonic tool ABCD-ER, explained in Box 24-4, outlines the principles.

In the case of suspected child abuse or neglect, it is better to ask about methods of disciplining children rather than to use the words *abuse* or *violence*. Questions that are open-ended and require a descriptive response can be less threatening and elicit

 RESEARCH HIGHLIGHT

Safety Planning Interventions for Intimate Partner Violence in Maternal Child Nursing Practice

Problem

Numerous barriers to screening for intimate partner violence (IPV) exist and include care provider discomfort, educational needs, attitudes, and time. Identifying supportive models and approaches to improve screening is necessary to increase longer-term health outcomes and well-being of those experiencing violence.

Purpose of Study

This study sought to discover if a nursing model focused on vulnerability (MOVE) would produce higher rates of screening, IPV disclosure, safety planning, and referrals compared with the comparison group (CG), and if increased screening would be sustained over the longer term (after 24 months).

Methods

A cluster randomized controlled trial tested the Improving Maternal and Child Health Care for Vulnerable Mothers (MOVE) nursing model of care. The aim of MOVE was to increase maternal child health (MCH) team screening rates, IPV disclosure, safety planning, and referrals over 12 months and program sustainability beyond 24 months. Mothers with babies up to age 12 months attending community-based MCH centres in Australia were included.

Key Findings

A gradual increase in routine screening was achieved, reaching its highest point of 56% at week 4 but not exceeding 36% over a year-long rate. Those in the MOVE intervention group scored higher than the control group, demonstrating a statistically significant increase in safety planning. The higher dose of domestic violence advocacy or liaison may have positively affected the team's confidence and uptake of referrals.

Implications for Nursing Practice

Nurses need to screen for domestic violence, particularly during pregnancy. It may be that models of care that specifically integrate and incorporate screening will address the barriers and, in particular, support safety planning for those experiencing IPV.

Source: Burnett, C., & Bacchus, L. (2016). Women find safety planning more useful than referrals in a maternal and child health IPV intervention. *Evidence-Based Nursing, 19*(2), 43–43. doi:10.1136/eb-2015-102201.

more relevant information than questions that are direct or can be answered with *yes* or *no* (see Chapter 10):
- What arrangements do you make when you have to leave your child alone?
- How do you discipline your child?
- When your infant cries for a long time, how do you get him or her to stop?
- What about your child's behaviour bothers you the most?

  Areas to include in any abuse assessment (child, older adult, IPV) include the following: (1) violence indicators, (2) levels of anxiety and coping responses, (3) family coping patterns, (4)

1. **Within the last year**, have you been hit, slapped, kicked, pushed, shoved, or otherwise physically hurt by someone? YES NO

   If YES, who? (Circle all that apply)

   Intimate partner   Care provider   Health professional   Family member   Other

   Please describe: _____   _____

2. **Within the last year**, has anyone forced you to have sexual activities? YES NO

   If YES, who? (Circle all that apply)

   Intimate partner   Care provider   Health professional   Family member   Other

   Please describe: _____   _____

3. **Within the last year**, has anyone prevented you from using a wheelchair, cane, respirator, or other assistive devices? YES NO

   If YES, who? (Circle all that apply)

   Intimate partner   Care provider   Health professional   Family member   Other

   Please describe: _____   _____

4. **Within the last year**, has anyone you depend on refused to help you with an important personal need, such as taking your medicine, getting to the bathroom, getting out of bed, bathing, getting dressed, or getting food or drink? YES NO

   If YES, who? (Circle all that apply)

   Intimate partner   Care provider   Health professional   Family member   Other

   Please describe: _____   _____

FIGURE 24-6 Abuse Assessment Screen. Source: McFarlane, J., Hughes, R. B., Nosek, M. A., et al. (2001). Abuse Assessment Screen—Disability (AAS-D): Measuring frequency, type, and perpetrator of abuse toward women with physical disabilities. *Journal of Women's Health & Gender-Based Medicine, 10,* 861–866. doi:10.1089/152460901753285750. The publisher for this copyrighted material is Mary Ann Liebert, Inc. publishers.

support systems, (5) suicide potential, (6) homicide potential, and (7) drug and alcohol use. The vignette illustrates the key points in assessing a woman in crisis at the initial interview, as well as suggested follow-up.

Maintaining Accurate Records

Documentation is an integral aspect of safe, effective nursing practice and must be comprehensive and legible and accurately reflect screening practice. For more information on documentation, refer to Chapter 7. According to the Registered Nurses' Association of Ontario (2005), the health care record needs to include the following related to aggression and interpersonal violence:

- A safety check
- Direct quotations of what the victim describes
- Direct observations made by the nurse
- Referrals discussed and made and information given

The record should be nonbiased and contain direct observations by the nurse. Nonbiased terms such as *chooses, declines,* or *patient states* are more appropriate than judgemental terms such as *alleges* or *victim* (Middlesex-London Health Unit, 2000). For

example, it would be better to record "Patient states, 'My partner beat me'" (nonjudgemental) than "Victim alleges he was assaulted by partner" (judgemental).

Referral services and secondary intervention would include more detailed documentation, such as the following (Middlesex-London Health Unit, 2000):

- Relevant health history
- History of abuse, including the first, worst, and most recent incident
- Where and when the abuse took place
- Name of and relationship to abuser
- Detailed description of injuries (e.g., a body map to indicate size, colour, shape, areas, and types of injuries, with explanations [see Figure 24-6] and photos, if taken)
- Physical evidence of sexual abuse, when possible
- All health care provided and information or referrals to resources provided

When no disclosure of abuse is made, the nurse should document "no disclosure to abuse screening."

Legal, ethical, and professional requirements guide the management of patient records, indicating that they must be

BOX 24-4 THE MNEMONIC TOOL ABCD-ER

A—Attitude and Approachability of the health care provider:
- Treat the patient with respect, dignity, and compassion.
- Be sensitive to differences in age, culture, language, ethnicity, and sexual orientation.
- State clearly that abuse is not the fault of the victim but the responsibility of the abuser.
- Reinforce that no one has the right to use physical, sexual, or emotional abuse to control another person's actions.
- Reinforce that physical and sexual abuse are against the law in Canada.
- Convey a nonthreatening, nonjudgemental stance in words, facial expressions, and body language.
- Express concern for the patient's safety.
- Acknowledge the strength the patient has shown in surviving abuse and disclosing it to you.
- Offer support.
- Avoid excessive criticism of the abuser.

B—Belief in the person's account of his or her own experience of abuse:
- Show by your words and your actions that you believe the patient's disclosure.
- Remember that the fear of not being believed silences many victims of abuse. Abusers may also convince victims that no one will believe them if they disclose the abuse.
- Help the patient to understand that most of us try to block out memories that are too painful to deal with. A patient disclosing retrospective abuse may not even be sure of exactly what happened or where it happened.
- Reassure and encourage the patient to have confidence in her or his own perceptions of the abuse.

C—Confidentiality is essential for disclosure:
- Interview in private, without the patient's partner or family members present.
- Use a professional interpreter if one is required, not a friend or family member.
- Tell the patient directly about the policies and procedures used in your practice or institution to protect patient confidentiality.
- Assure the patient that you will not release the information unless he or she gives written permission.
- Outline the exceptions to this pledge of confidentiality: (1) where child abuse or neglect is in question; (2) where the health care provider has reason to fear for the safety of a third party; and (3) where a file is subpoenaed by a court order.
- Let the patient know that you are documenting the information disclosed so that it will help you provide appropriate medical services and referrals and so that it will be available to help the patient later if she or he should provide you with permission to share it.

D—Documentation:
- Document consistently and legibly.

- Distinguish between your observations and the patient's reports.
- Record information on the first, the worst, and the most recent abusive incident.
- If more than one person has abused the patient, distinguish between the abusers and the specific injuries or health effects of each incident.
- Indicate the frequency of abusive incidents, as well as any increase or decrease in frequency and seriousness.
- Avoid subjective statements and speculations that might undermine the patient's credibility.
- Use the patient's own words, in quotation marks, as frequently as possible.
- Use diagrams and photographs where possible to document physical injuries.

E—Education:
- Educate about abuse and its health effects.
- Help the patient to understand that she or he is not alone.
- Attempt to engage the patient in long-term continuity of care by offering appropriate referrals and follow-up.
- Know about available community resources and help the patient choose the services he or she needs when ready to seek assistance.
- Display posters, brochures, and other available information about abuse in your office or institution.
- Provide the female patient with information about the abused women's helpline and the male patient with information about the crisis hotline.

R—Respect and Recognition:
- Respect the integrity and autonomy of the patient's life choices.
- Recognize that the patient must deal with the abuse at her or his own pace directed by her or his own decisions.
- Recognize that an abused person is an expert about his or her own abuse and abuser.
- Affirm the patient's strengths and survival skills.
- Do not try to tell the patient what to do but help him or her understand the options available; the patient must choose the options that will meet his or her own goals and priorities.
- Offer referrals to other specialized services and follow-up with you.
- Do not label the patient resistant or nonadherent if she or he decides not to accept your advice; make it clear you respect the patient's right to choose and will continue your support as her or his caregiver.
- Make sure any medications you offer to help the patient deal with stress or sleep problems do not impair the patient's ability to act appropriately on his or her own behalf.
- Help the patient to recognize that she or he cannot control the actions of others; the patient can choose only her or his own actions.

Source: Adapted from Middlesex-London Health Unit. (2000). *Task force on the health effects of woman abuse—Final report*. London, ON: Author.

carefully maintained (see Chapter 7). Policies and procedures concerning access to the patient's health information need to be developed as part of the screening protocol in all health care settings (Registered Nurses' Association of Ontario, 2005). The patient needs to be informed prior to screening that the interaction will be documented, that the record will be kept confidential, and that it can serve as evidence should legal action be initiated. Even if intervention or legal action does not occur at this time, the record is begun, and the next provider will be aware of the problem and be in a better position to offer support. The vignette illustrates some of the issues related to assessment that are

important for reporting and documentation related to a patient experiencing family violence.

Self-Assessment

Self-reflection assists nurses in all areas of practice to identify the values and biases that underscore their approach and interventions in response to those experiencing abuse (Registered Nurses' Association of Ontario, 2005). Strong negative feelings can cloud one's judgement and interfere with objective assessment and intervention, no matter how well we try to cover or deny personal bias. Common responses of health care providers to violence are listed in Table 24-2.

Since nursing is largely made up of women and women are more commonly the targets of abuse, it has been suggested that many nurses have experienced or are experiencing violence at the hands of their intimate partners (Registered Nurses' Association of Ontario, 2005). Nurses need to become aware of their reactions by gaining insight into their own somatic signals of distress (Unrau, Jakubec, & Jeske, 2017). Supervision and multidisciplinary team conferences can be especially helpful in clarifying reactions, neutralizing intense emotions, and reducing feelings of isolation and discomfort.

Level of Anxiety and Coping Responses

Nonverbal responses to the assessment interview can be indicative of the victim's anxiety level (see Chapter 12). Agitation and anxiety bordering on panic are often present in victims of violence. Abused individuals live under conditions of chronic stress, which can lead to health effects such as heart disease or heart attack, arthritis, fibromyalgia, asthma, stroke (Ford-Gilboe, Varcoe, & Merritt-Gray, 2010), and cervical cancer (Coker, Hopenhayn, DeSimone, et al., 2009). Coping mechanisms to endure living in violent and terrifying situations may take the form of flawed beliefs or myths (Table 24-3).

Family Coping Patterns

Consistent with a view of the intergenerational nature of the conditions and contexts of trauma, all forms of violence occurring in families of origin are predictive of future relationship violence (Franklin & Kercher, 2012). Altering the pattern of violence against women can affect child abuse because the main predictor of violence toward children is violence toward their mothers.

VIGNETTE

Petra is brought to the emergency department by ambulance in obvious distress with swollen eyes, lips, and nose and lacerations to her face. She tells the nurse that her husband had been in bed asleep for hours before she joined him. On getting into bed, she attempted to redistribute the blankets. Suddenly, he started punching her in the face and began to throw her against the wall. She called out to her 11-year-old son to call the police. The police arrived, called an ambulance, and took her husband, Dan, to jail. The nurse takes Petra to an individual examination room (to emphasize confidentiality) for a full assessment. She describes the relationship as "stormy" and "bad for a long time."

"Dan is always putting me down and yelling at me," she states. He started hitting her five years earlier when she became pregnant with her second and last child. The beatings have increased in intensity over the past year, and this emergency department visit is the fifth this year. Tonight is the first time she has ever called the police.

Petra has visibly lost control. Periods of crying alternate with periods of silence. She appears apathetic and depressed. The nurse remains calm and objective. After Petra has finished talking, the nurse explores alternatives designed to help her reduce the danger once she is discharged: "I'm concerned that you will be hurt again if you go home. What options do you have?" Acknowledging the escalating intensity of the violence, Petra is able to make arrangements with a shelter to take in her and her two children until after she has secured a restraining order. The nurse charts the abuse referrals. The keeping of careful and complete records helps to ensure that Petra will receive proper follow-up care and will assist her when and if she pursues legal action.

TABLE 24-2	COMMON RESPONSES OF HEALTH CARE PROVIDERS TO VIOLENCE
RESPONSE	**SOURCE**
Anger	Anger may be felt toward the person responsible for the abuse, toward those who allowed it to happen, and toward society for condoning its occurrence through attitudes, traditions, and laws.
Embarrassment	The victim may be a symbol of something close to home: the nurse may have experienced abuse.
Confusion	One's view of the family as a haven of safety and privacy is challenged.
Fear	A small percentage of perpetrators are dangerous to others.
Helplessness	The nurse may want to do more, eliminate the problem, or cure the victim, perpetrator, or both.
Discouragement	Discouragement may result if no long-term solution is achieved.
"Blame the victim" mentality	Health care workers can get caught up in "blaming the victim" for behaviours they see as provoking the abuse. There is never an excuse for abuse, and no one has the right to hurt another person. "Blaming the victim" can occur when health care providers feel overwhelmed. Supervision is essential for therapeutic intervention.

TABLE 24-3	MYTH VERSUS FACT: INTERPERSONAL VIOLENCE	
MYTH	**FACT**
Ninety-five percent of intimate partner violence victims are women.	In statistical self-reports, equal proportions of men and women reported being victims of spousal violence during the preceding 5 years—about 342 000 women and 418 000 men across the provinces (Statistics Canada, 2017).
The victim's behaviour often causes violence.	The victim's behaviour is *not* the cause of the violence. Violence is the perpetrator's pattern of behaviour, and the victim cannot learn how to control it.
Intimate partner abuse is a minor problem.	There is a *real* danger that victims may be killed by abusive partners.
Victims of intimate partner abuse could leave if they really wanted to.	Numerous factors influence a decision to stay or leave, including fear of injury or death, financial dependence, and welfare of children.
Interpersonal violence is most prevalent in poorly educated people from poor, working-class backgrounds.	Interpersonal violence occurs in all socioeconomic, religious, cultural, and educational backgrounds.
Family matters are private, and families should be allowed to take care of their own problems.	Intervention in interpersonal violence within families is justified; violence always escalates in frequency and intensity, can end in death, and is passed on to future generations.
Victims of violence tacitly accept the abuse by trying to conceal it, by not reporting it, or by failing to seek help.	When attempting to disclose their situation, many victims are met with disbelief, which discourages them from persevering.

Myths victims commonly believe include the following:
  "I can't live without him (her)."
  "If I hadn't done _____, it wouldn't have happened."
  "He (She) will change."
  "I stay for the sake of the children."
	These myths are coping mechanisms used to allay panic in a situation of random and brutal violence. They give the illusion of control and rationality.

Alcohol and stress are the major causes of physical and verbal abuse.	There are no excuses—violence is not acceptable behaviour. Aggression and violence are learned behaviours, not uncontrollable reactions. People are violent because they have acquired the belief that aggression is an acceptable and effective response to anger and a sense of lack of control.

However, it is important for the nurse to be nonjudgemental and to assess family strengths as well as styles of coping and stressors. Attitudes about child-rearing and discipline, including how parents were disciplined as children, may provide insight into violence and abuse in the home.

Living with and caring for children and older adults can cause frustration, anger, and stress. If there is no relief, the caregiver may become overwhelmed, lose control, and abuse the child or the older adult (Fulmer, Sengstock, Blankenship, et al., 2010; Public Health Agency of Canada, 2016). Box 24-5 is a useful guide for assessing the risk for child or older adult abuse in the home.

Support Systems

In the case of older adult abuse, risk factors include dependency on the caregiver for basic needs, isolation, limited or lack of access to support systems, and a history of intergenerational conflict between the older adult and the caregiver (Fulmer, Sengstock, Blankenship, et al., 2010). Assessment of the support system is crucial to identification of risk and resiliency factors. Children's support system options are especially limited, as are those of people who are physically and mentally challenged. Assessment for support systems should focus on intrapersonal, interpersonal, and community resources (e.g., the school system for school-aged victims).

Suicide Potential

A suicide attempt may be the presenting symptom in the emergency department. With sensitive questioning conducted in a caring manner, the nurse can elicit the history of violence. A person experiencing violence may feel desperate to leave yet be trapped in a detrimental relationship, and suicide may seem like the only option. The threat of suicide may also be used by an emotionally abusive person in an attempt to manipulate the victim into caving in to demands ("Don't leave me or I'll kill myself"; "I took all my pills…. I said I would the next time you were late").

Often the means of attempted suicide is overdose with a combination of alcohol and other central nervous system depressants, or sleeping medications that have been prescribed in previous visits to physicians' offices, clinics, or emergency departments. Refer to Chapter 22 for more on suicide.

Homicide Potential

At a minimum, the nurse should inquire about the patient's current safety risks and possible safety strategies. Because victims of abuse often underestimate the risk, using a tool such as the Danger Assessment (Campbell, Webster, & Glass, 2009) can be useful in helping victims to think about risk (for more information, see http://www.dangerassessment.org).

Individuals victimized by violence should be asked if they have ever felt like killing the perpetrator and, if so, whether they have the current desire and means to do so. If the answer is yes, intervention is required.

Drug and Alcohol Use

There is a high rate of co-occurrence of victimization and substance abuse among women (Macy, Renz, & Pelino, 2013). A person experiencing violence may self-medicate with alcohol or other drugs as a way of escaping an intolerable situation. The

BOX 24-5 FACTORS TO ASSESS DURING A HOME VISIT

For a Child

- Responsiveness to infant's signals
- Caregiver's facial expressions in response to infant
- Playfulness of caregiver with infant
- Nature of physical contact during feeding and other caretaking activities
- Temperament of infant
- Caregiver's history of harsh discipline or abuse as a child
- Parental attitudes:
  - Feelings of inadequacy as a parent
  - Unrealistic expectations of child
  - Fear of "doing something wrong"
  - Attribution of negative qualities to newborn
  - Misdirected anger
  - Continued evidence of isolation, apathy, anger, frustration
  - Adult conflict
- Environmental conditions:
  - Sleeping arrangements
  - Child management
  - Home management
  - Use of supports (formal and informal)
- Need for immediate services for situational (e.g., economics, child care), emotional, or educational information:
  - Information about hotlines, babysitters, homemakers, parent groups
  - Information about child development
  - Information about child care and home management services

For an Older Adult

- Absence of or lack of access to basic necessities (e.g., food, water, medications)
- Unsafe housing
- Lack of or inadequate utilities, ventilation, space
- Poor physical hygiene
- Lack of necessary assistive devices (e.g., hearing aids, eyeglasses, wheelchair)
- Medication mismanagement (outdated prescriptions, unmarked bottles)

TABLE 24-4 POTENTIAL NURSING DIAGNOSES FOR FAMILY VIOLENCE

SIGNS AND SYMPTOMS	POTENTIAL NURSING DIAGNOSES
Bruises, cuts, broken bones, lacerations, scars, burns, wounds in various phases of healing, particularly when explanations do not match injury or explanations are vague	*Risk for injury* *Acute pain* *Chronic pain* *Risk for infection* *Impaired skin integrity* *Risk for post-traumatic stress*
Isolation, fear, feelings of shame, low self-esteem, feelings of worthlessness, depression, feelings of helplessness	*Powerlessness* *Ineffective coping* *Fear* *Risk for self-directed violence* *Chronic low self-esteem* *Situational low self-esteem* *Hopelessness* *Spiritual distress*
Vaginal–anal bruises, sores, discharge, peritoneal pain, positive test results for sexually transmitted infections	*Rape-trauma syndrome* *Risk for infection*

the survivor and a primary support person. These outcomes should be continually reassessed and revised as new information about the survivor's needs emerges. A comprehensive plan can also guide the actions of the multidisciplinary team.

OUTCOMES IDENTIFICATION

The *Nursing Outcomes Classification (NOC)* (Moorhead, Johnson, Maas, et al., 2013) identifies the following indicators for the outcome of *Abuse cessation*, defined as "evidence that the victim is no longer hurt or exploited":

- Physical abuse has ceased.
- Emotional abuse has ceased.
- Sexual abuse has ceased.
- Financial exploitation has ceased.

NOC offers other abuse-specific outcomes, including *Abuse protection, Abuse recovery, Abuse recovery: Emotional, Abuse recovery: Financial, Abuse recovery: Physical,* and *Abuse recovery: Sexual.* In addition, outcomes focused on improved coping, self-esteem, social support, and pain control, to name a few, are appropriate for these patients.

Table 24-5 provides some specific outcome criteria, along with short-term and intermediate indicators for victims of child, intimate partner, and older adult abuse, as well as for the abuser.

PLANNING

Nurses and other health care workers encounter abuse frequently, not only in health care settings but also in their communities and families. Most hospitals and community centres provide protocols for dealing with child, intimate partner, or older adult abuse, but these protocols may or may not meet all the needs of a given patient.

drugs are usually central nervous system depressants (e.g., benzodiazepines) prescribed by physicians in response to the patient's presentation with vague complaints, which are often stress related (e.g., insomnia, gastrointestinal upsets, anxiety). The degree of intoxication can be determined by history, physical examination, and blood alcohol level. Refer to Chapter 18 for information on how to assess for a chronic alcohol or drug problem.

DIAGNOSIS

Nursing diagnoses are focused on the underlying causes and symptoms of family violence.

Table 24-4 lists potential nursing diagnoses for abuse.

The identification of desired outcomes and the design of nursing interventions that facilitate achieving those outcomes should be developed as much as possible in collaboration with

TABLE 24-5	*NOC* OUTCOMES FOR INTERPERSONAL VIOLENCE	
NURSING OUTCOME AND DEFINITION	**SHORT-TERM AND INTERMEDIATE INDICATORS**
Abuse cessation: Evidence that the victim is no longer hurt or exploited	Evidence that physical abuse has ceased
	Evidence that emotional abuse has ceased
	Evidence that sexual abuse has ceased
Abuse recovery: Physical: Extent of healing of physical injuries due to abuse	Timely treatment of injuries
	Healing of physical injuries
	Resolution of physical health problems
Abuse recovery: Financial: Extent of control of monetary and legal matters following financial exploitation	Control of social security and pension income
	Protection of financial resources
	Control of withdrawal of money from account(s)
Abusive behaviour self-restraint: Self-restraint of abusive and neglectful behaviours toward others	Obtains needed treatment
	Controls impulses
	Discusses the abusive behaviour

Source: Data from Moorhead, S., Johnson, M., Maas, M. L., et al. (2013). *Nursing outcomes classification (NOC)* (5th ed.). St. Louis: Elsevier.

Unless the case is one of child abuse in which the child has been removed from the home, most interventions performed after necessary emergency care will take place within the community. Plans should centre on the patient's safety first. The nurse must ascertain whether the survivor is in danger for his or her life, either from suicide or homicide, and, if there are children involved, whether they are in danger (Ford-Gilboe, Varcoe, & Merritt-Gray, 2010). Whenever it is possible or in the best interests of the patient, plans should be discussed with the patient. Planning should also take into consideration the needs of the abuser(s) (e.g., parents, caretakers, spouse, or partner), if they are willing to learn alternatives to abuse and violence.

IMPLEMENTATION

Interventions for those experiencing interpersonal violence are distinct from interventions for anger and aggression, though at times there may be overlapping concerns (reporting, debriefing, counselling, and so on). Anger management interventions concentrate on the distortions and misalignment of the expression of anger. In contrast, interventions for interpersonal violence focus on relationship power imbalances. Interventions for interpersonal violence are discussed below.

Reporting Abuse

There is no mandatory obligation to report abuse of a woman to the police. It is the woman's right to choose if she wishes to have police involvement, and she must consent to this involvement prior to the nurse's initiating contact with authorities (Registered Nurses' Association of Ontario, 2005). According to provincial or territorial legislation, any suspected or actual cases of child abuse must be reported to the official social service agency. For example, under Alberta's *Child, Youth and Family Enhancement Act* (2012), any person who has "reasonable and probable grounds" to believe that a child is being harmed or is in danger of being abandoned, neglected, physically injured, emotionally injured, or sexually abused must report the situation to authorities.

Child witnesses to abuse may be reportable to the provincial or territorial social service agency, as proximity to such events can represent a condition of harm for the child (Registered Nurses' Association of Ontario, 2005). Nurses are advised to consult their local social service agency to discuss individual situations, and all health care organizations need to have a protocol in place with their local social service agency.

The Canadian *Criminal Code* provides the legislation necessary to deal with physical, sexual, and financial abuse of older adults (Victims of Violence, 2017). In addition, provincial and territorial legislation addresses abuse and reporting. For example, some jurisdictions in Canada now enforce mandatory reporting of abuse of older adults, but several others do not. Nova Scotia and Newfoundland and Labrador have general mandatory reporting requirements in their adult protection legislation, placing a general social responsibility on all citizens to report suspected abuse or neglect. Alberta, Manitoba, and Ontario now have special legislation for the protection of persons in care, and laws in Prince Edward Island, New Brunswick, Saskatchewan, and British Columbia provide for voluntary reporting for specific forms of abuse and neglect of older adults. No provisions are available for reporting of adult abuse in the territories (Victims of Violence, 2017).

Competency may be a consideration in a situation of older adult abuse. Competent older adults have the right to self-determination. Unless the individual is found to be incompetent, help can be offered but cannot be forced on the person. In Canada, there is no general test of competency. The definition of competency varies across legislations, institutions, agencies, and provinces and territories (McDonald & Collins, 2000). However, it can be generally defined as a person's ability to understand the situation he or she is in and the decisions that have to be made about that situation (McDonald & Collins, 2000). The legal determination of incompetency is a last resort since it dramatically changes the rights of an individual. For this reason, it is important that the least restrictive approaches be taken before attempting to have an older adult declared incompetent.

Nurses must be cognizant of the cultural diversity of the populations with which they work (see Chapter 8). The term *cultural diversity* in this instance is used broadly and may be derived from one's race, ethnicity, class, religious or spiritual beliefs, age, ability, or sexual orientation (Registered Nurses' Association of Ontario, 2005). The nurse must be aware of the cultural issues of those experiencing abuse, as such issues may affect the survivor's response to violence and to intervention. The nurse is responsible for developing a communication plan to make the survivor an informed partner in the provision of care. Nurses need to check their provincial practice standards for the provision of culturally sensitive care.

Counselling

Counselling includes crisis intervention measures. It is important to emphasize that people have a right to live without fear of violence, physical harm, or assault. Powerful statements such as "Abuse is never right "and "No one deserves to be abused" will display unconditional acceptance and positive regard (Ford-Gilboe, Varcoe, & Merritt-Gray, 2010).

All individuals experiencing abuse should be counselled about developing a safety plan, a plan for a rapid escape when abuse recurs. Nurses should be aware that safety is never guaranteed, nor can the most detailed safety plan ensure that the violence will end (Registered Nurses' Association of Ontario, 2005). The victim experiencing violence is ultimately the only one who can reliably predict the risks and the likelihood for further violence, and therefore the best plan is the victim's own plan, one that is viewed by the victim as achievable and one that the victim has a personal commitment to follow (Middlesex-London Health Unit, 2000). The nurse should suggest packing the items listed in Box 24-6 ahead of time. The packed bag should be kept in a place where the perpetrator will not find it.

If the abused person chooses to leave, shelters or safe houses (for both sexes) are available in many communities in Canada. They are open 24 hours a day and can be reached through crisis hotline information numbers, hospital emergency departments, YWCAs, or the local office of the National Council of Women of Canada. Besides offering protection for individuals and families in crisis, many of these shelters and safe houses offer important education, counselling, and transitional housing services. Patients should be given the number of the nearest available shelter, even if they decide for the present to stay with their partners. Referral phone numbers may be kept for years before the decision to call is made. Having the number and a contact person during that time contributes to thinking about options.

Case Management

Nurses working in outpatient and community mental health settings have the opportunity to coordinate community, medical, criminal justice, and social services to provide comprehensive assistance to families in crisis. Strategies must encompass needs for household necessities, child care, stability in providing basic needs, economic stability, physical and emotional safety, counselling, legal protection, career development or job training, education, ongoing support groups, and health care. Safe and affordable housing is often crucial to the person's ability to break free (Daoud, Matheson, Pedersen, et al., 2016). A nurse functioning in a case manager role can assist the patient in choosing the best options and coordinating the interventions of several agencies. Box 24-7 lists selected *Nursing Interventions Classification (NIC)* interventions for *Abuse protection support* for children, intimate partners, and older adults (Bulechek, Butcher, Dochterman, et al., 2013).

Milieu Management

Interventions are geared toward stabilizing the home situation and maintaining an abuse-free environment. Some mental health programs have caseworkers or clinicians who visit the home

---

BOX 24-6   PERSONALIZED SAFETY GUIDE

Suggestions for Increasing Safety While in the Relationship

- I will have important phone numbers available to my children and myself.
- I can tell _____ and _____ about the violence and ask them to call the police if they hear suspicious noises coming from my home.
- If I leave my home, I can go to (list four places) _____, _____, _____, or _____.
- I can leave extra money, car keys, clothes, and copies of documents with _____.
- If I leave, I will bring items _____ (e.g., identification, birth certificates, social insurance card, school and medical records, health insurance card, money, bank books, credit cards).
- To ensure safety and independence, I can keep my cellphone battery charged or have another phone available, open my own savings account, rehearse my escape route with a support person, and review my safety plan on _____ (date).

Suggestions for Increasing Safety When the Relationship Is Over

- I can change the locks and install steel or metal doors, a security system, smoke detectors, and an outside lighting system.
- I will inform _____ and _____ that my partner no longer lives with me and ask them to call the police if he or she is observed near my home or my children.
- I will tell people who take care of my children the names of those who have permission to pick them up. The people who have permission are _____, _____, and _____.
- I can tell _____ at work about my situation and ask _____ to screen my calls.
- I can avoid stores, banks, and _____ that I used when living with my battering partner.
- I can obtain a restraining order from _____. I can keep it on or near me at all times, as well as have a copy with _____.
- If I feel down and ready to return to a potentially abusive situation, I can call _____ for support or attend workshops and groups to gain support and strengthen my relationships with other people.

Important Phone Numbers
- Police _____
- Crisis hotline _____
- Family _____
- Friends _____
- Shelter _____

BOX 24-7   INTERVENTIONS FOR ABUSE PROTECTION SUPPORT FOR CHILDREN, INTIMATE PARTNERS, AND OLDER ADULTS

Abuse Protection Support: Children

Definition of abuse protection support: children*:* Identification of high-risk, dependent child relationships and actions to prevent possible or further infliction of physical, sexual, or emotional harm or neglect of basic necessities of life.

Activities*:

- Identify mothers who have a history of late (4 months or later) or no prenatal care.
- Identify parents who have had another child removed from the home or have placed previous children with relatives for extended periods.
- Identify parents with a history of domestic violence or a mother who has a history of numerous "accidental" injuries.
- Determine whether a child demonstrates signs of physical abuse, including numerous injuries in various stages of healing; unexplained bruises and welts; unexplained pattern, immersion, and friction burns; facial, spiral, shaft, or multiple fractures; unexplained facial lacerations and abrasions, and so on.
- Encourage admission of child for further observation and investigation as appropriate.
- Monitor parent–child interactions and record observations.
- Report suspected abuse or neglect to proper authorities in compliance with mandatory reporting laws.

Abuse Protection Support: Intimate Partners

Definition of abuse protection support: intimate partners*:* Identification of high-risk, dependent domestic relationships and action to prevent possible or further infliction of physical, sexual, or emotional harm or exploitation of a domestic partner.

Activities*:

- Screen for risk factors associated with domestic abuse (e.g., history of domestic violence, abuse, rejection, excessive criticism, or feelings of being worthless and unloved; difficulty trusting others or feeling disliked by others; feeling that asking for help is an indication of personal incompetence; high physical care needs; intense family care responsibilities; substance abuse; depression; major psychiatric illness; social isolation; poor relationships between domestic partners; multiple marriages; pregnancy; poverty; unemployment; financial dependence; homelessness; infidelity; divorce; or death of a loved one).
- Document evidence of physical or sexual abuse using standardized assessment tools and photographs.
- Listen attentively to individual who begins to talk about own problems.
- Encourage admission to a hospital for further observation and investigation, as appropriate.
- Provide positive affirmation of worth.

Abuse Protection Support: Older Adults

Definition of abuse protection support: older adults*:* Identification of high-risk, dependent older adult relationships and actions to prevent possible or further infliction of physical, sexual, or emotional harm; neglect of basic necessities of life; or exploitation.

Activities*:

- Identify older patients who perceive themselves to be dependent on caretakers due to impaired health status, functional impairment, limited economic resources, depression, substance abuse, or lack of knowledge of available resources and alternatives for care.
- Identify family caretakers who have a childhood history of abuse or neglect.
- Monitor patient–caretaker interactions and record observations.
- Report suspected abuse or neglect to proper authorities in compliance with mandatory reporting laws.

Source: Adapted from Bulechek, G. M., Butcher, H. K., Dochterman, J. M., et al. (2013). *Nursing interventions classification (NIC)* (6th ed.). St. Louis: Mosby.
*Partial list.

instead of requiring the family to go to the agency. Providing and maintaining a therapeutic environment in the home ideally involves three levels of help for abusive families:

1. Provides the family with economic support, job opportunities, and social services
2. Arranges social support in the form of a public health nurse, day care teacher, schoolteacher, social worker, respite worker, or any other potential contact person who has a good relationship with the family
3. Encourages and provides family therapy

Promotion of Self-Care Activities

Nurses can help victims of abuse to find hope and view themselves as "survivors," which emphasizes agency and choices, identifies strengths, and attributes more responsibility to them over aspects of their lives that are under their control (Dunn & Powell-Williams, 2007). Reimagining their own capacities to choose and act may empower survivors to find options and ultimately take steps to leave the abusive relationship. Ford-Gilboe, Wuest, and Merritt-Gray (2005) found that women were able to promote the health of their families after leaving an abusive partner. Therefore offering hope, identifying strengths, and displaying confidence that the person can take care of him- or herself are important aspects of nursing care. Referrals regarding crisis counselling, emergency housing, or financial assistance, as well as legal and vocational counselling, should be made available to each patient. Referrals to parenting resources that explore alternative approaches to physical discipline of children in their care may also be appropriate.

Health Teaching and Health Promotion

Health teaching and health promotion include meeting with the individual, caregiver, and family to discuss the cycle of violence, associated risk factors, and situations that might trigger violence. Other nursing interventions can include teaching about healthy relationships and healthy sexuality, which may be especially important to children who have no role models.

Nurses who work on maternity units and in public health departments are often in a position to identify risk factors for abuse and initiate appropriate interventions, including education about effective parenting, caregiving, and coping techniques, as well as information for nurturing healthy relationships. Information about these interventions should be shared with the patient's health care team for appropriate monitoring and follow-up in the community. Assessment of risk and resiliency factors is essential to the implementation of health-promoting activities. For example, parents who are at particular risk for abusing a child include the following:

- New parents whose behaviour toward the infant is rejecting, hostile, or indifferent
- Teenage parents who require special help in handling the baby, have difficulty discussing their expectations of caring for the child, or lack support systems
- Parents with cognitive deficits, for whom careful, explicit, and repeated instructions on caring for the child and recognizing the infant's needs are indicated
- Parents who grew up watching their mothers being abused (a significant risk factor for perpetuation of family violence)

Nurses can often recognize when children are at risk and make referrals to community resources, including emergency child care facilities, emergency telephone numbers, numbers of 24-hour crisis centres or hotlines, and respite programs for parents to have some relief from child care. Community and public health nurses can make home visits to identify risk factors for abuse in the crucial first few months of life, during which the style of parent–child interactions is established. See Box 24-5 for important factors for the community health nurse to assess during a home care visit. Such observations made by nurses in clinic and public health settings are fundamental in case finding and evaluation.

Prevention of Abuse

Primary Prevention

Primary prevention consists of measures taken to prevent the occurrence of abuse. Identifying individuals and families at high risk, providing health teaching, and coordinating supportive services to prevent crises are examples of primary prevention. Specific strategies include (1) reducing stress, (2) reducing the influence of risk factors, (3) increasing social support, (4) increasing coping skills, and (5) increasing self-esteem. In particular, reducing the risk for the different forms of child abuse can contribute to reducing the repeated conditions and patterns of violence and abuse from generation to generation (Butchart, Harvey, & Fürniss, 2006). The most promising strategies for preventing child abuse include home visitation and parent education programs (Mikton & Butchart, 2009).

Community and public health nurses are in a unique position to assess family functioning in the home over time, which allows for assessment of changes. They are also in an excellent position

to connect those at risk (such as people with addictions) to appropriate resources in the community that can meet their needs. All nurses can advocate for social policy change to improve the coordination of health, justice, and social services, thereby enhancing the health care response to abuse (Registered Nurses' Association of Ontario, 2005).

Secondary Prevention

Secondary prevention involves early intervention in abusive situations to minimize their disabling or long-term effects. Nurses can establish universal screening programs in all health care settings for individuals at risk, assist in treating any injuries resulting from abuse, and coordinate community referrals to provide continuity of care (Registered Nurses' Association of Ontario, 2005). Stress, depression, low self-esteem, and social isolation can be addressed by providing supportive psychotherapy, psychoeducation, support groups, pharmacotherapy, and contact information for community resources. Caregiver burden can be reduced by arranging assistance in caregiving, nursing, or housekeeping or, if necessary, by placing the person in a different home or health care facility. For some, support through criminal proceedings may be important to prevent revictimization. Refer to the *Trauma-informed Practice Guide* from the BC Provincial Mental Health and Substance Use Planning Council (2013) at http://bccewh.bc.ca/wp-content/uploads/2012/05/2013_TIP-Guide.pdf. The Sheldon Kennedy Child Advocacy Centre, based in Calgary, Alberta, is another organization concerned with all levels of child abuse prevention, including community education and training to prevent revictimization and interrupt the potential cycle of violence from generation to generation. The vignette illustrates a successful secondary prevention effort.

Tertiary Prevention

Tertiary prevention, which often occurs in mental health care settings, involves nurses facilitating the healing and rehabilitative process by counselling individuals and families, providing support for groups of survivors, and assisting survivors of violence to achieve their optimal level of safety, health, and well-being. Examples of tertiary prevention include psychological therapies for abused children; screening and support services for victims of intimate partner, domestic, or family violence; and specific recognition of the needs of survivors of torture.

Advanced-Practice Interventions

Individual Psychotherapy

The goals of individual therapy for a survivor are empowerment, the ability to recognize and choose productive life options, and the development of a solid sense of self. Survivors of abuse may choose individual therapy to address symptoms of depression, anxiety, somatization, or PTSD. Many of the psychological symptoms shown by women who have been abused can be understood as complex survival strategies and responses to violence. This constellation of symptoms, such as fear and a perceived inability to escape, has been referred to as battered woman syndrome in legal proceedings (Ono, 2017).

VIGNETTE

George, age 4 years, is brought to the physician's office by 25-year-old Asha, the child's nanny, with second-degree burns on his right hand. Asha is the nanny for George and his younger brother, Tyrone, age 2, and older brother Logan, age 6. Asha appears apprehensive and says she is very concerned. Asha tells the nurse that the children have told her in the past that their mother has threatened them with burning if they do not behave. George told her that his mother once held his hands on a cold stove element and told him that if he was bad, she would turn it on and burn him. Asha is shocked that George's mother would do such a thing, but at the same time, she says she feels guilty for "telling on Ms. J."

Asha also states that the older brother, Logan, told her what happened to George but was afraid that if his mother found out, she would burn him also. Asha says she is aware that the mother hits the children, but she did not believe that anyone would burn her own child. The nurse reports the incident to the physician, and the mother is called and asked to come to the office. Meanwhile, the nurse asks Asha to stay with George while she examines him. George appears frightened and in pain.

Nurse: "Tell me about your hand, George." *(George looks down and starts to cry.)* "It's okay if you don't want to talk about it, George."

George: *(Does not look at the nurse and speaks softly.)* "My mommy burned my hand on the stove."

Nurse: "Tell me what happened before that."

George: "Mommy was mad because I didn't put my toys away."

Nurse: "What does your mommy usually do when she gets mad?"

George: "She yells mostly. Sometimes she hits us. Mommy is going to be so mad at Logan for telling."

Nurse: "Tell me about the hitting."

George: "Mommy hits us a lot since Daddy left." *(George starts to cry to himself.)*

On examination, the nurse notices on George's right palm a ringed pattern of burns resembling the burner on an electric stove. There are blisters on his fingers. George appears well nourished and properly dressed. He is at his approximate developmental age except for some language delay. Because of the physical evidence and history, there is strong suspicion of child abuse. The provincial social service agency is notified, and the family situation is evaluated for possible placement of George in foster care. The initial evaluation concludes that there is no indication of serious potential harm to the child and that George should return home. The mother, who is initially defensive, starts to cry and states, "I can't cope with being alone, and I don't know where to turn."

Nursing interventions centre on caring for George's immediate health needs, finding supports for the mother to help her cope with crises, providing a counselling referral for the mother to learn alternative ways of expressing anger and frustration, informing the mother of parents' groups, providing referrals to play groups or day care for the children to help increase their feelings of self-esteem and security, and providing a break and instruction in parenting for the mother.

Nurses must address the guilt, shame, and stigmatization experienced by survivors of abuse (Draucker, Martsolf, Ross, et al., 2009). It is helpful for nurses to understand that the patient's feelings and behaviours may reflect those of the grieving process since the survivor has experienced numerous losses as a result of the abusive relationship.

Programs for perpetrators of abuse are still associated with the justice system and are mandated interventions rather than voluntary and desirable community services for batterers. Although court-mandated treatment tends to be the most effective for perpetrators, it is critical that the domestic violence movement make assistance for perpetrators of abuse more readily available so as to shift societal norms to encourage and promote voluntary help-seeking behaviours (Campbell, Neil, Jaffe, et al., 2010). The perpetrator needs to seek help for issues concerning power and control. Refer to the Duluth model "Power and Control" wheel (Figure 24-4) and "Equality" wheel (Figure 24-7), which are standard frameworks for violence education.

Nurses engaged in therapy with perpetrators of abuse have a duty to warn potential victims if they conclude that the perpetrator is a danger. Refer to Chapter 7 for a more detailed discussion of the duty to warn and the duty to protect.

Family Psychotherapy

Because abuse is a symptom of a family in crisis, each member of the family system needs attention. Also, because change in one member of the family system affects the whole system, all members need support and understanding. Dialectical behaviour therapy (DBT) has been proven to be effective in treating individuals and families with histories of abuse by teaching emotion regulation, interpersonal skills, mindfulness, and distress tolerance skills (Feigenbaum, 2007). Family or marital therapy should take place *only* if the perpetrator has had individual therapy and has demonstrated change as a result and if both parties agree to participate.

Expected outcomes are that the perpetrator will recognize destructive patterns of behaviour and learn alternative responses. Intermediate goals are that members of the family will openly communicate and learn to listen to each other. Refer to the Duluth model "Nurturing Children" wheel (Figure 24-8), which is a standard framework for the care of children in families with histories of abuse. Refer to Chapter 34 for a more detailed discussion of family therapy.

Group Psychotherapy

Group therapy offers a powerful way to counter self-denigrating beliefs and to confront issues of secrecy and stigmatization while decreasing isolation, improving self-esteem, and increasing the potential for realistic problem solving (Draughon & Urbancic, 2010). Also, the therapeutic factor of universality, or the discovery that others have had similar experiences, may be beneficial, especially for child survivors. DBT has been used in groups with abusers to teach emotion regulation, interpersonal, mindfulness, and distress tolerance skills (Van Wel, Kockmann, Blum, et al., 2006).

Emotion regulation skills are taught to manage intense labile moods, interpersonal skills are taught to develop assertiveness

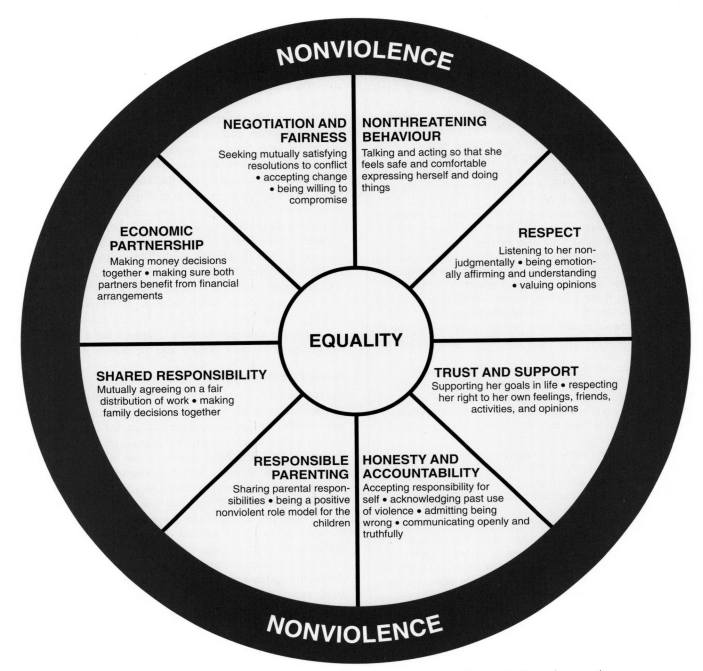

FIGURE 24-7 The Duluth "Equality" wheel. Source: Redrawn from Domestic Abuse Intervention Project, 202 East Superior Street, Duluth, MN 55802, Tel. 218-722-2781. Retrieved from http://www.theduluthmodel.org/training/wheels.html.

and problem-solving skills, mindfulness is taught for meditation, and distress tolerance skills are taught to learn how to tolerate and accept distress as a part of normal life (Feigenbaum, 2007). Group therapy can help create a community of healing and restoration. Refer to Chapter 33 for a more detailed discussion of group therapy.

EVALUATION

The failure of interventions with abusive families often are due to problems within the health, social, economic, and political systems. Nurses must act at all levels by lobbying for (1) better education about violence and abuse, (2) resources in health care

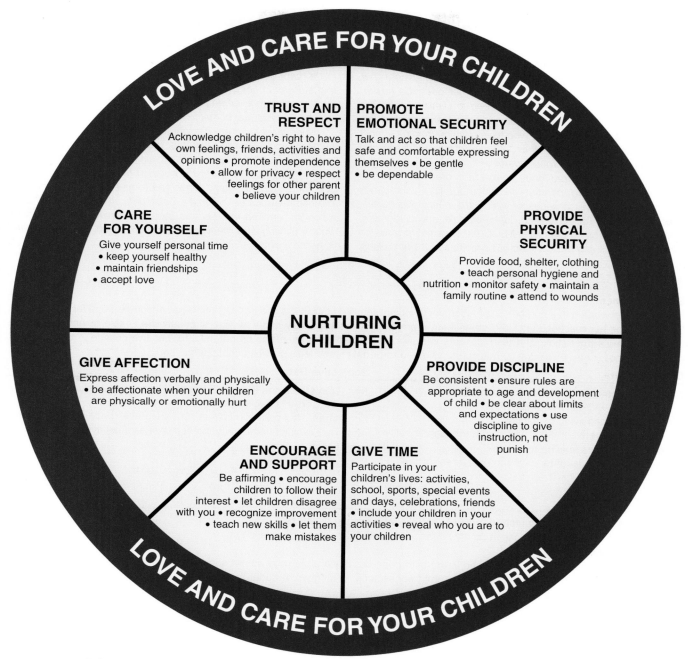

FIGURE 24-8 The Duluth "Nurturing Children" wheel. Source: Redrawn from Domestic Abuse Intervention Project, 202 East Superior Street, Duluth, MN 55802, Tel. 218-722-2781. Retrieved from http://www.theduluthmodel.org/training/wheels.html.

settings to support more effective responses to violence and abuse, (3) better collaboration across all sectors, and (4) the development of policies on understanding the dynamics of violence in such areas as social assistance and child welfare (Ford-Gilboe, Varcoe, & Merritt-Gray, 2010). Nurses can play a powerful role in lobbying against factors that promote violence (such as media that depict violence, gender or racial inequity, and devaluing of older adults).

The evaluation of brief interventions can be based on whether the survivor acknowledges the violence, is willing to accept intervention, and removes him- or herself from the abusive situation. The ultimate outcome of long-term interventions and follow-up is to end the violence and to empower the survivor to lead a productive and safe life without the haunting memories of abuse. Because abuse is a symptom of a family in crisis, diagnosis, interventions, and evaluation should be carried out by a multidisciplinary team that includes a physician, a nurse, a social worker, a lawyer, and perhaps a psychiatrist.

CASE STUDY AND NURSING CARE PLAN 24-1

Family Violence

Mrs. Tran, a recently widowed 84-year-old woman, moved into her son's apartment 3 months ago. She had been living in her third-floor walk-up in the city. Because of her declining health, crime in the neighbourhood, and the need to climb three flights of stairs, with her son Chien's encouragement, she went to live with him. He and his wife, Kim, who have been married for almost 20 years, have five children 6 to 18 years of age, all living in a rather cramped three-bedroom apartment.

Mrs. Tran is being cared for by a nurse from the Victorian Order of Nurses (VON), who monitors her blood pressure and adjusts her medication. Over a series of visits, the nurse, Ms. Grohl, notices that Mrs. Tran is looking unkempt, pale, and withdrawn. While taking her blood pressure, Ms. Grohl observes bruises on Mrs. Tran's arms and neck. When questioned about the bruises,

Mrs. Tran appears anxious and nervous. She says that she slipped in the bathroom. Mrs. Tran becomes increasingly apprehensive and stiffens in her chair when her daughter-in-law, Kim, comes into the room to ask when the next visit will be. The nurse notices that Kim avoids eye contact with Mrs. Tran.

When the injuries are brought to Kim's attention, she responds by becoming angry and agitated, blaming Mrs. Tran for causing so many problems. She will not explain the reason for the change in Mrs. Tran's behaviour or the origin of the bruises to the nurse. She merely comments, "I have had to give up my job since my mother-in-law came here. It's been difficult and crowded ever since she moved in. The kids are complaining. We are having trouble making ends meet since I gave up my job. And my husband is no help at all."

ASSESSMENT

Self-Assessment

Ms. Grohl has worked in a number of situations with violent families, but this is the first time she has encountered older adult abuse. She discusses her reactions with the other team members. She is especially angry at Kim, although she is able to understand the daughter-in-law's frustration. The team concurs with Ms. Grohl that there seems to be potential for positive change in this family. If abuse does not abate, more drastic measures will need to be taken and legal services contacted.

Objective Data	Subjective Data
Physical symptoms of violence (bruises, unkempt appearance, withdrawn attitude)	Mrs. Tran states she slipped in the bathroom, but physical findings do not support this explanation.
Stressful, crowded living conditions	Kim states, "It's been difficult and crowded ever since she moved in."
No eye contact between Mrs. Tran and her daughter-in-law	Mrs. Tran exhibits withdrawn and apprehensive behaviour in the presence of Kim.
Economic hardships leading to stress	
No support for the daughter-in-law from the rest of the family for care of Mrs. Tran	

DIAGNOSIS

On the basis of the data, the nurse formulates the following nursing diagnoses:

1. *Risk for injury* related to increase in family stress, as evidenced by signs of violence

Supporting Data
- Statement by Mrs. Tran that she slipped in the bathroom, but physical findings do not support this explanation
- Physical symptoms of violence (bruises, unkempt appearance, withdrawn attitude)
- Stressful, crowded living conditions

2. *Ineffective coping* related to helplessness, as evidenced by inability to meet role expectations

Supporting Data
- Unkempt, anxious, depressed
- Withdrawn and apprehensive behaviour

3. *Risk for other-directed violence* related to increased stressors within a short period, as evidenced by probable older adult abuse and feelings of helplessness verbalized by the primary caregiver

Supporting Data
- Kim states, "It's been difficult and crowded ever since she moved in."
- No eye contact between Kim and Mrs. Tran
- Signs and symptoms of physical abuse on Mrs. Tran
- Kim says, "My husband is no help at all."

4. *Caregiver role strain* related to extreme feelings of being overwhelmed and feeling helpless

Supporting Data
- Family not helping with care of mother-in-law; burden of care on Kim
- Economic hardships, leading to stress when Kim gave up her job to care for Mrs. Tran

CASE STUDY AND NURSING CARE PLAN 24-1—cont'd
Family Violence

OUTCOMES IDENTIFICATION

Abuse cessation: Evidence that the victim is no longer hurt or exploited
  Short-term indicators:
- Evidence that physical abuse has ceased
- Evidence that emotional abuse has ceased

PLANNING

Ms. Grohl discusses several possible outcomes with members of her team, giving attention to the priority of outcomes and to whether they are realistic in this situation. She also plans to report the older adult abuse to law enforcement and to work with Mrs. Tran, Kim, and the rest of the family to improve this situation for everyone.

IMPLEMENTATION

Mrs. Tran's plan of care is personalized as follows:
Nursing diagnosis: *Risk for injury* related to increase in family stress, as evidenced by signs of violence
Outcome: Abuse cessation

Short-Term Goal	Interventions	Rationale	Evaluation
1. On each visit made by the nurse, the patient will state that abuse has decreased, using a scale from 1 to 5 (1 being the least abuse).	1a. Follow provincial laws and guidelines for reporting older adult abuse.	1a. Provides maximum protection under the law. Provides data for future use	**Goal Met** Patient states that after family talked to the nurse and planned strategies, physical abuse no longer occurs.
	1b. Assess severity of signs and symptoms of abuse.	1b. Accurate charting (body map, pictures with permission, verbatim statements) helps follow progress and provides legal data.	
	1c. Do a careful home assessment to identify other areas of abuse and neglect. Identify community resources that could help the older adult and caregivers.	1c. Check for inadequacy of food, presence of vermin, blocked stairways, medication safety issues, and so on—all indicate abuse and neglect.	
	1d. Identify community resources that could help the older adult and caregivers to manage care at home.	1d. Determining the kinds of problems in the home and identifying available resources help with planning appropriate intervention.	
	1e. Discuss with patient factors leading to abuse and concern for safety.	1e. Allows for identification of family stressors and potential areas for intervention. Validates that situation is serious and increases patient's knowledge base	
2. Within 2 weeks, patient will be able to identify at least two supportive services to deal with emergency situations.	2. Discuss with patient supportive services such as crisis hotlines and 911 to call in case of emergency situations.	2. Maximizes patient's safety through use of support systems	**Goal Met** Patient has been talking to two old friends she had stopped talking to because of shame and depression. She has called the crisis hotline once to get information on transportation to the older adult centre in town.

Continued

CASE STUDY AND NURSING CARE PLAN 24-1—cont'd

Family Violence

Short-Term Goal	Interventions	Rationale	Evaluation
3. Within 3 weeks, family members will be able to identify difficult issues that increase their stress levels.	3. Discuss with family members their feelings, and identify at least four areas that are most difficult for the various family members.	3. Listening to each family member and identifying unmet needs helps both family and nurse identify areas that require changing and appropriate interventions.	**Goal Met** Family members identify areas of increased stress, such as overwork, lack of free time, lack of privacy, and financial difficulties.
4. Within 3 weeks, family will seek out community resources to help with anger management, need for homemaker support, and other needs.	4. Identify potential community supports, skills training, respite places, homemakers, financial aids, and so on that might help meet family's unmet needs.	4. When stressed, individuals solve problems poorly and do not know about or cannot manage to organize outside help. Finances may be controlled by the perpetrator or become unmanageable in the crisis stages of abuse.	**Goal Met** The daughter-in-law is glad to get out of the house for anger management classes, and the son states he will try to take on more responsibility, but he often feels guilty and angry, too. Reluctantly, the son and his wife agree to try a support group with other caregivers in similar situations.

EVALUATION

Eight weeks after Ms. Grohl's initial visit, Mrs. Tran appears well groomed, friendly, and more spontaneous in her conversation. She comments, "Things are better with my daughter-in-law." No bruises or other signs of physical violence are noticeable. She is considerably more outgoing and has even taken the initiative to contact an old friend. Mrs. Tran has talked openly to her son and daughter-in-law about stress in the family. Mrs. Tran says that she went for a walk when her daughter-in-law appeared tense and returned to find that the tension had lessened. Neither Mrs. Tran nor her family has initiated plans for alternative housing.

KEY POINTS TO REMEMBER

- Abuse can occur in any family and can be predicted with some accuracy by examining the risk and resiliency factors related to the characteristics of perpetrators, vulnerable people, and crisis situations in which violence is likely.
- Abuse can be physical, sexual, psychological or emotional, or economic or can be caused by deprivation or neglect.
- The cycle of violence includes three recurring phases of violence (tension building, acute battering, and honeymoon stages), which often increase in severity and frequency.
- Assessment includes identifying indicators of abuse, levels of anxiety, coping mechanisms, support systems, and suicide and homicide potential, as well as alcohol and drug abuse.

- Reporting abuse to the police is a matter of provincial legislation. Nurses should be aware that in cases involving abuse of adults, violence is something that competent adults must choose to self-report. Nurses are responsible for reporting abuse of children, dependent adults, and older adults to authorities, though the particular standards of reporting vary among provinces and territories. Awareness of these standards is the responsibility of the nurse.
- Interventions for victims or perpetrators of violence depend on the level of crisis and are focused on planning strategies to remove the individual and family members from violent situations and preventing abuse from recurring. Support and crisis intervention are key nursing interventions.

CRITICAL THINKING

1. A colleague who has witnessed a child being abused states, "I don't think it's any of our business what people do in the privacy of their own homes."
   a. What are you legally required to do?
   b. What are your ethical responsibilities?
2. Congratulations! You successfully convinced your colleagues to assess routinely for abuse. Now they want to know how

to do it. How would you go about teaching them to assess for child abuse? Intimate partner abuse? Older adult abuse?
3. Your health care organization's routine health screening form for adolescents, adults, and older adults has just been changed to include questions about family abuse. How would you respond to patients who indicate on this form that abuse occurs in their home?

4. Write out a safety plan that could be adopted by individuals who are being abused.
   a. Identify at least four referrals in your community for an abused person.

   b. Identify two referrals in your community for a violent person, partner, or parent.

5. What would the nurse screen for when a young, visibly upset pregnant woman attends a prenatal outpatient clinic with multiple bruises on her upper arms?

CHAPTER REVIEW

1. A man becomes frustrated when his children cry repeatedly and shoves his wife into the refrigerator. His wife explains to the neighbour, who witnessed this, that "I should have made the children go to bed earlier so they wouldn't be so cranky." This event is an example of:
   a. Masochism
   b. Emotional abuse
   c. Tension reduction
   d. Secondary prevention

2. Which statements about perpetrators and victims of abuse are accurate? Select all that apply.
   a. Approximately 40% of victims of intimate partner and family abuse are male.
   b. Abusive behaviour is usually the result of intoxication or stress.
   c. Perpetrators tend to respond best to treatment if it is court ordered.
   d. Victims do not report abuse because they tacitly are accepting of it.
   e. Victims of abuse stay in the relationship because they really do not want to leave.
   f. Disruptive behaviour may make older adults with dementia vulnerable to abuse.

3. A staff nurse, Chandra, is assisting a 30-year-old victim of domestic violence in the emergency department. The patient suffered numerous bruises and abrasions, is reluctant to be examined, seems very ashamed, and is very fearful that the Children's Aid Society will take custody of her young daughter, who has not been assaulted and is safe, if the police become involved. Which intervention is indicated?
   a. Report the assault to the police since reporting domestic violence is mandatory.
   b. Probe the patient for information to use as evidence in prosecuting the perpetrator.

   c. Press the patient to disrobe so that she can be examined for signs of hidden injuries.
   d. Guide and assist the patient to develop a safety plan for rapid escape should abuse recur.

4. Ms. Patel, a student nurse, is assigned to a patient recovering from injuries received during an episode of domestic violence, the third such assault for which she has received treatment. Ms. Patel left home at age 17 to escape an abusive father. Which statements about this situation are accurate? Select all that apply.
   a. Ms. Patel may be prone to blame the patient for her injuries and abuse.
   b. Ms. Patel's personal experiences give her special insight into the needs of this patient.
   c. Ms. Patel's experiences are likely to make her more empathic toward victims.
   d. Caring for victims of abuse will help Ms. Patel cope with her own abuse experiences.
   e. Ms. Patel may experience overwhelming anguish as a result of caring for abuse victims.
   f. Ms. Patel would likely benefit from clinical supervision related to caring for abuse victims.

5. Perpetrators of domestic violence tend to (select all that apply):
   a. Belong to lower socioeconomic groups and be poorly educated
   b. Have relatively poor social skills and have grown up with poor role models
   c. Believe that they, if male, should be dominant and in charge in relationships
   d. Force their mates to work and expect them to support the family
   e. Be controlling and willing to use force to maintain their power in relationships
   f. Prevent their mates from having relationships and activities outside the family

℮volve WEBSITE

Post-Test   interactive review

Visit the Evolve website for Chapter Review Answers and Rationales, Critical Thinking Answer Guidelines, and additional resources related to the content in this chapter: http://evolve.elsevier.com/Canada/Varcarolis/psychiatric/

REFERENCES

Allen, M. (2016). *Police reported crime statistics in Canada, 2015*. Retrieved from http://www.statcan.gc.ca/pub/85-002-x/2016001/article/14642-eng.htm.

Arkins, B., Begley, C., & Higgins, A. (2016). Measures for screening for intimate partner violence: A systematic review. *Journal of Psychiatric and Mental Health Nursing*, 23(3–4), 217–235. doi:10.1111/jpm.12289.

BC Provincial Mental Health and Substance Use Planning Council. (2013). *Trauma-informed practice guide*. Retrieved from http://bccewh.bc.ca/wp-content/uploads/2012/05/2013_TIP-Guide.pdf.

Bulechek, G. M., Butcher, H. K., Dochterman, J. M., et al. (2013). *Nursing interventions classification (NIC)* (6th ed.). St. Louis: Mosby.

Butchart, A., Harvey, A. H., & Fürniss, T. (2006). *Preventing child maltreatment: A guide to taking action and generating evidence*. Geneva: World Health Organization. Retrieved from http://www.who.int/violence_injury_prevention/violence/activities/child_maltreatment/en/index.html.

Campbell, J. C., Webster, D. W., & Glass, N. E. (2009). The danger assessment: Validation of a lethality risk assessment instrument for intimate partner femicide. *Journal of Interpersonal Violence, 24,* 653–674. doi:10.1177/0886260508317180.

Campbell, M., Neil, J. A., Jaffe, P. G., et al. (2010). Engaging abusive men in seeking community intervention: A critical research & practice priority. *Journal of Family Violence, 25,* 413–422. doi:10.1007/s10896-010-9302-z.

Canadian Medical Association. (2016). *Recognizing elder abuse and neglect*. Retrieved from http://www.demandaplan.ca/recognizing_elder_abuse_and_neglect.

Carter-Snell, C. J., & Jakubec, S. (2013). Exploring women's risks and resilience to mental illness after interpersonal violence. *International Journal of Child Youth and Family Studies, 4*(1), 72–99.

Coker, A. L., Hopenhayn, C., DeSimone, C. P., et al. (2009). Violence against women raises the risk of cervical cancer. *Journal of Women's Health, 18,* 1179–1185. doi:10.1089/jwh.2008.1048.

Coles, J., Lee, A., Taft, A., et al. (2015). Childhood sexual abuse and its association with adult physical and mental health: Results from a national cohort of young Australian women. *Journal of Interpersonal Violence, 30*(11), 1929–1944. doi:10.1177/0886260514555270.

Criminal Code. (1985). *Criminal Code (R.S.C., 1985, c. C-46): Assault*. Retrieved from http://laws-lois.justice.gc.ca/eng/acts/C-46/page-62.html.

Daoud, N., Matheson, F. I., Pedersen, C., et al. (2016). Pathways and trajectories linking housing instability and poor health among low-income women experiencing intimate partner violence (IPV): Toward a conceptual framework. *Women and Health, 56*(2), 208–225. doi:10.1080/03630242.2015.1086465.

Draucker, C., Martsolf, D., Ross, R., et al. (2009). The essence of healing from sexual violence: A qualitative metasynthesis. *Research in Nursing and Health, 32,* 366–378. doi:10.1002/nur.20333.

Draughon, J., & Urbancic, J. C. (2010). Childhood sexual abuse. In J. Humphrey & J. C. Campbell (Eds.), *Family violence and nursing practice* (2nd ed., pp. 319–346). New York: Springer.

Dunn, J. L., & Powell-Williams, M. (2007). Everybody makes choices. *Violence Against Women, 13,* 977–1001. doi:10.1177/1077801207305932.

Dutton, D. G. (1998). *The abusive personality*. New York: Guilford Press.

Dutton, D. G. (2007). *The abusive personality: Violence and control in intimate relationships* (2nd ed.). New York: Guilford Press.

Fallon, B., Chabot, M., Fluke, J., et al. (2013). Placement decisions and disparities among Aboriginal children: Further analysis of the Canadian Incidence Study Of Reported Child Abuse And Neglect Part A: Comparisons of the 1998 and 2003 surveys. *Child Abuse & Neglect, 37*(1), 47–60. doi:10.1016/j.chiabu.2012.10.001.

Feigenbaum, J. (2007). Dialectical behaviour therapy: An increasing evidence base. *Journal of Mental Health, 16,* 51–68. doi:10.1080/09638230601182094.

Ford-Gilboe, M., Varcoe, C., & Merritt-Gray, M. (2010). Intimate partner violence and nursing practice. In J. Humphrey & J. C. Campbell (Eds.), *Family violence and nursing practice* (2nd ed., pp. 115–153). New York: Springer.

Ford-Gilboe, M., Wuest, J., & Merritt-Gray, M. (2005). Strengthening capacity to limit intrusion: Theorizing family health promotion in the aftermath of woman abuse. *Qualitative Health Research, 15,* 477–501. doi:10.1177/1049732305274590.

Franklin, C. A., & Kercher, G. A. (2012). The intergenerational transmission of intimate partner violence: Differentiating correlates in a random community sample. *Journal of Family Violence, 27*(3), 187–199. doi:10.1007/s10896-012-9419-3.

Fulmer, T., Sengstock, M. C., Blankenship, J., et al. (2010). Elder mistreatment. In J. Humphrey & J. C. Campbell (Eds.), *Family violence and nursing practice* (2nd ed., pp. 347–365). New York: Springer.

Gill, A. K., Strange, C., & Roberts, K. A. (2014). *"Honour" killing and violence: Theory, policy and practice*. New York: Palgrave Macmillan.

Kendler, K. S., & Aggen, S. H. (2014). Clarifying the causal relationship in women between childhood sexual abuse and lifetime major depression. *Psychological Medicine, 44*(6), 1213. doi:10.1017/S0033291713001797.

Krug, E. G., Dahlberg, L. L., Mercy, J. A., et al. (Eds.). (2002). *World report on violence and health*. Geneva: World Health Organization. Retrieved from http://www.who.int/violence_injury_prevention/violence/world_report/en/.

MacIntosh, J., Wuest, J., Ford-Gilboe, M., et al. (2015). Cumulative effects of multiple forms of violence and abuse on women. *Violence and Victims, 30*(3), 502–521. doi:10.1891/0886-6708.VV-D-13-00095.

Macy, R. J., Renz, C., & Pelino, E. (2013). Partner violence and substance abuse are intertwined: Women's perceptions of violence–substance connections. *Violence Against Women, 19*(7), 881–902. doi:10.1177/1077801213498208.

McDonald, L., & Collins, A. (2000). *Abuse and neglect of older adults: A discussion paper*. Catalogue no. H72-21/162-1998E. Retrieved from http://dsp-psd.pwgsc.gc.ca/Collection/H88-3-30-2001/pdfs/violence/abuse_e.pdf.

McFarlane, J., Hughes, R. B., Nosek, M. A., et al. (2001). Abuse Assessment Screen—Disability (AAS-D): Measuring frequency, type, and perpetrator of abuse toward women with physical disabilities. *Journal of Women's Health & Gender-Based Medicine, 10,* 861–866. doi:10.1089/152460901753285750.

Mian, M., Shah, J., Dalpiaz, A., et al. (2015). Shaken baby syndrome: A review. *Fetal & Pediatric Pathology, 34*(3), 169–175. doi:10.3109/15513815.2014.999394.

Middlesex-London Health Unit. (2000). *Task force on the health effects of woman abuse—Final report*. London, ON: Author.

Mikton, C., & Butchart, A. (2009). Child maltreatment prevention: A systematic review of reviews. *Bulletin of the World Health Organization, 87,* 353–361. doi:10.2471/BLT.08.057075.

Moorhead, S., Johnson, M., Maas, M. L., et al. (2013). *Nursing outcomes classification (NOC)* (5th ed.). St. Louis: Elsevier.

Ono, E. (2017). Reformulating the use of battered woman syndrome testimonies in Canadian law: Implications for social work practice. *Affilia, 32*(1), 24–36. doi:10.1177/0886109916679862.

Papp, A. (2010). *Culturally driven violence against women: A growing problem in Canada's immigrant communities*. Retrieved from http://www.fcpp.org/files/1/Culturally-Driven%20Violence%20Against%20Women.pdf.

Paterno, M. T., & Draughon, J. E. (2016). Screening for intimate partner violence. *Journal of Midwifery & Women's Health, 61*(3), 370–375. doi:10.1111/jmwh.12443.

Pillemer, K., Burnes, D., Riffin, C., et al. (2016). Elder abuse: Global situation, risk factors, and prevention strategies. *The Gerontologist, 56*(Suppl. 2), S194–S205. doi:10.1093/geront/gnw004.

Podnieks, E., Rietschlin, J., & Walsh, C. A. (2012). Elder abuse in Canada— Reports from a national roundtable discussion: Introduction. *Journal of Elder Abuse & Neglect, 24*(2), 85.

Public Health Agency of Canada. (2016). *The chief public health officer's report on the state of public health in Canada 2016: A focus on family violence in Canada*. Retrieved from http://www.healthycanadians.gc.ca/publications/department-ministere/state-public-health-family-violence-2016-etat-sante-publique-violence-familiale/alt/pdf-eng.pdf.

Ramsey, S. H., & Abrams, D. E. (2010). A primer on child abuse and neglect law. *Juvenile and Family Court Journal, 61,* 1–31. doi:10.1111/j.1755-6988.2009.01036.x.

Raposo, S. M., Mackenzie, C. S., Henriksen, C. A., et al. (2014). Time does not heal all wounds: Older adults who experienced childhood adversities have higher odds of mood, anxiety, and personality disorders. *The American Journal of Geriatric Psychiatry: Official Journal of the American Association for Geriatric Psychiatry, 22*(11), 1241.

Registered Nurses' Association of Ontario. (2005). *Woman abuse: Screening, identification and initial response*. Toronto: Author.

Registered Nurses' Association of Ontario. (2014). *Best practice guidelines: Preventing and addressing abuse and neglect of older adults: Person-centred, collaborative, system-wide approaches*. Retrieved from http://rnao.ca/bpg/guidelines/abuse-and-neglect-older-adults.

Statistics Canada. (2017). *Family violence in Canada: A statistical profile, 2015.* Retrieved from http://www.statcan.gc.ca/daily-quotidien/170216/dq170216b-eng.htm.

Taillieu, T. L., Brownridge, D. A., Tyler, K. A., et al. (2016). Pregnancy and intimate partner violence in Canada: A comparison of victims who were and were not abused during pregnancy. *Journal of Family Violence, 31*(5), 567–579. doi:10.1007/s10896-015-9789-4.

Unrau, M., Jakubec, S. L., & Jeske, S. (2017). Somatics education for crisis intervention training. *Arts & Health, 9*(1), 91–96. doi:10.1080/17533015.2016.1233122.

Van Wel, B., Kockmann, I., Blum, N., et al. (2006). STEPPS group treatment for borderline personality disorder in the Netherlands. *Annals of Clinical Psychiatry, 18,* 63–67. doi:10.1080/10401230500464760.

Victims of Violence. (2017). *Research library: Duty to report abuse.* Retrieved from http://www.victimsofviolence.on.ca/research-library/duty-to-report-abuse/.

Walker, L. E. (1979). *The battered woman* (2nd ed.). New York: Springer.

Wallström, R., Persson, R. S., & Salzmann-Erikson, M. (2016). Working with children in families with parental substance abuse: Nurses' experiences and complexity in relationships. *Journal of Psychosocial Nursing and Mental Health Services, 54*(6), 38–44. doi:10.3928/02793695-20160518-06.

Wathen, C. N., Macgregor, J. C., Sibbald, S. L., et al. (2013). Exploring the uptake and framing of research evidence on universal screening for intimate partner violence against women: A knowledge translation case study. *Health Research Policy and Systems/BioMed Central, 11*(1), 13. doi:10.1186/1478-4505-11-13.

World Health Organization. (2017). *Health topics: Violence.* Retrieved from http://www.who.int/topics/violence/en/.

Sexual Assault

Jodie Flynn
Adapted by Sonya L. Jakubec

KEY TERMS AND CONCEPTS

aggravated sexual assault
blame
controlled style of coping
depersonalization
derealization
dissociative disorders
expressed style of coping
grounding techniques

intrusive thoughts
rape-trauma syndrome
secondary victimization
sexual assault
sexual assault nurse examiners (SANEs)
somatic therapies
vicarious trauma

OBJECTIVES

1. Define sexual assault and aggravated sexual assault.
2. Describe the profiles of the survivor and the perpetrator of sexual assault.
3. Distinguish between the acute and long-term phases of the rape-trauma syndrome, and identify some common reactions during each phase.
4. Discuss a trauma-informed approach and describe three related practices.

5. Reflect on one's own thoughts and feelings and consider the myths about sexual assault and its impact on survivors.
6. Identify five areas to assess and six overall guidelines for nursing interventions related to sexual assault.
7. Discuss the long-term psychological effects of sexual assault.
8. Identify three outcome criteria that would signify successful interventions for a person who has suffered a sexual assault.

ꬲvolve WEBSITE

Visit the Evolve website for Flashcards, Case Studies, and additional testing resources related to the content in this chapter: http://evolve.elsevier.com/Canada/Varcarolis/psychiatric/

Pre-Test | interactive review

In recent years, accounts of women being sexually assaulted by multiple perpetrators have garnered international attention. College and university campus sexual assaults of men and women have become the focus of recent study and interventions (Fedina, Holmes, & Backes, 2016; Voth Schrag, 2017). As many as 1 in 4 women will be sexually assaulted while obtaining a postsecondary education (Ending Violence Association of British Columbia, 2016). In some of these cases, further violation occurred through the display of electronic images of these assaults, and the resulting peer humiliation led to the hopelessness, desperation, and suicide

of the victims. While horrific and extreme, these outcomes have reinforced the seriousness and life-threatening consequences of sexual violence. These accounts demonstrate some of the most contemptible violations that can be perpetrated by one human being on another. In this chapter, we further explore the epidemiology, the consequences of, and the treatment approaches for sexual assault. Sexual assault, a legal term that refers to any sexual activity for which consent is not obtained or freely given, is also referred to as *sexual violence*. Sexual harassment and stalking, also criminal behaviours that are sexual in nature, are, however, not classified as assault. Sexual assault violates the sexual integrity of the victim and can result in a range of injury from no injury to serious injury. Using a weapon, threatening, or even endangering the life of the victim during a sexual attack are all defined as sexual assault; however, sexual assault or violence is more often much less extreme yet nonetheless can prove equally traumatic over time (Peter-Hagene & Ullman, 2015).

Sex offenders may commit acts of sexual violence against children, which are considered sexual abuse (see Chapter 24). These offences are termed *sexual interference, invitation to sexual touching, incest,* and *sexual exploitation* in the criminal justice system. Aggravated sexual assault is another legal term that is used when, during a sexual assault, the life of the survivor is endangered or the assault results in injury (*Criminal Code,* 1985).

Regardless of the descriptor or legal framework of a sexual assault, it is an act of violence. Research has demonstrated the significant mental health impacts of sexual assault (Carter-Snell & Jakubec, 2013). Sexual assault is not about sex but, rather, is an exertion of power and control over another individual. Children, older adults, women, and men can all be victims of sexual assault.

Nurses are often among the first to encounter patients who have been sexually assaulted and are instrumental not only in providing them with holistic care but also in helping to preserve evidence that could lead to prosecution of the perpetrator(s). It is essential that nurses be adequately informed about their roles and responsibilities with these patients.

Sexual assault is a multidimensional problem and calls for a public health approach that emphasizes the primary prevention of sexual violence (i.e., stopping it from occurring in the first place). Until recently, this approach has been relatively neglected in the field, with the majority of resources directed toward secondary or tertiary prevention (Mikton, Tanaka, Tomlinson, et al., 2017).

This chapter addresses issues surrounding sexual assault and the mental health impacts of this traumatic abuse of power and control. Throughout this chapter, survivors of sexual assault will be referred to using the female pronoun in recognition of the fact that women are significantly more frequently the victims of sexual assault. However, the principles discussed apply to anyone who has been sexually assaulted, male or female.

EPIDEMIOLOGY

Sexual assault is a topic people are reluctant to discuss because it is attached to much anguish, blame, shame, and desperation. The silence, however, has far-reaching impacts: it is estimated that more than 90% of sexual assaults in Canada go unreported. Nonetheless, more than 21 500 sexual assaults were reported nationwide in 2015, according to Statistics Canada (2016).

Everyone is at risk for sexual assault—it crosses all socio-economic groups; ages, from infant to older adult; genders; sexual orientations; abilities; and cultural groups (Association of Alberta Sexual Assault Services, 2017). Recent research studies, though, have identified particular risk and resiliency factors to mental health after an assault. In particular, it has been noted that rates of post-traumatic stress disorder (PTSD) are two to three times higher for survivors of sexual assault than for any other trauma,

including other crimes, motor vehicle accidents, and even disasters, and that cumulative traumas increase the impacts (LeBouthillier, McMillan, Thibodeau, et al., 2015). Further, a recent Canadian study points to pre-existing mental illness as a possible predisposing factor for sexual assault, findings that suggest a need for standardized screening tools and care for victims of sexual assault who also experience mental illness (Brown, Du Mont, Macdonald, et al., 2013).

Another important pattern of disease resulting from sexual assault is the concern for secondary victimization. Secondary victimization results when survivors experience further stress or trauma when seeking help, through practices such as victim blaming, insensitive communication techniques, delays in care, disbelief, shame, stigmatization, or minimization of the experience by others (Greeson, Campbell, & Fehler-Cabral, 2016). Social reactions to sexual assault contribute to increased PTSD and revictimization for victims of sexual assault, making public mental health interventions an important area of program implementation (Ullman & Peter-Hagene, 2016). Because of the high rate of the above-mentioned patterns, understanding sexual assault and its effects, prevention, and treatment is an important mental health and public health concern.

The *Criminal Code* of Canada was amended in 1983 to replace the crimes of rape and indecent assault with three new sexual assault offences, focusing on the violent rather than sexual aspects of sexual assault. These changes were in keeping with the view that sexual assault is an abuse of power and control and reinforced that a spouse could be charged with sexual assault and that both males and females could be considered victims of sexual assault. Separate categories of sexual assault are identified based on the severity of the incident. Level 1 is a term that describes assault of a sexual nature that violates the sexual integrity of a person. Sexual assault with a weapon or causing bodily harm is considered level 2. A level 3 sexual assault is characterized by an assault that wounds, maims, disfigures, or endangers the life of another person (*Criminal Code,* 1985).

Of the almost 21 500 police-reported sexual assaults recorded in 2015, the majority (98%) were classified as level 1 sexual assault. Although the majority of sexual assaults are considered less severe forms (as opposed to aggravated sexual assault), this descriptor does not lessen the anguish experienced following any sexual assault.

The rate of sexual assault level 1 increased between 2014 and 2015, up 3% to 58 per 100 000 population. The rates of sexual assault level 2 also increased 13%, with a total of 377 incidents reported in 2015, or a rate of 1 per 100 000 population. In contrast, the rate of the most serious sexual assaults (aggravated sexual assaults) declined 11% in 2015, with 104 incidents (12 fewer than in 2014).

Police-reported sexual assaults of all levels increased in most provinces and territories between 2014 and 2015, with the largest increases reported in Prince Edward Island (23% increase in rate) and Newfoundland and Labrador (21% increase in rate). Notable increases in rates were identified in the Northwest Territories (up 14%), Yukon (up 13%), and Quebec (up 9%). In contrast, Nunavut and Manitoba reported declines in rates of sexual assault (down 12% and 6%, respectively); however, despite these declines, these provinces are among those with the highest rates overall.

It is important to note that the number of sexual assaults reported by police is likely an underestimate of the true extent of sexual assault in Canada, as these types of offences often go unreported to police. For instance, self-reported data from the General Social Survey on Victimization showed that only 5% of sexual assaults experienced by Canadians age 15 years and older in 2014 were brought to the attention of police (Perreault, 2015).

The rate of reported sexual assault among Indigenous people is 70 incidents per 1000 people, compared to 23 per 1000 among non-Indigenous people. Indigenous women are almost three times as likely to experience violent victimization (physical or sexual violence) than non-Indigenous women (Perreault, 2015). Violence and sexual assault in Indigenous communities are unique from nation to nation, but share very complex issues involving historical trauma and childhood abuse that require multidimensional approaches, such as trauma and violence-informed practices (Centre for Research and Education on Violence Against Women & Children, 2017). Culture (see Chapter 8) is an important consideration of services provided, and without attention, patients may experience secondary victimization.

Profile of Sexual Perpetrators

Females are statistically more likely to be sexually assaulted, and males are most likely to be the perpetrator or perpetrators. Police-reported data state that 97% of persons accused of sexual offences were male. As mentioned, a large majority of reported sexual assaults were committed by a friend or acquaintance of the victim. Although we may think of the stranger lurking in the shadows in parking lots as the typical perpetrator, rape by a stranger is not typical: survivors typically know the person who sexually assaulted them. Police-reported data have indicated that 68% of aggravated sexual assaults occur at or near a residence (Statistics Canada, 2016), including at the victim's or perpetrator's home, at a house party, or in an outdoor party setting.

CLINICAL PICTURE

Relationships Between Victims and Perpetrators

The terms *intimate partner violence* and *spousal abuse* (see Chapter 24), *date rape*, *acquaintance rape*, and *drug-facilitated sexual assault* describe the relationship between the victim and perpetrator. In Canada, spousal sexual assault became against the law in 1983. Whether it is spousal abuse or date rape, in such cases the perpetrator is known to, and presumably trusted by, the person who is sexually assaulted.

The psychological and emotional outcomes of sexual assault seem to vary depending on the level of intimacy and the relationship between the victim and the perpetrator. Sexual distress (including postassault sexual problems such as dysfunction and pain) is more common among women who have been sexually assaulted by intimate partners; PTSD symptoms are common among those assaulted by someone they know; and fear and anxiety are more common in those assaulted by strangers. Depression has been found to be common among survivors,

whether the perpetrators were known to them or not (Carter-Snell & Jakubec, 2013).

Drug-facilitated sexual assault has been increasingly recognized over the past 15 to 20 years. Many drugs, including alcohol (the most commonly used date rape drug), can be used alone or in combination to facilitate sexual assault (Table 25-1). Often these drugs are given to an unknowing victim. Once the drugs are ingested, victims lose their ability to ward off attackers, develop amnesia, and become unreliable witnesses. Because the symptoms mimic those of alcohol intoxication, survivors are not always screened for these drugs, resulting in under-reporting of drug-facilitated sexual assault (Walsh, Zinzow, Badour, et al., 2016). As nurses, we must remember that whether a person willingly or unwillingly consumes alcohol or drugs and is subsequently sexually assaulted, it is not the victim's fault. The *Criminal Code* (1985) states that consent cannot be given by a person who is unconscious or intoxicated.

Psychological Effects of Sexual Assault

Most people who are sexually assaulted suffer severe and long-lasting emotional trauma. Long-term psychological effects of sexual assault may include depression, suicide, anxiety, and fear; difficulties with daily functioning; low self-esteem; sexual dysfunction; and somatic complaints. Survivors of incest may experience a negative self-image, depression, eating disorders, personality disorders, self-destructive behaviour, and substance abuse. A history of sexual abuse in psychiatric patients is associated with a characteristic pattern of symptoms that may include depression, anxiety disorders, chemical dependency, suicide attempts, self-mutilation, compulsive sexual behaviour, and psychosis-like symptoms (Carter-Snell & Jakubec, 2013). Reviews of the literature have summarized that timely intervention; trauma-informed approaches, such as having some control over the legal process; and the availability of positive support systems (both social and professional) provide resiliency to the psychological impacts of sexual assault (Carter-Snell & Jakubec, 2013).

Rape-Trauma Syndrome

Rape-trauma syndrome is a variant of PTSD and consists of an acute phase and a long-term reorganization process that occurs after an actual or attempted sexual assault. Each phase has separate symptoms, discussed below. See Chapter 12 for a more detailed discussion of PTSD.

Acute Phase

The acute phase of rape-trauma syndrome occurs immediately after the assault and may last 2 to 3 weeks. At this stage, patients usually are seen by emergency department personnel and, if available, the sexual assault nurse examiner (SANE), who are most involved in dealing with initial reactions. During this phase, there is a great deal of disorganization in the person's life, and somatic symptoms are common. This disorganization can be described in terms of impact, somatic, and emotional reactions (Box 25-1).

The survivor's most common initial reactions are shock, numbness, and disbelief. Outwardly, the person may appear

TABLE 25-1   DRUGS ASSOCIATED WITH DATE RAPE

DRUG, ALTERNATIVE NAMES, AND STATUS IN CANADA	FORM, MECHANISM OF ACTION, AND ONSET	EFFECT ON VICTIM	OVERDOSE SYMPTOMS AND TREATMENT
GHB (gamma-hydroxybutyrate) Also known as G, easy lay, liquid ecstasy, salty water, soap, cherry meth, and scoop Often made in illegal labs, resulting in the purity and strength of the final product being unpredictable	Liquid, white powder, or pill with a salty taste Schedule III central nervous system depressant A metabolite of gamma-aminobutyric acid (GABA) Onset within 5–20 minutes; duration, from 1–12 hours, is dose related	Produces relaxation, euphoria, and disinhibition Causes incoordination, confusion, deep sedation, and amnesia Tolerance and dependence exhibited by agitation, tachycardia, insomnia, anxiety, tremors, and sweating	*Symptoms:* Respiratory depression, seizures, nausea, vomiting, bradycardia, hypothermia, agitation, delirium, unconsciousness, and coma *Treatment:* Intubation for severe respiratory distress; atropine for bradycardia, and benzodiazepines for seizure activity; vomiting should be induced when possible
Rohypnol (flunitrazepam)* Also known as forget-me pill and roofies Mexico and other Latin American countries are the main illegal source of supply for North America	Pill that dissolves in liquids Schedule IV potent benzodiazepine; 10 times stronger than diazepam Impact is within 10–30 minutes and lasts 2–12 hours	More potent when combined with alcohol; causes sedation, psychomotor slowing, muscle relaxation, and amnesia Dependence and tolerance may develop	Overdose unlikely *Treatment:* Airway protection and gastrointestinal decontamination
Ketamine Also known as big K, kit-kat, Special K, wonk, and horsey P A rapid-acting anaesthetic drug used mainly by veterinarians and sometimes in human surgery	Liquid or a white powder An anaesthetic frequently used in veterinary practice; also a hallucinogenic substance related to phenylcyclohexyl piperidine (PCP) Onset within 30 seconds intravenously and 20 minutes orally; duration only 30–60 minutes; amnesia effects may last longer	Causes dissociative reaction, with a dreamlike state leading to deep amnesia and analgesia and complete compliance of the victim May become confused, paranoid, delirious, combative, with drooling and hallucinations	*Treatment:* Airway maintenance and use of anticholinergics such as atropine and benzodiazepines

*Two other benzodiazepines—clonazepam (Clonapam) and alprazolam (Xanax)—are also used.
Sources: Data adapted from Burchum, J., & Rosentha, L. (2016). *Lehne's pharmacology for nursing care* (9th ed.). Philadelphia: Elsevier; Health Canada. (2013). *Drugs of abuse and addiction.* Retrieved from http://healthycanadians.gc.ca/health-sante/addiction/index-eng.php; and U.S. Department of Health and Human Services. (2012). *Date rape drugs.* Retrieved from https://www.womenshealth.gov/a-z-topics/date-rape-drugs.

self-contained and calm and may make remarks such as "It doesn't seem real" or "I don't believe this really happened to me." Sometimes, cognitive functions may be impaired, and the traumatized person may appear extremely confused and have difficulty concentrating and making decisions. Alternatively, the person may become hysterical or restless or may cry or even smile. These reactions to crisis are typical and may shift in presentation and reflect cognitive, affective, and behavioural disruptions resulting from the trauma.

People who have experienced an emotionally overwhelming event may find it too painful to discuss. Examples of this response are found in statements such as "I don't want to talk about it" or "I just want to forget what happened." Behaviours that minimize the magnitude of the event include reluctance to seek medical attention and failure to follow up with legal counsel.

Long-Term Reorganization Phase

The long-term reorganization phase of rape-trauma syndrome occurs 2 or more weeks after the sexual assault. Nurses who care for survivors during the acute phase can help them anticipate and prepare for the reactions they are likely to experience during this later phase, which include the following:

- **Intrusive thoughts** of the sexual assault that break into the survivor's conscious mind both during the day and during sleep. These thoughts commonly include visions of violence toward the assailant, flashbacks (re-experiencing the traumatic event), or dreams with violent content contributing to insomnia and incite emotions such as anger.
- Increased activity, such as moving, taking trips, changing telephone numbers, and making frequent visits to old friends. This activity stems from the fear that the assailant will return.
- Increased emotional lability, including intense anxiety, mood swings, crying spells, and depression.

Fears and phobias develop as a defensive reaction to the sexual assault. Typical phobias include the following:

- Fear of the indoors if the assault occurred indoors
- Fear of the outdoors if the assault occurred outdoors
- Fear of being alone (common for most women after an assault)
- Fear of crowds (women may believe that any person in the crowd might be a rapist)
- Fear of sexual encounters and activities

Many women experience acute disruption of their sex lives with their partners. Sexual assault is especially disruptive for those with no previous sexual experience.

As mentioned, the consequences of sexual assault may be severe, debilitating, and long term. Intervention and support for the survivor can help prevent some of the complications of anxiety, depression, suicide, difficulties with daily functioning and interpersonal relationships, sexual dysfunction, and somatic complaints.

BOX 25-1 ACUTE PHASE OF RAPE-TRAUMA SYNDROME

Impact Reaction

Expressed Style

Overt behaviours:
- Crying, sobbing
- Smiling, laughing, joking
- Agitation, anger, hysteria
- Volatility, lability, restlessness
- Confusion, incoherence, disorientation
- Tenseness

Controlled Style

Ambiguous appearances and reactions:
- Confusion, incoherence, disorientation
- Lack of affective response
- Calm, subdued appearance
- Shock, numbness, confusion, freezing, disbelief
- Distractibility, difficulty making decisions

Somatic Reaction

Evidenced within first several weeks after a rape:
- Physical trauma
  - Bruises (breasts, throat, or back)
  - Soreness
- Skeletal muscle tension
  - Headaches
  - Sleep disturbances
  - Grimaces, twitches
- Gastrointestinal symptoms
  - Abdominal pains
  - Nausea
  - Loss of appetite
  - Diarrhea
- Genitourinary symptoms
  - Vaginal itching or discharge
  - Pain or discomfort

Emotional Reaction
- Fear of physical violence and death
- Denial
- Anxiety
- Shock
- Humiliation
- Fatigue
- Embarrassment
- Desire for revenge
- Self-blame
- Decreased self-esteem
- Shame
- Guilt
- Anger

Source: Adapted from Burgess, A. W. (1995). Rape trauma syndrome: A nursing diagnosis. *Occupational Health Nursing, 33*(8), 405; and Tannura, T. A. (2014). Rape trauma syndrome. *American Journal of Sexuality Education, 9*(2), 247–256. doi:10.1080/15546128.2014.883267.

BOX 25-2 PRACTICES USED IN A TRAUMA-INFORMED APPROACH

- Supporting patients in understanding the connections between their experience of trauma and their maladaptive or adaptive strategies for coping
- Ensuring that patients have choices about and control over their treatment options
- Using collaborative ways of determining needs and plans, and handling distress with sincere attempts to share power, decrease hierarchy, and build trust
- Adapting screening and intake procedures so that patients are not required to disclose trauma before they are ready or to repeatedly tell their stories
- Recognizing the range of emotional responses and symptoms that patients may experience, and identifying these as symptoms or adaptations to extreme life experiences rather than problem behaviours or extremes of personality
- Facilitating the development and use of coping skills, culturally safe healing strategies, and mechanisms for personal empowerment (which may or may not involve seeking police or legal action or survivor's support)

Source: Adapted from Canadian Centre on Substance Abuse. (2012). *The essentials of trauma informed care.* Retrieved from http://www.cnsaap.ca/SiteCollectionDocuments/PT-Trauma-informed-Care-2012-01-en.pdf.

APPLICATION OF THE NURSING PROCESS

A TRAUMA-INFORMED APPROACH

Trauma, such as a sexual assault, changes the world view of survivors so dramatically that it shifts the way they construct their sense of themselves and others. This trauma and the lasting effects then further inform other life choices and may guide the development of coping strategies that may help or hinder the growth and well-being of the patient. In this way, the impact of trauma may be felt throughout an individual's life in areas of functioning both related to and far removed from the trauma (Centre for Research and Education on Violence Against Women & Children, 2017).

Using a trauma-informed approach in the care of patients who have experienced sexual assault appropriately responds to the deep and profound impact of trauma (see Chapter 21). This approach emphasizes the physical, psychological, and emotional safety of both patients and caregivers and creates opportunities for patients to rebuild a sense of control and empowerment. A trauma-informed approach can include a range of specific practices (Box 25-2).

ASSESSMENT

Most sexual assault survivors do not report their sexual assault to the police, and few report it to doctors or nurses (Sheehy, 2012).

The Emergency Nurses Association (2010a) position statement on care of sexual assault victims suggests the following interventions:

- Using a nonjudgemental and empathic approach
- Rapidly assessing the needs and support required to prevent further trauma
- Treating and documenting injuries
- Providing a private environment (e.g., limiting personnel to those health care providers examining the patient, a translator if needed, and a specially trained advocate if indicated and consented to by the patient)
- Assisting with or conducting the physical examination
- Collecting evidence, with appropriate documentation and technique
- Assessing for sexually transmitted infections (STIs) (including obtaining pertinent laboratory tests such as human immuno-deficiency virus [HIV] testing, hepatitis profiles, and others) and treating STIs
- Conducting pregnancy risk evaluation and prevention
- Providing crisis intervention and arranging follow-up counselling

General Assessment

With consent, the SANE or nurse from the sexual assault response team (SART) should talk with the survivor, the family or friends who accompany the survivor, and the police to gather as much data as possible for assessing the crisis. The nurse then assesses the survivor's (1) level of anxiety, (2) coping mechanisms, (3) available support systems, (4) signs and symptoms of emotional trauma, and (5) signs and symptoms of physical trauma. Information obtained from the assessment is then analyzed, and nursing diagnoses are formulated.

Level of Anxiety

A patient experiencing severe to panic levels of anxiety will not be able to problem-solve or process information. Providing support, reassurance, and appropriate therapeutic techniques can lower the patient's anxiety and facilitate mutual goal setting and the assimilation of information. Refer to Chapters 12 and 20 for more detailed discussions of the levels of anxiety and therapeutic interventions for crises.

Coping Mechanisms

The same coping skills that have helped the survivor through other difficult problems in her lifetime will be used in adjusting to life after the sexual assault. In addition, new ways of getting through the difficult times may be developed for both the short-term and the long-term adjustment. Active and outwardly observable behavioural responses include crying; withdrawing; smoking; abusing alcohol and drugs; talking about the event; becoming extremely agitated, confused, disoriented, or incoherent; and even laughing or joking. These behaviours are examples of an **expressed style of coping** (see Box 25-1).

Cognitive coping mechanisms are the thoughts people have that help them deal with high anxiety levels. A positive cognitive response might be "At least I am alive and will get to see my children again." Not-so-positive responses may become generalized as a way to sum up the situation—"It's my fault this happened; my mother warned me about working in such a trashy place"—and may develop into an ego-damaging refrain. If such thoughts

are verbalized, the nurse will know what the survivor is thinking. If not, the nurse can ask questions such as "What are you thinking and feeling?" or "What can I do to help you in this difficult situation?" or "What has helped in the past?"

Available Support Systems

The availability, size, and usefulness of a survivor's social support system must be assessed. Often partners or family members do not understand the survivor's feelings about the sexual assault, and they may not be the best supports available. Pay careful attention to verbal and nonverbal cues of the survivor that may communicate the strength of her social network.

Signs and Symptoms of Emotional Trauma

Nurses work with sexual assault survivors most frequently in the emergency department soon after the sexual assault has occurred. Sexual assault is a psychological emergency and should receive immediate attention. Many emergency departments in urban areas

---

VIGNETTE

Sam, age 18, is brought to the emergency department by a concerned neighbour. She was found wandering aimlessly outside her house, sobbing and muttering, "He had no right to do that to me." Because of Sam's distraught appearance and her statement, the triage nurse suspects sexual assault and asks Sam if she would like to see the sexual assault nurse examiner (SANE). Sam agrees and is brought to a private area and introduced to the SANE, Ms. Davies. After respectful, nonjudgemental questioning, Sam divulges that her boyfriend forced her to have sex with him. Following the assessment and treatment, plans for discharge are discussed. Sam has nowhere to go because her family is away, and she does not want anyone called. Her neighbour, MaiLin, told the nurse earlier that Sam can stay with her family.

Nurse: "Earlier, your neighbour, MaiLin, told me that you are welcome to spend the weekend with her family."

Sam: (loudly, sharply, with eyes wide) "Oh no, I couldn't do that."

Nurse: "You don't like that idea?"

Sam: (wringing a tissue in her hands, head hanging, voice soft) "I can't go in her house anymore."

Nurse: "Something about being in that house disturbs you?"

Sam: "MaiLin's husband, Don" (deep sigh, pause) "used to … uh … take advantage of me when I would babysit their children."

Nurse: "Take advantage?"

Sam: "Yes …" (sobbing) "He used to try to get me to have sex with him. He said he'd blame it on me if I told anyone."

Nurse: "What a frightening experience that must have been for you."

Sam: "Yes."

Nurse: "I can see why you would not want to spend the night there. Let's explore other options."

A suitable place to stay is finally arranged. Sam is given counselling referrals that will help her deal with the process of reorganization after this current rape experience. Her counsellor will explore her feelings about past sexual abuse she has suffered at the hands of her neighbour when she is ready.

provide the services of **sexual assault nurse examiners (SANEs)** specially trained to meet the needs of sexual assault survivors. They are trained to assess the extent of psychological and emotional trauma that may not be readily apparent, especially if the person uses the **controlled style of coping**, a contained response, during the acute phase of the rape trauma (see Box 25-1).

Whether a SANE or another nursing or medical professional is conducting the assessment and evidence collection, a nursing history should be obtained and carefully recorded. When taking a history, the nurse determines only the details of the assault that will be helpful in addressing the immediate physical and psychological needs of the survivor. The nurse allows the survivor to talk at a comfortable pace; poses questions in nonjudgemental, descriptive terms; and refrains from asking "why" questions. The survivor frequently finds relating the events of the sexual assault traumatic and embarrassing.

If suicidal thoughts are expressed, the nurse assesses what precautions are needed by asking direct questions, such as "Are you thinking of harming yourself?" and "Have you ever tried to kill yourself before or since this attack occurred?" If the answer is yes, the nurse conducts a thorough suicide assessment, as described in Chapter 22.

Signs and Symptoms of Physical Trauma

It is essential that nurses provide psychological support while collecting and preserving legal evidence such as hair, skin, and semen samples that may be crucial for conviction of the perpetrator. The most characteristic physical signs of sexual assault are injuries to the face, head, neck, and extremities. Any physical injuries should be carefully documented, in both narrative and pictorial form using preprinted body maps, hand-drawn copies, or photographs. This assessment and all aspects must be conducted with the utmost respect for privacy and respect for the traumatic nature of the assault and potential for longer-term trauma and secondary victimization. The Ontario Coalition of Rape Crisis Centres (2017) provides a range of suggestions for supporting individuals who disclose that they have been sexually assaulted. These are listed in Box 25-3.

The nurse takes a brief gynecological history, including the date of the last menstrual period and the likelihood of current pregnancy, and assesses for a history of STIs. If the survivor has never undergone a pelvic examination, the steps of the examination will need to be explained. The nurse plays a crucial role in giving support and minimizing the trauma of the examination because the survivor may experience it as another violation of her body. Recognizing this, the nurse can explain the examination procedure in a way that will be reassuring and supportive. Allowing the survivor to participate in all decisions affecting care is essential to a trauma-informed approach and helps her to regain a sense of control over her life.

The survivor has the right to refuse either a legal or a medical examination. Consent forms must be signed before photographs are taken, a pelvic examination occurs, and any other procedures that might be needed to collect evidence and provide treatment are carried out. The correct preservation of body fluids and swabs is essential because DNA samples may identify the perpetrator. A shower and fresh clothing should be made available to

BOX 25-3	SUPPORTIVE PRACTICES FOR THE INTERVIEW AND ASSESSMENT OF VICTIMS OF SEXUAL ASSAULT

- Protect the patient's confidentiality and inform her that you will do so.
- Do not conduct an "investigation." Accept and believe what the client discloses.
- Listen emphatically and nonjudgementally.
- Tell the patient that that a sexual assault is never the victim's fault.
- Do not give personal advice (e.g., "If I were you, I would. ....").
- Do not call the police against the victim's wishes (unless you are specifically mandated to do so).
- Suggest options for action (e.g., legal, counselling, and other support), but let the client decide what action to take.
- Encourage the patient to seek medical help, including testing for unplanned pregnancy and sexually transmitted infections (STIs).
- Provide information (including in print) of the sexual assault services in the community that victims can access

Source: Adapted from Ontario Coalition of Rape Crisis Centres. (2017). *What can you do to support someone who has been sexually assaulted?* Retrieved from http://www.sexualassaultsupport.ca/whatyoucando.

the survivor as soon as possible after the examination and collection of specimens.

Providing prophylactic treatment for syphilis, chlamydia, and gonorrhea is common practice (Constantino, Crane, & Young, 2013). HIV exposure is often a concern of sexual assault survivors. This concern should always be addressed, and the sexual assault survivor should be given the information needed to evaluate the likelihood of risk. With this information, the person can make informed choices about HIV testing and safer-sex practices until testing can be done.

Depending on circumstances, the risk for pregnancy should be considered along with treatment options. Emergency contraception may be offered and prescribed; a few options are available in pill and intrauteriune device (IUD) methods (Constantino, Crane, & Young, 2013).

All data are carefully documented, including verbatim statements by the survivor, detailed observations of emotional and physical status, and all results of the physical examination. All laboratory tests performed are noted, and findings are recorded as soon as they are available. One of the greatest concerns is that crucial evidence may be lost or overlooked. The Emergency Nurses Association (2010b) position statement on forensic evidence collection underscores the role of the nurse in collecting and securing medical and legal evidence.

Self-Assessment

Nurses' attitudes influence the physical and psychological care received by sexual assault survivors. Knowing the myths and facts surrounding sexual assault can increase your awareness of your personal beliefs and feelings regarding sexual assault. If you examine personal feelings and reactions before encountering

TABLE 25-2 MYTH VERSUS FACT: RAPE

MYTH	FACT
Rape is caused by lust or uncontrollable sexual urges and the need for sexual gratification.	Rape is an act of physical violence and domination that is not motivated by sexual gratification.
Women fantasize about being raped.	No woman fantasizes about being raped. Fantasies about aggressive sex may be controlled and turned off if they become threatening. Sexual assault is a traumatic, painful, and terrifying experience.
Only "bad" women get raped.	Women of all ages, cultural backgrounds, social classes, and sexual orientations are equally likely to become victims of sexual assault.
When a woman dresses provocatively, she's inviting sexual attention and "asking for it."	Suggesting that women provoke sexual assault by the way they dress transfers blame from the perpetrator to the victim. If a woman is sexually assaulted, it is NOT her fault. No one ever "asks" or deserves to be sexually assaulted regardless of how she dresses or behaves.
Rape only occurs outside and at night.	Many rapes occur during the day and in the victims' homes. Eighty percent of sexual assaults occur in the home and 49% occur in broad daylight. Rape can and does occur anytime and anyplace.
Men cannot be sexually assaulted.	Men are sexually assaulted. Any man can be sexually assaulted regardless of size, strength, appearance, or sexual orientation.
Only homosexual men are sexually assaulted.	Heterosexual, gay, and bisexual men are equally likely to be sexually assaulted. Being sexually assaulted has nothing to do with your current or future sexual orientation.
Only homosexuals sexually assault other men.	Most men who sexually assault other men are heterosexual. This fact helps to highlight another reality that sexual assault is about violence, anger, and control over another person, not lust or sexual attraction.
Erection or ejaculation during sexual assault means "you really wanted it" or "enjoyed it" or consented to it.	Erection and ejaculation are physiological responses that may result from mere physical contact or even extreme stress. These responses do not imply that the victim wanted or enjoyed the assault and do not indicate anything about the victim's sexual orientation. Some rapists are aware how erection and ejaculation can confuse the sexual assault victim, manipulating their victims to the point of erection or ejaculation to increase their feelings of control and to discourage reporting of the crime.
It is impossible to sexually assault a man.	Young boys or adult males can be victims of rape or sexual assault.
Men do NOT experience the same degree of emotional pain associated with sexual assault as women. If a man experiences emotional pain, he should be able to deal with it.	All survivors may experience flashbacks, rage, depression, or anxiety when the traumatic experience is not acknowledged and treated. Survivors of trauma may turn to alcohol or drugs to cope with overwhelming feelings.

Sources: Created with data from http://www.d.umn.edu/cla/faculty/jhamlin/3925/myths.html; http://rwu.edu/campus-life/health-counseling/counseling-center/sexual-assault/rape-myths-and-fac; http://well.wvu.edu/articles/rape_myths_and_facts; http://www.secasa.com.au/pages/myths-about-male-rape/; and https://vsac.ca/myths/

a sexual assault survivor, you will be better prepared to give empathic and effective care. Examining your feelings about pregnancy termination is also important, because a patient might choose to terminate a pregnancy that results from assault. Table 25-2 compares sexual assault myths and facts. **Vicarious trauma**, a term used to describe the disruptions in thinking and perspectives of those who are exposed to the stories of those who are traumatized, is of concern for nurses and others working with sexual assault victims (Raunick, Lindell, Morris, et al., 2015). Supervision, reflection, and ongoing self-assessment are first steps to managing the effects of this trauma on nurses and on their nursing care.

DIAGNOSIS

The nursing diagnosis *Rape-trauma syndrome* applies to the physical and psychological effects of a sexual assault. It includes an acute phase of disorganization of the survivor's lifestyle and a long-term phase of reorganization. The syndrome is manifested by post-traumatic features such as:
- Alterations in concentration
- Anger

ASSESSMENT GUIDELINES
Sexual Assault

1. Assess psychological trauma, and document the patient's verbatim statements.
2. Assess level of anxiety. If in a severe to panic level of anxiety, the patient will not be able to problem-solve or process information.
3. Assess physical trauma and document per institutional, provincial or territorial, and Royal Canadian Mounted Police (RCMP) protocols. Use a preprinted body map, and ask permission and obtain written consent to take photographs.
4. Assess the survivor's available support system. Often partners or family members do not understand the trauma of sexual assault, and they may not be the best supports to draw on at this time.
5. Identify community supports (e.g., crisis centres, support groups, therapists) that work in the area of sexual assault.
6. Encourage the patient to talk about the experience, but do not press the patient to tell.

- Dissociative amnesia
- Headache
- Irritability
- Nightmares

The vignette describing the response of a male student highlights some of the symptoms at different stages following sexual assault.

Dissociative Disorders

Dissociative disorders occur after significant adverse experiences or traumas such as a sexual assault, and in these disorders individuals respond to stress with a severe interruption of consciousness. Dissociation is an unconscious defence mechanism that protects the individual against overwhelming anxiety through an emotional separation. However, this separation results in disturbances in memory, consciousness, self-identity, and perception.

Patients with dissociative disorders have intact reality testing. This means that although the person may have flashbacks or images, these are triggered by current events, relate to the past trauma, and are not delusions or hallucinations. Mild, fleeting dissociative experiences are relatively common to all of us. For example, we say we are on "auto pilot" when we drive home from work and cannot recall the last 15 minutes before reaching the house.

These common experiences are distinctly different from the processes of pathological dissociation. Dissociation is involuntary and results in failure of the normal control over a person's mental processes and normal integration of conscious awareness. Dimensions of a memory that should be linked are not and are fragmented. For example, a person may be aware of a sound or smell, but these sensations would not be linked to the actual event itself, leaving the person fearful or confused. Dissociation causes people to experience a distressing fragmentation of consciousness and a sense of separation from themselves. Disturbances of perception, sensation, autonomic regulation, and movement are common for those who have suffered significant trauma because trauma is often stored physically in the body. In addition, the person may re-enact, as well as re-experience, trauma without consciously knowing why.

Symptoms of dissociation may be either positive or negative. Positive symptoms refer to unwanted additions to mental activity such as flashbacks. Negative symptoms refer to deficits such as memory problems or the ability to sense or control different parts of the body. Dissociation decreases the immediate subjective distress of the trauma and also continues to protect the individual from full awareness of the disturbing event.

Dissociation can also be somewhat protective—for example, when a sexual assault victim from a small rural community or workplace regularly has contact with the perpetrator of the assault, or when a child is the victim of abuse by a close family member. This highlights the importance of attachments and relationships in allowing the child to grow socially, intellectually, and cognitively. If abuse or neglect has occurred, these memories become compartmentalized and often do not intrude into awareness until later in life when the person is in a stressful situation. Dissociative disorders include (1) depersonalization/derealization disorder, (2) dissociative amnesia, and (3) dissociative identity disorder.

Depersonalization/Derealization Disorder

Depersonalization/derealization disorder is found in both adolescents and adults, often in response to acute stress such as a sexual assault. In depersonalization the focus is on oneself. It is an extremely uncomfortable feeling of being an observer of one's own body or mental processes. In derealization the focus is on the outside world. It is the recurring feeling that one's surroundings are unreal or distant. The person may feel mechanical, dreamy, or detached from the body. Some people suffer episodes of these problems that come and go, whereas others have episodes that begin with stressors and eventually become constant. Patients describe these experiences as very distressing.

OUTCOMES IDENTIFICATION

The long-term outcome includes the absence of any residual symptoms after the trauma. The *Nursing Outcomes Classification (NOC)* identifies additional outcomes appropriate for the rape survivor: *Abuse protection*, *Abuse recovery: Emotional*, *Abuse recovery: Sexual*, *Coping*, *Personal resiliency*, *Sexual functioning*, and *Stress level* (Moorhead, Johnson, Maas, et al., 2013). Some of the suggested indicators for these outcomes include the following:

- Patient will demonstrate positive interpersonal relationships.
- Patient will demonstrate adequate social interactions.
- Patient will demonstrate healing of physical injuries.
- Patient will demonstrate evidence of appropriate opposite- or same-sex relationships.
- Patient will verbalize accurate information about sexual functioning.
- Patient will express comfort with body.
- Patient will express sexual interest.
- Patient will report increased psychological comfort.
- Patient will report a decrease in physical symptoms of stress.

PLANNING

Unless the survivor has sustained serious physical injury, treatment is offered, and the patient is released. However, because the ramifications of sexual assault are experienced for an extended

---

VIGNETTE

At a party, a male sexually assaults John, a 22-year-old university student. After John is brought to the emergency department by a friend, he describes feeling detached from his body. He cannot remember his surroundings during the assault: "It feels like it took place in a vacuum." He is agitated, irritable, and tells his friend to leave. John has difficulty concentrating on the examiner's questions. After a week, John still feels as though his mind is detached from his body. He reports having difficulty sleeping, nightmares, headaches, not being able to concentrate, and startling whenever anyone touches him.

time after the acute phase, the plan of care includes information for follow-up care. The survivor needs information about available community supports and how to access them. Nurses may also encounter sexual assault survivors in other settings when they are no longer in acute distress but still dealing with the aftermath of assault. Such settings include inpatient facilities, the community, and the home. A comprehensive plan of care addresses the continuing needs of the sexual assault survivor in any setting.

IMPLEMENTATION

The occurrence of sexual assault can be the most devastating experience in a person's life and constitutes an acute adventitious (unexpected) crisis. Comprehensive approaches to intervention address multiple levels and focus on leadership and policy, prevention, outreach, and interventions (Association of Alberta Sexual Assault Services, 2017; Regehr, Alaggia, Dennis, et al., 2013; Wells, Claussen, Aubry, et al., 2012). Typical crisis reactions reflect cognitive, affective, and behavioural disruptions. For survivors to return to their previous level of functioning, it is necessary for them to fully mourn their losses, experience anger, and work through their fears. Box 25-4 provides *Nursing Interventions Classification (NIC)* interventions for rape-trauma syndrome (Bulechek, Butcher, & Dochterman, 2013).

Counselling

The most effective approach for counselling in the emergency department or crisis centre is to provide nonjudgemental care and optimal emotional support. Confidentiality is crucial. The most helpful things the nurse can do are to listen and to let the survivor talk. A survivor who feels understood is no longer alone and feels more in control of the situation. It is especially important to help the survivor and significant others to separate issues of vulnerability from blame—attachment of personal responsibility for the assault onto the victim. Although the person may have made choices that made her more vulnerable, she is not to blame for the sexual assault. She may, however, decide to avoid some of those choices in the future (e.g., walking alone late at night, using alcohol excessively). Focusing on one's behaviour (which is controllable) allows the survivor to believe that similar experiences can be avoided in the future.

In many rural and urban communities across Canada, community-based organizations, health care providers, and grassroots organizations have brought forward concerns that the needs of survivors of sexual assault were not being met in emergency departments. Care provided was often delayed by long wait times, and nurses and physicians were not adequately trained to meet the unique needs of the survivor. Many communities have responded to these concerns. For instance, in 1984, Canada's first hospital-based sexual assault centre was opened at Women's College Hospital in Toronto. The mandate of such sexual assault and domestic violence treatment centres is to address the medical, emotional, social, forensic, and legal needs of women, men, and children who have been recently sexually assaulted or who are survivors of domestic abuse in a prompt, professional, and compassionate manner (Ontario Network of Sexual Assault/

BOX 25-4 INTERVENTIONS FOR RAPE-TRAUMA SYNDROME

Definition of interventions for rape-trauma syndrome: Provision of emotional and physical support immediately following a reported sexual assault.

Activities:
- Provide support person to stay with patient.
- Explain legal proceedings available to patient.
- Explain sexual assault protocol, and obtain consent to proceed through protocol.
- Document whether patient has showered, douched, or bathed since incident.
- Document mental state, physical state (clothing, dirt, and debris), history of incident, evidence of violence, and prior gynecological history.
- Determine presence of cuts, bruises, bleeding, lacerations, or other signs of physical injury.
- Implement forensic evidence collection kit (e.g., label and save soiled clothing, vaginal secretions, and vaginal hair combings).
- Secure samples for legal evidence.
- Implement crisis intervention counselling.
- Offer medication to prevent pregnancy, as appropriate.
- Offer prophylactic antibiotic medication against sexually transmitted infection (STI).
- Discuss human immunodeficiency virus (HIV) postexposure prophylaxis.
- Give clear, written instructions about medication use, crisis support services, and legal support.
- Offer follow-up services for STI results and counselling services.
- Document according to agency policy.

Source: Adapted from Bulechek, G. M., Butcher, H. K., & Dochterman, J. M. (Eds.). (2013). *Nursing interventions classification (NIC)* (6th ed.). St. Louis: Mosby.

Domestic Violence Treatment Centres, n.d.). Since the first one was opened, similar sexual assault care centres have been introduced in many different formats throughout Canada, including individual centres serving vast rural communities. Other examples of regional sexual assault organizations include the Northern Society for Domestic Peace in Smithers, British Columbia, and the Avalon Sexual Assault Centre in Halifax, Nova Scotia.

If the survivor consents, involve supportive family or friends and discuss with them the nature and trauma of sexual assault, as well as the possible delayed reactions that may occur. One survivor expressed the aftermath of her assault as follows: "It takes a few days to hit you. It was bad. It was really rough for my husband. I needed to be reassured. I needed to be told that there was nothing I could have done to prevent it. Understanding helps."

Social support effectively moderates somatic symptoms and subjective health ratings. The survivor who is able to confide comfortably in one or two friends or family members, especially immediately after the assault, is likely to experience fewer somatic manifestations of stress. In many cases, family and friends need support and reassurance as much as the survivor does. This is especially true for those from traditional cultures, particularly those cultures that believe that sexual assault brings shame to the entire family. The long-standing cultural myth that women are the property of men still prevents some people from empathizing with the woman's severe psychic injury and from being supportive. In these cases, the woman is devalued instead.

Promotion of Self-Care Activities

When preparing the survivor for discharge, the nurse provides a printout of all referral information and follow-up instructions, detailing potential physical concerns and emotional reactions, legal matters, referrals to community agencies and counselling, and ways that family and friends can help. Providing this information in print is important because the amount of verbal information the patient can retain will likely be limited due to high levels of anxiety. Written material can be referred to repeatedly over time.

Follow-Up Care

The emotional state and psychological needs of the survivor should be reassessed by telephone or personal contact within 24 to 48 hours of discharge from the hospital. Repeat referrals should be made for resources or support services. Effective crisis intervention and continuity of care require outreach activities and services beyond the emergency medical setting.

Survivors may avoid seeking treatment from psychiatric mental health care providers because medical treatment is more socially sanctioned, and they are likely to be experiencing physical symptoms of stress. Thus the outpatient nurse can make a more focused assessment of stress-related symptoms, depression, or both and ascertain the need for mental health referral. Reporting symptoms and seeking medical treatment are adaptive coping behaviours and can be reinforced as such.

Follow-up visits should occur at least 2, 4, and 6 weeks after the initial evaluation; however, this frequency requires the consent of the survivor. At each visit, the survivor should be assessed for psychological progress, the presence of an STI, and pregnancy. Follow-up treatments for potential HIV exposure may also be administered if required. Case Study and Nursing Care Plan 25-1 describes the care of a patient who has been sexually assaulted.

Advanced-Practice Interventions

Sexual Assault Nurse Examiners

Internationally, forensic nursing is becoming a specialty, and the largest subspecialty of forensic nursing is caring for the sexual assault survivor. This role is filled by the sexual assault nurse examiner. Training to become a SANE requires knowledge and skill in the areas of testing and treatment for STIs; collection of forensic evidence; assessment of injuries; documentation; typical survivor responses and crisis intervention; collaboration with community agencies, such as police and women's shelters; and physical assessment and examination to determine the effects of the sexual assault (Adams & Hulton, 2016).

Survivors. Most of those who have been sexually assaulted are eventually able to resume their previous lifestyle and level of functioning after supportive services and crisis counselling. However, many continue to experience emotional trauma, including flashbacks, nightmares, fear, phobias, and other

symptoms associated with the trauma and with the related PTSD (see Chapter 12). Some people who survive sexual assault may be susceptible to an acute stress response, dissociation, psychotic episode, or emotional disturbance so severe that hospitalization is required. Others whose emotional lives may be overburdened with multiple internal and external pressures may require individual psychotherapy.

Depression and suicidal ideation too frequently follow sexual assault. Depression is more common in those who do not disclose the assault to significant others because they have concerns about being stigmatized, have children living at home, or have a pending civil lawsuit. Any exposure to stimuli related to the traumatic event may activate a reliving of the traumatic state.

Evidence-based treatments include trauma-focused psychotherapy that may include components of exposure or cognitive restructuring and eye movement desensitization and reprocessing (EMDR) therapy. These modalities are often combined with anxiety management or stress reduction that focuses on alleviation of symptoms. Other helpful strategies include brief psychodynamic psychotherapy, imagery, relaxation techniques, and hypnosis. People who have been sexually assaulted are also likely to benefit from group therapy or support groups. These modalities may be particularly beneficial for survivors from cultures that are group oriented rather than individualistic and for women who derive much of their self-definition from cultural norms. Group therapy can make the difference between a person coming out of the crisis at a lower level of functioning and that person gradually adapting to the experience with an increase in coping skills.

Psychoeducation can benefit patients experiencing dissociative disorders following sexual assault or other traumatic events. There is a need to learn about these responses and to gain new coping skills and stress management to manage the symptoms that can be frightening. Normalizing experiences by explaining symptoms as adaptive responses to overwhelming events is important.

Grounding techniques promote awareness of in-the-moment real things and help counter dissociative episodes. For example, dissociation can be disrupted by stomping one's feet, taking a shower, holding an ice cube, exercising, deep breathing, or touching the upholstery on a chair. Patients can learn to keep a daily journal to increase awareness of feelings and to identify triggers to dissociation. If a patient has never written in a journal, the nurse should suggest beginning with a 5- to 10-minute daily writing exercise.

Somatic therapies or sensorimotor psychotherapy combines talk therapy with body-centred interventions and movement to address dissociative symptoms (Ogden, Minton, & Pain, 2006). This therapy is based on the premise that the body, mind, emotions, and spirit are interrelated and that a change at one level results in changes in the others. Awareness, focusing on the present, and recognizing touch as a means of communicating are some of the principles of this therapy. During psychotherapy sessions, the patient describes current physical sensations. The goal is to safely disarm the pathological defence mechanism of dissociation and replace it with other resources, especially body awareness and mindfulness.

Perpetrators. As stated previously, sexual assault is an act of violence and an abuse of power and control. This abuse is not necessarily indicative of a particular mental health problem; however, psychotherapy is essential for perpetrators of sexual assault to gain consciousness and change behaviours. Unfortunately, most perpetrators do not acknowledge the need for behavioural change, and no single method or program of treatment has been found to be completely effective. The nurse's awareness of his or her own feelings and reactions will be crucial to avoid interference with the therapeutic process.

EVALUATION

Sexual assault survivors are considered to be recovered if they are relatively free of any signs or symptoms of PTSD and dissociative disorders; that is, if they are

- Sleeping well, with very few instances of episodic nightmares or broken sleep
- Eating as they were before the assault (patients may respond to the crisis of rape by undereating or overeating)
- Calm and relaxed or only mildly suspicious, fearful, or restless
- Getting support from family and friends (some strain might still be present in relationships, but it should be minimal)
- Generally positive about themselves (on occasion, doubts about self-worth may occur)
- Managing stress adaptively, without dissociation and free from somatic reactions (if mild symptoms persist and minor discomfort is reported, the survivor should be able to talk about it and feel in control of the symptoms)
- Showing a return to pre–sexual assault sexual functioning and interest

In general, the closer the survivor's lifestyle is to the pattern that was present before the sexual assault, the more complete the recovery has been.

 RESEARCH HIGHLIGHT

Can Virtual Environments Mediate Post-Traumatic Stress Disorder (PTSD) for Sexual Assault Victims?

Problem
Most women who are victims of sexual assault report a post-traumatic response in the days and weeks following the event. In most cases, these manifestations fade away over time. Unfortunately, though, for about one quarter of victims of sexual assault, post-traumatic responses persist for months. Regardless, the effects can be disabling. Virtual reality has shown promising results in the treatment of PTSD for some traumatic experiences, but sexual assault has been understudied.

Purpose of Study
This study sought to examine the relevance and safety of a virtual environment intervention, allowing patients to be progressively exposed to a sexual assault scenario.

Methods
Thirty women (victims and nonvictims of sexual assault) were randomly assigned in a counterbalanced order to two immersions

in a virtual bar: a control scenario in which the encounter with the aggressor does not lead to sexual assault and an experimental scenario in which the participant is assaulted. Immersions were conducted in a fully immersive six-wall system. Questionnaires were administered, and psychophysiological measures were recorded. No adverse events were reported during or after the immersions.

Key Findings
Repeated-measures analyses of covariance revealed a significant time effect and significantly more anxiety and negative affect in the experimental scenario than in the control condition.

Implications for Nursing Practice
Given the safety of the scenario and its potential to induce emotions, it can be further tested to document its usefulness with sexual assault victims who suffer PTSD.

Source: Loranger, C., & Bouchard, S. (2017). Validating a virtual environment for sexual assault victims. *Journal of Traumatic Stress, 30*(2), 157–165. doi:10.1002/jts.22170.

CASE STUDY AND NURSING CARE PLAN 25-1

Sexual Assault

Jenna Smith is a 23-year-old Australian working at a Canadian ski hill hotel on a temporary work visa. One evening, when not on shift at the hotel, she goes out with some friends and workmates for a night of bowling and drinks at a club afterward. Later in the evening, Jenna is tired and ready to go home. A man, Ryan, who joined the group at the club, offers to take her home. She has seen Ryan at other parties before but does not know much about him, though he is fun to be around and is an acquaintance of one of her workmates. Not in the habit of going home alone with men she does not know, she hesitates. Their mutual friend, whom she trusts, encourages her to accept the ride, stating that he "seems like a nice man."

Ryan drives Jenna home. He then asks if he can come into her house to use the bathroom before driving the long distance back to his house. She reluctantly agrees and sits on the living room couch. After using the bathroom, Ryan sits next to Jenna and begins to kiss her and fondle her breasts. As she protests, Ryan becomes more forceful in his advances. Jenna is confused and frightened. She manages to get away from him briefly, but he begins grabbing, squeezing, and biting her. He tells her gruffly, "If you don't do what I say, I'll break your neck." She screams, but he proceeds to sexually assault her. Ryan becomes nervous that the noise will alert the neighbours and races out of the house.

Continued

CASE STUDY AND NURSING CARE PLAN 25-1—cont'd

Sexual Assault

A neighbour does in fact arrive just after Ryan flees. The neighbour calls the police and then brings Jenna to the local hospital emergency department for a physical examination, crisis intervention, and support. In the emergency department, Jenna is visibly shaken. She keeps saying, over and over, "I shouldn't have let him take me home. I should have fought harder; I shouldn't have let him do this."

The nurse takes Jenna to a quiet cubicle. She does not want Jenna to stay alone and asks the neighbour to stay with her. The nurse then notifies the doctor and the SANE. When the nurse comes back, she tells Jenna that she would like to talk to her before the doctor comes. Jenna looks at her neighbour and then down. The nurse asks the neighbour to wait outside for a while and says she will call her later.

Jenna: "It was horrible. I feel so dirty."
Nurse: "You have had a traumatic experience. Do you want to talk about it?"
Jenna: "I feel so ashamed. I never should have let that man take me home."
Nurse: "You think that if you hadn't gone home with a stranger this wouldn't have happened?"

Jenna: "Yes ... I shouldn't have let him do it to me anyway. I shouldn't have let him rape me."
Nurse: "You mentioned that he said he would break your neck if you didn't do as he said."
Jenna: "Yes, he said that ... he was going to kill me. It was awful."
Nurse: "It seems you did the right thing in order to stay alive."

As the nurse continues to talk with her, Jenna's anxiety level seems to lessen. The nurse talks to Jenna about the kinds of experiences survivors may have after a sexual assault and explains that the reactions she might have 2 or 3 weeks from now are normal in these circumstances. The nurse continues to collect the necessary information. She says that the doctor will want to examine Jenna and explains the procedure to her. She then asks Jenna to sign a consent form. While preparing Jenna for examination, the nurse notices bite marks and bruises on both breasts. She also notes Jenna's lower lip, which is cut and bleeding. The nurse keeps detailed notes on her observations and draws a body map of the injuries. After the examination, Jenna is given clean clothes and a place to shower.

ASSESSMENT

Self-Assessment

The nurse has worked with sexual assault survivors before and has helped develop the hospital protocol. It took a while for her to be able to remain both neutral and responsive, because her own anger at perpetrators had initially interfered. She also remembers a time when a woman came in stating that she was assaulted but was so calm, smiling, and polite that the nurse initially did not believe her story. She had not at that point examined her own feelings or dealt with the popular societal myths regarding sexual assault. It was only later, when she had talked to more experienced health care personnel, that she learned that crisis reactions can seem bizarre, confusing, and contradictory.

The nurse learned that staying with the survivor, encouraging her to express her reactions and feelings, and listening are effective methods of reducing feelings of anxiety. Once the nurse learned through supervision and peer discussion to let go of her personal anger at the attacker and her ambivalence toward the survivor, her care and effectiveness improved greatly. All of this growth took time and support from more experienced nurses and other members of the health care team.

Objective Data	Subjective Data
• Crying and sobbing	• "He was going to kill me."
• Bruises and bite marks on each breast	• "It was horrible. I feel so dirty."
• Lip cut and bleeding	• "I shouldn't have let him rape me."
• Sexual assault reported to the police	

DIAGNOSIS

The nurse formulates the following diagnosis:
Rape-trauma syndrome.

Supporting Data
• "I shouldn't have let him rape me."
• "He was going to kill me."
• Crying and sobbing
• Bruises and bite marks on both breasts
• Rape reported to the police
• "It was horrible. I feel so dirty."

OUTCOMES IDENTIFICATION

Overall outcome: *Abuse recovery: Emotional*
Short-term indicator: Jenna will demonstrate appropriate affect for the situation.
Intermediate indicator: Jenna will demonstrate confidence. Short-term and intermediate outcome indicators are measured on a five-point Likert scale from 1 (none) to 5 (extensive).

CASE STUDY AND NURSING CARE PLAN 25-1—cont'd

Sexual Assault

PLANNING

The nurse plans to provide emotional and physical support to Jenna while she receives care in the emergency setting and to make sure that Jenna is aware of the importance of follow-up care.

IMPLEMENTATION

Jenna's plan of care is personalized as follows.

Short-Term Goal	Intervention	Rationale
1. Jenna will demonstrate appropriate affect by discharge from the emergency department.	1a. Remain neutral and nonjudgemental, and assure survivor of confidentiality.	1a. Lessens feelings of shame and guilt and encourages sharing of painful feelings.
	1b. Do not leave survivor alone.	1b. Deters feelings of isolation and escalation of anxiety.
	1c. Allow patient negative expressions and behavioural self-blame while using reflective techniques.	1c. Fosters feelings of control.
	1d. Assure survivor she did the right thing to save her life.	1d. Decreases burden of guilt and shame.
	1e. When anxiety level is down to moderate, encourage problem solving, choice, and power in decision making.	1e. Increases survivor's feeling of control in her own life. (When in severe anxiety, a person cannot problem-solve.)
	1f. Tell survivor of common reactions experienced by people in long-term reorganization phase (e.g., phobias, flashbacks, insomnia, increased motor activity).	1f. Helps survivor anticipate reactions and understand them as part of recovery process.
	1g. Explain emergency department procedure to survivor.	1g. Lowers anticipatory anxiety.
	1h. Explain physical examination.	1h. Allows for questions and concerns; survivor may be too traumatized and may refuse.
	1i. Stay with survivor during physical examination. A SANE can perform examination.	1i. Physical examination may be experienced as a second assault. Nurse provides comfort and support.

EVALUATION

Jenna is able to express her feelings in the emergency department, as well as understand the feelings she may experience as she moves through the reorganization phase. The indicator is achieved at a level of 3 (moderate).

▌ KEY POINTS TO REMEMBER

- Sexual assault is a common and often under-reported crime of violence in Canada.
- Females are far more likely to be survivors of sexual assault and tend to know their perpetrators. Sexual assault of males tends to be under-reported, owing to the humiliation and stigma attached to such victimization.
- Psychoactive substances play a major role in sexual assault, and alcohol is the most commonly used date rape drug. Other disinhibiting and amnesic substances also play a role in forcible sex acts.
- A sexual assault survivor experiences a wide range of feelings, which may or may not be exhibited to others.
- Feelings of fear, degradation, anger and rage, helplessness, and nervousness; sleep disturbances; disturbed relationships;

flashbacks; depression; and somatic complaints are all common following sexual assault.
- The circumstances of the initial medical evaluation may be frightening and stressful. Police interrogation, repeated questioning by health care providers, and the physical examination itself all have the potential to add to the trauma of the sexual assault.
- The SANE can serve to minimize repetition of questions and support the survivor as she goes through the entire ordeal.
- Survivors require long-term health care that can include counselling to minimize long-term effects of the sexual assault and assist in early return to a normal living pattern.
- Telephone and online resources are available to assist sexual assault survivors.

CRITICAL THINKING

1. Isaac, 18 years of age, is brutally beaten and sexually assaulted by a group of young men at a university party where Isaac was intoxicated and unconscious. After he regained consciousness, he tried to walk home but fell and was found semiconscious by a passerby and taken to the emergency department. Isaac has three large bruises around the occipital area of his head and several on his chest and buttocks. He has sustained a cracked rib, which he splints when walking. In assessment, he has a visible 2-centimetre anal tear and is wincing in pain that he states is an 8 out of 10. Ms. Lynkowski, a SANE, works with Isaac using the hospital's sexual assault protocol. Isaac appears stunned and confused and has difficulty focusing on what the nurse says. He states repeatedly, "This is crazy, this can't be happening... . I can't believe this has happened to me... . Oh, my God, I can't believe this."

   a. What areas of Isaac's assessment should be given highest priority by Ms. Lynkowski and her staff while he is in the emergency department?

   b. Chart the signs and symptoms of Isaac's physical and emotional trauma and verbatim statements in as much detail as you can.

   c. What are some of the pivotal issues that need to be addressed in terms of assessing Isaac's signs and symptoms of physical trauma? Although the risk of pregnancy is not present, what other real physical risks need to be assessed?

   d. What are some of the signs and symptoms of rape-trauma syndrome? Of the controlled style of coping?

   e. Identify the short-term outcome criteria for Isaac that ideally would be met before he leaves the emergency department.

   f. What information does Isaac need to have regarding potential signs and symptoms that may occur in the near future? Why is this important for him to understand at present?

   g. Identify specific indicators that will be met if Isaac recovers with minimal trauma from the event. How would you evaluate these criteria?

CHAPTER REVIEW

1. The nurse is caring for a patient in the emergency department who was sexually assaulted just hours earlier. Which behaviours should the nurse expect if the patient was exhibiting controlled-style reactions?
   a. Shock, numbness
   b. Volatility, anger
   c. Crying, sobbing
   d. Smiling, laughing

2. The nurse is caring for a patient who has just been sexually assaulted. Which is the appropriate initial nursing response?
   a. "I will get you the number for the crisis intervention specialist."
   b. "May I get your consent to test you for pregnancy and HIV?"
   c. "You are safe here."
   d. "I need to look at your bruises and cuts."

3. A patient who has been sexually assaulted has chosen to accept pregnancy prophylaxis medication but states that she does not believe in abortion. What information can you, as a nurse, give that will help with her decision?
   a. "Emergency contraception is not an abortion pill and will not work if you are already pregnant. That is the reason we perform a pregnancy test."
   b. "Just take a few days to consider your options."

   c. "Here is the number to your local sexual health clinic. They can explain it to you."
   d. "I won't give you the pregnancy prophylaxis medication then."

4. The nurse is working at a telephone hotline centre when a sexual assault survivor calls. If the sexual assault survivor states that she is fearful of going to the hospital, what is the appropriate nursing response?
   a. "You don't need to go to the hospital if you don't want to."
   b. "I'm here to listen to you, and we can talk about your feelings."
   c. "Did you do something to make the other person attack you?"
   d. "Why are you afraid to seek medical attention?"

5. The nurse is caring for a patient who is in the long-term reorganization phase of rape-trauma syndrome. Which symptoms should the nurse anticipate? Select all that apply.
   a. Development of fear of locations that resemble the rape location
   b. Emergence of acceptance of the rape
   c. Dreams with violent content
   d. A shift from anxiety to calm
   e. Onset of phobia of being alone

℮volve WEBSITE

Post-Test   interactive review

Visit the Evolve website for Chapter Review Answers and Rationales, Critical Thinking Answer Guidelines, and additional resources related to the content in this chapter: http://evolve.elsevier.com/Canada/Varcarolis/psychiatric/

REFERENCES

Adams, P., & Hulton, L. (2016). The sexual assault nurse examiner's interactions within the sexual assault response team: A systematic review. *Advanced Emergency Nursing Journal, 38*(3), 213–227. doi:10.1097/TME.0000000000000112.

Association of Alberta Sexual Assault Services. (2017). *Sexual violence action plan.* Retrieved from https://aasas.ca/initiatives/sexual-violence-action-plan/.

Brown, R., Du Mont, J., Macdonald, S., et al. (2013). A comparative analysis of victims of sexual assault with and without mental health histories: Acute and follow-up care characteristics. *Journal of Forensic Nursing, 9*(2), 76.

Bulechek, G. M., Butcher, H. K., & Dochterman, J. M. (2013). *Nursing interventions classification (NIC)* (6th ed.). St. Louis: Mosby.

Carter-Snell, C., & Jakubec, S. L. (2013). Exploring influences on women's mental health after interpersonal violence. *International Journal of Child, Youth and Family Studies, 1,* 72–99. Retrieved from http://journals.uvic.ca/index.php/ijcyfs/article/view/11844/3413.

Centre for Research and Education on Violence Against Women & Children. (2017). *Trauma- and violence-informed care.* Retrieved from http://www.vawlearningnetwork.ca/knowledge-hub/trauma-and-violence-informed-care.

Constantino, R. E. B., Crane, P. A., & Young, S. E. (2013). *Forensic nursing: Evidence-based principles and practice.* Philadelphia: F. A. Davis.

Criminal Code. (1985). *Criminal Code (R.S.C., 1985, c. C-46): Assault.* Retrieved from http://laws-lois.justice.gc.ca/eng/acts/C-46/page-62.html.

Emergency Nurses Association. (2010a). *Emergency Nurses Association position statements: Care of sexual assault and rape victims in the emergency department.* Retrieved from http://www.ena.org/SiteCollectionDocuments/Position%20Statements/SexualAssaultRapeVictims.pdf.

Emergency Nurses Association. (2010b). *Emergency Nurses Association position statements: Forensic evidence collection.* Retrieved from http://www.ena.org/SiteCollectionDocuments/Position%20Statements/Forensic%20Evidence.pdf.

Ending Violence Association of British Columbia. (2016). *Campus sexual violence: Guidelines for a comprehensive response.* Retrieved from http://endingviolence.org/wp-content/uploads/2016/05/EVABC_CampusSexualViolenceGuidelines_vF.pdf.

Fedina, L., Holmes, J. L., & Backes, B. L. (2016). Campus sexual assault: A systematic review of prevalence research from 2000 to 2015. *Trauma, Violence and Abuse,* 152483801663112. doi:10.1177/1524838016631129.

Greeson, M. R., Campbell, R., & Fehler-Cabral, G. (2016). Nobody deserves this": Adolescent sexual assault victims' perceptions of disbelief and victim blame from police. *Journal of Community Psychology, 44*(1), 90–110. doi:10.1002/jcop.21744.

LeBouthillier, D. M., McMillan, K. A., Thibodeau, M. A., et al. (2015). Types and number of traumas associated with suicidal ideation and suicide attempts in PTSD: Findings from a U.S. nationally representative sample. *Journal of Traumatic Stress, 28*(3), 183–190. doi:10.1002/jts.22010.

Mikton, C. R., Tanaka, M., Tomlinson, M., et al. (2017). Global research priorities for interpersonal violence prevention: A modified delphi study/Priorités mondiales de recherche pour la prévention de la violence interpersonnelle: Une étude delphi modifiée/Prioridades de investigación globales para la prevención de la violencia interpersonal: Un estudio de delphi modificado. *Bulletin of the World Health Organization, 95*(1), 36. doi:10.2471/BLT.16.172965.

Moorhead, S., Johnson, M., Maas, M. L., et al. (2013). *Nursing outcomes classification (NOC)* (5th ed.). St. Louis: Elsevier.

Ogden, P., Minton, K., & Pain, C. (2006). *Trauma and the body: A sensorimotor approach to psychotherapy.* New York: Norton.

Ontario Coalition of Rape Crisis Centres. (2017). *What can you do to support someone who has been sexually assaulted?* Retrieved from http://www.sexualassaultsupport.ca/whatyoucando.

Ontario Network of Sexual Assault/Domestic Violence Treatment Centres. (n.d.). *Our centres: Mandate.* Retrieved from http://www.satcontario.com/en/home.php.

Perreault, S. (2015). *Criminal victimization in Canada, 2014. Juristat.* Statistics Canada Catalogue no. 85-002-X. Retrieved from http://www.statcan.gc.ca/pub/85-002-x/2016001/article/14631-eng.htm.

Peter-Hagene, L. C., & Ullman, S. E. (2015). Sexual assault-characteristics effects on PTSD and psychosocial mediators: A cluster-analysis approach to sexual assault types. *Psychological Trauma: Theory, Research, Practice and Policy, 7*(2), 162–170. doi:10.1037/a0037304.

Raunick, C. B., Lindell, D. F., Morris, D. L., et al. (2015). Vicarious trauma among sexual assault nurse examiners. *Journal of Forensic Nursing, 11*(3), 123–128. doi:10.1097/JFN.0000000000000085.

Regehr, C., Alaggia, R., Dennis, J., et al. (2013). Interventions to reduce distress in adult victims of rape and sexual violence: A systematic review. *Research on Social Work Practice, 23*(3), 257–265. doi:10.1177/1049731512474103.

Sheehy, E. A. (2012). *Sexual assault in Canada: Law, legal practice, and women's activism.* Ottawa: University of Ottawa Press.

Statistics Canada. (2016). *Police-reported crime statistics in Canada, 2015.* Retrieved from http://www.statcan.gc.ca/pub/85-002-x/2016001/article/14642-eng.htm.

Ullman, S. E. (2016). Sexual revictimization, PTSD, and problem drinking in sexual assault survivors. *Addictive Behaviors, 53,* 7–10. doi:10.1016/j.addbeh.2015.09.010.

Ullman, S. E., & Peter-Hagene, L. C. (2016). Longitudinal relationships of social reactions, PTSD, and revictimization in sexual assault survivors. *Journal of Interpersonal Violence, 31*(6), 1074–1094. doi:10.1177/0886260514564069.

Voth Schrag, R. J. (2017). Campus based sexual assault and dating violence. *Affilia, 32*(1), 67. doi:10.1177/0886109916644644.

Walsh, K., Zinzow, H. M., Badour, C. L., et al. (2016). Understanding disparities in service seeking following forcible versus drug- or alcohol-facilitated/incapacitated rape. *Journal of Interpersonal Violence, 31*(14), 2475–2491. doi:10.1177/0886260515576968.

Wells, L., Claussen, C., Aubry, D., et al. (2012). *Primary prevention of sexual violence: Preliminary research to support a provincial action plan.* Calgary: The University of Calgary & Shift: The Project to End Domestic Violence. Retrieved from https://aasas.ca/research/.

UNIT 6

Interventions for Distinct Populations

26. Sexuality and Gender

27. Disorders of Children and Adolescents

28. Psychosocial Needs of the Older Adult

29. Living With Recurrent and Persistent Mental Illness

30. Psychological Needs of Patients With Medical Conditions

31. Care for the Dying and for Those Who Grieve

32. Forensic Psychiatric Nursing

Sexuality and Gender

Erin Ziegler

KEY TERMS AND CONCEPTS

bisexual
cisgender
gay
gender
gender dysphoria
gender identity
heterosexual
homosexual

internalized homophobia
intersex
lesbian
queer
sexual orientation
sexuality
transgender
two-spirit

OBJECTIVES

1. Describe sexuality and gender, and be able to differentiate between the two.
2. Examine the importance of nurses being knowledgeable about and comfortable discussing topics pertaining to sexuality and gender. Explore your personal values and biases.
3. Apply assessment techniques for sexual and gender history.
4. Develop a plan of care for individuals diagnosed with gender dysphoria.
5. Describe the unique mental health issues in the LGBTQ (lesbian, gay, bisexual, transgender, and queer) population.

⊖volve WEBSITE

Visit the Evolve website for Flashcards, Case Studies, and additional testing resources related to the content in this chapter: *http://evolve.elsevier.com/Canada/Varcarolis/psychiatric/*

Pre-Test | interactive review

Everyday professional nursing practice requires us to engage in matter-of-fact discussions with patients on topics generally considered to be private. We perform head-to-toe assessments in which we inquire about everything from headaches and sore throats to difficulties urinating and problems with constipation. The realities of providing physical care necessitate becoming comfortable with several skills that relate to privacy and modesty—performing breast examinations, initiating urinary catheters, and inserting rectal medications.

Health promotion and disease prevention are key responsibilities for nurses. All nurses must assess a patient's sexuality and gender and be prepared to educate, dispel myths, assist with clarification, refer to appropriate care providers when indicated,

and share resources. As a nursing student, you are introduced to complex aspects of sexuality and gender that should facilitate thoughtful discussion of the topic, make you aware of your personal belief systems, and help you consider the broader perspective of sexuality and gender as they exist in contemporary society. This chapter addresses two general categories, sexuality and gender, followed by an exploration of relevant mental health issues.

SEXUALITY

Sexuality is the way that people experience and express themselves as sexual beings. Sexual orientation is a person's sexual identity

HOW A NURSE HELPED ME
Coming Out

As a little girl, I grew up in a loving family. My mom and dad were always very supportive of me, encouraging me to "be who I want to be." They would frequently make comments such as "when you get married and have kids" and "marry a good guy, just like your father." In high school I had a few boyfriends, nothing serious. I moved away to go to university when I was 18. It was at school that I met Stephanie. Stephanie, was great, funny, smart, and fun to be around. In fact, I wanted to spend all my time with her. Stephanie was gay. I started to think about what it would be like to be her girlfriend. These thoughts scared me. I had never had thoughts about my sexuality before. I just always assumed I would do what my parents said and marry a guy just like my father. But now, after meeting Stephanie, I began to question my sexuality.

I made an appointment to speak to the nurse at the health centre at school. I told the nurse all about my feelings and the thoughts that I was having. Over the course of a few meetings, the nurse helped me to explore my feelings and my sexuality. She provided me with guidance and resources, but most importantly she supported me. Through my conversations with the nurse I began to feel comfortable with my sexuality. She also helped me by providing me with resources to come out to my family and friends. The nurse helped me to realize who I was and provided me with the necessary tools I needed to explain my sexuality to my family and friends.

CONSIDERING CULTURE
Sexual Orientation and Gender Identity

When we think about culture, we often relate it to concepts such as language, ethnicity, and race. Yet culture can be an important consideration in our discussion of sexual orientation and gender identity. We live in a world where the idea of sexual relationships, marriage, and childbearing occur in the context of a monogamous male–female relationship. Having traditionally dominated the way that society is structured, these ideas have created a heteronormative culture within Canadian society. Heteronormativity assumes that heterosexuality is the only sexual orientation or the norm and is often associated with homonegativity and homophobia. Homonegativity is the disapproval of homosexuality, where homophobia is fear, aversion, or hatred toward homosexuality. It is important, however, to move beyond these traditional notions of sexuality and recognize that sexual orientation and gender identity can be diverse. Lesbian, gay, bisexual, and transgender issues are increasingly visible in our society. As nurses, we must recognize the dominance of our heterosexual culture and its shaping of our own values and beliefs when providing care for all patients.

Sources: Dean, J. J. (2011). The cultural construction of heterosexual identities. *Sociology Compass, 5,* 679–687. doi:10.1111/j.1751-9020.2011.00395.x; Eliason, M. J., Dibble, S., & Dejoseph, J. (2010). Nursing's silence on lesbian, gay, bisexual, and transgender issues: The need for emancipatory efforts. *Advances in Nursing Science, 33*(3), 206–218. doi:10.1097/ANS.0b013e3181e63e49; Mann, K., Gordon, J., & MacLeod, A. (2007). Reflection and reflective practice in health professions education: A systematic review. *Advances in Health Sciences Education, 14*(4), 595–621. doi:10.1007/s10459-007-9090-2.

in relation to the gender to which they are attracted. An individual's sexual orientation can be said to be heterosexual, homosexual, or bisexual. Sexual orientation is biological; people are born heterosexual, homosexual, or bisexual. People who identity as heterosexual are sexually attracted to people of the opposite sex. Those who identity as homosexual are sexually attracted to people of the same sex. Homosexuality can be further classified as gay and lesbian. Men who are sexually attracted to men often use the term *gay* to describe their sexual orientation, whereas women who are sexually attracted to women may use the term *lesbian. Gay* may be used interchangeably by both men and women to describe their sexual orientation. People who are attracted to both men and women use the term bisexual to describe their sexual orientation. Queer is often used as an umbrella term for individuals who do not identify as heterosexual. Statistics Canada (2015) reported that 1.7% of Canadians between the ages of 18 and 59 identified as gay or lesbian, whereas 1.3% of Canadians in the same age group identified as bisexual.

In this chapter, exploration of nursing care related to sexuality is for people who identify as homosexual or bisexual. To provide competent and compassionate nursing care to individuals who identify as homosexual or bisexual, it is important to also

understand the acronyms used to describe this population. Acronyms such as LGBT (lesbian, gay, bisexual, and transgender), LGBTQ (lesbian, gay, bisexual, transgender, and queer), and the full-inclusion LGBTTIQQ2SA (lesbian, gay, bisexual, transsexual, transgender, intersex, queer, questioning, two-spirited, and allies) have been used in the media, popular culture, and literature. Recently, the term *allies* was added to the community. *Allies* is a term used to describe someone who is supportive of LGBTQ people. It encompasses non-LGBTQ allies as well as those within the LGBTQ community who support each other. LGBTQ is the generally accepted acronym in Canada, and therefore it will be used to describe this population.

GENDER

When we inquire about the birth of a new infant, one of the first things we want to know is whether the baby is a boy or a girl. Actually, we are asking about the sex of the child (i.e., whether its chromosomes are XX or XY). Sometimes the gender of the individual is not known. Intersex is a set of medical conditions that features a congenital anomaly of the reproductive system or genitals. Intersex individuals are born with chromosomes, external genitalia, or internal reproductive systems that are not considered either male or female. However, biological assignment does not determine whether individuals think of themselves as male or female. **Gender** refers to a person's identity and social classifications, often based on masculine or feminine qualities and traits (Zunner & Grace, 2012). **Gender identity** refers to one's sense of self as male or female. Gender identity can be classified as cisgender or transgender. **Cisgender** refers to one's gender identity being aligned with the gender assigned at birth. A cisgender female is a person who was born female, identifies as female, and uses feminine pronouns such as *she* and *her*. **Transgender** refers to an incongruence in a person's gender identity with the gender assigned at birth. A transgender male is a person who was born female, identifies as male, and may use male pronouns such as *him* and *he* (LGBT Health Program, 2015). Recent estimates suggest that 1 in every 200 adults identifies as transgender (Scheim & Bauer, 2014). **Two-spirit** is used by some Indigenous people to describe their gender, sexual, or spiritual identity and refers to a person who embodies both a male and a female spirit.

Transgender is included within the acronym *LGBTQ*, which represents a sexual and gender minority. However, it is very important to distinguish that lesbian, gay, bisexual, and queer are related to sexual orientation, whereas transgender is related to gender identity. The sexual orientation of transgender individuals can be heterosexual, lesbian, gay, bisexual, or queer. As with cisgender people, sexual orientation should never be assumed. When asking a patient about sexual activities, avoid asking questions such as "Do you have a boyfriend?" or "In the last 6 months, how many women have you had sex with?" Such questions assume heterosexuality. For patients who do not identify as heterosexual, these types of questions may cause the patient to not fully disclose or discuss anything further, as they may feel that you are not open or may pass judgement. Instead, when asking about sexual activity or sexuality, make general statements such as "Do you have sex with men, women, or both?" By asking this question, the nurse is opening the door for further discussion and letting the patient know that sexuality is not an issue and that he or she can feel comfortable having these conversations.

VIGNETTE

Casey self-identifies as male. He prefers male pronouns and a masculine appearance. His family and friends are accepting and supporting of his transition. Casey still gets nervous in certain social situations and worries about his safety. His main concerns are having to use the men's washroom and showing his identification, which still has the name Cassandra and a female gender marker. What if someone questions or challenges him? What if this is not safe for him? For this reason, Casey tries his best to avoid anywhere he must show identification and using public washrooms.

Casey gets sick and needs to go to the clinic. He arrives at a new medical clinic to meet with the nurse. When he arrives, the first thing he notices is the large Safe Space poster on the door and in the reception area. He meets with the nurse, who right away asks him what name and pronouns he prefers. The nurse advises him that the clinic is a safe space and has gender-neutral washrooms for everyone's use. Because of these actions, Casey feels comfortable using this clinic and is able to talk with the nurse about his transition goals.

GENDER DYSPHORIA

When biological sex differs from gender identity, the individual may experience **gender dysphoria**, characterized by the strong feeling of being the wrong sex or the feeling that one's body is inconsistent with the internal sense of being either male or female (Walsh Brennan, Barnsteiner, de Leon Siantz, et al., 2012). Those with gender dysphoria experience some degree of incongruity between their anatomical sex and their gender identity. Gender dysphoria, as outlined in the *Diagnostic and Statistics Manual of Mental Disorders*, fifth edition (*DSM-5*), is a medical diagnosis often required prior to initiation of transgender medical or surgical transition. However, there has been great debate about the use of and appropriateness of using a psychiatric diagnosis with transgender individuals, within both the medical and the transgender communities. To stop pathologizing gender differences and validate gender identity, the *DSM-IV-TR* revised the diagnosis to gender dysphoria, a term previously referred to as gender identity disorder. For many health care providers, the diagnosis of gender dysphoria is used as a tool to defend medical interventions and treatments. It is important to be aware of the potential for stigmatization of transgender individuals when the diagnosis of gender dysphoria is perceived as a psychiatric illness (LGBT Health Program, 2015). Diagnostic criteria for gender dysphoria in children, adolescents, and adults are listed in the DSM-5: Criteria for Gender Dysphoria.

CLINICAL PICTURE

Gender dysphoria symptoms in children include expressions of a desire to be the opposite sex. Some children insist that they *are* the opposite sex and ask their families to call them by another name. Teenagers and adults may also verbalize a desire to be the other sex and to be treated as such. Adolescents may dread the appearance of secondary sexual characteristics. Individuals may seek hormones or surgery as part of their gender transition.

EPIDEMIOLOGY

It is estimated that there are approximately 25 million transgender individuals worldwide, with 0.5% of the adult population identifying as transgender. Specific Canadian data on the prevalence of transgender individuals are lacking. Statistics Canada currently collects gender data for only two categories: male and female.

NURSING CARE FOR GENDER DYSPHORIA

Nurses have a role in providing care and support for individuals with gender dysphoria. Nurses can help individuals in seeking social support, using healthy coping behaviors, and acknowledging and accepting sexual identity.

ADVANCED INTERVENTIONS

Pharmacological

Pharmacological interventions in adolescents may be used to delay puberty. Prevention of the secondary sex characteristic

DSM-5

Criteria for Gender Dysphoria

Gender Dysphoria in Children:

A. A marked incongruence between one's experienced or expressed gender and assigned gender, of at least 6 months' duration, as manifested by at least six of the following (one of which must be Criterion A1):

1. A strong desire to be of the other gender or an insistence that one is the other gender (or some alternative gender different from one's assigned gender).

2. In boys (assigned gender), a strong preference for cross-dressing or simulating female attire; in girls (assigned gender), a strong preference for wearing only typical masculine clothing and a strong resistance to wearing typical feminine clothing.

3. A strong preference for cross-gender roles in make-believe play or fantasy play.

4. A strong preference for the toys, games, or activities stereotypically used or engaged in by the other gender.

5. A strong preference for playmates of the other gender.

6. In boys (assigned gender), a strong rejection of typically masculine toys, games, and activities and a strong avoidance of rough-and-tumble play; in girls (assigned gender), a strong rejection of typically feminine toys, games, and activities.

7. A strong dislike of one's sexual anatomy.

8. A strong desire for the primary and/or secondary sex characteristics that match one's experienced gender.

B. The condition is associated with clinically significant distress or impairment in social, school, or other important areas of functioning.

Gender Dysphoria in Adolescents and Adults:

A. A marked incongruence between one's experienced or expressed gender and assigned gender, of at least 6 months' duration, as manifested by at least two of the following:

1. A marked incongruence between one's experienced or expressed gender and primary and/or secondary sex characteristics.

2. A strong desire to be rid of one's primary and/or secondary sex characteristics because of a marked incongruence with one's experienced or expressed gender (or in adolescents, a desire to prevent the development of the anticipated secondary sex characteristics).

3. A strong desire for the primary and/or secondary sex characteristics of the other gender.

4. A strong desire to be of the other gender (or some alternative gender different from one's assigned gender).

5. A strong desire to be treated as the other gender (or some alternative gender different from one's assigned gender).

6. A strong conviction that one has the typical feelings and reactions of the other gender (or some alternative gender different from one's assigned gender).

B. The condition is associated with clinically significant distress or impairment in social, occupational, or other important areas of functioning.

Specify if:

With a disorder of sex development (e.g., a congenital adreno-genital disorder such as 255.2 [E25.0] congenital adrenal hyperplasia or 259.50 [E34.50] androgen insensitivity syndrome).

Coding note: Code the disorder of sex development and gender dysphoria.

Specify if:

Post-transition: The individual has transitioned to full-time living in the desired gender (with or without legalization of gender change) and has undergone (or is preparing to have) at least one cross-sex medical procedure or treatment regimen—namely, regular cross-sex hormone treatment or gender reassignment surgery confirming the desired gender (e.g., penectomy, vaginoplasty in a natal male; mastectomy or phalloplasty in a natal female).

Source: Modified from American Psychiatric Association. (2013). *Diagnostic and statistical manual of disorders* (5th ed., pp. 452–453). Washington, DC: Author.

---

can provide adolescents with better self-esteem and improve their body image. Adults may choose to take hormones to help them in their gender transition. Female-to-male (FTM) transitions can include the use of testosterone. The testosterone allows for more muscle development, facial and body hair, clitoral enlargement, amenorrhea, and increased sex drive. Male-to-female (MTF) individuals may take estrogen and antiandrogens. These medications cause body fat redistribution, reduction in facial and body hair, breast growth, and loss of spontaneous erections and testicular volume.

Surgical

Gender-affirming surgery or sexual reassignment surgery may be the ultimate goal for transgender individuals, although it is important to note that not all transgender individuals have surgery. Surgical options for MTF individuals include the removal of the penis (penectomy) and testes (orchiectomy) and the addition of a vagina (vaginoplasty). Some MTF individuals also choose to have facial feminization surgery, including tracheal shaving, to have more feminine facial features and breast augmentation. In FTM individuals, surgical procedures may include the removal of the breasts (mastectomy) and chest re-contouring, removal of the uterus (hysterectomy) and ovaries (oophorectomy), and the construction of a neopenis (phalloplasty).

APPLICATION OF THE NURSING PROCESS

ASSESSMENT

Self-Assessment

Despite a learned fearlessness when it comes to addressing other intimate issues, nurses, as well as other health care providers, often find the topic of sexuality a source of discomfort. Nurses have a role in providing patients with support, education, and information, and by conducting a complete assessment, nurses will gather the information necessary to help their patients. By

📋 ASSESSMENT GUIDELINES
Sexuality and Gender Assessments

1. The interviewer should reflect on his or her personal biases and judgemental attitudes that could block open discussion of sexuality and gender.
2. A sexuality or gender assessment should be conducted in a setting that allows privacy and eliminates distractions.
3. Although note taking may be necessary for the beginner, it can be distracting to the patient and interrupt the flow of the interview. When note taking is necessary, it should be unobtrusive and kept to a minimum.
4. Good eye contact, relaxed posture, and friendly facial expressions communicate openness and receptivity on the part of the nurse and facilitate the patient's comfort.

legitimizing the topic of sexuality, nurses provide a clear message that it is okay to talk about these issues, and patients are often relieved when discussion is initiated by nurses (Quinn, Happell, & Welch, 2013). Yet there remains avoidance in talking about sexuality with patients. As a nurse, it is important for you to bring up this topic when assessing your patients. According to Quinn and Happell (2012), avoidance of discussing sexuality is not often related to the inability of the patient to discuss the issue, but to the nurse not making opportunities or giving permission to discuss the topic.

Remembering your position as a professional and addressing the topics in a tone and manner appropriate to a professional will increase your comfort, along with the patient's. Nurses can set the comfort level for discussion and foster opportunities to address feelings and concerns. Also, letting the patient know why you are asking such personal questions increases openness and cooperation. For example, you can say, "I am going to ask you some questions now that relate to your sexuality and gender. Your sexual health is important to your overall physical and emotional health."

Perhaps the most helpful consideration is that assessing sexuality is part of holistic nursing care. Your role and responsibility are to assist the patient in dealing with responses to illness or the treatment of the illness. Understanding your patient's concerns, acknowledging any discomfort or distress, and providing useful feedback will enhance your professional abilities to care for your patient and perhaps even improve self-understanding.

General Assessment

As a nurse, it is important to perform a comprehensive assessment, including a health history. When assessing a patient, it is important to ask questions about gender and sexuality as part of the health history. With some patients, a sexual or gender history may come up as part of the discussion initiated by the patient. However, the more likely scenario is that the nurse will need to start the conversation. Before bringing up the topic of sex, sexuality, or gender, it is extremely important to explain to the patient why you are asking these questions and that you ask all of your patients these questions. Patients may ask why you are asking these

questions, and it is important to provide them with answers that will further facilitate discussion. For example, if a patient asks why you are asking about his or her sexuality, you could say, "Your sexuality and sexual health are important aspects of your overall health and important to discuss."

When talking to patients about gender and sexuality, it is extremely important to avoid making assumptions. Making heterosexist and gender assumptions could jeopardize the nurse–patient relationship. For example, you are doing an initial assessment on a new female patient, and you want to know about her sexual history. If you ask the question, "Do you have a boyfriend?" you are assuming that this patient identifies as heterosexual. If the patient identifies as lesbian, she may answer "no." Not only could this affect the nurse–patient relationship, but it could also cause you to miss key points from her health history. Instead, you could ask, "Do you have a partner?" *Partner* is a gender-neutral term and is appropriate to use when questioning all patients to avoid assumptions. Similarly, to avoid assumption when asking about sexual activity, you should ask, "Do you have sex with men, women, or both?" Nurses can effectively obtain a complete sexual history using the algorithm in Box 26-1. Assessing gender can be approached along the same lines. When meeting a new patient, ask which gender pronoun the patients prefers you use. By asking these questions, you will be able to effectively communicate and assess your patients without making assumptions.

DIAGNOSIS

A comprehensive sexuality and gender assessment can reveal areas of concern or identify the need for patient support. This may determine the need for appropriate nursing diagnoses. Sexuality is the eighth domain of the North American Nursing Diagnosis Association International (NANDA-I) classification (Herdman, 2014). This domain includes sexual identity, sexual function, and reproduction. Priority nursing diagnoses, their definitions, and possible etiology follow from this NANDA-I domain. NANDA-I defines sexual identity as the state of being a specific person in regards to sexuality or gender. There are no nursing diagnoses included under the sexual identity domain. Domains of self-perception, perception/cognition, coping/stress tolerance, life principles, safety, growth and development, or other concurrent nursing diagnoses may be relevant for any patient. These are assessed accordingly.

OUTCOMES IDENTIFICATION

Some issues can effectively be managed for short-term outcomes using education as a nursing intervention. For example, frequently sexuality and gender misinformation can be corrected, giving the patient almost instant relief from perceived problems. The *Nursing Outcomes Classification (NOC)* (Moorhead, Johnson, Maas, et al., 2013) identifies outcomes related to sexuality, including *Sexual functioning* and *Sexual identity*. There are no outcomes related to gender. Table 26-1 provides selected intermediate and short-term indicators for *Sexual functioning* and *Sexual identity*.

BOX 26-1 ALGORITHM FOR TAKING A SEXUAL HISTORY

Set the Stage
- Bring up the sexual history as part of the overall history
- Explain that you ask these questions of all patients
- Ensure confidentially

Begin with Three Screening Questions
- Have you been sexually active in the last year?
- Do you have sex with men, women, or both?
- How many people have you had sex with in the last year?

Multiple Partners, New Partners
- Ask about
  - Partners
  - STI/HIV protection
  - Substance abuse
  - Sexual function and satisfaction
  - History of STIs
  - Other concerns

Long-Term Monogamous Partner
- Ask about
  - Pregnancy plans/protection
  - Trauma/violence
  - Sexual function and satisfaction
  - Other concerns

Not Sexually Active
- Ask about
  - Past partners
  - Any questions or concerns

Follow up as appropriate
- Counselling and education
- Referral
- STI or HIV testing

HIV, Human immunodeficiency virus; *STI*, sexually transmitted infection.
Source: Makadon, H., & Goldhammer, H. (2015). Taking a sexual history and creating affirming environments for lesbian, gay, bisexual, and transgender people. *The Journal of the Mississippi State Medical Association, 56*(12), 358–362.

PLANNING

Planning nursing care for patients may occur as part of care in any setting in which the patient seeks treatment for any of a variety of conditions. Once the assessment is completed, priority nursing diagnoses are developed and implemented in collaboration with the patient.

IMPLEMENTATION

All nurses need to be able to facilitate a discussion about sexuality and gender with the patient. To be a facilitator, the nurse must be nonjudgemental, have basic knowledge of sexuality and gender, and be able to conduct a basic assessment. Once the assessment is completed, the nurse may have the knowledge, skills, and judgement to address the patient's sexual health concern. Or, the nurse may need to know when and to whom to refer the patient. Depending on the nature of the problem, the patient may need a referral to a professional such as a nurse practitioner, physician, psychologist, or psychiatrist.

Box 26-2 provides sample interventions for sexual counselling from the *Nursing Interventions Classification (NIC)* (Bulechek, Butcher, Dochterman, et al., 2013).

MENTAL HEALTH ISSUES IN THE LGBTQ POPULATION

CLINICAL PICTURE

In the first part of this chapter, we examined the concepts of sexuality and gender. We now turn our attention to mental health issues within the LGBTQ population. Mental health literature has demonstrated an increased incidence of alcohol and drug abuse, depression, self-harm, suicide, low self-esteem, and eating disorders in the LGBTQ population. The higher risk for mental health issues is thought to be related to health disparities in the LGBTQ population. Health disparities in this population may include discrimination, prejudice, social stigma, and living in a heterosexist and homophobic environment (Rutherford, McIntyre, Daley, et al., 2012; Scott, Lasiuk, & Norris, 2016). Stigma and discrimination have a variety of negative effects on people. Experiences of stigma and discrimination may increase an individual's internalized homophobia. Internalized homophobia

TABLE 26-1 *NOC* OUTCOMES FOR SEXUAL DYSFUNCTION

NURSING OUTCOME AND DEFINITION	INTERMEDIATE INDICATORS	SHORT-TERM INDICATORS
Sexual functioning: Integration of physical, social, emotional, and intellectual aspects of sexual expression and performance	Expresses comfort with sexual expression Expresses knowledge of personal sexual needs	Expresses sexual interest Communicates comfortably with partner
Sexual identity: Acknowledgement and acceptance of own sexual identity	Integrates sexual orientation into life roles Challenges negative images of sexual self Reports healthy sexual functioning	Affirms self as a sexual being Exhibits clear sense of sexual orientation Exhibits comfort with sexual orientation Uses healthy coping behaviours to resolve sexual identity issues

Source: Data from Moorhead, S., Johnson, M., Maas, M., et al. (Eds.). (2013). *Nursing outcomes classification (NOC)* (5th ed.). St. Louis: Elsevier Mosby.

BOX 26-2 *NIC* INTERVENTIONS FOR SEXUAL COUNSELLING

Definition of sexual counselling: Use of an interactive helping process focusing on the need to make adjustments in sexual practice or to enhance coping with a sexual event or disorder
Activities*:
- Establish a therapeutic relationship based on trust and respect.
- Provide privacy and ensure confidentiality.
- Discuss the effects of changes in sexuality on significant others.
- Discuss the knowledge level of the patient about sexuality in general.
- Encourage the patient to verbalize fears and ask questions.
- Provide reassurance and permission to experiment with alternative forms of sexual expression, as appropriate.
- Provide referral or consultation with other members of the health care team, as appropriate.

*Partial list.
Source: Data from Bulechek, G. M., Butcher, H. K., Dochterman, J. M., et al. (Eds.). (2013). *Nursing interventions classification (NIC)* (6th ed.). Toronto: Elsevier.

is referred to as a set of negative beliefs and attitudes toward homosexuality and one's own homosexuality. Features of internalized homophobia include negative attitudes, discomfort with disclosing sexual orientation, and a feeling of disconnect toward other homosexuals. Internalized homophobia is a direct result of living in a homophobic society and is related to increased risk for depression (McLaren, 2016).

DEPRESSION

Depression is a highly prevalent, chronic illness with significant impact on quality of life. Identifying as lesbian, gay, or bisexual does not directly correlate with a higher risk for developing depression when compared to the heterosexual population. However, risk factors, including discrimination and homophobia, can increase the risk for depression within this population. Recent literature demonstrates an increased risk for depression in individuals who identify as bisexual, whereas individuals who identify as lesbian or gay have similar rates of depression when compared to the heterosexual population (Li, Pollitt, & Russell, 2016; Plöderl & Tremblay, 2015; Scott, Lasiuk, & Norris, 2016). Increased stress may be associated with a greater risk for depression in bisexual individuals, even when compared to gay and lesbian individuals. This increased stress could be due to the unique discrimination and stigma faced by bisexual people. An example of this stigma is the belief that bisexuality is not a real sexual identity. This additional stigma and discrimination, when combined with the generalized stress and discrimination associated with the LGBTQ community, may account for the increased risk for depression i individuals identifying as bisexual (Shearer, Herres, Kodish, et al., 2015).

The transgender population experiences high rates of depression and negative mental health outcomes when compared to cisgender, lesbian, gay, and bisexual individuals. The lifetime

RESEARCH HIGHLIGHT

Nursing Students' Knowledge, Attitude, and Cultural Competence

Problem
Lesbian, gay, bisexual, and transgender (LGBT) patients experience barriers to health care that include insensitivity, fear of discrimination, and lack of knowledge about LGBT-specific health needs. Nurses must ensure that they are knowledgeable and provide culturally competent care while eliminating health disparities and improving outcomes in the LGBT population.

Purpose of Study
The purpose of this study was to address the educational needs and determine whether undergraduate nursing students' knowledge, attitudes, and cultural competence toward LGBT patient care could be improved.

Methods
A convenience sample of 88 undergraduate nursing students was used for this study. Participants were provided with a 45-minute educational intervention focused on definitions, LGBT health disparities, cultural competence, and transgender-specific health care. The intervention was measured using a pretest and post-test.

Key Findings
- Attitudes toward LGBT individuals were significantly improved after the educational intervention.
- Although brief, the educational session demonstrated the potential to have a favourable impact on nursing students' knowledge and attitudes.
- Students identified that current undergraduate nursing curriculum is inadequate in addressing LGBT patient care.

Implications for Nursing Practice
Education sessions, even brief sessions, can improve attitudes and knowledge in LGBT health care. To promote nursing competence in providing health care to the LGBT population, education needs to be incorporated in undergraduate nursing curriculum.

Source: Strong, K. L., & Folse, V. N. (2015). Assessing undergraduate nursing students' knowledge, attitudes, and culture competence in caring for lesbian, gay, bisexual, and transgender patients. *Journal of Nursing Education, 54*(1), 45–49. doi:10.3928/01484834-20141224-01.

prevalence of depression within the transgender population has been reported to be as high as 50% to 67% (Carmel & Erickson-Schroth, 2016). This increased risk may be related to transphobia, gender discrimination, or abuse. Rates of depression significantly improve when transgender individuals begin their social and medical transition. The use of feminizing or masculinizing hormones is associated with a theoretical risk for depression, as well as for mania and aggression. However, evidence also suggests that use of the gender-affirming hormones improves quality of life and reduces depression. Transgender individuals who are experiencing an acute mental health decompensation should not be started on hormone therapy until their mental health status has stabilized. Transgender individuals already on hormone therapy, however, should not have their hormones discontinued because of an acute episode or hospitalization. The discontinuation of hormones may result in worsening the patient's mood.

SELF-HARM AND SUICIDE

It is a critical component of the nurse's role to assess patients and screen for risks for self-harm or suicidal ideation (refer also to Chapter 22). Self-harm involves the intentional act of causing personal injury to the body without the intent of suicide. Self-harm acts include cutting or burning the skin, hair pulling (trichotillomania), and ingestion of harmful substances or objects. Self-harm is most common in adolescents and young adults. Although of concern in the general population, rates of self-harm, suicide attempts, and suicides are alarming in the LGBTQ population. A survey of self-harm in the United States sampled 1 126 LGBTQ individuals ranging in age from 18 to 80 years. Results found that 21% of the sample had a history of self-harm (House, Van Horn, Coppeans, et al., 2011). Jackman, Honig, and Bockting (2016) reviewed the rates of self-harm in the LGBTQ population compared to the heterosexual population and found a prevalence of self-harm in the LGBTQ population as high as 47%, relative to prevalence in the heterosexual group of 15%. Within the LGBTQ population, they found that those who identified as bisexual or transgender were more likely to engage in acts of self-harm than those who identified as lesbian or gay.

Statistics on completed suicides in the LGBTQ community are not available, as sexual orientation is often not recorded. Therefore it is assumed that data on LGBTQ suicide are underestimated. In a meta-analysis, Bolton and Sareen (2011) found that lesbian, gay, and bisexual individuals were 2.4 times more likely to have attempted suicide than heterosexual individuals. Those who identified as bisexual were 3 times more likely to have attempted suicide compared to the heterosexual population. Rates of suicidal ideation and suicide attempts in the transgender population range from 25% to 76% (Carmel & Erickson-Schroth, 2016). A large study in Ontario found that 35% of transgender individuals seriously considered suicide and 11% had made a suicide attempt within the last year (Bauer, Scheim, Pyne, et al., 2015).

VIGNETTE

Ryan is a 19-year-old man who presents to the emergency department for the second time in a few weeks with superficial cuts to his forearm. He is seeing the nurse for his initial assessment. Ryan has been cutting his arm since the age of 15 at an average frequency of about once every 2 weeks. He states that doing so gives him relief from feelings of guilt and despair, which can become intense at times. He denies any episodes of low mood. The nurse starts to explore Ryan's feelings and asks him about his life, including his schooling, friends, sexual relationships, and sexual orientation. Ryan tells the nurse that no one has ever asked him about his sexuality before, and he feels comfortable telling the nurse that he identifies as bisexual. Through further discussion, Ryan discloses that his cutting is related to his feelings around his sexual orientation and fear of acceptance.

SUBSTANCE ABUSE

Substance use in the LGBTQ population has been reported at rates two to four times that in the general population. Substance use in the LGBTQ population, including use of alcohol, tobacco and drugs, has been well documented. LGBTQ individuals may use substances for the same reason as heterosexual individuals, but there also are some culturally specific reasons that may account for the higher rates of use in the LGBTQ population. Coping with stigma, discrimination, and trauma may be a cause of substance use. Substance use may be used to cope with stresses associated with coming out, homophobia, transphobia, or internalized homophobia.

Within the LGBTQ community, there may be some cultural acceptance of substance use. Historically, discrimination against the LGBTQ population caused there to be a lack of safe space for socialization. Bars, nightclubs, and parties were often considered safe places for LGBTQ individuals to socialize. Therefore there is an association of this community with socializing and use of alcohol and other substances. When bars, parties, or nightclubs are the main source of socialization, there is an increased risk of developing a social network that uses substances on a regular basis (Ritter, Matthew-Simmons, & Carragher, 2012).

Smoking in the LGBTQ population has been documented in the literature with rates as high as 59% for youth and 50% for adults. Clarke and Coughlin (2012) conducted a study in Toronto, Ontario, with a sample size of 3 140 LGBTQ individuals. Overall, 36% of respondents identified as smokers and 25% identified as former smokers. This was compared to the Canadian Community Health Survey, which identified 18.9% of the general population as smokers and 33.5% as former smokers. Rates of smoking varied within the LGBTQ population.

Alcohol and drug use within the LGBTQ community has been shown to be higher than that in the general population. A meta-analysis by Green and Feinstein (2012) showed that women who identified as lesbian were at a higher risk than heterosexual women for heavy drinking and alcohol-related problems. Men who identified as gay were more like than heterosexual men to use substances. Both men and women who identify as bisexual have a significantly higher rate of substance and alcohol use than heterosexual individuals or those who identify as lesbian or gay.

Substance use within the transgender population is also high. A large U.S. study of 1 229 transgender individuals explored substance use by gender. Heavy alcohol use on a regular basis was reported by 7% of transwomen and 12% of transmen. Binge drinking was reported within the last 3 months by 10% of both transmen and transwomen. Marijuana use was reported by 21% of transwomen and 32% of transmen. Illicit drug use was reported by 9% of transwomen and 13% of transmen (Horvath, Iantaffi, Swinburne-Romine, et al., 2014). Transgender individuals have reported high substance use rates to deal with negative experiences, transphobia, and depression.

EVALUATION

Evaluation of patients with mental health disorders related to gender dysphoria or discrimination and social factors related to sexual orientation or gender identity is based partly on determining whether the outcomes for the presenting problem were achieved. Respectful, frank, and open communication is central to this practice as a whole, as a part of both the general therapeutic relationship (see Chapter 9) and the nursing process related to any specific sexuality concerns or gender dysphoria.

KEY POINTS TO REMEMBER

- Sexual orientation is a person's sexual identity in relation to the gender to which they are attracted. An individual's sexual orientation can be said to be heterosexual, homosexual, or bisexual.
- Gender identity refers to one's sense of self as male or female.
- Health care workers are often uncomfortable asking questions related to sexuality and gender. Providing professional and holistic care requires that nurses include this vital area of assessment.
- There are distinctions between biological sex and gender identity. Gender dysphoria is the strong and persistent feeling of unease about one's maleness or femaleness.
- Health disparities in the LGBTQ population have been linked to higher rates of depression, self-harm, suicide, and substance abuse.

CRITICAL THINKING

1. To understand your own beliefs, answer these questions:
   a. Are you comfortable with your own sexuality? Are you comfortable with those who have a sexual orientation different from your own?
   b. Are you comfortable with your gender? Are you comfortable with those you identify as transgender?
   c. What factors have influenced your beliefs and values regarding sexuality and gender?
   d. How could you be helpful to someone who is questioning their sexuality or gender?
2. Kate, a 14-year old female, was admitted to the adolescent psychiatric mental health unit for depression and self-harm. Kate has asked to be referred to as Kyle and gets very upset if anyone, including family members and staff, uses the name Kate or female pronouns. What further information do you need from Kyle to complete a gender assessment? As a nurse, how can you advocate for Kyle on your unit and with Kyle's family.
3. As a nurse, you are constantly encountering adolescents who are misinformed about sexuality. What information would you include in a teaching session that would help these adolescents to acquire a greater understanding of sexuality?

CHAPTER REVIEW

1. A 27-year-old patient states that she is confused about her sexuality. Which response is most likely to be therapeutic?
   a. "What does your boyfriend think of this?"
   b. "Tell me more about what is confusing you."
   c. "Tell me about your sexual activities."
   d. "This is a common problem, which you shouldn't worry about right now."
2. Matthew, a 21-year old male, is meeting with the nurse for support and counselling. Matthew is questioning his sexuality. Which of the following are realistic short-term outcomes for Matthew? Select all that apply.
   a. Matthew displays a clear sense of his sexual orientation.
   b. Matthew accepts a negative self-image of his sexuality.
   c. Matthew develops healthy coping skills
   d. Matthew shows comfort with his sexual orientation.
3. A young male patient tells you that, somehow, he feels that he should not be a man, that inside he is a woman. This is likely an example of
   a. Confusion
   b. Gender dysphoria
   c. Borderline personality disorder
   d. Intersex
4. Farah is the nurse assigned to work with Mr. Roberts, a transgender male on a step-down unit. Farah is anxious at the prospect of working with Mr. Roberts and spends only the briefest periods of time possible responding to his needs. What are the best descriptions of what is occurring here? Select all that apply.
   a. Farah is failing to maintain professional objectivity because of her values and beliefs about this particular patient's decisions and behaviour.
   b. Farah is experiencing a common negative response to a situation about which she has limited knowledge and little understanding.
   c. Nurses have a right to have personal feelings about social issues, and as long as Mr. Roberts's minimal care needs are addressed, Farah is within her rights to respond in this way.
   d. Farah may be having difficulty looking beyond Mr. Roberts's gender issues and, as a result, is failing to see or respond to him simply as a person.

Ⓔvolve WEBSITE

Post-Test interactive review

Visit the Evolve website for Chapter Review Answers and Rationales, Critical Thinking Answer Guidelines, and additional resources related to the content in this chapter: http://evolve.elsevier.com/Canada/Varcarolis/psychiatric/

REFERENCES

Bauer, G., Scheim, A., Pyne, J., et al. (2015). Intervenable factors associated with suicide risk in transgender persons: A respondent driven sampling study in Ontario, Canada. *BMC Public Health, 15*, 525–540. doi:10.1186/s12889-015-1867-2.

Bolton, S., & Sareen, J. (2011). Sexual orientation and its relation to mental disorders and suicide attempts: Findings from a national representative sample. *Canadian Journal of Psychiatry, 56*(1), 35–43.

Bulechek, G., Butcher, H., Dochterman, J., et al. (2013). *Nursing interventions classification (NIC)* (6th ed.). Toronto: Elsevier.

Carmel, T., & Erickson-Schroth, L. (2016). Mental health and the transgender population. *Journal of Psychosocial Nursing, 54*(12), 44–48. doi:10.3928/02793695-20161208-09.

Clarke, M., & Coughlin, J. (2012). Prevalence of smoking among the lesbian, gay, bisexual, transsexual, transgender and queer (LGBTTQ) subpopulations in Toronto—The Toronto Rainbow Tobacco Survey (TRTS). *Canadian Journal of Public Health, 103*(2), 132–136.

Green, K., & Feinstein, B. (2012). Substance use in lesbian, gay, and bisexual populations: An update on empirical research and implications for treatment. *Psychology of Addictive Behaviours, 26*(2), 265–278. doi:10.1037/a0025424.

Herdman, T. H. (Ed.), (2014). *NANDA International nursing diagnoses: Definitions & classification* (pp. 2015–2017). Oxford, UK: Wiley-Blackwell.

Horvath, K., Iantaffi, A., Swinburne-Romine, R., et al. (2014). A comparison of mental health, substance use, and sexual risk behaviors between rural and non-rural transgender persons. *Journal of Homosexuality, 61*, 1117–1130. doi:10.1080/00918369.2014.872502.

House, A., Van Horn, E., Coppeans, C., et al. (2011). Interpersonal trauma and discriminatory events as predictors of suicidal and nonsuicidal self-injury in gay, lesbian, bisexual, and transgender persons. *Traumatology, 17*, 75–85. doi:10.1177/1534765610395621.

Jackman, K., Honig, J., & Bockting, W. (2016). Nonsuicidal self-injury among lesbian, gay, bisexual and transgender populations: An integrative review. *Journal of Clinical Nursing, 25*, 3438–3453. doi:10.1111/jocn.13236.

LGBT Health Program (2015). *Guidelines and protocols for hormone therapy and primary health care for trans clients.* Toronto: Sherbourne Health Centre.

Li, G., Pollitt, A., & Russell, S. (2016). Depression and sexual orientation during young adulthood: Diversity among sexual minority subgroups and the role of gender nonconformity. *Archives of Sexual Behaviors, 45*(3), 697–711. doi:10.1007/s10508-015-0515-3.

McLaren, S. (2016). The interrelations between internalized homophobia, depressive symptoms, and suicidal ideation among Australian gay men, lesbians, and bisexual women. *Journal of Homosexuality, 63*(2), 156–168. doi:10.1080/00918369.2015.1083779.

Moorhead, S., Johnson, M., Maas, M., et al. (2013). *Nursing outcomes classification (NOC)* (5th ed.). St. Louis: Elsevier Mosby.

Plöderl, M., & Tremblay, P. (2015). Mental health of sexual minorities: A systemic review. *International Review of Psychiatry, 27*(5), 367–385. doi:10.3109/09540261.2015.1083949.

Quinn, C., & Happell, B. (2012). Getting BETTER: Breaking the ice and warming to the inclusion of sexuality in mental health nursing care. *International Journal of Mental Health Nursing, 21*, 154–162. doi:10.1111/j.1447-0349.2011.00783.

Quinn, C., Happell, B., & Welch, A. (2013). Talking about sex as part of our role: Making and sustaining practice change. *International Journal of Mental Health Nursing, 22*, 231–240. doi:10.1111/j.1447-0349.2012.00865.

Ritter, A., Matthew-Simmons, F., & Carragher, N. (2012). *Monograph No. 23: Prevalence of and interventions for mental health and alcohol and other drug problems amongst the gay, lesbian, bisexual and transgender community: A review of the literature.* DPMP Monograph Series. Sydney, Australia: National Drug and Alcohol Research Centre. Retrieved from https://dpmp.unsw.edu.au/sites/default/files/dpmp/resources/DPMP%20MONO%2023.pdf.

Rutherford, K., McIntyre, J., Daley, A., et al. (2012). Development of expertise in mental health service provisions for lesbian, gay and transgender communities. *Medical Education, 46*, 903–913. doi:10.1111/j.1365-2923.2012.04272.x.

Scheim, A., & Bauer, G. (2014). Sex and gender diversity among transgender persons in Ontario, Canada: Results from a respondent-driven sampling survey. *The Journal of Sex Research, 52*(1), 1–14. doi:10.1080/00224499.2014.893553.

Scott, R., Lasiuk, G., & Norris, C. (2016). The relationship between sexual orientation and depression in a national population sample. *Journal of Clinical Nursing, 25*, 3522–3532. doi:10.1111/jocn.13286.

Shearer, A., Herres, J., Kodish, T., et al. (2015). Differences in mental health symptoms across lesbian, gay, bisexual, and questioning youth in primary care settings. *Journal of Adolescent Health, 59*, 38–43. doi:10.1016/j.jadohealth.2016.02.005.

Statistics Canada. (2015). *Canadian Community Health Survey.* Retrieved from http://www23.statcan.gc.ca/imdb/p2SV.pl?Function=getSurvey&SDDS=3226.

Zunner, B., & Grace, P. (2012). The ethical nursing care of transgender patients: An exploration of bias in health care and how it affects this population. *The American Journal of Nursing, 112*(12), 61–64. doi:10.1097/01.NAJ.0000423514.58585.a3.

Disorders of Children and Adolescents

Cheryl L. Pollard

KEY TERMS AND CONCEPTS

assent
attention-deficit/hyperactivity disorder (ADHD)
bibliotherapy
conduct disorder
consent
dissent
mutual storytelling
neurodevelopmental disorders (NDDs)

oppositional defiant disorder
pica
play therapy
principle of least restrictive intervention
rumination disorder
temperament
therapeutic games

OBJECTIVES

1. Explore factors contributing to child and adolescent mental disorders, and develop intervention strategies for this population.
2. Explain characteristics associated with resiliency.
3. Identify characteristics of positive mental health and development in children and adolescents.
4. Discuss holistic assessment of a child or adolescent.

5. Explore areas in the assessment of suicide for children and adolescents.
6. Compare and contrast at least six treatment modalities for children and adolescents.
7. Describe clinical features and behaviours of at least three child and adolescent mental disorders.
8. Formulate three nursing diagnoses, stating patient outcomes and interventions for each.

⊖volve WEBSITE

Visit the Evolve website for Flashcards, Case Studies, and additional testing resources related to the content in this chapter: *http://evolve.elsevier.com/Canada/Varcarolis/psychiatric/*

Pre-Test   interactive review

Many children and adolescents may struggle with a disabling mental illness, but most of these illnesses go unnoticed and unidentified (Mental Health Commission of Canada, 2012). Until *Changing Directions, Changing Lives: The Mental Health Strategy for Canada* was released by the Mental Health Commission of Canada (MHCC) in 2012, the mental health needs of young people in Canada had not received much attention.

Mental health disorders in children and adolescents are associated with disturbances in psychological, physiological, academic, and social functioning. The economic, social, and personal costs to society associated with childhood- and adolescent-onset mental disorders are tremendous because the

illness occurs during important developmental periods, has frequent recurrences, and persists into adulthood (Knapp, Snell, Healey, et al., 2015). Stigma and misconceptions can cause patients and families to attempt to conceal the conditions or even limit help seeking professional care (Polaha, Williams, Heflinger, et al., 2015). The MHCC also reports that stigma, a silent public health epidemic, can be addressed through "contact-based education" (Mental Health Commission of Canada, 2012)—that is, through meeting and talking with people and families who experience mental health problems.

Childhood and adolescence are distinct developmental periods during which significant changes in physical, cognitive, and social functioning occur. As such, childhood is defined in terms of early (1 to 4 years) and middle childhood (5 to 10 years), whereas adolescence is described in terms of the subphases of early (11 to 14 years), middle (15 to 17 years), and late (18 to 21 years) (Hagan, Shaw, & Duncan, 2017). Important mental disorders that can occur in children and adolescents include mood disorders, anxiety disorders, schizophrenia, and substance abuse. Anxiety and depression as they relate to this age group are discussed in this chapter. These disorders, as well as the others discussed in this chapter, are more difficult to diagnose in younger children because of limited language skills and cognitive and emotional development. In addition, children undergo more rapid psychological, neurological, and physiological changes over a briefer period than adults do. The rapidity and complexity of this development must be taken into consideration during assessment for mental health disorders. Clinicians and parents often wait to see whether symptoms are the result of a developmental lag or trauma response that will eventually correct itself; therefore intervention may be delayed—for instance, until the child reaches school age. Usually a number of factors influence a child's or adolescent's mental health, so a variety of interventions are needed to improve psychological, social, physical, educational, and spiritual well-being.

Meeting the mental health needs of youth and their families is a challenge for the nurse because need is steadily increasing while funding and access to care are decreasing and existing services remain fragmented or lacking in many communities. Considering all of the developmental changes and associated vulnerabilities and resiliencies that occur during childhood and adolescence, it is clear that this is an optimal time to target prevention and intervention.

This chapter describes the nurse's role in assessment and interventions for selected mental health disorders, as well as broad treatment modalities that are implemented through the nursing process with this population and their families.

EPIDEMIOLOGY

One in five children and adolescents in Canada suffers from a major mental illness that causes significant impairments at home, at school, with peers, and in the community. Some of these mental health disorders have a likelihood of recurrence and chronicity in young adulthood; in fact, 80% of adults with mental illness experienced problems in childhood or early adolescence. Epidemiology data suggest that about approximately 13% of Canadian children and youth may be experiencing a mental disorder at any given time (Waddell, Shepherd, Schwartz, et al., 2014). It is estimated that two thirds of young people with mental health problems are not receiving needed services. Suicide ranks as the second leading cause of death for youth ages 10 to 19 years, and suffocation was the predominant means of committing suicide among young Canadians. Suicide rates in Canada are increasing among female youth but decreasing among male children and adolescents (Skinner & McFaull, 2012).

Suicide is a significant problem for some Indigenous youth whose communities lack the necessary protective benefits and appropriate sources of support, including professional and nonprofessional help. It is reported that Indigenous youth have a suicide rate that is five to six times greater than that of non-Indigenous youth (Pollack, Mulay, Valcour, et al., 2016).

The Canadian government's recognition of childhood and adolescent mental health problems and efforts toward identifying effective treatments were reported in the Senate report *Out of the Shadows at Last* (Standing Senate Committee on Social Affairs,

---

🔍 RESEARCH HIGHLIGHT

Depression Impact on Adolescents

Problem

Adolescence itself can be a stressful time for youth. The presence of a mental health disorder during this developmental stage presents a major challenge for young people who are preparing for transition into adulthood. Understanding how depression affects the lives of young people will provide knowledge that aids development and implementation of nursing interventions specific to this population.

Purpose of Study

The purpose of this research study was to examine the lived experience of young people diagnosed with depression.

Methods

A phenomenological interpretative approach was used in semistructured, audio-recorded interviews with 26 youth ages 16 to 22 who described their experience of what it was like to have depression.

Key Findings

Four themes identified in the data reflecting the experience of living with depression were (1) struggling to make sense of their situation, (2) spiralling down, (3) withdrawing, and (4) contemplating self-harm or suicide. While *struggling to make sense of their situation*, the participants questioned why they were different and not the same as others in their peer group. The youth *spiralling down* expressed how the illness became more prominent and engulfed their lives. They described the onset of illness symptoms and not knowing what to do to reverse the situation. For the third theme, *withdrawing*, the adolescents reported distancing themselves from others because of the fear and stigma of being labelled mentally ill. This distancing allowed them time to reflect but contributed to their feelings of loneliness and isolation. The final theme, *contemplating self-harm or suicide*, involved how they reacted to their situation. Some youth reported engagement in risk-taking behaviours such as drug and alcohol use, suicidal behaviour, contemplation of suicide, and sexually promiscuous behaviours.

Implications for Nursing Practice

Nurses who have knowledge and understanding of how adolescents experience and cope with depression are better able to assess these patients' coping abilities and promote enhancement of healthy coping skills. They can also promote within this youth population initiatives to counteract stigma and to seek mental health care.

Source: McCann, T. V., Lubman, D. I., & Clark, E. (2012). The experience of young people with depression: A qualitative study. *Journal of Psychiatric and Mental Health Nursing, 19*(4), 334–340.

Science and Technology, 2006). Based on a key recommendation of this Senate committee, the MHCC was formed and—in close consultation with people living with mental health problems and illnesses, families, stakeholder organizations, governments, and experts—identified child and youth mental health services as a critical component to improving the mental health outcomes of Canadians. However, barriers to assessment, treatment, prevention, and early intervention remain, including the following:

- Lack of clarity about conditions for screening children
- Lack of coordination among multiple systems
- Lack of resources and long wait times for services
- Shortage of mental health care professionals
- Lack of a child and youth mental health framework

More research is needed to understand the reasons for the underuse and early termination of mental health care services, and funding is needed to improve access to and coordination among existing resources to provide programs for these young people (Government of Alberta, 2015).

COMORBIDITY

Children and adolescents with mental health disorders often meet the criteria for more than one diagnostic category. Attention-deficit/hyperactivity disorder (ADHD), a prominent comorbid condition, occurs in 90% of individuals with juvenile-onset bipolar disorder, 90% of children with oppositional defiant disorder, and 50% of those with conduct disorder. Childhood depression has a high incidence of comorbidity: 20% to 80% of children with depression have conduct or oppositional disorders, 30% to 75% have anxiety disorders, and 5% to 60% display symptoms of ADHD (Reinhardt & Reinhardt, 2013). Multiple services are often needed by those with coexisting diagnoses, such as special education evaluation and services, after-school services, family counselling, and behaviour management.

RISK FACTORS

Mental illness can become serious or severe and persistent if early detection and effective intervention are not implemented. A child with a parent with depression is at risk for developing an anxiety disorder, mood disorder, conduct disorder, or substance use disorder. The parent's inability to model effective coping strategies can lead to learned helplessness, the creation of anxiety or apathy, and an inability to master the environment. A child with a conduct disorder may develop an antisocial personality. In fact, two thirds of youth in the juvenile justice system have one or more diagnosable mental disorders (Teplin, Welty, Abram, et al., 2012).

Children who have been abused or neglected are at great risk for developing emotional, intellectual, and social problems as a result of their traumatic experiences (Akresh, 2016). Exposure to intimate partner violence and neglect are two of the most prevalent forms of child abuse in Canada. According to the Public Health Agency of Canada (2008), 235 842 child maltreatment–related investigations were conducted in Canada in 2008. Of those, 20% were related to physical abuse, 9% to emotional maltreatment, and 3% to sexual abuse. Although there has not been a national report since that time on child maltreatment–related investigations, Ontario researchers report that there has been no significant change in the rates in their province (Fallon, Van Wert, Trocmé, et al., 2015). Other studies suggest that more children suffer abuse and neglect than is reported to child protection services, with girls more frequently victims of sexual abuse. While boys are also sexually abused, the numbers are under-reported due to shame and stigma. The nurse must understand that sexual abuse ranges from fondling to forcing a child to observe or participate in lewd acts to sexual intercourse. All instances of sexual abuse are devastating to a child who lacks the mental capacity or emotional maturation to consent to this type of a relationship.

Witnessing violence also is traumatizing and a well-documented risk factor for many problems, including depression, anxiety, nightmares, intrusive thoughts, hypervigilance, aggressive and delinquent behaviour, drug use, academic failure, and low self-esteem (Whitson, Bernard, & Kaufman, 2015). Children who have been abused also are at risk for identifying with the aggressor, and they may act out, bully others, become abusers in adulthood, or otherwise develop dysfunctional patterns in close interpersonal relationships.

Among adolescents, gang involvement is a growing problem. Estimates from the Royal Canadian Mounted Police (2006) suggest that there are more than 300 gangs and 7 000 gang members across Canada. Primarily, youths ages 11 to 13, a time of particular vulnerability, are solicited to become gang members because their decision-making capacities are limited and they may look up to older peers for status and belonging. Certain risk factors seem to predispose a person to gang membership, including past trauma, learning disability, poor school performance, poverty, and family disorganization (Prowse, 2013). Gang members often inflict violence on others, including vandalism, theft, and aggression. Many end up in the juvenile court system, where they exhibit mental health problems that may remain untreated.

All Canadian provinces and territories have child protection legislation, and all instances of suspected abuse of a minor child are required to be reported to the local child protection services. Further, in 2001 the Government of Canada passed legislation that came into effect in 2008 to help protect youth from non-exploitative sexual activity by raising the age of consent for sexual activity from 14 to 16 years (Parliament of Canada, 2001). This legislation brought the age of consent in line with that of other countries such as the United States and Australia. Depending on the province or territory, a *child* is defined as a young person up to age 16 to 19, and the age of majority is 18 or 19 years. Box 27-1 discusses the decision-making terms *consent*, *assent*, and *dissent* as they relate to children.

It is important for nurses working in youth detention, school, and community settings to assess for post-traumatic stress disorder (PTSD) and safety of the environment for young people who have been traumatized or who have experienced abuse or a history of violence. Interventions should focus on teaching coping skills to deal with trauma, supporting efforts to achieve socially appropriate goals, and facilitating integration into healthy social support systems.

BOX 27-1	INCLUDING THE CHILD IN HEALTH CARE DECISION MAKING

Nurses working with children and youth need to recognize the young person's right to self-determination and participation in decision making related to health care and research. **Consent** is an expression of autonomy. It represents a person's capacity to understand information and voluntarily to act on this information. For example, a person may give consent (agree) to participate in a research study, or he or she may withhold consent (refuse) to participate in a particular health care treatment. Provincial and territorial legislation stipulates the age of majority—the age at which a person may give his or her own consent. Although not legally binding, including the child in the decision-making process shows respect for the child and gives the child a sense of ownership about what is happening. Despite children lacking the capacity to consent, they still may be able to express their wishes in a meaningful way (*assent* or *dissent*). **Assent** refers to the child's agreement to participate; **dissent** indicates a child's refusal to participate in the suggested health care or research study (Lambert & Glacken, 2011). Including the child in health care decision making supports the child's growth and development. However, a disagreement between the child and the legally recognized decision maker (i.e., parent or guardian) creates complex ethical dilemmas for members of the health care team. In these situations, requesting an ethics consult, often provided by a clinical ethicist, is appropriate.

Source: Lambert, V., & Glacken, M. (2011). Engaging with children in research: Theoretical and practical implications of negotiating informed consent/assent. *Nursing Ethics, 18*(6), 781–801.

ETIOLOGY

Mental illness in children and adolescents, as in adults, is caused by multiple factors, and distinguishing among the genetic, psychosocial, and environmental factors makes diagnosis challenging. Increasing numbers of children are born with or develop disordered brain function related to malnutrition, human immunodeficiency virus (HIV) infection, fetal alcohol syndrome, drug addiction, and brain injury. In addition, they are exposed to environmental stressors in the family, school, peer group, or community that have an impact on their social, emotional, cognitive, psychological, and spiritual development (Fryers & Brugha, 2013).

The degree of a child's vulnerability to mental illness changes over time. The resilience of the child and the presence of positive environmental factors (e.g., parental role models, a healthy school environment) enable a child to learn and adapt. Positive influences can decrease vulnerability to mental disorders or improve functioning to the fullest possible level if a disorder exists.

Biological Factors
Genetic
Hereditary factors are implicated in a number of mental disorders, including autism, bipolar disorders, schizophrenia, attention-deficit problems, and intellectual developmental disorder. Because not all genetically vulnerable children develop mental disorders, it is assumed that resilience and a supportive environment are key factors in avoiding the development of mental disorders. According to Lahiri, Sokol, Erickson, and colleagues (2013), some disorders (e.g., autism spectrum disorder [ASD], fragile X syndrome) have a direct genetic link.

Brain Development and Biochemicals
Dramatic changes occur in the brain during childhood and adolescence, including a declining number of synapses (they peak at age 5), myelination of brain fibres, changes in the relative volume and activity level in different brain regions, and interactions of hormones. Myelination increases the speed of information processing, improves the conduction speed of nerve impulses, and enables faster reactions to occur. Maturation of the cortex of the brain occurs most rapidly during childhood but continues until well after puberty (Barrasso-Catanzaro & Eslinger, 2016). The teen years are also marked by changes in the frontal and prefrontal cortex regions, leading to improvements in executive functions, organization and planning skills, and inhibiting responses (Sullivan, Pfefferbaum, Rohlfing, et al., 2011). These changes, including cerebellum maturation and hormonal changes, reflect the emotional and behavioural fluctuations characteristic of adolescence. Early adolescence is typically characterized by low emotional regulation and intolerance for frustration; emotional and behavioural control usually increase over the course of adolescence.

Alterations in neurotransmitters have also been implicated as playing a role in causing child and adolescent disorders. Decreased norepinephrine and serotonin levels are related to depression and suicide, and elevated levels are related to mania and pathological fear. Abnormalities in dopamine receptors and dopamine transporters are implicated in ADHD, certain addictions, and schizophrenia (Schatzberg, 2017).

Temperament
Temperament, according to Hanington, Ramchandani, and Stein (2010), is the style of behaviour habitually used to adapt to the demands and expectations of the environment. Varying temperaments are present in infants, are modified by maturation, and develop in the context of the social environment (Verhage, Oosterman, & Schuengel, 2015). All people have temperaments, and the fit between the child's and the parent's temperament is critical to the child's development. The parent's role in shaping that relationship is of primary importance, and, when needed, the nurse can teach parents ways to modify their behaviours to improve interactions with their children. If there is incongruence between parent and child temperament and the parent is unable to respond positively to the child, there is a risk for insecure attachment, developmental problems, and future mental disorders.

By the time children enter grade school, any inclination to use and abuse drugs in later life will show in their temperament and behaviour traits (e.g., traits such as shyness, aggressiveness, and rebelliousness). External risk factors for such abuse include substance use among peers, parental drug use, and involvement in legal problems such as truancy or vandalism. Researchers have also identified childhood protective factors that shield some children from drug use, including self-control, parental monitoring, academic achievement, anti–drug use policies, and strong neighbourhood attachment (Roffey, 2016).

Resilience

Most children with risk factors for the development of mental illness develop normally. The term *resilience* has been used to denote the relationship between a child's constitutional endowment and success negotiating stressful environmental factors. Studies have shown that a resilient child has the following characteristics (Cicchetti, 2010):

- Adaptability to changes in the environment
- Ability to form nurturing relationships with other adults when the parent is not available
- Ability to distance self from emotional chaos
- Good social intelligence
- Good problem-solving skills

Other studies have also identified the cushioning effects of family stability in the face of poverty and adversity. The nurse's role is to identify and foster these qualities to prevent at-risk children from developing emotional and mental problems.

Environmental Factors

To a greater degree than adults, children are dependent on others. During childhood, the main context is the family. Parents model behaviour and provide the child with a view of the world. If parents are abusive, rejecting, or overly controlling, the child may suffer detrimental effects at the developmental points at which the trauma occurs. There is strong evidence that a number of familial risk factors correlate with childhood psychiatric disorders, including severe marital discord, low socioeconomic status, large families and overcrowding, parental criminality, parental mental disorders, and foster care placement.

External factors in the environment can either support or put stress on children and adolescents and shape their development. Young people are vulnerable in an environment in which systems (e.g., schools, court systems) and people (e.g., parents, counsellors) have power and control (Gonzalez, Boyle, Kyu, et al., 2012).

Cultural Factors

Children and youth in ethnic minority groups may be at risk for a variety of mental health problems. Economics, service availability, cultural beliefs, values, and attitudes of health care providers toward young people may affect help seeking (Stewart, Simmons, & Habibpour, 2012). In addition, because of the lack of same-culture role models, children in some minority groups experience increased risk. Differences in the cultural expectations of family and peers, presence of stresses, and lack of support within the dominant culture may have profound effects on these children and increase the risk for mental, emotional, and academic problems. Nurses working with children and adolescents from diverse backgrounds require an increased awareness of their own biases, as well as the patient's needs. The social and cultural context of the patient and family, including factors as such as age, ethnicity, gender, sexual orientation, world view, religiosity, and socioeconomic status, should be taken into consideration when assessing and planning care.

CHILD AND ADOLESCENT PSYCHIATRIC MENTAL HEALTH NURSING

Child and adolescent psychiatric mental health nurses use evidence-informed knowledge to provide care that is responsive to the patient's and family's specific problems, strengths, personality, sociocultural context, and preferences.

Although the number of young people with acute mental illness in our society is increasing, inpatient and residential treatment time among this population has steadily decreased. Treatment for children often consists of brief hospitalization followed by interventions conducted in a wide spectrum of community support settings, including day treatment programs, partial hospitalization programs, clinics, schools, and psychiatric home care. To be considered eligible for inpatient hospitalization, the child or adolescent typically must be an imminent danger to self or others. In short-term inpatient facilities, the nurse has less time to form a therapeutic relationship with the child and family, making it more difficult to facilitate lasting behavioural changes. Residential and group home facilities for long-term placement are more difficult to secure because availability is often scarce, the cost is high, and consistent evidence of their effectiveness in reducing symptoms and improving long-term functioning is lacking (Edwards, Evans, Gillen, et al., 2015).

As psychiatric care moved from inpatient facilities to the community, child and adolescent psychiatric mental health nurses became an integral part of these programs. Advanced-practice registered nurses, including clinical nurse specialists, nurse counsellors, and nurse practitioners, have established outpatient practices, school-based primary prevention, and other innovative treatment programs for young people. Research on interventions for young people at risk for developing mental illness is also being carried out in nontraditional settings such as homeless shelters, group homes, and mentoring programs, as well as online.

Assessing Development and Functioning

A child or adolescent with mental illness is one whose progressive personality development and functioning is hindered or arrested due to biological, psychosocial, or spiritual factors, resulting in functional impairments. In comparison, a child or adolescent who does not have a mental illness matures with only minor regressions, coping with the stressors and developmental tasks of life. Learning and adapting to the environment and bonding with others in a mutually satisfying way are signs of mental health (Box 27-2). The degree of mental health or illness can be viewed on a continuum, with one's level on the continuum changing over time. Many mental illnesses are chronic but can be managed effectively with evidence-informed treatments.

Data Collection

Methods of collecting data include interviewing, screening, testing (neurological, psychological, intelligence), observing, and interacting with the child or adolescent. Histories are taken from multiple sources, including parents, other caregivers, the child

CONSIDERING CULTURE

Hostility Toward Lesbian, Gay, Bisexual, Transgender, and Queer Adolescents

How do nurses contribute to changing the social culture from intolerance to acceptance? Lesbian, gay, bisexual, transgender, and queer (LGBTQ) adolescents are not a specific cultural group; however, these individuals live within communities that have developed characteristics and attitudes in others that can manifest as discrimination and prejudice.

On October 18, 2011, in Ottawa, A.Y. Jackson High School student Jamie Hubley, 15 years of age, committed suicide. Jamie, who was openly gay, reported on his blog months before he died that he suffered continuous and constant bullying because of his sexuality. According to his father, an Ottawa city councillor, Jamie had been bullied throughout elementary school and into high school (Woods, 2011). At the time of his suicide, he was experiencing depression and receiving care from health care providers. Reaction to Jamie's death was brought forward in the House of Commons by members of Parliament, highlighting the need for bullying and other forms of intolerance toward others to end. This event illuminates the difficulties that schools and communities may have in coping with the needs of youth with emotional and behavioural difficulties and can open dialogue for nurses about how to increase community readiness to work with LGBTQ youth.

Statistics on hate crimes in Canada indicate that about 16% are related to sexual orientation, and two thirds of those crimes are marked by violence (Allen, 2015). Teenagers and children as young as 10 years of age may experience feelings of identification with or sexual attraction to the same gender. Young people often disclose these feelings to friends, and they may be met with social rejection, anger, ridicule, bullying, and violence. Studies have shown that LGBTQ youth are at risk for a variety of negative outcomes, including dramatically increased suicidality, mental health problems, high-risk behaviours, poorer school outcomes, and homelessness. Externally, LGBTQ youth are subject to higher rates of violence and victimization than heterosexual youth are.

A nursing diagnosis that may apply is *Readiness for enhanced community coping* related to adapting and problem solving to meet the demands or needs of the community (in this case, the school) for the management of current stressors. Better community adapting and problem solving would lead to improved communication among community members and larger organizations. In addition to providing counselling for LGBTQ youth, nurses could play a key role in the following:

- Educating schools and parents about the needs of LGBTQ youth in an effort to change attitudes
- Helping the community to apply for and obtain funds for additional programs for LGBTQ youth
- Encouraging communication and collaboration among community members on these issues
- Serving as advocates for LGBTQ youth

In its landmark document, *Changing Directions, Changing Lives: The Mental Health Strategy for Canada*, the Mental Health Commission of Canada (2012) identified this population as a priority. Stemming from one of the six key strategic directions was a recommendation for increased services and more knowledge and understanding among the public and among health care providers about the impact of discrimination and stigma for LGBTQ individuals.

Sources: Allen, M. (2015). *Police-reported hate crime in Canada, 2013*. Ottawa: Statistics Canada; Mental Health Commission of Canada. (2012). *Changing directions, changing lives: The mental health strategy for Canada*. Calgary: Author; and Woods, M. (2011). Bullied son of Ottawa city councillor commits suicide. *Toronto Star*, October 18. Retrieved from http://www.thestar.com/news/canada/2011/10/18/bullied_son_of_ottawa_city_councillor_commits_suicide.html.

BOX 27-2   CHARACTERISTICS OF A MENTALLY HEALTHY CHILD OR ADOLESCENT

- Trusts others and sees his or her world as being safe and supportive
- Correctly interprets reality—makes accurate perceptions of the environment and his or her ability to influence it through actions (e.g., self-determination)
- Behaves in a way that is developmentally appropriate and does not violate social norms
- Has a positive, realistic self-concept and developing identity
- Adapts to and copes with anxiety and stress using age-appropriate behaviour
- Can learn and master developmental tasks and new situations
- Expresses self in spontaneous and creative ways
- Develops and maintains satisfying relationships

nurses can use them to effectively monitor symptoms and behavioural changes.

The observation–interaction part of a mental health assessment begins with a semistructured interview in which the nurse meets with the child or adolescent alone and asks about the home environment, parents, and siblings and the school environment, teachers, and peers. In this format, the young person is free to describe current problems and give information about his or her developmental history. Play activities, such as games, drawings, and puppets, are used for younger children who cannot respond to a direct approach. The initial interview is key to observing interactions among the child, caregiver, and siblings (if available) and to building trust and rapport. The nurse needs to be cognizant of being nonthreatening in approach and using language appropriate to the young person's cognitive capabilities and verbal skills.

Assessment Data

The types of data collected to assess mental health depend on the setting, the severity of the presenting problem, and the availability of resources. Agency policies determine which data are collected, but a nurse should be prepared to make an independent judgement about what to assess and how to assess or adolescent, and other adults, such as teachers, when possible. Structured questionnaires and behaviour checklists can be completed by parents and teachers. A genogram can document family composition, history, and relationships (see Chapter 34). Numerous assessment tools are available, and with education, it. In all cases, a physical examination is part of a complete assessment for serious mental health problems. Box 27-3 identifies essential assessment data.

Developmental assessment. The developmental assessment provides information about the child or adolescent's maturational level. These data are then reviewed in relation to the child's chronological age to identify developmental strengths or deficits. The Denver II Developmental Screening Test is a popular assessment tool. For adolescents, tools may be tailored to specific areas of assessment, such as neuropsychological, physical, hormonal, and biochemical. One tool that can be used to assess risk is the Youth Risk Behavior Survey for children and adolescents.

Abnormal findings in the developmental and mental status assessments may be related to stress and adjustment problems or to more serious disorders. Children may outgrow a difficulty, but nurses need to evaluate behaviours indicative of stress or minor regressions, as well as those indicative of more serious psychopathology, and identify the need for further evaluation, intervention, or referral. Stress-related behaviours or minor regressions may be handled by working with parents or caregivers. However, as young people develop maladaptive coping behaviours and use these behaviours over time, they are at risk for developing mental health disorders. Serious psychopathology requires evaluation by an advanced-practice nurse in collaboration with clinicians specializing in child and adolescent health.

Mental status examination. Assessment of mental status of children and youth is similar to that of adults. It provides information about the mental state at the time of the examination and identifies problems with thinking, feeling, and behaving. Broad categories to assess include safety, general appearance, socialization, activity level, speech, coordination and motor function, affect, manner of relating, intellectual function, thought processes and content, and characteristics of play. It is also important to obtain information not only from the child or adolescent but also from others (e.g., parents, teachers, health care providers) who have been involved with the young person.

Risk assessment. Suicide is the second leading cause of death in adolescence (Statistics Canada, 2015); therefore assessment of suicidality is an essential nursing skill. Some children and youths make idle threats about killing themselves, but to determine the cause of the distress and the risk for violence, the nurse must use active listening when interacting with any young person expressing the wish to hurt self or others. The number-one

BOX 27-3 TYPES OF ASSESSMENT DATA

History of Present Illness
- Chief complaint
- Development and duration of problems
- Help sought and results
- Effect of problem on child's life at home and school
- Effect of problem on family and siblings' lives

Developmental History
- Pregnancy, birth, neonatal data
- Developmental milestones
- Description of eating, sleeping, and elimination habits and routines
- Attachment behaviours
- Types of play
- Social skills and friendships
- Sexual activity
- Spiritual beliefs

Developmental Assessment
- Psychomotor skills
- Language skills
- Cognitive skills
- Interpersonal and social skills
- Academic achievement
- Behaviour (response to stress, to changes in environment)
- Problem-solving and coping skills (impulse control, delay of gratification)
- Energy level and motivation
- Self-concept
- Drug and alcohol use

Neurological Assessment
- Cerebral functions
- Cerebellar functions

- Sensory functions
- Reflexes
  Note: Functions can be observed during developmental assessment and while playing games involving a specific ability (e.g., "Simon says touch your nose").

Medical History
- Review of body systems
- Traumas, hospitalizations, operations, and child's response
- Illnesses or injuries affecting central nervous system
- Medications (past and current)
- Allergies

Family History
- Illnesses in related family members (e.g., seizures, mental disorders, drug and alcohol abuse, diabetes, cancer)
- Background of family members (occupation, education, social activities, religion)
- Family relationship (separation, divorce, deaths, contact with extended family, communication, support system)

Mental Status Assessment
- General appearance
- Activity level
- Coordination and motor function
- Affect
- Speech
- Manner of relating
- Intellectual functions
- Thought processes and content
- Risk assessment
- Characteristics of play

predictor of suicidal risk is a past suicide attempt. Areas to explore when assessing suicidal risk include the following:

- Past and current suicidal thoughts, threats, or attempts
- Existence of a plan, lethality of the plan, and accessibility of any necessities for carrying out the plan
- Feelings of hopelessness; changes in level of energy
- Circumstances, state of mind, and motivation
- Viewpoints about suicide and death (e.g., Has a family member or friend attempted suicide?)
- Depression and other moods or feelings (e.g., anger, guilt, rejection)
- History of impulsivity, poor judgement, or decreased decision making
- Drug or alcohol use
- Prescribed medications and any recent adherence issues

Additional questions may be asked of teens, including those about risk-taking and acting-out behaviours, artwork with a violent theme, interests in music or books with morbid themes, and recent changes in behaviour or social life (e.g., eating, sleeping, isolating, loss of a relationship).

Assessing the lethality of a young child's suicide plan is complicated by the distorted concept of death, immature ego functions, and an immature understanding of lethality. For instance, a child who is highly suicidal may believe that a few aspirin will cause death. The incorrect judgement about the lethality does not diminish the seriousness of the intent. Another child simply seeking attention may threaten to jump off a bridge, believing that this action would not be fatal. Some teens may make a pact to kill themselves or become upset after a friend has committed suicide or died accidentally (Swanson & Colman, 2013). Early intervention is essential, and parents need to understand that suicidal thoughts or self-harming behaviour (e.g., burning, cutting, reckless driving, binge drinking) must be taken seriously and evaluated by mental health care providers as an emergency. Suicide prevention among children and youths is also reflected in several of the strategic directions in *Changing Directions, Changing Lives: The Mental Health Strategy for Canada* (Mental Health Commission of Canada, 2012).

Cultural factors. Mental health care providers recognize the importance of culture in evaluating psychiatric disorders, especially when working with families. The *Diagnostic and Statistical Manual of Mental Disorders*, fifth edition (*DSM-5*), identifies culture-bound syndromes of mental illness that are not diagnostic categories in Western medicine (see Chapter 8). Sensitivity to cultural influences in mental illness is a necessity to show respect for cultural preferences in providing individualized care and to avoid behaviour stereotyping and incorrect assessment. A translator should be used if there are any issues with understanding and communicating with the child, youth, or their guardians.

General Interventions

The interventions described in this section can be used by nurses in a variety of clinical and nonclinical settings. Many of the modalities can encompass activities of daily living, learning activities, multiple forms of play and recreational activities, and interactions with adults and peers.

Family Therapy

The family is seen as critical to improving the function of a young person with a psychiatric illness; therefore family counselling is often a key component of treatment used by nurses. There are many models of family therapy (see Chapter 34), but the focus of all models is on promoting, improving, and maintaining family functioning. Following assessment, the nurse works with family members to identify specific goals and provides education on ways to achieve the goals for the family or subunits within the family (e.g., parental, sibling). Homework assignments are often used for family members to practise newly learned skills outside the therapeutic environment.

In addition to therapy involving a single family, multiple-family therapy provides useful interaction for participants to learn how other families solve problems and build on strengths, develop insight and improve judgement about their own family, learn and practise new information, and develop lasting and satisfying relationships with other families (Wright & Leahey, 2012).

Group Therapy

Nurses use group therapy as an integral component of their practice to promote therapeutic change among children and adolescents. Group therapy (see Chapter 33) for younger children takes the form of play to introduce ideas and work through issues. For preschool and grade school children, it combines play, learning skills, and talk about the activity. The child learns social skills by taking turns and sharing with peers. For adolescents, group therapy involves learning skills and talking, focusing largely on peer relationships and working through specific problems. Adolescent group therapy might use a popular media event or personality as the basis for a group discussion. Groups have been used effectively to deal with specific issues in a young person's life (e.g., bereavement, depression, physical abuse, substance use, dating, chronic illnesses such as juvenile diabetes) (Jacobson & Mufson, 2012).

Behavioural Therapy

Behavioural therapy involves rewarding desired behaviour to reduce maladaptive behaviours. In a healthy relationship, a child's developmentally appropriate behaviours are validated by a significant adult (*operant conditioning*). Behaviour management in psychiatry is classified according to the level of restrictiveness and intrusiveness. To ensure that the civil and legal rights of individuals are not violated, and effective treatment is provided, techniques are selected according to the principle of least restrictive intervention. This principle requires that more restrictive interventions be used only after less restrictive interventions to manage the behaviour have been attempted. Intrusive techniques (such as physical restraints) are implemented to manage behaviour and maintain safety only when very severe or dangerous behaviours (i.e., those that may result in injury to the patient or others) are exhibited.

Most child and adolescent treatment settings use a behaviour modification program to motivate and reward age-appropriate behaviours. One popular method is the point or level system, in which points are awarded for desired behaviours and increasing levels of privileges can be earned. The value for specific behaviours and privileges for each level are spelled out, and points earned each day are recorded. Older youth can be made responsible for keeping their own point sheet and for requesting points for their behaviours. Children who work on individual behavioural goals (e.g., seeking help in problem solving) can earn additional points. Points are used to obtain a specific reward, which can be part of the system or be negotiated on an individual or group basis (Mohr, Martin, Olson, et al., 2009).

Cognitive Behavioural Therapy

As discussed in Chapter 4, cognitive behavioural therapy (CBT) is an evidence-informed treatment approach based on the premise that negative and self-defeating thoughts lead to psychiatric pathology and that learning to replace these thoughts with more accurate appraisals results in improved functioning. Researchers and clinicians have discovered that CBT is also useful in treating children and youth with depression, anxiety, obsessive-compulsive disorder, and self-harming tendencies (Benjamin, Puleo, Settipani, et al., 2011).

Milieu Management

Milieu management is the mechanism for structuring inpatient, residential, and day treatment programs. The nurse collaborates with other health care providers in structuring and maintaining the therapeutic environment to achieve the following:
- Provide physical and psychological security
- Promote growth and mastery of developmental tasks
- Ameliorate mental health disorders and promote well-being

The physical milieu for inpatient or residential care is designed to provide a safe, comfortable place to live, play, and learn, with areas for both private time and group activity. There may be a gym, outdoor playground, swimming pool, recreational facilities, and even pets. A daily schedule sets the structure for what activities will occur (e.g., school, therapy sessions, outings, family or home visits). The nurse and multidisciplinary team share and articulate a philosophy regarding how to provide physical and psychological security, promote personal growth, and work with problematic behaviours. This philosophy is reflected in the policies of the facility and is typically written in a handbook given to patients and families upon admission. The child or adolescent's behaviour, emotions, and cognitive processes are the focus of the therapeutic interventions in the milieu. The therapeutic factors operating in the milieu's structure, activities, and interactions with staff are listed in Box 27-4.

Seclusion and restraint. Hospitalized patients are often a high risk to themselves, and effective use of prevention strategies for dangerous behaviour begins at intake. Nurses have an important role in the promotion of a culture of patient safety through assessment and intervention. Promoting a therapeutic environment for all patients involves the following (De Hert, Dirix, Demunter, et al., 2011):
- Actively engaging the patient and family in treatment planning to avoid the use of seclusion or restraint
- Maintaining adequate staffing patterns with motivated staff experienced in working with patients who have been violent, abused, or both

---

BOX 27-4 THERAPEUTIC FACTORS IN THE MILIEU

- Safe, therapeutic environment with roles, boundaries, and limits
- Reduction of stressors
- Structure for coping with stress
- Ability to express feelings without fear of rejection or retaliation
- Availability of emotional support and comfort
- Assistance with reality testing and support for weak or missing ego functions
- Interventions for impulsive, aggressive, or inappropriate behaviours
- Opportunities for learning and testing new adaptive behaviours and mastering developmental tasks
- Consistent, constructive feedback from trained and supportive adult staff
- Reinforcement of positive behaviours and development of self-esteem
- Corrective emotional experiences
- Availability of role models for making healthy identifications and positive attachments
- Opportunities to develop peer relationships and practise handling peer pressure
- Opportunities to be spontaneous and creative
- Opportunities to explore issues related to self-esteem and identity formation

---

- Accurately assessing the acuity of the individuals and group makeup of the unit
- Using positive and less restrictive alternatives (e.g., de-escalation strategies, time-space interviews)

Although policymakers and advocates lobbied for a reduction or elimination of seclusion and restraint use over the past decade, a majority of inpatient treatment centres for children and adolescents report using such practices (Green-Hennessy & Hennessy, 2015). Evidence on the use of locked seclusion and physical restraint in managing dangerous behaviour suggests that both are psychologically harmful and can be physically harmful. Deaths have resulted, primarily by asphyxiation due to physical holds during restraints (De Hert, Dirix, Demunter, et al., 2011). However, at times a child's behaviour is so destructive or dangerous that physical restraint or seclusion is needed. All nurses who might be involved in therapeutic holding or physical restraint of children and adolescents must receive education and training to decrease the risk for injury to themselves and the child. This intervention requires prompt, firm, nonretaliatory protective restraint that is gentle and safe. Children are released as soon as they are no longer dangerous, usually after a few minutes, and most facilities strive to avoid all intensive interventions that restrict movement, such as holds and restraints.

The decision to restrain or seclude a child is made by the nurse who is working with the patient. A physician, nurse practitioner, or other advanced-level practitioner must authorize this action, either at the same time or after the fact. All patients in seclusion or restraints must be monitored constantly. Vital signs, including pulse and blood pressure, and range of motion in extremities must be monitored every 15 minutes. Hydration, elimination, comfort, and other psychological and physical needs should also be monitored. The patient's family should be informed of any incident of seclusion or restraint, and they should be encouraged to discuss the event with their child and reinforce the treatment plan to reduce the likelihood of future incidents.

Debriefings with staff after the incident help to strengthen the nurse–patient relationship, which may have been disrupted, and also enable staff to learn from the event to prevent it from happening in the future. Debriefings are important to determine if injury has occurred and identify whether the situation could have been avoided by using less restrictive alternatives. Research emphasizes the need for further reduction and eventual elimination of the use of restraints and seclusion as best practice in the clinical specialty of child and adolescent mental health (Azeem, Aujla, Rammerth, et al., 2011).

Quiet room. A unit may have an unlocked *quiet room* for a child who needs an area with decreased stimulation for regaining and maintaining self-control. Variations on the quiet room include the *feelings room*, which is carpeted and supplied with soft objects that can be punched and thrown, and the *freedom room*, which contains items for relaxation and meditation, such as music and yoga mats. The child is encouraged to express freely and work through feelings of anger or sadness in privacy and with staff support. When a child has difficulty being in touch with or expressing feelings, staff members provide practice sessions and act as role models.

Time out. Asking or directing a child or adolescent to take a *time out* from an activity is another method for intervening to halt disruptive behaviours or encourage self-control. It has been reported to be a less restrictive alternative to seclusion (Bowers, Ross, Owiti, et al., 2012). Taking a time out may require going to a designated room or sitting on the periphery of an activity until self-control is regained and the episode is reviewed with a staff member. The child's individual behavioural goals are considered in setting limits on behaviour and using time-out periods. If they are overused or used as an automatic response to a behavioural infraction, time outs lose their effectiveness.

Mind–Body Therapies

Mind–body therapies have been used in Western society for years as a treatment modality for a variety of physical and psychological disorders. These approaches focus on interactions between the mind and the body, using the mind to affect physical reactions and promote emotional health. Hypnotherapy, guided imagery, meditation, music therapy, and yoga have been shown to be effective for children and youth with mental health problems such as phobias, self-harming behaviour, anxiety, and eating disorders (Spinazzola, Rhodes, Emerson, et al., 2013). In a pilot study, Goldbeck and Ellerkamp (2012) reported that multimodal music therapy (MMT)—a combination of music therapy and CBT—was superior to treatment as usual for children with anxiety disorders.

Play Therapy

Play is often described as the work of childhood through which the child learns to master impulses and adapt to the environment.

🌀 INTEGRATIVE THERAPY

Yoga for Adolescents

Low self-esteem contributes to feelings of depression, suicide, teen pregnancy, and other health-related problems of adolescence. To live a healthy and safe life, teens need to feel good about themselves and be confident. This study involved a 20-session mindful yoga curriculum. The curriculum used the acronym *Be BOLD—Breathe, Observe, Let it go, and Do it again.* Sessions were provided to junior and senior high school students for 50 minutes 3 times a week for 7 weeks. Each session concluded with an affirmation of respect to self and others. Benefits of the program included decreased alcohol use, improved relationships, and improved attention spans.

Before teaching yoga, the nurse must assess for any physical limitation to yoga, obtain parental consent, and encourage children to progress safely, listening to their bodies and not forcing movements that might be painful.

Source: Fishbein, D., Miller, S., Herman-Stahl, M., et al. (2016). Behavioral and psychophysiological effects of a yoga intervention on high-risk adolescents: A randomized control trial. *Journal of Child and Family Studies, 25*(2), 518–529. doi:10.1007/s10826-015-0231-6.

A choice of play materials can be offered to the child to aid self-expression, assess developmental and emotional status, determine diagnosis, and institute therapeutic interventions. Clinicians can also use imaginary or pretend play with young children to gain an understanding of their world (Yanof, 2013). Melanie Klein (1955) and Anna Freud (1965) were the first to use play as a therapeutic tool in their psychoanalysis of children in the 1920s and 1930s. Axline (1969) identified the guiding principles of play therapy, which are still used by mental health care providers:

- Accept the child as he or she is and follow the child's lead.
- Establish a warm, friendly relationship that helps the child to express feelings.
- Recognize the child's feelings and reflect them back so that the child can gain insight into the behaviour.
- Accept the child's ability to solve personal problems.
- Set limits only to provide reality and security.

The many forms of play therapy can be used individually or in groups. The term *play therapy* usually refers to a one-to-one session the therapist has with a child in a playroom. Most playrooms are equipped with a range of developmentally appropriate toys, including art supplies, clay or play dough, dolls and dollhouses, hand puppets, toys, building blocks, and trucks and cars. The dolls, puppets, and dollhouse provide the child with opportunities to act out conflicts and situations involving the family, work through feelings, and develop more adaptive ways of coping. The following vignette shows how play therapy can help a child cope with a significant loss.

Mutual storytelling. Mutual storytelling is a psychodramatic technique developed by Gardner (1971) to help young children express themselves verbally. The child is asked to make up a story with a beginning, middle, and ending. At the end of the story, the child is asked to state the lesson or moral of the story. The nurse determines the psychodynamic meaning of the story

---

VIGNETTE

Hannah, a 6-year-old, begins having nightmares and refusing to go to school after her grandmother, who was also her babysitter, dies. Her parents do not let her attend the funeral, thinking it will upset her. Hannah becomes fearful and preoccupied with the death. In play sessions, she repeatedly uses dolls to act out her grandmother's hospitalization, death, and funeral. She then pretends to bury her grandmother in a small, coffinlike box. Her parents have told Hannah that "Grandma has gone to heaven." Hannah demonstrates the concept by removing "Grandma" from the box and placing her high up on a bookshelf in the playroom, looking down on the rest of the doll family.

VIGNETTE

Yotam, an intelligent 15-year-old with obsessive-compulsive behaviours and severe insecurity, lives with his parents and younger sister. In an art session, all family members are given paper on an easel and asked to draw themselves and the other members of the family. Yotam draws his parents and sister as being the same size and standing together shoulder to shoulder. He draws himself as a tiny figure in a box that appears to be suspended in space. When questioned, he reports feeling as though he were trapped in a falling elevator and disconnected from the family.

The family is surprised that he feels isolated (he is a normal size in their drawings). After completing a series of drawings and discussing them, the family is asked to draw a joint picture that requires them to work together. The picture they draw shows a smiling family standing by a house near a tree and a fence. The picture suggests that the family does view Yotam as separate and different, for although he is standing beside the family, he is placed behind the fence. This observation is discussed, and as an intervention, the family is given the task of finding ways to make Yotam feel included.

---

and selects one or two of its important themes. Using the same characters and a similar setting, the nurse retells the story, providing a healthier resolution. The lesson of the story is also reformulated to help the child become consciously aware of the better resolution. If the child has trouble starting a story, the nurse can assist by beginning the story with "Once upon a time in a faraway land there lived a …" and then asking the child to continue. After the child has identified the main characters, the nurse may need to keep prompting with comments such as "and then …" until the story is completed. The story can be recorded as audio or video, which allows for a review to reinforce the learning. A similar technique called multisensory storytelling is used with children and youth. This approach involves a combination of verbal and sensory technology (games, storytelling, video, computer animation) with an emphasis on sensory experience and social engagement (Penne, ten Brug, Munde, et al., 2012).

Therapeutic games. The use of therapeutic games is ideal for children who have difficulty talking about their feelings and problems. Playing a game with a child facilitates the development of a therapeutic alliance and provides an opportunity for conversation. The game might be as simple as checkers, but specific therapeutic games are more effective in eliciting children's fears and fantasies. Gardner (1979) developed a series of therapeutic games for children, one of which, Board of Objects, can be used with children 4 to 8 years of age. The game pieces are small items (people, animals, various objects) that are placed on a checkerboard. The players roll coloured dice. If a red side lands face up, the player selects an object. To get a reward chip, the player must say something about the object; if the player tells a story about the object, he or she gets two reward chips. The child's statement or story can be used in a therapeutic interchange (e.g., to communicate empathy or make a statement suggesting a more adaptive way to cope with a difficult situation). In the end, the player with the most chips (usually the child) wins.

A board game appropriate for latency-age children (6 to 12 years) is Gardner's (1986) Talking, Feeling, and Doing Game. The player throws dice to advance his or her playing piece along a pathway of different-coloured squares. Depending on the colour landed upon, the player draws a talking, feeling, or doing card, which gives instructions or asks a question. A reward chip is given when the player responds appropriately. For example, a feeling card might read, "All the girls in the class were invited to a birthday party except one. How did she feel?" If this game

is played with more than one child, the nurse can elicit additional responses and engage the whole group in the therapeutic interchange. The nurse may stack the deck to make sure that cards relating to the child's problems will be selected.

Bibliotherapy. Bibliotherapy involves using literature for children or adolescents to help the child express feelings in a supportive environment, gain insight into feelings and behaviour, and learn new ways to cope with difficult situations. When children listen to or read a story, they unconsciously identify with the characters and experience a catharsis of feelings. The books selected by the nurse should reflect the situations or feelings the child is experiencing. It is important to assess not only the needs of the child but also the child's readiness for the particular topic and the child's level of understanding. A children's librarian has access to a large collection of stories and knows which books are written specifically to help children deal with particular subjects; however, the nurse should read the book first to be sure that the content is age appropriate and fits with the treatment plan and be prepared to discuss it with the patient. Whenever possible, the nurse consults with the family to make sure the books do not violate the family's belief systems. A choice of several books is offered, and a book is never forced on the child.

Therapeutic drawing. Many children and adolescents love to draw and paint and will spontaneously express themselves in artwork. Their drawings capture the thoughts, feelings, and tensions they may not be able to express verbally, are unaware of, or are denying. For some, however, this modality may be too threatening or not engaging. Children and adolescents can be encouraged to draw themes, such as people, families, themselves, or more abstract themes, such as feelings. To use this modality, the nurse needs to be familiar with the drawing capabilities expected of children at particular developmental levels, and additional training is recommended. In the next vignette, the art therapist and the nurse use a family art session to identify family dynamics and begin interventions.

Psychopharmacology

Medication is usually not used as the first line of defence in treatment of children and youth with mental health disorders. Evidence of the safety and efficacy of medication use in this population is lacking (Egberts, Mehler-Wex, & Gerlach, 2011). Medicating children typically works best when combined with another treatment such as CBT (Schatzberg, 2017). Medications that target specific symptoms can make a real difference in a family's ability to cope and in quality of life, and they can enhance the child or adolescent's potential for growth. The Drug Treatment box lists some child and adolescent disorders and identifies some of the medications used in the treatment of these disorders.

NEURODEVELOPMENTAL DISORDERS

Neurodevelopmental disorders (NDDs) are a complex group of diseases that cause abnormal functions of the brain or central nervous system. Children and youth with these types of disorders show impairment in language, speech, learning, memory, and motor skills (Li, Zhao, & Gao, 2013). These attributes inhibit the child's ability to participate in age-appropriate activities and introduce the need for specific programs for the child and family. A population-based study reported that 5% of Canadian children had a disability, and, of these, 74% were classified as NDDs (Mâsse, Miller, Shen, et al., 2013). The disorders discussed in this section of the chapter are some of the most common child and adolescent NDDs.

✎ DRUG TREATMENT OF CHILD AND ADOLESCENT DISORDERS AND SYMPTOMS

DISORDER OR SYMPTOM	TYPE OF DRUG	EXAMPLES AND COMMENTS
Neurodevelopmental disorders	Antipsychotics	Risperidone (Risperdal) reduces hyperactivity, fidgetiness, and labile affect. Olanzapine (Zyprexa) reduces hyperactivity, social withdrawal, use of language, and depression.
Autism spectrum disorder	Antipsychotics	Haloperidol (Haldol) can reduce irritability and labile affect.
	Propranolol hydrochloride	Propranolol hydrochloride (Inderal) reduces rage outbursts, aggression, and severe anxiety.
	Selective serotonin reuptake inhibitors (SSRIs)	Clomipramine (Anafranil) may help treat anger and compulsive behaviour.
Attention-deficit/hyperactivity disorder (ADHD)	Stimulants	Methylphenidate hydrochloride (Ritalin, Biphentin) Amphetamine (Adderall XR) Both improve symptoms of ADHD.
	Antidepressants	Nortriptyline hydrochloride (Aventyl) Bupropion hydrochloride (Wellbutrin) Fluoxetine hydrochloride (Prozac) All produce improvements in issues of hyperactivity, attention, and global functioning.
	α-Adrenergic agonists	Clonidine hydrochloride (Catapres) can be used for aggressiveness, impulsivity, and hyperactivity in patients with ADHD.
Conduct disorders	Antipsychotics	Risperidone decreases aggression.
	Stimulants	Methylphenidate decreases antisocial behaviours.
	Antidepressants	Bupropion improves symptoms of conduct disorder.
	Mood stabilizers	Carbamazepine (Tegretol) and lithium both have demonstrated efficacy in decreasing aggression.
	α-Adrenergic agonists	Clonidine hydrochloride may help with impulsive and disordered behaviours.
Panic and school phobia	SSRIs	Citalopram (Celexa), fluoxetine, and paroxetine (Paxil) decrease symptoms of anxiety.
	Tricyclic antidepressants (TCAs)	Imipramine (Impril) is commonly used.
Obsessive-compulsive disorder (OCD)	SSRIs	Fluoxetine hydrochloride and paroxetine (Paxil) decrease symptoms of anxiety.
	TCAs	Clomipramine decreases symptoms of anxiety.
	Atypical anxiolytics	Buspirone hydrochloride (Bustab) is used as adjunct treatment for refractory OCD.
Separation anxiety disorder	TCAs	Imipramine decreases symptoms of anxiety.
	SSRIs	Fluoxetine hydrochloride decreases symptoms of anxiety.
Social phobia	TCAs	Imipramine decreases symptoms of anxiety.
	Anxiolytics	Buspirone hydrochloride decreases symptoms of anxiety.
Post-traumatic stress disorder (PTSD)	Atypical antipsychotics	Risperidone is used to control the flashbacks and aggression in PTSD.
Insomnia	Antihistamines	Diphenhydramine (Benadryl) causes the adverse effect of mild sedation.
Major depression and dysthymia	SSRIs	Fluoxetine is effective in decreasing depressive symptoms.
	TCAs	No significant differences have been found between responses to TCAs and placebo.
	Atypical antidepressants	Venlafaxine (Effexor XR): One small study reported no difference between venlafaxine and placebo.
Psychotic symptoms	Antipsychotics	Quetiapine (Seroquel) and risperidone are effective in reducing positive psychotic symptoms.

Source: Adapted from Schatzberg, A. F. (2017). *Textbook of psychopharmacology: DSM-5 ed.* Arlington, VA: American Psychiatric Association Publishing.

INTELLECTUAL DISABILITIES

Intellectual developmental disorder (intellectual disability), previously called *mental retardation*, is characterized by developmental deficits in intellectual and adaptive functioning. The young child's level of disability severity occurs on a continuum that ranges from mild to moderate, severe, and profound. Impairment in children includes deficits in problem solving, reasoning, judgement, communication, self-care activities, and social participation (Burack, Hodapp, Iarocci, et al., 2012).

COMMUNICATION DISORDERS

Communication disorders occur during the early developmental period of the child and are manifested by difficultly in language skills acquisition, which affects academic achievement, social achievement, and self-care activities. The main indicators of this condition are speech and language disorders, which affect a child's ability to communicate. The child has speech-related deficits in both expressive and receptive ability, which may be evident by the inability to make vocal sounds or a disturbance in fluency. As a result, the child may stutter. The child has little or no vocabulary growth, limiting the ability to initiate or maintain engagement with others (Carlsson, Norrelgen, Kjellmer, et al., 2013). Nurses who work in a variety of settings have knowledge of appropriate developmental milestones and can serve as an important resource for children and families in early identification and referral.

AUTISM SPECTRUM DISORDER

Autism spectrum disorder (ASD) is a complex neurobiological and developmental disability that is evident during a child's first three years of life. However, few children are diagnosed before reaching school age. It is reported that 1 in every 88 children born today has ASD (Autism Society Canada, 2013). This disorder affects the normal development of the brain in social interaction and communication skills. People with ASD typically have difficulties in verbal and nonverbal communication, social interactions, and leisure or play activities. These communication difficulties can include delays in babbling, echolalia (the pathological repeating of another's words), and nonmeaningful sentences. Severity is determined by the level of communication impairments and repetitive, stereotyped behaviours (Barbaro, Ridgway, & Dissanayake, 2011).

The concordance rate for identical twins is 70% to 80% (Wade, Prime, & Madigan, 2015), indicating a genetic component to ASD. Autism is four times more common in boys than in girls (Baio, 2014). It has no racial, ethnic, or social boundaries and is not influenced by family income, educational levels, or lifestyles.

Although there is currently no universally recommended screening program for detecting ASD, Autism Society Canada (2013) has advocated for screening to be made available in Canada. Early diagnosis, identification, and intervention for children with ASD are critical to promoting better developmental outcomes for affected children and their families (Barbaro, Ridgway, &

Dissanayake, 2011). Unfortunately, many families who have a child with ASD may not know it. Often symptoms are first noticed when the infant fails to be interested in others or to be socially responsive through eye contact and facial expressions. Some children show improvement during development, but puberty can be a turning point toward either improvement or deterioration.

Without intensive intervention, individuals with severe ASD may not be able to live and work independently, and only about one third achieve partial independence with restricted interests and activities. Managing the care of a child with ASD can be very stressful for parents and families. It is important for nurses to support and educate families in the provision of health care services that are critical in assessment, detection, and intervention for these young children. Nurses from a variety of practice settings may be involved in providing care and must use a family-centred approach.

The core presenting symptoms of ASD (Barbaro, Ridgway, & Dissanayake, 2011) include the following:
- Impairment in communication and imaginative activity
  - Language delay or absence of language
  - Stereotypical or repetitive use of language
  - Lack of spontaneous make-believe or imaginative play
  - Failure to imitate others' activities or words
- Impairment in social interactions
  - Lack of responsiveness to or interest in social activities
  - Limited eye-to-eye contact and facial responses
  - Indifference or aversion to affection and physical contact
  - Inability to share enjoyment, interest, or achievement with others
  - Failure to develop friendships or cooperative or imaginative play with peers
- Markedly restricted, stereotypical patterns of behaviour, interest, and activities
  - Rigid adherence to routines and rituals with catastrophic reactions to changes in the environment (e.g., eat only certain-textured foods)
  - Stereotypical and repetitive motor mannerisms (hand or finger flapping, spinning, head banging, hand biting)
  - Preoccupation with repetitive activities (flicking light switches, pouring water, twirling string)

ATTENTION-DEFICIT/HYPERACTIVITY DISORDER

Children with attention-deficit/hyperactivity disorder (ADHD) show an inappropriate degree of inattention, impulsiveness, and hyperactivity, all of which interfere with functioning or development. Some children can have attention-deficit disorder without hyperactivity (ADD). Preschoolers with ADHD exhibit excessive gross motor activity that becomes less pronounced as the child matures. The disorder is most often detected when the child has difficulty adjusting to elementary school. Attention problems and hyperactivity contribute to low frustration tolerance, temper outbursts, labile moods, poor school performance, peer rejection, and low self-esteem (Tarver, Daley, & Sayal, 2015).

For a diagnosis of ADHD or ADD, symptoms must be present in at least two settings (e.g., at home and school). Children with

ADHD often meet the diagnostic criteria for more than one mental disorder. They may also be diagnosed as having oppositional defiant disorder or conduct disorder. Presenting symptoms of ADHD include the following:

- Inattention
  - Has difficulty paying attention during tasks (especially those requiring sustained attention) or play, even if they are enjoyable activities
  - Has difficulty listening, even with prompts and redirection
  - Is easily distracted, loses things, and is forgetful in daily activities
  - Does not pay attention to social cues
- Hyperactivity
  - Fidgets, climbs, is unable to sit still or play quietly
  - Acts as if "driven by a motor" and is constantly "on the go"
  - Talks excessively
- Impulsivity
  - Blurts out answers before the question has been completed
  - Has difficulty waiting for own turn or being patient
  - Interrupts, intrudes in others' conversations and games

ADHD in adults is now well established as a recognized disorder (Jarrett, 2016), with a prevalence of 4.4% (Canadian Attention Deficit Hyperactivity Disorder Resource Alliance [CADDRA], 2011). Most adults who seek out a referral for assessment do so after the diagnosis of their own child or someone they know well (CADDRA, 2011). Adults with ADHD may present with a primary complaint that is an associated symptom, such as procrastination, disorganization, lack of motivation, insomnia, rage attacks, or labile moods (CADDRA, 2011). Currently, treatment of ADHD in adults is either not available or not adequate. Adult ADHD represents a significant health care need requiring physician and nursing education, the establishment of services within the health care system, and appropriate research on treatment and service delivery. The latest practice guidelines published by the CADDRA are available online at http://www.caddra.ca.

SPECIFIC LEARNING DISORDER (SLD)

Specific learning disorder (SLD) in children is identified during the school-aged years and varies in severity from mild to moderate to severe. One prominent feature is impairment in academic skills such as reading (dyslexia), mathematics (dyscalculia), and written expression (dysgraphia) acquisition. The prevalence of this disorder is 5% to 15% among school-aged children, and it is more common in males than in females (Peterson & Pennington, 2012). SLD is lifelong, so early assessment, intervention, and support are important for the child and the family. Nurses are instrumental in teaching parents and children how to manage and live with the disorder. Also, ongoing assessment will involve other professionals with expertise in the areas of SLD and psychological and cognitive assessment.

The educational and occupational outcomes for individuals with SLD include high dropout rates, low graduation rates, failure to attend postsecondary facilities, and higher rates of unemployment (Stein, Blum, & Barbaresi, 2011). Children and youth with SLD may require accommodation in school and their work environment. The Learning Disabilities Association of Canada, an important advocacy group for this population, provides education and support to families, teachers, and health care providers. These children and their families receive assistance through provincial and territorial school-based services and also through a disability tax credit offered by the federal government.

MOTOR DISORDERS

Motor coordination is important for children as they negotiate their world. These disorders present in the early developmental period, interfering with gross motor and fine motor skills. Developmental coordination disorder is diagnosed before 5 years of age when acquisition of motor skills or coordination is below what is expected for young children achieving motor milestones such as sitting, crawling, or walking (Zwicker, Missiuna, Harris, et al., 2012). These disorders are chronic and cause impairment in activities of daily living.

Two prevalent motor disorders are *stereotypic movement disorder* and *Tourette's disorder*. Stereotypic movement disorder is demonstrated by repetitive and stereotypic motor behaviour (e.g., body rocking, head nodding, hand shaking, waving). These movements are usually seen in young children during the first three years of life, and behaviours may occur many times during the day and last seconds, minutes, or longer. The stereotypic self-injury behaviours (e.g., head banging, self-biting, eye poking) may persist for years. The repetitive motor behaviour interferes with social, academic, or other daily activities (Jankovic & Kurlan, 2011). In assessment, the nurse needs to be aware that simple stereotypic movements are common in infancy and childhood (e.g., rocking) but usually resolve with age.

Interventions focus on changing behaviour, promoting safety, and preventing injury. Protective clothing (e.g., helmet, gloves) may be recommended for children who are prone to self-harm behaviour, as well as behaviour modification techniques including distraction and replacement. Psychotropic medications may be prescribed to reduce self-harm occurrences (Ougrin, Tranah, Leigh, et al., 2012).

Tourette's disorder (TD) usually presents itself before 18 years of age. The disorder is characterized by the presence of multiple motor tics (sudden, repetitive motor movements) and one or more vocal tics that repeat many times throughout the day. Tic disorders typically begin between 4 and 6 years of age, and diagnosis is based on the presence of motor or vocal tics or both for more than 1 year. Tics are classified as either simple (e.g., eye blinking, grunting) or complex (e.g., sexual or obscene gestures [copropraxia]). A child or adolescent with tics may experience impairment in social and academic relationships as a result of feeling ashamed and self-conscious and of being ridiculed or bullied by peers (Smith, Fox, & Trayner, 2015). Other symptoms associated with TD are obsessions, compulsions, hyperactivity, distractibility, and impulsivity.

Prevalence estimates in school-aged children range from 3 to 8 per 1 000, with males more commonly affected than females (Aldred & Cavanna, 2015). The disorder is usually permanent, but periods of remission may occur, and symptoms often diminish during adolescence and sometimes disappear by young adulthood. About 90% of people with TD have a comorbid disorder (Aldred & Cavanna, 2015). Common comorbidities include ADHD; obsessive-compulsive disorder; and depressive, bipolar, or substance use disorders.

The first-line treatment for TD is behaviour therapy rather than drug treatment. Pharmacological treatment is recommended only if tics are distressing and interfering with daily activities (Pringsheim, Doja, Gorman, et al., 2012). A comprehensive behavioural intervention for tics (CBIT) refers to habit-reversal training, which helps the patient to self-monitor current tics and then use a competing muscular response that is incompatible with the tic (Piacentini, Woods, Scahill, et al., 2010). The Canadian guidelines for treatment of tic disorders support the use of behavioural therapy, particularly habit-reversal therapy (HRT) and exposure and response prevention (ERP), for both adults and children. However, the use of deep brain stimulation or transcranial magnetic stimulation as treatment options is not recommended. Due to a lack of evidence to support their effectiveness, these treatments are considered experimental and are recommended only for adults in severe cases (Steeves, McKinlay, Gorman, et al., 2012).

APPLICATION OF THE NURSING PROCESS

ASSESSMENT

Assessment is the first stage of the nursing process. Assessing for developmental milestones, child–parent relationship, and mental status is critical when initiating care for patients with NDDs.

DIAGNOSIS

The child with an NDD has severe impairments in social interactions and communication skills, often accompanied by stereotypical behaviour, interests, and activities. The stress on the family can be severe, owing to the chronic nature of the disease. The severity of the impairment is evident in the degree of responsiveness to or interest in others, the presence of associated behavioural problems (e.g., head banging), and the ability to bond with peers. Table 27-1 lists potential nursing diagnoses.

OUTCOMES IDENTIFICATION

Nursing Outcomes Classification (NOC) (Moorhead, Johnson, Maas, et al., 2012) identifies a number of outcomes appropriate for the child with an NDD. Table 27-2 presents examples of *NOC* outcomes and supporting indicators that target developmental competencies and coping skills.

IMPLEMENTATION

Currently, two therapies reported to be effective interventions for ASD are applied behavioural analysis (ABA) and intensive behavioural intervention (IBI). These therapies are expensive, not available in all provinces and territories, and not routinely

 ASSESSMENT GUIDELINES
Neurodevelopmental Disorders

- Assess for developmental delays, uneven development, or loss of acquired abilities. Use baby books and diaries, photographs, films, or videotapes.
- Assess the quality of the parent–child relationship for evidence of bonding, anxiety, tension, and quality of caregiver–child temperaments.
- Be aware that children with behavioural and developmental problems are at risk for abuse, and be knowledgeable about community programs providing support services for parents and children, including parent education, counselling for parents and children, and after-school programs.

ASSESSMENT GUIDELINES
Attention-Deficit/Hyperactivity Disorder (ADHD)

- Observe for level of physical activity, attention span, talkativeness, frustration tolerance, impulse control, and the ability to follow directions.
- Assess social skills, friendship history, problem-solving skills, and school performance. Academic failure and poor peer relationships lead to low self-esteem, depression, and further acting out.
- Assess for associated comorbidities, such as depression.

publicly funded. However, the federal government offers a variety of income support for individuals with autism and their parents through the *Income Tax Act* and Canada Pension Plan Disability Benefits (Standing Senate Committee on Social Affairs, Science and Technology, 2007). These supports are usually insufficient to meet the demands of individuals with autism and their families.

Treatment plans include behaviour management plans with a reward system and education of parents for providing structure, rewards, consistency in rules, and expectations at home in order to shape and modify behaviour and foster the development of socially appropriate skills. It is important that the nurse recognize and capitalize on the individual's and family's strengths and incorporate them into the plan of care. Pharmacological agents such as risperidone (Risperdal), clomipramine (Anafranil), and desipramine are used with some success in conjunction with ongoing psychiatric medication management.

Interventions for ADHD include administration of pharmacological agents for the inattention and hyperactive-impulsive behaviours, behaviour modification, family counselling, and play therapy for young children. As the child ages, special education programs to address the academic difficulties and CBT may also be appropriate. Children and teens in specialized programs (e.g., day treatment programs) may receive additional services, such as recreational or art therapy.

Paradoxically, the mainstay of treatment for ADHD is the use of psychostimulant drugs. Responses to these drugs can be

TABLE 27-1   POTENTIAL NURSING DIAGNOSES FOR DISORDERS OF CHILDHOOD AND ADOLESCENCE

SIGNS AND SYMPTOMS	NURSING DIAGNOSIS
Lack of responsiveness or interest in others, lack of empathy, or unwillingness to share	*Impaired social interaction*
	Risk for impaired parent or child attachment
Severe behaviour problems, creating stress on family members	*Risk for caregiver role strain*
	Interrupted family processes
	Chronic sorrow
	Spiritual distress
Lack of cooperation or imaginative play with peers	*Activity intolerance*
Disruptive, hostile behaviour, leading to difficulty in making or keeping friends	*Situational low self-esteem*
Language delay or absence, stereotyped or repetitive use of language	*Impaired verbal communication*
Inability to feed, bathe, dress, or toilet self at age-appropriate level	*Delayed growth and development*
Head banging, face slapping, hand biting	*Risk for trauma*
Catastrophic reactions (e.g., severe temper tantrums, rage reactions)	*Risk for other-directed violence*
Impulsiveness, anger, and aggression	*Risk for self-mutilation*
Thoughts or verbalizations regarding self-harm	*Risk for self-directed violence*
Frequent disregard for bodily needs	*Self-care deficit (bathing, dressing, feeding, and toileting)*
	Risk for situational low self-esteem
Conflict with authority, refusal to comply with requests	*Powerlessness*
	Readiness for enhanced power
Failure to follow age-appropriate social norms	*Ineffective coping*
Blaming of others for problems or for causing his or her actions	*Defensive coping*
	Impaired individual resilience
Fear of being separated from parent (e.g., going to school or to a party)	*Anxiety*
	Relocation stress syndrome
Depression	*Stress overload*
	Spiritual distress
Refusal to attend school	*Ineffective coping*
	Readiness for enhanced parenting
Inability to concentrate, withdrawal, difficulty in functioning, feeling down, change in vegetative symptoms	*Risk for suicide*
Re-experiences of past trauma (dreams, illusions, flashbacks)	*Post-trauma syndrome*
	Rape-trauma syndrome
Fear of objects, people, or situations	*Anxiety*

TABLE 27-2   *NOC* OUTCOMES FOR NEURODEVELOPMENTAL DISORDERS

NURSING OUTCOME AND DEFINITION	INTERMEDIATE INDICATORS	SHORT-TERM INDICATORS
Child development: 3 Years: Milestones of physical, cognitive, and psychosocial progression by 3 years of age	Speech understood by strangers	Gives own first name
Child development: 4 Years: Milestones of physical, cognitive, and psychosocial progression by 4 years of age	Engages in creative play	Draws person with three parts
Child development: 5 Years: Milestones of physical, cognitive, and psychosocial progression by 5 years of age	Follows simple rules of interactive games with peers	Recognizes most letters of the alphabet
Communication: Expressive: Expression of meaningful verbal or nonverbal messages	Directs messages appropriately	Uses spoken language; vocal
Play participation: Use of activities by a child from 1 year through 11 years of age to promote enjoyment, entertainment, and development	Expresses emotions during play activities	Expresses satisfaction with play activities

Source: Moorhead, S., Johnson, M., Maas, M., et al. (2012). *Nursing outcomes classification (NOC)* (5th ed.). St. Louis: Mosby.

dramatic and can quickly increase attention and task-directed behaviour while reducing impulsivity, restlessness, and distractibility (Burchum & Rosenthal, 2016). Methylphenidate (Ritalin) is the most widely used psychostimulant because of its safety and simplicity of use. However, there is a risk for abuse and misuse. Unfortunately, the medication has gained a reputation as a street drug. A common adverse effect of stimulant ADHD medications is insomnia (Burchum & Rosenthal, 2016). To combat this effect, treating with the minimal effective dose is essential, as is administering the medication no later than 1600 hours.

Other adverse effects include headache, abdominal pain, and lethargy. Growth retardation secondary to appetite suppression has been associated with the use of stimulants, although studies have provided contradictory findings.

A nonstimulant serotonin–norepinephrine reuptake inhibitor (SNRI), atomoxetine (Strattera), is approved for childhood and adult ADHD. Although not as effective in improving symptoms as the stimulants, this drug eliminates the risk for abuse. Therapeutic responses develop slowly, and full improvement may take up to 3 weeks (Burchum & Rosenthal, 2016). The most common adverse effects are gastrointestinal disturbances, reduced appetite, weight loss, dizziness, fatigue, and insomnia. It may also cause a small increase in blood pressure and heart rate. Rarely, serious allergic reactions occur.

The dosing schedule of stimulant and nonstimulant medications is important. Drug preparations vary in their onset of action and duration of action, so dosing may be only once a day (in the morning) or up to three times a day. Because once-a-day dosing is easier and avoids the uncertainty and potential stigma of taking medications at school, long-acting medications tend to be more attractive. See Drug Treatment of Patients with ADHD for a summary of the Canadian-approved medications used to treat ADHD.

DISRUPTIVE, IMPULSE CONTROL, AND CONDUCT DISORDERS

OPPOSITIONAL DEFIANT DISORDER

Oppositional defiant disorder is a recurrent pattern of negativistic, disobedient, hostile, defiant behaviour toward authority figures without going so far as to seriously violate the basic rights of others (Winther, Carlsson, & Vance, 2013). Children with this disorder exhibit persistent stubbornness and argumentativeness, limit testing, unwillingness to give in or negotiate, touchiness and quick annoyance, and refusal to accept blame for misdeeds. The behaviours lead to significant impairment in home or social relationships and school or occupational functioning. Children and adolescents with oppositional defiant disorder justify their behaviour as a response to unreasonable demands or situations.

This disorder is usually evident before 8 years of age and, until puberty, is more common in males; after that point, the prevalence is equal for males and females. This disorder may vary in severity from mild to moderate to severe, and the severity is determined by the symptoms and setting (e.g., at home, at school, with peers, at work). Symptoms may be confined to only one setting (mild), be present in at least two settings (moderate), or appear in three or more settings (severe). Children and youth with this diagnosis have an increased risk for problems (e.g., antisocial behaviour, impulse control issues, substance use, anxiety, depression) as they transition to adulthood (Burke, 2012).

CONDUCT DISORDER

Conduct disorder is characterized by a persistent pattern of antisocial behaviour in which children and adolescents have no concern for the rights of others and a disregard for appropriate societal norms or rules. Children with this disorder also display callous–unemotional traits (e.g., lack of empathy or guilt, shallow affect) (American Psychiatric Association, 2013) and bullying, threatening, or intimidating behaviour. It is one of the most frequently diagnosed disorders of childhood and adolescence, and the behaviours associated with conduct disorder are commonly observed within settings frequented by this population (e.g., school, home, community). Complications associated with conduct disorder are academic failure, school suspensions and dropouts, juvenile delinquency, drug and alcohol abuse and dependency, and juvenile court involvement. Psychiatric disorders that frequently coexist with conduct disorder are anxiety, depression, ADHD, learning disabilities, and substance dependency.

There are four types of conduct disorder: (1) aggression toward people and animals, (2) property destruction, (3) theft, and (4)

💊 DRUG TREATMENT OF PATIENTS WITH ADHD

CLASSIFICATION	TRADE NAME	INDICATIONS	DURATION	SCHEDULE
Methylphenidate hydrochloride	Ritalin	Ages 6–12	3–5 hours	2 or 3 times a day
Extended or sustained release	Ritalin SR	Ages 6–12	6–8 hours	1 or 2 times a day
	Biphentin	Ages 6 and older	10–12 hours	Once a day
	Concerta	Ages 6–65	Up to 14 hours	Once a day
Dextroamphetamine sulphate	Dexedrine	Ages 3–16	4–6 hours	2 or 3 times a day
Short acting				
Intermediate acting	Dexedrine Spansule SRC	Ages 6–16	6–10 hours	1 or 2 times a day
Lisdexamfetamine dimesylate	Vyvanse	Ages 6–12	10–12 hours	Once a day
Amphetamine mixture	Adderall XR	Ages 6 and older	10–12 hours	1 or 2 times a day
Extended release				
Atomoxetine hydrochloride	Strattera	Ages 6–65	24 hours	Once a day
Extended release				

Source: Adapted from Burchum, J., & Rosenthal, L. (2016). *Lehne's pharmacology for nursing care* (9th ed.). Philadelphia: Saunders; Riddle, M. A. (2016). *Pediatric psychopharmacology for primary* care. Elk Grove Village, IL: American Academy of Pediatrics; and Schatzberg, A. F. (2017). *Textbook of psychopharmacology: DSM-5 ed.*. Arlington, VA: American Psychiatric Association Publishing.

serious violations of rules. There are two subtypes of conduct disorder—child onset and adolescent onset—both of which can occur in mild, moderate, or severe forms. Predisposing factors are ADHD, oppositional child behaviours, parental rejection, inconsistent parenting with harsh discipline, early institutional living, chaotic home life, large family size, absent mother or father, mother or father who abuses alcohol, antisocial and drug-dependent family members, and association with delinquent peers.

Childhood-onset conduct disorder occurs prior to age 10 years and is found mainly in males who are physically aggressive, have poor peer relationships, show little concern for others, and lack feelings of guilt or remorse. These children frequently misperceive others' intentions as hostile and believe that their aggressive responses are justified. Violent children also often display antisocial reasoning, such as "He deserved it," when rationalizing aggressive behaviours (Frick, 2012). Children with childhood-onset conduct disorder attempt to project a strong image, but they actually have low self-esteem. They also display limited frustration tolerance, irritability, and temper outbursts. Individuals with childhood-onset conduct disorder are more likely to have problems that persist through adolescence and, without intensive treatment, develop antisocial personality disorder in the adult years.

In *adolescent-onset conduct disorder*, youths tend to act out misconduct with their peer group (e.g., early onset of sexual behaviour, substance abuse, risk-taking behaviours). Males are apt to fight, steal, vandalize, and have discipline problems in school, whereas girls tend to lie, be truant, run away, abuse substances, and engage in prostitution. The male-to-female ratio is not as high as for the childhood-onset type, indicating that more girls become aggressive during this period of development (Thornton, Frick, Crapanzano, et al., 2013).

Bullying

Bullying, as a concept, is broadly defined in terms of behaviour and its impact on those who are bullied. Globally, the occurrence of child and adolescent bullying in society has become a universal concern and is recognized as a major public health problem. Children and youth with disruptive, impulse control, or conduct disorder may display aggressive behaviour toward others. Bullying is identified as an abuse of power that involves three components: harm, repetition, and unequal power. It is manifested in several ways, often called *physical* (e.g., hitting, kicking), *verbal* (e.g., threats, derogatory remarks or names), *relational* (e.g., social exclusion, spreading of rumours), and *cyberbullying* (i.e., bullying carried out through electronic means) (Klomek, Sourander, & Gould, 2010).

In Canada, the rates of bullying are reported to be higher than in many other countries (Lamb, Pepler, & Craig, 2009). Children who are victims of bullying experience low self-esteem, see themselves as socially incompetent, have more physical health problems, may go through depression, and may experience suicidal ideation. Research has also reported that the bullies themselves are more prone to substance misuse and to becoming involved in antisocial behaviours as teens and adults (van Noorden, Haselager, Cillessen, et al., 2015).

Nurses should be aware that children who are being bullied may not report problems unless asked directly (Vernberg, Nelson, Fonagy, et al., 2011). It is imperative that nurses and parents or other caregivers be knowledgeable of specific signs that may indicate bullying. Some reported behaviours are sleep disturbances, unexplained cuts or bruises, tearfulness, requesting to change schools, fear of walking to and from school, and self-harm behaviours (Klomek, Sourander, & Gould, 2010). Nurses play an important role in detecting early symptoms and signs through assessment and screening and need to work with the patient, family, and members of the school system to offset difficulties for these children and adolescents. A great resource for bullied children and their families is a government website that aims to stop bullying called Bullying Canada at https://www.bullyingcanada.ca/.

APPLICATION OF THE NURSING PROCESS

ASSESSMENT

When clinicians are assessing for the presence of a behavioural disorder, it is important to gather information from the perspective of the child and from that of the parent or guardian. Determining how the child and parent interact with each other as well as how the child interacts with peers, extended family, and authority figures yields valuable assessment data.

DIAGNOSIS

Children and adolescents with oppositional defiant disorder or conduct disorder display disruptive behaviours that are impulsive, angry or aggressive, and often dangerous. They are often in conflict with others, do not follow rules, do not follow age-appropriate social norms, and have inappropriate ways of meeting their needs. Refer to Table 27-1 for potential nursing diagnoses.

OUTCOMES IDENTIFICATION

NOC identifies a number of outcomes appropriate for the child experiencing hyperactivity, severe inattention, or difficulty controlling his or her impulses. These symptoms are most commonly seen in children with the neurodevelopmental disorder ADHD and in children who have any of the disruptive, impulse control, and conduct disorders (e.g., oppositional defiant disorder, conduct disorder, intermittent explosive disorder). Table 27-3 lists a sampling of *NOC* outcomes and supporting indicators that target hyperactivity, impulse self-control, the development of self-identity and self-esteem, positive coping skills, and family functioning.

IMPLEMENTATION

Interventions for severe oppositional defiant and conduct disorders focus on correcting the faulty personality (ego and superego) development, which includes firmly entrenched patterns such as blaming others and denial of responsibility for actions. Children and adolescents with these disorders also must generate more mature and adaptive coping mechanisms and prosocial

ASSESSMENT GUIDELINES

Disruptive, Impulse Control, and Conduct Disorders

- Assess the quality of the relationship between the child or adolescent and parents or caregivers for evidence of bonding, anxiety, tension, and quality of fit between temperaments, all of which can contribute to the development of disruptive behaviours.
- Assess parents' or caregivers' understanding of growth and development, effective parenting skills, and handling of problematic behaviours; a lack of knowledge and poor parenting contribute to the development of these problems.
- Assess cognitive, psychosocial, and moral development for lags or deficits because immaturity in developmental competencies results in disruptive behaviours.
- Assess for involvement in the justice system, which may suggest a lack of impulse control or a disregard for the rights of others.
- Assess parenting practices for rules, roles, and responsibilities in the family, relationships with siblings and extended family, history of conflict, and presence of support system (e.g., extended family members, clergy, after-school program).
- Assess the school history for problems and strengths in school, grades, occupational goals, disciplinary problems, and placements.

Oppositional Defiant Disorder

- Identify issues that result in power struggles and triggers for outbursts; note when they begin and how they are handled.

- Assess the child's or adolescent's view of his or her behaviour and its impact on others at home, at school, and with peers. Explore feelings of empathy and remorse.
- Explore how the child or adolescent can exercise control and take responsibility, problem-solve for situations that occur, and plan to handle things differently in the future. Assess barriers to change, motivation to change, and potential rewards to engage the patient.

Conduct Disorder

- Assess the seriousness, types, and initiation of disruptive behaviour and how it has been managed.
- Assess anxiety, aggression and anger levels, motivation, and the ability to control impulses.
- Assess moral development, problem solving, belief system, and spirituality for the ability to understand the impact of hurtful behaviour on others, to empathize with others, and to feel remorse.
- Assess the ability to form a therapeutic relationship and engage in honest and committed therapeutic work leading to observable behavioural change (e.g., signing a behavioural contract, drug testing, living according to "house rules").
- Assess for substance use (past and present).

TABLE 27-3 *NOC* OUTCOMES FOR ATTENTION-DEFICIT/HYPERACTIVITY DISORDER AND DISRUPTIVE, IMPULSE CONTROL, AND CONDUCT DISORDERS

NURSING OUTCOME AND DEFINITION	INTERMEDIATE INDICATORS	SHORT-TERM INDICATORS
Hyperactivity level: Severity of patterns of inattention of impulsivity in a child from 1 year through 17 years of age	Inappropriate aggressive behaviour decreases	Active listening
Impulse self-control: Self-restraint of compulsive or impulsive behaviours	Self-control maintenance without supervision	Identification of harmful impulsive behaviours
Self-esteem: Personal judgement of self-worth	Expression of feelings about self-worth	Acceptance of self-limitations
Coping: Personal actions to manage stressors that tax an individual's resources	Reports of psychological comfort increase	Identification of effective coping patterns
Family normalization: Capacity of the family system to maintain routines and develop strategies for optimal functioning when a member has a chronic illness or disability	Maintenance of usual parenting expectations for affected child; help sought from a health care provider as appropriate	Acknowledgement of impairment and its potential to alter family routines

Source: Data from Ackley, B., Ladwig, G., & Makic, B. F. (2017). *Nursing diagnosis handbook: An evidence-based guide to planning care* (11th ed.). St. Louis: Mosby; and Moorhead, S., Johnson, M., Maas, M., et al. (2012). *Nursing outcomes classification (NOC)* (5th ed.). St. Louis: Mosby.

goals, a process that is gradual and cannot be accomplished during short-term treatment. In the case of conduct disorder, inpatient hospitalization for crisis intervention, evaluation, and treatment planning, as well as transfer to therapeutic foster care, a group home, or long-term residential treatment, is often needed.

Oppositional youths are generally treated on an outpatient basis, using individual, group, and family therapy, with much of the focus on parenting issues.

Unfortunately, studies indicate that many children who are simply placed in group homes and in some residential programs do not maintain improvements following discharge. However, intensive programs such as multisystemic therapy and therapeutic foster care and the use of interprofessional, community-based treatment teams for children with serious emotional and behavioural disturbances have been found to improve outcomes and reduce offences over the long term (Besier, Fegert, & Goldbeck, 2009). These types of programs are more promising in improving positive adjustment, decreasing negative behaviours, and improving family stability. Unfortunately, many of these types of resources are limited to youth under the age of 18 years. Active case management strategies are required to assist youth transitioning into the adult system.

To control the aggressive behaviours, a wide variety of pharmacological agents have been tried, including antipsychotics, lithium, anticonvulsants, and antidepressants, with limited effect (Calles, 2011). CBT is used to change the pattern of misconduct by fostering the development of internal controls and working with the family to improve coping and support. Development of problem solving, conflict resolution, empathy, and social skills is an important component of the treatment program.

Families are actively engaged in therapy and given support in using parenting skills to provide nurturance and set consistent limits. They are taught techniques for behaviour modification, monitoring medication for effects, collaborating with teachers to foster academic success, and setting up a home environment that is consistent, structured, and nurturing and that promotes achievement of normal developmental milestones. If families are abusive, drug dependent, or highly disorganized, the child may require out-of-home placement. The following nursing interventions are helpful when working with parents and caregivers:

- Explore the impact of the child's behaviours on family life and the impact of the other members' behaviour on the child.
- Assist the immediate and extended family to access available and supportive individuals and systems.
- Discuss how to make home a safe environment, especially in regard to weapons and drugs; attempt to talk separately to family members whenever possible.
- Discuss realistic behavioural goals and how to set them; problem-solve potential problems.
- Teach behaviour modification techniques. Practise the techniques through role-play, with the parents in different problem situations that might arise with their child.
- Give support and encouragement as parents learn to apply new techniques.
- Provide education about medications.
- Refer parents or caregivers to a local self-help group.
- Advocate for special education services if needed.

Techniques for managing disruptive behaviours are listed in Box 27-5.

ANXIETY DISORDERS

The developmental period of childhood through adolescence poses many challenges. As a result, an anxiety disorder, such as separation anxiety disorder, specific phobia, social anxiety disorder, or adjustment disorder, may develop. Separation anxiety disorder and generalized anxiety disorder are discussed in more detail below.

The prevalence of anxiety disorders is higher than virtually all other mental disorders of childhood and adolescence (Butler-Jones, 2011). Not all anxiety is abnormal in childhood or adolescence, and a number of fears are a part of normal development. Young people may worry about grades, peer problems, or family issues. Anxiety becomes problematic when the child or adolescent fails to move beyond the fears associated with a particular problem or when the anxiety interferes with functioning over an extended period of time.

There is evidence of genetic contributions to anxiety disorders (Shimada-Sugimoto, Otowa, & Hettema, 2015). However, genetic predisposition does not mean that a disorder will develop. From a prevention standpoint, early intervention and support can be effective. Cognitive theorists propose that anxiety is the result of dysfunctional efforts to make sense of life events.

The physiological, behavioural, and cognitive characteristics of anxiety in youth are clinically similar to those in adults. Selective serotonin reuptake inhibitors (SSRIs) have demonstrated efficacy for the treatment of childhood social anxiety disorder (Masi, Pfanner, Mucci, et al., 2012). Studies have shown that CBT in combination with medication offers more benefit than either therapy alone (Lee, Dupuis, Jones, et al., 2013).

SEPARATION ANXIETY DISORDER

Separation anxiety disorder is recognized as one of the most common anxiety disorders in childhood. Children and adolescents with separation anxiety disorder become excessively anxious when separated from or anticipating separation from their home or parental figures. The fear or anxiety in children is usually persistent and excessive and results in impairment in social, academic, or occupational functioning (Allen, Lavallee, Herren, et al., 2010). Separation anxiety disorder may develop after a significant stress, such as the death of a relative or pet, an illness, a move or change in schools, or a physical or sexual assault. The prevalence in children is estimated to be 4%, with a higher incidence among females. It is common in first-degree biological relatives of an affected individual, and the incidence may be higher in children whose mothers have a panic disorder. Although remission rates are high, the disorder can persist and lead to panic disorder with agoraphobia. A depressed mood often accompanies the anxiety.

Characteristics of separation anxiety disorder identified in this population are the following (Allen, Lavallee, Herren, et al., 2010):

- Excessive distress when separated or anticipating separation from home or parental figures
- Excessive worries one will be lost, that parents will be harmed, or that the home will be violated or damaged
- Fear of being home alone or in situations without significant adults
- Refusal to sleep unless near a parental figure or refusal to sleep away from home

BOX 27-5 TECHNIQUES FOR MANAGING DISRUPTIVE BEHAVIOURS

Behavioural contract: A verbal or written agreement between the patient and nurse or other parties (e.g., family, treatment team, teacher) about behaviours, expectations, and needs. The contract is periodically evaluated and reviewed and typically coupled with rewards and other contingencies, both positive and negative.

Counselling: Verbal interactions, role-playing, and modelling to teach, coach, or maintain adaptive behaviour and provide positive reinforcement. It is most effective for motivated youth and those with well-developed communication and self-reflective skills.

Modelling: A method of learning behaviours or skills by observation and imitation that can be used in a wide variety of situations. It is enhanced when the modeller is perceived to be similar (e.g., age, interests) and attending to the task is required.

Role-playing: A counselling technique in which the nurse, the patient, or a group of youngsters act out a specified script or role to enhance the understanding of that role, learn and practise new behaviours or skills, and practise specific situations. It requires well-developed expressive and receptive language skills.

Planned ignoring: When behaviours are determined by staff not to be dangerous but are attention seeking, they may be ignored. Additional interventions may be used in conjunction (e.g., positive reinforcement for on-task actions).

Use of signals or gestures: Use a word, a gesture, or eye contact to remind the child to use self-control. To help promote behavioural change, this technique may be used in conjunction with a behavioural contract and a reward system. An example is placing your finger to your lips and making eye contact with a child who is talking during a quiet drawing activity.

Physical distance and touch control: You could move closer to the child for a calming effect, perhaps putting an arm around the child (with permission). Evaluate the effect of this, because some children may find such an action more agitating and may need more space and less physical closeness. This technique also may involve putting the nurse or a staff member between certain children who have a history of conflict.

Redirection: A technique used following an undesirable or inappropriate behaviour to engage or re-engage an individual in an appropriate activity. It may involve the use of verbal directives (e.g., setting firm limits), gestures, or physical prompts.

Additional affection: Giving a child planned emotional support for a specific problem or engaging in an enjoyable activity. It can be used to redirect a child away from an undesirable activity as well. This might be involvement in an activity, such as a game of basketball or working on a puzzle. This shows acceptance of the child while ignoring the behaviour and can increase rapport in the nurse–patient relationship.

Use of humour: Use well-timed, appropriate kidding about some external, nonpersonal (to the child) event as a diversion to help the child save face and relieve feelings of guilt or fear.

Clarification as intervention: Breaking down a problem situation that a child experiences can help the child understand the situation, other people's roles, and his or her own motivation for the behaviour. This technique can be done verbally or using worksheets, depending on the age and functional level of the child.

Restructuring: Changing an activity in a way that will decrease the stimulation or frustration (e.g., shorten a story, change to a physical activity). Restructuring requires flexibility and planning in advance to have an alternative in mind in case the activity is not going well.

Limit setting: Giving direction, stating an expectation, or telling a child what to do or where to go. Limit setting should be done firmly, calmly, without judgement or anger, preferably in advance of any problem behaviour occurring and consistently when in a treatment setting among multiple staff members. An example is "I would like for you to stop turning the light on and off."

Simple restitution: Refers to a procedure in which an individual is required or expected to correct the adverse environmental or relational effects of his or her misbehaviour by restoring the environment to its prior state, making a plan to correct his or her actions with the nurse, and implementing the plan (e.g., apologizing to the persons harmed, fixing the chairs that are upturned). Simple restitution is not punitive in nature, and there are typically additional activities involved (e.g., counselling).

Physical restraint: Therapeutic holding to control and protect the child from his or her own impulses to act out and hurt self or others.

- Refusal to attend school or other activities without parents
- Physical or somatic symptoms of anxiety

GENERALIZED ANXIETY DISORDER (GAD)

The child or youth with generalized anxiety disorder (GAD) has excessive worry or anxiety over routine activities such as school, family, or sports. The individual finds it difficult to control the worry and experiences physiological symptoms such as headache, muscle tension, sleep disturbance, fatigue, difficulty concentrating, heart palpitations, and restlessness. This disorder occurs in about 10% of children and adolescents, with an average age of onset of about 8.5 years. Children with GAD tend to need and seek

reassurance about all performance activities or other things they are worried about. In considering a diagnosis, a complete assessment is recommended to rule out other explanations for symptoms that may not be related to anxiety (Jarrett, Black, Rapport, et al., 2015).

APPLICATION OF THE NURSING PROCESS

ASSESSMENT

Children generally report their experiences of anxiety honestly but may be a bit hesitant to elaborate on their worries. The clinician needs to use a sensitive and caring approach with an anxious child.

TABLE 27-4 *NOC* OUTCOMES FOR ANXIETY DISORDERS

NURSING OUTCOME AND DEFINITION	INTERMEDIATE INDICATOR	SHORT-TERM INDICATOR
Anxiety level: Severity of manifested apprehension, tension, or uneasiness arising from an unidentifiable source *Anxiety self-control:* Personal actions to eliminate or reduce feelings of apprehension, tension, or uneasiness from an unidentifiable source	School achievement and performance in activities of daily living Controls anxiety response and demonstrates return of basic problem-solving skills	Problem behaviours (e.g., avoidance) with peers, family members, or other community members Monitors intensity of anxiety

Source: Data from Ackley, B., Ladwig, G., & Makic, B. F. (2017). *Nursing diagnosis handbook: An evidence-based guide to planning care* (11th ed.). St. Louis: Mosby; and Moorhead, S., Johnson, M., Maas, M., et al. (2012). *Nursing outcomes classification (NOC)* (5th ed.). St. Louis: Mosby.

ASSESSMENT GUIDELINES

Anxiety Disorders

- Assess the quality of the parent–child relationship for evidence of anxiety, conflicts, and quality of fit between their temperaments.
- Assess relationships among other family members.
- Observe parent–child interactions to determine patterns.
- Assess for recent stressors and their severity, duration, and proximity to the child.
- Assess parent or caregiver understanding of developmental norms, parenting skills, and handling of problematic behaviours.
- Assess the child's developmental level, and determine whether regression has occurred.
- Assess for symptoms of anxiety and coping style.

Separation Anxiety Disorder

Assess the child's previous and current ability to separate from parents or caregivers. (The separation or individuation process may not be completed, or the child may have regressed.)

DIAGNOSIS

The chief characteristic of anxiety disorders is disabling anxiety. Refer to Table 27-1 for potential nursing diagnoses.

OUTCOMES IDENTIFICATION

NOC identifies a number of outcomes appropriate for children with an anxiety disorder. The two most relevant outcomes focus on decreasing the anxiety level of the child or adolescent and increasing the child's ability to control anxiety (Table 27-4).

IMPLEMENTATION

The nursing interventions for an anxious child or adolescent include the following:

- Help prevent the child or adolescent from experiencing panic levels of anxiety by acting as a parental surrogate, providing a safe environment, and providing for biological and psycho-social needs.
- Accept regression, but give emotional support and praise to enable progression, healing, and reintegration into activities of daily living.
- Increase self-esteem and feelings of competence in the ability to perform, achieve, and influence the present and future.
- Help the child or adolescent to accept and work through traumatic events without the use of cognitive distortions or unrealistic fears.
- Teach and practise positive self-talk and reframing to reduce cognitive distortions.
- Teach coping skills (e.g., deep breathing, counting to 10, exercise, guided imagery, listening to music, distraction) to manage feelings.

Children and adolescents with anxiety disorders are most often treated on an outpatient basis, using cognitive behavioural techniques in individual, group, or family therapy. Medications such as antidepressants, antianxiety agents, and beta blockers are also used. Cognitive therapy focuses on the underlying fears and concerns, and behaviour modification is used to shape behaviour and reinforce self-control behaviours. Children who refuse to start school are introduced gradually into the school environment, with a supportive adult present for part of the day. When adolescents develop school phobia, the goal is to return them to the classroom at the earliest possible date and give parents support in setting limits on truancy.

Refer to the Drug Treatment box for a summary of medications used in the treatment of childhood and adolescent clinical and developmental disorders.

OTHER DISORDERS OF CHILDREN AND ADOLESCENTS

DEPRESSIVE DISORDERS AND BIPOLAR AND RELATED DISORDERS

The most frequently diagnosed mood disorders (disorders whose primary symptoms relate to changes in mood) in children and adolescents are major depressive disorder, persistent depressive disorder, and bipolar I or II disorder. Symptoms of depressive or bipolar disorders in young people may be similar to the symptoms in adults (see Chapters 13 and 14), with feelings of sadness, pessimism, hopelessness, and anhedonia (inability to experience happiness); social withdrawal; and suicidal ideation. Children may have somatic complaints, be critical of themselves and others, and feel unloved. Adolescents may have psychomotor agitation or retardation and hypersomnia (Maughan, Collishaw, & Stringaris, 2013). Both children and adolescents often manifest irritability leading to aggressiveness. They are less likely than adults to have psychotic symptoms.

Factors associated with child and adolescent depression are physical and sexual abuse or neglect; homelessness; parental problems, including marital discord, death, divorce or separation, or separation from parents; learning disabilities; chronic illness; and conflicts with others, such as peers. The complications of depression are school failure and dropout, substance abuse, sexual acting out, pregnancy, running away, illegal behaviour, and suicide.

POST-TRAUMATIC STRESS DISORDER (PTSD)

Children exposed to traumatic events such as receiving acute injuries from accidents or witnessing significant harm to others may develop a trauma- or stressor-related disorder (Carrion & Kletter, 2012). After an assessment for personal exposure to an extreme traumatic stressor, further information is needed about any evidence of internalized or externalized symptoms. These symptoms may include anxiety, dissociative symptoms, emotional re-experience of the trauma, and avoidance. It is also important to explore the child's understanding of the meaning of the event and feelings of safety and security. Children whose symptoms last longer than 1 month will be diagnosed with PTSD, a disorder that can occur at any age. Young children may engage in repetitive play in which themes of the traumatic event are expressed. The child may experience frightening dreams without recognizable content. Younger children with PTSD tend to exhibit behaviours indicative of internalized anxiety. In older children and adolescents, the anxiety is more often externalized. There may be comorbid disorders such as depression and anxiety and behaviours such as self-mutilation, depending on the severity and longevity of the trauma that precipitated the PTSD (Hornor, 2013).

FEEDING AND EATING DISORDERS

Feeding and eating disorders include pica, rumination disorder, and avoidant/restrictive food intake disorder (Bryant-Waugh, Markham, Kreipe, et al., 2010). Anorexia nervosa and bulimia nervosa, which also can occur in childhood and adolescence, are described in detail in Chapter 16. Pica is the persistent eating of non-nutritive substances without an aversion to eating food. Infants and toddlers may eat paint, plaster, string, or cloth. This behaviour is frequently associated with an intellectual disorder. Rumination disorder is the repeated regurgitation and rechewing of food without apparent nausea, retching, or gastrointestinal problems. In avoidant/restrictive food intake disorder, the child fails to eat adequate amounts of food, despite availability, and there is no medical condition or intellectual disability. However, because the child fails to gain weight or undergoes a significant weight loss, he or she can develop nutritional problems that lead to developmental delays.

Interventions for these disorders include working with the family to provide a safe and well-monitored environment that prohibits placing unsafe items in the child's mouth and ensures removal of unsafe items; working with associated care providers (e.g., pediatricians, nutritionists); and providing praise and support for parents and caregivers as they manage the child's behaviour.

▮ KEY POINTS TO REMEMBER

- One in five children and adolescents in Canada suffers from a major mental illness that causes significant impairments at home, at school, with peers, and in the community.
- Factors known to affect the development of mental and emotional problems in children and adolescents include genetic influences, biochemical (prenatal and postnatal) factors, temperament, psychosocial developmental factors, social and environmental factors, and cultural influences.
- The characteristics of a resilient child include an adaptable temperament, the ability to form nurturing relationships with surrogate parental figures, the ability to distance the self from emotional chaos in parents and family, and good social intelligence and problem-solving skills.
- Children experience a number of psychiatric disorders. The most commonly diagnosed child psychiatric disorders are anxiety disorders, depressive disorders, bipolar and related disorders, and impulse control disorders.
- Treatment of childhood and adolescent disorders requires a multimodal approach in almost all instances, and family involvement is seen as critical to improvement in outcomes.
- Nurses can be important advocates for children with severe emotional and behavioural disorders.
- Cognitive behavioural therapies, social skills groups, family therapy, parent training in behavioural techniques, and individual therapy focused on self-esteem issues have been found useful.
- Skills training may focus on a variety of areas, depending on the child's or adolescent's presenting symptoms, and require an individualized assessment to determine each child's need.

▮ CRITICAL THINKING

1. Owen, a 4-year-old boy, has been diagnosed with a neuro-developmental disorder—autism.
   a. Describe the specific behavioural data you would find on assessment in terms of (1) communication, (2) social interactions, (3) behaviours and activities.
   b. Name at least three realistic outcomes for a child with an NDD.
   c. Which interventions are the most important for a child with an NDD? Identify at least six.
   d. What kinds of support should the family receive?

2. Natasha is a 7-year-old girl in grade 2 who has been diagnosed with ADHD.
   a. What clinical behaviours might she be exhibiting at home and in the classroom? Give behavioural examples for her (1) inattention, (2) hyperactivity, and (3) impulsivity.
   b. Identify at least six intervention strategies one might use for Natasha, including medication management.
   c. Describe the concept of time out.
3. Saed is an 8-year-old boy who has been diagnosed with conduct disorder.
   a. Explain to one of your classmates his probable behaviours in terms of (1) aggression toward others, (2) destruction of property, (3) deceitfulness, and (4) violation of rules.
   b. What are three outcomes for this child? What is the overall prognosis for children with this disorder?
   c. What are four ways you could support Saed's parents? Where could you refer this family within your own community?
4. Jasmine is a 16-year-old who is attending an appointment with her nurse-therapist at the local community health clinic. Jasmine has been diagnosed with depression.
   a. Based on current research, what themes would you expect to hear as Jasmine describes her experiences of depression?
   b. As you complete a mental status exam, what area of assessment is essential?

CHAPTER REVIEW

1. The nurse is assessing a teenage patient for suicidal risk. Which patient response requires immediate further nursing assessment?
   a. "The idea of death really scares me."
   b. "I smoked only one time in my life."
   c. "My mom keeps a bunch of pills in her nightstand."
   d. "I've never tried to kill myself before."
2. The nurse meets with the parents of a child diagnosed with conduct disorder. What advice from the nurse is most appropriate?
   a. "Use time out as a way to control any unacceptable behaviour."
   b. "Ignore his head banging. He is just trying to get attention."
   c. "Allow the child to come up with a list of play activities."
   d. "Encourage the child to talk when he is around others."
3. The nurse is caring for a 9-year-old patient who will be entering a freedom room. Which activity should the nurse anticipate the child would engage in?
   a. Listening to a CD
   b. Throwing pillows
   c. Sitting in the periphery of the room
   d. Punching soft objects
4. A 7-year-old male who has not met earlier normal expectations in cognitive and language development and who has difficulty establishing friendships with other schoolchildren develops a fascination with the water fountain in his neighbourhood. Which condition should the nurse anticipate?
   a. Intellectual developmental disorder
   b. Major depressive disorder
   c. Tourette's disorder
   d. Autism spectrum disorder
5. The school nurse is assessing Than, who has been coming to the office over the past week with cuts and bruises for treatment. What must the nurse include in his assessment?
   a. Assess for suicidal ideation
   b. Offer professional advice about his reasons for the visits
   c. Question Than directly about bullying
   d. Anticipate the need for an antianxiety agent

Post-Test interactive review

⊖volve WEBSITE

Visit the Evolve website for Chapter Review Answers and Rationales, Critical Thinking Answer Guidelines, and additional resources related to the content in this chapter: http://evolve.elsevier.com/Canada/Varcarolis/psychiatric/

REFERENCES

Akresh, R. (2016). Climate change, conflict, and children. *Future of Children,* 26(1), 51–71. Retrieved from http://www.futureofchildren.org/.

Aldred, M., & Cavanna, A. E. (2015). Tourette syndrome and socioeconomic status. *Neurological Sciences,* 36(9), 1643–1649. doi:10.1007/s10072-015-2223-0.

Allen, J. L., Lavallee, K. L., Herren, C., et al. (2010). DSM-IV criteria for childhood separation anxiety disorder: Informant, age, and sex differences. *Journal of Anxiety Disorders,* 24(8), 946–952. doi:10.1016/j.janxdis.2010.06.022.

American Psychiatric Association. (2013). *Diagnostic and statistical manual of mental disorders* (5th ed.). Arlington, VA: Author.

Autism Society Canada. (2013). *What is autism spectrum disorder?* Retrieved from http://autismcanada.org/about-autism/.

Axline, V. (1969). *Play therapy.* New York: Ballantine Books.

Azeem, M. W., Aujla, A., Rammerth, M., et al. (2011). Effectiveness of six core strategies based on trauma informed care in reducing seclusion and restraints at a child and adolescent psychiatric hospital. *Journal of Child & Adolescent Psychiatric Nursing,* 24(1), 11–15. doi:10.1111/j.1744-6171.2010.00262.x.

Baio, J. (2014). *Prevalence of autism spectrum disorder among children aged 8 years—Autism and developmental disabilities monitoring network, 11 sites, United States, 2010: Surveillance summaries.* Atlanta: Centers for Disease Control and Prevention.

Barbaro, J., Ridgway, L., & Dissanayake, C. (2011). Developmental surveillance of infants and toddlers by maternal and child health nurses in an Australian community-based setting: Promoting the early identification of autism spectrum disorders. *Journal of Pediatric Nursing, 26*(4), 334–347. doi:10.1016/j.pedn.2010.04.007.

Barrasso-Catanzaro, C., & Eslinger, P. J. (2016). Neurobiological bases of executive function and social-emotional development: Typical and atypical brain changes. *Family Relations, 65*(1), 108–119. doi:10.1111/fare.12175.

Benjamin, C. L., Puleo, C. M., Settipani, C. A., et al. (2011). History of cognitive-behavioral therapy in youth. *Child and Adolescent Psychiatric Clinics of North America, 20*(2), 179–189. doi:10.1016/j.chc.2011.01.011.

Besier, T., Fegert, J. M., & Goldbeck, L. (2009). Evaluation of psychiatric liaison-services for adolescents in residential group homes. *European Psychiatry, 24*, 483–489. doi:10.1016/j.eurpsy.2009.02.006.

Bowers, L., Ross, J., Owiti, J., et al. (2012). Event sequencing of forced intramuscular medication in England. *Journal of Psychiatric and Mental Health Nursing, 19*(9), 799–806. doi:10.1111/j.1365-2850.2011.01856.x.

Bryant-Waugh, R., Markham, L., Kreipe, R. E., et al. (2010). Feeding and eating disorders in childhood. *International Journal of Eating Disorders, 43*(2), 98–111. doi:10.1002/eat.20795.

Burack, J. A., Hodapp, R. M., Iarocci, G., et al. (2012). *The Oxford handbook of intellectual disability and development.* New York: Oxford University Press.

Burchum, J., & Rosenthal, L. (2016). *Lehne's pharmacology for nursing care* (9th ed.). Philadelphia: Saunders.

Burke, J. D. (2012). An affective dimension within oppositional defiant disorder symptoms among boys: Personality and psychopathology outcomes into early adulthood. *Journal of Child Psychology and Psychiatry, 53*(11), 1176–1183. doi:10.1111/j.1469-7610.2012.02598.x.

Butler-Jones, D. (2011). *The chief public health officer's report on the state of public health in Canada, 2011: Youth and young adults—Life in transition.* Ottawa: Government of Canada.

Calles, J. L., Jr. (2011). Psychopharmacologic control of aggression and violence in children and adolescents. *Pediatric Clinics of North America, 58*, 73–84. doi:10.1016/j.pcl.2010.11.002.

Canadian Attention Deficit Hyperactivity Disorder Resource Alliance (CADDRA). (2011). *Canadian ADHS practice guidelines: CAP-Guidelines* (3rd ed.). Toronto: Author.

Carlsson, L. H., Norrelgen, F., Kjellmer, L., et al. (2013). Coexisting disorders and problems in preschool children with autism spectrum disorders. *Scientific World Journal, 2013*, 1–6. doi:10.1155/2013/213979.

Carrion, V. G., & Kletter, H. (2012). Posttraumatic stress disorder: Shifting toward a developmental framework. *Child and Adolescent Psychiatric Clinics of North America, 21*(3), 573–591. doi:10.1016/j.chc.2012.05.004.

Cicchetti, D. (2010). Resilience under conditions of extreme stress: A multilevel perspective. *World Psychiatry, 9*(3), 145–154.

De Hert, M., Dirix, N., Demunter, H., et al. (2011). Prevalence and correlates of seclusion and restraint use in children and adolescents: A systematic review. *European Child and Adolescent Psychiatry, 20*(5), 221–230. doi:10.1007/s00787-011-0160-x.

Edwards, D., Evans, N., Gillen, E., et al. (2015). What do we know about the risk factors for young people moving into, through and out of inpatient mental health care? Findings from an evidence synthesis. *Child & Adolescent Psychiatry & Mental Health, 9*(55), 1–17. doi:10.1186/s13034-015-0087-y.

Egberts, K. M., Mehler-Wex, C., & Gerlach, M. (2011). Therapeutic drug monitoring in child and adolescent psychiatry. *Pharmacopsychiatry, 44*(6), 249–253. doi:10.1055/s-0031-1286291.

Fallon, B., Van Wert, M., Trocmé, N., et al. (2015). *Ontario incidence study of reported child abuse and neglect—2013 (OIS-2013).* Toronto: Child Welfare Research Portal.

Freud, A. (1965). *Normality and pathology in childhood: Assessments of development.* New York: International Universities Press.

Frick, P. J. (2012). Developmental pathways to conduct disorder: Implications for future directions in research, assessment, and treatment. *Journal of Clinical Child & Adolescent Psychology, 41*(3), 378–389. doi:10.1080/15374416.2012.664815.

Fryers, T., & Brugha, T. (2013). Childhood determinants of adult psychiatric disorder. *Clinical Practice & Epidemiology in Mental Health, 9*, 1–50. doi:10.2174/1745017901309010001.

Gardner, R. A. (1971). *Therapeutic communication with children: The mutual story-telling technique.* New York: Jason Aronson.

Gardner, R. A. (1979). Helping children cooperate in therapy. In J. D. Noshpitz & S. I. Harrison (Eds.), *Basic handbook of child psychiatry: Therapeutic interventions* (pp. 414–432). New York: Basic Books.

Gardner, R. A. (1986). The talking, feeling and doing game. In C. E. Schaefer & S. E. Reid (Eds.), *Game play: Therapeutic use of childhood games* (pp. 41–72). New York: Wiley.

Goldbeck, L., & Ellerkamp, T. (2012). A randomized controlled trial of multimodal music therapy for children with anxiety disorders. *Journal of Music Therapy, 49*(4), 395–413.

Gonzalez, A., Boyle, M. H., Kyu, H. H., et al. (2012). Childhood and family influences on depression, chronic physical conditions, and their comorbidity: Findings from the Ontario child health study. *Journal of Psychiatric Research, 46*(11), 1475–1482. doi:10.1016/j.jpsychires.2012.08.004.

Government of Alberta. (2015). *Creating connections: Alberta's addiction and mental health strategy implementation—Interim report 2011–2014.* Edmonton: Author.

Green-Hennessy, S., & Hennessy, K. (2015). Predictors of seclusion or restraint use within residential treatment centers for children and adolescents. *Psychiatric Quarterly, 86*(4), 545–554. doi:10.1007/s11126-015-9352-8.

Hagan, J. F., Shaw, J. S., & Duncan, P. M. (Eds.), (2017). *Bright futures: Guidelines for health supervision of infants, children, and adolescents* (4th ed.). Elk Grove Village, IL: American Academy of Pediatrics.

Hanington, L., Ramchandani, P., & Stein, A. (2010). Parental depression and child temperament: Assessing child to parent effects in a longitudinal population study. *Infant Behavior & Development, 33*, 88–95. doi:10.1016/j.infbeh.2009.11.004.

Hornor, G. (2013). Posttraumatic stress disorder. *Journal of Pediatric Health Care, 27*(3), e29–e38. doi:10.1016/j.pedhc.2012.07.020.

Jacobson, C. M., & Mufson, L. (2012). Interpersonal psychotherapy for depressed adolescents adapted for self-injury (IPT-ASI): Rationale, overview, and case summary. *American Journal of Psychotherapy, 66*(4), 349–374.

Jankovic, J., & Kurlan, R. (2011). Tourette syndrome: Evolving concepts. *Movement Disorders : Official Journal of the Movement Disorder Society, 26*(6), 1149–1156. doi:10.1002/mds.23618.

Jarrett, M., Black, A., Rapport, H., et al. (2015). Generalized anxiety disorder in younger and older children: Implications for learning and school functioning. *Journal of Child & Family Studies, 24*(4), 992–1003. doi:10.1007/s10826-014-9910-y.

Jarrett, M. A. (2016). Attention-deficit/hyperactivity disorder (ADHD) symptoms, anxiety symptoms, and executive functioning in emerging adults. *Psychological Assessment, 28*(2), 245–250. doi:10.1037/pas0000190.

Klein, M. (1955). The psychoanalytic play technique. *American Journal of Orthopsychiatry, 25*, 223–237.

Klomek, A. B., Sourander, A., & Gould, M. (2010). The association of suicide and bullying in childhood to young adulthood: A review of cross-sectional and longitudinal research findings. *Canadian Journal of Psychiatry, 55*(5), 282–288.

Knapp, M., Snell, T., Healey, A., et al. (2015). How do child and adolescent mental health problems influence public sector costs? Interindividual variations in a nationally representative British sample. *Journal of Child Psychology & Psychiatry, 56*(6), 667–676. doi:10.1111/jcpp.12327.

Lahiri, D. K., Sokol, D. K., Erickson, C., et al. (2013). Autism as early neurodevelopmental disorder: Evidence for a sappa-mediated anabolic pathway. *Frontiers in Cellular Neuroscience, 21*, 1–17. doi:10.3389/fncel.2013.00094.

Lamb, J., Pepler, D. J., & Craig, W. (2009). Approach to bullying and victimization. *Canadian Family Physician, 55*, 356–360.

Lee, T. C., Dupuis, A., Jones, E., et al. (2013). Effects of age and subtype on emotional recognition in children with anxiety disorders: Implications for cognitive-behavioural therapy. *Canadian Journal of Psychiatry, 58*(5), 283–290.

Li, J., Zhao, G., & Gao, X. (2013). Development of neurodevelopmental disorders: A regulatory mechanism involving bromodomain-containing proteins. *Journal of Neurodevelopmental Disorders, 5*(5), 1–11.

Masi, G., Pfanner, C., Mucci, M., et al. (2012). Pediatric social anxiety disorder: Predictors of response to pharmacological treatment. *Journal of Child and Adolescent Psychopharmacology, 22*(6), 410–414. doi:10.1089/cap.2012.0007.

Mâsse, L. C., Miller, A. R., Shen, J., et al. (2013). Patterns of participation across a range of activities among Canadian children with neurodevelopmental disorders and disabilities. *Developmental Medicine & Child Neurology, 55*(8), 729–736. doi:10.1111/dmcn.12167.

Maughan, B., Collishaw, S., & Stringaris, A. (2013). Depression in childhood and adolescence. *Journal of the Canadian Academy of Child and Adolescent Psychiatry, 22*(1), 35–40.

Mental Health Commission of Canada. (2012). *Changing directions, changing lives: The mental health strategy for Canada.* Calgary: Author.

Mohr, W. K., Martin, A., Olson, J. N., et al. (2009). Beyond point and level systems: Moving toward child-centered programming. *American Journal of Orthopsychiatry, 79*(1), 8–18. doi:10.1037/a0015375.

Moorhead, S., Johnson, M., Maas, M., et al. (2012). *Nursing outcomes classification (NOC)* (5th ed.). St. Louis: Mosby.

Ougrin, D., Tranah, T., Leigh, E., et al. (2012). Practitioner review: Self-harm in adolescents. *Journal of Child Psychology and Psychiatry, 53*(4), 337–350. doi:10.1111/j.1469-7610.2012.02525.x.

Parliament of Canada. (2001). *Canada's legal age of consent to sexual activity.* Ottawa: Author. Retrieved from http://www.parl.gc.ca/content/LOP/researchpublications/prb993-e.htm.

Penne, A., ten Brug, A., Munde, V., et al. (2012). Staff interactive style during multisensory storytelling with persons with profound intellectual and multiple disabilities. *Journal of Intellectual Disability Research, 56*(2), 167–178. doi:10.1111/j.1365-2788.2011.01448.x.

Peterson, R. L., & Pennington, B. F. (2012). Developmental dyslexia. *Lancet, 379*(9830), 1997–2007. doi:10.1016/S0140-6736(12)60198-6.

Piacentini, J., Woods, D. W., Scahill, L., et al. (2010). Behavior therapy for children with Tourette disorder: A randomized controlled trial. *Journal of the American Medical Association, 303*(19), 1929–1937. doi:10.1001/jama.2010.607.

Polaha, J., Williams, S. L., Heflinger, C. A., et al. (2015). The perceived stigma of mental health services among rural parents of children with psychosocial concerns. *Journal of Pediatric Psychology, 40*(10), 1095–1104. doi:10.1093/jpepsy/jsv054.

Pollack, N., Mulay, S., Valcour, J., et al. (2016). Suicide rates in Aboriginal communities in Labrador, Canada. *American Journal of Public Health, 106*(7), 1309–1315. doi:10.2105/AJPH.2016.303151.

Pringsheim, T., Doja, A., Gorman, D., et al. (2012). Canadian guidelines for the evidence-based treatment of tic disorders: Pharmacotherapy. *Canadian Journal of Psychiatry, 57*(3), 133–143.

Prowse, C. E. (2013). *Defining street gangs in the 21st century: Fluid, mobile, and transnational.* New York: Springer-Verlag.

Public Health Agency of Canada. (2008). *Canadian incidence study of reported child abuse and neglect 2008.* Retrieved from http://www.phac-aspc.gc.ca/cm-vee/csca-ecve/2008/.

Reinhardt, M. C., & Reinhardt, C. A. U. (2013). Attention deficit–hyperactivity disorder, comorbidities, and risk situations. *Jornal de Pediatria, 89*(2), 124–130. doi:10.1016/j.jped.2013.03.015.

Roffey, S. (2016). Building a case for whole-child, whole-school wellbeing in challenging contexts. *Educational & Child Psychology, 33*(2), 30–42. Retrieved from http://www1.bps.org.uk/.

Royal Canadian Mounted Police. (2006). *RCMP environmental scan: Feature focus: Youth gangs and guns.* Retrieved from http://publications.gc.ca/collections/collection_2012/grc-rcmp/PS64-99-2006-eng.pdf.

Schatzberg, A. F. (2017). *Textbook of psyhopharmacology: DSM-5 ed.* Arlington, VA: American Psychiatric Association Publishing.

Shimada-Sugimoto, M., Otowa, T., & Hettema, J. M. (2015). Genetics of anxiety disorders: Genetic epidemiological and molecular studies in humans. *Psychiatry and Clinical Neurosciences, 69*(7), 388–401. doi:10.1037/t07557-000.

Skinner, R., & McFaull, S. (2012). Suicide among children and adolescents in Canada: Trends and sex differences, 1980–2008. *Canadian Medical Association Journal, 184*(9), 1029–1034. doi:10.1503/cmaj.111867.

Smith, H., Fox, J. R., & Trayner, P. (2015). The lived experience of individuals with Tourette syndrome or tic disorders: A meta-synthesis of qualitative studies. *British Journal of Psychology, 106*(4), 609–634. doi:10.1111/bjop.12118.

Spinazzola, J., Rhodes, A. M., Emerson, D., et al. (2013). Application of yoga in residential treatment of traumatized youth. *Journal of the American Psychiatric Nurses Association, 17*(6), 431–444. doi:10.1177/1078390311418359.

Standing Senate Committee on Social Affairs, Science and Technology. (2006). *Out of the shadows at last: Transforming mental health, mental illness and addiction services in Canada.* Retrieved from http://www.parl.gc.ca/39/1/parlbus/commbus/senate/com-e/soci-e/rep-e/rep02may06-e.htm.

Standing Senate Committee on Social Affairs, Science and Technology. (2007). *Pay now or pay later: Autism families in crisis.* Retrieved from http://www.parl.gc.ca/Content/SEN/Committee/391/soci/rep/repfinmar07-e.htm.

Statistics Canada. (2015). *Leading causes of death, total population, by age group and sex, Canada: Annual.* Retrieved from http://www5.statcan.gc.ca/cansim/a26?lang=eng&retrLang=eng&id=1020561&&pattern=&stByVal=1&p1=1&p2=31&tabMode=dataTable&csid=#F6.

Steeves, T., McKinlay, B. D., Gorman, D., et al. (2012). Canadian guidelines for the evidence-based treatment of tic disorders: Behavioural therapy, deep brain stimulation, and transcranial magnetic stimulation. *Canadian Journal of Psychiatry, 57*(3), 144–151.

Stein, D. S., Blum, N. J., & Barbaresi, W. J. (2011). Developmental and behavioral disorders through the life span. *Pediatrics, 128*(2), 364–373. doi:10.1542/peds.2011-0266.

Stewart, S. M., Simmons, A., & Habibpour, E. (2012). Treatment of culturally diverse children and adolescents with depression. *Journal of Child and Adolescent Psychopharmacology, 22*(1), 72–79. doi:10.1089/cap.2011.0051.

Sullivan, E. V., Pfefferbaum, A., Rohlfing, T., et al. (2011). Developmental change in regional brain structure over 7 months in early adolescence: Comparison of approaches for longitudinal atlas-based parcellation. *Neuroimage, 57*(1), 214–224. doi:10.1016/j.neuroimage.2011.04.003.

Swanson, S. A., & Colman, I. (2013). Association between exposure to suicide and suicidality outcomes in youth. *Canadian Medical Association Journal, 185*(10), 870–877. doi:10.1503/cmaj.121377.

Tarver, J., Daley, D., & Sayal, K. (2015). Beyond symptom control for attention-deficit hyperactivity disorder (ADHD): What can parents do to improve outcomes. *Child: Care, Health & Development, 41*(1), 1–14. doi:10.1111/cch.12159.

Teplin, L. A., Welty, L. J., Abram, K. M., et al. (2012). Prevalence and persistence of psychiatric disorders in youth after detention: A prospective longitudinal study. *Archives of General Psychiatry, 69*(1), 1031–1043. doi:10.1001/archgenpsychiatry.2011.2062.

Thornton, L. C., Frick, P. J., Crapanzano, A. M., et al. (2013). The incremental utility of callous–unemotional traits and conduct problems in predicting aggression and bullying in a community sample of boys and girls. *Psychological Assessment, 25*(2), 366–378. doi:10.1037/a0031153.

van Noorden, T. H., Haselager, G. J., Cillessen, A. H., et al. (2015). Empathy and involvement in bullying in children and adolescents: A systematic review. *Journal of Youth & Adolescence, 44*(3), 637–657. doi:10.1007/s10964-014-0135-6.

Verhage, M. L., Oosterman, M., & Schuengel, C. (2015). Linkage between infant negative temperament and parenting self-efficacy: The role of resilience against negative performance feedback. *British Journal of Developmental Psychology, 33*(4), 506–518. doi:10.1111/bjdp.12113.

Vernberg, E. M., Nelson, T. D., Fonagy, P., et al. (2011). Victimization, aggression, and visits to the school nurse for somatic complaints, illnesses, and physical injuries. *Pediatrics, 127*(5), 842–848. doi:10.1542/peds.2009-3415.

Waddell, C., Shepherd, C., Schwartz, C., et al. (2014). *Children and youth mental disorders: Prevalence and evidence-based interventions—A research report for the British Columbia Ministry of Children and Family Development.* Vancouver: Children's Health Policy Centre, Simon Fraser University.

Wade, M., Prime, H., & Madigan, S. (2015). Using sibling designs to understand neurodevelopmental disorders: From genes and environments to prevention programming. *BioMed Research International, 2015,* 1–16. doi:10.1155/2015/672784.

Whitson, M., Bernard, S., & Kaufman, J. (2015). The mediating role of parenting stress for children exposed to trauma: Results from a school-based system of care. *Journal of Child & Family Studies, 24*(4), 1141–1151. doi:10.1007/s10826-014-9922-7.

Winther, J., Carlsson, A., & Vance, A. (2013). A pilot study of a school-based prevention and early intervention program to reduce oppositional defiant disorder/conduct disorder. *Early Intervention in Psychiatry,* 1–9. doi:10.1111/eip.12050.

Wright, L. M., & Leahey, M. (2012). *Nurses and families: A guide to family assessment and intervention* (6th ed.). Philadelphia: F. A. Davis.

Yanof, J. A. (2013). Play technique in psychodynamic psychotherapy. *Child and Adolescent Psychiatric Clinics of North America, 22*(2), 261–282. doi:10.1016/j.chc.2012.12.002.

Zwicker, J. G., Missiuna, C., Harris, S. R., et al. (2012). Developmental coordination disorder: A review and update. *European Journal of Paediatric Neurology, 16*(6), 574–578. doi:10.1016/j.ejpn.2012.05.005.

Psychosocial Needs of the Older Adult

Leslie A. Briscoe
Adapted by Cheryl L. Pollard

KEY TERMS AND CONCEPTS

adult support program
ageism
caregiver burden
medication reconciliation

OBJECTIVES

1. Discuss facts and myths about aging.
2. Describe mental health disorders that may occur in older adults.
3. Analyze how ageism may affect attitudes and willingness to care for older adults.
4. Explain the importance of a comprehensive geriatric assessment.
5. Describe the role of the nurse in different settings of care.
6. Discuss the importance of pain assessment, and identify three tools used to assess pain in older adults.

⊖volve WEBSITE

Visit the Evolve website for Flashcards, Case Studies, and additional testing resources related to the content in this chapter: *http://evolve.elsevier.com/Canada/Varcarolis/psychiatric/*

Pre-Test interactive review

The aging of the population is a global phenomenon that is occurring at a record-breaking rate, especially in developing countries around the world. In 2015 the number of Canadians age 65 years and older exceeded the number of Canadian children ages 0 to 14 years (Statistics Canada, 2015). The Canadian economy, as well as health and social services, is affected by this marked increase in the proportion of older adults in the population. Among older adults, the fastest-growing subgroups are minorities, the poor, and those age 85 years and older. Of the G7 countries, the United States (15%) and Canada (16.1%) have the lowest proportions of persons age 65 years and older. Conversely, Japan's population is among the oldest in the world, with the highest proportion of persons age 65 years and older (26%) among the G7 countries (Statistics Canada, 2015).

Providing "person-centered nursing care in partnership with persons experiencing a mental health condition and/or addiction, along the continuum of care and across the lifespan" (Canadian Association of Schools of Nursing [CASN] & Canadian Federation of Mental Health Nurses [CFMHN], 2017, p. 14) is an essential competency for nurses. As nurses therapeutically engage with older persons with mental illness or addiction, they must also demonstrate professional responsibility and accountability to recognized and reduce the detrimental impact of these attitudes (CASN & CFMHN, 2017).

The chapter begins with a summary of the major developmental theories relevant to providing mental health care to an aging population. This is followed by a brief discussion highlighting mental health issues related to aging. As people age, distinguishing between psychiatric and physical symptoms can be even more challenging than with the general adult population. Pain is one area where an overlap of symptoms can make assessment and treatment less straightforward, particularly if there are also cognitive impairments. Therefore assessment of pain in individuals with a major neurocognitive disorder is presented. The chapter concludes with a discussion of the nursing care of older adults.

DEVELOPMENTAL THEORIES OF AGING

An outline of some major developmental theories of aging is provided in Box 28-1. Although these theories provide the framework for formulating appropriate nursing interventions for caring for older adults, there is no specific theory that encompasses all developmental stages.

In addition to dealing with the developmental milestones associated with aging, as people live longer, they are more likely to deal with chronic illness and disability. In 2012, 85% of seniors ages 65 to 79 years and 90% of seniors age 80 years and older reported having at least one chronic condition. About 24% of seniors have three or more chronic diseases and account for 40% of all health care use among seniors (Taylor, 2014).

Statistics indicate that women generally outlive men. This disparity has significant ramifications for society at large and for the health care system in particular. Not only do women constitute the largest proportion of older adults, but they also use health care services more frequently than men and seek services earlier, even for minor conditions. Most provincial governments recognize an impending crisis as health care costs soar, resources dwindle, and the baby boomers age (Statistics Canada, 2015).

Chronological age is considered an arbitrary indicator of function because there are significant variables that contribute to the capabilities of adults. Surveys focusing on how older adults see themselves reveal that nearly half of people age 65 years and older consider themselves to be middle-aged or young. There is a significant difference between a person who is 65 years old and a person who is 90 years old. Imagine this same age range in younger people. A person who is 25 years old has different experiences and expectations than a person who is 50 years old.

Aging is accompanied by increased rates of medical and psychiatric illnesses. This increase is brought about in part by increasingly stressful life events (e.g., the loss of a spouse, family members, and independence) and comorbid illness. Polypharmacy also contributes to health problems, especially since there is a gradual reduction in renal, hepatic, and gastric function—all of which are needed to metabolize and degrade medications.

Aging is a complex psychological and physical process. Box 28-2 provides some facts and myths about aging that influence how society perceives the older adult.

BOX 28-1 MAJOR THEORIES OF AGING

Biological

Aging is influenced by molecular, cellular, or physiological systems and processes.

- *Gene theory:* Harmful genes become active in later life.
- *Error theory:* Error in protein synthesis results in impaired cellular function.
- *Free radical theory:* Reactive molecules damage DNA.
- *Wear-and-tear theory:* Internal and external stressors harm cells.
- *Programmed aging theory:* Biological or genetic clock plays out on genes.
- *Neuroendocrine theory:* There is neurohormonal regulation of life until death.
- *Immunological theory:* Immune system diversifies with age.

Psychological

- *Kohlberg's theory:* Crises and turning points in adult life are moral dilemmas.
- *Piaget's theory:* Cognitive operations in youth influence aging.
- *Erikson's theory:* Integrity is built on morality and ethics.
- *Bandura's theory:* Self-efficacy is essential for longevity.
- *Sullivan's theory:* Interpersonal responses influence behaviour.
- *Freud's theory:* Control of instinctual responses decreases with age.
- *Psychobiological theory:* Neurotransmitters modulate behaviours, emotions, and thoughts.
- *Dialectical theory:* Crises and transitions release positive and negative forces that lead to developmental progress.
- *Behavioural theory:* Learning determines the organization of behaviour.

Psychosocial

- *Maslow's theory:* Self-actualization and the evolution of developmental needs occur as the individual ages.
- *Disengagement theory:* Mutual withdrawal occurs between the aging person and others.
- *Activity theory:* Actions, roles, and social pursuits are important for satisfactory aging.
- *Continuity theory:* Life satisfaction and activity are expressions of enduring personality traits.

Source: Touhy, T. A., & Jett, K. F. (Eds). (2016). *Ebersole & Hess' toward healthy aging: Human needs and nursing response* (9th ed.). St. Louis: Mosby.

BOX 28-2 FACTS AND MYTHS ABOUT AGING

Facts

- The senses of vision, hearing, touch, taste, and smell decline with age.
- Muscular strength decreases with age. Muscle fibres atrophy and decrease in number.
- Regular sexual expressions are important to maintain sexual capacity and effective sexual performance.
- At least 50% of restorative sleep is lost as a result of the aging process.
- Older adults are major consumers of prescription drugs because of the high incidence of chronic diseases in this population.
- Older adults have a high incidence of depression.
- Many individuals experience difficulty when they retire.
- Older adults are prone to become victims of crime.
- Older widows appear to adjust better than younger ones.

Myths

- Most adults past the age of 65 have dementia.
- Sexual interest declines with age.
- Older adults are unable to learn new tasks.
- As individuals age, they become more rigid in their thinking and more set in their ways.
- The aged are well off and no longer impoverished.
- Most older adults are infirm and require help with daily activities.
- Most older adults are socially isolated and lonely.

🌐 CONSIDERING CULTURE
Chinese Immigrants Growing Old in Canada

Canada has a rapidly aging population, and this population is becoming more ethnically diverse. People who come to Canada in later life have unique challenges that have typically been overlooked. Nearly a third of the Canadian population identifies themselves as Chinese, accounting for the second largest visible-minority population in the country. It is critical that nurses recognize the diversity among the Chinese in Canada. These individuals come from diverse origins and speak many different dialects. Nurses need to avoid making broad-based cultural assumptions.

Chow (2010) investigated the health care needs, general well-being, and life satisfaction of older-adult Chinese immigrants and explored the views of Chinese Canadians on various health-related issues. A sample of 147 Chinese older adults was drawn from residential complexes located in Calgary, Alberta, that were occupied exclusively by older adults of Chinese origin. Interviews using a structured questionnaire were conducted by trained bilingual interviewers. The interviews took an average of 30 minutes to complete.

The results suggest that higher levels of physical well-being are significantly associated with increased physical mobility, country of origin (Hong Kong emigrants), increased education, and a self-perception of financial security. Better reports of psychosocial health are significantly associated with being female, being married, having a higher level of education, and having resided in Canada longer.

Several areas have been suggested for further research, including comparing the health status of foreign-born Chinese older adults to those who were born in Canada and comparing the health status of Chinese older adults who co-reside with adult children.

Source: Chow, H. P. (2010). Growing old in Canada: Physical and psychological well-being among elderly Chinese immigrants. *Ethnicity & Health, 15*(1), 61–72.

MENTAL HEALTH ISSUES RELATED TO AGING

Changing Directions, Changing Lives: The Mental Health Strategy for Canada (Mental Health Commission of Canada, 2012) has made several recommendations that relate to mental health issues in Canada's aging population. These strategies include identifying and treating mental illnesses early, decreasing age discrimination, and helping older adults to continue to engage in meaningful activities.

Late-Life Mental Illness

Older adults who develop late-life mental illness are less likely than young adults to be accurately diagnosed and receive mental health treatment. Psychiatric issues such as depression, memory loss, and prolonged grieving are not a normal part of aging and should be diagnosed and treated. Treating psychiatric disorders prolongs the individual's ability to remain independent and increases his or her ability to take the lead in personal decision making.

Depression

Depression is not a normal part of aging and is often under-identified because of comorbid medical conditions. Depression is often confused with a neurocognitive disorder, and delirium is often misdiagnosed as a neurocognitive disorder. A careful, systematic assessment is necessary to properly distinguish among the three.

This assessment must determine the following:
- Onset of mental-status change and course of illness
- Level of consciousness
- Attention span

All three illnesses are treatable if properly identified. Delirium and major neurocognitive disorders are discussed in significantly more detail in Chapter 17; therefore they are not discussed further in this chapter. Chapter 17 also provides more information on distinguishing among depression, dementia, and delirium.

Selective serotonin reuptake inhibitors (SSRIs) are the first-line treatment for depression; this category of drug is often helpful if anxiety, worry, or rumination is problematic. If pain or diabetic neuropathy is a comorbid condition, serotonin–norepinephrine reuptake inhibitors (SNRIs) are often prescribed. Tricyclic antidepressants (TCAs) are used for those with chronic pain. Treatment-resistant depression can be treated with psychostimulants such as methylphenidate (Concerta); such monoamine oxidase inhibitors (MAOIs) are older treatments but remain effective.

Depression and suicide risk. Death by suicide is a significant consideration when working with Canadians between the ages of 80 and 84 years. Within this category men are the highest risk of taking their own life. The factors that affect the risk for suicide within this demographic are mental illness and addictions, personality factors, medical illness, negative life events, difficult transitions, lack of social support, and functional impairment (Canadian Coalition for Seniors' Mental Health, 2006). Approximately 70% of people who commit suicide suffer with depression. Early identification of and treatment for depression, therefore, are key measures for suicide prevention. Other factors that can lead to suicide are feelings of hopelessness, uselessness, and despair. For older adults, suicide may be seen as a final gesture of control at a stage when independence is at risk or activities are limited. Severe medical illness, functional disability, alcohol abuse, history of suicide attempts, comorbid anxiety, and psychotic depression are added risk factors for suicide (Szanto, 2017). Unlike younger persons, whose suicidal gestures may be a cry for help, older adults more frequently have a real desire to die.

Even though the suicide rate among older adults is high, suicide in this group is probably under-reported. Suicide is often not listed on the death certificate, even if it is suspected. The numbers also do not reflect those who passively or indirectly die by suicide by abusing alcohol, starving themselves, overdosing or mixing medications, stopping life-sustaining drugs, or simply losing the will to live. Unfortunately, primary care providers continue to under-recognize and undertreat depression; many are slow to refer older adults to mental health care providers despite evidence that treatment of depression is cost effective and decreases the amount of health care expenditures used (Canadian Coalition for Seniors' Mental Health, 2006). Review Chapter 22 for an in-depth discussion of suicide.

Anxiety Disorders

Disabling anxiety disorders are twice as prevalent as dementia and four to eight times as common as major depressive disorders. Again, accurate diagnosis of the anxiety disorder is difficult. The most common sources of anxiety are phobias and generalized anxiety disorder (Kishita & Laidlaw, 2017). One unique anxiety-related problem in older adults is the fear of falling. Its impact on keeping individuals homebound is similar to agoraphobia because fear of falling results in activity restriction (Denkinger, Lukas, Nikolaus, et al., 2015). Comorbid conditions, including depression, bipolar disorder, dementia, and alcoholism, may contribute to anxiety.

Psychosocial risk factors for anxiety include childlessness, low socioeconomic status, and having experienced trauma. Other risk factors include being female, being single, and having multiple medical conditions. Protective factors include social support, spiritual beliefs, physical activity, cognitive stimulation, and having coping strategies. Anxiety disorders may have been present earlier in life, but they did not significantly impaired functioning. Once the stress of aging, retirement, loss, or physical frailty occurs, the previous coping strategies may no longer be effective. Older adults with anxiety often have physical complaints or describe fears of illness.

Treatment for anxiety disorders typically includes an SSRI. Antianxiety agents are also used, but they should be used cautiously since they may result in confusion, oversedation, and paradoxical agitation. Anxiety disorders are discussed in greater detail in Chapter 12.

Substance Use Disorders

People of any age can abuse any type of substance. Regardless of age, substance abuse has social, psychological, and physical consequences. Almost 80% of Canadians consume alcohol at least once a year (Health Canada, 2011). Although heavy drinking tends to decline with age, it continues to be a serious problem that can create particular difficulties for older adults. The risk factors for heavy drinking among older adults are being male and single, having less than a high school education, having a low income, and smoking (Sorrell, 2017). Identifying alcohol and substance abuse is often difficult because personality and behavioural changes frequently go unrecognized in older adults.

The stressful or reactive factors that precipitate late-onset substance abuse are often related to environmental conditions and may include retirement, widowhood, and loneliness. These stressors in the older adult, who may have retired, may not drive, and may be isolated from family and friends, are often greater than the problems faced by the middle-aged adult, who has to manage a job or career and care for a family and household. Work and family responsibilities may help keep a potential alcoholic from drinking too much. Once these demands are gone and the structure of daily life is disrupted, there is little impetus to remain sober. Another factor that may lead to

late-onset substance abuse is chronic pain. Chronic pain is discussed in more detail later in this chapter.

Caution is required when medicating the older adult who abuses alcohol or other substances. Central nervous system toxicity from psychoactive drugs increases with aging. Ingestion of antidepressants or tranquillizers can be particularly harmful because their effect is further potentiated by alcohol. The toxicity of other drugs (e.g., acetaminophen) is enhanced by alcohol and by the age-related decrease in clearance (Lehne, 2013).

Whenever there is a suspicion or indication that an older adult is abusing alcohol, the health care provider should conduct a screening test. The CAGE-AID screening tool (Wagenaar, Mickus, & Wilson, 2001) (Box 28-3) and the MAST-G (Box 28-4) are instruments commonly used to assess high-risk drinking in older adults.

Signs of alcohol abuse in younger individuals (e.g., alcohol-induced pancreatitis or liver disease, blackouts, major trauma) occur infrequently in older adults. Instead, the older adult who abuses alcohol displays vague geriatric syndromes of contusions, malnutrition, self-neglect, depression, and falls (Sorrell, 2017). Diarrhea, urinary incontinence, decreased functional status, failure to thrive, and apparent dementia may also be present. Although confusion and disorientation in an older patient are often associated with dementia or Alzheimer's disease, they could be caused by other factors, including alcohol abuse. Assessment of these conditions is necessary to differentiate the normal physiological changes of aging from those caused by excessive drinking.

Although the older adult with alcohol or substance abuse issues is difficult to treat, the prognosis for a person who has lived to this point without recourse to substances—and their use being precipitated by losses and stressors—is excellent. This individual often responds very positively to a recovery program, especially if it is accompanied by environmental interventions. It is important that health care providers recognize this recovery potential. Treatment plans should emphasize social therapies. Older people respond well to emotional and social support, and family therapy should be encouraged (Sorrell, 2017). Group therapy with other middle-aged and older adults with alcoholism,

---

BOX 28-3 CAGE-AID SCREENING TOOL

C—Have you ever felt you ought to **C**ut down on your drinking (drug use)?

A—Have people **A**nnoyed you by criticizing your drinking (drug use)?

G—Have you ever felt bad or **G**uilty about your drinking (drug use)?

E—Have you ever had a drink (used drugs) first thing in the morning (**E**ye-opener) to steady your nerves or get rid of a hangover?

AID—**A**dapt to **I**nclude **D**rugs.

One positive answer indicates a possible problem; two positive answers indicate a probable problem.

Source: Ewing, J. A. (1984). Detecting alcoholism: The CAGE questionnaire. *Journal of the American Medical Association, 252*(14), 1905–1907. Copyright © 1984 American Medical Association. All rights reserved.

BOX 28-4 **MICHIGAN ALCOHOLISM SCREENING TEST—GERIATRIC VERSION (MAST-G)**

Please answer "Yes" or "No" to each question by marking the line next to the question. When you finish answering the questions, please add up how many "Yes" responses you checked, and put that number in the space provided at the end.

1. After drinking, have you ever noticed an increase in your heart rate or beating in your chest?	___ Yes	___ No
2. When talking to others, do you ever underestimate how much you actually drank?	___ Yes	___ No
3. Does alcohol make you sleepy so that you often fall asleep in your chair?	___ Yes	___ No
4. After a few drinks, have you sometimes not eaten or been able to skip a meal because you didn't feel hungry?	___ Yes	___ No
5. Does having a few drinks help you decrease your shakiness or tremors?	___ Yes	___ No
6. Does alcohol sometimes make it hard for you to remember parts of the day or night?	___ Yes	___ No
7. Do you have rules for yourself that you won't drink before a certain time of the day?	___ Yes	___ No
8. Have you lost interest in hobbies or activities you used to enjoy?	___ Yes	___ No
9. When you wake up in the morning, do you ever have trouble remembering part of the night before?	___ Yes	___ No
10. Does having a drink help you sleep?	___ Yes	___ No
11. Do you hide your alcohol bottles from family members?	___ Yes	___ No
12. After a social gathering, have you ever felt embarrassed because you drank too much?	___ Yes	___ No
13. Have you ever been concerned that drinking might be harmful to your health?	___ Yes	___ No
14. Do you like to end an evening with a nightcap?	___ Yes	___ No
15. Did you find your drinking increased after someone close to you died?	___ Yes	___ No
16. In general, would you prefer to have a few drinks at home rather than go out to social events?	___ Yes	___ No
17. Are you drinking more now than in the past?	___ Yes	___ No
18. Do you usually take a drink to relax or calm your nerves?	___ Yes	___ No
19. Do you drink to take your mind off your problems?	___ Yes	___ No
20. Have you ever increased your drinking after experiencing a loss in your life?	___ Yes	___ No
21. Do you sometimes drive when you have had too much to drink?	___ Yes	___ No
22. Has a doctor or nurse ever said they were worried or concerned about your drinking?	___ Yes	___ No
23. Have you ever made rules to manage your drinking?	___ Yes	___ No
24. When you feel lonely, does having a drink help?	___ Yes	___ No
TOTALS:	___ **Yes**	___ **No**

Scoring: A score of 3 points or less is considered to indicate no alcoholism; a score of 4 points is suggestive of alcoholism; a score of 5 points or more indicates alcoholism.
Source: Blow, F., Brower, K., Schulenberg, J. E., et al. (1992). The Michigan Alcoholism Screening Test–Geriatric Version: A new elderly specific screening instrument. *Alcoholism: Clinical and Experimental Research, 16*, 372. Michigan Alcoholism Screening Test-Geriatric Version (MAST-G). © The Regents of the University of Michigan, 1991.

---

as well as self-help groups like Alcoholics Anonymous, can also be effective. Nurses can be pioneers in the developing need for substance abuse rehabilitation focused on older adults. Refer to Chapter 18 for more information on treatment approaches for people with a substance use disorder.

Trauma

Older adults are also susceptible to the effects of psychological trauma. Chapter 24 discusses interpersonal violence in more detail. Refer to Chapter 25 for more information on the consequences of sexual assault.

Caregiver Burden

Another phenomenon with the aging population is the increase in caregiver burden. Although there is not a consistent definition of caregiver burden, most researchers and clinicians view this concept as the physical, psychological, emotional (e.g., increased depression, increased stress, increased fatigue), social, and financial (e.g., increased costs associated with caring, decreased work hours) stresses that individuals experience as a result of providing care (Bastawrous, 2013). A common scenario is the two-income family in the middle of raising children and planning for their future retirement that is now faced with aging parents in need of help. Shorter lengths of stay for hospitalization, limited home care options, and complicated procedures to access care have increased the need for adult children to advocate for and provide care to aging parents. Unfortunately, this scenario is different for older adults who have lived with a chronic mental illness. Schizophrenia and bipolar disorders take a toll on family members and intimate relationships, and it is not uncommon for those with severe mental illness to have no family support available as they age. Grown children may be estranged because of a parent's frequent hospitalization, poor parenting ability, or paranoid symptoms. The support system of those aging with chronic mental illness often becomes case managers, community nurses, and mental health care providers.

Access to Care

The disparity of mental health services in Canada has led to a complicated and fragmented system of care (Mental Health Commission of Canada, 2014). Nurses may feel powerless to change shortfalls in the health care system; however, they can take advantage of their numbers and the respect given to the profession to be strong advocates for improving health care.

RESEARCH HIGHLIGHT

Trauma: The Potential Impact of Canadian Residential Schools Among Indigenous People in Canada

Problem

Currently, four generations of Indigenous people in Canada have been exposed to the Canadian residential school system. Tens of thousands of Indigenous children were sent to residential schools, whose primary mandate was to Christianize, civilize, and resocialize them. The last Canadian residential school closed in 1996. The children in residential schools experienced a loss of culture, language, traditional values, family bonding, parenting skills, and community connections. Survivors of residential schools may have transmitted the trauma that they experienced to their own children and grandchildren and to other community members through indirect trauma effects.

Purpose of Study

The purpose of the study was to investigate whether direct or indirect exposure to the mass trauma linked to being in a residential school was associated with trauma and suicidal behaviour of the residential school survivors, their offspring, and broader community members.

Methods

Ethical approval for the study was obtained from a research ethics board at the University of Manitoba. A multistage stratified random sampling method was used to identify potential participants. An in-person interview was used to collect information on the lifetime history of abuse, suicidal thoughts and behaviour, relationship status, residential school attendance, and general health and well-being. Bivariate testing was conducted, with all covariate explanatory variables using logistic regression modelling.

Key Findings

- Residential school experiences have resulted in multigenerational trauma that has had a negative impact on these individuals, their family members, and their communities.
- Older adults who were the first generation to attend residential schools and who do not have a complex trauma history appear to be more resilient.
- The chronic stress experienced by older Indigenous people in Canada may predispose them to ineffectively cope (i.e., experience suicidal ideation) as they age.
- Some survivors of residential schools have been resilient to the effects of the trauma they experienced.

Implications for Nursing Practice

- The experience of trauma can have multigenerational effects.
- When providing nursing care to Indigenous people, assessment of the individual, family, and community is needed to determine the direct and indirect effects of historical trauma. Useful frameworks to conceptualize the traumas experienced include describing the trauma in terms of connectedness, collectivity, and relationships.
- People who have experienced historical and contemporary trauma have increased rates of suicidal thoughts and attempts; therefore thorough risk assessments are required.
- Although mental and emotional support services are provided to survivors of residential schools and their families through Health Canada, First Nations and Inuit Health's Indian Residential Schools Resolution Health Support Program, the effects of this multigenerational trauma need to be recognized when and where Indigenous people in Canada access health services.

Source: Elais, B., Mignone, J., Hall, M., et al. (2012). Trauma and suicide behaviour histories among a Canadian indigenous population: An empirical exploration of the potential role of Canada's residential school system. *Social Science & Medicine, 74*(10), 1560–1569. doi:10.1016/j.socscimed.2012.01.026.

Access to care is also affected by the availability of financial resources. Although every Canadian has access to all medically necessary services, regardless of ability to pay, "all medically necessary services" is typically interpreted within an illness- or disease-focused paradigm. As a result, health promotion activities and many factors associated with the social determinants of health—for example, housing—are not included within the delivery of "all medically necessary services." People therefore are individually responsible for the costs associated with meeting their overall health care needs.

Ageism

In Western culture, growing older is not viewed as a privilege, and old age does not tend to confer a revered social status on those who have attained it. Ageism has been defined as a bias against older people because of their age. It is based on erroneous beliefs that older adults are unattractive, unintelligent, asexual, unemployable, and senile. Ageism affects not only employment opportunities for the older population but also the quality of health care this population receives (Stall, 2012). For example, most older people present with several comorbid conditions,

yet the Canadian health care system is organized into single diagnostic specialties (e.g., psychiatry, endocrinology, hematology, surgery). This division poses the risk that patients with diagnoses in several areas may not receive the best possible care because of the complexity of their presentation. In addition, a decreasing number of health care providers is choosing geriatrics as a specialty area (Eymard & Douglas, 2012).

Ageism is not limited to the way the young view the old, though; it can also be exhibited by older adults themselves. Indeed, the attitudes of older adults toward their contemporaries, particularly those with mental disabilities, are often negative—perhaps because the threat of contagion by association with the frail and infirm raises feelings of vulnerability. Ageism differs from other forms of discrimination in that it cuts across gender, race, religion, and socioeconomic status to reach the majority of those over age 65.

Ageism and Public Policy

The results of ageism can be observed in every level of society. Financial and political support for programs for older adults is difficult to obtain. The needs of this population often are addressed only after those of younger, albeit smaller, population groups. However, the Canadian Association for Retired Persons (CARP), a powerful lobbying group, is fighting to change this trend.

Ageism and Drug Testing

Clinical drug trials often exclude people over the age of 65 on the assumption that they already take multiple medications or have an existing chronic illness. Information about medications for the general population has to be generalized for older adults, and appropriate (generally lower) doses may not have been tested or even be available (Shepherd, Nuttall, Hood, et al., 2015).

DISTINGUISHING BETWEEN PSYCHIATRIC AND PHYSICAL SYMPTOMS

Older adults are the fastest growing segment of the world's population. As people age, there is an increased incidence and prevalence of pain. The pain that older adults experience may be related to many medical conditions, such as arthritis, peripheral vascular disease, diabetic neuropathy, or musculoskeletal disease. Like many mental health disorders, pain may be under-reported and incorrectly believed to be a normal part of the aging process. Pain and mental health problems affect an older adult's sense of well-being and quality of life.

Pain

Pain is often associated with depression (Hung, Bounsanga, Voss, et al., 2017). There are three categories of depressive symptoms: emotional (mood, motivation, apathy, anxiety), cognitive (concentration, memory), and physical (insomnia, fatigue, headache, and pain). When experiencing pain, your emotional, cognitive, and physical functioning can also be affected. Pain can lead to increased stress, delayed healing, decreased mobility, disturbances in sleep, decreased appetite, and agitation with accompanying aggressive behaviours. Nurses must be able to determine what the presenting symptoms are related to in order to make an accurate nursing diagnosis and an effective treatment plan.

Principles of Pain Management

Assessment tools. When pain is suspected, the nurse begins with a physical assessment for the origins of the pain and assesses characteristics of the pain itself. To aid older adults who may have sensory deficits or cognitive impairments, simply worded questions and simple drawings may be necessary. The Wong-Baker FACES Pain Rating Scale (Figure 28-1) is an assessment instrument currently in use. The FACES scale shows facial expressions

on a scale from 0 (a smile) to 5 (crying grimace). Respondents are asked to choose the face that depicts the pain they feel.

The present pain intensity (PPI) rating from the McGill Pain Questionnaire (MPQ) (Powell, Corbo, Fonda, et al., 2015) is another tool accepted for use with older patients. Patients are asked to respond by selecting the description (from "no pain" [0] to "excruciating pain" [5]) that they believe identifies the pain they feel.

The Pain Assessment in Advanced Dementia (PAINAD) scale is used to evaluate the presence and severity of pain in patients with advanced dementia who no longer have the ability to communicate verbally (Figure 28-2). The scale evaluates five domains: breathing, negative vocalization, facial expression, body language, and consolability (Box 28-5). The score guides the caregiver in the appropriate pain intervention.

Barriers to accurate pain assessment. There are a number of beliefs and misconceptions that may interfere with appropriate assessment and treatment. Older adults may believe that pain is a punishment for past behaviours, an inevitable part of aging, indicative of pending death, related to serious illness, or a sign of weakness. External obstacles include inadequate assessment by health care providers, complicated clinical presentation, assumptions by health care providers that pain is part of aging, and communication deficits due to cognitive impairment.

Changes in behaviour may indicate pain and should be assessed, especially in people who have difficulty verbally communicating their needs (e.g., those with dementia). Unlike younger adults, older adults may understate their pain using words such as *discomfort, hurting,* or *aching.* Multiple painful problems may occur together, making it difficult to differentiate new pain from pre-existing pain. Sensory impairments, memory loss, dementia, and depression can add to the difficulty of obtaining an accurate pain assessment. An interview with family members, caregivers, or friends is vital.

Pain treatment. There are three essential features of treating pain:
1. Do a thorough assessment and establish an accurate diagnosis.
2. Recognize that pain reduction, rather than complete elimination of pain, may be the treatment goal.
3. Treat symptoms of coexisting disorders, such as depression, anxiety, or other physical conditions, that exacerbate the pain.

Pharmacological pain treatments. The cause of the pain should be addressed along with treatment of the pain itself. Pain should be managed with pharmacological or alternative measures. Pharmacological pain management relies on the use of

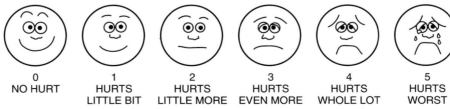

| 0 | 1 | 2 | 3 | 4 | 5 |
| NO HURT | HURTS LITTLE BIT | HURTS LITTLE MORE | HURTS EVEN MORE | HURTS WHOLE LOT | HURTS WORST |

FIGURE 28-1 Wong-Baker FACES Pain Rating Scale. Source: Hockenberry, M. J., & Wilson, D. (2013). *Wong's essentials of pediatric nursing* (9th ed.). St. Louis: Mosby. Used with permission. Copyright Mosby.

	0	1	2	Score
Breathing Independent of vocalization	Normal	Occasional laboured breathing; short period of hyperventilation	Noisy, laboured breathing; long period of hyperventilation; Cheyne-Stokes respirations	
Negative Vocalization	None	Occasional moan or groan; low-level speech with a negative or disapproving quality	Repeated troubled calling out; loud moaning or groaning; crying	
Facial Expression	Smiling or inexpressive	Sad; frightened; frown	Facial grimacing	
Body Language	Relaxed	Tense; distressed pacing; fidgeting	Rigid; fists clenched; knees pulled up; pulling or pushing away; striking out	
Consolability	No need to console	Distracted or reassured by voice or touch	Unable to console, distract, or reassure	
			TOTAL	

FIGURE 28-2 Pain Assessment in Advanced Dementia (PAINAD) scale. Source: Reprinted from Warden, V., Hurley, A. C., & Volicer, L. (2003). Development and psychometric evaluation of the Pain Assessment in Advanced Dementia [PAINAD] scale. *Journal of the American Medical Directors Association*, *4*(1), 9–15. Copyright 2003, with permission from Elsevier.

prescription and nonprescription medications, frequently based on the recommendation of the health care provider. These include analgesics, opioid analgesics, and adjuvant medications. When administering and teaching patients about these types of medication, information should be provided about their potentially addictive nature. Consultation with a pain-management specialist is often helpful with chronic pain syndromes. Some considerations for pharmacological pain management in older adults are listed in Box 28-6.

As an individual ages, the body's ability to eliminate drugs via the kidney decreases. Nurses must be aware of this change, which can result in overdosing. On the other hand, fear of narcotic overmedication, which can cause respiratory depression and falls, may lead the nurse to give out less pain medication to older adults than is needed for effective treatment (Lehne, 2013). It is critical for nurses to evaluate the effectiveness of pain interventions at regular intervals and to be attentive to behavioural changes or verbal responses that indicate that the patient is experiencing pain. It is a common misconception that the ability to perceive pain decreases with aging. No physiological changes in pain perception in older adults have been demonstrated. In fact, older adults may feel pain even more keenly than younger persons do. Careful and continuing assessments and an understanding of pain physiology are necessary for effective pain management of older adults.

In older adults, it is important to perform a systematic review of current medication use known as medication reconciliation. Medication reconciliation is the process of developing the most accurate list possible of all medication a patient is taking. This list should include drug name, dose, frequency, and route. The purpose of this process is to reduce adverse incidents, side effects, and potentially lethal combinations.

Assessing the use of multiple medications (polypharmacy) includes prescription, over-the-counter drugs, and herbal agents. Adverse drug reactions or negative responses to drugs are common among the older adult. Older adults are at greater risk for these events due to multiple medical problems and memory issues that may result in taking too little or too much medication. Renal and liver impairment affect excretion and are associated with dose-related adverse reactions.

Metabolic changes and decreased drug clearance compound the risk of drug–drug interactions. The risk for adverse drug reactions doubles for people taking five to seven medications as compared to those taking fewer than five medications (Onder, Petrovic, Tangiisuran, et al., 2010). For people taking eight or more medications, the risk for adverse drug reactions increases by four times. The American Geriatrics Society (2015) recently updated the criteria for and list of potentially inappropriate medications for older adults. Many psychiatric medications appear on the list, including benzodiazepines, anticholinergics, antipsychotics, antidepressants, antiepileptics, and antiparkinson drugs. Nurses must be diligent in reviewing older adults' medication lists for completeness.

Prescribing cascades happen when drug-induced symptoms are treated with another drug. The health care provider may assess the side effect of the first drug as part of the original

BOX 28-5	THE FIVE ELEMENTS OF THE PAIN ASSESSMENT IN ADVANCED DEMENTIA (PAINAD) SCALE

1. Breathing

   Normal breathing is effortless breathing characterized by quiet, rhythmic respirations.

   Occasional laboured breathing is characterized by episodic bursts of harsh, difficult, or wearing respirations.

   Short period of hyperventilation is characterized by intervals of rapid, deep breaths lasting a short period of time.

   Long period of hyperventilation is characterized by excessive rate and depth of respirations lasting a considerable time.

   Cheyne-Stokes respirations are characterized by rhythmic waxing and waning of breathing from very deep to shallow respirations with periods of apnea.

2. Negative Vocalization

   None is characterized by speech or vocalization that has a neutral or pleasant quality.

   Occasional moan or groan: Occasional moaning is characterized by mournful or murmuring sounds, wails, or laments. Occasional groaning is characterized by louder than usual inarticulate involuntary sounds, often abruptly beginning and ending.

   Low-level speech with negative or disapproving quality is characterized by muttering, mumbling, whining, grumbling, or swearing in a low volume with a complaining, sarcastic, or caustic tone.

   Repeated, troubled calling out is characterized by phrases or words being used over and over in a tone that suggests anxiety, uneasiness, or distress.

   Loud moaning or groaning: Loud moaning is characterized by mournful or murmuring sounds, wails, or laments in a much louder than usual volume. Loud groaning is characterized by louder than usual inarticulate involuntary sounds, often abruptly beginning and ending.

   Crying is characterized by an utterance of emotion accompanied by tears. There may be sobbing or quiet weeping.

3. Facial Expression

   Smiling or inexpressiveness: Smiling is characterized by upturned corners of the mouth, brightening of the eyes, and a look of pleasure or contentment. Inexpressiveness refers to a neutral, at ease, relaxed, or blank look.

   Sad is characterized by an unhappy, lonesome, sorrowful, or dejected look. Eyes may be teary.

   Frightened is characterized by a look of fear, alarm, or heightened anxiety. Eyes may appear wide open.

   Frowning is characterized by a downward turn of the corners of the mouth. Increased facial wrinkling in the forehead and around the corners of the mouth may appear.

Facial grimacing is characterized by a distorted, distressed look. The brow is more wrinkled, as is the area around the mouth. Eyes may be squeezed shut.

4. Body Language

   Relaxed is characterized by a calm, restful, mellow appearance. The person seems to be taking it easy.

   Tense is characterized by a strained, apprehensive, or worried appearance. The jaw may be clenched.

   Distressed pacing is characterized by activity that seems unsettled. There may be a fearful, worried, or disturbed element present. The rate may be faster or slower.

   Fidgeting is characterized by restless movement. Squirming about or wiggling in the chair may occur. The person might be hitching a chair across the room. Repetitive touching, tugging, or rubbing body parts can also be observed.

   Rigid is characterized by stiffening of the body. The arms and/or legs are tight and inflexible. The trunk may appear straight and unyielding (exclude contractures).

   Fists clenched is characterized by tightly closed hands. They may be opened and closed repeatedly or held tightly shut.

   Knees pulled up is characterized by flexing the legs and drawing the knees upward toward the chest (exclude contractures).

   Pulling or pushing away is characterized by resistiveness upon approach or to care. The person is trying to escape by yanking or wrenching himself or herself free or by shoving you away.

   Striking out is characterized by hitting, kicking, grabbing, punching, biting, or other forms of personal assault.

5. Consolability

   No need to console is characterized by a sense of well-being. The person appears content.

   Distracted or reassured by voice or touch is characterized by a disruption in the behaviour when the person is spoken to or touched. The behaviour stops during the period of interaction, with no indication that the person is at all distressed.

   Unable to console, distract, or reassure is characterized by the inability to soothe the person or stop a behaviour with words or actions. No amount of verbal or physical comforting will alleviate the behaviour.

Scoring: (See Figure 28-3 for point allocation.)

0–1 = No significant pain

2–3 = Mild to moderate pain

4–6 = Moderate to severe pain

7–10 = Severe to very severe pain

Source: Lane, P., Kuntupis, M., MacDonald, S., et al. (2003). A pain assessment tool for people with advanced Alzheimer's and other progressive dementias. *Home Healthcare Nurse, 21*(1), 36.

medical problem or a new one. Prescribing cascades are particularly problematic and complicated. One of the most common examples is when a person begins antiparkinson therapy for symptoms brought about by antipsychotics. Antiparkinson drugs may bring about new and dangerous symptoms such as delirium and orthostatic hypotension. Anticholinesterase inhibitor drugs used to treat dementia (e.g., donepezil, rivastigmine, galantamine) may cause urinary incontinence and diarrhea. These symptoms

may result in a prescribing cascade with use of an anticholinergic such as oxybutynin, which can cause cognitive dulling and confusion.

Pharmacists have begun to play a critical role in reviewing and advising on matters of prescribing for the older adult. The American Geriatrics Society (2015) has updated the Beers List and Criteria, which was developed in 1991 to identify inappropriate medications for the older adult. Maher, Hanlon, and Hajjar

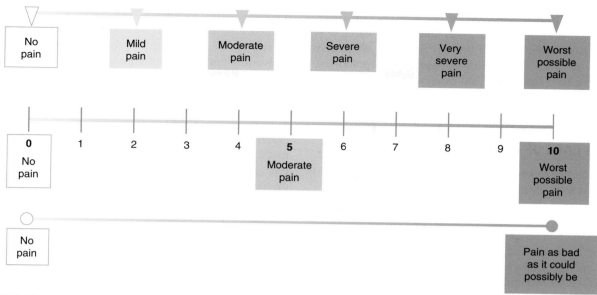

FIGURE 28-3 Visual analogue scales used in the management of cancer pain. Source: Jacox, A., Carr, D. B., Payne, R., et al. (1994). *Management of cancer pain (Clinical Practice Guideline No. 9, AHCPR Publication No. 94-0952)*. Rockville, MD: U.S. Department of Health and Human Services, Public Health Service, Agency for Health Care Policy and Research.

BOX 28-6 TIPS FOR PHARMACOLOGICAL PAIN MANAGEMENT IN OLDER ADULTS

- Remember that many older adults receive pain medication less often than younger adults because their pain is often considered a natural part of aging. As a result, many older adults receive inadequate pain relief.
- Safe administration of analgesics is complicated because of possible interactions with drugs used to treat certain chronic disorders, as well as because of nutritional alterations and altered pharmacokinetics in older adults.
- Analgesics reach a higher peak and have a longer duration of action in older adults than in younger individuals. Start with one-fourth to one-half the adult dose, and titrate up carefully.
- Give oral analgesics around the clock at the beginning. Administer on an as-needed basis later on, as indicated by the patient's pain status.
- If acute confusion occurs, assess for other contributing factors before changing the medication or stopping analgesic use. Confusion in postoperative patients has been found to be associated with unrelieved pain rather than with opiate use.

- Acetaminophen is an effective analgesic in older adults. Although there is an increased risk of end-stage renal disease with long-term use, it does not produce the gastrointestinal bleeding seen with nonsteroidal anti-inflammatory drugs (NSAIDs).
- Analgesics and adjuvants, such as anticholinergics and pentazocine, may produce increased confusion in older adults. NSAIDs can have the same effect during their initial period of administration.
- Opiates have a greater analgesic effect and longer duration of action than nonopioid analgesics. Avoid the use of meperidine, whose active metabolite may stimulate the central nervous system and lead to confusion, seizures, and mood alterations. If this drug is selected, do not use it for more than 48 hours. Avoid intramuscular administration in the older adult because of tissue irritation and poor absorption. Morphine is a safer choice than meperidine because its duration of action is longer, so a smaller overall dose is required.
- Assess bowel function daily, because constipation can be a frequent adverse effect of opiates.

Source: Lehne, R. A. (2013). *Pharmacology for nursing care* (8th ed.). St Louis: Elsevier.

(2014) identify how polypharmacy affects the older adult. They cite nine negative clinical consequences of inappropriate drug use:

1. Increased health care costs
2. Adverse drug reactions
3. Drug interactions
4. Nonadherence
5. Decline in functional status
6. Increased cognitive impairment
7. Increased falls
8. Increased urinary incontinence
9. Increased risk for malnutrition

Common problems associated with medication include confusion, which can be caused by anticholinergics, antihistamines, and benzodiazepines. Psychosis has been linked to levodopa, steroids, and even cholesterol-lowering medications. Depressive symptoms have been linked with α-adrenergic agonists and opiates.

Nonpharmacological pain treatments. Nonpharmacological treatments for pain include vagal nerve stimulation, exercise, hydrotherapy, heat and cold packs, chiropractics, and transcutaneous electrical nerve stimulation (TENS). Yoga, biofeedback, hypnosis, acupuncture, massage, shiatsu, reiki, guided imagery, reflexology, and therapeutic touch are integrative therapies for managing pain. Herbal remedies include cayenne, capsaicin, ginger extract, echinacea, kava kava, and willow bark. It is important to ask older adults if they are using any alternative treatments for pain relief. Pain-management education is important for both the patient and caregivers. The key to successful pain management lies in the application of a variety of techniques that the patient must learn and practise.

NURSING CARE OF OLDER ADULTS

Nurses encounter older adults in a variety of settings, and in each of these settings, the nurse is responsible for applying the nursing process to the individual patient's situation.

Studies suggest that because nursing students are not given enough information about older adults and often are not exposed to older patients, they may hold ageist views when they begin their nursing careers. Such biases have significant implications for practice, education, and research (Kagan & Melendez-Torres, 2015). It is important for all nurses to gain a better understanding of the aging process. Adequate theory and principles of practice are needed to provide safe and excellent care for older adults. The Canadian Gerontological Nursing Association (2010) has developed practice standards to define the uniqueness and scope of gerontological nursing. The standards are organized into six categories: (1) physiological health, (2) optimizing functional health, (3) responsive care, (4) relationship care, (5) health system, and (6) safety and security.

Positive attitudes toward older adults and their care need to be instilled during basic nursing education. Education programs must include the following:

- Information about the aging process
- Discussion of attitudes relating to the care of older adults
- Sensitization of participants to their patients' needs
- Exploration of the dynamics of nurse–patient and staff–patient interactions
- Respect for older patients and appreciation of their wisdom and life experience

Assessment Strategies

Nurses who work with older adults benefit from specific knowledge about normal aging, drug interactions, and chronic disease. Those who work with older patients who have mental health problems need to have specific skills in interviewing and assessing and special knowledge of effective treatment modalities. The Canadian Gerontological Nursing Association (2010) has recommended a comprehensive geriatric assessment, which includes the following areas: physiological, functional, cognitive, psychological, sociocultural, spiritual, environmental, risk factors, response to pharmacological intervention and drug use patterns, and diagnostic results and implications related to treatment. Specific assessment questions should also be asked regarding pain in older adults. Figure 28-4 shows what is considered in a comprehensive geriatric assessment.

A thorough assessment, including a physical assessment and diagnostic testing, must precede any treatment or diagnosis of a mental illness in older adults. Common tests include thyroid, kidney, and liver function; complete blood count; comprehensive metabolic panel; vitamin B_{12}, folic acid, and therapeutic drug levels; urinalysis; syphilis serology (RPR); B-type natriuretic peptide (BNP); and computed tomography (CT) of the head. A review of current medications and possible adverse reactions or drug–drug interactions must also occur (Lehne, 2013). Confusion can be caused by anticholinergics, antihistamine, and benzodiazepines. Psychosis has been linked to steroids and even to cholesterol-lowering medications, and depression has been linked to beta blockers, α-adrenergic agonists, and opiates. Serious medical conditions such as cancer, anemia, diabetes, infections, electrolyte imbalance, malnutrition, dehydration, and cardiac disease can manifest in symptoms such as fatigue or anorexia before more specific physical manifestations occur. Nurses are in a unique position to advocate for and coordinate appropriate medical evaluation for older adults.

An examination and interview of an older adult conducted in unfamiliar surroundings can produce anxiety. Unlike younger patients, who may be comfortable discussing personal issues—family conflicts, feelings of sadness, sexual practices, finances, and bodily functions—older adults may view such topics as private or taboo and be uncomfortable discussing them. It is important to respect these feelings while reviewing essential history by doing the following:

- Conducting the interview in a private area
- Introducing oneself and asking the patient what he or she would like to be called (use of the first name is rarely appropriate unless one is invited to use it)
- Establishing rapport and putting the patient at ease by sitting or standing at the same level as the patient
- Ensuring that lighting is adequate and noise level is low in recognition of the fact that hearing and vision may be impaired
- Using touch (with permission) to convey warmth, while at the same time respecting the patient's comfort level with personal touch
- Summarizing the interaction, inviting feedback and questions, and thanking the patient for giving his or her time and information

Assessment of the cognitive, behavioural, and emotional status of the older adult is very important in managing the nursing care of the patient and is particularly vital for detecting dementia, delirium, and depression, whose prevalence increases with age (Prince, Wimo, Guerchet, et al., 2015). The Geriatric Depression Scale (Short Form) (Box 28-7) is a subjective questionnaire (Sheikh & Yesavage, 1986), and the Cornell Scale for Depression in Dementia is an objective screening tool for caregivers to help identify the presence of depressive symptoms (Alexopoulos, Abrams, Young, et al., 1988). The periodic repetition of these assessments serves to evaluate the effectiveness of intervention.

It is also essential to assess for suicidal thoughts and suicidal intent by asking specific questions such as these:

- Have you ever thought about killing yourself?
- Have you ever felt that life is not worth living?
- Have you ever tried to hurt yourself in the past?

Thoughts of harming others also must be assessed. Interventions for the prevention of suicide in older adults are discussed in greater depth later in this chapter. Also see Chapter 22 for a more detailed discussion of suicide assessment and intervention.

COMPREHENSIVE GERIATRIC ASSESSMENT					
Name:		Date of birth:		Gender:	

Physical Health

Chronic disorder					
Vision	Adequate Inadequate	Eyeglasses: Y N		Needs evaluation	
Hearing	Adequate Inadequate	Hearing aids: Y N			
Mobility	Ambulatory: Y N	Assistive device:			
	Falls: Y N			Needs evaluation	
Nutrition	Albumin:	TLC:	HCT:		
	Weight:	Weight loss or gain: Y N		Needs evaluation	
Incontinence	Y N	Treatment:	Y N	Needs evaluation	
Medications	Total number:	Reviewed & revised: Y N			
	Adverse effects/allergy:				
Screening	Cholesterol:	TSH:	B12:	Folate:	
	Colonoscopy: Date:		N/A		
	Mammogram: Date:		N/A		
	Osteoporosis: Date:		N/A		
	Pap smear: Date:		N/A		
	PSA: Date:		N/A		
Immunization	Influenza: Date:				
	Pneumonia: Date:				
	Tetanus: Date:		Booster:		
Counselling	Diet	Exercise	Calcium	Vitamin D	
	Smoking	Alcohol	Driving	Injury prevention	

Mental Health

Dementia	Y N	MMSE score:	Date:	Cause (if known):	
Depression	Y N	GDS score:	Date:	Treatment: Y N	

Functional Status

ADL	Bathing: I D		Dressing: I D		Toileting: I D
	Transferring: I D		Feeding: I D		Continence: Y N

FIGURE 28-4 Comprehensive geriatric assessment. *ADL,* Activities of daily living; *B12,* vitamin B$_{12}$; *D,* dependent; *GDS,* Geriatric Depression Scale; *HCT,* hematocrit; *I,* independent; *MMSE,* Mini-Mental State Examination; *N,* no; *PSA,* prostate-specific antigen; *TLC,* total lymphocyte count; *TSH,* thyroid-stimulating hormone; *Y,* yes.

Older adult abuse is another area to explore during a nursing assessment and is discussed in depth in Chapter 24. Questions about being hit, pushed, kicked, and slapped are important, but it is also imperative to inquire about care being withheld. Not being fed, cleaned, helped, or cared for are critical issues. Asking initially, "How are you being treated at home?" or "Are you afraid of anyone?" may encourage further exploration. Financial exploitation is another issue that is difficult to uncover. Older adults may feel ashamed or embarrassed to admit that they have been taken advantage of by family, friends, or strangers.

BOX 28-7 GERIATRIC DEPRESSION SCALE (SHORT FORM)

1. Are you basically satisfied with your life?	Yes/No
2. Have you dropped many of your activities and interests?	Yes/No
3. Do you feel that your life is empty?	Yes/No
4. Do you often get bored?	Yes/No
5. Are you in good spirits most of the time?	Yes/No
6. Are you afraid that something bad is going to happen to you?	Yes/No
7. Do you feel happy most of the time?	Yes/No
8. Do you often feel helpless?	Yes/No
9. Do you prefer to stay at home rather than going out and doing new things?	Yes/No
10. Do you feel you have more problems with memory than most?	Yes/No
11. Do you think it is wonderful to be alive now?	Yes/No
12. Do you feel pretty worthless the way you are now?	Yes/No
13. Do you feel full of energy?	Yes/No
14. Do you feel that your situation is hopeless?	Yes/No
15. Do you think that most people are better off than you are?	Yes/No

Source: Sheikh, J. I., & Yesavage, J. A. (1986). Geriatric Depression Scale (GDS): Recent evidence and development of a shorter version. In Brink, T. (Ed.), *Clinical gerontology: A guide to assessment and intervention*. New York: The Haworth Press.

BOX 28-8 MAKING THE INTERVIEW MORE EFFECTIVE

- Gather preliminary data before the session, and keep questionnaires relatively short.
- Ask about often-overlooked problems, such as difficulty sleeping, incontinence, falling, depression, dizziness, and loss of energy.
- Pace the interview to allow the patient to formulate answers; resist the tendency to interrupt prematurely.
- Use yes-or-no or simple-choice questions if the person has trouble coping with open-ended questions.
- Begin with general questions such as "How can I help you most at this visit?" or "What's been happening?"
- Be alert for information about the patient's relationships with others, thoughts about families or co-workers, typical responses to stress, and attitudes toward aging, illness, occupation, and death.
- Assess mental status for deficits in recent or remote memory, and determine if confusion exists.
- Be aware of all medications the patient is taking, and assess for adverse effects, efficacy, and possible drug interactions.
- Determine how fast the condition of the patient has been changing to assess the extent of the patient's concerns.
- Include the family or significant other in the interview process for added input, clarification, support, and reinforcement.

Box 28-8 provides helpful interview techniques to use with older adults.

Intervention Strategies

Certain psychotherapeutic methods are especially useful for older adults:

- Applying crisis intervention techniques (see Chapter 21)
- Providing empathic understanding and active listening
- Encouraging ventilation of feelings and normalizing emotional responses
- Re-establishing emotional equilibrium when anxiety is moderate to severe
- Providing health education and explaining alternative solutions
- Assisting in the use of problem-solving approaches
- Allowing adequate time to process information
- Ensuring that hearing aids are working or using an amplifier to facilitate good communication

An older adult may require acute inpatient mental health care for signs and symptoms of severe psychiatric conditions, such as nondementia psychiatric illnesses, major depression with suicidal thoughts, bipolar disorder, and schizophrenia. Just as in the general adult population, with the shift to community-based service delivery models, the number of patients with psychiatric illnesses treated on an inpatient basis is declining. Regardless of the person's age, inpatient treatment is recommended when the patient is at high risk for self-harm (whether intentional or unintentional) or poses a risk for harm to other people.

Specialized geropsychiatric units provide a comprehensive and specialized approach to care. These units use a multidisciplinary approach to assessment, treatment planning, implementation, and evaluation of care. Ideally, the team consists of a geriatric psychiatrist, geriatrician, social worker, nurses, a pharmacist, psychologist, dietitian, occupational therapist, physiotherapist, and other specialists as indicated. Nurses play the major role in providing continuous care from admission to discharge.

Psychosocial Interventions

The basic-level nurse uses counselling skills to assist the patient in talking about present problems, examining his or her present situation, looking at alternatives, and planning for the future. Sometimes counselling is provided through group therapy, which helps to decrease the sense of disorientation and isolation. Remotivation therapy (Box 28-9) and reminiscence therapy are also appropriate interventions for the basic-level nurse.

The advanced-practice nurse may provide individual or group psychotherapy to older adults with depression. Groups are useful because they can diminish social isolation and loneliness and help the members understand that they are not alone in their situation. Group members can learn creative ways to improve their mood and increase quality of life (Yalom, 2005). Table 28-1 outlines the purpose, format, and desired outcomes for each type of psychotherapeutic group. Individual therapies, specifically cognitive behavioural, interpersonal, and psychodynamic therapy, are also useful. The best outcomes result from combining some kind of therapy with medication. Primary care providers therefore must acquire the skills to enable sensitive assessment for depression and suicide risk and must be knowledgeable about methods

BOX 28-9 EXAMPLE OF REMOTIVATION SESSION (BODIES OF WATER)

Step 1: Climate of Acceptance

The leaders personally welcomed each participant as he or she arrived at the group session. After the leaders introduced themselves, each group member made a self-introduction. The leader used a calendar to orient the members to the date and time of the current remotivation session. The theme for session four was introduced by the leader as "Bodies of Water—Rivers, Lakes, and Oceans." All group members had some familiarity with bodies of water because of their residence in Seattle.

Step 2: Creating a Bridge to Reality

The world globe was used as a visual aid to stimulate discussion on bodies of water. The leader asked questions such as "How are bodies of water formed from glaciers?" Pictures of glaciers, rivers, and lakes were shown.

The leader read poems about tide pools, seashells, and fishing written by anonymous grade-school children. Discussion was stimulated by the leader's asking, "What can we do at the ocean?" Visual aids and props were provided for direct sensory stimulation. Some examples of these aids and props were (1) different types of seashells, (2) fishing tackle and bait, (3) suntan lotion, (4) sun hat, and (5) sunglasses.

An anonymous author's poem about fishing was read to the group, followed by recorded music with lyrics about fishing experiences.

Step 3: Sharing the World We Live In

Group discussion focused on jobs related to bodies of water. Topics the participants discussed in regard to self or others included crabbing, clamming, shrimping, and fishing. Visual aids, such as pictures of river rafting, canoeing, scuba diving, and sailing, stimulated further discussions of past related experiences involving bodies of water.

Step 4: An Appreciation of the World of Work

This time was used for the members to think about work in relation to others. More experiences in past work roles, as well as hobbies and pastimes, were discussed. The group then participated in singing a familiar old song, "Love Letters in the Sand," written in 1931 by J. Fred Coots and revived in 1957, when sung by Pat Boone.

Step 5: Climate of Appreciation

The leaders thanked the group members individually for coming to the group and sharing their experiences. The next remotivation session theme and meeting date were announced prior to terminating the session.

Group Response to Session Four

Most members of the group appeared to enjoy discussing their experiences in relation to bodies of water. Many members recalled fishing and boating experiences. Other members expressed interest in this topic by their nonverbal participation in touching and smelling some physical props and observation of visual aids. All but two participants touched the seashells and smelled the fish eggs. One lady in the group stood up and modelled the sun hat and glasses, while a man demonstrated how to reel in the line on a fishing pole. Several participants remarked on how beautiful the pictures of the glaciers were. All but a couple of group members sang to the recorded lyrics on fishing. One member stood up and danced to the music while many others clapped to her movements.

Source: Reprinted with permission from SLACK Incorporated: Janssen, J. A., & Giberson, D. L. (1988). Remotivation therapy. *Journal of Gerontological Nursing, 14*(6), 31–34.

---

of intervention. Collaboration with other mental health care providers is best practice.

Pharmacological Interventions

Evidence about the biology of mental illness and the discovery of new psychotropic medications have expanded the role of the geropsychiatric nurse. Nurses play a vital role in monitoring, reporting, and managing medication adverse effects such as acute dystonia, akathisia, pseudoparkinsonism, neuroleptic malignant syndrome (NMS), serotonin syndrome, and anticholinergic effects. Physical assessment of response to medication is also important and includes monitoring vital signs, pain, laboratory work, elimination (bowel and bladder), changes in gait, prevention of falls, and neurological checks when appropriate. The nurse assesses for underlying medical problems. Often patients with chronic persistent mental illnesses, such as schizophrenia, misinterpret or do not report visceral cues, pain, and vital symptoms of illness. As a result, the nurse needs to be vigilant to assess and appropriately treat theses symptoms.

Health Teaching and Health Promotion

The nurse provides health teaching to both patient and caregiver on a variety of issues, including the nature of the patient's illness, symptom management, maintenance of safety, self-care strategies, management of medications (see Patient and Family Teaching: Drug Safety), coping skills, steps necessary for recovery, and resources that will support recovery. When information is printed, providing a large-print version is often helpful.

Promotion of Self-Care Activities

Hospitalization may result in regression that ranges from needing assistance to requiring total care in accomplishing the activities of daily living. A goal for nurses is to encourage the patient to regain independence in the realm of personal care. Hospitalization may be an opportunity for the patient to receive much-needed assessment of the skin, feet, hair, mouth, and perineal areas. These assessments can often uncover hidden infections, unhealed wounds, and growths that may otherwise have been missed and lead to needed medical attention.

Milieu Management

The major roles of the nurse in terms of milieu management are to assist the patient in adjusting to the environment, keep the patient safe at all times (e.g., make sure roommates are compatible, call lights are within reach, patients at risk for falling are placed close to the nurses' station), minimize the adverse effects of hospitalization on functional capacity (e.g., encourage patients to walk and to do so as independently as possible),

TABLE 28-1	USEFUL GROUP THERAPY MODALITIES FOR OLDER ADULTS		
	REMOTIVATION THERAPY	**REMINISCENCE THERAPY (LIFE REVIEW)**	**PSYCHOTHERAPY**
Purpose of Group	Resocialize regressed and apathetic patients Reawaken interest in the environment	Share memories of the past Increase self-esteem Increase socialization Increase awareness of the uniqueness of each participant	Alleviate psychiatric symptoms Increase ability to interact with others in a group Increase self-esteem Increase ability to make decisions and function more independently
Format	Groups are made up of 10 to 15 people. Meetings are held once or twice a week. Meetings are highly structured in a classroom-like setting. Group uses props. Each session discusses a particular topic. See Box 28-9 for the five basic steps used in each session.	Groups are made up of 6 to 8 people. Meetings are held once or twice weekly for 1 hour. Topics include holidays, major life events, birthdays, travel, and food.	Group size is 6 to 12 members. Group members should share similar: • Problems • Mental status • Needs Groups should be mixed (both men and women). Group meets at regularly scheduled times (certain number of times a week, specific duration of session) and place.
Desired Outcomes	Increases participants' sense of reality Offers practice of health roles Realizes more objective self-image	Alleviates depression in institutionalized older adults Through the process of reorganization and reintegration, provides avenue by which members: • Achieve a new sense of identity • Achieve a positive self-concept	Decreases sense of isolation Facilitates development of new roles and re-establishes former roles Provides information for other types of groups Provides group support for effecting changes and increasing self-esteem

Source: Touhy, T. A., & Jett, K. F. (Eds). (2016). *Ebersole & Hess' toward healthy aging: Human needs and nursing response* (9th ed.). St. Louis: Mosby.

PATIENT AND FAMILY TEACHING

Drug Safety

- Learn about your medicines:
  - Read medicine labels and package inserts, and follow the directions.
  - If you have questions, ask your doctor or other health care providers.
- Talk to your team of health care providers about your medical conditions, health concerns, and all the medicines you take (both prescription and over-the-counter), as well as dietary supplements, vitamins, and herbal supplements.
  - The more they know, the more they can help.
  - Do not be afraid to ask questions.
- Keep track of adverse effects or possible drug interactions, and let your doctor know right away about any unexpected symptoms or changes in the way you feel.
- Make sure to go to all doctor appointments and to any appointments for monitoring tests done by your doctor or at a laboratory.

- Use a calendar, pillbox, or something to help you remember what medications you need to take and when.
- Write down information your doctor gives you about your medicines or your health condition.
- Take a friend or relative to your doctor's appointments if you think you need help to understand or remember what the doctor tells you.
- Have a "medicine checkup" at least once a year.
  - Go through your medicine cabinet to get rid of old or expired medicines.
  - Ask your doctor or pharmacist to go over all the medicines you now take. Remember to include all over-the-counter medicines, vitamins, dietary supplements, and herbal supplements you take.
- Keep all medicines out of the sight and reach of children.

provide reality orientation, and engage in therapeutic communication with the patient. It helps to know that reorienting a patient is not always therapeutic, especially if the patient has dementia and reorientation causes agitation. Using distraction techniques is often the intervention of choice.

Another vital aspect of milieu management is the prevention and reduction of agitation by maintaining a visible presence on the unit and anticipating the patient's needs. Crisis intervention techniques may be used if an agitated patient does not respond to redirection or verbal attempts to de-escalate agitation. As a crisis situation unfolds, staff response will largely determine the outcome, and a well-trained crisis team improves these outcomes. The crisis team leader is usually a nurse for several reasons:

- Nurses provide professional care 24 hours a day, 7 days a week and have detailed knowledge of patients.
- The nurse is aware of the patient's medical condition.
- The nurse is able to guide the team and help prevent injury of a patient who needs physical restraint but has osteoporosis.

After the crisis has been de-escalated, the team leader, the team, and other patients (as indicated) help to restore a sense of safety and calm. As the agitated patient gains control, it is important to help the individual ease back into the milieu with dignity.

Care Settings

As discussed in Chapter 3, the mental health system has increasingly become focused on the goal of community living rather than institutional living, but resources necessary to meet this goal have been chronically underfunded. Patients who would benefit from residential care are often moved from the most structured environment (inpatient care) to unstructured and unsupervised living situations in the community.

Long-Term Care Facilities

Some long-term care settings provide specialized psychiatric mental health care, but most do not. There may be little consistency in the education of nurses and nursing assistants in appropriate psychiatric assessment and intervention. Clinicians may believe that patients who refuse personal hygiene, medication, or wound care are exercising their right to refuse care, rather than recognizing the negative symptoms of schizophrenia. Nurses who accept these refusals may inadvertently contribute to a patient's deterioration.

A geriatric psychiatric unit can be a stabilizing environment for a person with severe mental illness who thrives within the structure of a therapeutic environment. Providing a documented plan of care and intervening when behavioural symptoms increase are as important as monitoring and intervening when a resident has signs of infection. Specialized geropsychiatric units provide a comprehensive and specialized approach to care. These units use a multidisciplinary approach to assessment, treatment planning, implementation, and evaluation of care. Ideally the team consists of registered nurses, geriatric psychiatrists, geriatricians, social workers, pharmacists, psychologists, dietitians, occupational therapists, and physical therapists.

There now is much greater awareness of and focus on the use of nonpharmacological interventions for the treatment of agitation, wandering, confusion, yelling, and aggression. Drugs often deemed "unnecessary" are generally antipsychotics, antianxiety agents, and sedatives. Patients with a history of depression, schizophrenia, obsessive-compulsive disorder, generalized anxiety disorder, or bipolar disorder need ongoing treatment to prevent relapse and re-emergence of symptoms. Nurses can play an important role in advocating for psychiatric evaluation and intervention to assist with (1) managing medications, (2) monitoring and documenting behavioural changes, (3) notifying the physician of behavioural changes, and (4) planning care for the needs of those residents with mental illness.

One of the major roles of the nurse is milieu management. This involves assisting in adjustment to the environment and keeping the unit safe by making sure roommates are compatible, call lights are within reach, and patients at risk for falling are close to the nurses' station.

Recognizing the tone of the unit and making modifications when needed, such as reducing noise levels and decluttering areas, is a critical role of the staff nurse. Another vital aspect of nursing is the prevention and reduction of agitation by maintaining a visible presence on the unit and anticipating the patient's needs. Crisis intervention techniques may be necessary if an agitated patient does not respond to redirection or verbal attempts to de-escalate agitation. As a crisis situation unfolds, staff response will largely determine the outcome, and a well-trained crisis team improves these outcomes. The crisis team leader is usually a nurse for several reasons:

1. Nurses provide professional care 24 hours a day, 7 days a week, and have detailed knowledge of patients and the milieu.
2. The nurse is aware of the patient's medical condition.
3. The nurse is able to guide the team and help prevent injury to patients who may need physical restraint.

After the crisis has been de-escalated, the team leader, the team, and other patients (as indicated) need to discuss the situation; this will help restore a sense of safety and calm. As the agitated patient gains control, it is important to help the individual ease back into the milieu with dignity.

Should the services provided within a long-term care setting be required, the move may often trigger a sense of loss for both the patient and the caregiver. Family members of people admitted to long-term care will often go through a grieving process as they accept the changing needs of their loved ones. Many family members describe feeling guilty despite knowing that they can no longer care for their loved one at home. Nurses are in an excellent position to support both the person admitted and the caregivers in taking on a less physically demanding role but remaining involved in providing care.

Partial Hospitalization

Partial hospitalization, or an acute psychiatric day hospital program, is sometimes recommended for ambulatory patients who do not need 24-hour nursing care but require and would benefit from intensive, structured psychiatric treatment. Health services provided in these programs include symptom monitoring and management, medication education and management, relapse and stress prevention, and problem solving of health maintenance issues to enable the patient to adapt to active functioning in the community. The nurse also reviews with the team, in collaboration with the patient and family or caregiver, additional referrals for needed services (e.g., Meals on Wheels, transportation services, church activities, home care services).

Day Treatment Programs

Multipurpose centres for older adults provide a broad range of services, including (1) health promotion and wellness programs; (2) health screening; (3) social, educational, and recreational activities; (4) meals; and (5) information and referral services. For those in need of nursing care and custodial care services, an adult support program is an appropriate choice. There are three types of adult support programs: (1) social care, (2) adult health or medical treatment programs, and (3) maintenance care. In each type, older adults are cared for during the day and stay in a home environment at night. The boundaries of these programs blend and overlap. All three models are meant to provide a safe, supportive, and nonthreatening environment and fulfill a vital function for older adults and their families. The programs allow older adults to continue their present living arrangements and maintain their social ties to the community; they also relieve families of the burden of 24-hour-a-day care for older adult dependants. If institutionalization becomes necessary, adult day care staff can work with patients and their families to assess the situation and make recommendations for placement.

Behavioural Health Home Care

Older adults typically prefer that the continuum of services be delivered in the least restrictive setting, which is usually their homes. Home-based behavioural health care is particularly recommended to assist the homebound older adult adjust to and manage illness and disability either before or after hospitalization. It is often the role of the behavioural health home care nurse to help a person affected by a cognitive brain disorder or a severe and persistent mental illness to remain in the home or to facilitate a transfer to a temporary or permanent facility, if necessary. Local home care agencies can assist with providing nursing and rehabilitation services; home health care aide services to provide assistance with activities of daily living; homemaking services, such as housekeeping and meal preparation (although many provincial health care plans do not cover homemaking costs); or a combination of services. The goal of all of these services is to increase the older adult's ability to live independently.

The target population for behavioural health home care includes older adults who need help with activities of daily living, have behavioural issues related to their physical illness, or have an enduring mental illness. Nursing services are usually provided by a basic-level practitioner, a certified generalist nurse in community health or home health care, or an advanced-practice registered nurse certified in adult psychiatric mental health nursing.

Respite Care

Family caregivers are at great risk for burnout. Respite care is designed to allow caregivers to have a break for a specific number of days. During this time, the patient is admitted to a nursing facility for a planned number of days. Family can then go on vacation, travel, or just have a needed break from caregiving. Respite care can also be provided in the home as well.

Community-Based Programs

The hazards of institutionalization are numerous: increased risk for health care–associated infections, which may result in increased mortality; injuries occurring due to initial disorientation to a new setting; and patients developing learned helplessness and losing interest in self-care activities. (Chapter 2 provides a historical overview of deinstitutionalization.) There also may be fewer opportunities for socialization in an institutional setting. In contrast, community-based programs aim to promote the older adult's independent functioning and reduce the stress on the family system.

Community-based programs that provide specialized case-management services assist older adults with coordination of care and assistance (e.g., Meals on Wheels, transportation). Constant assessment of the changing needs of older adults requires frequent contact and rapid intervention when they become sick or need additional services. Hospitalization can be averted if aggressive and skilled case management is in place, and nurses are uniquely qualified to fulfill the role of case manager.

Older adults living in the community may still be driving, which can become a safety concern for caregivers, family, and the public. If there is evidence that the older adult can no longer safely drive a vehicle (e.g., failing visual acuity, hearing loss, memory deficits, impaired mobility, movement disorders such as Parkinson's disease), or if there have been frequent small collisions, it is appropriate to notify the provincial or territorial ministry of motor vehicles for a driving evaluation to determine the older adult's capacity for safe operation of a vehicle.

▌ KEY POINTS TO REMEMBER

- The older adult population continues to increase exponentially.
- The increase in the number of older adults poses a challenge not only to nurses but also to the entire health care system to be prepared to respond to the special needs of this population.
- Attitudes toward older adults are often negative, reflecting ageism—a bias against older adults based solely on age.

- Ageism is found at all levels of society and even among health care providers and can affect the quality of care of older patients.
- Nurses who care for older adults in various settings may function at different levels. All should be knowledgeable about the process of aging and be cognizant of the differences between normal and abnormal aging changes.

- Older adults face increasing problems of substance abuse and suicide.
- Adequate pain assessment is important, and the nurse must bear in mind that older adults tend to understate their pain. Sufficient pain medication should be administered and drugs should be carefully titrated.

- Nurses working with mentally ill patients must know psychotherapeutic approaches relevant for the older adult. Advanced-practice nurses may offer psychotherapy groups geared toward the special needs of this population.

CRITICAL THINKING

1. Mr. Abbott has received treatment for alcohol withdrawal. He is a very quiet, religious man who refuses to eat, does not sleep at night, admits to thoughts of desperation, and wishes he could die. He also confides that he attempted suicide when his wife died 5 years earlier, which is when he started drinking heavily.
   a. What cultural considerations may be helpful to know about religious people's response to depression?
   b. Which depression assessment tool is appropriate to use in assessing the severity of Mr. Abbott's condition? Explain your answer.

2. Mrs. Bélanger is 75 years old and lives with her daughter's family. She has moderate to advanced Alzheimer's disease. Although Mrs. Bélanger's family wants to keep her at home for as long as possible, they are overwhelmed by her needs and by being unable to leave her alone. What community placements might be best for Mrs. Bélanger? Explain your answer.

3. How should the nurse frame the multigenerational effects of historical trauma among Indigenous people in Canada? Useful frameworks should describe the trauma in terms of connectedness, collectivity, and relationships.

CHAPTER REVIEW

1. The nurse is caring for an older adult patient. Which symptom should the nurse recognize as a normal part of aging?
   a. Depression
   b. Memory loss
   c. Situational grieving
   d. Dementia

2. The nurse is caring for an older adult patient with depression. Which nursing response is appropriate when the patient's daughter asks, "Will he ever stop acting like this?"
   a. "I'm sorry, your father will likely be in this state from now on."
   b. "Although older adults have a high incidence of depression, it is treatable and your father will improve on the antidepressants."
   c. "Depression is caused by infections or electrolyte imbalances, and the damage is permanent."
   d. "A benzodiazepine will help alleviate the depression."

3. The nurse is caring for an older adult patient with pain. What is one myth about pain held by health care providers?
   a. Pain is an inevitable part of aging.
   b. Older adults may understate their pain using words such as *discomfort*, *hurting*, or *aching*.
   c. Dementia and depression can add to the difficulty of obtaining an accurate pain assessment.
   d. An interview with family members, caregivers, or friends is vital.

4. An older adult patient experiencing pain states that she is going to use kava kava, which she has heard provides pain relief. Which nursing response is appropriate?
   a. "Kava kava is an appropriate herb to use for pain relief."
   b. "Older adults should not use herbal preparations."
   c. "Willow bark would be a better herbal supplement to use."
   d. "Are you using any other treatments for pain relief?"

⊖volve WEBSITE

Post-Test   interactive review

Visit the Evolve website for Chapter Review Answers and Rationales, Critical Thinking Answer Guidelines, and additional resources related to the content in this chapter: http://evolve.elsevier.com/Canada/Varcarolis/psychiatric/

REFERENCES

Alexopoulos, G. S., Abrams, R. C., Young, R. C., et al. (1988). Cornell scale for depression in dementia. *Biological Psychiatry, 23*, 271–284. doi:10.1016/0006-3223(88)90038-8.

American Geriatrics Society. (2015). Updated Beers criteria for potentially inappropriate medication use in older adults. *Journal of American Geriatric Society, 63*, 2227–2246.

Bastawrous, M. (2013). Caregiver burden: A critical discussion. *International Journal of Nursing Studies, 50*(3), 431–441. doi:10.1016/j.ijnurstu.2012.10.005.

Canadian Association of Schools of Nursing (CASN) & Canadian Federation of Mental Health Nurses (CFMHN). (2017). *Entry-to-practice mental health and addiction competencies for undergraduate nursing education in Canada.* Ottawa: CASN.

Canadian Coalition for Seniors' Mental Health. (2006). *National guidelines for seniors' mental health: The assessment of suicide risk and prevention of suicide.* Toronto: Author.

Canadian Gerontological Nursing Association. (2010). *Gerontological nursing competencies and standards of practice 2010.* Vancouver: Author.

Denkinger, M. D., Lukas, A., Nikolaus, T., et al. (2015). Factors associated with fear of falling and associated activity restriction in community-dwelling older adults. *The American Journal of Geriatric Psychiatry, 23*(1), 72–86.

Eymard, A., & Douglas, D. (2012). Ageism among health care providers and interventions to improve their attitudes toward older adults: An integrative review. *Journal of Gerontological Nursing, 38*(5), 26–35. doi:10.3928/00989134-20120307-09.

Health Canada. (2011). *Canadian alcohol and drug use monitoring survey: Summary of results for 2011.* Ottawa: Author.

Hung, M., Bounsanga, J., Voss, M. W., et al. (2017). The relationship between family support: Pain and depression in elderly with arthritis. *Psychology, Health & Medicine, 22*(1), 75–86. doi:10.1080/13548506.2016.1211293.

Kagan, S. H., & Melendez-Torres, G. J. (2015). Ageism in nursing. *Journal of Nursing Management, 23*(5), 644–650. doi:10.1111/jonm.12191.

Kishita, N., & Laidlaw, K. (2017). Cognitive behaviour therapy for generalized anxiety disorder: Is CBT equally efficacious in adults of working age and older adults? *Clinical Psychology Review, 52*(1), 124–136. doi:10.1016/j.cpr.2017.01.003.

Lehne, R. A. (2013). *Pharmacology for nursing care* (8th ed.). St. Louis: Elsevier.

Maher, R., Hanlon, J., & Hajjar, E. (2014). Clinical consequences of polypharmacy in older adult. *Expert Opinion on Drug Safety, 13*(1), 57–65.

Mental Health Commission of Canada. (2012). *Changing directions, changing lives: The mental health strategy for Canada.* Calgary: Author.

Mental Health Commission of Canada. (2014). *Addressing the mental health needs of Canadians.* Ottawa: Presentation at HealthPartners.

Onder, G., Petrovic, M., Tangiisuran, B., et al. (2010). Development and validation of a score to assess risk of adverse drug reactions among in-hospital patients 65 years or older: The GerontoNet ADR risk score. *Archives of Internal Medicine, 170*(13), 1142–1148.

Powell, M., Corbo, V., Fonda, J., et al. (2015). Sleep quality and re-experiencing symptoms of PTSD are associated with current pain in U.S. OEF/OIF/OND/ veterans with and without mTBIs. *Journal of Traumatic Stress, 28*(4), 322–329. doi:10.1002/jts.22027.

Prince, M., Wimo, A., Guerchet, M., et al. (2015). *World Alzheimer report 2015: The global impact on dementia: An analysis of prevalence, in cadence, cost and trends.* London, UK: Alzheimer's Disease International.

Sheikh, J. I., & Yesavage, J. A. (1986). Geriatric Depression Scale (GDS): Recent evidence and development of a shorter version. In T. Brink (Ed.), *Clinical gerontology: A guide to assessment and intervention.* New York: The Haworth Press.

Shepherd, V., Nuttall, J., Hood, K., et al. (2015). Setting up a clinical trial in care homes: Challenges encountered and recommendations for future research practice. *BioMedCentral Research Notes, 8*(1), 1–4. doi:10.1186/s13104-015-1276-8.

Sorrell, J. M. (2017). Substance use disorders in long-term care settings: A crisis of care for older adults. *Journal of Psychosocial Nursing and Mental Health Services, 55*(1), 24–27. doi:10.3928/02793695-20170119-08.

Stall, N. (2012). Time to end ageism in medical education. *Canadian Medical Association Journal, 184*(6), 728. doi:10.1503/cmaj.112179/-/DC1.

Statistics Canada. (2015). *Canada's population estimates: Age and sex, July 1, 2015.* Retrieved from http://www.statcan.gc.ca/daily-quotidien/150929/dq150929b-eng.htm.

Szanto, K. (2017). Cognitive deficits: Underappreciated contributors to suicide. *The American Journal of Geriatric Psychiatry, 25*(6), 630–632. doi:10.1016/j.jagp.2017.02.012.

Taylor, G. (2014). *Chief public health officer's report on the state of public health in Canada, 2014: Public health in the future.* Ottawa: Public Health Agency of Canada.

Wagenaar, D., Mickus, M., & Wilson, J. (2001). Alcoholism in late life: Challenges and complexities. *Psychiatric Annals, 31*(11), 665–672.

Yalom, I. D. (2005). *The theory and practice of group psychotherapy* (5th ed.). Cambridge, MA: Basic Books.

Living With Recurrent and Persistent Mental Illness

Edward A. Herzog
Adapted by Sonya L. Jakubec

KEY TERMS AND CONCEPTS

community treatment orders (CTOs)
institutionalized
psychoeducation
rehabilitation
social skills training

stigma
supported-employment model
supportive psychotherapy
vocational rehabilitation

OBJECTIVES

1. Discuss the effects of serious mental illness on daily functioning, interpersonal relationships, and quality of life.
2. Describe three common problems associated with serious mental illness.
3. Discuss five evidence-informed practices for the care of the person with serious mental illness.
4. Explain the role of the nurse in the care of the person with serious mental illness.
5. Develop a nursing care plan for a person with serious mental illness.
6. Discuss the causes of treatment nonadherence, and plan interventions to support treatment adherence.

℮volve WEBSITE

Visit the Evolve website for Flashcards, Case Studies, and additional testing resources related to the content in this chapter: *http://evolve.elsevier.com/Canada/Varcarolis/psychiatric/*

Pre-Test | interactive review

The term *mental illness* encompasses a wide range of human illness experience, from acute and time-limited reactions to stress to severe disruptions in cognitive functioning. The terms *serious mental illness* and *biologically based mental illness* refer to a small but significant group of mental illnesses. In Canada, there is no uniform definition of serious mental illness (SMI) or *serious and persistent mental illness* (SPMI), but many Canadian researchers and clinicians use *serious mental illness* to refer to schizophrenia, mood disorders, and other psychotic disorders. In the United States, categorizing mental illnesses according to levels of severity has tremendous implications for setting mental health policy and facilitating access to appropriate care. In Canada, where health care is funded through a comprehensive government-sponsored health insurance plan, strict categorization of levels of severity is less critical. That said, in Canada, there is considerable variation

in spending on mental health services among the provinces (Canadian Institute for Health Information, 2016); the understanding that mental illness exists on a continuum of severity can help clinicians and policymakers set priorities in ongoing efforts to develop a national and comprehensive mental health policy.

SMI is a significant health care challenge: the estimated lifetime prevalence of mental illness in Canada suggests that at least 1 in 3 Canadians will experience a mood disorder, generalized anxiety disorder, or substance dependence in their lifetime, with the majority of people reporting serious mental illnesses also enduring other chronic health conditions comorbidly (Government of Canada, 2015). Individuals with SMI usually have difficulties in multiple areas, including activities of daily living, relationships, social interaction, task completion, communication, leisure activities, safe movement about the community, finances and budgeting, health maintenance, vocational and academic activities, and coping with stressors.

SMIs are chronic or recurrent. Some patients experience remissions interrupted by exacerbations of varying lengths; the remissions may be essentially symptom-free but in most cases involve some degree of residual symptoms. Other patients experience illness as a chronic and sometimes deteriorating experience, during which symptoms wax and wane but never remit.

People with SMI are at risk for multiple physical, emotional, and social problems: they are more likely to be victims of crime, be medically ill, have undertreated or untreated physical illnesses, die prematurely, be homeless, be incarcerated, be unemployed or underemployed, engage in binge substance abuse, live in poverty, and report lower quality of life and social satisfaction than persons without such illnesses (Manseau, 2014; Sederer, 2016).

The impairments associated with SMI, along with related factors such as poverty, stigma, unemployment, and inadequate housing, can significantly affect quality of life. While these factors, increasingly described as social determinants of mental health, have tremendous impact on people, the necessary social and political intervention are still placed well in the background, eclipsed by the largely individual treatment focus of interventions for SMI (Larsson, 2015).

Serious Mental Illness Across the Lifespan

SMI occurs in persons of any gender, age, culture, or geographical location. However, the population of people currently living with SMIs can be separated into two groups that have had different experiences with the mental health care system: (1) those old enough to have experienced long-term institutionalization, and (2) those young enough to have been hospitalized only for acute care during exacerbations of their disorders.

Older Adults

Until the second half of the twentieth century, most psychiatric inpatient treatment took place in large institutions uniquely dedicated to the care of the severely mentally ill. During this time, psychiatric hospitals were the long-term residences for many people (see Chapter 2). Medical paternalism, in which the health care provider made all decisions for patients with SMIs, was a pervasive philosophical stance at that time. Thus patients became institutionalized (i.e., they became dependent on the services and structure of institutions and unable to function independently outside such institutions). It was difficult to distinguish whether behaviours were the result of the disease process or altered responses that resulted from institutionalization.

Some of today's older adults with SMI have experience with this system of care. They have learned that they are expected to accept the treatment team's decisions. Today's emphasis on patient-centred care, which requires the patient to express his or her opinions and wishes, challenges some older adults who grew up in the paternalistic institutions of the past.

It was between 1960 and 1980 that all Canadian provinces began to make changes in the inpatient treatment of SMI by closing beds in large mental hospitals and opening inpatient units in general hospitals. The 1990s heralded further deinstitutionalization of psychiatric services as the total number of inpatient days for mental health care in psychiatric hospitals and general hospitals declined (Spagnolo, 2014).

> **VIGNETTE**
>
> At the age of 19, Marian was admitted to a facility that cares for people with serious mental illnesses. She is now 79, and with the exception of living in a group home for 2 years in her thirties, she has been an inpatient at the SMI facility. Marian's symptoms have been stable, and the treatment team discusses discharge with her. She accepts their recommendation that she no longer needs inpatient treatment. She is discharged to a community supportive-living home. At her new home, she spends long periods sitting in front of the living room window. Marian does not ask to go out into the garden she watches for so many hours. Indeed, she rarely asks for anything, including snacks or recreational activities. The caregivers work with Marian for several months to help her to recognize her needs of the moment and then to articulate or act on them. There is a major celebration on the day she walks into the kitchen and makes a peanut butter sandwich of her own volition. Some of the dependency caused by the institutionalization is being positively altered.

Younger Adults

People young enough never to have been institutionalized usually do not have problems of passivity and dependency. However, treatment via a series of short-term hospitalizations has given them limited experience with formal treatment and has contributed to some patients not truly believing that a problem exists. Individuals who do not understand that they are ill, perhaps because of the impairment of the illness itself (poor insight, possibly related to *anosognosia*), are at particular risk for additional problems. Young adults with SMI, for example, are at particular risk for additional problems such as legal difficulties, substance abuse, and unemployment.

> **VIGNETTE**
>
> After graduating from high school, Christopher enlists in the armed forces and serves for 5 years. Afterward, he settles in Nova Scotia and takes a job in a security firm. In his first psychotic break, Christopher becomes paranoid and threatening at work and is hospitalized briefly. Upon discharge, Christopher refuses aftercare and will not take medication. He quits his job and moves to another city. For the next 15 years, Christopher works intermittently, is homeless off and on, and drinks heavily whenever he has money. He is hospitalized only when his behaviour is threatening to others. He consistently resists aftercare recommendations, showing no insight into his illness. One day, Christopher simply disappears.

DEVELOPMENT OF SERIOUS MENTAL ILLNESS

SMI has much in common with chronic physical illness: the original problem increasingly overwhelms and erodes basic coping mechanisms and increases the use of compensatory processes. As the disorder extends beyond the acute stage, more and more of the neighbouring systems are involved. For example, a person with schizophrenia may experience disturbed thought processes and social skills, which cause interactions with others to become increasingly awkward and anxiety provoking for both parties. This awkwardness, in turn, results in others becoming increasingly hesitant to interact with the affected person and in the affected person's self-esteem weakening.

REHABILITATION VERSUS RECOVERY: TWO MODELS OF CARE

For many years, the concept of rehabilitation, which focused on managing patients' deficits and helping patients learn to live with their illnesses, dominated psychiatric care. Staff directed the treatment and concentrated on helping patients function in their daily roles. Advocates for improved mental health care and people with SMI (many of whom prefer to call themselves *consumers* to emphasize the choices they have, or seek to have, over their treatment, or *survivors* to indicate a separation or survival from the formal psychiatric system) have increasingly sought a different treatment approach.

The recovery model developed out of the consumer movement. The recovery model is patient or consumer centred, involves active partnership with care providers, and is integrated within broader social and political agendas (Frost, Tirupati, Johnston, et al., 2017). It is a hopeful, empowering, strengths-focused model whereby staff assist the consumer to achieve the highest quality of life possible. This model of care encourages a high degree of patient independence and self-determination, focusing on achieving goals of the patient's choosing and leading increasingly productive and meaningful lives (Frost, Tirupati, Johnston, et al., 2017). The emphasis is on the person and the future rather than on the illness and the present.

Although it has been suggested that the recovery philosophy has been slower to take hold in Canada (Mulvale & Bartram, 2015), the Mental Health Commission of Canada (MHCC, 2015) identified recovery as central to mental health care reform. According to the MHCC, a recovery-oriented system creates the possibility for people with severe mental illness to gain more control over their lives and make choices about treatments, while being supported by professionals, families, and other people who are significant in their lives. A recovery community model of housing and support is discussed in the Research Highlight box.

ISSUES CONFRONTING THOSE WITH SERIOUS MENTAL ILLNESS

Establishing a Meaningful Life

Finding meaning in life and establishing goals can be difficult for people living with SMI, particularly if they also experience

 RESEARCH HIGHLIGHT

Recovery Communities for People With Serious Mental Illness

Problem

Housing is an issue of crucial concern for people with serious mental illnesses given high rates of homelessness among this population.

Purpose of Study

This study sought to examine the housing environment, in particular intentional communities or recovery communities, as it relates to recovery among people with serious mental illnesses.

Methods

Focus groups were conducted with recovery community residents at 4-month intervals to inquire into day-to-day life in these communities. Focus group transcripts were reviewed and thematic analysis was conducted to identify prominent and emergent themes relating to the recovery community and recovery.

Key Findings

Three identified domains highlight how recovery communities were contributing to the recovery of residents with serious and persistent mental illness. These themes were (1) service environment, (2) physical environment, and (3) social environment. Recovery communities were found to be embedded in a complementary service system; the physical environment provides a refuge from homelessness, drug activity, and violence; and the social environment offers a place to "belong" amid peer support for mental health and sobriety.

Implications for Nursing Practice

Recovery-oriented communities are identified in this study to encompass multiple, complex needs that include more than clinical efforts to reduce psychiatric symptomatology, substance use, and the impact of trauma. People with serious mental illnesses living in recovery communities identified support needs for fundamental security, connection, and belonging. Recovery communities may offer support for psychiatric concerns as well as a refuge from poverty, homelessness, and isolation.

Source: Carpenter-Song, E., Hipolito, M. M. S., & Whitley, R. (2012). Right here is an oasis: How "recovery communities" contribute to recovery for people with serious mental illnesses. *Psychiatric Rehabilitation Journal, 35*(6), 435–440. doi:10.1037/h0094576.

poor self-esteem or apathy. Patients may struggle with the possibility that they may never be the person they once expected to be. Finding a way to "reset" one's goals so that meaning can be found in new ways (e.g., helping others, volunteering, or simply surmounting a significant illness) is important to achieving a satisfactory quality of life and avoiding despair.

Those who cannot work or attend school have a significant amount of free time to fill. If these people do not own a car or have easy access to public transit, lack money for movies or other pastimes, are afraid to go outside, or do not have enough confidence to join peers, options can be very limited.

Comorbid Conditions

Physical Disorders

One of the strategic directions of the MHCC is to achieve an "increase [in] the life expectancy of people living with severe mental illnesses" (MHCC, 2012, p. 129). People with SMI are at greater risk for co-occurring physical illnesses and die prematurely (on average, 15 years prematurely for women and 20 years for men). Furthermore, the conditions of this premature mortality are increasingly understood to result from a combination of socioeconomic, health care, and clinical risk factors, and not from higher rates of suicide (Thornicroft, 2013).

Contributing factors include failing to provide for their own health needs, inability to access or pay for care, and other obstacles, such as stigma or stereotyping. Expressing health care needs in an eccentric or unclear manner, for example, can influence the quality of care received. One patient with schizophrenia experienced a detached retina and sought assistance at a local health clinic. She told the nurse that she had "the sun in (her) eye." Because the nurse knew the patient's history, she decided that the patient was hallucinating and delusional and did not perform a physical examination. It wasn't until the next morning, after an antipsychotic had been administered and the patient reported that the visual disturbance persisted, that the nurse examined the patient's eye more carefully. Staff bias or inadequate understanding of mental illness had resulted in a less thorough evaluation and a delay in treatment. Inequalities in access and delivery of health care may also be related to the separation of mental health programs from other health care programs (Thornicroft, 2013).

Depression and Suicide

Persons with SMI may experience a profound sense of loss. This loss can lead to acute or chronic grief, which, along with the chronicity of the illness and its demands and impact on daily life, can contribute to despair, depression, and a lifetime risk for suicide of 5% for persons with schizophrenia (Hor & Taylor, 2010); however, it is estimated that many more people with SMI engage in self-harming behaviours, which are strongly associated with substance use (Dharmawardene & Menkes, 2017).

Substance Abuse

People who experience SMI are at much higher risk for substance abuse than people in the general population (McKee, 2017). A person who experiences both a mental disorder and a substance use disorder is said to have a *concurrent disorder*. People with mental illnesses are twice as likely to have a substance use problem compared to the general population. It is estimated that 20% of people with a mental illness have a concurrent disorder, and the rate may be as high as 50% for people with schizophrenia. Similarly, those with substance use problems are three times as likely to have a mental illness as the general population. It is estimated that more than 15% of those with substance use disorders have a comorbid mental illness (Centre for Addiction and Mental Health, 2017).

Substance abuse may be a form of self-medication, countering the dysphoria or other symptoms caused by illness or its treatment (e.g., the sedation caused by one's medications). Nicotine use has always been higher among those with SMI and is not declining as it has been in the general population (Tidey, 2016). Substance abuse contributes to comorbid physical health problems, reduced quality of life, incarceration, relapse, and reduced effectiveness of medications (Centre for Addiction and Mental Health, 2017).

Social Problems

Stigma

Stigma has been described as negative attitudes or behaviours toward a person or group based on a belief that they possess negative traits (Gaebel, Rössler, & Sartorius, 2017). The MHCC (2012) reported that stigma and discrimination of all kinds "are the major reasons that mental health issues have remained in the shadows for so long" (pp. 22–23). Stigma stems from a lack of understanding of mental illness that causes others to make assumptions about those with SMI. Stigma can result in discrimination and cause shame, anger, and further isolation (Patten, Williams, Lavorato, et al., 2016). It is perpetuated by stereotypical images in North American culture. Meeting and talking with someone with an SMI can help the general public to reduce their stigmatizing behaviours and attitudes toward people with SMIs. A member of the public stated:

People assume that an oddly behaving person sitting on a street corner has to be on drugs or is some crazy loser that is a discard of our society: someone that cannot get better. Next time you look at a young person on the street or an older adult, think of them as your son or daughter, or maybe your sister or brother. They could be. (MHCC, 2009, p. 84)

Initiatives such as the Opening Minds project seek to improve understanding and acceptance through education and reduction of stigma (MHCC, 2009).

Isolation and Loneliness

Social isolation and loneliness are concerns of many people with chronic illnesses, not just those with SMI. Stigma reduces the social contact of persons with SMI, and individual factors such as poor self-image, poverty (which interferes with recreational and social activities), passivity, and impaired hygiene also interfere with relationships. Romantic relationships and opportunities for sexual expression, usually desired among persons with SMI just as in any population, are also affected by isolation (and often by sexual dysfunction from medications). In response to this challenge, dating services specifically for persons with disabilities or mental illness have been created.

Victimization

Stereotypes would have us believe that people with SMI are more likely to be violent than people who do not have mental illness. However, the reverse is actually true: mentally ill people are more likely to be victims of violence than perpetrators of it (Centre for Addiction and Mental Health, 2013). Sexual assault or coerced sexual activity also commonly occurs within this vulnerable population. Impaired judgement, impaired interpersonal skills (e.g., unknowingly acting in ways that might provoke others, such as standing too close or not leaving when told to), passivity, poor self-esteem, dependency, residence in high-crime neighbourhoods, and an appearance of vulnerability may contribute to this significant problem.

Economic Challenges
Unemployment and Poverty

Most people derive at least part of their identity and sense of value from the work they do. Many people with SMI would like to work, but symptoms such as cognitive slowing or disorganization interfere with obtaining or succeeding at work. According to the MHCC (2013), between 70% and 90% of people with SMI are unemployed, and 50% of those with SMI do not receive sufficient income from their disability entitlements. It can be difficult to find an employer open to hiring a person with SMI, and laws to prevent discrimination do not guarantee a job.

Atypical antipsychotic medications can be extremely expensive. Each province administers its own prescription drug plan, and patients with SMI may be able to obtain coverage under these plans. However, not every medication is covered. Because people with SMI are less likely to be employed, they are less likely to have private insurance coverage to cover the additional costs of medication. In addition to the challenges of obtaining pharmacological treatment, in many cases those with SMI do not have private or public insurance to cover treatment from other mental health care providers (e.g., psychologists), which may be a significant barrier to mental health treatment in Canada (Dezetter, Duhoux, Menear, et al., 2015).

Housing Instability

Even though stable, safe, and affordable housing is very important for people living with SMI, homelessness is unfortunately prevalent (Goering & Streiner, 2015). Many people with SMI have limited funds, which equates to limited options for housing. Obtaining an affordable apartment may require one to live far from needed resources (e.g., stores, health care centres, support persons) or in unsafe neighbourhoods. An episode of behaviour deemed inappropriate could lead to eviction and a negative reputation among landlords, closing doors to future housing. Living with family can produce interpersonal strains and conflict about patient behaviour (e.g., nonadherence, impaired self-care), which in turn often lead to estrangement and loss of housing with family.

Symptoms can cause behaviour that leads to police arrest. For example, one patient asked a store clerk if he could pay him later for a bottle of pop and, thinking concretely, mistook the clerk's sarcastic "Oh, sure" as genuine approval, only to leave with the pop and find himself charged with theft an hour later. A single bad decision caused an arrest that could leave the person ineligible for housing subsidies or public housing. Even with a subsidy, however, waiting lists can be up to 2 years long. Finding and keeping good housing can be very challenging for these patients.

Caregiver Burden

Caregivers, particularly family members, provide important support for people with SMI. However, coping with the persistent and challenging needs of people with SMI can be extremely challenging and requires significant emotional, physical, and, at times, financial resources. Caregivers also age, become ill, and may require care themselves, depleting their ability to provide support for the person with SMI. When caregivers are no longer able to provide the needed support for the person with SMI, a very difficult adjustment can result, leading to crises such as homelessness, conflict between caregiver and patient, and even exacerbation of the SMI symptoms.

Treatment Issues
Nonadherence

At any point in time, nearly half of all people with mental illness are not receiving treatment or are nonadherent to treatment, thereby potentially increasing the likelihood of relapse (Weiden, 2016). Most health care providers address this problem with medication education, but patients faced with repetitive medication groups and exhortations to take medications often become more resistant rather than insightful. Other obstacles, such as adverse effects, drug costs, interruptions in treatment, and rotating treatment providers, increase the risk for nonadherence and threaten stability and prognosis. Box 29-1 describes nursing interventions that promote adherence.

Anosognosia

Many people assume that people with mental illness who do not understand that they are mentally ill must be in denial (i.e., they know they are ill but cannot accept it). Although denial is a possibility, another is *anosognosia* (ă-nō′sog-nō′sē-ă), the inability to recognize one's deficits due to one's illness. Anosognosia is a lack of awareness of neurological and neuropsychological deficits associated with frontotemporal-parietal damage, observed in some patients with dementia or who have had a stroke. There is some evidence linking the phenomenon to core pathophysiology of schizophrenia, which justifies extension of the construct of anosognosia to schizophrenia-related insight deficits (Lehrer & Lorenz, 2014). As yet, however, there is debate about application of the term to schizophrenia where the neurobiological markers are not confirmed (Osatuke, Ciesla, Kasckow, et al., 2008).

What is known is that individuals who do not understand that their symptoms are illness related will find it difficult to recognize that they have an illness. Others may believe or hope that the illness will go away on its own (Morris, Johns, & Oliver, 2013). People who do not perceive themselves to be mentally ill are unlikely to seek or accept treatment. It can take months or years for a person with SMI to acknowledge having a mental illness. The best approach of mental health nurses should be empathic, supportive, and focused on harm reduction rather than punitive (Weiden, 2016).

It is important for mental health nurses to listen and assess carefully where there may be high risk or potential for harm to self or others and to build a trusting helping relationship to support safety and optimal recovery. For others, who are functioning and may simply hold understandings of their distress or preferences that differ from the medical approach to treatment, assessment and support must be provided through building trust and understanding.

BOX 29-1   INTERVENTIONS TO IMPROVE ADHERENCE TO TREATMENT

- Select treatments and dosages that are most likely to be effective and well tolerated by each patient.
- Actively manage adverse effects to avert or minimize patient distress, which could result in nonadherence.
- Simplify treatment regimens to make them more acceptable and understandable to the patient (e.g., once-a-day dosing instead of twice-daily dosing).
- Tie treatment adherence to achieving the patient's goals to increase motivation. Point out and reinforce improvements, connecting them to treatment adherence.
- To improve patient insight and motivation, provide **psychoeducation** (an approach to care that emphasizes helping a person to gain the knowledge necessary to manage the illness) about SMI and the role of treatment in recovery. Take care not to assume that nonadherence means that the patient does not understand. There are many reasons for nonadherence; applying psychoeducation when the problem is something other than a lack of knowledge is unlikely to succeed.
- Assign consistent, committed caregivers who have (or are skilled at building) positive therapeutic bonds with the patient and who will be able to work with the patient for extended periods of time.
- Involve the patient in support groups with members who have greater insight and first-hand experience with illness and treatment—people whose viewpoints the patient may be more likely to accept.
- Provide culturally safe, trauma-informed care. Cultural beliefs and practices (e.g., suspicious attitudes or traumatic histories with health care and authority figures, valuing self-sufficiency or privacy above health care) can be a barrier to therapeutic relationships and result in rejection of treatment.
- Carefully monitor medication decreases or changes to control adverse effects and improve the therapeutic effect.
- When other interventions have not been successful, use medication monitoring, long-acting forms of medication (depot injections or sustained-release formats), motivational interviewing, and other techniques as indicated to increase adherence.
- Never reject, blame, or shame the patient when nonadherence occurs. Instead, label it as simply an issue for continuing focus, and work toward harm reduction.

Sources: Weiden, P. J. (2007). Discontinuing and switching antipsychotic medications: Understanding the CATIE schizophrenia trial (Supplemental material). *Journal of Clinical Psychiatry, 68,* 12–19; and Weiden, P. J. (2016). Redefining medication adherence in the treatment of schizophrenia: How current approaches to adherence lead to misinformation and threaten therapeutic relationships. *The Psychiatric Clinics of North America, 39*(2), 199.

Medication Adverse Effects

Psychotropic medications, especially antipsychotic agents, can produce a range of distressing adverse effects, from involuntary movements to increased risk for diabetes. Some adverse effects are treatable; others may diminish over time or can be compensated for via behavioural changes (e.g., changing position slowly to reduce dizziness from hypotension). Addressing adverse effects in an evidence-informed, humble, and honest manner is essential to gaining an understanding of a patient's situation and struggles with diagnosis, treatment, and side effects. Although some people respond well to medication, psychiatric drugs can sometimes induce or exacerbate illness.

Some people with schizophrenia may pursue alternative treatments or select to refrain from long-term psychiatric medication use, and many with stronger social support and coping strategies ultimately fare better (Harrow, Jobe, & Faull, 2012). It is the work of careful and attentive professionals to ensure that those who are most at risk for nonadherence and who lack the support and coping skills needed to overcome potential triggers of relapse are supported and that their safety is secured.

The approach of motivational interviewing is suggested as a way to explore the values and personal goals of individuals and to assess readiness for participating more actively in the treatment. Motivational interviewing can also be employed to develop strategies for obstacles specific to symptoms of schizophrenia, such as cognitive deficits and negative symptoms with associated motivational problems (Rusch & Corrigan, 2002). Research Highlight: Motivational Interviewing and Medication Adherence describes recent research validating this approach. Regardless of therapeutic strategies or approach, a strong helping relationship can support understanding and perhaps a realistic and sustained treatment that can promote equilibrium and recovery and maximize quality of life (Thompson & McCabe, 2012). See Chapter 9 for more on the therapeutic relationship and Chapter 11 for a detailed discussion of antipsychotic drugs.

Treatment Inadequacy

It has been suggested that there are significant gaps between the quality of mental health care provided and optimal care (Addington, Kyle, Desair, et al., 2010). Often discontinuation of treatment is precipitated by poor treatment response. Patients must be informed and diligent in ensuring that they are receiving the most effective treatment, and agencies and staff must be diligent in updating their programs and practice. A strong therapeutic alliance and commitment to a recovery model are pivotal in staying the course and persevering through setbacks, ineffective treatments, and patient choices (Symanski-Tondora, Miller, Slade, et al., 2014).

Residual Symptoms

Residual symptoms are those that do not improve completely or consistently with treatment. They can be very frustrating, and patients may feel that these symptoms mean they will not get better or that treatments are not working (promoting helplessness and hopelessness). The patient may then discontinue treatment, worsening the illness. Residual symptoms can also cause or worsen associated issues (e.g., inappropriate social behaviour and

RESEARCH HIGHLIGHT

Motivational Interviewing and Medication Adherence

Problem

Nonadherence to antipsychotic medication is common among patients and contributes to high relapse rates. Little is known, however, about interventions to support medication adherence.

Purpose of Study

This study was designed to test and evaluate the effectiveness of an adherence therapy for outpatients with schizophrenia spectrum disorders, based on a motivational interviewing approach over a 6-month follow-up period.

Methods

A single-blind, randomized controlled trial with a repeated-measures, two-parallel-groups design was conducted using a random sample of 114 participants with schizophrenia spectrum disorders in one community psychiatric nursing service. After pre-test, the participants were randomly assigned to either an eight-session course of motivational interviewing treatment plus usual care or usual psychiatric care (n = 57 per group). The main outcomes, including medication adherence, symptom severity, insight into treatment, hospitalization rate, and functioning, were measured at baseline and immediately and 6 months after intervention.

Key Findings

A total of 110 participants completed this trial, an attrition rate of 3.5%. Results indicated that the treatment participants reported significantly greater improvements in their insight into illness or treatment, psychosocial functioning, symptom severity, number of rehospitalizations, and medication adherence over a 6-month follow-up, when compared with usual care.

Implications for Nursing Practice

Motivational interviewing approaches for people with schizophrenia can be effective to reduce symptom severity and rehospitalizations and to improve medication adherence, functioning, and insight into illness or treatment over a medium-term (6 months) period of follow-up.

Source: Chien, W. T., Mui, J. H. C., Cheung, E. F. C., et al.. (2015). Effects of motivational interviewing-based adherence therapy for schizophrenia spectrum disorders: A randomized controlled trial. *Trials, 16*(1), 270. doi:10.1186/s13063-015-0785-z.

impulsiveness that can add to stigmatization and isolation). Psychoeducation about both symptoms and treatment has been found to be effective in reducing stigma related to aspects of treatment (Choe, Sung, Kang, et al., 2016).

Relapse, Chronicity, and Loss

The majority of patients with SMI face the possibility of relapse even when adhering to treatment, which may contribute to hopelessness and helplessness. Living with SMI paradoxically requires more effort and emotional resources from people who are less able to cope with such demands. Each relapse can cause loss of relationships, employment, and housing, adding that much more loss to the patient's life and making discharge planning significantly more complicated.

RESOURCES FOR PEOPLE WITH SERIOUS MENTAL ILLNESS

Comprehensive Community Treatment

Community services, particularly for those with serious mental illness, have been described as fragmented and inefficient, with blurring of responsibility among agencies, programs, and levels of government (Addiction and Mental Health Collaborative Project Steering Committee, 2014). Ideally, the community-based mental health care system provides comprehensive, coordinated, and cost-effective (from the perspective of the government) care for the patient with mental illness. Interventions at the individual, family, community, and societal or political levels must all be part of the complex coordination of all levels of prevention for those with serious and persistent mental illness.

The overall goal of community psychiatric treatment is to improve the patient's ability to function independently in the community. Community services vary according to local needs and resources. Patients sometimes find that needed services are not locally available or have long wait lists, and they may have difficulty identifying the best programs for their needs amid the maze of agencies and services. When people with SMI are unable to access community-based services, they are often forced to rely on institution-based care (Davis, 2013).

Community Services and Programs

A case-management program is a comprehensive service provided by a multidisciplinary team. The team coordinates the patient's overall care, brokers access to services, and provides psychosocial education, guidance, and support (Davis, 2013). Case managers can provide medication monitoring, wherein they observe and facilitate the patient's use of medications. Intensive case management has been strongly linked to improved consumer engagement, psychological functioning, and adaptation to the demands of everyday living (Goldner, Jenkins, & Bilsker, 2016). Assertive community treatment (ACT), discussed later in this chapter, is one model of case management. Other community services and programs that may be available include social skills training, crisis intervention services, emergency psychiatric services, and community outreach programs.

Substance Abuse Treatment

A variety of services exist for those who have a concurrent diagnosis of SMI and alcohol- or drug-related problems. Chemical dependency clinics provide therapeutic and rehabilitative services, including medical and psychosocial assessment, detoxification, crisis intervention, and medication such as methadone. Most clinicians endorse treatment that is integrated (i.e., delivered by a single provider rather than split between a mental health agency and a drug or alcohol agency), using personnel with dual areas of expertise, but this standard has not yet been met in some settings (Centre for Addiction and Mental Health, 2009). See Chapter 18 for a detailed discussion of treatment settings for patients with substance abuse issues.

> **VIGNETTE**
>
> After 3 years of living on his own, Christopher returns home to his parents. He is soon arrested for threatening a police officer with a steel pipe, is found "not criminally responsible," and is released on the condition that he receive psychiatric treatment. Because of his history of nonadherence, he goes to a clinic and receives intramuscular depot medication. He is also enrolled in a day program and is assigned a case manager, who helps him apply for income assistance and refers him to a group home when his aging parents state that he can no longer live with them. Because he wants to work, he is referred to a supported-employment program. He gets a job unloading delivery trucks and stays in that job for the next 5 years. When the requirements of his conditional release are completed, he continues in treatment and continues working nearly full time. Because he is stable, his medication is changed to an oral atypical antipsychotic, and he continues to receive supervision in his group home.

> **VIGNETTE**
>
> Christopher, now age 50, has schizophrenia. He has lived in a group home since his late twenties. He has been stable for the past 10 years and has had a steady girlfriend for the past 3 years. He announces that he wants to move out on his own and maybe get married. Despite respectful disagreement from his nurse therapist, he finds himself a room to rent. Over the next 2 months, his mental status remains stable: he is polite, quiet, and guarded as usual. However, his psychiatrist, who weighs him monthly, notices that he has lost 10 kilograms. Christopher cannot identify any change in his eating habits, and he is referred to his primary care provider for an evaluation. He does not follow up with the primary care provider, and over the next 4 weeks, he loses another 5 kilograms. His nurse therapist calls his work supervisor, who reports that Christopher is behaving differently: he is talking out loud to himself, becoming more isolated, and, one morning, smelled of alcohol. She is supportive of Christopher and hopes he will get treatment. At his next clinic appointment, the psychiatrist and therapist discuss these changes and recommend that Christopher go into the partial hospital program for medication re-evaluation. He reluctantly agrees, denying that he has any problem.

EVIDENCE-INFORMED TREATMENT APPROACHES

Assertive Community Treatment

Assertive community treatment (ACT) is an approach to caring for the person with severe mental illness in the community. ACT teams provide multidisciplinary, comprehensive, and, in some cases, intensive treatment services. The ACT model of care is a structure of treatment and rehabilitative and supportive services that enhance the ability of the person with SMI to live successfully in the community. ACT serves individuals who have not been able to successfully manage their illnesses in traditional outpatient or rehabilitation services. Key principles of ACT include maintaining small patient-to-staff ratios, engaging in a proactive approach, and establishing highly individualized treatment plans. ACT has been shown to improve symptoms of SMI and reduce inpatient admissions, incarceration, and homelessness among persons with mental illness in urban and rural communities (Pope & Harris, 2014).

Cognitive Behavioural Therapy

Cognitive behavioural therapy (CBT) has been shown to be effective in helping patients with SMI to cope with symptoms such as auditory hallucinations, to address defeating beliefs and self-stigma, and to contemplate recovery (Dopke & Batscha, 2014; Nowak, Sabariego, Świtaj, et al., 2016). The cognitive component of CBT focuses on patterns of thinking and "self-talk" (i.e., what one says to oneself internally). It identifies cognitive distortions and guides patients to substitute more effective forms of thinking. The behavioural component of CBT uses natural consequences and positive reinforcers to shape the person's behaviour in a more positive or adaptive manner.

Cognitive Enhancement Therapy

Cognitive enhancement therapy (CET) is based on the principle that the brain is able to change and that compromised neurological functions can be assumed by healthier areas of the brain. CET involves many hours (i.e., 60 or more) of computer-based drills and exercises that incrementally challenge functions, such as focusing attention, processing and recalling information, and interpreting social and emotional information (e.g., inferring a person's mood from his or her expression or tone of voice). Research has shown that CET leads to sustained improvement in these functional areas and improves social and vocational functioning (Eack, 2012).

Family Support and Partnerships

Families and significant others can face considerable stresses related to the mental illness of a loved one and may suffer as a result of insufficient empathy and understanding (Park & Seo, 2016). Having sound family support and partnerships is one of the strongest predictors of recovery; treatment is enhanced and conflict is reduced when treatment providers work as empathic partners with both patients and their significant others. The Canadian Mental Health Association (CMHA) partners with a variety of public and private agencies to provide family support programs that are tailored to the specific needs of a community or region. Provincial branches of the CMHA serve as an excellent source of information, support, and practical guidance for patients and their significant others.

Social Skills Training

Social skills training focuses on the teaching of a wide variety of social and activities of daily living (ADL) skills. People with SMI often have social deficits that cause functional impairment; for example, those unable to respond assertively may respond aggressively instead. Complex interpersonal skills, such as negotiating or resolving a conflict, are broken down into subcomponents, which are then taught in a step-by-step fashion (Lyman, Kurtz, Farkas, et al., 2014).

Supportive Psychotherapy

Although definitions vary, supportive psychotherapy is generally understood to be an approach that stresses empathic understanding, a nonjudgemental attitude, and the development of a therapeutic alliance (Dulmus & Nisbet, 2013). Supportive psychotherapy has been shown to enhance the therapeutic alliance and improve long-term recovery prospects in patients with serious mental illness (Harder, Koester, Valbak, et al., 2014).

Vocational Rehabilitation and Related Services

Vocational rehabilitation and related services vary widely but can include vocational training, financial support for attaining employment, or supported-employment services. Like most people, those with SMI want to feel as though they contribute and therefore want to be engaged in meaningful employment (Khare, Mueser, & McGurk, 2016). The benefits of employment (or volunteer work) are enhanced self-esteem, improved organizational abilities, and increased socialization and income.

Vocational rehabilitation programs using a clubhouse model, in which patients jointly run their own business, such as a coffee shop or housekeeping service, teach all members to perform a job in order to make the business work. Such programs have led to the supported-employment model, which has been shown to be one of the most effective evidence-informed interventions for helping people with SMI to achieve employment. The model includes rapid job placement, on-the-job support, and provision of a job coach who is linked to the mental health team (Mueser & McGurk, 2014).

OTHER POTENTIALLY BENEFICIAL SERVICES OR TREATMENT APPROACHES

While not yet evidence-informed practices, research to date supports use of the following services and treatment approaches.

Consumer-Run Programs

The CMHA and other organizations offer training that enables consumers to assist peers in the recovery process. Consumer-run programs range from informal "clubhouses"—which offer socialization, recreation, and sometimes other services, such as educational programs—to competitive businesses—which are often part of a vocational rehabilitation program.

Wellness and Recovery Action Plans

Wellness and recovery action plans (WRAPs) and similar programs are psychoeducational programs that empower and train patients in skills that promote recovery and prepare them to deal with stressors and crises (Olney & Emery-Flores, 2017). Training focuses on daily maintenance plans (i.e., things that must be done and resources needed to maintain wellness), identification and management of triggers that could provoke a relapse, early identification of impending relapse, and crisis plans (i.e., plans for managing crises or impending relapse). Typically a wide variety of useful tools, templates, and techniques are provided, and the programs lead to developing practical and concrete action plans for promoting recovery.

Exercise

Exercise holds many benefits for persons with SMI, including improved activity tolerance and ability to cope with symptoms, reduced anxiety and depression, enhanced self-esteem, weight control or loss (important for patients with weight-related comorbidities, such as diabetes and hypertension), and cost effectiveness (Pearsall, Smith, Pelosi, et al., 2014).

NURSING CARE OF PATIENTS WITH SERIOUS MENTAL ILLNESS

Nurses encounter patients with SMI in a variety of inpatient and community settings. All roles and techniques used by psychiatric mental health nurses in inpatient psychiatric settings also apply in the community and other settings.

Assessment Strategies

Important assessments include the following:
- Signs of risk to self or others (suicidality or homicidality)
- Depression or hopelessness
- Signs of relapse (especially increased impulsivity or paranoia, diminished reality testing, increased delusional thinking or command hallucinations)
- Inadequate attention to proper nutrition, adequate clothing or medical care and carelessness while driving, smoking, or cooking (e.g., leaving pots on the stove and becoming distracted or falling asleep)
- Signs of treatment nonadherence or impending relapse (early detection and correction of relapse reduces its intensity and duration and prevents hospitalization, loss of housing, arrest, and loss of entitlements)
- Physical health problems, such as brain tumours or drug toxicity, that can cause psychiatric symptoms and be mistaken for mental illness or relapse
- Comorbid illnesses (ensuring that the patient provides appropriate self-care and receives adequate health care)

Table 29-1 lists potential nursing diagnoses that apply to the patient with SMI. Table 29-2 lists examples of specific nursing outcomes.

TABLE 29-1	POTENTIAL NURSING DIAGNOSES FOR THE PATIENT WITH SERIOUS MENTAL ILLNESS
SIGNS AND SYMPTOMS	**NURSING DIAGNOSES**
Speaking too softly to be heard	Communication, impaired verbal
Verbalization incongruent with the setting	Social interaction, impaired
Silence in groups or withdrawal when approached	Social isolation
Failure to keep appointments	Noncompliance
Admitted missing of medication or observed return of symptoms	
Self-negating verbalization	Chronic low self-esteem
Fear of trying new things or situations	Powerlessness
Nonassertiveness or passivity	
Distortion of patient's health problem, often denial	Disabled family coping
	Caregiver role strain
Neglect of other members of family	
Excessive concern for and supervision of patient	

TABLE 29-2	NOC OUTCOMES RELATED TO SERIOUS MENTAL ILLNESS	
NURSING OUTCOME AND DEFINITION	**INTERMEDIATE INDICATORS**	**SHORT-TERM INDICATORS**
Self-care: Instrumental activities of daily living (IADL): Ability to perform activities needed to function independently in the home or community, with or without assistive device	Manages medications Manages money	Shops for groceries Prepares meals Uses phone Travels on public transportation
Family coping: Family actions to manage stressors that tax family resources	Uses available social support Cares for needs of all members	Involves family members in decision making Establishes family priorities Plans for emergencies

Source: Moorhead, S., Johnson, M., Maas, M. L., et al. (2013). *Nursing outcomes classification (NOC)* (5th ed.). St Louis: Mosby.

BOX 29-2	*NIC* INTERVENTIONS FOR SERIOUS MENTAL ILLNESS SELF-CARE ASSISTANCE: IADL

Definition of self-care assistance: IADL: Assisting and instructing a person to perform instrumental activities of daily living (IADL) needed to function in the home or community
  Activities:
* Instruct individual on appropriate and safe storage of medications.
* Instruct individual on alternative methods of transportation (e.g., buses and bus schedules, taxis, city or county transportation for disabled people).
* Assist individual in establishing methods and routines for cooking, cleaning, and shopping.

Family Support
Definition of family support: Promotion of family values, interests, and goals
  Activities*:
* Listen to family concerns, feelings, and questions.
* Accept the family's values in a nonjudgemental manner.
* Identify congruence between patient, family, and health professional expectations.

*Partial list.
Source: Bulechek, G. M., Butcher, H. K. & Dochterman, J. M. (2013). *Nursing interventions classification (NIC)* (6th ed.). St. Louis: Mosby.

Intervention Strategies

Basic nursing interventions for patients with SMI include the following:
* Empowering the patient by involving him or her in goal setting and treatment selection increases the likelihood of treatment adherence and success.
* Emphasizing quality-of-life issues conveys an interest in the person (rather than in the illness) and reflects the patient's best interests (rather than the staff's preferences).
* Developing and maintaining relationships are keys to overcoming anosognosia and achieving treatment adherence. People with SMI often require extended periods of working with staff to form these connections.
* Supportive psychotherapy aids in maintaining therapeutic rapport and helps the patient to maintain positive self-esteem and cope effectively.

* Impaired reality testing is the hallmark of SMI and contributes to hallucinations and delusional thinking. Encouraging the patient to seek independent information on whether experiences are real or not can help the patient to identify these experiences as part of the illness and respond accordingly.
* SMIs predispose people to isolation due to stigma, impaired social skills, and social discomfort. Isolation contributes to loneliness and reduces access to support. Activities that increase skill and comfort with interaction, reduce aloneness, or provide opportunities for socialization (especially with supportive persons and positive role models, such as other patients who are further along in recovery) contribute to improved functioning and a higher quality of life.
* Support groups such as the Schizophrenia Society of Canada expose the patient to members who "have been there." In addition to providing support and socialization opportunities, such groups often have practical suggestions for issues and

problems that patients and significant others face. Involvement in support groups is often empowering for the patient.

- Education and reinforcement are essential, since SMI may result in impaired judgement, desperation for connectedness, or other vulnerabilities that increase the risk for victimization, sexually transmitted infections, and undesired pregnancies.
- Care for the whole person is especially important with SMI patients, who have higher burdens of physical illness, poorer hygiene and health practices, less access to effective medical treatment, and more premature mortality than the general population. Exercise has also been found to reduce cardiometabolic risk, negative symptoms, and cognitive deficits, which often go untreated in patients with SMI (Firth, Cotter, Elliott, et al, 2015).
- Involving people with co-occurring substance abuse in Alcoholics Anonymous or Narcotics Anonymous and other services for people with concurrent disorders is important, since substance abuse rates are high in SMI populations and such abuse increases relapse and interferes with recovery.

Box 29-2 outlines two relevant *Nursing Interventions Classification (NIC)* interventions for the management of serious mental illness (Bulechek, Butcher, & Dochterman, 2013).

Evaluation

Identified outcomes serve as the basis for evaluation. Each *NOC* outcome has a built-in rating scale (immediate, short-term, and potentially long-term indicators) that helps the nurse to measure improvement.

CURRENT ISSUES

Involuntary Treatment

Involuntary treatment involves treatment mandated by a court and delivered without the patient's consent. Traditionally, this situation involved involuntary inpatient admissions, but beginning in the 1990s, provinces began to experiment with community treatment orders (CTOs), which provide mandatory treatment in a less restrictive setting. It has been suggested that implementation of a CTO may facilitate patient engagement with community services and improve access to supportive housing (Swigger & Heinmiller, 2014). One difficulty in implementing CTOs is determining how to respond if the person does not follow the ordered outpatient treatment: rehospitalization is an expensive option and may not have any positive impact on a patient's desire to participate in treatment (Dawson, 2016; Kisely, 2016).

Criminal Offences and Incarceration

In Canada, the number of incarcerated offenders with mental illness continues to increase. Research from Correctional Services Canada over several years shows that 62% of incoming female offenders in the criminal justice system required further mental health evaluation. For incoming male offenders, 50% required further mental health assessment, and 40% of male offenders met the criteria for a current mental illness diagnosis other than substance abuse or antisocial personality disorder (Correctional Services Canada, 2015). People with SMIs may commit crimes out of desperation, impaired judgement, or impulsivity; most often they are nonviolent crimes, such as disorderly conduct. Police may also become involved with patients who seem unable to care for themselves and cannot be persuaded to accept treatment but who do not meet the criteria for involuntary treatment (usually imminent danger to self or others). Consider a patient with impaired judgement who does not dress adequately for cold weather and spends time in laundromats and libraries for warmth, causing disruption. When expelled, the individual is at risk for hypothermia. In such cases, the risk to self may not be "imminent," and therefore hospitalization may not be possible. Loved ones or police may then seek arrest simply to get the person off the street for his or her own safety.

Many advocates for the mentally ill feel that incarceration, even if considered "for the patient's own good," is harmful. Imprisonment can lead to victimization, increased hopelessness, relapse due to increased stress and isolation, or overstimulation. Also, mental health care in correctional settings is usually both expensive and inadequate, and a criminal record can reduce future access to housing or employment. Advocates instead seek diversion from jail to clinical care. Two interventions to achieve this end are as follows:

1. Educating police so they can identify mental illness, distinguish it from criminal intent, and connect persons with SMI to help instead of jailing them
2. Establishing mental health courts that are designed to intercept persons whose crimes are secondary to mental illness and that feature specially trained officials with the authority to order treatment instead of imprisonment

▌ KEY POINTS TO REMEMBER

- Patients with SMI suffer from multiple impairments in thinking, feeling, and interacting with others.
- The course of SMI involves exacerbations and remissions, as do many chronic medical illnesses.
- Coordinated, comprehensive community services help the SMI patient to function at his or her optimal level.
- People with SMI often suffer complications due to insufficient housing, nonadherence to treatment, comorbid medical or substance use problems, and the stigma of mental illness.

- The family and support systems play a major part in the care of many persons with SMI and should be included as much as possible in planning, education, and treatment activities.
- The recovery model stresses hope, strengths, quality of life, patient involvement as an active partner in treatment, and eventual recovery.

CRITICAL THINKING

1. John Yang, age 42, concurrently diagnosed with schizophrenia and alcohol and marijuana abuse, is brought to the clinic by his mother, Mrs. Yang. During this initial assessment, Mrs. Yang reports that she has been caring for her son at home since he was 15 years old; however, since recently moving to town, she is at a loss about what is available in the community. John has been prescribed haloperidol (Haldol), but Mrs. Yang says that he rarely takes it because of muscle rigidity and sexual adverse effects. They have tried many of the traditional antipsychotic drugs without success.

   a. Given your understanding of the problems faced by a person with a severe mental illness, what are some areas of John's life you might want to explore in your assessment? Consider relationships, employment history, cognitive abilities, social skills, and behaviour. How would knowledge in these areas help your long-term planning?

   b. After you assess John's medication history, how can you be an advocate in terms of his nonadherence to traditional antipsychotics? What are some of the obstacles to adherence for a person with a concurrent disorder? What approach or change in treatment would offer the best chance of success?

   c. Of the resources mentioned in this chapter, which might be appropriate for John?

   d. Identify three basic aims of psychoeducation for John and his mother.

   e. What would recovery mean to John?

2. You are doing your psychiatric rotation in a psychiatric inpatient unit where many of the patients are diagnosed with schizophrenia. Although you had been apprehensive about this rotation, you are surprised to realize that patients respond well to you and that you are fascinated by this specialty area and may consider it as a career. A fellow student remarks, "You must be crazy to want to work with these people."

   a. What social problem is represented by this student's remark?

   b. Identify other social prejudices that have been significant problems in Canada. What responses were effective in reducing and eliminating their impact?

3. During your mental health rotation, you notice that there are several patients with other chronic physical illnesses. When assessing a person with SMI, why is it important to include a comprehensive physical assessment?

4. Competitive employment is an important factor in recovering from a psychotic episode. Identify the factors related to work that contribute to its importance in recovering from mental illness.

CHAPTER REVIEW

1. A patient with schizophrenia does not feel that he needs medication because "there is nothing wrong with me." This response is most likely an example of:

   a. Denial
   b. Projection
   c. Anosognosia
   d. Paranoid ideation

2. Sarah, a young woman with schizophrenia who has struggled with hygiene and other activities of daily living, has been on a 4-hour pass. She is tearful and reports that when she sat down on the bus to return to the hospital, the woman she sat next to immediately moved to another seat. Which responses would most likely be therapeutic? Select all that apply.

   a. Acknowledge Sarah's distress, and remind her that dinner will be ready in 30 minutes so that she has time to settle in before eating.

   b. State, "You sound discouraged. Sometimes people who do not understand mental illness can be hurtful," and offer to sit with her.

   c. Advise Sarah that the woman's behaviour was simply rude and can be ignored because it is something people with mental illness have to get used to.

   d. Suggest to Sarah that perhaps her hygiene would benefit from improvement, and offer to help her improve her hygiene so that others will be less likely to reject her.

3. Christopher is a 25-year-old male who has been hospitalized three times for exacerbations of schizophrenia. Each time he was discharged, he became homeless and relapsed. Typically he is very disorganized, does not spend his money responsibly, loses his housing when he does not pay the rent, and, in turn, cannot be located by his case manager, leading to treatment nonadherence and relapse. Which response would be most therapeutic in this situation?

   a. Advise Christopher that if he does not pay his rent, he will be placed in a group home instead of independent housing.

   b. Discuss with Christopher the option of having a guardian who will ensure that the rent is paid and that his money is managed to meet his basic needs.

   c. Suggest to Christopher's prescribing clinician that he be placed on a long-acting injectable form of antipsychotic medication to address the issue of treatment nonadherence.

   d. Encourage Christopher's case manager to hold him responsible for the outcomes of his poor decisions by allowing such periods of homelessness to serve as a natural consequence.

4. Pia has experienced repeated episodes of severe depression and mania. These episodes and related hospitalizations have disrupted her full-time employment and created discord within her marriage. She argues with the outpatient staff about medications, does not believe that she has a mental illness, and—although she takes her medications while hospitalized—stops taking them after discharge. She will be discharged in 2 weeks. Which intervention is most likely to increase her adherence to medications?

a. Advise Pia that she will be assigned to new outpatient staff to reduce the conflicts she is experiencing with her current providers.

b. Explain to Pia that the medications will help her and that all medications have adverse effects she can learn to live with in time.

c. Involve Pia in a medication education group that will help her learn the types and names of psychotropic medications, their purpose, and possible adverse effects.

d. Explore with Pia her perceptions of the medications and her experiences with them, and guide her to connect use of the medications with achieving her goals.

5. Which interventions would be appropriate to promote recovery for persons with serious mental illness who live in the community? Select all that apply.

a. Meet regularly with the patients, and encourage them to make steady progress toward complete independence.

b. Introduce patients to others with similar illnesses, and encourage participation in social activities with peers.

c. Support the development of advance directives and involvement in social and employment activities run by other patients.

d. Use public transportation to take patients to a museum, and share a nutritious dinner with them at an inexpensive restaurant.

e. Instruct them to develop written plans that identify resources to maintain stability and steps to take when faced with unusual stressors.

f. Over time, guide the patients to identify and switch to sources of support outside the family to reduce dependence on their loved ones as their primary support resource.

⊖volve WEBSITE

Post-Test interactive review

Visit the Evolve website for Chapter Review Answers and Rationales, Critical Thinking Answer Guidelines, and additional resources related to the content in this chapter: http://evolve.elsevier.com/Canada/Varcarolis/psychiatric/

REFERENCES

Addiction and Mental Health Collaborative Project Steering Committee (2014). *Collaboration for addiction and mental health care: Best advice.* Ottawa: Canadian Centre on Substance Abuse.

Addington, D., Kyle, T., Desair, S., et al. (2010). Facilitators and barriers to implementing quality treatment in primary mental health care. *Canadian Family Physician, 56,* 1322–1331.

Bulechek, G. M., Butcher, H. K., & Dochterman, J. M. (2013). *Nursing interventions classification (NIC)* (6th ed.). St. Louis: Mosby.

Canadian Institute for Health Information. (2016). *National health expenditure trends.* Retrieved from https://www.cihi.ca/en/national-healt h-expenditure-trends.

Centre for Addiction and Mental Health. (2009). *Partnering with families affected by concurrent disorder: Facilitators guide.* Retrieved from http://www.camh.net/Publications/Resources_for_Professionals/Partnering_ with_families/app1_references.html.

Centre for Addiction and Mental Health. (2013). *Mental health and criminal justice policy framework.* Retrieved from https://www.camh.ca/en/hospital/ about_camh/influencing_public_policy/Documents/MH_Criminal_ Justice_Policy_Framework.pdf.

Centre for Addiction and Mental Health. (2017). *Mental illness and addictions: Facts and statistics.* Retrieved from http://www.camh.ca/en/hospital/ about_camh/newsroom/for_reporters/Pages/ addictionmentalhealthstatistics.aspx.

Choe, K., Sung, B., Kang, Y., et al. (2016). Impact of psychoeducation on knowledge of and attitude toward medications in clients with schizophrenia and schizoaffective disorders. *Perspectives in Psychiatric Care, 52*(2), 113–119. doi:10.1111/ppc.12106.

Correctional Services Canada. (2015). *Research results—Mental health.* Retrieved from http://www.csc-scc.gc.ca/ publications/005007-3030-eng.shtml.

Davis, S. (2013). *Community mental health in Canada: Theory, policy, and practice* (revised and expanded ed.). Vancouver: UBC Press.

Dawson, J. (2016). Doubts about the clinical effectiveness of community treatment orders. *The Canadian Journal of Psychiatry, 61*(1), 4–6. doi:10.1177/0706743715619436.

Dezetter, A., Duhoux, A., Menear, M., et al. (2015). Reasons and determinants for perceiving unmet needs for mental health in primary care in Quebec.

The Canadian Journal of Psychiatry, 60(6), 284–293. doi:10.1177/070674371506000607.

Dharmawardene, V., & Menkes, D. B. (2017). Violence and self-harm in severe mental illness: Inpatient study of associations with ethnicity, cannabis and alcohol. *Australasian Psychiatry, 25*(1), 28–31. doi:10.1177/1039856216671650.

Dopke, C. A., & Batscha, C. L. (2014). Cognitive-behavioral therapy for individuals with schizophrenia: A recovery approach. *American Journal of Psychiatric Rehabilitation, 17*(1), 44–71. doi:10.1080/15487768.2013.876458.

Dulmus, C. N., & Nisbet, B. C. (2013). *Person-centered recovery planner for adults with serious mental illness* (1st ed.). Hoboken, NJ: Wiley.

Eack, S. M. (2012). Cognitive remediation: A new generation of psychosocial interventions for people with schizophrenia. *Social Work, 57*(3), 235–246. doi:10.1093/sw/sws008.

Firth, J., Cotter, J., Elliott, R., et al. (2015). A systematic review and meta-analysis of exercise interventions in schizophrenia patients. *Psychological Medicine, 45*(7), 1343–1361. doi:10.1017/ S0033291714003110.

Frost, B. G., Tirupati, S., Johnston, S., et al. (2017). An integrated recovery-oriented model (IRM) for mental health services: Evolution and challenges. *BMC Psychiatry, 17*(1), doi:10.1186/s12888-016-1164-3.

Gaebel, W., Rössler, W., & Sartorius, N. (2017). *The stigma of mental illness: End of the story?* Cham, Switzerland: Springer.

Goering, P. N., & Streiner, D. L. (2015). Putting housing first: The evidence and impact. *The Canadian Journal of Psychiatry, 60*(11), 465–466. doi:10.1177/070674371506001101.

Goldner, E., Jenkins, E., & Bilsker, D. (2016). *A concise introduction to mental health in Canada* (2nd ed.). Toronto: Canadian Scholars Press.

Government of Canada. (2015). *Report from the Canadian Chronic Disease Surveillance System: Mental illness in Canada, 2015.* Retrieved from https://www.canada.ca/en/public-health/services/publications/ diseases-conditions/report-canadian-chronic-disease-surveillance-system- mental-illness-canada-2015.html.

Harder, S., Koester, A., Valbak, K., et al. (2014). Five-year follow-up of supportive psychodynamic psychotherapy in first-episode psychosis: Long-term outcome in social functioning. *Psychiatry, 77*(2), 155. doi:10.1521/psyc.2014.77.2.155.

Harrow, M., Jobe, T. H., & Faull, R. N. (2012). Do all schizophrenia patients need antipsychotic treatment continuously throughout their lifetime? A 20-year longitudinal study. *Psychological Medicine, 42*(10), 1–11. doi:10.1017/S003329171200022.

Hor, K., & Taylor, M. (2010). Review: Suicide and schizophrenia: A systematic review of rates and risk factors. *Journal of Psychopharmacology, 24*(Suppl. 4), 81. doi:10.1177/1359786810385490.

Khare, C., Mueser, K. T., & McGurk, S. R. (2016). Vocational rehabilitation for individuals with schizophrenia. *Current Treatment Options in Psychiatry, 3*(2), 99–110. doi:10.1007/s40501-016-0082-9.

Kisely, S. (2016). Canadian studies on the effectiveness of community treatment orders. *The Canadian Journal of Psychiatry, 61*(1), 7–14. doi:10.1177/0706743715620414.

Larsson, P. (2015). What can be done about the social determinants of mental health? *Perspectives in Public Health, 135*(1), 16–17. doi:10.1177/1757913914561713.

Lehrer, D. S., & Lorenz, J. (2014). Anosognosia in schizophrenia: Hidden in plain sight. *Innovations in Clinical Neuroscience, 11*(5–6), 10.

Lyman, D. R., Kurtz, M. M., Farkas, M., et al. (2014). Skill building: Assessing the evidence. *Psychiatric Services, 65*(6), 727–738. doi:10.1176/appi.ps.201300251.

Manseau, M. W. (2014). Economic inequality and poverty as social determinants of mental health. *Psychiatric Annals, 44*(1), 32. doi:10.3928/00485713-20140108-06.

McKee, S. A. (2017). Concurrent substance use disorders and mental illness: Bridging the gap between research and treatment. *Canadian Psychology, 58*(1), 50. doi:10.1037/cap0000093.

Mental Health Commission of Canada (MHCC) (2009). *Toward recovery and well-being: A framework for a mental health strategy for Canada.* Ottawa: Author.

Mental Health Commission of Canada (MHCC) (2012). *Changing directions, changing lives: The mental health strategy for Canada.* Calgary: Author.

Mental Health Commission of Canada (MHCC) (2013). *The aspiring workforce: Employment and income for people with serious mental illness.* Calgary: Author.

Mental Health Commission of Canada (MHCC). (2015). *Guidelines for recovery-oriented practice.* Retrieved from http://www.mentalhealthcommission.ca/sites/default/files/MHCC_RecoveryGuidelines_ENG_0.pdf.

Morris, E. M. J., Johns, L. C., & Oliver, J. E. (2013). *Acceptance and commitment therapy and mindfulness for psychosis* (1st ed.). West Sussex, UK: Wiley-Blackwell.

Mueser, K. T., & McGurk, S. R. (2014). Supported employment for persons with serious mental illness: Current status and future directions. *L'Encéphale, 40*(Suppl. 2), S45.

Mulvale, G., & Bartram, M. (2015). No more "us" and "them": Integrating recovery and well-being into a conceptual model for mental health policy. *Canadian Journal of Community Mental Health, 34*(4), 31.

Nowak, I., Sabariego, C., Świtaj, P., et al. (2016). Disability and recovery in schizophrenia: A systematic review of cognitive behavioral therapy interventions. *BMC Psychiatry, 16*(1), 228. doi:10.1186/s12888-016-0912-8.

Olney, M. F., & Emery-Flores, D. S. (2017). I get my therapy from work: Wellness recovery action plan strategies that support employment success. *Rehabilitation Counseling Bulletin, 60*(3), 175–184. doi:10.1177/0034355216660059.

Osatuke, K., Ciesla, J., Kasckow, J. W., et al. (2008). Insight in schizophrenia: A review of etiological models and supporting research. *Comprehensive Psychiatry, 49*(1), 70–77. doi:10.1016/j.comppsych.2007.08.001.

Park, K., & Seo, M. (2016). Care burden of parents of adult children with mental illness: The role of associative stigma. *Comprehensive Psychiatry, 70*, 159–164. doi:10.1016/j.comppsych.2016.07.010.

Patten, S. B., Williams, J. V. A., Lavorato, D. H., et al. (2016). Perceived stigma among recipients of mental health care in the general Canadian population. *The Canadian Journal of Psychiatry, 61*(8), 480–488. doi:10.1177/0706743716639928.

Pearsall, R., Smith, D. J., Pelosi, A., et al. (2014). Exercise therapy in adults with serious mental illness: A systematic review and meta-analysis. *BMC Psychiatry, 14*(1), 117. doi:10.1186/1471-244X-14-117.

Pope, L. M., & Harris, G. E. (2014). Assertive community treatment (ACT) in a rural Canadian community: Client characteristics, client satisfaction, and service effectiveness. *Canadian Journal of Community Mental Health, 33*(3), 17.

Rusch, N., & Corrigan, P. W. (2002). Motivational interviewing to improve insight and treatment adherence in schizophrenia. *Psychiatric Rehabilitation Journal, 26*(1), 23.

Sederer, L. I. (2016). The social determinants of mental health. *Psychiatric Services, 67*(2), 234–235. doi:10.1176/appi.ps.201500232.

Spagnolo, J. (2014). Improving first-line mental health services in Canada: Addressing two challenges caused by the deinstitutionalization movement. *Healthcare Quarterly, 17*(4), 41.

Swigger, A., & Heinmiller, B. T. (2014). Advocacy coalitions and mental health policy: The adoption of community treatment orders in Ontario. *Politics & Policy, 42*(2), 246–270. doi:10.1111/polp.12066.

Symanski-Tondora, J. L., Miller, R., Slade, M., et al. (2014). *Partnering for recovery in mental health: A practical guide to person-centered planning* (2nd ed.). West Sussex, UK: Wiley-Blackwell.

Thompson, L., & McCabe, R. (2012). The effect of clinician-patient alliance and communication on treatment adherence in mental health care: A systematic review. *BMC Psychiatry, 12*(1), 87. doi:10.1186/1471-244X-12-87.

Thornicroft, G. (2013). Premature death among people with mental illness. *BMJ (Clinical Research Ed.), 346*, f2969. doi:10.1136/bmj.f2969.

Tidey, J. W. (2016). A behavioral economic perspective on smoking persistence in serious mental illness. *Preventive Medicine, 92*, 31–35. doi:10.1016/j.ypmed.2016.05.015.

Weiden, P. J. (2016). Redefining medication adherence in the treatment of schizophrenia: How current approaches to adherence lead to Misinformation and threaten therapeutic relationships. *The Psychiatric Clinics of North America, 39*(2), 199.

Psychological Needs of Patients With Medical Conditions

Cheryl L. Pollard

KEY TERMS AND CONCEPTS

coping skills
holistic approach

psychiatric consultation liaison nurse (PCLN)
stigmatized persons with medical conditions

OBJECTIVES

1. Assess a person with a general medical condition and a psychiatric condition.
2. Formulate a nursing diagnosis appropriate for an individual with a nonpsychiatric and psychiatric diagnosis.
3. Consider the impact of stress on general medical conditions.
4. Describe two psychosocial interventions that would be appropriate for a patient with a nonpsychiatric and psychiatric diagnosis.
5. Explain the importance of nurses being knowledgeable about and comfortable discussing topics pertaining to the relationship between nonpsychiatric and psychiatric illnesses.
6. Identify two instances in which a consultation with a psychiatric consultation liaison nurse might have been useful for your medical-surgical patients.

ꞔvolve WEBSITE

Visit the Evolve website for Flashcards, Case Studies, and additional testing resources related to the content in this chapter: http://evolve.elsevier.com/Canada/Varcarolis/psychiatric/

Pre-Test   interactive review

There are two separate though related classifications of the relationship between physical conditions and psychological factors: (1) somatic symptom disorders—distressing somatic symptoms with abnormal thoughts, feelings, and behaviours in response to these symptoms—(discussed in Chapter 12), and (2) the influence of psychological factors or psychiatric disorders on nonpsychiatric disorders. The latter more fully recognizes the relationships among health, health care, the determinants of health, and well-being.

This chapter helps to prepare nurses to use a holistic approach, which addresses both the psychological and the physiological needs of patients. Despite the unfortunate reality that the health care delivery system is fragmented for people with both medical and mental health problems, psychiatric mental health nurses must provide holistic care for patients with physical illnesses, and nurses who work outside of psychiatric settings must be aware of the influence of psychological factors and psychiatric disorders on the course of general medical conditions and plan for care accordingly.

PSYCHOLOGICAL FACTORS AFFECTING MEDICAL CONDITIONS

Psychological factors have been found to influence a variety of physical illnesses. The presence of psychiatric disorders along with general medical conditions increases the patient length of stays and also may negatively affect care outcomes (Wu, Suk, Dekker, et al., 2017). As a result of the interrelationships between psychiatric and medical comorbidities, collaboration among providers of primary health care and mental health care can lead to more accurate diagnoses and effective treatments.

Hans Selye (1956) was the first to introduce the concept of stress into the fields of medicine and physiology. Stress can lead to changes in physical and mental health in many ways (see Chapter 5). Cannon's (1914) identification of the fight-or-flight response and Selye's description of the general adaptation syndrome provided insight into the biological and molecular reactions to stressors in the sympathetic nervous system, the hypothalamic-pituitary-adrenal axis, and the immune system. Researchers have continued to increase our understanding of the basic physiological responses to stress (see Chapter 5), and there is deep interest in improving both the outcomes and the efficiency of health care delivery.

Without conflating health with well-being, a key determinant of health is how individuals promote self-care, cope with challenges, develop self-reliance, solve problems, and make choices. The psychological impact of medical illness can be severe and can account for a higher rate of disruption in functional ability than just the medical illness alone would indicate.

Among the most common psychological responses to physical illness are depression, anxiety, substance use, denial, hopelessness, and anger. A psychological condition, however, may supersede or be comorbid with a medical condition. In general, individuals with medical disorders and psychological symptoms have poorer outcomes than those with the same medical disorders but without psychological problems (Wu, Suk, Dekker, et al., 2017). Table 12-7 identifies some common medical conditions, such as cardiovascular disease, ulcers, cancer, and headaches, that are negatively affected by stress and would benefit from stress reduction and support. However, anyone experiencing a serious medical condition needs a variety of psychological supports and may benefit from learning new coping skills.

 RESEARCH HIGHLIGHT

When Fear of Cancer Recurrence Becomes a Clinical Issue

Problem
Cancer is a life-threatening illness. Cancer survivors with low levels of fear of recurrence may be motivated to take care of their health and follow the advice of their health care team. However, when this fear escalates and is difficult to manage, it is associated with anxiety and depression and tends not to decrease over time. As a result, these cancer survivors experience a lower quality of life and impaired physical, social, occupational, and cognitive functioning.

Purpose of Study
Currently there is no agreed-upon definition of the fear of cancer recurrence or agreement on when this phenomenon becomes "clinical" and should be a focus of treatment. The goal of this study was to investigate the potential hallmarks of clinical fear of cancer recurrence.

Methods
After receiving ethics approval, semistructured interviews were conducted with cancer survivors of both genders, of various cancer types, and experiencing a range of fear of cancer recurrence severity. Study participants met the following inclusion criteria: (1) had been diagnosed with breast, prostate, lung, or colorectal cancer; (2) had received treatment from the Ottawa Hospital Cancer Centre within the last 13 years; (3) were under 85 years of age to help ensure that participants did not have significant cognitive deficits; and (4) were able to comprehend and speak English. Forty interviews were completed. The analysis reflected this combination of approaches, as the interviews were analyzed with an understanding of the features of clinical fear of cancer recurrence, such as intrusive thoughts, impairment in functioning, the role of coping strategies, intolerance of uncertainty, and triggers of fear of cancer recurrence.

Key Findings
The 9 most commonly reported features associated with clinical fear of cancer recurrence were death-related thoughts; feeling alone; experiencing fear of cancer recurrence–related thoughts and imagery that lasted 30 minutes or more; experiencing fear of cancer recurrence–related thoughts and imagery that were daily, recurrent, and difficult to control; experiencing more fear of cancer recurrence–related thoughts as time goes on; feeling certain that the cancer will return; experiencing distress; impairment in functioning; and intolerance of uncertainty. Participants experiencing nonclinical and clinical fear of cancer recurrence reported similar coping strategies and triggers of fear of cancer recurrence, thereby suggesting that the simple occurrence of coping strategies or triggers of fear of cancer recurrence may not indicate clinical fear of cancer recurrence.

Implications for Nursing Practice
While features of clinical fear of cancer recurrence such as intrusive thoughts, distress, and impact on functioning found in this analysis confirmed previous fear of cancer recurrence research, other features including death-related thoughts, feeling alone, and belief that the cancer will return spontaneously emerged from the interviews. The participants' descriptions of cancer-specific fear and worry suggest that fear of cancer recurrence is a distinct phenomenon related to cancer survivorship, despite its similarity to psychological disorders (e.g., anxiety, depressive disorders). Although a distinct phenomenon, nurses should consider using cognitive reframing and thought monitoring techniques, which may help those who believe that a cancer recurrence will inevitably happen by reframing thoughts to include the idea that the return of cancer is only one possible outcome. The "feeling alone" symptom may respond to therapeutic techniques that establish connection with others who have had similar experiences, including social support, therapy, or self-help groups. Future research investigating the construct of fear of cancer recurrence and the distinguishing features of clinical fear of cancer recurrence across a range of cancer types and genders is required.

Source: Mutsaers, B., Jones, G., Rutowski, N., et al. (2016). When fear of cancer recurrence becomes a clinical issue: A qualitative analysis of features associates with clinical fear of cancer reoccurrence. *Support Care Cancer, 24*(10), 4207–4218. doi:10.1007/s00520-016-3248-5.

Caregivers of those with a chronic illness also experience psychological sequelae. Often this includes depression and anxiety. HealthPartners (2015) reports that 20% of caregivers experience depression as a result of their caregiving responsibilities. Many caregivers attempt to balance their caregiving responsibilities with other family duties while continuing to work.

PSYCHOLOGICAL RESPONSES TO SERIOUS MEDICAL CONDITIONS

The diagnosis of a medical problem or condition is stressful for nearly everyone. However, the degree of stress depends on the person's perception of the illness. People's questions can be many and varied when they find themselves faced with a serious medical problem:

- Will I be disfigured?
- Will I have a long-term disability?
- Will I be able to function as a wife or husband, parent, and member of society?
- Will I be able to continue to work?
- Will I suffer pain?
- Will I be stigmatized?

When strong emotional supports and social ties are not available, other questions may arise:

- How will I cope?
- How will this affect my life?
- Will I retain a reasonable quality of life?

Depression

A strong body of evidence suggests that depression is more common in patients with physical disorders, particularly in those with multiple physical disorders. The Mental Health Commission of Canada (2014) suggests that up to 50% of people living with a chronic illness also suffer from depression. People with a chronic medical condition are three times as likely to experience depression than those without one. Often depression is masked by the medical condition itself and goes unrecognized and thus untreated. For example, uremic symptoms in patients who have renal disease may mask the somatic and neurovegetative symptoms of depression. Just a few of the medical illnesses that typically are associated with depression are cancer, human immunodeficiency virus (HIV), diabetes, hypertension, and stroke.

If not recognized and treated, depression can affect the severity of the medical disorder, increase personal distress, impair functioning, and interfere with adherence to a prescribed medical regimen. Patients with depression have been found to be three times more likely to be nonadherent to medical treatment than are patients without depression (Volpato, Banfi, & Pagnini, 2017). This is because people with depression are less motivated, or able, to follow self-care regimens. They may have poor diet, neglect exercise routines, smoke, overindulge in substances, all of which take away from recovery (HealthPartners, 2015). However, people with medical conditions who are treated for co-occurring depression often experience improvement in their overall medical condition, show better adherence to recommendations for general medical care, and experience a better quality of life.

VIGNETTE

Candace is a single, 30-year-old head administrative paralegal who recently arrived in emergency with nausea, vomiting, and abdominal pain. She reports having no energy, a lack of interest in her usual hobbies, and difficulty concentrating. She states, "I feel very scared and alone. I don't know where I would get the money to live if I need to miss work." These observations were reported to the nurse practitioner. After a thorough assessment and medical workup, it is determined that Candace has prerenal acute renal failure and depression.

Anxiety

Acute anxiety can influence a person's coping capacity, defensive structure, adaptive capacity, and resilience. Illnesses that evoke sympathetic nervous system responses, such as nervousness, insomnia, breathlessness, palpitations, jitteriness, high blood pressure, and high cholesterol, are complicated when the individual also has a comorbid anxiety disorder. Anxiety leads to heightened awareness of physical symptoms, as well as to physiologically caused medical symptoms because of increased muscle tension and autonomic nervous system and hypothalamic–pituitary–adrenal axis dysregulation. Recognizing treatable anxiety disorders that are highly concurrent with medical comorbid conditions is important in alleviating distress and improving the course of the illness.

Verbalization can be an effective outlet for anxiety. However, the ability to effectively communicate one's feelings may be compromised by cultural expectations, disability, or lack of a listener. A sense of helplessness often accompanies anxiety in the person who feels a loss of control over events, such as when awaiting surgery or undergoing invasive treatments. In this case, defence mechanisms (e.g., denial, regression) may be used with greater frequency, or compulsive behaviours may surface. Unreasonable requests of caregivers (e.g., demanding that the nurse sit with a patient throughout the night) may be a cover for feelings of inadequacy.

VIGNETTE

Pat is 19 years old. He has been diagnosed with Crohn's disease. He knows that there is no known cure for his illness. He belongs to an online "Gutsy Peer Support Group." The bloating, nausea, cramping, and loss of appetite he experiences are constant. Sometimes the symptoms are better, and sometimes they are worse. Final exams are approaching, and Pat always finds exams stressful. When he is stressed, the symptoms always get worse. He finds it hard to concentrate when he is always worrying about having to go to the bathroom.

The nurse at student counselling services talks to Pat about the power of the mind–body connection. The nurse works with Pat to explore practical ways of managing the urgency of his diarrhea, nausea, and cramping during the exams. Stress-management practices are taught to help him cope with stress in a helpful and empowering way. Assertiveness techniques are also practised to reduce the chances of becoming overcommitted and overscheduled, as it is difficult to feel healthy when one is drained and at the end of one's rope.

Possible nursing diagnoses for Pat in the vignette above include the following:

- *Risk for ineffective coping* related to high levels of anxiety that are interfering with his ability to study.
- *Ineffective role performance* related to diagnosis of Crohn's disease as evidenced by fatigue and lack of energy.

Substance Use

Long-term abuse of various substances can lead to a variety of medical complications; for example, alcohol use is associated with hepatic conditions, marijuana use with lung disease, cocaine use with cardiac toxicity, and ecstasy (3,4-methylenedioxymethamphetamine, or MDMA) use with neurotoxicity (e.g., problems with memory, reasoning, impulse control). However, patients who are diagnosed with serious medical conditions often turn to alcohol or other substances to cope with overwhelming feelings of hopelessness, fear, anxiety, depression, or pain.

Thus health care providers need to be diligent in their initial assessments and identify any coexisting or resulting psychological responses or disorders. In most cases of physical illness, the focus is on the complaints of physical symptoms, and minimal attention is given to the psychological responses of the patient.

Grief and Loss

Serious medical illnesses are nearly always accompanied by grief. As well, any type of treatment or procedure intended to treat a physical illness that creates a major permanent change is accompanied by feelings of loss. The dynamics involved in coping with these feelings are similar to those in a person who is dealing with his or her own impending death or the death of a loved one. The person must grieve for the loss, just as the dying person must work through confusion and darkness until a degree of acceptance and relative peace is achieved. Negotiating the loss of physical well-being involves moving through feelings of frustration, vulnerability, and sadness to become a whole person once again. This journey encompasses both spiritual and emotional changes and, for this reason, requires spiritual assessment of the patient, as well as a focus on psychosocial issues.

VIGNETTE

Candace's kidney damage continues. Her kidneys have failed, and she is being treated with hemodialysis. She has been complaining of frequent tension headaches and occasional stomach upsets before her treatment appointments. The hemodialysis nurse has always been impressed by Candace's patience and compliant attitude despite her debilitating illness, which has robbed her of a normal family life. For this reason, the nurse suspects that Candace's physical complaints could be a way of dealing with her emotions, so the nurse makes a point to spend more time with Candace to allow her to talk about her frustrations. Candace expresses anger and some feelings of hopelessness. She resents others who are healthy, including the people who care for her. Frequent opportunities to verbalize these feelings gradually result in the lessening of her somatic complaints and a decrease in her sense of powerlessness and isolation.

Possible nursing diagnoses for Candace in the vignette above include the following:

- *Hopelessness* related to chronic illness as evidenced by verbal comments and feelings of resentment toward others who are healthy
- *Ineffective individual coping* related to chronic illness as evidenced by expressions of anger and feelings of hopelessness.

Denial

Bodily changes affect individuals' identities in important ways, and some chronically ill patients work very hard at maintaining their pre-illness identity, sometimes to the detriment of their health. Common responses to the initial symptoms of illness, the diagnosis, and functional limitations and impairments evoke the complicated process of denial, acceptance, and adaptation (although not necessarily in that order). Denial, an unconscious defence mechanism, may be evident when the diagnosed person and the family seem to have little knowledge or interest in learning about the condition or define the illness as acute rather than chronic. Nurses and other health care providers may actually foster such beliefs by withholding information about the meaning and likely consequences of a particular problem. Initial illness crises support explanations of the illness as acute and can be so overwhelming for patients and families as to prevent consideration of a long-term course of illness.

As symptoms and acute crises repeat over time, individuals begin to accept the chronicity of their illnesses and the effects of the illnesses on their daily lives. People begin to experience their bodies as altered and come to think of illness as real in ways that allow them to relate symptoms to the changes in their lives. They compare their present condition with that of the past, weighing the risks of continuing their regular activities and activity levels and then adapting those activity levels. Patients may feel estranged from the persons they have become, betrayed by their own bodies, or guilty for not meeting standards of activity levels, functioning, and appearance. Patients can also distance themselves from their illness, diagnosis, and body, objectifying their symptoms as a way of coping.

VIGNETTE

After a car accident, Katya is being assessed by the triage nurse in the emergency department for possible injuries. She complains of a slight headache and dizziness but denies having any other pain or symptoms. Katya is preoccupied with ensuring that her 2-year-old son, who was also in the car, is being examined, so she denies her own need for medical attention. Katya's blood pressure is 86/50 mm Hg, and her body posture indicates that she is guarding her abdomen. These observations are reported to the examining physician immediately because they indicate possible internal bleeding and danger of shock. Katya is eventually taken to the operating room so that the bleeding may be stopped.

Possible nursing diagnoses for Katya in the vignette above include the following:

- *Acute pain* related to recent car accident as evidenced by headache, dizziness, and body posture indicating she is guarding her abdomen

- *Anxiety* related to concern for her child as evidenced by being preoccupied with seeing her 2-year-old son.

Fear of Dependency

Responses to being dependent may be exhibited as an inability to accept warmth, nurturing, or tenderness from caregivers or as a refusal to accept treatment or medical advice. This reaction is strongest in those who have unmet dependencies and those who have had negative experiences when seeking help in the past. Anger may mask acute embarrassment over being in a dependent position or may be used by the patient who feels the need to project an independent image. Others are fearful of not having their dependency needs met and do not express any negative feelings to caregivers. These people strive to be "good" patients out of fear that they will be abandoned if they are perceived to be difficult. Suppressed anxiety or anger, however, could be exhibited through increased somatic complaints.

> **VIGNETTE**
> Rebecca, a 25-year-old with multiple sclerosis, worked as a home attendant until she fractured her leg and sustained a severe elbow injury when a patient she was assisting fell on her. The resultant disabilities and flare-up of her multiple sclerosis have prevented her from resuming her job as a home attendant. Prior to this incident, she was independent, hard working, self-supporting, and able to manage a mild anxiety disorder through cognitive reframing and controlled breathing. Her injuries forced her to apply for financial support and rely on her boyfriend for assistance with transportation and care of her apartment. She began to experience shortness of breath, palpitations, and impaired concentration.

A possible nursing diagnosis for Rebecca in the vignette above is the following: *Anxiety* related to recent change in health status as evidenced by impaired concentration and palpitations.

HUMAN RIGHTS ABUSES OF STIGMATIZED PERSONS WITH MEDICAL CONDITIONS

Some consumers of health care and some health care providers have voiced the need to examine human rights abuses in the health care system—specifically, the inadequate care of people who are stigmatized by health care providers. These **stigmatized persons with medical conditions** are assumed by health care providers to be bad, disgusting, or even just unusual and often include those who have mental illnesses, those who are HIV positive, and those who have undergone transgender surgeries or treatments. The abuses that many of these patients endure can result in inadequate care and lead to undue stress, worsening of physical illness, and even death. By making assumptions about these patients, health care workers fail to acknowledge and understand that these patients' psychosocial issues are similar to those of other patients and that the same nursing interventions for anger, anxiety, and grief are applicable. Examples of human rights abuse include the following:

- Failure to fully investigate somatic complaints made by emergency department patients with a history of psychiatric illness

- Avoidance of contact with, or refusal to care for, persons who are stigmatized, which results in worsening illness or death
- Hastily labelling with a psychiatric diagnosis and giving a prescription of antipsychotic drugs to persons who are experiencing normal emotional responses (e.g., sadness, anger) to chronic physical illness
- Inappropriate psychiatric admission of persons who are on medical units or in nursing homes, based on the financial needs of the institution or on the staff's inability to manage emotional responses to physical illness or the aging process

Such situations may occur more frequently to individuals who lack family support or the personal resources to advocate for themselves (e.g., those from lower socioeconomic classes, newly arrived immigrants, those living socially "unacceptable" lifestyles). The key to increasing awareness of human rights issues in psychiatric mental health care may be the integration of these concepts into nursing curricula. Humanitarian values are at the very heart of our profession and practice. Nurses are in a unique position to advocate for equal patient treatment, but many hesitate to confront employers about violations of basic patient rights, fearing reprisal. A committee composed of nurses and other hospital employees could be formed to review such cases and make recommendations to the hospital administration. In this age of managed care and cuts to hospital budgets, upholding human rights is one of nursing's greatest challenges.

APPLICATION OF THE NURSING PROCESS

ASSESSMENT

Assessment of patients is a complex process that requires careful and complete documentation. Assessment should begin with the collection of data about the nature, location, onset, character, and duration of the symptom or symptoms. A thorough medical, emotional, and psychosocial history is also essential. Assessment of nutrition, fluid balance, and elimination needs should be a high priority in patients with complaints relating to gastrointestinal distress, diarrhea, constipation, and anorexia.

Psychosocial Assessment

Psychosocial factors are relevant to the course of an illness, and the way a person thinks and feels can have a profound effect on how the disease progresses. Struggling with illness evokes a range of difficult emotions, such as fear, anger, sadness, confusion, and guilt. Patients may feel overwhelmed and alone, whereas family members may feel helpless and at a loss emotionally. The elements of a thorough psychosocial assessment are described in detail in Chapter 10.

Quality of Life Assessment

For interventions to be most effective, the nurse must understand how a person's medical condition affects his or her quality of life. For example, how is the medical illness affecting the ability to function in the home, at work, or in school? How are the patient's feelings about the illness (e.g., depression, anxiety, hopelessness) affecting his or her relationships and ability to function? There are a number of quality of life assessment tools,

ASSESSMENT GUIDELINES

Psychological Needs of Patients With Medical Conditions

1. Assess for nature, location, onset, characteristics, and duration of the physical and psychological symptoms.
2. Assess the patient's ability to meet basic needs and quality of life.
3. Determine availability and capacity of social supports.
4. Assess risks to safety and security needs of the patient, including self-harm and suicide, as a result of all symptoms.
5. Assess for substance use (i.e., prescription and nonprescription medication, alcohol consumption, nicotine and caffeine consumption).
6. Explore the patient's cognitive style and ability to communicate feelings and needs.
7. Determine current level of psychological symptoms (mild, moderate, severe, or panic).
8. Perform a psychosocial assessment. Always ask the person, "What is going on in your life that may be contributing to your health issues?" The patient may identify a problem that should be addressed by counselling (e.g., stressful marriage, recent loss, stressful job or school situation).
9. Remember that culture can affect how psychological symptoms are manifested.

TABLE 30-1	ASSESSMENT OF COPING SKILLS	
EFFECTIVE COPING SKILLS	**INEFFECTIVE COPING BEHAVIOURS**
Has optimistic attitude (sees glass as half full)	Has pessimistic attitude (sees glass as half empty)
Confronts the issues; acts accordingly	Minimizes critical health status or signals
Seeks information; gets guidance	Shows tendency to escape or withdraw
Shares concerns; finds consolation	Blames someone or something else
Has capacity for healthy denial	Denies as much as possible; shows prolonged denial
Redefines the situation, reviews alternatives, examines consequences	Feels things are hopeless, were meant to be; has attitude of "What's the use?"
Constructively uses distractions: keeping busy; maintaining positive emotional ties with family, friends, community	Withdraws; broods; is overwhelmed with self-pity, anger, envy, guilt about having caused the illness

ranging from self-assessment rating scales to lengthy questionnaires. Different organizations use different tools. One example of an assessment tool is the World Health Organization's (2004) Quality of Life—BREF (WHOQOL-BREF), which can be used to examine an individual's perceptions about quality of life in the context of culture, value systems, and personal goals, standards, and concerns. The development of this tool was based on statements made by patients from a variety of cultures and with a range of diseases. This tool is available in English and French. The most useful assessment tool is a simple one: ask the patient how the illness or disease is affecting the quality of his or her life.

Coping Skills

Assessing how a patient has dealt with adversity in the past provides information about the person's coping skills available for use now and in the future. Health care providers can also support the patient in gaining additional coping skills that may help him or her to better manage a serious medical or surgical situation.

A person who has a life-threatening disease or chronic illness often deals with distressing physical adverse effects and changes in body image. For example, a patient who is given a colostomy to avoid death from cancer or ulcerative colitis is left with complex emotional and physical issues. The patient must learn techniques for dealing with not only the stoma but also the lifelong consequences and their effects on body image, appearance, and relationships. Concerns such as the following may arise:

- Will my partner still be attracted to me?
- Will I continue to be interested in sexual relationships?

Breast cancer survivors, for example, have been helped by camaraderie with other survivors who openly share their techniques for dealing with appliances or prostheses. Other survivors can also show patients how to respond to well-intended but probing or embarrassing questions. People who have previously travelled the same path are the best resources for helping those newly diagnosed to establish how to manage inevitable questions about their illness.

Table 30-1 highlights some of the characteristics that allow people to cope well and some of the characteristics that may be changed or improved through psychosocial interventions or cognitive behavioural approaches.

Social and Spiritual Support

Medical conditions initially may elicit strong support from friends and family, but as time wears on, this support may begin to wane. Knowing who is there for the patient will be helpful in planning for later interventions. Does the patient have sufficient social supports (e.g., family, friends, elders, religious or spiritual help) to enable him or her to share thoughts and feelings? Would the patient benefit from a medical support group?

Nurses and other health care workers are becoming increasingly aware of the role that spirituality or religion plays in many patients' lives and its importance as a source of peace. Support from a priest, pastor, rabbi, or other religious leader may be indicated, especially in a case of spiritual distress. Beliefs and practices are forces that promote resilience; practising healthy coping depends on the capacity to create meaning.

Self-Assessment

Nurses and other health care professionals can find it difficult to work with individuals who have strong emotional reactions.

They feel more confident dealing with patients' physical needs. Many worry that they may say something wrong and make the patient more upset. However, connection, mutuality, vulnerability, and respect are used to establish a therapeutic relationship, wherein teaching, coaching, and modelling are most effective.

It is helpful for health care providers, no matter the setting, to discuss emotional reactions to patients in conferences with other members of the health care team. Sharing these feelings facilitates critical reflections and helps the clinician to develop an awareness of counter-transference issues that will negatively affect patient care.

DIAGNOSIS

Patients will present with many different diseases, illnesses, and disorders. *Ineffective coping, powerlessness, interrupted family processes,* and *self-care deficit* are frequently diagnosed. Causal statements might include the following:
- Suppression of feelings
- Caregiver burnout
- Inability to meet role expectations
- Dependence on others
- Inability to meet basic care needs

OUTCOMES IDENTIFICATION

Some of the *Nursing Outcomes Classification (NOC)*–recommended outcomes related to anxiety include *Anxiety self-control, Anxiety level, Stress level, Coping, Social interaction skills,* and *Symptom control* (Moorhead, Johnson, Maas, et al., 2012). Additional outcomes may be developed through a shared decision-making process that helps the patient and the nurse to see concrete evidence of progress. The following are examples of possible outcomes:
- Patient will identify ineffective coping patterns.
- Patient will make realistic appraisal of strengths and weaknesses.
- Patient will assertively verbalize feelings such as anger, shame, or guilt.

PLANNING

Because patients with primary nonpsychiatric disorders are rarely admitted to psychiatric care settings for treatment, treatment is initiated in other settings. In primary care settings, providers are generally less confident about managing psychological symptoms. Because of the frequency of comorbidities between nonpsychiatric and psychiatric illnesses in primary care, an integrated model of care among mental health and medical clinicians is essential. In an ideal situation, a multidisciplinary team of clinicians would include an advanced-practice nurse who could provide consultation to health care providers outside of psychiatry.

The following are some highlights that can help the nurse plan necessary interventions. When working with someone who is medically ill, it is important to know if the person has any of the following:

- Someone who can share his or her concerns and who cares for him or her
- Friends and supports in the community
- Any coexisting conditions that could negatively affect adjustment to the illness, the course of the illness, adaptation to the illness, or ability to heal (e.g., depression; personality disorder; substance abuse; compulsive behaviours such as gambling, eating, or cybersex)
- Risky health behaviours (e.g., sedentary lifestyle, smoking, engaging in unsafe sex practices, abusing alcohol or drugs)
- A cultural view of health and illness that helps or impedes the process of seeking adequate care

IMPLEMENTATION

People who have a medical condition are vulnerable to a variety of psychosocial stresses. These influences affect lifestyle choice through at least five areas: personal life skills, stress, culture, social relationships and belonging, and a sense of control. Interventions that support the creation of supportive environments will enhance the capacity of individuals to make healthy lifestyle choices in a world where many choices are possible. As a result, how individuals cope with these stresses may be the difference between living with an acceptable quality of life and giving in to despair, withdrawal, helplessness, or hopelessness.

Nurses are in a position to assess and understand patients' psychosocial stressors, identify needed coping skills, and teach stress-management techniques (for more information, refer to Chapters 12 and 13). Nurses can play an important role not only in providing and managing patients' immediate medical care but also in helping patients to improve their ability to cope and increase their quality of life during the course of a chronic medical illness.

Health Teaching and Health Promotion

The type and depth of teaching is determined by the information the patient already understands about their illnesses and coping strategies. The Patient and Family Teaching box provides guidelines for teaching patients and their families about how to adapt to a major medical illness.

Coping Skills

Effective coping skills are healthier ways of looking at and dealing with illness (e.g., assertiveness training, cognitive reframing, problem-solving skills, social supports). They are many and varied and can be taught. A nurse is in a key position to assess patients' ability to cope, educate patients about coping skills, or provide referrals to patients to learn healthier ways of looking at and dealing with illness. Consider referring the patient for instruction in a variety of relaxation techniques, such as meditation, guided imagery, or breathing exercises, or teach the patient such techniques yourself. Behavioural techniques are useful, and nurses with special training can offer their patients progressive muscle relaxation or biofeedback. Relaxation techniques, stress management, and supportive education should be part of the care of the patient with a medical condition, regardless of the medical diagnosis. Other beneficial approaches include cognitive

PATIENT AND FAMILY TEACHING
Coping With a Major Medical Illness

Learn all you can about your illness. Knowledge can help reduce anxiety. Keeping your anxiety at manageable levels helps you understand your options and helps you make decisions you believe are right for you.

Practise healthy behaviours. Good sleep hygiene, diet, and exercise are good policies. Even if you are physically limited, exercise promotes a positive state of well-being. Lack of sleep can increase pain, irritability, and fatigue. Proper nutrition in the face of a medical illness can preserve or promote a healthy immune system.

Take advantage of support groups that help you manage your medical condition. Support groups that focus on your medical issue can provide you with information, help you learn how to handle difficult situations related to your illness, reduce isolation, and offer a safe place to share difficult thoughts and feelings.

Consider entering psychotherapy. There is growing evidence that psychotherapy helps people endure medical illness. Benefits include less pain, better coping skills, and even longer survival in some situations.

Find a way to express your feelings. Studies have examined the profound healing power of putting upsetting experiences into words (e.g., writing them down, keeping a journal). Acknowledging thoughts and feelings can help your nervous system relax.

Seek additional help if you become depressed, demoralized, anxious, or panicky or have unremitting pain. Your clinician might not be aware of these changes, and there are approaches (e.g., acupuncture, acupressure, biofeedback) that can give people control over their physiological responses and reduce the need for higher doses of medication.

Find a creative outlet. Doing anything creative—writing poetry or prose, painting or making collages, playing an instrument or singing—is a powerful tool in working with the feelings of fear, anger, and loss that are stirred up by illness.

If you are a caregiver, do not neglect your own self-care. Take time for rest and restoration and time to renew important life interests and activities. If you become depleted, you cannot give to another what is depleted and what you no longer possess.

Source: Adapted from Zerbe, K. J. (1999). *Women's mental health in primary care.* Philadelphia: Saunders.

behavioural psychotherapy, guided imagery, biofeedback, acupressure, and psychodynamic psychotherapy.

Although medical procedures may extend or promote life, they often take a toll on the patient's physical state because of the high degree of anxiety they evoke. Research has shifted the focus from patients' knowledge of the disease and its treatment to their confidence and skills in managing their condition. Interventions now support patients and their support systems being active participants in managing their condition (Hillebregt, Vlonk, Bruijnzeels, et al., 2017). The following have all been shown to affect a patient's recovery positively:

- Educating the patient regarding the specific medical treatment
- Referring the patient to community support groups (or systems)
- Teaching patients more effective coping skills that take into consideration patients' values, preferences, and lifestyle
- Focusing on a patient's strengths and reinforcing coping skills that work (e.g., prayerfulness, participation in hobbies, relaxation techniques).

Advanced-Practice Interventions

When working as part of nonpsychiatric multidisciplinary teams, the advanced-practice nurse is often referred to as a psychiatric consultation liaison nurse (PCLN). Within this role, the PCLN functions as a consultant to other nurses in managing psychological concerns and symptoms of psychiatric disorders and also works directly with patients as a clinician to help them deal more effectively with physical and emotional problems. The PCLN is a resource for members of a nursing staff who feel unable to intervene therapeutically with a patient who presents a management problem or has problems that impede care. The PCLN first meets with the nurse who initiated the consultation and then reviews the patient's medical records, talks with the physicians, and interviews the patient. After the patient interview, the PCLN discusses the assessment and suggestions for care with the referring nurse.

EVALUATION

Interventions are determined to be effective when patients remain safe, new coping strategies have improved quality of life, and stress is handled more adaptively. Evaluation of patients with comorbid disorders is a simple process when measurable behavioural outcomes have been written clearly and realistically.

▐ KEY POINTS TO REMEMBER

- There is irrefutable evidence that psychiatric disorders and psychological responses influence general medical conditions.
- A bidirectional effect exists between physical and emotional states of health. Physical illnesses are often accompanied by a spectrum of emotional responses, particularly anxiety and depression. Likewise, adverse emotional states often increase the severity of physical symptoms.

- The holistic philosophy of nursing dictates that all nurses, regardless of their roles or specialties, assess patients' psychosocial needs as well as their strengths.
- Health care personnel in the medical and mental health communities recognize the need to target both the psychological and the physical problems of a patient to increase adherence to the care regimen, maximize quality of life, and promote healing.

- Understanding a patient's psychosocial needs and knowing when to intervene and where to refer the patient are essential for the nurse who practises holistic care and more effectively promotes health.
- Identifying the existence of depression, anxiety, and substance abuse and getting the patient treatment can help promote a positive outcome of the medical disorder and improve the patient's quality of life.
- A holistic approach to patient care includes assessment of physical, psychosocial, social, and spiritual needs.

- A growing concern about patients is the state of their spiritual lives. Including this dimension in the holistic nursing assessment allows nurses to see inner strengths in their patients that might be overlooked when using a more traditional approach.
- The psychiatric consultation liaison nurse is a nurse clinician who is in the key position of being able to help other health care personnel look at their patients in a holistic manner and help those who care for these patients understand nonmedical issues that are impeding medical progress.

CRITICAL THINKING

1. Marie Vaudrie is a 45-year-old woman who has had a partial hysterectomy. Although she is asymptomatic and has a normal physical examination, her laboratory results indicate that she is HIV positive. Marie was unaware that her boyfriend of 2 years was engaging in unprotected sex with men. She and her ex-husband have been divorced for 5 years but maintain a good relationship and share custody of their three teenage children. Marie has a supportive extended family and several close friends, and she belongs to a church. After her diagnosis, Marie is encouraged to talk about her feelings and see a therapist. Marie states, "I will be able to do everything I did before. I feel healthy." The nurse has several concerns, including Marie's focus on self-care, her acceptance and understanding of her HIV-positive status, and her willingness to disclose her status to sexual or intimate partners.
   a. How would you evaluate Marie's social support system?
   b. What other information about Marie's situation would be helpful in your assessment (e.g., cultural beliefs about illness)?
   c. What recommendations or referrals could you make to Marie, and how would you approach her with these recommendations? Would you include contact data for any medically related or HIV-related support groups in the information you would give her?

2. Discuss how you would approach the physician regarding Marie's need to be evaluated for depression. What are some of the compelling reasons why depression (and any coexisting mental condition) should be treated in any and all seriously ill medically patients?
3. What cognitive behavioural coping skills have proven useful for a patient who is HIV positive?
4. What important areas should the nurse assess with an Indigenous woman with a past history of intimate partner violence who is attending an outpatient clinic and expressing a fear that she may be HIV positive?

CHAPTER REVIEW

1. Which statement about the psychological impact of medical illnesses is accurate?
   a. An experience of grief and loss is not typical of most serious medical illnesses.
   b. Depression is a significant issue in more than 60% of persons with cancer or heart disease.
   c. Psychological responses to medical illnesses can delay recovery but do not worsen the outcome.
   d. Patients often have significant concerns regarding the impact a medical illness can have on their ability to function.

2. While taking the vital signs of a patient about to undergo surgery, you notice that she is tearful. When asked, she tells you that her mother had the same surgery and later died of a postoperative infection. Which response is most likely to be therapeutic?
   a. Ask the patient if she would like to speak with the chaplain before surgery.
   b. Reassure the patient that she has an excellent surgeon and that complications for her surgery are rare.
   c. State, "Surgery can be very frightening," and sit down next to the patient to convey your availability to talk.
   d. State, "Many people become anxious before surgery, but this is a normal reaction. You will be fine."

3. An older adult male with heart disease feels both angry and guilty about his illness, blaming himself for becoming obese and inactive and feeling anger toward tobacco and fast-food companies. He presented in the emergency department today 4 hours after the onset of unrelenting chest pain, reporting that it "didn't hurt that much" and that, given his prior experiences with chest pain, he "did not think it would matter much" whether he came in quickly or tried to "wait it out." Now awaiting the results of his electrocardiogram (ECG), he is reading magazines and talking about the likelihood that a new stent will once again give him a new lease on life. Based on this information, how well would you expect this patient to be able to cope with his illness?
   a. Poorly
   b. Inadequately
   c. Adequately
   d. Exceptionally
4. A nurse on a medical-surgical unit is admitting a patient with a history of bipolar disorder and alcohol abuse. Which action would be most appropriate for ensuring that this patient receives the best possible nursing care?
   a. Consult with the psychiatric consultation liaison nurse regarding assessment skills and interventions likely to benefit this patient.
   b. Review online, textbook, or journal resources pertaining to the patient's mental health and substance abuse disorders.
   c. Consult more experienced colleagues and the head nurse for tips on assessing and caring for persons with comorbid psychiatric disorders.
   d. Focus primarily on the patient's physical health needs, and refer the patient for outpatient psychiatric care at discharge if the patient requests it.

5. Which statements about persons with mental illness who present with serious medical conditions are most accurate? Select all that apply.
   a. Such patients are at higher risk for receiving inadequate care, owing to failure to fully assess somatic complaints.
   b. Patients who have both a medical and a mental illness tend to receive more care and more costly care because of their concurrent disorders.
   c. Staff are more likely to minimize their time with such patients compared to medically ill patients without mental illness.
   d. Such patients risk being admitted to psychiatric settings instead of needed medical-surgical units, owing to staff's anxiety about caring for them.
   e. Emotional responses to medical conditions may be mistakenly attributed to psychiatric illness rather than being addressed as normal responses to medical conditions.

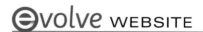 WEBSITE

Post-Test   interactive review

Visit the Evolve website for Chapter Review Answers and Rationales, Critical Thinking Answer Guidelines, and additional resources related to the content in this chapter: http://evolve.elsevier.com/Canada/Varcarolis/psychiatric/

REFERENCES

Cannon, W. B. (1914). The emergency function of the adrenal medulla in pain and the major emotions. *American Journal of Physiology, 33,* 356–372.

HealthPartners. (2015). *Chronic disease and mental health report.* Ottawa: Author.

Hillebregt, C. F., Vlonk, A. J., Bruijnzeels, M. A., et al. (2017). Barriers and facilitators influencing self-management among COPD patients: A mixed methods exploration in primary and affiliated specialist care. *International Journal of Chronic Obstructive Pulmonary Disease, 12,* 123–133. doi:10.2147/COPD.S103998.

Mental Health Commission of Canada. (2014, July). *Addressing the mental health needs of Canadians.* Ottawa, ON: Presentation at HealthPartners.

Moorhead, S., Johnson, M., Maas, M., et al. (2012). *Nursing outcomes classification (NOC)* (5th ed.). St. Louis: Mosby.

Selye, H. (1956). *The stress of life.* New York: McGraw-Hill.

Volpato, E., Banfi, P., & Pagnini, F. (2017). A psychological intervention to promote acceptance and adherence to non-invasive ventilation in people with chronic obstructive pulmonary disease: Study protocol of a randomized controlled trial. *Trials, 18*(59), 1–9. doi:10.1186/s13063-017-1802-1.

World Health Organization. (2004). *World Health Organization Quality of Life—BREF.* Retrieved from http://www.who.int/substance_abuse/research_tools/en/english_whoqol.pdf.

Wu, J., Suk, K., Dekker, R., et al. (2017). Prehospital delay, precipitants of admission, and length of stay in patients with exacerbation of heart failure. *American Journal of Critical Care, 26*(1), 62–69. doi:10.4037/ajcc2017750.

Care for the Dying and for Those Who Grieve

Sonya L. Jakubec

KEY TERMS AND CONCEPTS

anticipatory grief
bereavement
complicated grief
disenfranchised grief
Four Gifts of Resolving Relationships

grief
hospice palliative care (HPC)
mourning
palliative care

OBJECTIVES

1. Compare and contrast specific goals of end-of-life care inherent in the hospice palliative care model with those of the medical model.
2. Analyze the effects of specific interventions nurses can implement when working with a dying person and his or her family and loved ones.
3. Analyze how the Four Gifts of Resolving Relationships (forgiveness, love, gratitude, and farewell) can be used to help people respond to a dying loved one.
4. Explain the distinction between the terms *grief* and *mourning* as presented in this chapter and how the effectiveness of a holistic approach can be beneficial to the person.

5. Differentiate among some of the characteristics of normal bereavement and complicated grieving.
6. Explain how various models of understanding grieving (dual process, four tasks of mourning) can enhance your care of those who grieve.
7. Discuss at least five guidelines for dealing with catastrophic loss, and identify appropriate support for someone in acute grief.

⊖volve WEBSITE

Visit the Evolve website for Flashcards, Case Studies, and additional testing resources related to the content in this chapter: http://evolve.elsevier.com/Canada/Varcarolis/psychiatric/

Pre-Test   interactive review

Caring for patients who have terminal illnesses or are near death due to other conditions challenges and rewards nurses in deep and personal ways. In caring for the dying, nurses may grow personally, both by accepting their patients' deaths and by developing a richer understanding of their own mortality. Nurses also have an opportunity to bring dignity to the dying and help shape an enduring positive memory for family members and caregivers. At times of crisis (e.g., traumatic death such as death

by suicide), mental health nurses may work closely as witnesses and companions in the grief process of those surviving.

Nurses continue to provide care for dying patients primarily in medical institutions, despite evidence supporting care in the home and the overwhelming wish of most Canadians to die at home, surrounded by loved ones (Stajduhar, 2013). Although 70% of Canadian deaths occur in hospital (Canadian Hospice Palliative Care Association, 2017), alternatives for community-based palliative care and grief support are emerging across the country. Patient-centred palliative care is an interdisciplinary and collaborative effort aimed at relieving pain and suffering and involving various health care providers at all levels of interventions (Canadian Hospice Palliative Care Association, 2016) and in which nurses play an integral and important role. In addition to using the necessary assessment and management skills, nurses are often the entry point into the system for patients and their families.

Health care providers in all settings must be advocates for the chronically and terminally ill and their often overburdened caregivers. The Canadian hospice palliative care treatment model (Canadian Hospice Palliative Care Association, 2013) and the advance care planning national framework (Canadian Hospice Palliative Care Association, 2010a) provide tools that promote patient- and family-centred care for people facing potentially life-threatening situations. The tools support basic human rights, including having control over decisions affecting health and living situations; having advance directives, such as instructions to suspend or withhold curative efforts, completed and followed; and receiving excellent palliative care that promotes optimum comfort.

HOSPICE PALLIATIVE CARE

In 1967, in response to a system in which dying people were often neglected, isolated, and left to die in pain, Dame Cicely Saunders, a nurse, social worker, and physician, established St. Christopher's Hospice in London, England. Dame Cicely received universal recognition as the founder of the modern hospice movement. Central to her work was an aggressive pursuit of effective pain management that contributed to optimal quality of life (Clarke, 2010).

During the same period, in the United States, Dr. Elisabeth Kübler-Ross, also a nurse, began actively listening to the terminally ill. In her groundbreaking work, Kübler-Ross (1969) identified distinctive phases, or cycles, in people's responses to terminal illness: denial, anger, bargaining, depression, and acceptance. She also realized that personal growth actually accelerated in the last stages of life. Encouraged by the work of Kübler-Ross, those working with the dying adapted the St. Christopher's comprehensive model, and the multidisciplinary care team evolved to include a physician, a nurse, a social worker, a pastor or chaplain, and an aide.

The term *palliative care* was coined in the mid-1970s by Canadian physician Balfour Mount, who was inspired by the work of Kübler-Ross and Dame Cicely Saunders (Cahill, 2010). Like those before him, Dr. Mount found that treatments for the terminally ill were abysmally inadequate, so he set up a hospital-based palliative care unit at the Royal Victoria Hospital in Montreal, taking the name *palliative* from its meaning, "to improve the quality of something." Dr. Balfour is known as "the father of palliative care," an approach that evolved into a pan-Canadian movement, with goals of relieving suffering and improving quality of life for those who are living with or dying from an illness (Canadian Hospice Palliative Care Association, 2013). This movement eventually led to the development of the

Canadian Hospice Palliative Care Association (CHPCA), established in 1991, which is the national voice for hospice palliative care (HPC) in Canada. HPC is defined as whole-person health care aimed at relieving suffering and improving quality of life rather than aimed at a cure (Canadian Hospice Palliative Care Association, 2017).

Death is considered a natural and inevitable part of life. Using an interdisciplinary approach, the national HPC model is appropriate for patients and families of all ages living with or at risk for developing a life-threatening illness of any kind or magnitude, for whom HPC may complement therapy or be the total focus of care (Canadian Hospice Palliative Care Association, 2013). The goals of HPC are to address all needs (physical, psychological, social, cultural, spiritual, and practical), prepare for and manage self-determined life closure and the dying process, and help with coping with loss and grief during illness and bereavement (Canadian Hospice Palliative Care Association, 2013). Historically, the terms *hospice* and *palliative care* were often used interchangeably; however, the CHPCA has brought the two terms together to form HPC. One of the central themes of HPC in Canada is the belief that each of us has the right to die pain-free and with dignity (Canadian Hospice Palliative Care Association, 2017).

> **VIGNETTE**
>
> Mr. Spence contracted amyotrophic lateral sclerosis (ALS) at the age of 52. He lived at home until his care overwhelmed his family, and he has now been in a care centre for 9 months. He is almost completely paralyzed but can still use a letter board with a head-mounted laser pointer. He has a warm smile and a pleasant gaze. He is experiencing shooting pains in his legs and has increasing difficulty with swallowing and breathing. Despite being barely able to eat, he has refused a feeding tube. The staff feel helpless. How can they just stand by while he starves to death? Will he starve to death? One of the aides has decided to quit working with him because caring for Mr. Spence has become so emotionally difficult for her.
>
> An HPC referral was made. A nurse and social worker visited the care facility and offered practical help and guidance for staff, patient, and family in treating Mr. Spence. They talked with him about what to expect as his condition declines. Comfort-oriented medication and nonpharmacological care were reviewed, and Mr. Spence was offered as many choices as possible. Emotional, spiritual, and educational support were offered to the family and staff concerning the course of the illness, anticipatory grieving, and ways of using the remaining time to meet goals and nurture relationships. Mr. Spence, assisted by his family and an HPC volunteer, chose to work on a memoir about his illness and its impact on his growth as a person.

Quality palliative care is identified as a human right in a growing literature and global action items (Brennan, Gwyther, Lohman, et al., 2015; Rosa, 2017). Although palliative care is widely available to all Canadians, regardless of age or diagnosis, access to high-quality integrated care is not the same across the county. Despite the progressive move toward an integrated, streamlined system, many Canadians, unlike Mr. Spence, are still dying without adequate supports (Canadian Hospice Palliative Care Association, 2010b). Among the reasons for this lack of supports are geography, lack of patient-centred care, lack of knowledge and policy leadership, cultural diversity, and funding. Although HPC grew from the concept of caring for the dying, it is now used to guide care at any point during an acute, chronic, or life-threatening illness or bereavement (Canadian Hospice Palliative Care Association, 2013).

Palliative care is a philosophy of care as opposed to a treatment. Because Canadians are living longer with chronic health conditions, bringing this philosophy into being through access to quality care is necessary at earlier points in the continuum of life, not just at the end of life. Patients can receive HPC in hospital, at home, in community care homes (e.g., long-term care), or in hospice programs. Respite beds are also available in some centres. Innovative programs in Ottawa and Toronto to provide palliative care to marginalized populations, particularly the homeless, have emerged over the past decade, highlighting a number of systemic challenges (Huynh, Henry, & Dosani, 2015). Calgary's Allied Mobile Palliative Program also demonstrates the challenges of merging complex street-level care and harm reduction with palliative care principles (Colgan, Edwards, & Jakubec, 2017). Several factors need to be considered when determining the best place for providing care, such as personal choice, a balance between patient and family needs, and the availability of resources to meet those needs.

Regardless of setting, the HPC approach is interprofessional and cross-sector in nature. In addition to access to health care providers, this approach also requires spiritual care, volunteer services, bereavement services, medical equipment, medications, and supplies related to the illness. A personalized plan of care is developed with the patient, reflected in the care, and regularly reviewed and updated.

NURSING CARE AT THE END OF LIFE

End-of-life (EOL) care is a term that describes care to assist people as they progress through the final stage of life. Hospice and palliative care may be part of the EOL care that patients and families receive at that time (Nicol & Nyatanga, 2014).

Hospice Palliative Care Nursing

Although nurses are educated to provide holistic care, few are prepared to deal with the death and dying trajectory they will ultimately face at some point in their careers. The Canadian Association of Schools of Nursing (CASN, 2011) has developed entry-to-practice competencies and indicators for registered nurses. In addition to providing practical care, nurses need to demonstrate enhanced communication, coordination, and management skills; self-care; and the ability to attend to the compassion and dignity needs of those suffering loss. Nurses working in HPC settings should pursue additional certification.

The Art, Presence, and Caring of Nursing

Caring for patients at the end of life requires a shift in professional expectations. It involves not only curing but also healing concepts of care (Chochinov, 2016; Nicol & Nyatanga, 2014), the demand

for genuine human presence toward the patient while using evidence-informed knowledge, the management of pain and symptom control, and other technical aspects of care. "Whole-person care" involves seeing the patient first as a human being while being attentive to all aspects of suffering. The Canadian Hospice Palliative Care Association (2006) developed gold standards for nurses providing HPC and EOL care, with the following five dimensions of nursing to help guide their work in any setting.

- **Valuing**—believing in the intrinsic value of others, in the value of life, and that death is a natural process
- **Connecting**—establishing a therapeutic relationship with the person and the family through making, sustaining, and closing the relationship
- **Empowering**—providing care that is empowering for the person and the family
- **Doing for**—providing care based on best practice in pain and symptom management, coordination of care, and advocacy
- **Finding meaning**—helping the person and family to find meaning in their lives and their experiences of illness

Inherent in these dimensions is the ability to engage in therapeutic relationships with people who are grounded in the *art*, *presence*, and *caring* concepts of nursing. Previously, these three were considered individual concepts, but Finfgeld-Connett (2008c) proposed their convergence into one theoretical framework based on their similarities. Interactions with patients are characterized by openness and honesty, while also demonstrating vulnerability, kindness, compassion, and empathy (Finfgeld-Connett, 2006, 2008a, 2008b). Positive outcomes are experienced by the nurse as well as the patient, with enhanced physical well-being for the patient and enhanced emotional well-being for both (Finfgeld-Connett, 2008c).

To approach nursing work with art, presence, and caring, two essential skills you can practise are listening and observing (see Chapters 9 and 10). Reflect back to the speaker what you heard by restating or summarizing the message. Observe the patient's nonverbal communications. Do you sense well-being? Sorrow? Suffering? Ask the patient and family open-ended questions such as the following:

- Would you tell me what this is like for you?
- How do you see your condition right now?
- Where do you see things going?
- Are you worried about anything?
- What are you hoping for?

Practise staying silent and giving the patient or family member all the time needed to respond. Offer a reassuring touch. The artful, present, and caring nurse can invite and permit the patient to discover new dimensions of his or her own experiences, bringing greater wholeness.

Assessment for Spiritual Issues

Spirituality, the dimension of human experience that can provide meaning for life, is integral to EOL care. Conducting a comprehensive spiritual assessment is important to understanding how a patient's spirituality may enhance comfort. Charbonneau and Bélanger (2013), in their study of home palliative patients in

Quebec City, found that, much like physical care, spiritual care was something felt by patients. They want to feel genuinely cared about and have the opportunity to talk about their fears, hopes, issues, and despair in everyday language. Nurses, then, must focus on presence, listening, connecting, creating openings, and engaging in reciprocal sharing as they make the journey with their patients. Time spent with the patient and family and genuine expressions of compassion (Sinclair, Norris, McConnell, et al., 2016) are considered essential for successful outcomes. Assessment of spirituality can be guided by an appropriate spirituality assessment tool such as SHARE (Kramer-Howe & Huls, 2004), FICA (Puchalski, 2007), or HOPE (Anandarajah & Hight, 2001), although no stand-alone tool is validated for spirituality in palliative care. Regardless of the tool used, it is important to use unbiased, open language and ensure appropriate timing in the relationship, having already established trust and rapport as a companion and witness in the palliative experience (Chochinov, 2016; Chochinov, McClement, Hack, et al., 2013). Some examples of questions are: Tell me how you are doing spiritually. What gives your life meaning? What role do your beliefs play in regaining your health? Spiritual caring is a huge part of holistic care and can be interwoven with the nurse's daily work through the process of self-awareness, empathy, and commitment to EOL care (Sansó, Galiana, Oliver, et al., 2015). In addition to thoroughly assessing connections to a specific religion, nurses can become skilled at listening for the patient's intrinsic spirituality. For many patients, religion and spiritual practices provide context, community, and comfort when facing EOL challenges.

Awareness and Sensitivity of Cultural Contexts

Spiritual and cultural contexts and care are often inextricably intertwined. Although it is impossible for the nurse to know all things about all cultures, it is imperative as professionals to be aware of the need to explore cultural practices that affect care at all times across the health care continuum (see Chapter 8). Canada is a multicultural nation, but in particular it has a growing older adult Indigenous population (Bourassa, Hampton, Baydala, et al., 2010). As Indigenous people age, they suffer even higher burdens of chronic disease and illness than do non-Indigenous Canadians. In addition, many Indigenous people live in rural communities, which often do not have the same access to health care services (palliative care among these) as their urban counterparts (Pesut, McLeod, Hole, et al., 2012). Like other Canadians, the majority of Indigenous people living in remote communities would prefer to die at home (Fruch, Monture, Prince, et al., 2016). However, unlike many other Canadians, they are not often given this opportunity, due to a lack of services and resources (Duggleby, Kuchera, MacLeod, et al., 2015). In addition to this difference, even when HPC is available, it is often not safe for or sensitive to Indigenous or other cultures. The Canadian Virtual Hospice (2016) developed a curriculum for health care providers that is inclusive of culturally sensitive and appropriate protocols for providing support to Indigenous families in need of HPC services. Many cultural practices of Indigenous persons (e.g., respect for elders, the special gifts of elders, the role of sacred items such as feathers, ceremonies) are rooted in culture and grounded in spirituality (Canadian Virtual Hospice, 2016).

Research on palliative care for Indigenous communities is a priority (see Research Highlight box).

 RESEARCH HIGHLIGHT

First Nations Communities and Palliative Care

Problem

Many elders were dying in hospital and long-term care homes outside their communities due to a lack of palliative care programs for First Nations.

Purpose of Study

The purpose of the study was to develop a framework to help guide the development and implementation of palliative care programs in 12 First Nations communities in northwestern Ontario and to evaluate the interventions and resources used.

Methods

Partnerships were formed with Indigenous health organizations; 12 First Nations communities composed of elders, chiefs, and residents; and the researchers. A needs assessment—including questionnaires, interviews, and focus groups—helped to identify values and beliefs related to death and dying and EOL care issues. Each community then identified and developed culturally appropriate educational materials.

Key Findings

The integrative palliative care framework included the development of strong partnerships, using a participatory action research approach that adhered to research ethics, embraced ownership and control, and celebrated cultural competence and safety across all cultural groups encountered, including the research team. Three of the 12 communities involved in the study followed up by developing local palliative care teams, and regional palliative care experts further supported the development of protocols for home death.

Implications for Nursing Practice

Nurses can and should be a part of culturally sensitive palliative care research. Strategies from the framework provide useful approaches for nurses, who—as part of their professional practice competencies—are responsible for demonstrating sensitivity to and respect for diversity in health practices and beliefs (e.g., spirituality, culture) and for advocating for improved services.

Source: Prince, H., & Kelley, M. L. (2010). An integrative framework for conducting palliative care research with First Nations communities. *Journal of Palliative Care, 26*(1), 47–53.

Palliative Symptom Management

Excellent symptom management is a hallmark of HPC nursing (Canadian Hospice Palliative Care Association, 2013). The patient or substitute decision maker has the right to be informed and make decisions about all aspects of care, including the right to a dignified and comfortable death (Canadian Hospice Palliative Care Association, 2013; Canadian Nurses Association, 2008). Nurses can offer a wide spectrum of interventions to alleviate symptoms, guided by patients' own reports and careful assessment. The most commonly reported EOL symptoms are pain, constipation, dyspnea, fatigue, depression, and delirium (Kreher, 2016). It is gratifying to relieve pain or nausea or to give patients control over bowel medications and breathing treatments. For symptoms such as worry, fear, sadness, and low energy, however, better approaches might include education, normalization, counselling, integrative therapies (e.g., massage, music), and stress-reduction practices.

Each symptom should be assessed individually. Treatable, reversible, and temporary conditions can be mistakenly attributed to the terminal diagnosis. For example, if a patient reports feeling depressed, it is important not to assume that the feelings are due to the dying process. If the patient becomes confused or lethargic, it is essential to rule out causes such as medication effects, dehydration, delirium, urinary tract infections, and constipation before attributing the symptom to terminal decline.

Care of the patient and family can be viewed through the lens of Roger Woodruff's total suffering model (Figure 31-1). This model can also be used to describe guidelines when caring for the dying (Box 31-1). The use of such a model can help guide the practice of nurses throughout the nursing process when working with palliative care patients.

The Importance of Effective Communication

Nurses need excellent communication skills when working in all settings, at all times, and with all members involved in the HPC experience (Matzo & Sherman. 2014). Nurses have a role even at the beginning of the EOL continuum. The value of simply asking patients and their families, "Do you have any concerns?" followed by strong encouragement to seek out their support system while waiting for news cannot be understated.

During stressful periods, two factors seem to make things more bearable: (1) the ability to have—or believe one can have—some control over the situation, and (2) the ability to predict changes. Information and education from nurses can improve a family's sense of control. Information should be conveyed slowly, given repeatedly, written down, and reviewed often. People tend to need several reiterations of information when under stress (see Chapter 12). Effective communication skills are at the heart of developing a therapeutic relationship, assessing the patient, and providing holistic care to the patient and family. A strong therapeutic relationship will guide discussions and decision making for patients and families in times of loss (see Chapter 9). In addition, effective communication helps to decrease distress and total pain and suffering (Canadian Hospice Palliative Care Association, 2009b). Through their relationship and communication practices, psychiatric mental health nurses have a profound influence on how patients experience end of life and on patients' sense of dignity. Canadian palliative care psychiatrist Harvey Chochinov and colleagues have developed and tested a model of dignity-conserving care with an ABCD mnemonic that serves as a guide for effective care (Chochinov, 2007). Guidelines for Communication: Dignity-Conserving Care highlights practical approaches in more detail.

The balance of kindness and respect through empathy and information is always at the front of mind in care of the dying. The following vignette illustrates the confusion and misery that can result from lack of information, the desire to take control of one's life situation, and the inadequacy of the term *dying* to describe living with a terminal disease.

BOX 31-1 GUIDELINES WHEN CARING FOR THE DYING

Pain—Remember that patients' pain is what they say it is, and they have the right to have their pain needs met effectively, using the simplest route. Reassure them that you will provide relief from their pain to help decrease their anxiety.

Physical—Intervene quickly to manage symptoms that may affect other organ systems (e.g., nausea, constipation or diarrhea, incontinence, air hunger, inadequate nutrition) in order to promote and maintain the highest level of comfort possible.

Psychological—Keep patients and their families informed about the disease and its symptoms. Invite them to deal with their emotions, acknowledging the losses and changes in their lives. Practise the art of presence and caring through active listening, genuine empathy, and personal sharing.

Social—Many people at the end of life are afraid of dying alone and need reassurance that they are not alone. Promote this sense of security by verbalizing this reassurance, and demonstrate it by responding to their needs quickly and spending time with them. Provide companionship for them by supporting their visitors, engaging in conversations with them and their families, and providing privacy when appropriate or when requested.

Cultural—Ask questions to discover the person's cultural background and meaningful practices used during EOL care to promote a peaceful journey. Explore appropriate language used (are there any taboo words?), and inquire about whom to share information with first. Explore the role of the family in care, and explore care practices other than science-based medicine, such as alternative medicines or other therapies.

Spiritual—By asking appropriate questions, offer the opportunity to patients to discuss what is meaningful in their lives, such as relationships, any faith or spiritual practices they use to keep themselves calm, and who or what they turn to when dealing with the challenges of life. Exploring spirituality can offer the opportunity to assess and promote effective coping skills based on past behaviours.

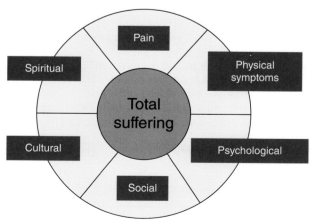

FIGURE 31-1 Woodruff's total suffering model. **Source:** Woodruff, R. (2004). *Palliative medicine: Evidence-based symptomatic and supportive care for patients with advanced cancer* (4th ed.). New York: Oxford University Press.

GUIDELINES FOR COMMUNICATION

Dignity-Conserving Care

Attitudes

Reflective Questions

- How would I be feeling in this patient's situation?
- What is leading me to draw those conclusions?
- Have I checked whether my assumptions are accurate?
- Am I aware how my attitude toward the patient may be affecting him or her?
- Could my attitude toward the patient be based on something to do with my own experiences, anxieties, or fears?
- Does my attitude as a nurse enable or disenable me to establish open and empathic professional relationships with my patients?

Actions to Be Taken

- Consciously and routinely make these questions a part of your reflection on the care of each and every patient
- Discuss attitudes in regular clinical supervision and debriefings
- Embrace learning opportunities and experiences that challenge and question your attitudes and assumptions as they might affect patient care
- Support the acknowledgement and discussion of these issues with others in the workplace to support a growing culture of dignity-conserving care

Behaviours

General Disposition

- Treat contact with patients as you would any potent and important clinical intervention
- Professional behaviours toward patients must always include respect and kindness
- Lack of curative options should never rationalize or justify a lack of ongoing patient contact

Assessment Practices

- Always ask the patient's permission to engage in any clinical assessment or intervention
- Always ask the patient's permission to include others in the assessment or interventions
- Although assessment and interventions may be part of routine care, it is rarely routine for the patient, so always, as much as possible, take time to set the patient at ease and show that you have some appreciation for what he or she is about to go through (e.g., "I know this might feel a bit uncomfortable"; "I'm sorry that we have to do this to you"; "I know this is an inconvenience"; "This should only hurt for a moment"; "Let me know if you feel we need to stop for any reason"; "Asking these questions again is necessary because ...")
- Limit conversations with patients during medical interventions (aside from providing them with instruction or encouragement) until they have dressed or been covered appropriately and are rested

Facilitating Communication

- Demonstrate to your patient that he or she has your full and complete attention

- Always invite the patient to include people from his or her support network present, particularly when you plan to discuss complex or "difficult" information
- All personal issues should be raised in ways that respect the patient's need for privacy
- When speaking with the patient, try to be seated at a comfortable distance for conversation, at the patient's eye level when possible
- Offer patients and families repeated explanations as requested
- Present information free of jargon, using only language that the patient will understand
- Ask if the patient has questions and allow time for questions to arise and be recalled

Compassion

Getting in touch with one's own feelings requires the consideration of human life and experience, through a number of avenues, such as:

- Reading and discussing stories and novels and experiencing films, theatre, expert talks, and art that portray the depth and despair of the human condition
- Reflect on the personal stories that accompany illness
- Experiencing some degree of identification with those who are ill or suffering—be with your vulnerability

Ways to Show Compassion

- An understanding look
- A gentle touch on the shoulder, arm, or hand
- Honest communication, spoken or unspoken, that acknowledges the person beyond his or her illness

Dialogue

Acknowledging Personhood

- "This must be frightening for you."
- "I can only imagine what you must be going through."
- "It's natural to feel pretty overwhelmed at times like these."

Knowing the Patient

- "What should I know about you as a person to help me take the best care of you that I can?"
- "What are the things at this time in your life that are most important to you or that concern you most?"
- "Who else (or what else) will be affected by what's happening with your health?"
- "Who should be here to help support you?" (friends, family, spiritual or religious support network, etc.)
- "Who else should we get involved at this point, to help support you through this difficult time?" (psychosocial services, group support, chaplaincy, complementary care specialists, etc.)

Psychotherapeutic Approaches

- Dignity therapy
- Meaning-centred therapy
- Life review/reminiscence

Source: Adapted from Chochinov, H. M. (2007). Dignity and the essence of medicine: The A, B, C, and D of dignity conserving care. *BMJ, 335*(7612), 184–187. doi:10.1136/bmj.39244.650926.47.

Anticipatory Grief

Patients and families can experience "grief ahead of time," known as anticipatory grief, when they receive a life-limiting diagnosis or when they are threatened with loss of ability to function independently, loss of identity, and changes in role definition (Shore, Gelber, Koch, et al., 2016). Future loss is mourned as people acknowledge the importance of the impending loss, adjust their lives to accommodate the intervening time, and anticipate how their futures will be altered by the loss. Sensitive communication and support can help family members process this information (Overton & Cottone, 2016). The experience of anticipatory grief varies by individual, family, and culture (Box 31-2). Nurses can help patients and loved ones understand that their feelings are common and assist them with developing coping strategies and with redefining their roles within the family and in the outside world (Matzo & Sherman, 2014). Nurses must also remind those in their care to keep in mind that, although they are experiencing loss, there is always hope.

As with all types of grieving, nurses need to recognize that people can experience symptoms of grief physically, cognitively, emotionally, socially, and spiritually (Canadian Hospice Palliative Care Association, 2008) and intervene appropriately.

The Four Gifts of Resolving Relationships

An important role of the nurse during EOL care is to invite families to accept the dying of their loved one and say goodbye. Taking the opportunity to say goodbye has been correlated with more positive bereavement outcomes (Zisook, Iglewicz, Avanzino, et al., 2014). The Four Gifts of Resolving Relationships is one means of opening conversations about the coming separation. The concept of the Four Gifts was interpreted from the writings of Elisabeth Kübler-Ross and used with her permission by Beverly Ryan of the Hospice of the Twin Cities in Minnesota. In her workshops for the terminally ill, Dr. Kübler-Ross witnessed many couples and families shift from being distant, cold, or angry to becoming warm, loving, and close. She observed that this change resulted from a predictable sequence of communications, which were later formulated into the Four Gifts. People often intuitively recognize the gifts as processes they have already been

experiencing. Perhaps these processes are innate within human relationships, but anxiety, sorrow, and denial can obstruct their expression.

The nurse can describe the Four Gifts in simple terms and encourage families and patients to express them in their own ways. The gifts—forgiveness, love, gratitude, and farewell—can work for both giver and receiver. When given with sincerity and simplicity, they can precipitate a healing shift in relationships.

Forgiveness. The first step in forgiveness is to admit to wrongs and hurts experienced in the relationship. The intention is to forgive, seek forgiveness, and release the hurt so that healing can occur. Sometimes a face-to-face encounter is not possible (e.g., when the patient is sedated, comatose, or experiencing dementia), and sometimes it is not advisable (e.g., when it would cause more distress than it would relieve). Reconciliation requires two people who wish to heal a broken relationship. Forgiveness is a one-sided act, which can be given unilaterally. Granting forgiveness does not mean condoning or accepting a truly injurious or abusive action. It does not make a wrong right. What it does is signal a desire to let go of blame and anger, to release one's own heart from the chains of resentment. As such, it is a gift to the one who offers forgiveness, whether reconciliation is possible or not.

Love. The second gift is to express love to each other. Many adult children wish to hear their parent say, "I love you, and I am proud of you." Between spouses, in some long-term marriages, these words have faded away to be replaced by daily togetherness and the practical caring of a shared life. It is not uncommon in bereavement for survivors to regret that they did not hear or say the words "I love you" and long for that final recognition of the relationship's value. Ultimately, the message we need to hear at the end of life is that we are loved for being who we are, not for what we have done or achieved.

Gratitude. Expressions of love naturally flow into gratitude for what each has been in the other person's life. People look back over life together and remember the good times and the tough times. They can take out photograph albums, show videotapes, reminisce, and listen again to favourite stories. It is especially gratifying to acknowledge the things that were taken for granted. Parents or caregivers may never have been thanked for going to work every day for 30 or 40 years, caring for the home, or offering nurturance, support, or guidance. Similarly, acknowledgement of the love and attention of caregivers or dependants can be important expressions of gratitude. Many exhausted caregivers weep when they are told they really are doing a good job and are appreciated.

Farewell. Many people say they hate goodbyes because they bring up feelings of grief at the finality of parting. Also, it is awkward to say goodbye before someone is actually leaving. It may appear to be rushing the person or even causing the departure. Yet when the final separation of death awaits us, the act of saying goodbye is deeply appropriate and meaningful. In cases when there is no chance to say goodbye, or when the opportunity to say goodbye is not taken, survivors may express long-term regret. The words or gestures used do not matter as long as the meaning is adequately expressed.

BOX 31-2 SIGNS OF ANTICIPATORY GRIEF

- Feelings of emptiness or of being lost
- A sense of being numb and fatigued
- A feeling of unreality and disbelief
- Periods of weeping or raging
- The desire to run away from the situation
- The need to protect the patient from suffering or death by overseeing every detail of care
- Worry about the future and the unknown
- Anger at the patient, health care providers, or both
- Pronounced clinging to or dependency on the patient or other family members
- Fear of going crazy

VIGNETTE

Susan, a 74-year-old divorced woman living alone, is told by her doctor that she is dying of liver cancer. Upon hearing that she cannot be cured, she assumes that she will die in a few days or weeks. She goes home, settles all her affairs, calls everyone she cares about and says goodbye, accepts hospice care, and begins to await death. As weeks and then months go by, Susan feels betrayed by her doctor, embarrassed to be alive, unsure how to behave, and uncomfortable with her friends and relatives. She has time to begin worrying about how her death will be, how much control she will lose, and how she can afford care at the end. She is confused and even disoriented by the unexpected apparent improvement in her symptoms.

Susan shares her feelings with the nurse. The nurse educates Susan about her cancer and how to interpret her symptoms. The HPC team addresses her emotions and needs in many ways. They encourage her to take a trip she had postponed and to begin seeing friends again. They educate her on the concept of "living with terminal illness" rather than dying from it. Susan needs to learn new approaches to living meaningfully with an uncertain future. When Susan finally enters the end stage of her disease, she is comfortable and cared for by her relatives at home.

BOX 31-3 GUIDELINES FOR SELF-CARE WHEN CARING FOR THE DYING

1. Remind yourself that what is happening to your patients and their families is not happening to you. This is their life drama right now but not your own.
2. When you notice that you are having a particularly strong emotional reaction, either positive or negative (counter-transference), take it as a signal to explore your deeper issues or needs by talking with a trusted friend, counsellor, or colleague.
3. Protect your private life by practising time management, avoiding working outside of normal hours, protecting your pager or telephone number, and taking regular days off and vacations.
4. Clearly state what you can and cannot do for your patients so that your human and professional limitations are known up front.
5. Practise humility. There is much you can do, but there is also much that is unknown and unknowable.
6. Do your own mourning when your heart is touched and you need to acknowledge the importance of others in your life. Even after a person has died, you can honour the relationship you had in your memory. Attend funerals or create grieving rituals when someone you felt close to dies.
7. Create a healthy, balanced private life by releasing stress. Working with patients who are dying creates stresses at many levels. The challenge is to work them into your busy schedule and stay on course. Foremost among these methods are regular exercise, a balanced diet, adequate rest, vacations, fun and laughter, loving and accepting relationships, and a connection to higher meaning in life.

In the preceding vignette, Trent did not rehearse, resist, or complicate the Four Gifts but used the sequence to express the full range of his feelings. His story illustrates how simple and natural this process can be. Many families need no encouragement to forgive, cherish, thank, and release a loved one. The Four Gifts can be a helpful contribution, however, to families whose members are overwhelmed, cling to false hope, or are emotionally reticent.

Self-Care

As front-line medical caregivers, nurses are educated to help patients get better, stronger, and more independent. Supporting patients at the end of life, as they grow weaker, sicker, and ultimately die, can be overwhelming, challenging the nurse's sense of competency and professionalism. The demands inherent in EOL nursing lead to increased vulnerability to emotional attachments and compassion fatigue. These experiences, along with daily exposure to grief and dying, require nurses to practise conscious self-care in both their professional and their private lives. Health care providers naturally grow attached to some patients and may experience both anticipatory grieving and bereavement. To maintain emotional balance and health, it is essential to rely on the support of others and practise good self-care. This is a journey that promotes greater self-understanding, wisdom, and compassion (Chochinov, McClement, Hack, et al., 2013; Sansó, Galiana, Oliver, et al., 2015). The multidisciplinary team approach of supportive supervision is helpful in this process.

Caring for patients who are dying and those who grieve can bring up personal reactions, which may be triggered by a patient who is younger than the nurse, one who resembles a significant person in the nurse's own life, one who is experiencing symptoms reminiscent of other difficult deaths, or one who offends the nurse's sense of fairness or acceptability. Workplace conditions such as complex caseloads, rapid turnover in office staff, several losses in a short period, or too many demands for on-call time or overtime can intensify a nurse's vulnerability to feeling overwhelmed. Box 31-3 provides guidelines to help the health care provider maintain emotional health when working with death and the dying.

NURSING CARE FOR THOSE WHO GRIEVE

Loss is part of the human experience, and grieving is the response that enables people to accept and reconcile the loss and adapt to change. We grieve the commonplace losses in our lives, be they loss of a relationship (e.g., divorce, separation, death, abortion); health (e.g., a body function or part, mental or physical capacity); friendship, status, or prestige; security (e.g., occupational, financial, social, cultural); or a dream. Other normal losses include changes in circumstances, such as retirement, promotion, marriage, and aging. These losses can promote growth through adaptation or may result in apathy, anger, and resentment.

Losing a significant person through death is a major life crisis. Long-term relationships deeply bond us to each other, shaping our world and our identity in it. Their loss can diminish aspects of our own self-concept and tear apart our assumptive world. Grief is experienced holistically, affecting us emotionally, cognitively, spiritually, and physically. Those who grieve sometimes describe the death of a loved one as an amputation.

GRIEF REACTIONS, BEREAVEMENT, AND MOURNING

Grief encompasses all of an individual's reactions to loss and is defined as sorrow experienced in anticipation of, during, and after a loss (Canadian Hospice Palliative Care Association, 2013). Normal grief reactions include depressed mood, insomnia, anxiety, poor appetite, loss of interest, guilt, dreams about the deceased, and poor concentration. Psychological states include shock, denial, and yearning or searching for the deceased. **Bereavement**, derived from the Old English word *berafian*, meaning "to rob," is the period of grieving following a death. **Mourning** refers to things people do to cope with their grief, including shared social expressions of grief, such as attending funerals and other ceremonies or rituals, as well as participating in bereavement groups. Everyone grieves, but not everyone engages in the work of mourning. The length of time, degree, and rituals for mourning are often typically determined by cultural, religious, and familial factors. Despite a wide variation in experiences of duration and intensity, grief becomes a serious physical and mental health concern for relatively few people (Gray, 2014).

The study of human grief and bereavement has evolved over the past 40 years. Research examines questions such as: What constitutes normal, healthy grieving? What are predictors of complicated grief? What interventions, if any, benefit different populations of grieving people? When is medication useful for the bereaved person? What is the impact of losses on family systems? What are cultural mediators of delivering grief support? How does complicated or unresolved grief affect public and private health care usage? What are best practices to intervene in special types of loss, such as traumatic loss, genocidal loss, societal loss, and wartime loss?

Types of Grief

Grief is a multifaceted, deeply personal human response to loss. The time it takes to grieve is individual and unique to each person. Even each family member affected grieves differently. Many variables, such as how the death occurred, coping skills, previous losses, other life stressors, and support systems, affect how people grieve. The nature of the relationship with the person who has died is of particular importance (Mortell, 2015). Nurses are in a position to provide appropriate assessment to help differentiate disenfranchised grief, anticipatory grief, and complicated grief from the normal grieving process (Canadian Hospice Palliative Care Association, 2008).

Disenfranchised grief can occur when losses are not always openly acknowledged, supported, or recognized as significant, such as a loss through suicide, the loss of a friend, the loss of a pet, or the grief of someone thought incapable of grieving (e.g., a child, a person with dementia). A sense of isolation can occur, and nurses need to recognize the grief as real and intervene by acknowledging the loss, supporting feelings, and encouraging the person grieving to reach out to supportive networks. Disenfranchised grief has numerous psychological components that

> ## VIGNETTE
>
> Trent is a 28-year-old man with developmental disabilities and bipolar disorder. He arrives at his dying father's home to see him for the last time. Trent lives in a group home and has not seen his family for many months. The last time he visited, he had not taken his medication, and his behaviour caused his family to avoid him. The HPC nurse tells Trent that his father is dying and explains the Four Gifts. The young man sadly enters his father's bedroom and sits on the bed. He says, "Dad, I know you are going to die, and I want you to know that I am so sorry for the ways I have acted and the trouble I have caused. Please forgive me, Dad. You have always looked out for me, and I shouldn't have gone off my meds. I love you, Dad. You've never given up on me. Thank you for finding me the place where I live and people to love me and look after me. Thanks for being my dad. I know I have to say goodbye. I promise I will keep taking my meds so I will behave right. I promise I'll listen to my counsellors and have a good life. I love you so much, Dad. Goodbye." He weeps with his father, who holds him for a little while. Then he comes out of the room with a tear-streaked face, knowing he will never see his father alive again. He feels complete, however. He has said the important things with courage and taken proper leave of his father.

can create the conditions for dysregulation and confusion and that have been associated with complicated grief (McNutt & Yakushko, 2013).

Nurses also need to recognize when grief becomes **complicated grief**, a term applied to grief that remains unresolved and is thought to affect between 3% and 25% of those who grieve. With complicated grief, bereavement symptoms can at times evolve into other mental health concerns, such as substance abuse or chronic depression (Shear, Ghesquiere, & Glickman, 2013). Taken together, these grief presentations warrant careful assessment and appropriate levels of psychiatric mental health nursing intervention (Mortell, 2015).

In the past, there was debate about how best to recognize and manage more severe reactions to grief, with some supporting the need to consider complicated grief a separate entity under the *Diagnostic and Statistical Manual of Mental Disorders (DSM-5)* and others arguing the need to stop trying to pathologize varied grief experiences (Bandini, 2015; Stroebe, Stroebe, Schut, et al., 2017). The newly revised *DSM-5* has addressed this debate and cautions clinicians to differentiate normal grieving from a mental health diagnosis of major depressive or adjustment disorder, following clear criteria for these distinct disorders. The goal is to ensure that those who need intervention receive an accurate diagnosis.

With appropriate supports, patients should be allowed to experience grief as a normal process of life in their own unique and personal way. Nurses should also consider *Chronic sorrow*, the presence of enduring lifelong feelings of grief, as a potential nursing diagnosis (Alligood, 2018).

Nurses are expected to identify those at risk for complicated grief and differentiate between grief and depression (Canadian Hospice Palliative Care Association, 2009a), intervening in timely and appropriate ways, such as providing counselling and coordinating referrals.

Assessment may include validated screening inventories for depression and other specific grief measures such as the Brief Grief Questionnaire (Ito, Nakajima, Fujisawa, et al., 2012). Identification of risk factors that can complicate grieving is another place to begin the assessment and would include a number of factors, such as the following:
- Heavy emotional dependence on the deceased
- Unresolved conflicts between the bereaved person and the deceased

- Young age of the deceased (often the most profound loss) or of the bereaved person
- Lack of a surviving meaningful relationship or support system
- A history of losses
- A lack of sound coping skills
- A death that was associated with a cultural stigma (e.g., acquired immune deficiency syndrome [AIDS], suicide)
- A death that was unexpected or associated with violence (e.g., murder, suicide)
- A history of depression, drug or alcohol abuse, or other psychiatric illness

Prolonged depression is the most common response to unresolved grief, and assessment of mood should follow the practices described in Chapter 13. Disturbances in mood are associated with biological changes in the body during stress-related depressive illness. Some examples are electrolyte disturbance, nervous system alterations, and faulty regulation of the autonomic nervous system. Always assess the potential for suicide.

Table 31-1 identifies common grief experiences and describes the pathological intensification of these phenomena that indicates the need for psychotherapy.

Models for understanding grief are being clinically tested and refined so that health care systems can understand grieving, best use limited health care resources, and relieve suffering whenever possible.

Theories

The psychoanalytic model of grieving posits a distinct psychological process that involves disengaging strong emotional ties from a significant relationship and reinvesting those ties in a new and productive direction. This process requires engaging

TABLE 31-1	COMMON EXPERIENCES DURING GRIEF AND THEIR PATHOLOGICAL INTENSIFICATION	
PHENOMENON	**TYPICAL RESPONSE**	**PATHOLOGICAL INTENSIFICATION**
Dying	Emotional expression and immediate coping with the dying process	Avoidance; feeling of being overwhelmed, dazed, confused; self-punitive feelings; inappropriately hostile feelings
Death and outcry	Outcry of emotions with news of the death and turning to others for help or isolating self with self-soothing	Panic; dissociative reactions, reactive psychoses
Warding off (denial)	Avoidance of reminders and social withdrawal, focusing elsewhere, emotional numbing, not thinking of implications to self or of certain themes	Maladaptive avoidance of confronting the implications of death, drug or alcohol abuse, promiscuity, fugue states, phobic avoidance, feeling of being dead or unreal
Re-experience (intrusion)	Intrusive experiences, including recollections of negative experiences during relationship with the deceased, bad dreams, reduced concentration, compulsive re-enactments	Flooding with negative images and emotions; uncontrolled ideation, self-impairing compulsive re-enactments, night terrors, recurrent nightmares, distraught feelings resulting from the intrusion of anger, anxiety, despair, shame, or guilt; physiological exhaustion resulting from hyperarousal
Working through	Recollection of the deceased and a contemplation of self with reduced intrusiveness of memories and fantasies and with increased rational acceptance, reduced numbness and avoidance, more "dosing" of recollections, and a sense of working through it	Feeling of inability to integrate the death with a sense of self and continued life; persistent warding-off of themes that may manifest as anxious, depressed, enraged, shame-filled, or guilty moods and psychophysiological syndromes
Completion	Reduction in emotional swings and a sense of self-coherence and readiness for new relationships; ability to experience positive states of mind	Failure to complete mourning, which may be associated with inability to work or create or to feel emotion or positive states of mind

Source: Horowitz, M. J. (1990). A model of mourning: Change in schemas of self and others. *Journal of the American Psychoanalytic Association, 38*(2), 297–324. doi:10.1177/000306519003800202. Copyright © 1990 by SAGE. Reprinted by Permission of SAGE Publications.

in "grief work" that is thought to progress through predictable stages and phases. Since Kübler-Ross's groundbreaking work with the dying in the 1960s, her phases of denial, anger, bargaining, depression, and acceptance (Kübler-Ross, 1969) have been identified by many with the stages of grieving. Other models of grieving emphasize dual processes of coping with bereavement stressors, the potential for personal growth and coping skills, and adaptive tasks (Stroebe, Stroebe, Schut, et al., 2017).

The goals of mourning have evolved from "doing the grief work, getting over it, and moving on with life." Many now regard mourning as a complex, individual, culturally embedded process of accepting the death, confronting the painful experience of grief, constructing an identity and a life in a transformed environment, and finding an enduring relationship with the deceased, based not on physical presence but on accurate memory. Depending on many factors, this process can take many months

to a number of years. Our losses transform our lives, and we are never quite the same person again. Over time, people move from pain defining who they are, and constant preoccupation with their loss, to living with the residual pain and forever carrying the memory of the loved one.

Dual Process Model of Coping With Bereavement

Bereavement is an enormously challenging life stressor (Table 31-2). Healthy adaptation is crucial for long-term health and re-engagement in life. In a review of the dual process model (DPM), Stroebe and colleagues (2017) identify adaptive versus maladaptive coping activities using three central constructs: loss-oriented coping, restoration-oriented coping, and oscillation. The DPM attempts to address inadequacies in the "grief work" concept, such as a lack of specificity about grief stressors, cultural bias, the favouring of intuitive or female expressions of grief

TABLE 31-2 PHENOMENA EXPERIENCED DURING BEREAVEMENT	
SYMPTOMS	**EXAMPLES**
Sensations of Somatic Distress The bereaved person may experience tightness in the throat, shortness of breath, sighing, mental pain, or exhaustion; food may taste like sand; things may feel unreal. Pain or discomfort may be identical to the symptoms experienced by the dead person. Normally, symptoms are brief.	A woman whose husband died of a stroke complains of weakness and numbness on her left side.
Preoccupation With the Image of the Deceased The bereaved person brings up, thinks about, and talks about numerous memories of the deceased. The memories are positive. This process goes on with great sadness. The idealization of the deceased lets the bereaved person relive the gratifications associated with the deceased and helps resolve any guilt she or he feels concerning the deceased. The bereaved person may also take on many of the mannerisms of the deceased through identification—identification serves the purpose of holding on to the deceased. Preoccupation with the dead person can continue for many months before it lessens.	A man whose wife recently died states, "I just can't stop thinking about my wife. Everything I see reminds me of her. We picked up this seashell on our honeymoon. I remember every wonderful moment we had together. The pain is so great, but the memories just keep coming." His friends notice that when he talks, his hand gestures and expressions are like those of his recently deceased wife.
Guilt The bereaved person reproaches himself or herself for real or fancied acts of negligence or omissions in the relationship with the deceased.	"I should have made him go to the doctor sooner." "I should have paid more attention to her, been more thoughtful."
Anger The anger the bereaved person experiences may not be toward the object that gives rise to it. Often the anger is displaced onto the medical or nursing staff. Other times, it is directed toward the deceased. The anger is at its height during the first month but is often intermittent throughout the first year. The overflow of hostility disturbs the bereaved person, resulting in the feeling that he or she is "going insane."	"The doctor didn't operate in time. If he had, Mary would be alive today." "How could he leave me like this … how could he?"
Change in Behaviour: Depression, Disorganization, Restlessness The bereaved person may exhibit marked restlessness and an inability to organize his or her behaviour. A depressive mood during routine activities is common, decreasing as the year passes and the intensity of the grief declines. Absence of depression is more abnormal than its presence. Loneliness and aimlessness are most pronounced 6 to 9 months after the death.	Six months after her husband died, Mrs. Faye states, "I just can't seem to function. I have a hard time doing the simplest tasks. I can't be bothered with socializing. I feel so down … so, so empty."
Reorganization of Behaviour Directed Toward a New Object or Activity Gradually, the bereaved person renews his or her interest in people and activities. The grieving thus releases him or her from one interpersonal relationship, and new ones are free to take its place.	Twenty months after her husband's death, Mrs. Faye tells a friend, "I'll be away this weekend. I am going fishing with my brother and his friend. This is the first time I've felt like doing anything since Harry died."

over instrumental styles (Stroebe, Stroebe, Schut, et al., 2017), and the discounting of the value of denial and distraction in grieving.

Using the DPM as a guide, Stroebe and colleagues (2017) identified *loss-oriented stressors*, which include concentrating on the loss experience, feeling the pain of grief, remembering, and longing. *Restoration-oriented stressors* re-engage the mourner with the outer world, as in overcoming loneliness (seeking social support), mastering skills and roles once performed by the deceased person, finding a new identity, and facing many practical details of life. By identifying specific coping activities on both sides of the model, the nurse can strengthen a grieving person's skills and reinforce positive meanings.

Both orientations assert that denial, avoidance, and distraction from grief are beneficial, as long as they are not excessive. The process of alternating between the two spheres of coping results in the third construct called *oscillation*, wherein confronting and avoiding various stressors of bereavement are an indication of healthy adaptation. However, a prolonged moving back and forth between these poles can be seen as an indication of complicated grieving (Stroebe, Stroebe, Schut, et al., 2017).

Four Tasks of Mourning

Many theorists who have studied the grief process, including George Engel, Colin Parkes, Erich Lindemann, John Bowlby, and J. William Worden, have identified similar, commonly experienced psychological and behavioural phenomena, including the following:

- Shock and disbelief
- Sensation of somatic distress
- Preoccupation with the image of the deceased
- Guilt
- Anger
- Change in behaviour (e.g., depression, disorganization, restlessness)
- Reorganization of behaviour directed toward a new object or activity

Worden organizes aspects of mourning into four tasks: (1) accept the reality of the loss, (2) experience the pain of grief, (3) adjust to an environment without the loved one (externally, internally, and spiritually), and (4) relocate and memorialize the loved one. He emphasizes that every loss must be assessed according to mediating factors such as the nature of the person who died, the nature of the attachment, the circumstances of the death, personality factors, family history, social circumstances, and concurrent changes resulting from the death (Worden, 2009). His model can be readily understood by the mourner as empowering and hopeful and serves as a specific guide for the nurse providing counselling or therapy.

Helping People Cope With Loss

The majority of people who suffer bereavement are resilient and recover from the experience. However, Zisook and colleagues (2014) are concerned that the emphasis on understanding the consequences of bereavement and the protective qualities that help people cope with loss has shifted focus from early interventions for those at risk for mental health problems or complicated grief. Many risk factors for mental health problems associated with grief cannot be changed (e.g., gender, unexpected death) or might be difficult to change (e.g., a negative change in finances), but it is important to identify those risk factors that can be changed with appropriate interventions. Some people who are grieving are resilient, and limited counselling support, focusing on grief education, normalizing of experiences, and skilled supportive presence, seems to be helpful for them (Sandler, Tein, Cham, et al., 2016; Zisook, Iglewicz, Avanzino, et al., 2014). A deeper understanding of the grief process can provide reassurance for those grieving (Baier & Buechsel, 2012). Social support is also instrumental in natural helping through the grief process (Hoy, 2016). Other helpful interventions include writing letters (both to and from the deceased), performing simple rituals and ceremonies, "dosing" times of grieving throughout the day or week, working on projects to memorialize the deceased (e.g., planting a tree, creating a website), walking and time in nature, and planning ahead for holidays and anniversary dates. Table 31-3 provides guidelines for helping people to grieve, and the Guidelines for Communication box offers advice for communicating with a person suffering a profound loss.

Box 31-4 offers guidelines that can help people and their families to cope with bereavement.

📖 GUIDELINES FOR COMMUNICATION WITH A BEREAVED PERSON

Situation	Sample Response
When you sense an overwhelming sorrow	"This must hurt terribly."
When you hear anger in the bereaved person's voice	"I hear anger in your voice. Most people go through periods of anger when their loved one dies. Are you feeling angry now?"
If you discern guilt	"Are you feeling guilty? This is a common reaction many people have. What are some of your thoughts about this?"
If you sense a fear of the future	"It must be scary to go through this."
When the bereaved person seems confused	"This can be a bewildering time."
In almost any painful situation	"This must be very difficult for you."

Source: GOOD INTENTIONS by Duke Robinson. Copyright © 1996 by Reverand Andrew (Duke) Robinson. By permission of Grand Central Publishing. All rights reserved.

CURRENT TOPICS AND FUTURE DIRECTIONS

Medically Assisted Death Legislation

The Supreme Court of Canada has decriminalized medically assisted death, and existing international legislation suggests that psychiatrists will be asked to play a role in this practice. The new law (also discussed in Chapter 22) provides the framework, but how this legislation will be fully implemented remains to be seen. The role of psychiatric mental health professionals will continue to evolve in key related areas of capacity assessment, the perception of suicide, and the assessment of suffering. These are challenges described by Duffy (2015) as opportunities for

TABLE 31-3	GUIDELINES FOR HELPING PEOPLE IN ACUTE GRIEF
INTERVENTION	**RATIONALE**
Give your full presence: Use appropriate eye contact, attentive listening, and appropriate touch.	Talking is one of the most important ways of dealing with acute grief. Listening patiently helps the bereaved person express all feelings, even ones he or she feels are "negative."
	Appropriate eye contact helps to convey that you are there and are sharing the person's sadness.
	Suitable human touch can express warmth and nurture healing. Inappropriate touch can leave a person confused and uncomfortable.
Be patient with the bereaved person in times of silence. Do not fill silence with empty chatter.	Sharing painful feelings during periods of silence is healing and conveys your concern.
Know about and share with the bereaved person information about the phenomena that occur during the normal mourning process because they may concern some people (e.g., intense anger at the deceased, guilt, symptoms the deceased had before death, unbidden floods of memories). Give the bereaved person support during the occurrence of these phenomena and a written handout to refer to.	Although the knowledge will not eliminate the emotions, it can greatly relieve a person who is thinking that there is something wrong with having these feelings.
Encourage the support of family and friends. If no supports are available, refer the person to a community bereavement group. (Bereavement groups are helpful even when a person has many friends or much family support.)	Friends can help with routine matters—for example: • Bringing food into the house • Making phone calls • Driving to the funeral home • Taking care of the bereaved person's children or other family members
Offer spiritual support and referrals when needed. When intense emotions are in evidence, show understanding and support (see Guidelines for Communication box).	Dealing with an illness or catastrophic loss can cause the most profound spiritual anguish. Empathic words that reflect acceptance of a bereaved individual's feelings are healing.

the development of new skills in EOL care. Certainly, future case studies and other research will lead to new guidelines in capacity assessment and suicide and suffering assessment, as well as to new areas of therapy and intervention in the field of death and dying.

Palliative Care for Patients With Dementia

The incidence of Alzheimer's disease and related dementias in Canada continues to grow at a staggering rate (Alzheimer Society, 2017), a trend that is expected to continue. It is difficult to determine survival or time until death, often leaving those with dementia to die without appropriate palliative care services or, as some researchers suggest, to receive aggressive interventions to the detriment of their quality of life (Ryan, Ingleton, Gardiner, et al., 2009). As with other chronic illnesses, HPC should be considered at the time of a dementia diagnosis and assessed regularly for changes in status. Enhanced educational opportunities for nurses and other caregivers about the unique elements of palliative dementia care are essential to promote increased comfort and enhanced quality of life for this population. The Registered Nurses' Association of Ontario (2016) best practice guideline for older adults with dementia, although not specifically from an HPC perspective, can help guide nursing practice.

People with advanced dementia experience significant impairments in insight, language, and judgement, limiting their ability to communicate unmet needs and desires. Difficult behaviours such as irritability or refusal to cooperate with care are often a form of communication, indicating discomfort in body, mind, or spirit. Caregivers who use an anticipatory approach to care can frequently prevent or reduce behaviours that result

when a person with dementia is unable to communicate important unmet needs. Caregivers must remember to focus on the person, rather than the disease, and recognize the numerous opportunities that arise with every interaction to affirm the meaning of the individual's life, uphold dignity, and provide pleasurable sensory and spiritual experiences. The goal is to create meaningful connections for these patients. One effective method for customizing care that honours the unique preferences and lifelong interests of the patient is to use some form of life story or About Me form (Dougherty, Gallagher, Cabral, et al., 2007). This abbreviated biography guides and informs care to enhance the patient's enjoyment of life's simple pleasures. Dignity therapy is another approach suited to older adults and to adults with dementia at end of life (Goddard, Speck, Martin, et al., 2013).

Best practice recommendations for palliative care in dementia are to ensure that people with advanced dementia are included in the provision of palliative care; they remain in familiar surroundings whenever possible; restraint-free policy and staff education programs are developed; and quality of EOL experiences for those with dementia and their families are evaluated (Joanna Briggs Institute, 2011). More specifically, it is also important to address health care decisions for those with advanced dementia, such as resuscitation, hospitalizations, antibiotics, and nutrition and hydration. Health care providers should (1) identify the patient's goals for care and consider educating the family to minimize aggressive medical interventions, (2) eliminate medications that may detract from safety or quality of life, and (3) proactively manage issues such as pain and depression. Families and friends spend a significant amount of time, finances, and emotions caring for a loved one with dementia. It is important

BOX 31-4 GUIDELINES FOR DEALING WITH BEREAVEMENT

Global effect of loss. The death of someone close can be life-changing, affecting all areas of your life. It can feel as though your world has shattered. Grieving is a journey between how things were and how they will be. It is your personal journey.

Grief as a natural process. The grief you feel is because of living, loving, and having a connection with your loved one. Grief is a normal response to loss. Understanding how you respond can help.

Individual differences in grieving styles. How you grieve is a reflection of your personality, past losses, and the relationship you had with the person who died. Each person grieves in his or her own way and on his or her own timetable. Some people openly express their emotions, whereas others control their thoughts and emotions. Neither is right or wrong; each can be effective.

Children and grief. Children look to the adults in their lives to learn how to grieve. They are sensitive to the moods and behaviour of adults and will not talk about their thoughts and feelings unless the adults do. Children are frightened by what they do not know or understand. Simple information about death and grief is most helpful.

Social connections and support. You want and need support from others now more than ever. Some people may not be able to provide the understanding and caring you expect from them because of their own experience with grief or for other reasons. Because all of the relationships in your life will be altered in some way, it is normal to look at, change, or sometimes even end certain relationships. You may find the company of other bereaved people particularly comforting.

Experiences you might have in grief. You may feel very different from your usual self as your emotions, mind, and reactions seem unreliable. You may feel intense pain and emotions not felt before. You are not going crazy; these feelings are natural. Symptoms and emotions like fatigue, forgetfulness, and irritability are common.

Fluctuations in the grief process. As you journey through grief, your feelings and responses will vary at different times. There will be ups and downs; there may be good days and bad days. Understand and value the good days as a rest in your journey.

Self-care and what helps. There are things you can do to help yourself. Information about grief can help you understand. Be gentle, patient, and forgiving with yourself. Do what you can to keep some normal routine for health and social contact. Support may come from different sources (e.g., family, friends, bereavement groups, chat rooms). If you are concerned about yourself and your grief, seek professional help.

Time for grief. Despite what you may hear about "getting over it" or "the first year," there are no timelines for grief; it takes as long as it takes. Often the journey is longer than you or others expected, and you may feel pressured to "move on." This loss will continue to be part of your life, and you will always have times when you think about, miss, and grieve for your loved one.

Grief as a spiritual journey of healing. Your life has changed, putting you on a different path. Nothing will ever be the same, yet you must somehow go on and find meaning in your changed life. As the journey continues, you may experience healing and personal growth as a result of the suffering you have endured and the lessons you have learned about what you truly value.

Source: Adapted from Victoria Hospice Bereavement Services. (2011). *Ten things to know about grief.* Retrieved from http://www.victoriahospice.org/sites/default/files/imce/VicHospTenThings.pdf.

to recognize and support the role of family caregivers as they navigate the day-to-day challenges and cope with many losses.

Areas for Future Discovery

We are emerging from a time when many people who are grieving have been pathologized and treated with psychotropic drugs for depression, anxiety, and sleep disorders. A study found that compassionate primary caregivers, seeing symptoms of acute grief such as crying and sleep disturbances in their older adult patients, spontaneously prescribed benzodiazepines, contrary to all major guidelines on the subject (Cook, Marshall, Masci, et al., 2007). On the other end of the spectrum, grief has been overlooked by many health care providers as a possible underlying contributor to their patients' presenting problems (Stroebe, Stroebe, Schut, et al., 2017). Current diagnostic categories intend to address the issues of overdiagnosis and underdiagnosis; however, the classification system can never stand in for compassion and genuinely meeting patients and families with a shared humanity (Bandini, 2015; Fox & Jones, 2013). Internationally, grief recovery models are being adapted to diverse cultures to assist traumatized people, especially children and youth, to begin to heal and re-engage with life, hope, and the future. There is a growing urgency for practitioners to become knowledgeable about and skilled at supporting human mourning in all health care settings. The realization of full human health and happiness may depend on it.

KEY POINTS TO REMEMBER

- The HPC movement offers compassionate care for those who are dying. HPC focuses on patients' physical and emotional comfort and offers holistic support for people who are dying and their families.
- More hospitals are offering palliative expertise for EOL care, but in many hospitals conflict continues to exist between the wishes of people who are dying and their families and the medical model of treatment that focuses on the prolongation of life.
- In work with HPC patients, nursing goals include providing physical, emotional, cultural, and spiritual support and helping with adjustments in lifestyle and relationships. Nurses need to understand the value of providing a caring human presence even in the face of helplessness.

- People with dementia may exhibit challenging behaviours during EOL care that may communicate discomfort in mind, body, or spirit. Care should focus on providing meaningful connections with patients and between family members and patients.
- Those who work with people who are dying need to maintain their own emotional health. EOL care is usually delivered by multidisciplinary teams so that no one discipline bears too much responsibility. Nurses need to learn to draw on team support, protect their private lives by setting clear personal boundaries, and recognize their human and professional limitations.
- Providing timely and ongoing information about the disease and its effects and about physical and psychological signs of death can help the family deal with anticipatory mourning.
- Health care workers involved in care of the dying can teach families communication skills, such as the Four Gifts of Resolving Relationships, that will help them to express love, share memories, say goodbye, and provide a sense of peace.

- Family members may experience anticipatory grief, and it is helpful for them to understand that this grief is normal, although difficult.
- Common phenomena are evident during the experience of grief, and mourning is greatly influenced by cultural norms. However, everyone's experience of grieving is shaped by many mediating factors, such as the relationship to the person who died and the capacities of the mourner.
- Indicators of the potential for complicated grief include social isolation, extensive dependency on the deceased person, unresolved interpersonal conflicts, loss of a child, violent and senseless death, and catastrophic loss.
- Grief work is successful when the relationship to the deceased person has been restructured, energy is available for new relationships and life pursuits, and the mourner can remember realistically both the pleasures and the disappointments of the lost relationship. Outcomes for successful grief work have been identified.

CRITICAL THINKING

1. George is dying of pancreatic cancer. His wife and adult children are asking about using HPC services. Help George's family to make an informed decision by comparing and contrasting the HPC model of care with the medical model of care for someone who is dying.
2. How can you use the Four Gifts of Resolving Relationships in working with the families of dying people in your practice of nursing? Do you think you would find this tool useful for a personal family member in the future?
3. What are some concrete ways in which you can help another person to cope with a loss? Identify specific components in the following areas:

a. How can you let the person tell his or her story, and what is the potential therapeutic value of doing so?
b. Avoiding banal (overused or trite) advice, what are some things you might say that could offer comfort? Use the guidelines in Table 31-3 and the Guidelines for Communication box to describe how you would help a person who is suffering a profound loss.
4. What practices would demonstrate a culturally safe and sensitive approach for Indigenous people in Canada seeking palliative care?

CHAPTER REVIEW

1. The nurse is caring for a patient who is grieving. The patient has stated that she is angry that she has been diagnosed with terminal cancer. Which behaviour should the nurse anticipate next as the patient reconciles her anger?
a. Denial that she has cancer
b. Depression over the diagnosis of cancer
c. Acceptance that her cancer is a reality
d. Begging God to remove the cancer from her body
2. The nurse is planning hospice palliative care for a dying patient. Which outcome is most appropriate?
a. Patient will regain health
b. Patient will remain pain-free
c. Patient will not fear death
d. Patient will decline all medications
3. Which patient statement regarding spirituality would require further nursing teaching?
a. "I am not religious, so therefore I am not spiritual."
b. "Death scares me."
c. "My family is what gives my life meaning."
d. "I believe in a higher power."

4. The nurse identifies that a patient is experiencing complicated grief related to the loss of her spouse. Which evaluation finding would indicate that a treatment plan is appropriate? The patient:
a. No longer thinks of her spouse
b. Copes without the need for a support system
c. States that she should have taken her spouse to the doctor more often
d. Laughs occasionally with her grandchildren
5. The nurse is caring for a patient whose partner—with whom she was having an affair—died suddenly after a myocardial infarction. The patient had told no one about the affair, so no friends or family are aware that she experienced a loss. How should the nurse document the patient's grieving?
a. Disenfranchised grief
b. Dysfunctional grief
c. Maladaptive grief
d. Normal bereavement

℮volve WEBSITE

Post-Test   interactive review

Visit the Evolve website for Chapter Review Answers and Rationales, Critical Thinking Answer Guidelines, and additional resources related to the content in this chapter: http://evolve.elsevier.com/Canada/Varcarolis/psychiatric/

REFERENCES

Alligood, M. R. (2018). *Nursing theorists and their work* (9th ed.). Philadelphia: Elsevier.

Alzheimer Society. (2017). *About dementia.* Retrieved from http://www.alzheimer.ca/en/About-dementia.

Anandarajah, G., & Hight, E. (2001). Spirituality and medical practice: Using the HOPE questions as a practical tool for spiritual assessment. *American Family Physician, 63*(1), 81–88. Retrieved from http://www.aafp.org/afp/2001/0101/p81.pdf.

Baier, M., & Buechsel, R. (2012). A model to help bereaved individuals understand the grief process. *Mental Health Practice, 16*(1), 28–32.

Bandini, J. (2015). The medicalization of bereavement: (Ab)normal grief in the DSM-5. *Death Studies, 39*(6), 347–352. doi:10.1080/07481187.2014.951498.

Bourassa, C., Hampton, M., Baydala, A., et al. (2010). *Completing the circle: End of life care with Aboriginal families. Canadian Virtual Hospice.* Retrieved from http://www.virtualhospice.ca/en_US/Main+Site+Navigation/Home/For+Professionals/For+Professionals/The+Exchange/Current/Completing+the+Circle_++End+of+Life+Care+with+Aboriginal+Families.aspx.

Brennan, F., Gwyther, L., Lohman, D., et al. (2015). Palliative care as a human right. In B. R. Ferrell, N. Coyle, & J. A. Paice (Eds.), *Oxford textbook of palliative nursing* (4th ed., pp. 1174–1178). New York: Oxford University Press.

Cahill, G. (2010). *Whole person care: The legacy of Balfour Mount. Social Innovation Generation.* Retrieved from http://sigeneration.ca/blog/?p=52.

Canadian Association of Schools of Nursing. (2011). *Palliative and end-of-life care: Entry-to-practice competencies and indicators for registered nurses.* Retrieved from http://casn.ca/wp-content/uploads/2014/12/PEOLCCompetenciesandIndicatorsEn1.pdf.

Canadian Hospice Palliative Care Association (2006). *The Pan-Canadian Gold Standard for Palliative Home Care.* Ottawa: Author. Retrieved from http://www.chpca.net/media/7652/Gold_Standards_Palliative_Home_Care.pdf.

Canadian Hospice Palliative Care Association (2008). *Certification Examination: List of Assumptions and Competencies.* Ottawa: Author. Retrieved from http://www.chpca.net/media/7511/Canadian_HPC_Nursing_Assumptions_and_Competencies.pdf.

Canadian Hospice Palliative Care Association (2009a). *Canadian Hospice Palliative Care Nursing Standards of Practice.* Ottawa: Author. Retrieved from http://www.chpca.net/media/7505/Canadian_Hospice_Palliative_Care_Nursing_Standards_2009.pdf.

Canadian Hospice Palliative Care Association (2009b). *Nursing Competencies Case Examples.* Ottawa: Author. Retrieved from http://www.chpca.net/media/7502/Canadian_Hospice_Palliative_Care_Nursing_Competencies_Case_Examples_Revised_Feb_2010.pdf.

Canadian Hospice Palliative Care Association (2010a). *Advance Care Planning in Canada: A National Framework.* Ottawa: Author. Retrieved from http://www.chpca.net/media/7449/acp_synopsis_of_the_framework_sept_16_10.pdf.

Canadian Hospice Palliative Care Association (2010b). *Policy Brief on Hospice Palliative Care: Quality End-Of-Life Care? It Depends on Where You Live and Where You Die.* Ottawa: Author. Retrieved from http://www.chpca.net/media/7682/HPC_Policy_Brief_-_Systems_Approach_-_June_2010.pdf.

Canadian Hospice Palliative Care Association. (2013). *A Model to Guide Hospice Palliative Care.* Retrieved from http://www.chpca.net/media/319547/norms-of-practice-eng-web.pdf.

Canadian Hospice Palliative Care Association (2016). *Fact Sheet: Hospice Palliative Care in Canada.* Ottawa: Author. Retrieved from http://www.chpca.net/media/481407/Fact_Sheet_HPC_in_Canada%20Fall%202016%20-%20EN.pdf.

Canadian Hospice Palliative Care Association (2017). *About the Canadian Hospice Palliative Care Association.* Ottawa: Author. Retrieved from http://www.chpca.net/Home.

Canadian Nurses Association (2008). *Code of Ethics for Registered Nurses.* Ottawa: Author.

Canadian Virtual Hospice. (2016). *Living my culture.* Retrieved from http://livingmyculture.ca/culture/.

Charbonneau, C., & Bélanger, B. (2013). Identification of spiritual and religious needs of terminally ill patients receiving palliative home-care. *Journal for the Study of Spirituality, 3*(1), 33–45. doi:10.1179/2044024313Z.0000000003.

Chochinov, H. M. (2007). Dignity and the essence of medicine: The A, B, C and D of dignity conserving care. *British Medical Journal, 335,* 184–187.

Chochinov, H. M. (2016). Health-care provider as witness. *Lancet, 388*(10051), 1272–1273. doi:10.1016/S0140-6736(16)31668-3.

Chochinov, H. M., McClement, S. E., Hack, T. F., et al. (2013). Health care provider communication: An empirical model of therapeutic effectiveness. *Cancer, 119*(9), 1706–1713. doi:10.1002/cncr.27949.

Clarke, D. (2010). *Dame Cicely biography. Cicely Saunders International.* Retrieved from http://www.cicelysaundersfoundation.org/about-us/dame-cicely-biography.

Colgan, S., Edwards, R., & Jakubec, S. L. (2017). *Death and dignity have no address: Calgary's Allied Mobile Palliative Program. Calgary Homeless Foundation Research Symposium 2017.* Retrieved from http://calgaryhomeless.com/content/uploads/11-CAMPP-talk.pdf.

Cook, J. M., Marshall, R., Masci, D., et al. (2007). Physicians' perspectives on prescribing benzodiazepines for older adults: A qualitative study. *Journal of General Internal Medicine, 22*(3), 303–307.

Dougherty, J., Gallagher, M., Cabral, D., et al. (2007). About me: Knowing the person with advanced dementia. *Alzheimer's Care Quarterly, 8*(1), 12–16.

Duffy, O. A. (2015). The Supreme Court of Canada ruling on physician-assisted death: Implications for psychiatry in Canada. *The Canadian Journal of Psychiatry, 60*(12), 591–596. doi:10.1177/070674371506001211.

Duggleby, W., Kuchera, S., MacLeod, R., et al. (2015). Indigenous people's experiences at the end of life. *Palliative & Supportive Care, 13*(6), 1721–1733. doi:10.1017/S147895151500070X.

Finfgeld-Connett, D. (2006). Meta-synthesis of presence in nursing. *Journal of Advanced Nursing, 55,* 708–714. doi:10.1111/j.1365-2648.2006.03961.x.

Finfgeld-Connett, D. (2008a). Meta-synthesis of caring in nursing. *Journal of Clinical Nursing, 17,* 196–204. doi:10.1111/j.1365-2702.2006.01824.x.

Finfgeld-Connett, D. (2008b). Qualitative comparison and synthesis of nursing presence and caring. *International Journal of Nursing Terminologies and Classifications, 19,* 111–119. doi:10.1111/j.1744-618X.2008.00090.x.

Finfgeld-Connett, D. (2008c). Qualitative convergence of three nursing concepts: Art of nursing, presence and caring. *Journal of Advanced Nursing, 63,* 527–534. doi:10.1111/j.1365-2648.2008.046?.x.

Fox, J., & Jones, K. D. (2013). DSM-5 and bereavement: The loss of normal grief? *Journal of Counseling and Development, 91*(1), 113. doi:10.1002/j.1556-6676.2013.00079.x.

Fruch, V., Monture, L., Prince, H., et al. (2016). Coming home to die: Six nations of the grand river territory develops community-based palliative care. *International Journal of Indigenous Health, 11*(1), 50. doi:10.18357/ijih111201615303.

Goddard, C., Speck, P., Martin, P., et al. (2013). Dignity therapy for older people in care homes: A qualitative study of the views of residents and recipients of "generativity" documents. *Journal of Advanced Nursing, 69*(1), 122–132. doi:10.1111/j.1365-2648.2012.05999.x.

Gray, B. (2014). The use of rituals, primarily related to grief, in a hospital setting: How are they helpful and how can they be most effective? *Critical Horizons, 2*(2), 165–177. doi:10.1558/hscc.v2i2.23838.

Hoy, W. G. (2016). *Bereavement groups and the role of social support: Integrating theory, research, and practice.* New York: Routledge/Taylor & Francis Group.

Huynh, L., Henry, B., & Dosani, N. (2015). Minding the gap: Access to palliative care and the homeless. *BMC Palliative Care, 14*(1), 62. doi:10.1186/s12904-015-0059-2.

Ito, M., Nakajima, S., Fujisawa, D., et al. (2012). Brief measure for screening complicated grief: Reliability and discriminant validity. *PLoS ONE, 7*(2), e31209. doi:10.1371/journal.pone.0031209.

Joanna Briggs Institute. (2011). Palliative approach to care for people with advanced dementia. Best Practice: Evidence-based information sheets for health professionals. *Best Practice, 15*(5), 1–4. Retrieved from http://connect.jbiconnectplus.org/ViewSourceFile.aspx?0=7116.

Kramer-Howe, K., & Huls, P. T. (2004). *A spiritual assessment tool.* Phoenix: Hospice of the Valley.

Kreher, M. (2016). Symptom control at the end of life. *The Medical Clinics of North America, 100*(5), 1111.

Kübler-Ross, E. (1969). *On death and dying.* New York: Macmillan.

Matzo, M., & Sherman, D. W. (2014). *Palliative care nursing: Quality care to the end of life* (4th ed.). New York: Springer.

McNutt, B., & Yakushko, O. (2013). Disenfranchised grief among lesbian and gay bereaved individuals. *Journal of LGBT Issues in Counseling, 7*(1), 87–116. doi:10.1080/15538605.2013.758345.

Mortell, S. (2015). Assisting clients with disenfranchised grief: The role of a mental health nurse. *Journal of Psychosocial Nursing and Mental Health Services, 53*(4), 52–57. doi:10.3928/02793695-20150319-05.

Nicol, J., & Nyatanga, B. (2014). *Palliative and end of life care in nursing.* London, UK: Learning Matters.

Overton, B. L., & Cottone, R. R. (2016). Anticipatory grief: A family systems approach. *The Family Journal, 24*(4), 430–432. doi:10.1177/1066480716663490.

Pesut, B., McLeod, B., Hole, R., et al. (2012). Rural nursing and quality end-of-life care: Palliative care, palliative approach, or somewhere in-between? *ANS. Advances in Nursing Science, 35*(4), 288.

Puchalski, C. M. (2007). Spirituality and the care of patients at the end-of-life: An essential component of care. *OMEGA: Journal of Death and Dying, 56*(1), 33–46.

Registered Nurses' Association of Ontario (RNAO). (2016). *Delirium, dementia and depression in older adults: Assessment and care* (2nd ed.). Retrieved from http://rnao.ca/bpg/guidelines/assessment-and-care-older-adults-delirium-dementia-and-depression.

Rosa, W. (2017). The economics of palliative care as a human right: A global action item. *Nursing Economics, 35*(1), 5.

Ryan, T., Ingleton, C., Gardiner, C., et al. (2009). Supporting people who have dementia to die with dignity. *Nursing Older People, 21*(5), 18–23.

Sandler, I., Tein, J., Cham, H., et al. (2016). Long-term effects of the family bereavement program on spousally bereaved parents: Grief, mental health problems, alcohol problems, and coping efficacy. *Development and Psychopathology, 28*(3), 801–818. doi:10.1017/S0954579416000328.

Sansó, N., Galiana, L., Oliver, A., et al. (2015). Palliative care professionals' inner life: Exploring the relationships among awareness, self-care, and compassion satisfaction and fatigue, burnout, and coping with death. *Journal of Pain and Symptom Management, 50*(2), 200–207. doi:10.1016/j.jpainsymman.2015.02.013.

Shear, M. K., Ghesquiere, A., & Glickman, K. (2013). Bereavement and complicated grief. *Current Psychiatry Reports, 15*(11), 1–7. doi:10.1007/s11920-013-0406-z.

Shore, J. C., Gelber, M. W., Koch, L. M., et al. (2016). Anticipatory grief: An evidence-based approach. *Journal of Hospice & Palliative Nursing, 18*(1), 15–19. doi:10.1097/NJH.0000000000000208.

Sinclair, S., Norris, J. M., McConnell, S. J., et al. (2016). Compassion: A scoping review of the healthcare literature. *BMC Palliative Care, 15*(1), 6. doi:10.1186/s12904-016-0080-0.

Stajduhar, K. I. (2013). Burdens of family caregiving at the end of life. *Clinical and Investigative Medicine/Médecine clinique et experimentale, 36*(3), E121.

Stroebe, M., Stroebe, W., Schut, H., et al. (2017). Grief is not a disease but bereavement merits medical awareness. *The Lancet, 389*(10067), 347–349. doi:10.1016/S0140-6736(17)30189-7.

Worden, J. W. (2009). *Grief counseling and grief therapy* (4th ed.). New York: Springer.

Zisook, S., Iglewicz, A., Avanzino, J., et al. (2014). Bereavement: Course, consequences, and care. *Current Psychiatry Reports, 16*(10), 1–10. doi:10.1007/s11920-014-0482-8.

Forensic Psychiatric Nursing

Sonya L. Jakubec

⊝volve WEBSITE

Several high-profile incidents involving people with mental illness and criminal activity, police shootings, and suicides in prison have brought attention to the relationship of the mental health and criminal justice systems in Canada and elsewhere. Individuals living with mental health challenges are over-represented in the Canadian criminal justice system as both victims and offenders (Mental Health Commission of Canada, 2012). Societal factors such as access to treatment, substance use, poverty, inadequate housing, and trauma all increase risk. There are also instances when mental illnesses actually cause people to behave in ways that lead to a criminal justice response. Whatever the reason, the over-representation of people with mental illness in the criminal justice system is often referred to as the "criminalization" of mental illness. This criminalization of people with mental illness can be viewed through a social justice lens for clinical practice, so that individuals receive the support, care, and treatment they need and to which they are entitled (Centre for Addiction and Mental Health, 2013).

In many respects, it is not surprising that there is such a high incidence of antisocial personality disorder in corrections populations, both in institutions and in the community. Clinically, the disorder is characterized by behaviours that involve failure to conform to social norms that constitute grounds for arrest, such as rule breaking, deceitfulness, impulsivity or failure to plan ahead, irritability and aggressiveness, and disregard for the safety of self or others (refer to Chapter 19 for more on personality disorders). By definition, the majority of people in the criminal justice system meet many of these criteria. However much of the concern about over-representation relates to those with a serious mental disorder, primarily schizophrenia or other psychosis, for whom social-ecological issues, rather than specific pathology, are key contributing factors in their criminal involvement (MacPhail & Verdun-Jones, 2013).

Another population of concern is Indigenous peoples, who are significantly over-represented in the Canadian criminal justice system as both victims and offenders. The rate of violent victimization among Indigenous people was more than double that among non-Indigenous people (163 incidents per 1 000 people versus 74 per 1 000). In particular, in 2014 Indigenous females had an overall rate of violent victimization that was double that of Indigenous males and close to triple that of non-Indigenous females. When controlling for various risk factors, Indigenous males were no more at risk for violent victimization than their non-Indigenous counterparts (Department of Justice Canada, 2017).

The over-representation of Indigenous peoples is also observed within the custody of Canadian correctional services. In 2015 the proportion of Indigenous adults in custody relative to their proportion in the population was 8 times higher for Indigenous men, 12 times higher for Indigenous women, 5 times higher for Indigenous male youth, and 7 times higher for Indigenous female youth. Indigenous people accounted for 33% of people accused of homicide, at a rate 10 times that of non-Indigenous people. The greatest proportion of these homicide offenders were Indigenous females (Department of Justice Canada, 2017). Gutierrez and colleagues (2013) note that Indigenous offenders are more likely than non-Indigenous offenders to have experienced historical and intergenerational trauma, poverty, family violence, and substance abuse in their home environment, and as children, they were more likely to have been involved with child welfare services. Refer to Chapter 8 for more on the impact of culture on mental health and trauma-informed practice.

A number of other factors have contributed to the over-representation of all people with mental health problems in the criminal justice system, including the deinstitutionalization of people challenged by mental illness without adequate community mental health services, a lack of affordable housing, and inadequate income-support programs. These factors increase the vulnerability of individuals with mental illnesses, leading to greater victimization of this population. The media often portray individuals living with mental illness as violent and unpredictable; however, the reality is that people who have a mental illness are much more likely to be the victims of violence than are people in the general population. In fact, 1 in 4 individuals with a mental illness is likely to be a victim of violence in a given year. Experiencing victimization intensifies feelings of anxiety and vulnerability and can lead to an exacerbation of one's illness and a lower quality of life (Canadian Mental Health Association, 2013).

At times, people experiencing mental illness, crisis, or the effects of substance use have interactions that result in police violence. Improving police interactions with people with mental illness requires adhering to best practices in this area, such as specialized training for police officers and employing the least restrictive and forceful measures. In addition, mobile crisis teams and accessible community-based mental health and social services are also needed (Kara, 2014). Collaborative intersectoral collaboration among criminal justice and mental health systems is necessary. No one sector can be solely responsible for dealing with the response.

Demonstration of procedural systems in police interactions with persons experiencing mental health crises (and other marginalized groups) has the potential to profoundly change the nature of these police encounters. If people with mental illness and others perceive that they are treated fairly by police and in a procedural manner with decency and respect, they are more likely to acknowledge the legitimacy of police authority and cooperate with investigations or arrests if necessary. If, however, persons with mental illness experience a police interaction in which they believe they are not treated according to procedures, they are more likely to resist authority (Kara, 2014).

This increased risk for victimization continues during incarceration. Both male and female inmates with a mental illness are more likely than other inmates to have been physically assaulted by their peers or correctional staff. In addition, individuals with a mental illness may be more likely to engage in acts of self-harm while incarcerated. Self-harm behaviour among federal inmates is increasing, as individuals struggle with a stressful and often dehumanizing environment and limited assistive services. Among those incarcerated in Canada, death by suicide is reported to be seven times greater than the national average (Centre for Addiction and Mental Health, 2013).

Mental health support must not end when a person is released from incarceration, however. The transition back into society is difficult for many individuals, who often receive little to no support in obtaining housing, employment, and other services upon their release. Transition and reintegration programs are, as yet, not well evaluated, and few best practices are identified (Centre for Addiction and Mental Health, 2013). Individuals with a mental illness who have been involved in the criminal justice system tend to have higher rates of homelessness, difficulty adhering to treatment, lower rates of social support, and greater incidence of substance abuse in comparison to other adults with a mental illness (Simpson, McMaster, & Cohen, 2013). Without adequate services and a treatment plan in place, the likelihood of further victimization and recidivism among this population is high. Mental health care in the criminal justice system serves, in this way, as a crime prevention strategy.

Canada's National Crime Prevention Strategy (NCPS) is based on the premise that well-designed interventions can have a positive influence on behaviours: by addressing risk factors associated with offending, crimes can be reduced or prevented. Successful interventions have been shown to reduce not only victimization but also the social and economic costs that result from criminal activities and the costs related to processing cases in the criminal justice system. The Government of Canada has focused on key project areas in the crime prevention strategy, with evidence-informed interventions and evaluations currently being expanded across the country (Public Safety Canada, 2015). Box 32-1 outlines the key elements of the NCPS.

Forensics (an abbreviation derived from *forensic science*) is an umbrella term that refers to legal issues or working with the courts. In recent years, nurses formalized a broad category called *forensic nursing*, which brings together components of traditional nursing care and legal issues to serve victims of violence and individuals who have committed acts that have brought them into contact with the criminal justice system. In this chapter, we explore a variety of roles that registered nurses assume within the legal system, identify competencies and challenges associated with the forensic nursing role, and profile the priority health care needs of patients who have committed an offence.

FORENSIC NURSING

Forensic nursing is the application of nursing science to public or legal proceedings and the combination of the forensic and biopsychosocial aspects of health care in the scientific investigation of trauma or death of victims and perpetrators of abuse, violence, criminal activity, and traumatic accidents (International Association of Forensic Nurses, 2016). Unlike most nursing specialties, forensic nursing includes several different areas of nursing practice: *forensic nurse examiners* work with sexual assault survivors; *forensic nurse death investigators* work with the deceased; *forensic psychiatric mental health nurses* work with mentally ill offenders; *clinical forensic nurses* work with victims of interpersonal violence; *forensic correctional nurses* work with offenders; and *forensic geriatric* or *pediatric nurses* work with victims of abuse and neglect (Kent-Wilkinson, 2009, 2010). Forensic nurses provide direct services to victims of crime and individuals who have committed crimes; consultation services to colleagues in nursing-, medical-, and law-related agencies; and expert court testimony in cases of trauma or questioned death, adequacy of service delivery, and specialized diagnoses of specific conditions related to nursing. Forensic nurses also work with families or significant others and the community (International Association of Forensic Nurses, 2016), for instance, in the death investigation and care of survivors of a workplace fatality (Harris, 2017).

The International Association of Forensic Nurses (IAFN), formed in 1992 by 74 nurses, most of whom were sexual assault nurse examiners (SANEs), represents nurses whose practice overlaps with key areas of forensic science and law. The group currently represents nurses who are forensic nurse generalists, SANEs, forensic psychiatric nurses, death investigators, coroners, correctional nurse specialists, and those in other forensic nursing specialties that continue to evolve (International Association of Forensic Nurses, 2016). The American Nurses Association (ANA)

officially recognized forensic nursing as a specialty practice area in 1995 and combined efforts with the IAFN to develop the *Scope and Standards of Forensic Nursing* in 1997 and update it in 2015 (American Nurses Association & International Association of Forensic Nurses, 2015). While these standards may be useful guidelines for forensic nursing practice, they may not be directly applicable in Canada. Each provincial or territorial practice site and the federal Correctional Service of Canada (CSC) has unique guidelines that nurses in Canada must follow.

The goals of the IAFN (2016) are paraphrased as follows:
- To incorporate primary prevention strategies into nurses' work at every level in an attempt to eliminate violence
- To establish and improve standards and ethics for forensic nursing practice
- To promote and encourage the exchange of ideas and the transmission of knowledge among members and related disciplines
- To create and facilitate educational opportunities for forensic nurses and related disciplines

Although the Canadian Nurses Association (CNA) has endorsed psychiatric mental health nursing as a specialty area of practice and offers certification for nurses who meet the criteria, it has not yet recognized forensic nursing as a distinct specialty area of practice. However, in July 2007, the CNA did approve the Forensic Nurses' Society of Canada (FNSC) as a special interest group. The goal of the FNSC is to provide a network for forensic nurses and a platform for sharing ideas and discussing evidence-informed practice in the area of forensics (Canadian Forensic Nurses Association, 2017).

Education

In 2001, certification in forensic nursing became available for the subspecialty of sexual assault nurse examiners. At the same time, the IAFN called for the incorporation of forensic content at all levels of nursing education. In Canada, however, many nurses are involved in forensic nursing without having any specialized training. Some topics relevant to forensic nursing may be covered at the undergraduate level as part of psychiatric mental health nursing or community nursing courses; however, more often forensic nursing is taught as a certificate program following the completion of a basic nursing program or as a course at the postgraduate level, where the core fundamentals of nursing are already established. Canada was first in the world to offer an online forensic studies certificate program. Currently there are no specific forensic nursing master's or doctoral programs (Kent-Wilkinson, 2009, 2010), but a master of nursing program with the specialty of forensic nursing is offered at the University of Saskatchewan.

Roles and Functions

In forensic nursing, it is not the role of the forensic nurse to make a decision as to guilt or innocence or to determine whether a victim is being candid in his or her reporting of what happened. The roles of the forensic nurse centre on the identification of victims; creation of appropriate treatment plans; and collection, documentation, and preservation of potential evidence. The forensic nurse possesses expertise in assessment and treatment roles related to competency, risk, and danger. Forensic nurses are educated in nursing science and may have taken additional courses in theories of violence and victimology and legal issues, enabling them to objectively assess the circumstances of the case.

An understanding of both the victim and the offender enhances evidence collection. Forensic nurses may apply medical-surgical knowledge to the care of victims and offenders, and they may function in a legal role as they collect evidence, testify in court, or collaborate with law practitioners with relation to a forensic patient.

Nurse Examiner or Sexual Assault Nurse Examiner

The sexual assault nurse examiner (SANE) was the first specialized forensic role for nurses that required advanced education. The largest group of self-identified forensic nurses, SANEs are registered nurses who seek training in the care of adult and pediatric victims of sexual assault (*SANE-A* and *SANE-P*, respectively).

The IAFN has established clear guidelines for the preparation of SANEs and provides SANE certification for nurses, although not all nurses who work in this capacity have certification. The training is relatively brief: the course is typically 5 days and 40 contact hours and is available online or in a classroom setting. The course may also include a clinical component. Currently 7 of the 10 provinces in Canada offer SANE programs.

Nurses recognize the need to provide consistent care for all victims; therefore nurses and leaders in many communities in Canada have set standards for educating the public on sexual assault prevention techniques and establishing comprehensive care for victims through sexual assault response teams (SARTs), which use a multidisciplinary model in providing care. SANEs are involved in the formation of SARTs in many communities across Canada. Along with SANEs, members of a SART may include representatives from the health department, police services, advocacy groups, the local department of children and family services, Crown attorneys' offices, local hospitals, victim assistance programs, and other service areas, as pertinent (Sekula, Colbert, Zoucha, et al., 2012). The multidisciplinary approach provides a standard of care that includes expert care in the acute setting, advocacy for the acute and long-term needs of the victim, and referral for counselling for survivors to decrease long-term effects resulting from the assault. The Research Highlight box describes the findings of a research study on survivors' satisfaction with nurse-led sexual assault and domestic violence care in Ontario.

Nurse Coroner or Death Investigator

This forensic nursing subspecialty is recognized internationally as having its historical roots in Alberta. Passage of the *Fatalities Inquiries Act* led to the formation of the Medical Examiners' Office in 1977 in Alberta. Subsequently, the medical examiners system for investigation of all deaths (unnatural, unexpected, or unexplained) was adopted, and nurses were hired as death investigators or medical examiner nurse investigators (Constantino, Crane, & Young, 2013). Currently, the medical examiner system operates in Alberta, Manitoba, Nova Scotia, and Newfoundland. Other provinces have a coroner system or a

---

 RESEARCH HIGHLIGHT

Survivors' Satisfaction With Nurse-Led Sexual Assault and Domestic Violence Care

Problem

Respect for confidentiality and an ethical responsibility not to retraumatize victims of sexual assault challenge the ability to conduct research on or evaluation of survivors' experiences of and satisfaction with services. As a result, little is known about the impact of comprehensive nursing-led, hospital-based sexual assault and domestic violence treatment programs.

Purpose of Study

The study sought out the views and opinions of survivors of sexual assault on their experiences with nurse-led sexual assault care in Ontario.

Methods

This study surveyed clients or guardians who presented to 30 of 35 of Ontario's Sexual Assault/Domestic Violence Treatment Centres on seven key domains: presentation characteristics, client characteristics, assailant characteristics, assault characteristics, health consequences, service use, and satisfaction with services.

Key Findings

Participation rates were high, with 1 484 people participating in the study, 96% of whom were women or girls. Participants were mostly White (75.3%), 12 to 44 years old (87.8%), and living with family (69.6%); 97.9% of clients used at least one service. The most commonly used service was assessment and/or documentation of injury (84.8%), followed by on-site follow-up care (73.6%). Nearly all of the clients or guardians reported that they received the care needed (98.6%) and rated the overall care as excellent or good (98.8%). Most (95.4%) stated that the care had been provided in a sensitive manner. Concerns about and recommendations to improve care expressed by a small proportion of clients or guardians focused on broader systemic and institutional issues of long wait times, negative attitudes of emergency department staff, issues of privacy and confidentiality, and difficulty with accessing services.

Implications for Nursing Practice

Based on their findings, recommendations for cross-training and attention to broader systemic issues can be made. The high uptake and overwhelmingly positive evaluation of services provided by Ontario's Sexual Assault/Domestic Violence Treatment Centre programs confirm the value of nursing-led, hospital-based care in the aftermath of sexual assault and domestic violence. Ongoing evaluation of such services will ensure the best care possible for this patient population.

Source: Du Mont, J., Macdonald, S., White, M., et al. (2014). Client satisfaction with nursing-led sexual assault and domestic violence services in Ontario. *Journal of Forensic Nursing, 10*(3), 122.

---

combination of both system types (Kent-Wilkinson, 2009, 2010). Over the years, registered nurses have also held the position of coroner in some territories and provinces. This nursing role involves assessing the deceased through understanding, discovery, preservation, and use of evidence.

As a representative of the medical examiner's or coroner's office, the forensic nurse death investigator is in charge of the body at a scene and works in collaboration with police services and other officials involved in the case. This nurse interviews witnesses, collects evidence, and documents findings. He or she may also notify the next of kin of the death (Baumann & Stark, 2015). Such nurses are able to expand the role of the coroner and improve services provided to families, health care agencies, and communities by employing the basic principles of holistic nursing care.

The Forensic Mental Health System in Canada

An increasing number of individuals struggling with mental illness and living in the community without adequate mental health services and resources are coming into contact with the law. This phenomenon is frequently referred to as the *criminalization of the mentally ill*. According to Stall (2013), the psychiatric deinstitutionalization movement, which started in the 1960s, and changes to civil law that rendered involuntary treatment and hospitalization more difficult (both part of the movement toward the promotion of the self-determination of individuals with mental illness) have contributed to the criminal justice system becoming the new entry point to mental health services for many individuals with mental illness. Peternelj-Taylor and Panosky (2013) point to the continuing lack of adequate mental health policies for individuals living with chronic mental illness and the lack of community-based services, resulting in a fragmented mental health care system.

The Canadian forensic mental health system provides mental health services (inpatient and community) to individuals who have a mental illness and have come into contact with the justice system. Although health care in Canada receives financial support from the federal government and the *Criminal Code* dictates some degree of consistency, the forensic mental health systems in the provinces and territories have evolved separately because the Constitution grants each jurisdiction authority over health matters (Library of Parliament, 2008). The provincial and territorial forensic mental health systems therefore reflect the uniqueness of each jurisdiction—geography, climate, existing services, population needs, and available resources and expertise.

FORENSIC PSYCHIATRIC NURSING

Forensic psychiatric mental health nurses "seek the truth about when, what, where, how and who in a traumatic or catastrophic event" (Zalon, Constantino, & Crane, 2013, p. 3). Devnick (2010, p. 48) describes forensic mental health nursing as multifaceted, calling for the balancing of competing philosophies of caring and containment; inciting contradictory emotions in response to possibly heinous behaviours and trauma; and requiring complex skills of collaborating with interdisciplinary health, legal, and security staff in the management of clinical interventions to address potentially dangerous behaviours. This specialty requires skills in psychiatric mental health nursing assessment, evaluation, and treatment of forensic clients diagnosed with a mental illness.

Evidence collection is central to the role of the forensic psychiatric nurse. For example, evidence is collected by a careful evaluation of a forensic patient's mental status at the time of an offence. This evaluation aids in determining the individual's fitness to stand trial and may later influence the sentence. Forensic psychiatric nurses may spend many hours with an accused individual collecting evidence and carefully documenting the dialogue. In this capacity, the role of the forensic psychiatric nurse is not to determine guilt or innocence but to provide assessment data that can help make a final diagnosis within the multidisciplinary forensic team (Sekula, Colbert, Zoucha, et al., 2012).

Roles and Functions

The role of the forensic psychiatric nurse formally began in Canada in the 1970s, when mentally disordered offenders were separated from the general inmate population and forensic psychiatric services were provided federally by the CSC. The role subsequently evolved with the establishment of forensic psychiatric inpatient units (Kent-Wilkinson, 2009, 2010). The role has continued to evolve, and forensic psychiatric nurses may now function as forensic nurse examiners, expert witnesses, and consultants to the criminal justice system, law enforcement, or health care agencies. These roles may involve providing nursing services to forensic clients and victims of violence, expert court testimony, and services to a Crown attorney or defence lawyer.

Roles of the forensic psychiatric nurse may be examined in relationship to the settings in which the nurse is employed. The forensic psychiatric nurse, as a member of an interprofessional team, may work on a forensic assessment unit in a mental health facility, conducting court-ordered evaluations of criminal responsibility and court-ordered treatment to determine if individuals are fit to stand trial or may work on a forensic rehabilitation unit providing treatment, care, and rehabilitation for patients who have been found to be unfit or not criminally responsible on account of mental disorder (NCRMD).

Canadian law specifies that a person cannot be tried for a criminal offence if, because of a mental disorder, he or she is unable to provide a defence. The *Criminal Code* defines "unfit to stand trial" as unable on account of mental disorder to conduct a defence at any stage of the proceedings before a verdict is rendered or to instruct counsel to do so and, in particular, unable on account of mental disorder to:

1. understand the nature or object of the proceedings,
2. understand the possible consequences of the proceedings, or
3. communicate with counsel. (*Criminal Code*, 1985, s. 2)

It is the accused individual's capacity *at the time of trial* that is in question in determining fitness to stand trial. The court may decide that an individual found unfit to stand trial is to be treated for the purpose of making the individual fit to do so. Before rendering this decision, the court must be satisfied, based on medical evidence, that the proposed treatment is likely to make the individual fit to stand trial and that without treatment the individual is likely to remain unfit; that any potential harm associated with the treatment does not outweigh the anticipated benefits; and that the specified treatment is the least restrictive and least intrusive given the circumstances. Then every 2 years, until the person is either acquitted or tried, a review board holds a hearing to determine if the person has become fit to stand trial (Department of Justice Canada, 2015a). Although there continues to be much debate, Canadian law currently requires only that individuals be able to provide a factual account to their lawyers, not necessarily an analytical or rational analysis.

Criminal responsibility refers to the mental state of a defendant at the time of the offence. A person is not criminally responsible (NCR) if he or she has a mental disorder that makes him or her unable to judge the nature or quality of the criminal act or to understand that the act was wrong at the time it was committed (*Criminal Code*, 1985, s. 16). Merely having a mental disorder does not automatically exempt a person from criminal responsibility. The courts make the decision based on a thorough legal and psychiatric review to determine the person's state at the time of the offence. If the person is tried, the verdict will then be guilty, not guilty, or not criminally responsible on account of mental disorder.

A literature review of the role of the forensic psychiatric mental health nurse identified a series of competencies (Box 32-2).

The forensic psychiatric nurse must be highly skilled in interpersonal communications and able to develop collegial relationships with those in other disciplines. The ability to be self-reflective and objective is also critical (Sekula & Amar, 2016).

One of the most challenging aspects of forensic psychiatric nursing is balancing the custodial role with the therapeutic role. The forensic psychiatric nurse must be able to look beyond the index offence and see forensic patients as human beings with specific needs (Dhaliwal & Hirst, 2016).

Forensic psychiatric nursing appeals to a particular type of nurse, one who thrives in a stimulating intellectual environment, seeks out opportunities to apply clinical skills to complex legal problems, and enjoys pushing the limits of traditional boundaries. Because of the value placed on tradition by the nursing profession, the forensic psychiatric nurse is sometimes viewed with scepticism in nursing and with caution in the legal system. These responses must be met with professionalism by forensic psychiatric nurses in their practice, research, and education.

Correctional Nursing in Canada

The number of incarcerated individuals (both men and women) in Canada has remained stable over recent years. In Canada in 2015–2016, there were 120 568 offenders in prison or in the community. Of that population, 22 956 adult offenders were being supervised through the federal prison system; the rest were involved in provincial and territorial systems (Statistics Canada, 2017). Incarcerated individuals are significantly more likely than those in the general public to have infectious diseases, chronic health conditions such as diabetes, cardiovascular conditions, and asthma, as well as to experience mental illness and substance use disorders (Kouyoumdjian, Schuler, Matheson, et al., 2016).

Offenders are guaranteed the right to treatment as well as the right to refuse treatment (Department of Justice Canada, 2015b). Therefore correctional facilities are required to provide "adequate and reasonable" health services to inmates, either directly or through community health services organizations.

BOX 32-2   COMPETENCIES ASSOCIATED WITH THE ROLE OF A FORENSIC PSYCHIATRIC MENTAL HEALTH NURSE

Specific Task-Oriented Areas
- Safety and security
- Assessment and management of risk
- Monitoring of patients and their property
- Management of violent and aggressive behaviour
- Therapies
- Practical skills (e.g., first aid)
- Escorting patients within and outside of the secure environment
- Visitor-related issues (e.g., observation, communication)
- Management of hostage situations and other security breaches
- Report writing

Knowledge
- Mental health and criminal justice systems
- Appreciation of physical, legal, emotional, and spiritual consequences of being legally detained
- Mental health wellness and illness
- Public attitudes, moral values, ignorance and stigma, empowerment, and paternalism

Skills
- Self-awareness, reflection, and honesty
- Therapeutic use of self
- Clinical risk assessment and management
- Planning of therapeutic interventions
- Development and maintenance of independent living skills
- Facilitation of meaningful relationships
- Help in the identification of behavioural boundaries and the development of self-control
- Addressing of socially unacceptable behaviours

Personal Qualities (Values and Attitudes)
- Ability to be nonjudgemental (e.g., ensuring that principles of equality, fairness, and confidentiality are maintained)
- Ability to be detached (i.e., not personalizing negative events)
- Ability to appear calm and relaxed (i.e., never being threatening)
- Understanding and setting boundaries in therapeutic relationships
- Ability to make decisions effectively

Source: Adapted from Bowering-Lossock, E. (2006). The forensic mental health nurse: A literature review. *Journal of Psychiatric & Mental Health Nursing, 13*, 780–785. doi:10.1111/j.1365-2850.2006.00993.x. Copyright © 2006, John Wiley and Sons.

Correctional nursing is defined by the location of the work or the legal status of the patient rather than by the role or functions being performed by the nurse. In fact, the role of nurses in correctional settings involves all aspects of nursing practice, including emergency care, medication administration, comprehensive mental and physical health assessments, infection control, health teaching, provision of treatments such as wound care, management of acute and chronic mental and physical illnesses, and collaboration with other health care providers (Constantino, Crane, & Young, 2013).

As mentioned, today's inmates experience a disproportionately greater number of chronic illnesses and infectious diseases than the general population. Treatment and services for inmates with chronic mental health diagnoses are a significant part of the job for nurses working in correctional facilities. Research from the CSC over several years shows that 62% of incoming female offenders in the criminal justice system required further mental health evaluation. For incoming male offenders, 50% required further mental health assessment, and 40% of male offenders met the criteria for a current mental illness diagnosis other than substance abuse or antisocial personality disorder (CSC, 2015). Lifetime substance use was particularly notable for male and female offenders. The rate of mental illness among offenders is several times higher than the rate of mental health disorders in the general Canadian population.

Correctional nurses provide care for many individuals with serious mental illness who are caught in a cycle of homelessness, psychiatric hospitals, and prison. Unfortunately, only some will end up being admitted to either a regional hospital or a regional mental health treatment centre, where they can receive comprehensive psychiatric mental health services. Frequently, these individuals instead become incarcerated as a result of psychiatric emergencies that generally include threats made to others. Because psychiatric resources to help manage such emergencies are scarce, these individuals often end up in prison instead of in a hospital. Once they are in a correctional facility, their psychiatric condition often worsens because of the lack of adequate psychiatric intervention.

Another issue that must be considered in the treatment of those who are incarcerated is substance use and abuse. In Canada, some 80% of offenders serving prison sentences of 2 years or more have problems with drugs, alcohol, or both (CSC, 2015). Drug courts, mandatory drug treatment, and drug or alcohol treatment within correctional facilities have all been shown to decrease the likelihood of recidivism and to increase the likelihood of abstinence from drugs or alcohol after release.

Because of the impacts of mental health and addiction problems on recidivism (repeat offences) and on resource allocation, policymakers and legislators are beginning to recognize the importance of providing treatment for individuals who are incarcerated. In Canada, the *Corrections and Conditional Release Act* (1992) actually references the fact that inmates receiving mental health treatment alongside correctional programming (in prison and in the community) demonstrate functional improvement. The correctional setting, however, is not conducive to the intensive therapy required to adequately treat mental health issues; therefore the needs of the vast majority of people with mental illnesses or concurrent disorders in the correctional system are not appropriately addressed.

There are more than 700 nurses at the CSC working in a variety of settings, including correctional remand, psychiatric assessment, and prison facilities; regional hospitals; mental health treatment centres; and Indigenous healing lodges (Box 32-3). They can specialize in a wide range of areas, from mental disorders

---

BOX 32-3 TYPES OF HEALTH CARE SETTINGS IN THE CORRECTIONAL SERVICE OF CANADA

Institutional Health Units (Ambulatory Care Centres)
Every CSC institution has a health services centre with varying hours of operation based on factors such as level of security and proximity to community services. The primary care providers in these units are nurses. Each institution provides a variety of routine and emergency psychology services to offenders.

CSC Regional Hospital
Each region has a hospital located within the compound of a multilevel or maximum security level institution that provides more specialized or comprehensive health care services on a 24-hour basis. Services include but are not limited to postoperative care, trauma care, observation, dialysis, palliative care, and any condition requiring 24-hour nursing services.

CSC Reception Centre
Each region has at least one reception centre that conducts the CSC standardized admission process (both health and security) for all newly sentenced federal offenders. The admission process involves various health assessments, such as a mental status assessment, comprehensive health assessment, and tuberculosis assessment.

CSC Regional Treatment Centre (Mental Health)
An inpatient mental health treatment facility is located in each region to provide treatment to inmates with psychiatric disorders that are too severe to allow them to remain in the general inmate population.

---

to substance abuse to chronic care (CSC, 2013). Alongside drug and alcohol treatment interventions, nurses working with incarcerated patients with mental illness employ biological treatments as well as psychoeducation, cognitive behavioural therapies, and other integrative therapies to promote coping (for instance, yoga therapy, which has a strong evidence base for this population) (Maruca & Shelton, 2016).

The CSC has recognized that correctional nurses face a number of challenges, including a high level of stress associated with the correctional environment, demanding work hours, caring for individuals who have a substance use disorder, and concerns for personal safety expressed by family and friends. In response to these challenges, the CSC has implemented extensive education and training for newly hired nurses as well as for those who have been working in corrections for a number of years (CSC, 2013).

Correctional nurses perform psychiatric mental health nursing role functions, including completing comprehensive mental status examinations and implementing psychiatric care plans. The vignette illustrates a challenging situation facing a nurse working in the health services centre of a correctional facility.

> **VIGNETTE**
>
> Suzanne is a 45-year-old woman incarcerated at a federal institution in the general inmate population. She was convicted of assault with a deadly weapon following a confrontation with a "friend." Her psychiatric diagnoses include major depression and post-traumatic stress disorder (PTSD; resulting from severe abuse in her childhood and from an intimate partner during her early twenties). Although she is not on a locked forensic unit, she is being treated with medication and being seen by one of the institution's nurses for medication management.
>
> While watching television in the common area one morning, Suzanne attacked a fellow inmate for no apparent reason, screaming and clawing at anyone who approached her. The staff was unable to control her physically. She was placed in solitary confinement
>
> with mechanical restraints; these actions did nothing to control her screaming. She was seen by the nurse on call, who reported that Suzanne was having a flashback related to her PTSD. The solitary confinement and mechanical restraints were only worsening these flashbacks. The staff and the nurse were facing a common dilemma in correctional health care: custody versus caring. While the nurse was focused on the needs of the individual inmate, the correctional staff was focused on the goals of the correctional facility related to custody of violent offenders and protection of the environment. The successful correctional treatment team seeks to balance the two sides of this debate: creating an environment in which the potential rehabilitation of offenders is possible without compromising the compulsory "punitive" aspects of incarceration.

KEY POINTS TO REMEMBER

- Forensic nursing is an emerging specialty area of practice that combines elements of traditional nursing, forensic science, and criminal justice.
- The IAFN was established in 1992 as the professional association representing this specialty internationally.
- Forensic nurses fulfill a variety of roles, including that of sexual assault nurse examiner, nurse coroner or death investigator, forensic psychiatric mental health nurse, and correctional nurse.
- Incarcerated individuals have higher rates of serious and chronic physical and mental illnesses than the general population.

CRITICAL THINKING

1. How would you describe the nurse–patient relationship in forensic nursing? In what ways does it differ from the nurse–patient relationship in other areas of nursing?

2. Respect is an essential component of any therapeutic nurse–patient relationship; however, nurses often find it challenging to respect patients who have committed serious offences. Is it possible for nurses working in a forensic or correctional setting to respect every patient? Explain your answer.

CHAPTER REVIEW

1. Which statement regarding forensic nursing is accurate?
   a. Forensic nurses must all be prepared at the doctoral level.
   b. Forensic nurses perform only sexual assault examinations.
   c. Forensic nurses may participate in death investigations.
   d. Forensic psychiatric mental health nurses work only in correctional facilities.

2. What is one of the most challenging aspects of forensic psychiatric nursing?
   a. Working independently instead of as a member of an interdisciplinary team
   b. Balancing the custodial role with the therapeutic role
   c. Spending time in maximum security settings
   d. Determining the guilt or innocence of forensic patients

3. What does it mean for an individual to be found unfit to stand trial?
   a. The individual is unable to understand the court proceedings.
   b. The individual has a life-threatening physical illness.
   c. The individual has a chronic mental illness.
   d. The individual does not demonstrate insight into his or her mental illness.

4. Which type of patients would a correctional nurse typically see?
   a. Students
   b. Police officers
   c. Teachers
   d. Inmates

5. The nurse is caring for an incarcerated patient. Based on an understanding of the health profile of incarcerated individuals, what health care challenge may the nurse most anticipate working on with this patient?
   a. Drug or alcohol issues
   b. Autoimmune diseases
   c. Eating disorders
   d. Anxiety

Evolve WEBSITE

Post-Test interactive review

Visit the Evolve website for Chapter Review Answers and Rationales, Critical Thinking Answer Guidelines, and additional resources related to the content in this chapter: http://evolve.elsevier.com/Canada/Varcarolis/psychiatric/

REFERENCES

American Nurses Association & International Association of Forensic Nurses. (2015). *Forensic nursing: Scope and standards of practice.* Retrieved from http://c.ymcdn.com/sites/www.forensicnurses.org/resource/resmgr/Docs/SS_Public_Comment_Draft_1505.pdf?hhSearchTerms=%222015protect%20$elax%20pm%20$andprotect%20$elax%20pm%20$draft%22.

Baumann, R., & Stark, S. (2015). The role of forensic death investigators interacting with the survivors of death by homicide and suicide. *Journal of Forensic Nursing, 11*(1), 28–32. doi:10.1097/JFN.0000000000000058.

Canadian Forensic Nurses Association. (2017). *About.* Retrieved from http://forensicnurse.ca/about/.

Canadian Mental Health Association. (2013). *Violence and mental illness.* Retrieved from http://www.cmha.ca/mental_health/violence-and-mental-illness/.

Centre for Addiction and Mental Health. (2013). *Mental health and criminal justice policy framework.* Retrieved from https://www.camh.ca/en/hospital/about_camh/influencing_public_policy/Documents/MH_Criminal_Justice_Policy_Framework.pdf.

Constantino, R. E. B., Crane, P. A., & Young, S. E. (2013). *Forensic nursing: Evidence-based principles and practice.* Philadelphia: F. A. Davis Co.

Correctional Services of Canada (CSC). (2013). *Careers at CSC—Nurses.* Retrieved from http://www.csc-scc.gc.ca/careers/003001-1301-eng.shtml.

Correctional Services of Canada (CSC). (2015). *Research results—Mental health.* Retrieved from http://www.csc-scc.gc.ca/publications/005007-3030-eng.shtml.

Corrections and Conditional Release Act, S.C. 1992, c. 20.

Criminal Code, R.S.C. 1985, c. C-46.

Department of Justice Canada. (2015a). *The review board systems in Canada: An overview of results from the mentally disordered accused data collection study.* Retrieved from http://www.justice.gc.ca/eng/rp-pr/csj-sjc/jsp-sjp/rr06_1/p1.html.

Department of Justice Canada. (2015b). *Canada's system of justice.* Retrieved from http://www.justice.gc.ca/eng/csj-sjc/just/img/courten.pdf.

Department of Justice Canada. (2017). *Indigenous overrepresentation in the criminal justice system: JustFacts.* Retrieved from http://www.justice.gc.ca/eng/rp-pr/jr/jf-pf/2017/jan02.html.

Devnick, B. R. (2010). *The forensic mental health nurse: Confusion, illusion, or specialization? A scoping literature review.* (Dissertation). University of Victoria, Victoria, BC. Retrieved from http://dspace.library.uvic.ca:8080/bitstream/handle/1828/4092/Devnick_Betty_MN_2010.pdf?sequence=1&isAllowed=y.

Dhaliwal, K., & Hirst, S. (2016). Caring in correctional nursing: A systematic search and narrative synthesis. *Journal of Forensic Nursing, 12*(1), 5.

Gutierrez, L., Wilson, H. A., Rugge, T., et al. (2013). The prediction of recidivism with aboriginal offenders: A theoretically informed meta-analysis. *Canadian Journal of Criminology and Criminal Justice, 55*(1), 55–99. doi:10.3138/cjccj.2011.E.51.

Harris, C. (2017). Forensic nursing provides closure in workplace fatality. *Journal of Forensic Nursing, 13*(1), 35–38. doi:10.1097/JFN.0000000000000137.

International Association of Forensic Nurses. (2016). *About forensic nursing.* Retrieved from http://www.forensicnurses.org/?page=WhatisFN.

Kara, F. B. (2014). Police interactions with the mentally ill: The role of procedural justice. *Canadian Graduate Journal of Sociology and Criminology, 3*(1), 79–94.

Kent-Wilkinson, A. E. (2009). An exploratory study of forensic nursing education in North America: Constructed definitions of forensic nursing. *Journal of Forensic Nursing, 5*(4), 201–211. doi:10.1111/j.1939-3938.2009.01055.x.

Kent-Wilkinson, A. E. (2010). Forensic psychiatric/mental health nursing: Responsive to social need. *Issues in Mental Health Nursing, 31*(6), 425.

Kouyoumdjian, F., Schuler, A., Matheson, F. I., et al. (2016). Health status of prisoners in Canada: Narrative review. *Canadian Family Physician/Médecin de famille Canadien, 62*(3), 215.

Library of Parliament. (2008). *The federal role in health and health care.* Retrieved from https://lop.parl.ca/content/lop/researchpublications/prb0858-e.pdf.

MacPhail, A., & Verdun-Jones, S. (2013*). Mental illness and the criminal justice system.* Retrieved from http://icclr.law.ubc.ca/sites/icclr.law.ubc.ca/files/publications/pdfs/Mental%20Illness%20and%20the%20Criminal%20Justice%20System%20%5BFinal%20VS%5D.pdf.

Maruca, A. T., & Shelton, D. (2016). Correctional nursing interventions for incarcerated persons with mental disorders: An integrative review. *Issues in Mental Health Nursing, 37*(5), 285.

Mental Health Commission of Canada. (2012). *Changing directions, changing lives: The mental health strategy for Canada.* Calgary: Author.

Peternelj-Taylor, C., & Panosky, D. (2013). Advancing forensic correctional nursing. *Journal of Forensic Nursing, 9*(1), 1.

Public Safety Canada. (2015). *Crime prevention information, project descriptions and summaries.* Retrieved from https://www.publicsafety.gc.ca/cnt/cntrng-crm/crm-prvntn/tls-rsrcs/nfrmtn-dscrptns-smmrs-en.aspx.

Sekula, K., & Amar, A. F. (2016). Forensic mental health nursing. In A. F. Amar & L. K. Sekula (Eds.), *A practice guide to forensic nursing: Incorporating forensic principles into forensic practice* (pp. 1–15). Indianapolis: Sigma Theta Tau International.

Sekula, L. K., Colbert, A. M., Zoucha, R., et al. (2012). Strengthening the science of forensic nursing through education and research. *Journal of Forensic Nursing, 8*(1), 1–2.

Simpson, A. I. F., McMaster, J. J., & Cohen, S. N. (2013). Challenges for Canada in meeting the needs of persons with serious mental illness in prison. *Journal of the American Academy of Psychiatry and the Law Online, 41*(4), 501.

Stall, N. (2013). Imprisoning the mentally ill. *CMAJ : Canadian Medical Association Journal = Journal de l'Association Medicale Canadienne, 185*(3), 201–202. doi:10.1503/cmaj.109-4390.

Statistics Canada. (2017). *Adult correctional statistics 2015/2016.* Retrieved from http://www.statcan.gc.ca/pub/85-002-x/2017001/article/14700-eng.htm.

Zalon, M. L., Constantino, R. E., & Crane, P. A. (2013). Fundamentals of contemporary forensic nursing practice, education and research. In R. E. B. Constantino, P. A. Crane, & S. E. Young (Eds.), *Forensic nursing: Evidence-based principles and practice* (pp. 2–26). Philadelphia: F. A. Davis Co.

Advanced Intervention Modalities

33. Therapeutic Groups

34. Family Interventions

35. Integrative and Complementary Therapies

33

Therapeutic Groups

Donna Rolin, Sandra Snelson Yaklin
Adapted by Cheryl L. Pollard

KEY TERMS AND CONCEPTS

conflict
group
group content
group norms
group process
group psychotherapy

group themes
group work
psychoeducational groups
self-help groups
support groups
therapeutic factors

OBJECTIVES

1. Identify basic concepts related to group work.
2. Describe the phases of group development.
3. Define task and maintenance roles of group members.
4. Discuss the therapeutic factors that operate in all groups.

5. Discuss four types of groups commonly led by nurses.
6. Describe a group intervention for (1) a member who is silent or (2) a member who is monopolizing the group.

Evolve WEBSITE

Visit the Evolve website for Flashcards, Case Studies, and additional testing resources related to the content in this chapter: http://evolve.elsevier.com/Canada/Varcarolis/psychiatric/

Pre-Test | interactive review

We all live among and interact with groups throughout our lives. We are born into a family group and grow up with various peer groups, such as those at school, at work, within religious or spiritual affiliations, and so on. As adults, we establish our own family group. A group consists of two or more people who come together for the purpose of pursuing common goals, interests, or both. A group's progress and outcomes are influenced by the group's characteristics, including the following:

- Size
- Defined purpose
- Degree of similarity among members
- Rules
- Boundaries
- Content (what is said in the group)
- Process (underlying dynamics among group members)

Box 33-1 defines terms related to types of groups and group work. Group work is a method whereby individuals with a common purpose come together and benefit by giving and receiving feedback within the context of group life.

There are advantages and disadvantages of the group approach for people living with mental illness. Advantages include the following:

- Engaging multiple people in treatment at the same time, thereby saving costs
- Enabling participants to benefit from the feedback not only of the nurse leader but also of peers, who may possess a unique understanding of the issues
- Providing a relatively safe setting to try out new ways of relating to other people and practising new communication skills
- Promoting a feeling of belonging

BOX 33-1	TERMS CENTRAL TO THERAPEUTIC GROUPS

Terms Describing Group Work

Group content—all that is said in the group

Group process—the dynamics of interaction among the members (e.g., who talks to whom, facial expressions, body language)

Group norms—expectations for behaviour in the group that develop over time and provide structure for members (e.g., starting on time, not interrupting)

Group themes—members' expressed ideas or feelings that recur and have a common thread (The leader can clarify a theme to help members recognize it more fully.)

Conflict—open disagreement among members (Positive conflict resolution within a group is key to successful outcomes.)

Terms Describing Types of Groups

Heterogeneous group—a group in which there is a range of differences among members

Homogeneous group—a group in which all members share central traits (e.g., men's group, group of people with bipolar disorder)

Closed group—a group in which membership is restricted; no new members are added when others leave

Open group—a group in which new members are added as others leave

Subgroup—an individual or a small group that is isolated within a larger group and functions separately (Members of a subgroup may have greater loyalty, more similar goals, or more perceived similarities to one another than they do to the larger group.)

BOX 33-2	THERAPEUTIC FACTORS IN GROUPS

Instillation of hope—The leader shares optimism about group treatment, and members share their improvements.

Universality—Members realize that they are not alone in their problems, feelings, or thoughts.

Imparting of information—Participants receive formal teaching by the leader or advice from peers.

Altruism—Members feel a reward from giving support to others.

Corrective recapitulation of the primary family group—Members repeat patterns of behaviour in the group that they learned in their families; with feedback from the leader and peers, they learn about their own behaviour.

Development of socializing techniques—Members learn new social skills based on feedback from others.

Imitative behaviour—Members may copy behaviour from the leader or peers and can adopt healthier habits.

Interpersonal learning—Members gain insight into themselves based on feedback from others. This process is complex and occurs later in the group, after trust is established.

Group cohesiveness—This powerful factor arises in a mature group, when each member feels connected to the other members, the leader, and the group as a whole; in a cohesive group, members can accept positive feedback and constructive criticism.

Catharsis—Intense feelings, as judged by the member, are shared.

Existential resolution—Members learn to accept painful aspects of life (e.g., loneliness, death) that affect everyone.

Source: Data from Yalom, I. D. (2005). *The theory and practice of group psychotherapy* (5th ed.). New York: Basic Books.

Disadvantages include the following:

- Time constraints in which an individual member may feel cheated of floor time, particularly in large groups
- Concerns that private issues may be shared outside the group
- Disruptive member behaviour during an emotionally vulnerable point

Not everyone benefits from group treatment. People who are acutely psychotic, acutely manic, or intoxicated have difficulty interacting effectively in groups and may interfere with other members' ability to remain focused on group goals and progress.

THERAPEUTIC FACTORS COMMON TO ALL GROUPS

Irvin D. Yalom (2005), one of the most noted researchers on group psychotherapy, is credited with identifying the factors that make groups therapeutic (Box 33-2). Therapeutic factors are aspects of the group experience that facilitate therapeutic change. For example, as group members begin to share life experiences, feelings, and concerns, they may recognize for the first time that they are not "alone in the world"—their experiences may be more universal than they initially thought, allowing them to connect with others. Yalom calls this factor *universality*—the recognition that other people feel the same way or have had the same experiences. Recognizing universality can provide a

validation of the person's experiences and, subsequently, a profound sense of relief. Different therapeutic factors operate at different phases of a group, and during the initial phase, the leader may role-model several behaviours, such as instilling hope and imparting information. Just as with other types of treatment, each person's response to a group is highly individualized, based on past experiences and level of participation.

PLANNING A GROUP

Planning a group should include developing a description of its specific characteristics—for example:

- Name and objectives of the group
- Common concerns or diagnoses of members
- Group schedule (frequency, times of meetings, etc.)
- Descriptions of leader's and members' responsibilities
- Methods or means of evaluating outcomes of the group

Planning and structure is especially important when group leaders are likely to change (e.g., in inpatient settings, where staffing patterns change) or when several groups are running at the same time with a common goal (e.g., in a research study).

PHASES OF GROUP DEVELOPMENT

All groups go through developmental phases similar to those identified for individual therapeutic relationships (see Chapter 9).

In each phase, the group leader has specific roles and challenges to address in support of positive interaction, growth, and change.

In the *orientation phase*, the group leader's role is to structure an atmosphere of respect, confidentiality, and trust. The purpose of the group is stated, and members are encouraged to get to know one another. Group rules such as confidentiality or avoidance of potentially inflammatory topics such as politics are reviewed. Initially, members may be overly silent or over-bearing because they have not yet established trust with one another. Therapeutic interaction is supported when the group leader points out similarities between members, encourages them to talk directly to each other rather than to the leader, and reminds members about ground rules for respectful interaction.

In the *working phase*, the group leader's role is to encourage a focus on problem solving consistent with the purpose of the group. As group members begin to feel safe within the group, conflicts may be expressed, which should be viewed by the group leader as a positive opportunity for group growth. It is important for the leader to guide and support conflict resolution. Through successful resolution of conflicts, group members are empowered to develop confidence in their problem-solving abilities and better support one another in their individual efforts to grow and change.

In the *termination phase*, the group leader's role is to encourage members to reflect on the progress they have made and identify post-termination goals. Members may experience feelings of loss or anger about the group ending; at times, these feelings can be directed toward other group members or the leader. It is important to openly address such feelings as part of the group's work toward successful termination.

Evaluation and follow-up are fundamental aspects of a therapeutic group. Objective measures are an important way to demonstrate group effectiveness. Questionnaires can be helpful in refining what patients found helpful. The Therapeutic Factors Inventory-19 (Joyce, MacNair-Semands, Tasca, et al., 2011) is a questionnaire that asks patients to identify which of the thera-peutic factors were present in therapy. The Group Questionnaire (Burlingame, 2010) is another tool that evaluates the climate, cohesion, empathy, and alliance of the group. Regardless of the scale or instrument used, group leaders should evaluate all groups to determine if goals set in the planning phase were accomplished and to re-evaluate or redesign future groups.

GROUP MEMBER ROLES

We each have a unique style of interacting with others, and we gravitate toward specific comfort zones within groups. Consider your own behaviours within groups. You may tend to sit back and mainly observe, giving your opinion only after careful consideration. Or perhaps you feel that it is important to keep everyone moving in a common direction or to help maintain order and actively urge people to continue working. The way we behave in groups is a function of our innate personalities, our socialization, and the specific context of the group.

Studies of group dynamics have identified informal roles that group members often assume and that may or may not be helpful in the group's development. The classic descriptive categories for these roles are *task*, *maintenance*, and *individual* roles (Benne & Sheats, 1948). Task roles serve to keep the group focused on its main purpose and get the work done. Maintenance roles function to help each person feel worthwhile and create a sense of group cohesion. Individual roles have nothing to do with helping the group but instead relate to specific personalities, personal agendas, and a desire to have needs met by shifting the group's focus to them. Awareness of roles can assist the group leader to identify behaviours that need to be confronted or reinforced. Table 33-1 describes the informal roles of group members.

GROUP LEADERSHIP

Responsibilities

The group leader has multiple responsibilities in initiating, maintaining, and terminating a group.

The first responsibility is to determine the purpose, parameters, and membership of the group. Will the group be open, accepting new members regularly, or closed to new members after it begins? How often will the group meet, where, and for how long? It is also advisable in many instances to choose a co-leader to help facilitate the group and, especially on inpatient units, one or more observers.

The leader and co-leader should base selection of group members on clear criteria, depending on the type of group. Group members need to have a certain degree of cognitive functioning in order to participate in an insight-oriented psychotherapy group.

The styles of group leadership vary depending on the type of group and on the stage of group development. For example, the leader is often most direct in the orientation phase. During this phase, the structure, size, composition, purpose, and timing of the group are defined. Task and maintenance functions may be discussed and demonstrated. During the working phase, the leader facilitates communication and ensures that meetings begin and end on time. In the termination phase, the leader ensures that each member summarizes individual accomplishments and gives positive and negative feedback regarding the group experience.

Maintenance of cultural safety for individual members is a key responsibility of the group leader. The leader initially sets a foundation for open communication by defining the importance of mutual respect and rules for group conduct. As group members begin to engage with one another, the leader's sensitivity to issues that may have a cultural basis can be pivotal in facilitating efforts to maintain open communication and mutual respect.

Diversity may exist in many forms, including racial, ethnic, economic, and sexual orientation. Encouraging members to share and explore their cultural foundations and beliefs promotes genuine communication and provides the group with the opportunity to share similarities and differences in an environ-ment of mutual respect.

Consider the example of a woman who came to group after seriously harming herself. She remained silent and withdrawn until the leader encouraged her to explore her feelings about

TABLE 33-1	INFORMAL ROLES OF GROUP MEMBERS	
	ROLE	**FUNCTION**
Task roles	Coordinator	Tries to connect various ideas and suggestions
	Elaborator	Gives examples and follows up meaning of ideas
	Energizer	Encourages group to make decisions or take actions
	Evaluator	Measures the group's work against a standard
	Information giver	Shares facts or own experience as an authority figure
	Information seeker	Tries to clarify the group's values
	Initiator–contributor	Offers new ideas or a new outlook on an issue
	Opinion giver	Shares opinions, especially to influence group values
	Orienter	Notes the progress of the group toward goals
	Procedural technician	Supports group activity by distributing papers, arranging seating, etc.
	Recorder	Keeps notes and acts as the group's memory
Maintenance roles	Compromiser	In a conflict, yields to preserve group harmony
	Encourager	Praises and seeks input from others
	Follower	Agrees with the flow of the group
	Gatekeeper	Monitors the participation of all members to keep communication open
	Group observer	Keeps records of different aspects of group process and reports to the group
	Harmonizer	Tries to mediate conflicts between members
	Standard setter	Verbalizes standards for the group
Individual roles	Aggressor	Criticizes and attacks others' ideas and feelings
	Blocker	Disagrees with group issues; oppositional
	Dominator	Tries to control other members of the group with flattery or interruptions
	Help seeker	Asks for sympathy of group excessively
	Playboy	Acts uninterested in group process
	Recognition seeker	Seeks attention by boasting and discussing achievements
	Self-confessor	Verbalizes feelings or observations unrelated to group
	Special-interest pleader	Advocates for a special group, usually with own prejudice or bias

Source: Data from Benne, K., & Sheats, P. (1948). Functional roles of group members. *Journal of Social Issues, 4*, 41–49. doi:10.1111/j.1540-4560.1948.tb01783.x.

the group. The woman revealed that she "wasn't smart like everyone else" and that she was "basically just trailer trash." Other group members began to share their similarities and differences in backgrounds, with a focus on their common needs, fears, and insecurities. When this woman finished the group, she acknowledged having learned an important lesson: she could give and get help from people she saw as different from her, and not everyone would treat her as though she was "less than them."

Styles of Leadership

There are three main styles of group leadership, and a leader selects the style that is best suited to the therapeutic needs of a particular group—the therapeutic needs of the group are determined by the type of group and by the stage of group development. The *autocratic leader* exerts control over the group and does not encourage much interaction among members. For example, staff leading a community meeting with a fixed, time-limited agenda may tend to be more autocratic. In contrast, the *democratic leader* supports extensive group interaction in the process of problem solving. Psychotherapy groups most often employ this leadership style. In this style, the leader and co-leader take a facilitative role, redirecting questions or issues to group members rather than providing answers or solutions. A *laissez-faire leader* allows the group members to behave in any way they choose and does not attempt to control the direction of the

group. In a creative group, such as an art or horticulture group, the leader may choose a laissez-faire style.

In any group, the leader must be thoughtful about communication techniques since these can have a tremendous impact on group content and process. Table 33-2 describes communication techniques frequently used by group leaders. It is also important to note that inpatient groups have significant differences from outpatient groups (Table 33-3), and consequently the role of the leader must be adapted accordingly.

Clinical Supervision

Clinical supervision, sometimes referred to as *peer supervision* or *clinical consultation*, is important for group leaders, as it provides feedback about performance and enhances professional growth of the nurse. Transference and counter-transference issues occur in groups just as in individual treatment (see Chapter 4), and a more objective input supports a focus on therapeutic goals. Feedback related to the functioning of the group and the leadership style being used can also help further develop the skills related to respect and engagement. Another strategy used to support group leader development is co-leadership. Co-leadership is a common practice and has several benefits, including (1) providing training for less experienced staff, (2) allowing for immediate feedback between leaders after each session, and (3) offering two role models for teaching communication skills to members.

TABLE 33-2   GROUP LEADER COMMUNICATION TECHNIQUES

TECHNIQUE	EXAMPLE
Giving information—provides resources and information that support treatment goals	"Antidepressants may take as long as 4 weeks or more to show real therapeutic effects."
Clarification—asks group members to expand and clarify what they mean	"What do you mean when you say 'I can't go back to work'?"
Confrontation—encourages group members to explore inconsistencies in their communication or behaviour	"Jane, you're saying 'nothing's wrong,' but you're crying."
Reflection—encourages group members to explore and expand on feelings (rather than on thoughts or events)	"I noticed you're clenching your fists. What are you feeling right now?" "It sounds like that really upset you."
Summarization—closes a discussion or group session by pointing out key issues and insights	"We've talked about different types of cognitive distortions, and everyone identified at least one irrational thought that has influenced his or her behaviour in a negative way. In the next group, we'll explore some strategies for correcting negative thinking."
Support—gives positive feedback and acknowledgement	"It took a lot of courage to explore those painful feelings. You're really working hard on resolving this problem."

TABLE 33-3   COMPARISON OF OUTPATIENT AND INPATIENT GROUPS

OUTPATIENT GROUPS	INPATIENT GROUPS
The group has a stable composition.	The group is rarely made up of the same members for more than one or two meetings.
Members are carefully selected and prepared.	Members are admitted to the group with little prior selection or preparation.
The group is homogeneous with regard to ego function.	The group has a heterogeneous level of ego function.
Motivated, self-referred people make up the group; therapy is growth oriented.	Members are ambivalent, and often therapy is compulsory; therapy is relief oriented.
Treatment proceeds as long as required: it may continue for 1 to 2 years.	Treatment is limited to the hospital period, with rapid member turnover.
The boundary of the group is well maintained, with few external influences.	Whatever happens on the unit affects the group.
Group cohesion develops normally, given sufficient time in treatment.	There is no time for cohesion to develop spontaneously; group development is limited to the initial phase.
The leader allows the process to unfold; there is ample time to set up group norms.	The group leader structures time and is not passive.
Members are encouraged to avoid extra-group contact.	Members eat, sleep, and live together outside of the group; extra-group contact is endorsed.

Source: Adapted from Mackenzie, K. R. (1997). *Time-managed group psychotherapy: Effective clinical applications.* Washington, DC: American Psychiatric Press.

Group Observation

In some groups, it is useful—and even essential—to assign staff as observers. In some cases, the use of an observer may occur for the purpose of clinical supervision. Another reason would be for staff to observe how group members interact and then share their observations with the leaders in order to assess and plan for modifications to the group or individual patient care plans. In inpatient groups or day programs, there may be concern about patients leaving the group in a fragile emotional state; one role of the observer is to maintain safety. The observer follows and tends to the needs of any group member who left the session before it was over.

It is useful for the group observer to monitor not just content but also process—that is, not only *what* is talked about but *how* it is talked about. A simple method is to draw a diagram of who is sitting where and, while observing, draw lines between members to indicate who speaks to whom. This diagram can give instant feedback as to patterns of behaviour in group members.

NURSE AS GROUP LEADER

Psychiatric mental health nurses are involved in a variety of therapeutic groups in acute care and long-term treatment settings. Nurses are able to provide strong leadership skills in a variety of basic groups, such as activity, psychoeducational, task, and support groups, and, with support, they may co-lead more advanced groups, such as cognitive behavioural therapy or counselling groups. More complex skills are necessary for leading psychotherapy groups, and only advanced-practice nurses or nurse therapists are qualified to lead these and other specialized groups.

For all group leaders, a clear theoretical framework is necessary to provide a foundation for analyzing the group interaction. Table 33-4 describes several theoretical frameworks commonly used in group work.

Ethical Issues in Group Therapy

The Canadian Federation of Psychiatric Mental Health Nurses (2014) and Canadian Nurses Association (2008) provide the

TABLE 33-4	THEORETICAL FOUNDATIONS FOR GROUP THERAPY	
THEORY	**CONCEPTS**	**ROLE OF THERAPIST**
Psychodynamic/ psychoanalytic	Applies Freud's concepts of psychoanalysis to individual members and to the group itself; focus is on unconscious conflicts and transference; goal is insight	Helps members to recognize unconscious conflicts and encourages peer feedback
Interpersonal	Applies Sullivan's theories about interpersonal learning; focus is on understanding how current relationships repeat early significant relationships; goal is to rebuild individual's personality	Helps to reduce anxiety and encourages members to validate feelings and thoughts with each other
Communication	Applies a systems model, holding that the whole (group) is greater than the sum of its parts (members); focus is on subgroups and communication, both verbal and nonverbal; goal is to learn clear, congruent communication skills	Helps point out confusing or contradictory messages; acts as a role model for clear communication
Group process	Analyzes the group with a focus on individual roles and group patterns of behaviour (phases, norms, etc.); goal is to resolve authority and intimacy issues	Helps develop a mature group in which members trust each other and give supportive feedback
Existential/gestalt	Applies theories of Maslow and Rogers to encourage individuals to develop to full potential; focus is on the here and now to increase members' awareness of feelings; goal is self-actualization, in which individual takes full responsibility for choices	Helps focus members on here-and-now experiences to promote self-learning; promotes emphasis on the "what" of behaviours, not the "why"
Cognitive behavioural	Applies concepts of learning theory and Ellis's cognitive therapy; focus is on behaviour and thinking patterns, with the group used to reinforce adaptive behaviour and extinguish maladaptive patterns; usually time limited; goal is to change behaviour or thinking patterns	Helps develop a trusting group in which members give supportive feedback to reinforce healthier behaviour; may provide formal teaching, including homework assignments

Sources: Data from Dies, R. (1992). Models of group psychotherapy: Sifting through confusion. *International Journal of Group Psychotherapy, 42*(1), 1–17; and Scheidlinger, S. (1997). Group dynamics and group psychotherapy revisited: Four decades later. *International Journal of Group Psychotherapy, 47*(2), 141–159.

definition for professional ethical conduct for registered nurses. The nurse group leader has an ethical obligation to inform participants of risks and benefits of group participation (informed consent). They must also discuss both confidentiality and exceptions to confidentiality. Because a group contains individuals who are not bound by a professional code of ethics, there is no way to guarantee confidentiality. Other topics the group leader must address are "Who is free to leave the group?" and "What are the rules about group members socializing outside the group?"

A member is only removed from the group as a last resort. One obvious reason is if one member were to become violent or aggressive toward another member. This would necessitate temporary or permanent removal. Other reasons that might require temporary or permanent removal from the group include (1) a member who is consistently unwilling or unable to participate or (2) a member who violates the agreements created for group membership.

Group leaders should obtain appropriate training or credentialing to practise and must work within their regulatory body's defined scope of practice. The best way to help patients is for the group leader to consistently follow the ethical guidelines and professional standards of practice.

To protect the integrity of the group therapy process, nurse clinicians should use evidence-based practice. For instance, brief cognitive behavioral therapy (CBT) has proven beneficial for depression and anxiety (Bernhardsdottir, Vilhjalmsson, & Champion, 2013). Staying current with research helps nurse clinicians to select the best therapeutic modality for the target group audience. Evidence-based practice helps ensure that the therapeutic group maximizes benefit and minimizes harm.

Basic Groups
Psychoeducational Groups

Psychoeducational groups aim to increase knowledge or skills about a specific subject and allow members to communicate emotional concerns. These groups may be time limited or may be supportive for long-term treatment. Generally, written handouts or audiovisual aids are used to focus on specific teaching points. Nurses are prepared to teach a variety of health subjects.

Medication education. The most common psychoeducational group led by a nurse is the medication education group. These groups are designed to teach patients about their medications, answer their questions, and prepare them for self-management. When patients have concerns about taking medications, it is often the group members themselves who are in the position to respond to these questions: "Yes, I got a dry mouth when I first started taking that, but it got better. Hang in there." Box 33-3 outlines an example of a medication education group protocol, and Figure 33-1 provides a means of evaluating the effectiveness of this type of nursing intervention.

Health education. Nurses also frequently lead health education groups, including groups on sex education. For instance, people who have used poor judgement in sexual behaviour because of mental illness are at high risk for sexually transmitted infections.

Family education. Nurses may also facilitate family psycho-educational groups, usually as part of an interdisciplinary team. Individual relapse rates decrease significantly when families are educated about mental illness, treatments, and recovery, as well

BOX 33-3 EXAMPLE OF MEDICATION EDUCATION GROUP PROTOCOL

Description of Group

A group for all patients, regardless of level of concentration, that prepares them for self-management of medication on discharge

Criteria for Member Selection

Open to all inpatients except those who are displaying suicidal or homicidal behaviours or the potential for assault

Visual Aids

PowerPoint slides, transparencies, flip charts, films, patient medication education sheets

Purpose

1. To educate members on the primary function of their medications
2. To provide information on adverse effects (that benefits can outweigh risks)
3. To describe a mechanism to negotiate relationships with health care workers
4. To enhance a sense of self-control over treatment

Procedure

1. Orientation and introduction to the group
2. Brief description of major symptoms in a diagnosis
3. Overview of antipsychotic drugs or antidepressants
4. Use of medication education sheets
5. Specific open question period

Behavioural Objectives

At the end of the 45-minute session, members will be able to:

1. State one of their symptoms that is treated by their medication
2. Ask at least one question about their medication
3. Identify one mechanism that helps in adhering to the medication regimen

Theoretical Justification

Even people who think they are adherent take only 80% of doses. Counselling and therapy are always adjuncts to drug therapy.

Source: Adapted from Ott, C. A. (2000). *Pediatric psychopharmacology.* South Easton, MD: American Healthcare Institute.

Criteria	Strongly Agree	Somewhat Agree	Agree	Disagree	Strongly Disagree
1. I know the name(s) of the medication(s) I am taking.					
2. I know what symptoms the medication(s) can help me with.					
3. I know the common adverse effects of my medication(s).					
4. I feel comfortable talking to my prescriber if I am having problems with my medication(s).					
5. It is important to take my medication(s) at the same time every day.					

FIGURE 33-1 Medication group evaluation tool.

as strategies for interacting with an ill family member and managing crises. Family psychoeducation is a recognized evidence-informed practice in psychosocial rehabilitation (Niemelä, Marshall, Kroll, et al., 2016).

Concurrent disorders. Concurrent disorder groups integrate learning about coexisting mental illnesses and substance abuse. Since treatment issues for people with a concurrent disorder can be complex, group leaders must have demonstrated competency in both mental health and chemical dependence treatment. The goal is to engage people in treatment and decrease their use of substances in a step-by-step process. Research has shown that combined treatment for people with serious mental illness produces improved outcomes (Gamble & O'Lawrence, 2016).

Symptom management. For people with a common symptom such as anger or anxiety, symptom management groups are ideal. The focus is on sharing positive and negative experiences so that members learn coping skills from each other. A primary goal is

to increase self-control or prevent relapse by helping members develop an individualized plan for action at the first appearance of symptoms.

Stress management. Often, time-limited stress management groups teach members about various relaxation techniques, including deep breathing, exercise, music, and spirituality. One such technique that is increasingly demonstrating efficacy in stress management is mindfulness (Kahnen, 2016). Mindfulness groups focus on developing awareness of the present moment, with the intent of inducing relaxation and promoting insight into thoughts, emotions, and physical responses.

Support and self-help groups. Support groups (often facilitated by a professional) and self-help groups (facilitated by the group itself) are structured for the purpose of providing members with the opportunity to maintain or enhance personal and social functioning through cooperation and shared understanding of life's challenges (Yalom, 2005). Examples include support groups for survivors of cancer, bereavement support, or support groups for families who have lost a loved one to suicide. Supportive group therapy can also benefit those with severe mental illness.

The nurse may serve as a resource for individuals and families and must be aware of the wide array of self-help groups available. One of the most important functions of such groups is to demonstrate to individuals and families that they are not alone in having a particular problem. Participants in these types of group report feeling as though their experiences and feelings have been validated. Thus, these groups provide members with support, and their members help each other by telling their stories and providing alternative ways to view and resolve problems. Box 33-4 describes characteristics of support and self-help groups.

Advanced-Practice Nurse or Nurse Therapist
Group Psychotherapy
Group psychotherapy is a specialized treatment intervention in which a trained leader (or co-leaders) establishes a group for the purpose of treating people with psychiatric disorders. Expertise is necessary since the group is used as a tool to bring about change. Often group psychotherapy is done in conjunction with individual psychotherapy as part of an ongoing plan. The Canadian Group Psychotherapy Association provides standards and training for mental health professionals, including nurses, to develop skills in this specialty.

Psychodrama groups. Psychodrama groups are specialized groups in which members are encouraged to act out life experiences or situations for the purpose of learning and insight. Leaders should have graduate-level education and training specific to this approach.

Dialectical behaviour treatment. Dialectical behaviour treatment (DBT) is a type of group psychotherapy in which people are seen each week with the goal of improving interpersonal, behavioural, cognitive, and emotional skills and reducing self-destructive behaviours (Linehan, 1993). Unlike in other types of group therapy, DBT group members are discouraged from making observations about others in the group. This treatment also requires specialized training and advanced education.

Integrative groups. An integrative group program consists of a number of sessions with a particular theme or purpose, in which individual group sessions may draw from any of the aforementioned approaches. An example is a group intervention for vulnerable children, which is reported in the Research Highlight box. Integrative groups may also be used to support and treat psychological symptoms that survivors of interpersonal trauma or abuse may experience. Chapter 24 further describes support and treatment approaches for people who have experienced interpersonal trauma.

Dealing With Challenging Member Behaviours
Research has identified certain behaviours of individual members that are challenging to manage within a group. Defensive behaviours interfere with people's ability to function or achieve satisfaction in their lives. Group therapy is about working through problem behaviours, but some behaviours can be especially

---

BOX 33-4 SUPPORT AND SELF-HELP GROUPS

Target Population
- People who have shared the experience of a common problem, illness, crisis, or tragedy

Group Leader Activities
- May or may not be defined; may rotate among members
- Role is often more task oriented

Examples of Support Groups
- Bereavement groups for those who have experienced the loss of a loved one
- Suicide survivor groups for those who have lost a loved one to suicide
- Canadian Mental Health Association (CMHA) groups for patient or family support (or both), education, and advocacy
- Cancer support groups for families and individuals coping with the ramifications of this illness
- Internet support groups for a growing number of people, providing online, real-time interaction and support

Examples of Self-Help Groups and Resources
- Twelve-step groups that use a common model for recovery:
  - Alcoholics Anonymous (AA)—the prototype for other 12-step groups
  - Gamblers Anonymous (GA)
  - Overeaters Anonymous (OA)
  - Narcotics Anonymous (NA)
  - Co-Dependents Anonymous
  - Adult Children of Alcoholics (ACOA)
- Online listings of self-help resources in Canada:
  - eMentalHealth.ca (listing of national self-help and mutual aid groups): http://www.ementalhealth.ca/canada/en/_Self-help_mutual_aid_and_support_groups_a1_b44.html?filterLocalOnly=1
  - National Network for Mental Health (NNMH): http://nnmh.ca/
  - Self-Help Connection: http://www.selfhelpconnection.ca
  - Canadian Coalition of Alternative Mental Health Resources: http://ccamhr.ca/memberslist.html

Goals of Support and Self-Help Groups
- To provide health education and networking for resources
- To reduce anxiety and decrease feelings of isolation
- To provide support and encouragement of positive coping behaviours:
  - Decrease feelings of isolation
  - Provide mutual support
  - Provide psychoeducation and health education
  - Reduce stress
  - Help people cease self-destructive behaviours or come to terms with an overwhelming event or situation

Frequency and Duration
- Meets one or more times per week for an indefinite period of time
- Ongoing and open membership

RESEARCH HIGHLIGHT

Benefits of an Arts-Based Mindfulness Group Intervention for Vulnerable Children

Problem

Vulnerable children, such as those who have experienced deleterious effects of abuse, neglect, loss, trauma, and family dysfunction on their physical, cognitive, emotional, social, and behavioural development face greater risks for experiencing behaviour problems that can create a myriad of difficulties in later life. It is unclear how teaching vulnerable children mindfulness-based skills and concepts would improve aspects of their resilience and self-concept such as emotion regulation and self-esteem.

Purpose of Study

To explore the effects of a 12-week arts-based mindfulness group program for vulnerable children (children who were involved with the child welfare or mental health system and experienced a variety of challenges) on their level of resiliency and self-concept.

Methods

Interpretive thematic qualitative analysis was conducted using transcribed interview data from postgroup individual interviews with children or guardians. Pre- and postintervention self-report data (using the Piers-Harris Children's Self-Concept Scale and the Resiliency Scales for Children and Adolescents) quantitative analysis was completed.

Key Findings

Qualitative analysis revealed two primary themes. The first theme had to do with the children's perceptions of Holistic Arts-Based Program (e.g., that it's a lot of fun and involves playing games, creating arts and crafts, learning mindfulness, gaining support, and making friends). Most of the children would not change anything about the group except to make it a longer duration and to conduct more activities outside. The second theme involved perceived benefits of participating in the group. Participants reported improved (a) emotion regulation, (b) mood, (c) coping and social skills, (d) confidence and self-esteem, (e) empathy, and (f) ability to pay attention and focus.

The quantitative analysis used self-report data from the participating children. There were issues with gaps in the data collected, which affected the statistical validity of the analysis. Despite these gaps, there was a significant improvement to the perceptions of self-concept. However, factors related to resiliency did not significantly differ before and after intervention.

Implications for Nursing Practice

With increased understanding of one's feelings and thoughts, a child can make better choices regarding his or her emotional expression, which can lead to improved functioning at school, home, and with peers. Nurses can use a group-delivered intervention to decrease the sense of isolation and improve a child's self-concept. Further research is needed regarding effective strategies to increase resilience.

Source: Coholic, D. A., & Eys, M. (2016). Benefits of an arts-based mindfulness group intervention for vulnerable children. *Child and Adolescent Social Work Journal, 33*(1), 1–13. doi:10.1007/s10560-015-0431-3.

disruptive to the group process and difficult for the leader to manage. The person who monopolizes the group, the person who complains but continues to reject help, the demoralizing person, and the silent person are examples (Yalom, 2005).

In dealing with any problematic behaviours in groups, members may appreciate help disclosing their own feelings and responses. The leader encourages the use of statements such as "When you speak this way, I feel …" The leader helps by noting that feelings are not right or wrong but simply exist. People tend to feel less defensive when "I feel" statements rather than "you are" statements are used. This approach helps members feel like part of the group, not alienated from it.

Monopolizing Member

The person who monopolizes the group may be attempting to deal with anxiety. As group tension grows, the person's level of anxiety rises, and the tendency to speak increases. Some people are just extremely talkative or may be hypertalkative due to hypomania or mania. In any case, no one else gets a chance to be heard, and other group members eventually lose interest and begin to withdraw.

VIGNETTE

Holly is the most talkative member of the group until the nurse intervenes. Initially, Holly talks at length about her early experiences related to losing both of her parents and having to live with her grandparents. The other members of the group become bored with the same old story, and they drift off. They have heard these stories many times, not only in group therapy but also during other activities.

There are several useful strategies for dealing with an overly talkative group member. One strategy is to request a response from group members who have not had a chance to talk about the day's topic. If the behaviour continues, it may be necessary to speak directly to the monopolizing group member, either privately or in the group setting. In private, you can share your observations and suggest that perhaps nervousness may be a factor causing the talkativeness. Asking for clarification may lead to a greater understanding of what the group member is experiencing. You may then ask him or her to limit contributions to a specific number of times (e.g., two or three). In the group setting, the leader may ask the group members if they would like to share observations or feedback about other members, thereby offering a chance for growth. This strategy is probably the most challenging but potentially the most rewarding in that members feel empowered and the real therapeutic forces of groups are realized.

Complaining Member Who Rejects Help

The person who complains but continues to reject help brings problems to the group, often describing them in a manner that makes the problems seem insurmountable. In fact, the person appears to take pride in the insolubility of his or her problems. He or she comes across as entirely self-centred, and the group's attempts to help are continually rejected.

The person who uses these tactics generally has highly conflicting feelings about his or her own dependency; any notice from the leader temporarily increases the person's self-esteem. On the other hand, the person has a pervasive mistrust of all authority figures. Most people who complain but continue to reject help have been subjected to severe deprivation early in their lives and may have experienced emotional or physical abuse or both.

VIGNETTE

Shamaila is always complaining about how horrible her relationship with her boyfriend is, and she manages to get the entire group worked up over the situation. Members tell her to leave him, not to spend all her time with him, and not to spend all her money on him, but each week she reports a new incident or crisis. In every session, the group members become concerned and offer encouragement, advice, and solutions. Each time, the group becomes angry at her lack of change, and she is frustrated by her own inability to change. She asserts that the group is not helpful.

The leader should acknowledge the person's pessimism but maintain a neutral affect. If the person stays in the group long enough, and the group develops a sense of cohesion, this individual can be helped to recognize relationship patterns. The leader should encourage the person to look at the habitual "yes … but" behaviour objectively.

Demoralizing Member

Some people whose behaviour is self-centred, angry, or depressed may lack empathy or concern for other members of the group. They refuse to take any personal responsibility and can challenge the group leader and negatively affect the group process.

VIGNETTE

Dina comes to the support group on the inpatient psychiatric unit. She is very angry, stating, "I don't know why I come to these groups anyway! They don't help." Dina is to be discharged the next day to a 28-day alcohol rehabilitation program. She has a previously scheduled dental appointment before the rehabilitation intake interview, and she is being strongly encouraged by her therapist to reschedule the appointment. The therapist fears that Dina is at high risk for drinking again, because she states that she constantly has the urge to drink. When a group member who is an addictions therapist confronts Dina about not being flexible and prioritizing her need for alcohol treatment, she explodes. "I thought this group was for support. This is outrageous!" Group members are obviously uncomfortable with her anger.

In this case, the group leader should listen to the comments objectively. Again, the leader may choose to speak to the group member in private and ask what is causing the anger. Sometimes this simple exchange can make the person feel a greater connection with the nurse and more important as a member of the group, which likely will decrease hostile behaviour and increase the

group's benefit. In the group setting, the leader can focus on positive group members, whose comments may reduce the hostility of the negative group member.

Remember that angry people may be extremely vulnerable, and devaluing or demoralizing keeps others at a distance and maintains the person's own precarious sense of safety. Leaders must empathize with the member in a matter-of-fact manner, such as "You seem angry that the group wants to support you in putting sobriety ahead of your dental needs."

Silent Member

Members who are silent in the group may be observing intently until they decide that the group is safe for them, or they may believe that they are not as competent as other, more assertive group members. Silence does not mean that the member is not engaged or involved, but it should be addressed, for several reasons. The person who does not speak cannot benefit from others' feedback, and other group members are deprived of this group member's valuable insights. Furthermore, a silent group member may make others uncomfortable and create a sense of mistrust.

VIGNETTE

Anne has attended three group sessions for survivors of childhood sexual abuse. Although she appears to be listening, she rarely makes eye contact with the leader or other group members. She responds to yes or no questions, but when it comes to open-ended questions such as "What do you think, Anne?" she tends to shrug her shoulders and respond with "I don't know." Other group members have tried to draw Anne out, as has the leader. Katia, another group member, is beginning to exhibit frustration with Anne: "Look, I have shared some of the most private and painful memories of my childhood. I feel like you think you're too good to share what happened to you."

There are several techniques that may help in this case, including allowing the person to have extra time to formulate his or her thoughts before responding. Saying, "I'll give you a moment to think about that" and then waiting or coming back to the group member later is often helpful. Another tactic is to make an assignment that every person in the group respond to a certain topic or question. For example, "Let's all think of a positive and assertive response to something that you generally feel helpless about. I'll give you a minute or so to think this topic over, and then I'm going to ask each of you to share."

Sometimes partnering with another group member will give the silent member the courage she or he needs to participate. You may break the group into pairs and ask them to discuss a certain topic and then each report back to the group what they heard the other person say.

EXPECTED OUTCOMES

Expected outcomes of group participation will vary, depending on the type and purpose of the group. For education groups, such as a medication education group, the expected outcome would be demonstration of knowledge. For therapy groups, the expected outcomes will focus more on insights, behaviour changes, and reduction in symptoms. For example, in an alcohol treatment group, an expected outcome might be that the person develops insight into the connection between drinking and negative consequences. An expected behavioural outcome could be abstinence from alcohol use. In groups that focus primarily on emotional issues such as depression or anxiety, standardized tests can be used to measure symptom reduction as an outcome of group participation.

KEY POINTS TO REMEMBER

- Research has identified 11 therapeutic factors that operate in groups and lead to therapeutic change for members. Yalom's therapeutic factors identify specific positive aspects of groups, such as universality of experience, imparting information, altruism, corrective recapitulation of the primary family group, development of socializing techniques, imitative behaviour, interpersonal learning, group cohesiveness, catharsis and existential resolution, and the instillation of hope.
- When a new group is formed, similarities and differences in many dimensions, including diagnosis, age, gender, and culture, must be considered.
- A group format has advantages over individual therapy, including cost savings, increased feedback, an opportunity to practise new skills in a relatively safe environment, and instillation of a sense of belonging.
- Groups develop through predictable phases over time.
- For a group to continue and be productive, members must fulfill specific functions known as *task* or *maintenance roles*.

- Individual roles are not productive and are based on individual personalities and needs.
- Clinical supervision is important so that group leaders can objectively analyze group interactions and leadership techniques.
- Nurses have opportunities to lead or co-lead therapeutic groups, some in the hospital but primarily in community settings.
- Psychoeducational groups, activity groups, task groups, and support groups are often led by nurses and provide significant treatment as part of the multidisciplinary treatment plan.
- Advanced-practice nurses and nurse therapists may lead psychotherapy groups based on various theoretical models.
- Challenging member behaviours, such as silence, complaining, or demoralizing, can be especially difficult. A variety of interventions are recommended to minimize the disruption to the group and maximize the benefit to the person engaging in these behaviours.

CRITICAL THINKING

1. You are assigned to work with Malia, a 30-year-old woman who was admitted to the psychiatric unit with major depression after recently harming herself. Her nurse has told her she needs to attend group therapy. While lying in bed and staring at the ceiling, Malia tells you that she is a private person and that listening to other people's problems will not help and will only make her more depressed.
   a. How would you describe the benefits of group therapy to Malia?
   b. What interventions might make it easier for Malia to attend group therapy?
2. Construct an outline for a medication teaching group that would cover information useful for your patients. If possible, co-lead this group with a staff member, with guidelines from your instructor.

3. Ms. Joseph is a 22-year-old Haitian-born nursing student admitted to the psychiatric unit after a nearly lethal overdose of acetaminophen (Tylenol). She admits to drinking excessively for the past 6 months. She is at risk for failing school. She complains of depressed mood, a loss of interest in her studies, decreased concentration, and social isolation. In the concurrent disorders group, she has been silent for the past two sessions and sits staring at the floor.
   a. What is your evaluation of Ms. Joseph's situation?
   b. What might Ms. Joseph's nonverbal behaviour mean?
   c. What approach would you use to involve her more in the group?
   d. What criteria could you use to evaluate the effectiveness of your intervention?
   e. What cultural implications should you consider?

CHAPTER REVIEW

1. The nurse is caring for four patients. Which patient would not be appropriate to consider for group therapy?
   a. The patient with limited financial resources
   b. The patient who is acutely manic
   c. The patient who has few friends on the unit
   d. The patient who does not speak up often, yet listens to others

2. The nurse tells group members that they will be working on expressing conflicts during the current group session. Which phase of group development is represented?
   a. Formation phase
   b. Orientation phase
   c. Working phase
   d. Termination phase

3. Group members are having difficulty deciding what topic to cover in today's session. Which nurse leader response reflects autocratic leadership?
   a. "We are talking about fear of rejection today."
   b. "Let's go around the room and make suggestions for today's topic."
   c. "I will let you come to a conclusion together about what to talk about."
   d. "I'll work with you to find a suitable topic for today."

4. The nurse is planning care that includes a concurrent disorders group. A patient with which of the following disorders would be appropriate for this group?
   a. Depression and suicidal tendencies
   b. Anxiety and frequent migraine headaches
   c. Bipolar disorder and anorexia nervosa
   d. Schizophrenia and alcohol abuse

5. A member continues to dominate the group conversation despite having been asked to allow others to speak. What is the most appropriate nursing response to address this behaviour?
   a. "You are monopolizing the conversation."
   b. "When you talk constantly, it makes everyone feel angry."
   c. "You are supposed to allow others to talk also."
   d. "When you speak out of turn, I feel concerned that others cannot participate equally."

℮volve WEBSITE

Post-Test interactive review

Visit the Evolve website for Chapter Review Answers and Rationales, Critical Thinking Answer Guidelines, and additional resources related to the content in this chapter: http://evolve.elsevier.com/Canada/Varcarolis/psychiatric/

REFERENCES

Benne, K. D., & Sheats, P. (1948). Functional roles of group members. *Journal of Social Issues, 4*, 41–49. doi:10.1111/j.1540-4560.1948.tb01783.x.

Bernhardsdottir, J., Vilhjalmsson, R., & Champion, J. D. (2013). Evaluation of a brief cognitive behavioral group therapy for psychological distress among female Icelandic university students. *Issues in Mental Health Nursing, 34*(7), 497–504.

Burlingame, G. (2010). Small group treatments: Introduction to special section. *Psychotherapy Research: Journal of the Society for Psychotherapy Research, 20*, 1–7.

Canadian Federation of Psychiatric Mental Health Nurses (2014). *Canadian standards for psychiatric-mental health nursing* (4th ed.). Toronto: Author.

Canadian Nurses Association (2008). *Code of ethics for registered nurses* (2008 centennial ed.). Ottawa: Author.

Gamble, J., & O'Lawrence, H. (2016). An overview of the efficacy of the 12-step group therapy for substance abuse treatment. *Journal of Health and Human Services Administration, 29*(1), 142–160. Retrieved from http://jhhsa.spaef.org/.

Joyce, A. S., MacNair-Semands, R., Tasca, G. A., et al. (2011). Factor structure and validity of the Therapeutic Factors Inventory–Short Form. *Group Dynamics: Theory, Research, and Practice, 15*(3), 201.

Kahnen, D. (2016). How does decreasing stress impact the healthy practice environment. *Medsurg Nursing, 25*(4), 12–17. Retrieved from http://www.medsurgnursing.net/cgi-bin/WebObjects/MSNJournal.woa.

Linehan, M. M. (1993). *Cognitive behavioral treatment of borderline personality disorder.* New York: Guilford.

Niemelä, M., Marshall, C. A., Kroll, T., et al. (2016). Family-focused preventive interventions with cancers cosurvivors: A call to action. *American Journal of Public Health, 106*(8), 1381–1387. doi:10.2105/AJPH.2016.303178.

Yalom, I. D. (2005). *The theory and practice of group psychotherapy* (5th ed.). New York: Basic Books.

Family Interventions

Laura G. Leahy, Laura Cox Dzurec
Adapted by Sonya L. Jakubec

KEY TERMS AND CONCEPTS

behavioural family therapy
boundaries
clear boundaries
enmeshed boundaries
family systems theory
family triangle
flexibility

genogram
insight-oriented family therapy
intergenerational issues
nuclear family
psychoeducational family therapy
rigid boundaries
sociocultural context

OBJECTIVES

1. Define the concept of family.
2. Differentiate between functional and dysfunctional family patterns of behaviour as they relate to the five family functions.
3. Compare and contrast insight-oriented family therapy and behavioural family therapy.
4. Identify family theorists and their contributions to the family therapy movement.
5. Incorporate the family's sociocultural context when assessing and planning intervention strategies.
6. Construct a genogram using a three-generation approach.

7. Formulate outcome criteria that a nurse counsellor and family might develop together.
8. Identify strategies for family intervention in specific psychiatric clinical situations.
9. Distinguish between the nursing intervention strategies of a basic-level nurse and those of an advanced-practice nurse with regard to counselling and psychotherapy and psychobiological issues.
10. Explain the importance of the nurse's role in psychoeducational family therapy.

⊖volve WEBSITE

Visit the Evolve website for Flashcards, Case Studies, and additional testing resources related to the content in this chapter: http://evolve.elsevier.com/Canada/Varcarolis/psychiatric/

Pre-Test | interactive review

Although family structure and function have changed dramatically over the years, the Canadian family remains central to the fabric of Canadian society. Same-sex marriages, recognition of common-law relationships, and blended families have influenced family structure and roles. In addition, Canada is a multicultural society with diverse cultural expectations of family roles, all of which are subject to societal influences. As the second-wave feminist movement of the 1960s advocated for gender equality, more women began working outside the family home, moving toward emancipation. As a result, today's family frequently consists of a range of configurations of one, two, or more people leading the household, with children and without, as well as working inside and outside of the home (Evans & Chamberlain, 2015).

As another example of the numerous societal influences on Canadian families, in the late nineteenth century, the Canadian government's assimilation policies toward Indigenous peoples significantly influenced the erosion of Indigenous traditional family structure and values. The residential school system policies severely affected family structure, parenting roles, and traditions, which contributed to intergenerational trauma and cultural loss. Children were removed from their homes and lost their culture, language, and connection to family and the land. Furthermore, adoption policies allowed for the removal of Indigenous children from their homes to be adopted by White families. These events have inserted patterns affected by intergenerational trauma into the lives of many families. The consequences of intergenerational trauma have inextricably changed the way people view themselves; their children, parents, and leaders; and their relationship to society (Bellamy & Hardy, 2015; Kirmayer, Tait, & Simpson, 2009; Klinic Community Health Center, 2013). The Truth and Reconciliation Commission of Canada (TRC, 2015) and The United Nations Declaration on the Rights of Indigenous Peoples (United Nations, 2007) have established awareness and recognition of Indigenous history and culture. Expanded awareness and strength is compelling action toward healing destructive family patterns through innovative family programs such as Indigenous family court, healing programs, and Indigenous family therapy that recognize the effects of trauma and create cultural safety and growth (Ontario Centre of Excellence for Child and Youth Mental Health, 2017).

Canadian families are experiencing rapid change in these functions, and there is a growing diversity in family configurations within a rapidly changing, globalized, fast-paced society. Alongside these changing family structures, environments, and societal organization, more is being demanded of families in all facets of functioning. For example, caregiving for and support of family members who are experiencing physical illness, mental illness, and aging continue to expand, with implications for family functioning. Nearly half of all Canadians (13 million) have provided care to a family member or friend with a long-term health condition, disability, or aging-related need at some point in their lives, and 8 million do so each year (Turcotte, 2013).

Family in its ideal form may provide security, kinship, a means to maintain traditions and culture, and a place of belonging. As such, family is a positive force in assisting its members through crises and the life cycle. Alternatively, family experiences may include difficulties such as all manner of crises, differences and interpersonal conflict, mental illness, poverty, or violence. It is within these diverse and challenging social and family contexts that nurses strive to provide *family-centred care*, an approach that is characterized by dignity and respect, information sharing, patient and family participation, and family–professional collaboration (Registered Nurses' Association of Ontario, 2015).

Family intervention may assist such families to gain healthy ways to adjust to change, to grow, and to gain skills for stronger ways of being. Some families may need psychotherapeutic intervention during the early years of a child's development to assist the child and family to correct maladaptive patterns. The impact of conflict, crisis, and violence on children and their longer term mental health and functioning has been well documented (Layne, Abramovitz, Stuber, et al., 2017), as explored in Chapters 24 and 27. During times of crisis, inclusive of health crises, many families require psychological, emotional, and practical supports to restore their equilibrium. Family interventions may minimize psychological impairment and build on the strengths of the family. To facilitate nonjudgemental and sensitive practice to assist families to grow with change or heal from particularly overwhelming circumstances, nurses require education in and understanding of diverse family experiences, economics, emotions, and context (Varcoe & Doane, 2015). This chapter explores the definitions and boundaries of families, examines sites of family conflict, and identifies specific family therapies for both entry-level and advanced practice.

FAMILY

What is a family? The Registered Nurses' Association of Ontario (2015) and Wright and Leahey (2013) state that families are self-defined—in other words, a family is made up of the people the patient identifies as family and can include neighbours and significant people in the community. When working with families, nurses must be sensitive about and honour the patient's identification of family (Wright & Leahey, 2013).

The family is the primary system to which a person belongs. Birth, puberty, marriage, and death occur within the context of the family experience. The family can be a source of love or hate, pride or shame, and security or insecurity. Although individual family members have roles and functions, the over-riding value in families lies in the relationships among family members. It is these family relationships that provide the primary context of human development. Many family theorists consider the intergenerational connectedness of the family to be one of our greatest human resources.

VIGNETTE

Anna Lowen is a 54-year-old Hutterite Canadian woman who has been admitted to the acute psychiatric ward for an episode of mania. She had been diagnosed with bipolar disorder several years before and has had two previous episodes of mania. Anna lives in a Hutterite colony with her three children and her husband, Jake, and is respected for her hard work and good nature with older adults and children.

Before being admitted to the hospital, she had been unable to sleep or eat for 1 week. In the mornings she was loud and irritable in the community kitchen and insisted on serving all of the children large bowls of porridge with eggs that she had collected from the henhouse. She was wandering the colony grounds, singing loudly in the middle of the night, when her family brought her to the hospital in the city. Currently, she is on a medication to stabilize her mood and help her to sleep and eat.

Her husband, sisters, and several community members are visiting her at the hospital. The children have been left at the colony and do not understand what has happened to their mother. The nurse assesses the situation and adopts a family-centred nursing care approach inclusive of the community members. First, he identifies his own need to increase his understanding of the Hutterite culture, adapts psychoeducational materials to meet the family's needs, and encourages the family to bring the children to a meeting to have their questions about their mother answered.

Family Functions

Families are unique, each having its own strengths, resources, and challenges (Varcoe & Doane, 2015; Wright & Leahey, 2013). However, some general characteristics of a family include future obligations and caregiving functions, such as protection, nourishment, and socialization of its members (McGoldrick, Garcia Preto, & Carter, 2016). The Vanier Institute of the Family (2017) identified the following as functions of a Canadian family:

- Provision of love and nurturance
- Socialization of children
- Social control of members
- Production and consumption of goods and services
- Addition of new family members through birth or adoption
- Physical care and maintenance of family members

These functions take place within a societal context, which also influences family members.

Families play a significant, often unrecognized, role as caregivers (Turcotte, 2013). In certain contexts the burden of caregiving is considerable—for example, with additional barriers for the care of older parents or elders in rural and remote Indigenous communities (Habjan, Prince, & Kelley, 2012). Not all caregivers, however, are adults. It is estimated that 10% of children have a parent with a mental illness, largely undiagnosed and untreated (Gladstone, Boydell, Seeman, et al., 2011). These children are often invisibly caregivers of their parents. Assuming too much responsibility in childhood could interfere with attainment of children's developmental needs. Stigma also affects these children's experiences and well-being throughout their lives (Murphy, Peters, Wilkes, et al., 2017), as it does for parents supporting adult children who are experiencing mental illness (Park & Seo, 2016; Raymond, Willis, & Sullivan-Bolyai, 2017). Respite, education, and support are important interventions for both of these types of family members supporting other family members with mental illness experiences.

Families and Mental Illness

Historically, when mental illness occurred, health care providers often cast blame on the family. Blame was particularly predominant in the mental illness of children, especially those with autism, eating disorders, or schizophrenia. Theories charged that mothers' ways of interacting with their children were the root cause of child disturbance. Today, theories suggest holistic, complex explanations for illness (Mental Health Commission of Canada, 2013), but self-stigma and blame persist for many parents (Eaton, Ohan, Stritzke, et al., 2016). Nurses need to be aware of this history and pattern of parental blame, as remnants of these ideas linger.

An important component of nursing practice is to advise family members of appropriate support groups. Those experiencing a first psychotic break of a child are particularly vulnerable to being overwhelmed by the situation. Parental support groups such as the Prevention and Early Intervention Program for Psychoses (www.PEPP.ca) in London, Ontario, were founded to assist such families. In addition, family support programs through the Schizophrenia Society of Canada and Canadian Mental Health Association assist all family members, parents, children, spouses, friends, and other loved ones in a number of educational, social support, and recreational program options.

CANADIAN MODELS OF FAMILY NURSING CARE AND ASSESSMENT

Three esteemed Canadian models of family care are the McGill Model of Nursing, developed by Dr. Moyra Allan, and the Calgary Family Assessment Model and Calgary Family Intervention Model, both based on the work of Wright and Leahey (2013). These models guide both beginning and advanced-level nurses to practise from a family nursing perspective.

McGill Model of Nursing

The McGill Model of Nursing (http://www.mcgill.ca/nursing/about/model/) focuses on family health, collaboration, learning, and health promotion. It was developed in response to health care system changes that occurred when universal health care was introduced in Canada. It has been widely adopted in Canada within many diverse nursing areas. Its main assumption is that families possess strengths, motivations, and resources. These serve to assist families to move toward health promotion, which will result in improved health outcomes. Because health behaviour is predominantly learned within the family context, it is imperative that nurses focus on working with the family by setting goals and establishing learning environments to share knowledge, build on existing knowledge, and assist in making changes in behaviours. Family members become active learners in the implementation phase of the nursing process. The processes of coping and development are dynamic (i.e., they occur in any phase). Family health is achieved by building on the strengths of the family and its individual members and using external resources, such as nurses and other health care providers. Ultimately, however, it is patients and families who are deemed experts in their own care in this model (Gottlieb, 2013).

Calgary Family Assessment Model (CFAM) and Calgary Family Intervention Model (CFIM)

The basic assumptions underlying CFAM and CFIM are derived from systems, communication, differing views of reality, and change theories. The models are multidimensional and consider structure, development, and function to guide a nurse's interventions with families (Wright & Leahey, 2013). The assessment and intervention approaches focus on promoting and improving family functioning in three domains: cognitive, affective, and behavioural. The CFIM recommends many relational nursing practices that promote family health and functioning, including asking interventive questions, offering commendations, providing information, validating emotional responses, encouraging illness narratives, supporting family caregivers, and encouraging respite. Within a nurturing and nonhierarchical relationship, this approach to family nursing interventions privileges family expertise and is anchored by a commitment to listen deeply to the concerns, suffering, and questions of family members.

The guidance provided by Varcoe and Doane (2015) in their discussion of relational inquiry is another helpful guide for relational engagement with the families encountered in a nurse's practice.

FAMILY THERAPY

Family therapy is a psychotherapeutic process that focuses on changing the interactions among the people who make up the family or marital unit. It serves to improve the family, the subsystems within the family, and the individuals who make up the family. It focuses on evaluating these relationships and the communication patterns, structure, and rules that govern the family interactions (Sadock, Sadock, & Ruiz, 2017). Although novice nurses do not engage in family therapy, nurses may take additional educational courses to develop family therapy skills.

Every day, in every family, decisions are made regarding the functions of power, rule making, provision of financial support, future planning, and goods allocation. Families may address these functions in a variety of ways, but most commonly the adults in the family determine how these functions are to be performed. In lone-parent families, these functions may sometimes become overwhelming, highlighting the need for additional supports. In chaotic families, a family member not well prepared to make decisions, such as a teenager, may be the decision maker. Although children learn decision-making skills as they mature and increasingly make choices about their own lives, they should not be expected to take on responsibility for the family. Cultural expectations and norms affect the allocation of roles and perspectives on how families negotiate these tasks.

Boundaries are the distinctions made between individuals in the family. Boundaries may be clear, enmeshed, rigid, or inconsistent (Box 34-1). Most families exhibit several combinations of the various boundary types (Goldenberg, Stanton, & Goldenberg, 2017). When boundaries are functioning properly, family members work out arrangements by compromise based on an understanding of appropriate roles. Each generation is made aware of how decisions will be made and clearly understands who is in charge and when. Blurred boundary function results in family members interfering with each other's goals, creating tension and anxiety between family members. Children in these families may become confused, manipulative, and insecure.

Issues Associated With Family Therapies
Communication

Communication patterns are important in family life. Healthy communication patterns are characterized by clear and comprehensible messages (e.g., "I would like to go now"; "I don't like it when you interrupt what I'm saying"). Families with healthy communication are encouraged to ask for what they want and to express their feelings appropriately. In these families, both affection and conflict are openly expressed, and members have no need to resort to manipulation. When communication is unclear, solving problems or resolving conflicts becomes difficult; therefore the cardinal rule for effective and functional communication is "Be clear and direct in saying what you want and need."

As simple as this concept may seem, it may be difficult to activate in a family system. To be direct, individuals must first have a sense that the self is respected and loved; they then will

---

BOX 34-1 TYPES OF BOUNDARIES

- **Clear boundaries**: Boundaries that are well understood by all members of the family and give family members a sense of "*I*-ness" and also "*we*-ness." They help define family members' roles and allow members to function without unnecessary interference from other members. However, they are not so rigid as to restrict contact among family members. For example, a mother tells her 14-year-old daughter, "You don't need to worry whether your little brother eats his breakfast. Your father and I will handle that." This boundary may be redefined: "I want you to make sure that your little brother gets his homework done while your father and I are at the movies."
- **Enmeshed boundaries** (also called *diffuse boundaries*): Boundaries that result from a blending together of the roles, thoughts, and feelings of the individual family members so that clear distinctions fail to emerge. The members of a family that operates with enmeshed boundaries are more prone to psychological or psychosomatic symptoms. A common phenomenon within families with enmeshed boundaries is that individuals expect other members of the family to know what they are thinking (e.g., "Why did you take that? You know I wanted it!") and believe they know what other family members are thinking (e.g., "I know exactly why you did that!").
- **Rigid boundaries** (also called *disengaged boundaries*): Boundaries in which the rules and roles are consistently adhered to no matter what; thus, rigid boundaries prevent family members from trying out new roles or, in some cases, from taking on more mature functions as time goes on. In families in which rigid boundaries predominate, isolation may be marked. Family members are often cut off from the community and outside influences and even from each other.

VIGNETTE

Liz would like to spend more time on the weekends with her husband, Michael; however, Michael always seems to be busy around the house or talking with friends on the telephone. Liz feels that he does not notice her or maybe is not interested in her, so she spends a lot of time working out. Michael figures that Liz is doing what she wants to do and that it makes her happy, so he contents himself with finding things to do alone. The result is that Liz and Michael spend little time together. Liz finally confronts Michael clearly and directly about his "lack of interest" in her and tells him what she wants and needs—to spend more time together on the weekends. Michael replies that he had no idea she felt that way. He had thought she enjoyed the way things were, and he would like to have more time together too.

---

be confident to set healthy boundaries with others. The consequences of being clear and direct may be unpleasant when boundaries are enmeshed and confusion is the norm. Changing a family pattern will cause discomfort in the system. Explicitly stating what one wants and needs is especially difficult when one believes that family members should already know—especially if the family member is a spouse, a parent, or a close sibling. No one is able to mind-read, but emotionally undifferentiated

BOX 34-2   EXAMPLES OF DYSFUNCTIONAL COMMUNICATION

Manipulating: Instead of asking directly, family members manipulate others to get what they want. A family member makes requests with "strings attached" so that the other person has a difficult time refusing the request: "If you do this for me, I won't tell Daddy you are getting poor grades in school."

Distracting: To avoid functional problem solving and resolve conflicts within the family, family members introduce irrelevant details into problematic issues (e.g., asking who picked up the dry cleaning when discussing communication problems).

Generalizing: When dealing with problematic family issues, members use global statements like *always* and *never* instead of dealing with specific problems and areas of conflict. Family members may say "Adem is always angry" instead of "Adem, what is upsetting you?"

Blaming: Family members blame other family members for failures, errors, or negative consequences of an action to keep the focus away from themselves. Blaming is a response to fear of being blamed by others.

Placating: Family members pretend to be inadequate but well meaning to keep peace in the family at any price: "Don't yell at the children, dear. I'll put the shoes on the stairs."

members may believe that family members can. The following vignette describes a spousal situation that shows how easily communication can be misunderstood when clear and direct messages are not sent. See Box 34-2 for examples of unhealthy communication patterns.

Emotional Support

All families encounter conflicts during their life journeys. However, in a healthy family, feelings of affection are generally uppermost, and anger and conflict do not dominate the family's pattern of interaction. Healthy families are concerned about each other and consistently meet family members' emotional and physical needs. Members feel supported and free to grow and explore new roles and facets of their personalities. A family that is dominated by conflict and anger alienates its members, leaving them isolated, fearful, and emotionally fragile. It is important for the nurse to note that patterns of family crises, including issues arising from substance use, may have underlying links to intergenerational trauma, historical oppression, and colonization.

Socialization

Within families, each member learns socialization skills. People learn coping skills and how to interact, negotiate, and plan for the future. Children learn to socialize effectively within the family and then apply their skills in society.

Family Life Cycle

The life cycle of individuals takes place within the family life cycle, the primary context of human development. Family life takes place within relationships, and changes within the relationships affect the roles of the parents. For example, as children mature and leave home, parents may renegotiate the pattern of their lives together. "Boomerang children" may unexpectedly return home, causing yet another change in family roles. Later, parents may need their adult children's help as they become less able to care for themselves. As the Canadian population ages, more family members will be providing care to older adult parents.

In the traditional Canadian family type, there are six main phases of the family life cycle: (1) launching the single young adult, (2) joining families through couple formation, (3) becoming parents and caring for young children, (4) parenting adolescents, (5) launching children and moving on, and (6) experiencing later life, often encompassing the role of grandparent. Families may experience some of the phases and not others. In addition, with the increased cultural diversity of Canadian society, nurses may expect to see diverse interpretations of family tasks.

The family system moves through time, with potential for family stress at transition points (e.g., birth of a child, employment changes, children leaving home, retirement) or during an interruption in the life cycle (e.g., untoward events such as an unexpected death by suicide, first psychotic break of a young adult, imprisonment, divorce). At these times, therapy may be required to assist family members to proceed in the life cycle. For family members who feel trapped within a dysfunctional family system, extreme pressures can lead to distress or even suicide. Symptoms can be perceived as a response to an interruption in the family life cycle. This family life cycle assumes a traditional family organization and requires modification for increasingly nontraditional family structures (McGoldrick, Garcia Preto, & Carter, 2016).

Working With the Family

Many concepts are used when working with families. The concepts of the *identified patient*, the *family triangle*, and the *nuclear family emotional system* are discussed here. Box 34-3 describes other concepts relevant to family work.

The Identified Patient

The *identified patient* is the individual in the family whom everyone regards as "the problem." A descriptive term for this person is the "family symptom-bearer." This family member is generally the focus of most of the family system's anxiety. She or he may serve to divert the attention from other more serious and debilitating problems within the family, such as a crumbling marriage, substance abuse, or infidelity. Furthermore, the symptoms of the identified patient may serve as a stabilizing mechanism to bring about customary behaviour in a distressed family (Goldenberg, Stanton, & Goldenberg, 2017). The identified patient may even be aware at some level of the role he or she serves in "saving" the family. For example, adult children may sacrifice their autonomy by staying in the home to hold the parents together.

When a family comes for treatment, the presenting problem, which is usually related to one member of the family, must be addressed before the underlying systemic problem. The family

BOX 34-3 CENTRAL CONCEPTS OF FAMILY SYSTEMS THEORY

Triangulation: The tendency, when two-person relationships are stressful and unstable, to draw in a third person to stabilize the system through the formation of a coalition in which the two join the third. Triangles often occur with low differentiation and high anxiety and tend to draw in the third person but freeze the conflict as irresolvable.

Scapegoating: A form of displacement in which a family member (usually the least powerful) is blamed for another family member's distress. The purpose is to keep the focus off the painful issues and problems of the blamers. In a family, the blamers are often the parents, and the scapegoat is a child.

Double bind: A situation in which a positive command (often verbal) is followed by a negative command (often nonverbal), which leaves the recipient confused, trapped, and immobilized because there is no appropriate way to act. A double bind is a "no win" situation in which you are "darned if you do, darned if you don't."

Hierarchy: The function of power and its structures in families, differentiating parental and sibling roles and generational boundaries.

Family life cycle: The family's developmental process over time; refers to the family's past course, its present tasks, and its future course.

Differentiation: The ability to develop a strong identity and sense of self while at the same time maintaining an emotional connectedness with one's family of origin.

Sociocultural context: The broader social and ecological framework for viewing the family in terms of the influence of gender, race, ethnicity, religion, economic class, and sexual orientation.

Mino-Pimatisiwin (an Indigenous approach to helping): Seeking the good life with a focus on the interconnections between individual, family, community and nations. Key concepts are wholeness, balance, harmony, and healing (Debassige, 2010).

Intergenerational issues: The continuation and persistence from generation to generation of certain emotional interactive family patterns. Various patterns of behaviour (e.g., involving geographical distance between members, suicide, divorce, addiction, affairs, grief, triangles, historical colonization, loss) that continue to affect successive generations.

Family Triangles

Bowen's (1985) focus was on patterns that develop in families in order to defuse anxiety. A key generator of anxiety in families is the perception of either too much closeness or too great a distance in a relationship. The degree of anxiety in any one family will be determined by the current levels of external stress and the sensitivities to particular themes that have been transmitted down the generations. If family members do not have the capacity to think through their responses to relationship dilemmas, but rather react anxiously to perceived emotional demands, a state of chronic anxiety or reactivity may be set in place. Bowen described an important and common relationship process in families; it can be seen as a system of interlocking triangles. When tension in a family is low, the dyad or two-person system may interact comfortably, although some tension lies in the struggle between closeness and independence. When the tension in a close twosome builds, a third person (child, friend, or parent) may be brought in to help lower the tension. The family triangle (Figure 34-1) then becomes the basic building block of interpersonal relationships. All triangles contain a close side, a distant side, and a side in which conflict or tension exists between two people (Ramisch & Nelson, 2014).

The intensity of the triangulation process varies among families and within the same family over time because triangles create emotional instability. The lower the level of differentiation in a family, the higher the tension is and the more important the role of triangulation is to lowering tension and preserving emotional stability. As the family becomes stressed for whatever reasons, the anxiety in the system is triggered, and the triangles become more active.

A common problem that occurs in families is the setting up of a triangle among two parents and a child; one parent is overinvolved with the child, and the other plays a more peripheral role. In this situation, the child eventually becomes the means by which the parents communicate with each other about issues they cannot deal with directly. In other words, spousal conflicts may be brought into the parental arena, where they do not belong.

---

member who is the identified patient may or may not be the one who initially seeks help from inpatient or outpatient services.

When working with families, it is important to consider not only the family as a system in a particular stage of life cycle development but also the individual developmental stage of each family member. For example, a family may present with parents in Erikson's stage of generativity vs. stagnation, adolescent children dealing with identity vs. role confusion issues, a school-aged child facing challenges of industry vs. inferiority, and grandparents dealing with ego integrity vs. despair. Thus there is more than one perspective to be considered when looking at the identified patient in terms of the family system. The focus is on the family system's anxiety.

VIGNETTE

Six-year-old Kami is having trouble making friends. Her mother, Makayla, has been feeling anxious and helpless as she tries to find ways to engage Kami with other youngsters. Makayla develops an overprotectiveness that further inhibits Kami from making friends. Makayla feels that her husband, Leon, is uncaring and disinterested because he thinks that she should be more relaxed about Kami's social life and let things develop naturally. Leon's job requires that he travel most of the week, so he is not involved with Makayla's daily experiences and struggles with Kami.

Makayla and Leon have been avoiding intimacy for almost a year. Makayla is angry with Leon for spending so much time with his parents, which further casts him in a peripheral role in their nuclear family, and Leon is angry with Makayla, sensing her rejection of him. Both are feeling isolated and alienated and are consequently angry with each other. Neither Leon nor Makayla addresses this issue directly. Instead, they play out their anger in the parental arena as they battle over how to handle Kami's social isolation.

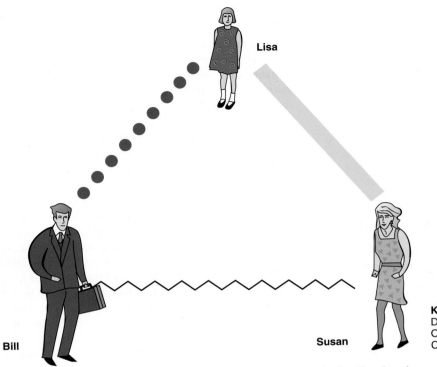

Key:
Distance ....
Overinvolvement ▬▬▬▬
Conflict ∿∿∿∿

FIGURE 34-1 Example of a family triangle.

The nurse's response to triangulation. The main goal of Bowenian therapy is to reduce chronic anxiety by first facilitating awareness of how the emotional system functions and then increasing levels of differentiation, where the focus is on making changes for the self rather than on trying to change others. Although basic-level nurses do not provide family therapy, they do interact with patients and families and can assist families in awareness and insight around their patterns in relationship to one another. Nurses should also be aware of their own differentiation process and family-of-origin issues, which may affect their responses. When personal reactions interfere, the nurse may become "triangulated" into the family's system. The nurse's continued self-assessment is necessary to maintain emotional stability in the face of a chaotic family situation, in which the nurse's own issues may arise.

For advanced-practice nurses who engage in family therapy, holding family members accountable for themselves—making clear that the responsibility for change is theirs and not the nurse's—is a way of remaining clear of triangles. For example, the nurse therapist could become triangulated into a family system in any number of ways: perhaps the nurse recently experienced the loss of a family member; the nurse may belong to an enmeshed family system, in which the children are regularly drawn into spousal arguments; or perhaps stubbornness is an unresolved issue for the nurse. Any of these possibilities could allow the nurse to become triangulated into a family system, making therapeutic intervention difficult. Engaging in personal family-of-origin therapy and regular supervision is recommended when nurse therapists work with individuals, couples, or families. Supervision can be conducted with peer professionals, in groups,

or privately with a more experienced clinician. One indication that a nurse is being triangulated is that his or her level of anxiety is greater than the situation warrants.

The Nuclear Family Emotional System

The term nuclear family refers to parents and the children under the parents' care. Bowen (1985) developed the concept of a *nuclear family emotional system*, defined as the flow of emotional processes within the nuclear family. This concept views symptoms as belonging to the nuclear family emotional system rather than to an individual. Bowen made a distinction between conventional medical (psychiatric) diagnosis and family diagnosis: Rather than viewing a symptom as reflecting a disease that is confined to a patient, Bowen identified an emotional process that transcends the boundaries of a patient and encompasses the family relationship system. The example in the vignette of 8-year-old Luca, whom family members and others believed had attention-deficit/hyperactivity disorder (ADHD), illustrates how Luca's symptoms could be viewed as reflecting the family's conflicts and changes.

Refer to Box 34-3 for a summary of concepts central to family life.

FAMILY THERAPY THEORY

Family therapy emerged from the early child guidance clinics and marriage counselling efforts in the early twentieth century, stemming from social work movements in the United Kingdom and the United States. Psychotherapists began to consider the effects of the social milieu on their patients and included the family in clinical observations and practice. The formal development of family therapy occurred in the 1940s and 1950s and was propelled by a focus on communication, which shifted the previous focus on individual pathology to a more systemic perspective (Becvar & Becvar, 2013). An *interactive* (interpersonal) rather than *indwelling* (intrapsychic Freudian) model of mental illness was becoming more widely accepted. These influences paved the way for an interest in the family system as it related to psychiatric disorders.

Leading theorists such as Virginia Satir (1972, 1983) and Jay Haley (1980, 1996) shifted the focus from the patient's symptoms (*indwelling*) to the patient's position and relationships within the family (*interactive*). Further work by Salvador Minuchin (1974, 1996), a structural therapist, established the legitimacy of family therapy within psychiatry. Bowen (1975, 1985) was a leading proponent of the family systems theory, a theory that downplays problem resolution, focusing instead on the long-term awareness of family patterns and differentiation of individual family members. *Differentiation* is a term introduced by Bowen (1975) that describes the ability of an individual to make autonomous choices while separating out feelings and cognitions. Decisions are not driven by emotionality, but the individual remains emotionally connected to a significant relationship system (e.g., the family). Extreme lack of differentiation and rigid cultural expectations are reflected in honour killings, in which young women are killed by family members—usually fathers or brothers—because of so-called dishonouring of the family. Canadian cases generally result from these girls engaging in relationships deemed inappropriate by the family or dressing and behaving in ways that male members of their families consider disrespectful (Gill, Strange, & Roberts, 2014).

The aims of the family systems theory are to decrease emotional reactivity and encourage differentiation among individual family members. Parents or adults in the system are encouraged to recognize emotional patterns from their family of origin and to use resources from members of the extended family to re-engage in more mature interaction patterns. Children who are identified as the "problem" receive counselling and behavioural therapy but are not the focus of the therapy. Instead, parents are encouraged to consider system factors contributing to the child's emotional or behavioural problems.

The terms *strategic* and *structural* are used to identify the frameworks adopted by specific therapists. A *strategic model of family therapy* assumes that change in any single element in the family system will bring about change in the entire system. The aim of strategic therapy is to change the patterns, rules, and meaning of family interactions.

In the vignette about the De Santis family, the family's communication patterns and decision making, partly for cultural reasons, exclude any discussion with the children. Children in such families often feel powerless and act out. Using the strategic model, the family therapist works with the family to change rigid communication patterns so that children are informed earlier in the decision-making process and so as to ease the emotional turmoil of the parents. This change provides children with an opportunity to comment or offer suggestions about how issues could be resolved. Being given a sense of control over

---

VIGNETTE

Eight-year-old Luca De Santis, who is hyperactive and disruptive at school and at home, is brought to the community mental health clinic to be evaluated for attention-deficit/hyperactivity disorder (ADHD). The nurse clinician performs an assessment and finds that a great deal of turmoil exists within the De Santis family. The family is composed of Luca's married parents, their other two children, and a grandmother. Luca's father has just lost his job, and his grandmother was recently diagnosed with bladder cancer. Luca's mother is considering filing for separation because of constant, unresolved arguments with her husband. She was raised a strict Roman Catholic and is unsure of this plan. Because of the family's communication patterns and cultural background, none of these issues have been discussed with Luca. Viewing this family from a strategic model, the nurse clinician sees Luca's symptoms as a function of many difficult losses and transitions that are stressing the entire family's coping mechanisms.

The nurse considers the multiple family stressors and their potential influence on Luca's symptoms of acting out and hyperactivity. Once the family issues are addressed, perhaps Luca's symptoms will subside. She refers the couple to a family therapist and, in the meantime, encourages them to focus more on their own issues and less on Luca's behaviour. An appointment is made to return to the clinic in 1 month, at which time Luca will be re-evaluated.

---

some aspects of one's life can alleviate anxiety and reduce behavioural problems. This intervention would result in a systemic change in the way the family communicates.

The *structural model of family therapy* explains family problems from the perspective of dysfunctional boundary and role structure. These problems become evident when the family is exposed to a stressor or a transition point and is unable to adapt to the changing conditions (Goldenberg, Stanton, & Goldenberg, 2017). A therapist using the structural model with the De Santis family in the vignette would highlight the importance of boundaries between the parental and sibling (child) subsystems rather than focus on changing a specific pattern. At the same time, the therapist would emphasize the importance of flexibility, which would allow for the changes inherent in normal growth and development.

In family therapy, there is no single accepted model for treating families. Not all techniques are applicable to all problems, so the experienced clinician must be discerning. Most of the theoretical schools of marital and family therapy fall into two broad classifications: insight-oriented family therapy (a combination of behavioural therapy and education of families so that they better understand their power struggles, defence mechanisms, and other negative behaviours) and behavioural family therapy (a collection of psychological techniques for modifying maladaptive behaviours). Table 34-1 summarizes some of the types of therapy in each classification, describes their basic concepts and approaches, and lists the major theorists.

The Family as a System

Every family can be viewed as a unique system with its own structure, rules, and history of handling life problems and crises.

TABLE 34-1	INSIGHT-ORIENTED AND BEHAVIOURAL FAMILY THERAPIES	
TYPE OF THERAPY	**CONCEPTS**	**MAJOR THEORISTS**
Insight-Oriented Family Therapy		
Psychodynamic therapy	Problems arise from: • Developmental arrest • Current interactions • Projections • Current stresses Improvement through insight into problematic relationships originating in the past	Nathan Ackerman James Framo Ivan Boszormenyi-Nagy
Family-of-origin therapy	Family viewed as an emotional relationship system: • Goal of fostering differentiation and decreasing emotional reactivity • Concept of triangulation • Emphasis on the family of origin	Murray Bowen
Experimental–existential therapy	Goal of therapy is to encourage the growth of family: • Symptoms express family pain • Family is responsible for its own solutions • Therapist uses nurturing and identifies dysfunctional communication patterns	Carl Whitaker Virginia Satir Leslie Greenberg Susan Johnson
Behavioural Family Therapy		
Structural therapy	Focus is on organizational patterns, boundaries, systems and subsystems, and use of scapegoating: • Restructures dysfunctional triangles • Clarifies boundaries • Looks at enmeshment and disengagement (excessive distance) issues	Salvador Minuchin
Strategic therapy	Goal is to change repetitive and maladaptive interaction patterns: • Identifies inequality of power, life cycle perspectives, and use of double-bind messages • Uses paradox • Prescribes rituals	Jay Haley Chloe Madanes Milan group (Mara Palazzoli, Gianfranco Cecchin, Giuliana Prata)
Cognitive behavioural therapy	Based on learning theory; focuses on changing cognition and behaviour: • Problem solving and solutions focused on present situations • Skills training emphasized	Gerald Patterson Richard Stuart Robert Liberman

Focusing on family patterns and interactions is fundamental to marital family therapy. The focus is *not* on an individual, as it is in traditional therapy, but rather on the interpersonal process of the family group (Nichols & Davis, 2016).

APPLICATION OF THE NURSING PROCESS

ASSESSMENT

Intervention is designed based on the initial assessment of family issues and adjusted with ongoing assessment throughout the nursing process. The Calgary Family Assessment Model (CFAM) (Figure 34-2) has multiple focuses, including but not limited to the following (Nichols & Davis, 2016):

- Family system
- Family subsystems
- Individual members of the family
- Sociocultural context of family
- Past medical and mental health illness
- Family interactions and communication styles
- Stressors within the family system

Varcoe and Doane (2015) identified a number of issues that should be assessed in family therapy, nursing practice, and counselling environments:

- Phases of the family life cycle
- Sociocultural context, beliefs
- Multigenerational issues, inclusive of historical oppression
- Relational practice

Sociocultural Context

Rather than being viewed as an isolated unit, the family is viewed in a sociocultural context, wherein issues of gender, race, ethnicity, class, sexual orientation, and religion are considered equally. Each of these contextual issues affects the family's values, norms, traditions, roles, and rules. For example, the way the family relates to a terminally ill family member may be decidedly different in a first-generation Filipino Canadian Catholic family than in a traditional Indigenous family. The nurse assesses how the family's cultural and religious beliefs affect acceptable care options.

Gender is often related to status and diverse cultural perspectives. In addition, beliefs about mental illness and their etiology and treatment have culturally diverse family interpretations. Cultural sensitivity prepares the nurse to provide culturally competent family intervention in all nursing practice settings (refer to Chapter 8 for further information on culture and mental health). A holistic assessment will include pertinent information on sexual orientation, religious and spiritual beliefs, and trauma

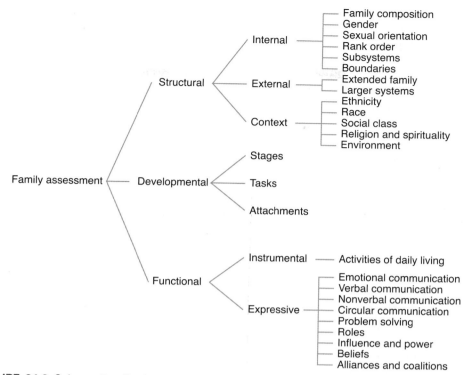

FIGURE 34-2 Calgary Family Assessment Model. Source: Wright, L. M., & Leahey, M. (2013). *Nurses and families: A guide to family assessment and intervention* (6th ed., p. 52, Fig. 3-1). Philadelphia: F. A. Davis.

histories so as to provide an understanding of influencing factors on the current situation.

Intergenerational Issues

The influence of family is not restricted to the immediate family. Family is composed of the entire emotional system of at least three and sometimes four generations, meaning that the family is affected by intergenerational issues. Various patterns of behaviour (e.g., involving geographical distance between members, suicide, divorce, addiction, affairs, grief, triangles, historical colonization, loss) may affect successive generations. The legacy of the multigenerational family may relate to the patient's presenting problem. For example, in working with the family of an Indigenous teenager who has engaged in nonsuicidal self-injurious behaviours, nurses will consider the historical and current context of the family life. A history of residential school attendance may contribute to the family's current parenting problems due to the lack of culturally appropriate role models, loss of identity, and loss of traditional way of life (Wilk, Maltby, & Cooke, 2017). An astute nurse therapist will also be aware of the potential for mistrust of health care providers and authority figures related to historical oppression and incorporate this knowledge into management of the current situation. This family may deal with grief by using silence and little outward expression of painful feelings. The nurse therapist would respect the family's way of expressing feelings. Indigenous families often bring extended family to the hospital to support the ill family member. Accommodation for this cultural expression of support is helpful for the family to resolve hospitalization issues. More important,

Indigenous people are seeking to understand colonialism and history through their own perspectives and interpretation of current problems of poverty, suicide, addictions, and injustice. A trauma-informed therapy approach is a universal approach to draw on in all family therapy practice (see Chapters 8 and 21 for more on trauma-informed practices).

Constructing a Genogram

The genogram is a tool for efficiently providing a clinical summary of information and relationships across generations of a family. It provides a graphic display of complex patterns and serves as a source of hypotheses as to how the presenting problem connects to the family context and the evolution of the family. It may help the family to understand patterns of behaviours.

Information for the genogram should be gathered in an empathic and caring manner. Bowen (1985) provided the conceptual framework for the analysis of genogram patterns that have been further developed by McGoldrick (2016). Bowen proposed that the family is organized according to generation, age, sex, roles, functions, and interests and suggested that where each individual fits into the family structure influences the family functioning, relational patterns, and type of family formed in the next generation. Sex and birth order shape sibling relationships and characteristics. Some issues are played out from generation to generation through persisting interactive emotional patterns (Bowen, 1975).

By using a genogram, nurses may map family structure and record family information inclusive of location, occupation, and educational level; functional information regarding medical, emotional, and behavioural status; and critical events such as moves, job changes, separations, abortions, imprisonment, illnesses, and deaths. Some health centres have standardized genogram forms, but genograms can also be sketched onto other forms, such as admission forms and patient care records. The genogram can be a useful tool to initiate assessment and for the family members to gain shared understanding and insight about patterns within the family.

The abilities required to do the genogram include a strong understanding of therapeutic relationships, communication, and interviewing skills. In particular, the following are needed: listening with respect, a nonjudgemental attitude, empathy, capacity to reformulate and reframe responses, respect for hesitance and resistance, and ability to ask open-ended questions. Time and place are crucial considerations in the interview, and to complete this assessment and discovery intervention, a private and quiet location, ideally one with a writing surface, is selected. Since the scope of constructing a family genogram is large, it is necessary to ensure that there is sufficient time. It is acceptable, and may be practical, to complete the genogram in stages, over more than one session.

The interview may include the discussion or disclosure of difficult events, such as the death by suicide of a family member, or the experience of isolation or rejection, or specific life habits of certain family members that they would prefer not to have revealed, such as alcoholism, incest, or imprisonment. In this way, it is recommended that the questions start with the more ordinary and lead later to the more delicate so that the individual or family gets used to the exploration process and gains comfort with the nurse therapist or interviewer. To put the person at ease, a simple conversational style of interview gives the best results (McGoldrick, 2016).

Practically, it is best to construct the skeleton of the genogram first—that is, to draw up the graphic representation of the various family members using the symbols of the genogram. Start systematically at fits, by couples for each of the maternal and paternal ancestors, then for the descendants on both sides in chronological order by birth, for three generations, if possible. Gather the demographic information: dates of birth, death, and if helpful the place of residence, urban or rural; occupation; level of education; religion; cultural or ethnic groups; and so on.

Functional information is then explored to give information about the physical and mental health of the members of the family. Then, finally, information concerning critical events in chronological order is obtained—for example, important changes such as relationship status (separations, divorce), adoption, emigration, moves or changes in work, and finally health crises or other significant events (McGoldrick, 2016).

The specific questions required to create the genogram must be adapted to the context and the age of the person and will vary if the person is single, married, has children, and so on. The following are just some of numerous examples of questions:

- Tell me about your present family situation.
- What is the occupation of each of member, their dates of birth, their religious affiliation, and their nationality?
- How many children do you have? What are their ages and sex? Their order of birth?
- Have there been any child deaths? When? Were there any stillborn children, abortions, or miscarriages? Adoptions? A child with a particular difficulty?
- Who lives at the same home with you?
- Where do the other members of the family live?
- What was the reason for their relocation?
- What recent events have happened in your family? What happened exactly? What was the reaction of each family member to this event?
- Were there any changes in the relationship between family members?
- What other types of changes occurred: moves, work changes?
- Are your children married? Tell me about their spouses. What are their religions, their nationalities, the dates of their marriage? How many children do they have? What are their ages, sexes, and order of birth? Have there been any deaths among them? When? Stillborn infants, abortions, or miscarriages? Adoptions? A child with a particular difficulty?
- Tell me about the bonds that unite your children to their spouses.
- Have there been any separations or divorces?
- Has there been a break in the relationship with your brothers and sisters? What might have precipitated that?

When in process or once completed, the genogram becomes part of the documentation about individual patients and family members. Figure 34-3 provides an example of a genogram derived from data about the family in the vignette.

VIGNETTE

Hank (of Polish Jewish descent) and Catherine Schneider (of Irish Catholic descent) are both university educated, and each suffers from intermittent depression. Hank is an only child whose father died of a heart attack at age 55, Hank's present age. Hank's mother killed herself at age 35. Her death by suicide is a toxic subject in Hank's family of origin. In Catherine's family of origin, she is the eldest, born after three miscarriages. Much pressure and many expectations were placed on her. Catherine's brother, Mike, was born 4 years after Catherine, and their mother died during Mike's birth. Mike never finished high school. He is now 50 years old, has a serious substance use disorder, and has had three marriages that ended in divorce. One can speculate about the level of guilt Mike may feel regarding the loss of his mother.

Hank and Catherine have two children, Keith and Jennifer. Keith, the identified patient, is 35 years old, has a university degree, but has not been able to hold down a job. He has an addiction to alcohol. In 2009, Keith made a suicide attempt. In November 2010, Keith experienced a psychotic episode for which he was hospitalized, and he was diagnosed as having schizophrenia. His younger sister, Jennifer, 31, has a university degree and is a practising pediatric nurse. She married William, a stockbroker the same age as she, in 2009, the year Keith attempted suicide. Jennifer and William have two young children, Ethan and Jackson, ages 4 and 2, respectively.

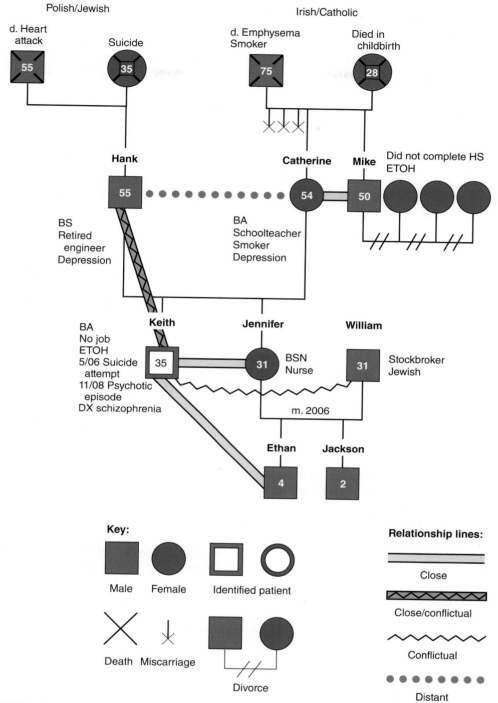

Polish/Jewish

Irish/Catholic

d. Heart attack

Suicide

d. Emphysema Smoker

Died in childbirth

55

35

75

28

Hank

Catherine

Mike

Did not complete HS ETOH

55

54

50

BS
Retired engineer
Depression

BA
Schoolteacher
Smoker
Depression

BA
No job
ETOH
5/06 Suicide attempt
11/08 Psychotic episode
DX schizophrenia

Keith

Jennifer

William

35

31

BSN Nurse

31

Stockbroker Jewish

m. 2006

Ethan

Jackson

4

2

Key:

Male   Female   Identified patient

Death   Miscarriage

Divorce

Relationship lines:

Close

Close/conflictual

Conflictual

Distant

FIGURE 34-3 Genogram of the Schneider family. *BA,* Bachelor of Arts; *BS,* Bachelor of Science; *BSN,* Bachelor of Science in Nursing; *d.,* deceased; *DX,* diagnosis; *ETOH,* alcohol; *HS,* high school; *m.,* married.

Self-Awareness

Nurses frequently interact with families in hospital and community-based settings. Nurses who are aware of their personal family-of-origin issues and who practise ongoing self-awareness are most effective. Common defence mechanisms of nurses may contribute to issues in nurse–family relationships: the formation

of triangles to reduce anxiety, defensive reactions when personal family-of-origin issues arise, and role blurring when sensitive personal issues and conflicts are triggered. Inexperienced nurses without supervision are particularly at risk for boundary violations.

An advanced-practice nurse educated at the master's level, with special training in family work, is best qualified to conduct

> ### BOX 34-4 POSSIBLE NURSING DIAGNOSES FOR FAMILY INTERVENTIONS
>
> - *(Risk for) Caregiver role strain*
> - *Sexual dysfunction*
> - *Interrupted family processes*
> - *Altered family processes*
> - *Spiritual distress*
> - *Risk for compromised resilience*
> - *Ineffective denial*
> - *Deficient knowledge*
> - *Impaired verbal communication*
> - *Defensive coping*
> - *Relocation stress syndrome*
> - *(Risk for) Impaired parenting*

family therapy. Nurses may experience intense reactions to alcohol or drug use, family abuse, codependency, rescue fantasies, and lifestyles choices. Clinical supervision is necessary to ensure that the nurse remains neutral and is not drawn into the client–family dynamics.

DIAGNOSIS

Families have unique needs at different times in their developmental stages. Family life involves new members, deaths, mental and physical illnesses, economic challenges, developmental crises, and unanticipated blows of life. Severe dysfunctional patterns (e.g., marked relational conflict, sexual misconduct, abuse, violence, suicide) exist within many families and cause significant physical or mental anguish to family members. Upon entering into a therapeutic relationship with a family, to promote health and wellness, nurses need to consider the economic, social, historical, and geographical context of the family. As well, nurses must understand how their own views were formed, consider their position in society and the privilege associated with that position, and then begin to understand how other people may be in different positions (Varcoe & Doane, 2015). In line with the above, words such as *dysfunctional* need to be carefully considered prior to use. Nursing diagnoses useful in working with families are identified in Box 34-4.

OUTCOMES IDENTIFICATION

Different therapists adhere to various theories and use a wide variety of methods; however, the goals of family therapy are basically the same (Nichols & Davis, 2016):

- To reduce *dysfunctional* behaviour of individual family members (Recognize the power of language and recall that families also have strengths. Root causes of dysfunction may be related to circumstances that are difficult to rise above.)
- To resolve or reduce intrafamily relationship conflicts
- To mobilize family resources and encourage adaptive family problem-solving behaviours

- To improve family communication skills
- To heighten awareness of other family members' emotional needs and help family members to meet those needs
- To strengthen the family's ability to cope with major life stressors and traumatic events, including chronic physical or psychiatric illness
- To improve integration of the family system into the societal system (i.e., especially the extended family but also school, medical facilities, workplace, and so on)
- To promote appropriate individual psychosocial development of each member of the family
Family psychoeducational teaching is often provided by nurses. Goals for the family include these:
- Learning to accept a family member's illness
- Learning to deal effectively with an ill member's symptoms (e.g., hallucinations, delusions, poor hygiene, physical limitations, paranoia, aggression)
- Understanding the role of medications and when to seek medical advice
- Learning about community resources and how to access them
- Feeling less anxiety and regaining control and balance in family life

PLANNING

The immediate and long-term needs of the family should be determined. For example, is the family in crisis—related to a member being severely ill, homicidal, suicidal, abusive, or a victim of abuse? Is hospitalization necessary to protect the family member? What are the family's coping mechanisms? What new skills can be used to help the family facilitate resolution of normal life cycle crises? Is there a need for psychoeducational family interventions? Nurses are adept at educating family about the illness of one of the members (e.g., severe mental illness, dementia), providing information about medications and potential adverse effects, and identifying support groups and community resources to help the family cope with the crisis and improve quality of life for family members.

A careful analysis of assessment data helps the nurse and other health care team members to identify the most appropriate family interventions.

IMPLEMENTATION

Family therapy has been applied to virtually every type of clinical disorder among children, adolescents, and adults and has demonstrated efficacy for each population studied (Nichols & Davis, 2016). Family therapy appears to be effective in the treatment of substance abuse disorders, child behavioural problems, marital relationship distress, and as an element of the treatment plan for schizophrenia (Nichols & Davis, 2016).

Counselling and Communication Techniques

The basic-level nurse may provide counselling through the use of a problem-solving approach to address an immediate-family difficulty related to health. Developing and practising strong listening skills and viewing family members in a positive, nonjudgemental way are critically important qualities for nurses.

Nurses respond to family members' cues that indicate the degree and amount of stress the family system is experiencing. Indicators of stress in a family system include the following:

- Inability of the family or a family member to understand and act on certain recommended treatment directives
- Various somatic complaints among family members
- High degree of anxiety
- Depression
- Problems in school
- Drug use

Promoting and monitoring a family's mental health can occur in any setting and often requires maximizing an opportune moment, rather than holding a formal meeting. Sometimes an informal conversation (*therapeutic encounter*) can have a significant effect on the family.

Nurses can convey a nonjudgemental approach through the way information is presented, their tone of voice, and how they ask questions. For example, the question "Don't you think you should at least try to comply with your medical regimen?" would probably cause the patient to become defensive, whereas the invitation statement "Tell me what your medical regimen is like" invites collaborative problem solving.

This nonjudgemental approach promotes open communication among professionals and family members and respects everyone's viewpoint. Information imparted in a clear, understandable manner to all family members assists discussion and decision making regarding the patient's care. Family decision making empowers families by indicating that they are accountable and responsible for how they choose to use the information. Families also possess strengths that may be manifested in forms of resilience. Families use their skills to prevent the deterioration of their family units, oppose threats to the family, and keep their families intact (Becvar, 2013; Walsh, 2016). Refugee and immigrant families often provide examples of extraordinary efforts to keep their families together. In working with family strengths in this way to expand resilience, the perspective of each family member must be elicited and heard. Often family members hear another member's view for the first time and may be surprised (e.g., "I didn't know you felt that way"). This approach defines the family as the central psychosocial unit of care. The following vignette provides an example of maintaining neutrality, building strengths and not assigning blame, and hearing from all members.

Further possible interventions for the situation in the vignette above would be to problem-solve with Aaron and his mother what is realistic for each of them regarding visiting and to organize regular telephone contact. Perhaps an extended family member or a friend can visit when the mother cannot. Long-range discharge planning for Aaron will include the identification of family supports.

Unfortunately, negative comments about family members by staff occur all too often. Hearing these comments can present a difficult situation for the nursing student, who is entering the unit as an outsider and who realizes the negative effect this

> **VIGNETTE**
>
> Doris, the head nurse on the adolescent psychiatric unit, is concerned about the negative comments staff members are making regarding the fact that none of Aaron's family has visited him for 10 days. Doris is concerned that Aaron is picking up the staff's feelings as well. After many attempts, Doris reaches Aaron's mother by phone and begins to assess the situation. She discovers that Aaron's mom is divorced and is working double shifts to meet the family's expenses. There is a 2-year-old at home and a set of twins in grade 4.
>
> Aaron's mother had been planning to visit on the weekend, but her babysitter cancelled.
>
> Once Doris understood the situation from another perspective and learned that this family has young children and is struggling to make ends meet, she called a staff meeting to address the situation.

behaviour has on family members. The student should seek supervision from the instructor so that the most effective approach can be planned. One useful technique is for the student to ask questions of the head nurse and staff in such a manner that alternative ways of viewing the family are embedded in the questions. An example of this is "Has anyone had a chance to contact Aaron's mother to see if there are any problems?" or "I wonder what it's like for Aaron's mother to have her son in a psychiatric unit."

Family Therapy

The advanced-practice nurse who has graduate or postgraduate training in family therapy may conduct private family therapy sessions. Family therapy is viewed by professionals as appropriate for most situations, although it may be contraindicated in the following circumstances (Nichols & Davis, 2016):

- The therapeutic environment is unsafe, and harm results from information, anxiety, or hostility.
- Family members demonstrate an unwillingness to be honest.
- Family members demonstrate an unwillingness to maintain confidentiality.
- A parental conflict involves issues of sexuality that are inappropriate for the children.

In most other situations, traditional family therapy is useful, especially when combined with psychopharmacology in the treatment of bipolar disorder, depression, or schizophrenia. Other options that may be less costly and time consuming are psychoeducational family therapy and self-help groups.

Traditional Family Therapy

Family therapists use diverse theoretical philosophies and techniques to bring about change in dysfunctional behaviours and interactions. Some therapists focus on the here and now; others rely more heavily on a family's history and reports of happenings between sessions. Most family therapists use an eclectic approach, drawing on a variety of techniques to fit the particular personality and strengths of the family.

Multiple-family group therapy is used with families who have a family member in an inpatient setting. These groups can help family members gain insight into their problems, as they are reflected in the problems of other families. Several families meet in one group with one or more therapists, usually once a week until their ill family member is discharged; these groups often continue for a specific period of time after discharge.

Psychoeducational Family Therapy

Psychoeducational family therapy provides families with the information they need about mental illness and the coping skills that will help them deal with their family member's psychiatric disorder. Psychoeducational family training has been applied successfully in treatment of patients with schizophrenia. Family work supports families in coping with a family member with a severe mental illness.

The primary goal of psychoeducational family therapy is the sharing of mental health information. Family education groups help family members to understand their member's illness, prodromal symptoms (symptoms that may appear before a full relapse), medications, and ways to access community resources. Psychoeducational family meetings encourage the expression of feelings and identify strategies to manage problems. For example, parents may learn how to work with a child with a conduct disorder. Feelings of anger, loss, stigmatization, sadness, and helplessness can be shared and put in a perspective that the family and individual members can manage more satisfactorily.

Self-Help Groups

Self-help groups are led by laypeople who have the illness or a family member of someone who has the illness. They assist people with a personal problem or social deprivation and families with a member who has a specific diagnosis. Some groups focus on families with healthy members, whereas others offer assistance to families whose members are experiencing a health disorder or crisis. Nurses help patients and their families to find appropriate support groups. For many people, self-help groups provide healing and ongoing therapeutic support.

Case Management

Case managers coordinate services for patients and families and monitor the patient's condition. The patient's and family's culture, ethnicity, socioeconomic status, stage of family life cycle, and beliefs about illness combine to affect an individual's response to case management. Case management entails teaching, giving appropriate referrals, and offering emotional support.

Pharmacological Interventions

The nurse is often the first to explain to the family the purpose of a prescribed medication, the desired effects, and potential adverse reactions. Generally, the more information family members have, the less likely it is that anxiety will distort their observations and decision making after discharge. The nurse

---

 RESEARCH HIGHLIGHT

Problem

Often referred to as "family burden" or "carer burden," numerous problems are reported by people supporting a person with depression, including financial difficulties, feelings of isolation, reduction in social activities, relationship distress, feeling confused and overwhelmed by depressive symptoms, worry about stigma, worry about the future, and being able to access treatment. There is considerable evidence demonstrating that family interventions for mental disorders lead to improved outcomes for both patient and carer, though most of these studies have focused on caregivers of family members with schizophrenia.

Purpose of Study

The first aim of this systematic review was to evaluate the evidence for family psychoeducation (FPE) interventions for major depressive disorder (MDD). A second aim was to compare the efficacy of different modes of delivering face-to-face FPE interventions.

Methods

Ten studies (based on nine distinct samples) were identified comprising four single-family studies, four multifamily studies, one single versus multifamily comparative study, and one peer-led, mixed-diagnosis study. Seven studies measured patient functioning and six reported positive outcomes. Six studies measured carer's well-being and four reported positive outcomes. All studies

examined face-to-face psychoeducation groups for people ages 14 to 85 that were specifically focused on psychoeducation for family members of people with the diagnosis of MDD.

Key Findings

Results provide preliminary evidence that FPE leads to improved outcomes for patient functioning and family-carer's well-being for persons with depression, In particular, the outcomes suggest that FPE needs to be specifically tailored to the needs of patients with MDD and their families and carers.

Findings also reveal a number of gaps in this field of study, as only 50% of trials identified (i.e., n = 5) were based on a randomized control design. Also, no studies reported level of session attendance by participants; hence it cannot be determined whether results were influenced by treatment dosage effect. Only two studies measured follow-up outcomes beyond 6 months to determine treatment retention effects. Finally, there was little consistency in the measures used across studies, limiting a more comprehensive analysis.

Implications for Nursing Practice

For those planning psychoeducation groups, the evidence shows that the more focused the topic of psychoeducational groups, the better. The value of psychoeducational groups appears promising, but longer term follow-up studies are needed.

Source: Brady, P., Kangas, M., & McGill, K. (2017). "Family matters": A systematic review of the evidence for family psychoeducation for major depressive disorder. *Journal of Marital and Family Therapy, 43*(2), 245–263. doi:10.1111/jmft.12204

VIGNETTE

David Gilbert, age 21 years, is leaving the hospital after experiencing his first psychotic episode while taking his final examinations before graduation from university. David is being discharged back to his family, consisting of his mother and father; his maternal grandfather, who is bedridden; and a younger brother, Louis, who is 17 years of age. David's diagnosis is schizophrenia.

While David is hospitalized and later, in postdischarge family therapy, the nurse meets with the family and takes a psychoeducational approach with them. Through reading materials and discussion, initial interventions convey information about David's mental illness and recovery. The nurse identifies psychosocial support groups and how to access them. The nurse performs ongoing assessment of the family's strengths and weaknesses, including community support. She identifies areas that require discussion. Issues include the following:

- Reorganizing family roles related to a newly diagnosed serious mental illness
- Managing the bedridden grandfather

- Attending to Louis's probable fears that he may develop this illness
- Dealing with potential parental guilt feelings
- Planning how to mobilize should David experience another psychotic episode
- Managing medication and adherence
- Dealing with concerns about David's future
- Formulating realistic expectations
- Coping with feelings of loss for what was and what was hoped for
- Maintaining the spousal subsystem

The nurse discusses these issues with the family and how they can best be addressed. For example, a visiting nurse will evaluate the grandfather's situation and need for home care, and a multiple-family psychoeducation group is contacted to increase the family's understanding of David's illness, help the family learn to cope with common problems, and provide a safe place for family members to share feelings of loss and grief.

reviews David's medication with him and his family during his hospitalization and before discharge. The nurse monitors David to determine if adverse effects are interfering with his functioning. The nurse may consult with a physician to titrate medications based on the efficacy of the medications and David's toleration of any adverse effects.

EVALUATION

Evaluation focuses on whether family members have improved functioning, reduced or resolved conflicts, improved communication skills, and strengthened coping and whether the family is more integrated into the societal system.

KEY POINTS TO REMEMBER

- Family therapy is based on a variety of theoretical concepts.
- Family therapy aims to decrease emotional reactivity and to encourage differentiation among family members.
- The primary characteristics of healthy family functioning are flexibility and clear boundaries.
- Family-oriented approaches that help family members gain insight and make behavioural changes are most successful.
- The genogram is an efficient clinical summary for providing information and defining relationships across at least three generations.

- The family's culture, ethnicity, socioeconomic status, and life cycle phase, as well as its unique beliefs about illness, affect the individual patient's progress and response to case management.
- Assessment of the family includes a focus on the family life cycle phase, multigenerational issues, the individual's developmental stage, and the family's sociocultural status.
- Nurses with basic education frequently conduct psychoeducation with families.
- Nurses with specialized education and certification provide family therapy using diverse theoretical approaches.

CRITICAL THINKING

1. Select a family with whom you've worked during your clinical experience. Evaluate this family's status in terms of functionality or dysfunctionality with reference to the family functions described in the text (i.e., provision of love and nurturance, socialization of children, social control of members, production and consumption of goods and services, addition of new family members through birth or adoption, and physical care and maintenance of family members).

2. Create your own personal genogram, including at least three generations.
   a. Be sure to include the following:
      - Location, occupation, and educational level
      - Critical events such as births, marriages, moves, job changes, separations, divorces, illnesses, and deaths
      - Relationship patterns, if possible, such as emotional cutoffs, distancing, overinvolvement, and conflict
   b. Analyze and reflect on patterns of behaviour that may have been transmitted through the generations within your family. These may be positive patterns or more painful patterns.

3. A family has just found out that their young son is going to die. The parents have been fighting and blaming each other for ignoring the child's ongoing symptom of leg pain, which was eventually diagnosed as advanced cancer. There are two other siblings in the family.
   a. How would you apply family concepts to help this family?
   b. What would be your outcome criterion?

4. A mother of a 6-year-old girl has recently been diagnosed with schizophrenia. How would you address her mother's diagnosis with the 6-year-old?

CHAPTER REVIEW

1. Jeff is a single, noncustodial parent recently divorced. He will be hospitalized for several days following surgery. Which primary concern of Jeff's should the nurse anticipate during this time?
   a. Mourning the loss of his nuclear family
   b. Wondering how to deal with his spouse's extended family
   c. Attempting to restructure the relationship with his former spouse
   d. Finding ways to continue to effectively parent his child

2. While the nurse works with a family, the father—with a smirk on his face—states, "I love my wife, and she's a good woman who would do anything for her family" and rolls his eyes. Which behaviour should the nurse recognize?
   a. Triangulation
   b. Scapegoating
   c. Double-binding
   d. Differentiation

3. Which family member should the nurse refer to individual therapy rather than family therapy?
   a. The mother who has anxiety controlled by medication
   b. The father who is questioning his sexual orientation
   c. The brother who is verbally angry with his parents
   d. The sister who has consented to maintaining confidentiality

4. The nurse is evaluating the family therapy experience. Which behaviour would indicate that further family therapy is indicated?
   a. The wife has set aside 15 minutes daily to connect with her husband.
   b. The son's grades have risen from a "D" average to a "C" average.
   c. The daughter's headaches have subsided.
   d. The mother has stopped using illicit substances, and the father's use has decreased.

5. The nurse is conducting family therapy. Which nursing intervention would be appropriate for an advanced-practice nurse?
   a. Mobilizing family resources and encouraging adaptive family problem-solving behaviours
   b. Improving family communication skills
   c. Explaining what medications can and cannot do
   d. Working with the underlying dynamics and structure of the family group

Post-Test interactive review

℮volve WEBSITE

Visit the Evolve website for Chapter Review Answers and Rationales, Critical Thinking Answer Guidelines, and additional resources related to the content in this chapter: http://evolve.elsevier.com/Canada/Varcarolis/psychiatric/

REFERENCES

Becvar, D. S. (2013). *Handbook of family resilience.* New York: Springer.

Becvar, D. S., & Becvar, R. J. (2013). *Family therapy: A systematic integration* (8th ed.). New York: Pearson.

Bellamy, S., & Hardy, C. (2015). *Understanding depression in Aboriginal communities and families.* Prince George, BC: National Collaborating Centre for Aboriginal Health (NCCAH).

Bowen, M. (1975). Family therapy after 20 years. In S. Ariti, D. Freedman, & J. Dyrud (Eds.), *American handbook of psychiatry* (2nd ed., pp. 379–391). New York: Gardner Press.

Bowen, M. (1985). *Family therapy in clinical practice.* New York: Jason Aronson.

Debassige, B. (2010). Re-conceptualizing Anishinaabe Mino-Bimaadiziwin (the good life) as research methodology: A spirit-centered way in Anishinaabe research. *Canadian Journal of Native Education, 33*(1), 11.

Eaton, K., Ohan, J. L., Stritzke, W. G. K., et al. (2016). Failing to meet the good parent ideal: Self-stigma in parents of children with mental health disorders. *Journal of Child and Family Studies, 25*(10), 3109. doi:10.1007/s10826-016-0459-9.

Evans, E., & Chamberlain, P. (2015). Critical waves: Exploring feminist identity, discourse and praxis in Western feminism. *Social Movement Studies, 14*(4), 396–409. doi:10.1080/14742837.2014.964199.

Gill, A. K., Strange, C., & Roberts, K. A. (2014). *"Honour" killing and violence: Theory, policy and practice.* New York: Palgrave Macmillan.

Gladstone, B. M., Boydell, K. M., Seeman, M. V., et al. (2011). Children's experiences of parental mental illness: A literature review. *Early Intervention in Psychiatry, 5*(4), 271–289. doi:10.1111/j.1751-7893.2011.00287.x.

Goldenberg, H., Stanton, M., & Goldenberg, I. (2017). *Family therapy: An overview* (9th ed.). Boston: Cengage Learning.

Gottlieb, L. N. (2013). *Strengths-based nursing care: Health and healing for person and family.* New York: Springer.

Habjan, S., Prince, H., & Kelley, M. L. (2012). Caregiving for elders in First Nations communities: Social system perspective on barriers and challenges. *Canadian Journal on Aging, 31*(2), 209. doi:10.1017/S071498081200013X.

Haley, J. (1980). *Leaving home*. New York: McGraw-Hill.

Haley, J. (1996). *Learning and teaching therapy*. New York: Guilford.

Kirmayer, L., Tait, C., & Simpson, C. (2009). The mental health of Aboriginal peoples in Canada: Transformations of identity and community. In L. K. Kirmayer & G. Guthrie Valaskakis (Eds.), *Healing traditions: The mental health of Aboriginal peoples in Canada* (pp. 3–35). Vancouver: UBC Press.

Klinic Community Health Center (2013). *Trauma-informed: The trauma toolkit* (2nd ed.). Winnipeg: Author.

Layne, C. M., Abramovitz, R., Stuber, M., et al. (2017). *The core curriculum on childhood trauma: A tool for preparing a trauma-informed mental health workforce. Traumatic StressPoints, January 31*, 1–8. Retrieved from http://sherwood-istss.informz.net/informzdataservice/onlineversion/ind/bWFpbGluZ2luc3Rhbmc9NjI1MTUwNCZzdWJzY3JpYmVya2V5WQ9MTA0NDYxODQ0MQ.

McGoldrick, M. (2016). *The genogram casebook: A clinical companion to genograms: Assessment and intervention*. New York: W. W. Norton & Company.

McGoldrick, M., Garcia Preto, N., & Carter, B. (Eds.), (2016). *The expanded family life cycle: Individual, family, and social perspectives* (5th ed.). Boston: Allyn & Bacon.

Mental Health Commission of Canada. (2013). *National guidelines for a comprehensive service system to support family caregivers of adults with mental health problems and illnesses*. Retrieved from http://www.mentalhealthcommission.ca/sites/default/files/Caregiving_MHCC_Family_Caregivers_Guidelines_ENG_0.pdf.

Minuchin, S. (1974). *Families and family therapy*. Cambridge, MA: Harvard University Press.

Minuchin, S. (1996). *Mastering family therapy*. New York: John Wiley & Sons, Inc.

Murphy, G., Peters, K., Wilkes, L., et al. (2017). Adult children of parents with mental illness: Navigating stigma. *Child & Family Social Work, 22*(1), 330–338. doi:10.1111/cfs.12246.

Nichols, M. P., & Davis, S. (2016). *Family therapy: Concepts and methods* (11th ed.). New York: Pearson.

Ontario Centre of Excellence for Child and Youth Mental Health. (2017). *Working with Indigenous families: An engagement bundle for child and youth mental health agencies*. Retrieved from http://www.excellenceforchildandyouth.ca/sites/default/files/docs/bundle_working_with_indigenous_families.pdf.

Park, K., & Seo, M. (2016). Care burden of parents of adult children with mental illness: The role of associative stigma. *Comprehensive Psychiatry, 70*, 159–164. doi:10.1016/j.comppsych.2016.07.010.

Ramisch, T., & Nelson, T. S. (2014). Transgenerational family therapies. In J. L. Wetchler & L. L. Hecker (Eds.), *An introduction to marriage and family therapy* (2nd ed., pp. 319–356). New York: Routledge.

Raymond, K. Y., Willis, D. G., & Sullivan-Bolyai, S. (2017). Parents caring for adult children with serious mental illness. *Journal of the American Psychiatric Nurses Association, 23*(2), 119–132. doi:10.1177/1078390316685404.

Registered Nurses' Association of Ontario. (2015). *Person and family centred care*. Retrieved from http://rnao.ca/bpg/guidelines/person-and-family-centred-care.

Sadock, B. J., Sadock, V. A., & Ruiz, P. (2017). *Concise textbook of clinical psychiatry* (4th ed.). Philadelphia: Lippincott Williams & Wilkins.

Satir, V. (1972). *Peoplemaking*. Palo Alto, CA: Science and Behaviour Books.

Satir, V. (1983). *Conjoint family therapy*. Palo Alto, CA: Science and Behaviour Books.

Truth and Reconciliation Commission (TRC) of Canada (2015). *Honouring the truth, reconciling for the future: Summary of the final report of the Truth and Reconciliation Commission of Canada*. Winnipeg: Author. Retrieved from www.trc.ca.

Turcotte, M. (2013). *Family caregiving: What are the consequences?* (Catalogue no. 75-0006-X). Retrieved from http://www.statcan.gc.ca/pub/75-006-x/2013001/article/11858-eng.pdf.

United Nations. (2007). *The United Nations declaration on the rights of Indigenous peoples*. Retrieved from http://www.un.org/esa/socdev/unpfii/documents/DRIPS_en.pdf.

Vanier Institute of the Family. (2017). *Definition of family*. Retrieved from http://vanierinstitute.ca/definition-family/.

Varcoe, C., & Doane, G. (2015). Relational nursing and family nursing in Canada. In J. Rowe, V. Gedaly-Duff, D. P. Coehlo, et al. (Eds.), *Family health care nursing: Theory, practice, & research* (5th ed., pp. 167–186). Philadelphia: F. A. Davis.

Walsh, F. (2016). Family resilience: A developmental systems framework. *European Journal of Developmental Psychology, 13*(3), 313–324. doi:10.1080/17405629.2016.1154035.

Wilk, P., Maltby, A., & Cooke, M. (2017). Residential schools and the effects on Indigenous health and well-being in Canada: A scoping review. *Public Health Reviews, 38*, doi:10.1186/s40985-017-0055-6.

Wright, L. M., & Leahey, M. (2013). *Nurses and families: A guide to family assessment and intervention* (6th ed.). Philadelphia: F. A. Davis.

Integrative and Complementary Therapies

Cheryl L. Pollard
with Contributions from Karen Scott Barss

KEY TERMS AND CONCEPTS

acupuncture
aromatherapy
chiropractic medicine
conventional health care
healing touch
holistic nurse
homeopathy
integrative health care

natural health products (NHPs)
naturopathy
reflexology
Reiki
therapeutic touch
traditional, complementary, and alternative medicine
(TCAM)

OBJECTIVES

1. Define the terms *integrative, traditional, complementary*, and *alternative health care therapies*.
2. Identify trends in integrative health care.
3. Discuss how to help educate the public in the safe use of integrative modalities.
4. Explore information resources available through literature and online sources.

5. Explore five aspects of integrative care: whole medical systems, mind–body–spirit approaches, biologically based interventions, manipulative approaches, and energy therapies.
6. Discuss the techniques used in major traditional, complementary, and alternative modalities and potential applications to psychiatric mental health nursing practice.

⊝volve WEBSITE

Visit the Evolve website for Flashcards, Case Studies, and additional testing resources related to the content in this chapter: http://evolve.elsevier.com/Canada/Varcarolis/psychiatric/

Pre-Test interactive review

This chapter considers *integrative care* as part of a holistic nursing philosophy. **Integrative health care** is an interdisciplinary model of health care with the intent to synergistically blend the best of conventional health care and traditional, complementary therapies in a nonhierarchical manner.

In Western countries, **conventional health care** is also referred to as *biomedicine, allopathic medicine*, or *mainstream medicine* and is based largely on highly controlled, evidence-informed scientific research (Rakel & Jonas, 2012). Meanwhile, *traditional medicine (TM)* is defined by the World Health Organization

(WHO, 2000) as the "sum total of the knowledge, skills and practices based on the theories, beliefs and experiences indigenous to different cultures, whether explicable or not, used in the maintenance of health, as well as in the prevention, diagnosis, improvement or treatment of physical and mental illnesses. The terms complementary/alternative/non-conventional medicine are used interchangeably with traditional medicine in some countries" (p. 1). This type of therapy is of interest and used by many individuals outside of indigenous cultures. This chapter will use the WHO terminology of traditional, complementary,

	TRADITIONAL, COMPLEMENTARY, AND ALTERNATIVE MEDICINE USED IN PSYCHIATRIC DISORDERS
TABLE 35-1	
DISORDER	**EXAMPLES OF TRADITIONAL, COMPLEMENTARY, AND ALTERNATIVE MEDICINE USED (NOT ALL INCLUSIVE)**
Anxiety	Exercise, yoga, mindfulness-based stress reduction, music, acupuncture, homeopathy, Reiki
Bipolar disorder	Exercise, mindfulness/meditation, yoga
Depression	Exercise, nutrition, chiropractic, bright-light therapy, music, Reiki, religious/spiritual, healing touch, qigong, massage
Post-traumatic stress disorder	Guided imagery, yoga, acupuncture
Schizophrenia/psychosis	Exercise, yoga, acupuncture
Substance use disorder	Exercise, mindfulness/meditation, yoga, qigong

Sources: Lake, J. (2009) *Integrative mental health care: A therapist's handbook.* New York: Norton; and Wynn, G. H. (2015). Complementary and alternative medicine approaches in the treatment of PTSD. *Current Psychiatry Reports, 17*(8), 600.

and alternative medicine (TCAM). The term *TCAM* recognizes that many of the philosophical underpinnings for the approaches presented are derived from both non-Western cultural traditions and studies in the nature of energy and reality, which have not historically been a part of conventional health care delivery. However, TCAM will be discussed in the broader context of integrative health care. With the increased use of integrative mental health therapies, it is essential that nurses have a knowledge base in this area in order to meet provincial or territorial regulatory entry-to-practice competencies (Canadian Association of Schools of Nursing & Canadian Federation of Mental Health Nurses, 2017). Refer to Table 35-1 for traditional, complementary, and alternative medicine concurrently used to help treat the symptoms of selected psychiatric disorders.

INTEGRATIVE HEALTH CARE IN CANADA

Many Canadians seek assistance from alternative and conventional providers at the same time and believe that using both conventional and alternative therapies is better than using either one alone. A 2006 Fraser Institute survey found that more than half (54%) of Canadians used at least one alternative therapy the year prior, an increase from the rate of use in 1997 (50%) (Esmail, 2007). Seventy-three percent of Canadians had used at least one alternative therapy at some time in their lives and had used alternative therapies an average of 8.6 times the year prior. The five most commonly used modalities were massage, spiritual practice, chiropractic, relaxation, and herbal therapies. The term **natural health products (NHPs)** is used in Canada to describe substances such as vitamins and minerals, herbal medicines,

homeopathic preparations, energy drinks, probiotics, and many alternative and traditional medicines (Health Canada, 2012b). A Health Canada consumer survey on NHPs also suggests an attitudinal trend toward integration of conventional care and TCAM (Health Canada, 2012c). A majority of Canadians agreed that NHPs can be used to maintain or promote health (77%) or to treat illness (68%). Fewer (43%) agreed that NHPs were better than conventional medicine. At the same time, 81% of Canadians thought it was important to respect the role that NHPs play in some cultures. They also expressed the belief that Canadians have the right to use any NHP they choose. This attitude highlights the importance of psychiatric mental health nurses being aware of the risks and benefits of these various therapies.

Health Canada responded to integrative health care trends by establishing the Natural Health Products Directorate (NHPD) in 1999. The NHPD's mandate is "to ensure that Canadians have ready access to natural health products that are safe, effective and of high quality while respecting freedom of choice and philosophical and cultural diversity" (Ramsay, 2009). The directorate's Natural Health Products Regulations (NHPR) came into effect on January 1, 2004. Under the NHPR, NHPs require a product licence to be legally sold in Canada. To receive a licence to be sold as an NHP, products must be appropriate for consideration as over-the-counter products and not need a prescription. Products that need a prescription are regulated as drugs (Health Canada, 2012b). Controversy has been associated with the NHPR over concerns about increased cost and decreased access to NHPs (Health Canada, 2012d).

Jurisdiction over Canadian practitioners of TCAM is currently at the provincial and territorial level, resulting in a mosaic of relevant registrations, certifications, and licensures (Ramsay, 2009). In this context, various TCAM practitioners are working toward achieving professional status for their respective modalities and practices. Those who have been successful, such as massage therapists, chiropractors, and naturopathic doctors (NDs), are increasingly becoming part of mainstream health care (Canadian Association of Naturopathic Doctors, 2011; Canadian Chiropractic Association, 2011). For example, legislation requiring licensure for naturopathic doctors currently exists in British Columbia, Saskatchewan, Manitoba, Ontario, and Nova Scotia, and new regulations for NDs in Alberta have been prepared and await government approval; other provinces and territories are actively pursuing regulation (Canadian Association of Naturopathic Doctors, 2011). Many conventional health care practitioners, including those in mental health services, are integrating evidence-informed TCAM practices into their professional practice (Canadian Holistic Nurses Association, 2011). For example, acupuncture is being integrated by a variety of health care providers as an adjunct to the other techniques and treatments within their scopes of practice (Acupuncture Canada, 2011). These practitioners are not called acupuncturists but rather use acupuncture as a tool and are regulated accordingly by their professional regulating body (Acupuncture Canada, 2011). Further information about the current status of regulation across provinces and territories for various integrative modalities can be obtained by contacting applicable professional associations.

BOX 35-1   INTEGRATIVE HEALTH CARE RESOURCES

- Acupuncture Canada: https://www.acupuncturecanada.org/
- Canadian Association of Naturopathic Doctors: http://www.naturopathicassoc.ca/
- Canadian Chiropractic Association: https://www.chiropractic.ca/
- Canadian Federation of Aromatherapists: http://cfacanada.com/
- Canadian Foundation for Trauma Research & Education: http://www.cftre.com/
- Canadian Holistic Nurses Association (CHNA): http://www.chna.ca/
- International Society for Complimentary Medicine Research (ISCMR): http://www.iscmr.org/
- Canadian Research Institute of Spirituality & Healing: http://www.crish.org/
- The Center for Contemplative Mind in Society: http://www.contemplativemind.org/
- Health Canada: Natural and Non-prescription Health Products: http://www.hc-sc.gc.ca/dhp-mps/prodnatur/index-eng.php
- International Network of Integrative Mental Health: http://www.inimh.org/
- Massage.ca: http://massage.ca/
- Native Mental Health Association of Canada (NMHAC): http://www.nmhac.ca/
- Role of the Registered Psychiatric Nurse in Relation to Complementary and Alternative Healing: http://www.rpnas.com/about/position-statements/alternative-healing/
- World Health Organization (WHO): http://www.who.int/en (Search "Traditional, Complementary, and Alternative Healing" for various guidelines and updates.)

(Box 35-1 highlights several national associations; numerous related provincial and territorial associations also exist.)

Because of the growing interest in and use of TCAM, the United States government's National Institutes of Health (NIH) established the National Center for Complementary and Alternative Medicine (NCCAM) in 1998. Since no equivalent Canadian organization has been established to date, NCCAM is an essential resource for Canadian health care providers and patients. The NCCAM supports fair and scientific evaluation of integrative therapies and dissemination of information that allow health care providers and patients to make good choices regarding the safety and appropriateness of various TCAM modalities (NCCAM, 2011f).

Research

Research on the efficacy of TCAM is increasing in the field of mental health, most notably concerning anxiety and depression (Sarris, Moylan, Camfield, et al., 2012). However, studies in the field are minimal when compared to those of conventional medicine (Khorsan, Coulter, Crawford, et al., 2011). Reasons for this lack of research include (1) the relatively recent use of some of these therapies in Western countries, (2) the lack of financial incentive to support the research, and (3) the difficulties encountered when researching these modalities. These difficulties include personality, belief systems, spiritual practices, and temperament of both the researcher and participants; difficulty trying to standardize modalities; and the influence of studying a phenomenon or person within a naturalistic setting.

PATIENTS AND INTEGRATIVE CARE

Patients are attracted to integrative care for a variety of reasons, including the following:

- A desire to be an active participant in their health care and to engage in holistic practices that can promote health and healing
- A desire to find therapeutic approaches that seem to carry lower risks than medications
- Dissatisfaction with the practice style of conventional medicine (e.g., rushed office visits, short hospital stays)
- A need to find modalities and remedies that provide comfort for chronic conditions for which no conventional medical cure exists, such as anxiety, chronic pain, and depression (Young & Koopsen, 2011).

It is essential that nurses maintain up-to-date knowledge of these modalities, continue to evaluate the evidence supporting the effectiveness and safety of TCAM, and be able to help patients make safe choices about the use of these treatments for their mental health and recovery.

Safety

People who use TCAM therapies often do so without informing their conventional health care providers, which poses some risk. In a 2010 survey, 15% of Canadians who used NHPs reported that they had experienced unwanted adverse effects; this number is up from 12% in a 2005 survey (Health Canada, 2012c). Some patients may believe that a natural substance from a health food store must be safe and effective; however, "natural" does not mean "harmless." Herbal products and supplements may contain powerful active ingredients that can cause damage if taken inappropriately or in combination with pharmaceutical preparations (Ulbricht, 2011). Health Canada (2012a) consumer guidelines for safe use of NHPs are listed in Box 35-2.

Nurses have a professional responsibility to provide patient education that protects patients from unscrupulous practices. The Registered Psychiatric Nurses Association of Saskatchewan's (2011) *Position Statement on the Role of the Registered Psychiatric Nurse in Relation to Complementary and Alternative Healing* recommends that the patient choosing TCAM be encouraged to select practitioners who address the following:

- Can provide documentation regarding their credentials, educational preparation, and experience that demonstrate that they have the necessary qualifications to practise the modality professionally
- Can identify whether or not their modality is regulated by a professional organization and, if so, can provide documentation of membership in that organization and show that they practise in accordance with its code of ethics, standards of practice, and any other appropriate guidelines
- Facilitate informed consent by outlining potential risks, benefits, and limitations of the modality
- Support a multidisciplinary approach

BOX 35-2 HOW CAN I USE ALTERNATIVE OR NATUROPATHIC HEALTH PRODUCTS SAFELY?

- Talk to a health care professional like a doctor, pharmacist, or naturopath before choosing a product. This is especially important for children, pregnant or breastfeeding women, older adults, and people with serious medical conditions.
- To prevent interactions, make sure your health care provider knows what other drugs and natural health products you are using.
- Use approved products. Look for NPN/DIN-HM numbers that identify licensed products.
- Be sceptical of health-related claims that seem too good to be true. Don't rely on ads: do your own research and talk to your health care provider.
- Read and follow all instructions on the product label.
- Report unwanted side effects (adverse reactions) to your health care provider and Health Canada.

Source: Health Canada. (2012). *About natural health products: How can I use natural health products safely?* Retrieved from http://www.hc-sc.gc.ca/dhp-mps/prodnatur/about-apropos/cons-eng.php#a3. Reproduced with permission from the Minister of Health, 2013.

Another concern regarding TCAM therapies that nurses need to address with their patients is that diagnosis and treatment may be delayed while patients try alternative interventions, which is common with mental health disorders such as major depression and anxiety. On the other hand, many TCAM and conventional health care practitioners are aware of patients who have been injured by an uncaring conventional medical system or have suffered consequences from the use of conventional pharmaceuticals. Nurses, in consultation with all relevant practitioners, can play a key role in assisting patients to carefully and safely weigh the risks and benefits of all treatments under consideration.

Efficacy

Some people make the claim that integrative therapies work through a mechanism known as the *placebo effect*. The term *placebo effect* refers to a treatment that actually does nothing, yet the condition for which it is used improves (Rakel & Jonas, 2012); the improvement comes about because of the power of suggestion and a belief that the treatment works. Research on this phenomenon continues and is necessary to deepen our understanding of it. In the meantime, it is known that integrative care is based on optimism; a positive approach and the use of positive suggestion, no matter what treatment modality is being implemented, offer a greater chance of success than does communication that is negative or fosters a poor response. The placebo effect can be most powerful when the need is greatest and a trusting relationship has been established between patient and health care provider. In fact, the literature on integrative health care increasingly refers to this positive placebo effect as "the healing response" that should intentionally be activated within holistic care to enhance healing outcomes (Rakel & Jonas, 2012).

INTEGRATIVE NURSING CARE

The Canadian Holistic Nurses Association (CHNA) recognizes holistic nursing as a specialty that supports holistic health and a philosophy of holistic nursing encompassing self-care and responsibility, humanizing health care, and wellness promotion (Canadian Holistic Nurses Association, 2011). The CHNA is affiliated with the American Holistic Nurses Association (AHNA), which defines the holistic nurse as one who recognizes and integrates body–mind–emotion–spirit–environment principles into practice; attends to self-awareness and personal healing; removes barriers to the healing process; facilitates growth in others; and assists illness recovery or transition to a peaceful death (Mariano, 2013, pp. 60–61).

Regardless of their practice philosophy, nurses need to have a basic knowledge of treatments used in integrative care since they care for patients who increasingly use a variety of unconventional modalities to meet their health needs. In addition, nurses need to respond to the reality that patients are looking to nurses and other health care providers to offer holistic health care (Willison, 2008). Nursing education programs are beginning to include basic integrative modalities such as relaxation, imagery, and contemplative practices in their curricula, and some may include energy-based approaches such as therapeutic touch (Barrere, 2013).

To fully understand and respond to the needs of patients, nurses must ask questions about the use of TCAM as part of a holistic assessment. Such inquiry can be naturally integrated into holistic exploration of the mental, emotional, physical, spiritual, social, and cultural dimensions of the person's life and healing process.

CLASSIFICATION OF INTEGRATIVE THERAPIES

NCCAM has developed a system of classification for TCAM therapies. These classifications are adapted in this chapter to include the following: (1) whole medical systems, (2) mind–body–spirit approaches, (3) biologically based practices, (4) manipulative approaches, and (5) energy therapies. It is important for readers to keep in mind that these classifications are interrelated; many of the modalities discussed could fit into more than one such classification. Furthermore, many modalities are increasingly being classified as "conventional" in light of ever-expanding research and usage. It is essential for nurses to regularly revisit the literature on the effectiveness of a given modality in relation to a specific mental health issue.

Whole Medical Systems

NCCAM (2011a) defines a whole medical system as a complete system of theory and practice that has evolved over time in a variety of cultures and apart from biomedical and allopathic medicine. Whole medical systems addressed in this chapter are traditional Indigenous medicine, Ayurvedic medicine, traditional Chinese medicine, homeopathy, and naturopathy.

Traditional Indigenous Medicine

Traditional Indigenous medicine is central to integrative health care in Canada, given the large number of Canadians who are of Indigenous ancestry. In this healing system, mental, emotional, spiritual, social, cultural, and physical health are inseparable (Binda, 2011). Discussed in more detail in Chapter 8, Indigenous medicine wheel teachings are increasingly being integrated into mental health treatment approaches for those of Indigenous and non-Indigenous ancestry. Specific teachings vary, depending on the affiliation of Indigenous peoples. Traditional Indigenous elders and healers combine such narrative with a variety of spiritual and healing practices such as ceremonies (e.g., sweat lodges), vibrational medicine (e.g., chanting and drumming), and use of traditional medicines (e.g., native herbs) to restore balance and harmony (Binda, 2011). Further information about Indigenous mental health and healing, as well as practices to acknowledge the elders and keepers of traditional knowledge, can be obtained from the Native Mental Health Association of Canada (2008).

Ayurvedic Medicine

Ayurvedic (pronounced i•yur•vay•dik) medicine originated in India around 5000 BC and is one of the world's oldest medical systems. *Ayurveda* means "the science of life" and is a philosophy that emphasizes individual responsibility for health. It is holistic, promotes prevention, and recognizes the uniqueness of the individual. Ayurvedic practitioners offer a variety of natural treatments such as herbs, dietary adjustments, contemplative practices, cleansing techniques, and ways of balancing the individual's *chakras*. According to Jackson and Keegan (2013), a chakra is the "specific centre of consciousness in the human energy system that allows for the inflow and directing of energy from outside, as well as for outflow from the individual's energy field" (p. 347). Seven major chakras relate to the spine, alongside many minor energy systems throughout the body.

Ayurvedic treatments aim to eliminate impurities and balance the individual's unique constitution (*prakriti)* and life forces (*doshas)* (NCCAM, 2011a).

Traditional Chinese Medicine

Traditional Chinese medicine (TCM) provides the basic theoretical framework for many TCAM therapies, including acupuncture, acupressure, transcendental meditation, tai chi, and qigong. TCM comes from the Eastern tradition, specifically the philosophy of Taoism, and emphasizes the promotion of harmony (health) or to bring order out of chaos (illness).

The main concept in TCM is the movement of life energy or essence, *qi*, which maintains an individual's health and wellness. If this life energy is disrupted, it can seriously affect the mind, body, and spirit (Shields & Wilson, 2016). TCM is a vast medical system based on a constellation of concepts, theories, laws, and principles of energy movement within the body. Therapy addresses the patient's illness in relation to the complex interaction of mind, body, and spirit.

Adherents of TCM say that it addresses not only physiological and psychological symptoms but also cosmological events that relate to the dynamics of the universe. These meridians become significant in the practice of acupuncture, touch therapy, and the more recent energy-based therapies used to treat emotional symptoms and promote mental health. Forms of movement such as qigong and tai chi may be used, as well as yoga. Viewed as a stressor itself, movement seems to mediate the effects of other stressors.

In TCM, health is the balance between *yin* and *yang*, and illness emanates from imbalances. The TCM practitioner uses the history and physical examination to understand the imbalances of mind, body, and spirit that have caused the patient's illness. Diagnosis involves both questioning and observing body structure, skin colour, breath, body odours, nail condition, voice, gestures, mood, and pulse. Eastern goals, perspectives, and stages of healing are useful in treating mental illnesses, many of which are long term. The goals of healing in Eastern medicine include the following:

- Being in harmony with one's environment and with all of creation in mind, body, and spirit
- Reawakening the spirit to its possibilities
- Reconnecting with life's meaning

Acupuncture. Given that acupuncture is an integral part of TCM, it is discussed within this context, although it has also become an increasingly popular therapy in Western countries as a healing modality in and of itself. **Acupuncture** involves the placement of needles into the skin at meridian points to modulate the flow of energy (*qi*). Sometimes acupuncture needles are inserted and removed immediately, and at other times they are twirled, attached to electrodes for stimulation, or allowed to remain in place for a time. Sensations are described as rushing, warm, tingling, or, occasionally, painful. Acupuncture is thought to stimulate physical changes such as in brain activity, blood chemistry, endocrine function, blood pressure, heart rate, and immune system response. Acupuncture can play a role in regulating blood cell counts and in relieving pain and emotional distress by triggering endorphin production (NCCAM, 2011b).

Acupuncture has been used to manage symptoms of withdrawal from substances, reduce hallucinations in schizophrenia, and treat mood disorders and post-traumatic stress disorder (PTSD), with mixed results according to the literature to date (Zhang, Chen, Yip, et al., 2010). A 2009 systematic review suggests that acupuncture is effective in the treatment of insomnia (Cao, Pan, Li, et al., 2009). Risks identified relate to improper technique in sterilization or placement of needles (NCCAM, 2011b).

Homeopathy and Naturopathy

Homeopathy and naturopathy are examples of Western whole medical systems. Developed in Germany more than 200 years ago, **homeopathy** uses small doses (dilutions) of specially prepared plant extracts, herbs, minerals, and other materials to stimulate the body's defence mechanisms and healing processes. Infinitesimally small doses of diluted preparations that produce symptoms mimicking those of an illness are used to help the body heal itself. Homeopathy is based on the Law of Similars ("like cures like"), and dilutions are prescribed to match the patient's illness or symptom (or both) and personality profile (NCCAM, 2011c).

Homeopathy has been difficult to study using current scientific methods because its highly diluted solutions cannot be readily measured and homeopathic treatments are highly individualized. A systematic review found that homeopathic remedies in high dilution, taken under the supervision of trained professionals, are generally considered safe and unlikely to cause severe adverse reactions. They are not known to interact with conventional drugs. Patients with addictions should be informed that some homeopathic remedies contain alcohol. Patients should also be informed that there may be a temporary worsening of symptoms before they improve (NCCAM, 2011c).

There is mixed evidence on the effectiveness of homeopathic treatments for different mental illnesses. For instance, the breadth of evidence does not currently support homeopathic treatments for anxiety disorders (Sarris, Moylan, Camfield, et al., 2012).

Naturopathy emphasizes health restoration rather than disease treatment and combines nutrition, homeopathy, herbal medicine, hydrotherapy, light therapy, massage therapy, therapeutic counselling, and other treatments. It is a whole medical system that has evolved from a combination of traditional practices and health care approaches popular in Europe during the nineteenth century. Naturopathic practitioners, guided by a philosophy that emphasizes the healing power of nature, now use a variety of traditional and modern therapies. Practitioners view their role as supporting the body's inherent ability to maintain and restore health and prefer to use treatment approaches they consider the most natural and least invasive. Such holistic concepts are useful in considering the body–mind–spirit nature of mental health and illness (NCCAM, 2011e).

Mind–Body–Spirit Approaches

Mind–body–spirit (MBS) approaches make use of the continuous interaction between mind, body, and spirit. Most of these techniques emphasize facilitating the mind and spirit's capacity to affect bodily function and symptoms; however, a reciprocal relationship is also part of the equation (i.e., physical illness affects mental and spiritual health). These approaches are based on the recent research advances in psychoneuroimmunology and psychoneuroendocrinology (Lloyd & Dunn, 2007).

The MBS relationship is well accepted in conventional medicine and likely to be the domain most familiar to psychiatric mental health nurses and nurses in general. Many of the MBS interventions, such as cognitive behavioural therapy, relaxation techniques, guided imagery, hypnosis, and support groups, are now considered mainstream and have been the subject of considerable research. Research substantiates that these approaches dampen the parasympathetic responses in trauma that can lead to chronic health problems, PTSD, anxiety, and depression (Anselmo, 2013). Meditation, prayer, spiritual healing, and therapies using creative outlets such as dance, music, and art have been researched less and often continue to be categorized as TCAM.

Guided Imagery

The use of guided imagery has been in nursing literature for at least three decades. In her seminal work, Zahourek (2002) describes imagery as a holistic phenomenon that is a "multidimensional mental representation of reality and fantasy that includes not only visual pictures, but also remembrance of situations and experiences such as sound, smell, touch, movement and taste" (p. 113). As such, it can be used to promote the healing response in all dimensions of health. The clinical effectiveness of imagery has been well documented in the treatment of anxiety, depression, and a variety of stress-related illnesses (Schaub & Burt, 2013). Nurses can actively assist patients to explore what health-promoting images they can integrate into their self-care practices.

Principles of imagery have been integrated with new expressions of MBS therapy, such as somatic experiencing (SE) and self-regulation therapy (SRT), as a way of holistically processing and releasing trauma (Levine, 2010). Specialized preparation is required for practice of these modalities.

Biofeedback

Biofeedback is the use of some form of external equipment or method of feedback (some as simple as a handheld thermometer; others as complex as cardiac monitoring) that informs a person about his or her psychophysiological processes and state of arousal (Anselmo, 2013). This process enables the person to begin to voluntarily control reactions that were previously outside conscious awareness. Biofeedback has been extensively practised and researched since the 1960s to treat anxiety, substance abuse, and a variety of stress-related health challenges (Anselmo, 2013).

Hypnosis and Therapeutic Suggestion

Hypnosis is both a state of awareness (consciousness) and an intervention. As a state of consciousness, hypnosis is a natural focusing of attention that may range in susceptibility to suggestion. In stress states, people are more susceptible to suggestion because their focus of attention is narrowed. People who dissociate in traumatic situations are in a trancelike state. When relaxation and imagery techniques are used, individuals frequently will enter a similarly altered state of awareness, or trancelike state, that can promote a healing response (Gurgevich, 2012).

Meditation

Several forms of meditation have become popular self-help methods to reduce stress and promote wellness. Meditation practices include such simple behaviours as consciously breathing and focusing attention while walking, sitting, or engaging in other contemplative activity such as yoga (Fortney & Bonus, 2012). Other forms of meditation have arisen from scientifically based work such as that done by Benson in relation to "the relaxation response" and by Kabat Zinn in relation to mindfulness-based stress reduction (MBSR) (Anselmo, 2013). Whatever its origins, meditation practice cultivates a contemplative state of mind that can induce an experience of deep relaxation and calm (Anselmo, 2013). Nurses may guide patients toward individual teachers, meditation books, audio recordings, or group classes, with religious (e.g., Hindu, Buddhist) or nonreligious (e.g., MBSR) approaches, depending on patients' preferences and interests.

Recent meta-analyses have demonstrated the effectiveness of meditation, in particular in the treatment of anxiety (Sedlmeier, Eberth, Schwartz, et al., 2012). A literature review by Hofmann and colleagues (2010) suggests that mindfulness-based therapy is a particularly promising intervention for treating anxiety and mood problems (see Research Highlight). An Australian research synthesis showed strong evidence for moderate exercise and

🔍 RESEARCH HIGHLIGHT

Animal-Assisted Therapy

Problem
Animal-assisted interventions are not well understood within the psychiatric community. It is believed that this poses a barrier to the recognition and acceptance of this complementary therapy.

Purpose of Study
The purpose of the present Australian-based qualitative study was to examine equine-assisted psychotherapy (EAP) facilitators' perspectives on the biopsychosocial benefits and therapeutic outcomes of EAP for adolescents experiencing depression or anxiety.

Methods
A qualitative research design was used to gain an in-depth understanding of how therapists experience and create meaning in relation to EAP. Individual interviews were conducted. Themes developed from this data, and the lived experience was reported by the researchers.

Key Findings
The findings suggest a range of improvements within adolescent clients, including increases in confidence, self-esteem, and assertiveness, as well as a decrease in undesirable behaviours. The effectiveness of the therapy was thought to be due to the experiential nature of involving horses in therapy.

Implications for Nursing Practice
These results suggest that EAP is a promising intervention for treating anxiety and mood problems in adolescents experiencing depression or anxiety. Nurses are advised to be aware of the approaches and referral sources. Further research in this area is required.

Source: Wilson, K., Buultjens, M., Monfries, M., et al. (2017). Equine-assisted psychotherapy for adolescents experiencing depression and/or anxiety: A therapist's perspective. *Clinical Child Psychology and Psychiatry, 22*(1), 16–33. doi:10.1177/1359104515572379.

mindfulness meditation in the management of anxiety disorders. The trials reviewed found significant oxygenation and neuro-chemical changes as a result of even brief meditation practices (Sarris, Moylan, Camfield, et al., 2012).

Such meditative practices are increasingly being integrated with neuroscience by such innovators as University of Toronto psychiatrist Dr. Norman Doidge, who has pioneered their use in promotion of brain neuroplasticity and "re-wiring" in relation to anxiety, mood symptoms, and other mental health challenges (Doidge, 2007). Numerous recent studies featured by NCCAM reveal that meditation is, indeed, associated with structural changes in the brain, opening the door to further study of specific applications to treat specific mental health challenges (NCCAM, 2011d).

Rhythmic Breathing

While breathing is an integral part of meditation practice, Kitko (2007) describes rhythmic breathing as an easy-to-learn and easy-to-implement MBS intervention in its own right. The nurse helps the patient focus on purposeful breath and usually breathes alongside the patient. This activity enhances the relaxation response in both nurse and patient and has implications for psychiatric mental health nurses working with agitated patients.

Spirituality

Historically, there are many precedents for the inclusion of spirituality in mental health care (Koenig, 2011). Today, there is increasing interest in the use of spiritual interventions in all aspects of health (Kalish, 2012). Their positive influence on mental health has been well documented in the interdisciplinary literature in terms of enhanced coping, improved quality of life, and faster recovery (Balbuena, Baetz, & Bowen, 2013). Integration of spiritual care has been associated with fulfilled spiritual needs (such as connectedness, trust, hope, meaning, mastery, and calm), which are observed to promote enhanced overall physiological functioning and openness to mental, emotional, spiritual, and relational transformation, whether or not chronic psychiatric symptoms persist (Rakel & Jonas, 2012).

One challenge in meeting the spiritual needs of psychiatric patients is maintaining appropriate boundaries. Patients may experience difficulty in knowing where their own beliefs stop and those of the health care provider begin. Patients are in a vulnerable position of potentially being unfairly influenced by someone with strong beliefs, particularly if their functioning is compromised by psychiatric symptoms (Koenig, 2011). In meeting the spiritual needs of psychiatric patients, it is imperative that nurses be continually aware and respectful of boundary issues and never impose their beliefs on patients. This awareness is particularly important in the pluralistic Canadian context, wherein a great diversity of spiritual world views coexist (Bibby, 2011). As such, it is important for the nurse to avoid the assumption that tending to spiritual needs involves connection to religious activity.

To address the spiritual needs of patients, we explore their spiritual practices, concerns, beliefs, questions, and resources. The assessment itself is a powerful intervention. When we ask patients about the importance of spirituality in their lives, we are helping them to mobilize their spiritual resources to promote healing (Young & Koopsen, 2011). In the mental health setting, such inquiry must always be done in a way that does not reinforce any religious delusions that may be present.

The Canadian-based T.R.U.S.T. Model for Inclusive Spiritual Care draws on the interdisciplinary literature to offer guidelines for a nonintrusive, integrative approach to spiritual assessment and intervention in a pluralistic context (Scott Barss, 2012) (Figure 35-1). Inclusive spiritual care is defined as relevant, nonintrusive care that tends to the spiritual dimension of health by addressing universal spiritual needs, honouring unique spiritual world views, and helping individuals to explore and mobilize factors that can help them gain or regain a sense of trust in order to promote optimal healing. The spiritual dimension of health is defined as the dimension of health associated with "matters of the spirit," as ultimately defined by each individual (Scott Barss, 2012). The spiritual dimension may or may not involve a sense of connection to a divine presence or to religious structures or

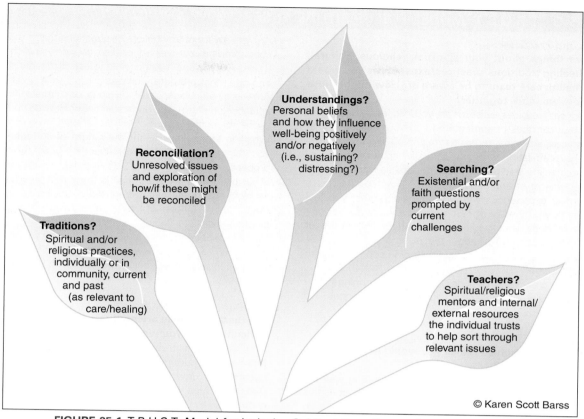

FIGURE 35-1 T.R.U.S.T. Model for Inclusive Spiritual Care. Source: Scott Barss, K., 2008.

traditions, and it is associated with universal spiritual needs such as trust, hope, meaning, purpose, interconnection, reconciliation, inspiration, and creativity (Kalish, 2012). Box 35-3 includes sample questions to inform patient-centred spiritual exploration should patients wish to have it included in their holistic health care (Scott Barss, 2012). The box highlights initial assessment questions to help nurses meet minimum standards for spiritual care that emphasize that all patients are to be invited to receive spiritual care in keeping with their individual world view (Pinto, March, & Pravikoff, 2008). The initial assessment questions are closed-ended to ensure that such inquiry is nonintrusive. They need to be accompanied by explicit statements establishing their relevance and affirming the availability of related exploration at a later time if the patient is not currently interested. Any such inquiry may need to be postponed if the patient is actively psychotic or unable to focus on such exploration (Koenig, 2011). Deep listening is essential for health care providers to be able to discern which, if any, questions are currently relevant to explore with the patient; of course, such questions are just one dimension of the therapeutic dialogue (Scott Barss, 2012). In the process, patients can integrate spiritual and cultural practices and resources to support their healing. Those individuals specifically trained to offer therapy and counselling from a religious and spiritual perspective (e.g., leaders with shamanic training, Islamic imams, Christian pastors or priests, spiritual or cultural care leaders or hospital chaplains, Catholic or Buddhist nuns) may be an important resource at times of illness and crisis. Certain

religious communities offer informal or formal community outreach and events that may be an important part of ongoing recovery and inclusion into community life for patients as well as families.

Biologically Based Therapies

Biologically based therapies include the use of dietary supplements such as vitamins, minerals, herbs, or other botanicals; amino acids; and substances such as enzymes, organ tissues, and metabolites. With the proliferation of literature on natural health products, many people are purchasing over-the-counter products and bypassing a visit to a health care provider. Open discussions and ongoing literature reviews on the associated risks and benefits are a must within the nurse–patient relationship. The NCCAM and Natural Standard websites and publications offer ongoing research updates in this rapidly expanding area (Ulbricht, 2011). This chapter briefly introduces dietary and herbal supplements that have been used in relation to various mental health challenges and directs readers to engage in additional ongoing research in order to promote patient safety. Consultation with all relevant members of the patient's integrative health care team is also essential in accessing accurate, up-to-date information.

Diet and Nutrition

It is essential that nurses assess the patient's nutritional status and practices and address these areas in health teaching. Assess

BOX 35-3 T.R.U.S.T. MODEL FOR SPIRITUAL ASSESSMENT AND CARE

Traditions and Practices

- **Are there things about your spiritual, religious, cultural, and/or healing traditions/practices/experiences you would like the health care team to be aware of? How might these affect how we work together?**
- What practices, activities, or issues are you inspired by/passionate about? How can these be integrated into your healing? What new practices, activities, or issues might you like to explore?
- Do you have affiliation with any particular spiritual, religious, cultural or healing traditions? If so, do you see it/them as a current source of strength? Of distress? How so? Are there aspects of or experiences with your tradition(s) that you feel contribute to your well-being? Compromise your well-being?
- What do or does your tradition(s) say about the nature of suffering? How do you feel about that?
- What gives you hope? How can we help you connect to your sources of hope?
- How are you creative in your daily life? In your coping? How can this creativity be applied to your current challenges? To your life in general?

Reconciliation

- **Are there any unresolved issues you would like support in exploring at this time?**
- Are there situations, choices, or actions of others in your life with whom you cannot currently make peace? How does this influence your sense of well-being? What do you wish to do with this awareness?
- Do you find yourself focusing on past choices or actions that you regret? How does this focus influence your sense of well-being? What do you wish to do with this awareness?
- What does "reconciliation" mean to you? What would "reconciliation" look and feel like to you? What might be the benefits of reconciliation?
- Do your current spiritual/religious/cultural traditions play a role in finding reconciliation? What do their teachings say about "reconciliation," "forgiveness," "non-attachment," or "re-balancing"? Do they assist/interfere? How so?
- Have you found anything positive arising from your painful experiences? (e.g., development of inner strengths you didn't know you had; closer relationships; deeper trust; lessons learned; deeper appreciation for the good times; a sense of purpose or meaning, more creative coping?) If so, how does/can this enhance your daily life amidst the difficulties you face? If not, does it feel okay, for now, to grieve the losses associated with your difficulties?
- What/who can sustain you until you feel more hopeful/peaceful? Do you see yourself being able to feel more hopeful/peaceful?

Understandings

- **Are there particular personal beliefs or practices sustaining you/offering you comfort at this time? How can we help you draw upon these for strength?**

- Are you aware of any beliefs or questions that are distressing/compromising your well-being? If so, how do you wish to address these? Do you see it as possible to eventually transform them into ones that promote wellness?
- Are there particular spiritual, religious, or cultural influences that influence or inform your understandings? How do you feel about these influences?
- What do you believe about the nature of suffering? How do you think these beliefs are influencing your current healing process?
- What gives your life meaning? Is there any meaning that you make in relation to your current difficulties? If so, what? How does this influence the way you navigate your circumstances?
- Has this experience prompted you to ponder your overall life's purpose(s)? If so, what is your sense about it/them? How does this influence your well-being/your approach to life/your healing process?

Searching

- **Are there spiritually oriented questions about your current difficulties that you would like an opportunity to explore?**
- How have your current difficulties influenced your beliefs? Are there any of your previously held beliefs that you are currently questioning? How do you feel about questioning these beliefs? Does this type of questioning feel safe/unsafe? What/who contributes to this sense of safety/risk?
- What answers about life/death/spirituality are you currently seeking? How difficult is this searching?
- What/who is a source of disillusionment for you? Have you had an opportunity to grieve associated losses? If not, how might you do so?
- Has the imposition of others' beliefs added to your distress? If so, how? How can you gain protection from these intrusions?

Teachers

- **Are there people/groups/resources you find helpful in exploring spiritual questions? How can they be involved in your healing process?**
- Who do you consider to be your spiritual teachers/mentors/leaders/companions?
- What readings and activities do you find personally inspiring or comforting? How might they contribute to your healing? How can you draw these resources into your regular routine?
- What new mentors, readings, activities, and events would you like to access?
- What resources within yourself can you name and draw upon? What new internal resources would you like to develop?

Note: Bolded questions have been identified as suitable for initial assessment/trust-building.
Source: Scott Barss, K. (2012). T.R.U.S.T.: An affirming model for inclusive spiritual care. *Journal of Holistic Nursing, 30*(1), 24–34. doi:10.1177/0898010111418118. Copyright © 2011 by SAGE. Reprinted by Permission of SAGE Publications.

for the use of nutrients such as vitamins, protein supplements, herbal preparations, enzymes, and hormones that are considered dietary supplements. Since some nutritional supplements interact with medications, nurses should specifically ask about the use of supplements during the assessment and should not expect patients to share this information without being asked (Ulbricht, 2011). Nurses can review the use of the supplements and the potential interactions with foods, drugs, and other supplements to reduce risks and maximize benefits.

Nutritional therapies are used to treat a variety of mental health disorders, including depression, anxiety, attention-deficit/hyperactivity disorder (ADHD), menopausal symptoms, dementia, and addictions (NCCAM, 2011d). The efficacy of omega-3 fatty acids continues to be studied in the treatment of mood, impulse control, and psychotic disorders (NCCAM, 2011d). B vitamins, especially vitamin B_6 and folic acid, appear to improve anxiety and depression (Schneider & Lovett, 2007). According to Lake (2009), these vitamins often augment conventional care with antipsychotic, antidepressant, and mood-stabilizing medications. The literature supports combining such approaches with exercise and meditative practices (NCCAM, 2011d).

Megavitamin therapy, also called *orthomolecular therapy*, is a specific approach to nutritional therapy used in integrative mental health care that involves taking large amounts of vitamins, minerals, and amino acids. The theory is that the inability to absorb nutrients from a proper diet alone may lead to the development of different illnesses (Ford, Flicker, Thomas, et al., 2008). The earliest use of megavitamin therapy was for the treatment of schizophrenia, for which a high dosage of niacin was recommended. Canadian psychiatrist Dr. Abram Hoffer pioneered this controversial approach in 1952 and continued to study and promote it throughout his career (Hoffer, 1999).

Herbal Therapy

As with dietary and nutritional supplements, health care providers need to be aware of their patients' use of herbal therapies and any potential adverse effects, interactions, and benefits. Related information can be obtained through NCCAM and Natural Standard websites and publications. Increasingly, pharmacists are able to provide additional information and resources. Each herbal preparation needs to be researched in the same manner as a medication in order to provide safe care. To facilitate this process, it is helpful for nurses to be aware of herbal therapies most frequently used in relation to mental health challenges.

St. John's wort has been used for centuries to improve mood and alleviate pain. It has been extensively researched and generally found to be as effective as antidepressants in the treatment of mild to moderate depression. Results are inconclusive in relation to severe depression, prompting ongoing research. St. John's wort should not be taken in tandem with antidepressant pharmaceuticals due to its serotonergic effects. Caution is also warranted with bipolar disorder, as cases of mania have been reported with its use (Ulbricht, 2011).

Ginkgo biloba has been used and studied in relation to prevention and treatment of cognitive decline, depression, and memory loss associated with electroconvulsive therapy. Overall, results are inconclusive, and studies are ongoing (Ulbricht, 2011).

Kava kava is an herb from the South Pacific taken for anxiety. Kava was considered both safe and effective until 2002, when at least 25 cases of liver toxicity—including hepatitis, cirrhosis, and liver failure—were linked to its use. According to Lake (2009), the cases of liver failure were associated with a processing error in the production of a single batch of kava. In response to this controversial information, much confusion has arisen as to its legal status in Canada. However, kava kava is currently not legal for sale through Canadian businesses.

Valerian is used as an antianxiety agent and has also been reported to have antidepressant and sedative properties (NCCAM, 2011d). Results about its efficacy are mixed, but it is generally recognized as safe for the short-term treatment of insomnia when taken at the recommended dosages and not taken in combination with other sedative medications.

Herbal teas have long been used for their sedative–hypnotic effects. Common ingredients in these teas (in addition to valerian) are hops, lemon balm, chamomile, and passionflower. The most studied of these is chamomile, a tea widely used as a folk remedy. Chamomile extract has been found to bind with gamma-aminobutyric acid (GABA) receptors. These teas, along with improving sleep hygiene, may be part of a set of interventions for insomnia; they are generally safely recommended but should be used with awareness of their individual potential effects, adverse effects, and interactions (Ulbricht, 2011). Table 35-2 provides examples of herbal and dietary supplements used with psychiatric symptoms and disorders.

Aromatherapy

Aromatherapy, the use of essential oils for enhancing physical and mental well-being and healing, is a popular therapy. Essential oils, often derived from herbs and plants, may be applied directly to the skin by carrier oil or diffused into the atmosphere through a diffuser. Essential oils are believed to stimulate the release of neurotransmitters in the brain. The sense of smell connects with the part of the brain that controls the autonomic (involuntary) nervous system. Depending on the essential oil used, the resulting effects are calming, pain reducing, stimulating, sedating, or euphoria producing (Smith & Kyle, 2008).

Smith and Kyle (2008, p. 7) provide a convenient chart on how various classifications of oils affect people, as follows:
- Rooty oils such as patchouli and valerian affect calming, grounding, and stabilizing.
- Floral oils such as ylang-ylang and jasmine create mood uplifting, relaxation, and sensuality.
- Green herbaceous oils such as lavender and chamomile create balance, regulation, and clarification.

Aromatherapy has been used to treat anxiety and mood disorders. Several recent research studies featured by NCCAM report positive results in this regard. Some individuals, particularly those with pulmonary disease, may be sensitive or allergic to essential oils when they come into contact with the skin or are inhaled. To prevent an allergic reaction, always dilute oils, administer a small amount, and perform a 24-hour skin patch test before massaging any essential oil into the skin. Ongoing consultation with a trained aromatherapist is essential, keeping

TABLE 35-2	TRADITIONAL, COMPLEMENTARY, AND ALTERNATIVE MEDICINE USED IN PSYCHIATRIC DISORDERS	

HERBAL SUPPLEMENT	USES	CAUTIONS
St. John's wort	Depression	• Interaction with other medications • Photosensitivity • Increased risk of serotonin syndrome when combined with pro-serotonergic medications such as antidepressants, triptans, and methadone
Kava (Kava kava)	Insomnia Fatigue Anxiety	• Warnings against use due to the link to severe liver damage
Golden Root (Rhodiola)	Anxiety Fatigue Depression	• Dizziness, dry mouth, and headaches may occur • Allergic reactions can occur
Valerian Root	Insomnia Anxiety Depression	• Generally considered safe for short time periods • Mild side effects could include morning fatigue, headaches, dizziness, upset stomach
Chamomile	Sleeplessness Anxiety	• Allergic reactions can occur, particularly in those allergic to the daisy family of plants
Lavender	Anxiety Restlessness Insomnia Depression	• Topical use generally considered safe if diluted properly, although breast growth in young boys has been reported • Oil taken by mouth may be poisonous • Teas and extracts may cause side effects including GI complaints and headache • Use with medications with sedative properties may cause drowsiness to increase
Melatonin	Insomnia Jet lag Night shift	• May worsen mood in dementia • Side effects uncommon, but possibly drowsiness, dizziness, headache, nausea • Long-term use may affect the body's ability to produce melatonin on its own
SAMe	Depression	• May interact with certain medications • Increased risk of serotonin syndrome when combined with pro-serotonergic medications such as antidepressants, triptans, and methadone • Side effects are uncommon
Fish Oil (Omega-3 Fatty Acids)	Depression Bipolar disorder	• Possible GI effects, like belching, indigestion • Caution with those having fish/shellfish allergies • May increase bleeding time

GI, Gastrointestinal.
Source: National Center for Complementary and Integrative Health (NCCIH). Retrieved from https://nccih.nih.gov.

in mind that the training and practice of aromatherapists currently remains unregulated (Canadian Federation of Aromatherapists, 2011).

Manipulative Practices

Manipulative practices are based on physically touching another person. (Therapeutic touch is included among the energy therapies since it technically does not involve physical touching of a patient.) The use of any physical touch in psychiatric mental health nursing practice continues to be controversial. Some believe it is not used enough, but most believe it should be used sparingly, with clear intent, recognizing that maintenance of therapeutic boundaries is extremely important, particularly with patients who have psychiatric disorders and might misinterpret touch (Jackson & Latini, 2013).

Chiropractic Medicine

Chiropractic medicine is one of the most widely used integrative therapies. The term *chiropractic* comes from the Greek words *praxix* and *cheir*, meaning "practice" or "treatment by hand." Chiropractic medicine focuses on the relationship between the body's structure (mainly the spine) and function and the way that relationship affects the preservation and restoration of health, using manipulative therapy as a treatment tool. Many chiropractors treat patients with depression, anxiety, and chronic pain (NCCAM, 2011h). Limited formal research is evident in this regard.

Massage Therapy

Massage therapy includes a broad group of practices and techniques that press, rub, and manipulate muscles and soft tissues of the body. There are more than 80 different types of massage therapy (Esmail, 2007). It is intended to promote relaxation and circulation in order to promote healing. Massage has been used in the mental health context to enhance mood and reduce anxiety associated with a variety of diagnoses; as such, it is considered an appropriate adjuvant therapy for those who are so inclined (Schneider & Lovett, 2007). Shiatsu massage, which stimulates similar points to those in acupuncture, may be a favourable alternative to acupuncture for patients with an aversion to the use of needles. Shiatsu has shown promise in reducing both psychopathology and pharmaceutical adverse effects in schizophrenia when used as an adjuvant therapy (Lichtenberg, Vass, Ptaya, et al., 2009).

Reflexology

Reflexology is a type of manipulative practice that focuses on the feet, hands, or ears. This approach is based on the understanding that zones and points on these areas of the body (most commonly the feet) correspond to other parts of the body. The purpose of treatments is to improve circulation in the feet to promote optimal function elsewhere in the body (Jackson & Latini, 2013). Research on this intervention is sparse at present. Morris (2006) completed a pilot study with perimenopausal and postmenopausal women using hand, ear, and foot reflexology. Results indicated that women were more relaxed and had more sleep after a 50-minute reflexology session once a week.

Energy Therapies

Energy therapies are based on the belief that nonphysical bioenergy forces pervade the universe and people. Explanations vary as to the nature of this energy, the form of the therapies, and the rationale for how healing is believed to occur, depending on the affiliated world view. The energy is referred to as *qi* in TCM, *prana* in Indian Ayurvedic medicine, *ki* in Japanese medicine, and a variety of other names in other cultures, including *biofield energy* in contemporary Western cultures (Slater, 2013). This energy takes a particular form in each person, called the *human energy field* or *aura*. This energy field is said to contain a number of layers, each with energy of different frequencies. Energy is transferred between layers and eventually into the physical body through *chakras*. Disturbances of the energy field are seen as the cause of illness, and healing is understood to occur when the human energy field is balanced and energy is flowing freely (Slater, 2013).

Practitioners of energy medicine believe that they are able to increase their awareness of the human energy field and enhance healing through meditation and centring (or other practice to access a sense of inner calm) (Zahourek, 2002). Practitioners believe that they can then detect problems in others' energy fields and adjust the quality or create balance. This detection is accomplished by placing one's hands in or through these fields to direct the energy through visualized or actual pressure or manipulation (or both) of the body. Energy-based modalities currently have uncertain biomedical research support (Anderson & Taylor, 2011). Engebretson and Wardell (2007) explain that such research on energy therapies presents particular challenges. First, determining a method to measure the success of energy therapies is difficult since their success is based on restoring balance and total healing, which are not easily quantified. Further, establishing the appropriate time for an intervention to take effect and the dosage of an energy therapy is currently impossible. Finally, establishing control groups and dealing with personality variables with individual healers and patients confound results. Still, several recent qualitative studies report positive results of the biofield therapies in terms of patients' self-reported sense of well-being, specifically in relation to reduced anxiety, depression, and pain. In addition, no adverse effects have been documented, warranting ongoing investigation and use as relevant

to patients' world views and preferences (Jackson & Latini, 2013).

Therapeutic touch, healing touch, and Reiki are the most common energy therapies practised by nurses, and in many provinces and territories, the integration of such therapies into nursing practice is regulated by standards of nursing practice, alongside institutional guidelines, and always with patient consent. The CHNA, the AHNA, and Healing Touch International offer certificate courses in therapeutic touch and healing touch (Slater, 2013). These modalities are sometimes blended with thought field therapy (TFT) and emotional freedom technique (EFT), which are discussed below.

Therapeutic Touch

Therapeutic touch was developed in the 1970s by Dolores Krieger, a nursing professor at New York University, and Dora Kunz, a Canadian healer. The premise for therapeutic touch is that healing is promoted by balancing the body's energies. In preparation for a treatment session, practitioners focus completely on the person receiving the treatment, without any other distraction. Practitioners then assess the energy field, clear and balance it through hand movements, and direct energy in a specific region of the body. The therapist does not physically touch the patient. After undergoing a session of therapeutic touch, patients report a sense of deep relaxation (Jackson & Latini, 2013).

Healing Touch

Healing touch is a derivative of therapeutic touch developed by a registered nurse, Janet Mentgen (Anderson & Taylor, 2011). Healing touch combines several energy therapies and is based on the belief that the body is a complex energy system that can be influenced by another through that person's intention for healing and well-being. Healing touch is related to therapeutic touch in the belief that working energetically with people to achieve their highest level of well-being, and not necessarily to relieve a specific symptom, is the goal. Healing touch involves gentle "laying of the hands" on a clothed body or moving over the body in the energy field. The practitioner may focus on a specific problem area or the full body (Jackson & Latini, 2013).

Reiki

The Japanese spiritual practice of Reiki has become an increasingly popular modality for nurses to learn and practise. Reiki is an energy-based therapy in which the practitioner's energy is connected to a universal source (*chi, qi, prana,* and *ki*) and is transferred to a recipient for physical or spiritual healing (NCCAM, 2011g). Numerous hospitals, hospices, cancer support groups, and clinics are now offering Reiki in complementary programs. Research has been conducted on such topics as reducing anxiety, depression, and pain and on promoting self-care for caregivers (vanderVaart, Gijsen, de Wildt, et al., 2009). It has thus been used as an adjunct in psychotherapy (Jackson & Latini, 2013).

Thought Field Therapy and Emotional Freedom Technique

Thought field therapy (TFT) was first developed by Roger Callahan in the 1980s and then modified in the 1990s by Gary

Craig, who called his version the *emotional freedom technique* (EFT). The basis for these interventions is the idea that negative emotions are the result of energy imbalances and blocks in the body. The goal is to release these blocks and view the problem with less distress by tapping specific acupuncture points and meridians and repeating a positive mantra (Borgatti, 2008).

Bioelectromagnetic-Based Therapies

In contrast, bioelectromagnetic-based therapies involve the unconventional use of electromagnetic fields, such as pulsed fields, magnetic fields, or alternating-current or direct-current fields. Transcranial magnetic stimulation (TMS) and vagus nerve stimulation (VNS) treatments for depression are in this category.

Pulsating magnetic fields are sent through a metal coil attached to the person's scalp using these techniques (see Chapter 13). High-frequency pulses stimulate, and low-frequency pulses dampen, neural impulses. TMS has been used to treat depression and to decrease auditory hallucination in schizophrenia (see Chapter 13). VNS was originally developed for epilepsy and showed some promise in treating medication-resistant depression. Its effectiveness is still being evaluated (see Chapter 13). Similarly, transcutaneous electrical acupoint stimulation is being evaluated as an adjunctive treatment for opioid detoxification (Meade, Lukas, McDonald, et al., 2010).

Note: The NCCAM website (http://nccam.nih.gov) provides detailed information, reviews, and updates about these and other traditional, complementary, and alternative modalities.

KEY POINTS TO REMEMBER

- A philosophy of holism and the promotion of a therapeutic relationship are at the heart of psychiatric mental health nursing and are important no matter what healing modality is used.
- Traditional, complementary, alternative, and integrative approaches are in demand as patients seek a broader range of therapies than those offered by biomedical approaches.
- With the availability of online information, patients are more likely to have researched their symptoms or conditions and identified potential TCAM treatments.
- Nurses are in an ideal position to guide patients to reliable resources, such as NCCAM, that provide up-to-date information for health care providers and patients.
- Nurses need to keep abreast of current research about major TCAM therapies so that they can (1) identify those that could be beneficial, affordable, and safe; (2) help patients avoid incurring unnecessary costs on ineffective therapies; (3) guide patients in discerning which therapies could be harmful; and (4) assist patients to maximize the benefits of TCAM therapies.

CRITICAL THINKING

1. As a nurse, you may have patients who use integrative therapies in conjunction with the conventional therapies prescribed by the health care provider. Identify issues that are important to assess, and discuss how you would ask about the use of these nonconventional practices.
2. Choose and research a healing modality that you would like to use for self-care. Reflect on your experience of accessing evidence-informed studies and how they improve your nursing practice.
3. Since mindfulness-based approaches demonstrate good effects for patients with anxiety and depression, consider what the nurse can do to support the patient's efforts in using these strategies.

CHAPTER REVIEW

1. A patient has questioned the nurse about the safety of a herbal supplement. Which nursing response is most appropriate?
   a. "Herbal supplements are regulated by the provinces and territories."
   b. "Since they are natural products, herbal supplements are harmless."
   c. "I know of a couple of websites and a pharmacist that can help us address your question."
   d. "If your supplement was available over the counter, it should be safe."
2. Which of the following is true of integrative health care?
   a. It is synonymous with complementary and alternative healing.
   b. It is being widely offered in the Canadian health care system.
   c. It requires nurses to focus solely on the patient.
   d. It encourages nurses to adopt an overall holistic lifestyle.
3. A patient with schizophrenia has asked the nurse about replacing prescribed antipsychotic medications with meditation and shiatsu massage. Which nursing response is most appropriate?
   a. "Both modalities may have benefits as adjuncts to your antipsychotic medication, but likely not as replacements. How can I help you find out more?"
   b. "You shouldn't even consider it. They're not safe."
   c. "I'm concerned that your illness is affecting your judgement. I think we should talk with your doctor about a medication adjustment."
   d. "I've read that they're very promising. It's worth a try."

4. In facilitating spiritual care in a mental health setting, it is important for nurses to do which of the following:
   a. Avoid facilitating spiritual care with patients who are psychotic
   b. Explicitly share personal beliefs so patients know where they stand
   c. Address spiritual needs without reinforcing any delusional thinking present
   d. Rely on referral to clergy since their expertise is needed to approach the topic

5. Contemplative practices are an important aspect of integrative mental health care because of which of the following:
   a. They have the potential to positively enhance brain structure and function.
   b. They promote a sense of calm and trust.
   c. They reduce symptoms of anxiety and depression.
   d. All of the above are important aspects of integrative mental health care.

⊖volve WEBSITE

Post-Test interactive review

Visit the Evolve website for Chapter Review Answers and Rationales, Critical Thinking Answer Guidelines, and additional resources related to the content in this chapter: http://evolve.elsevier.com/Canada/Varcarolis/psychiatric/

REFERENCES

Acupuncture Canada. (2011). *Regulation in Canada*. Retrieved from https://www.acupuncturecanada.org/.

Anderson, J., & Taylor, A. (2011). Effects of healing touch in clinical practice: A systematic review of randomized clinical trials. *Journal of Holistic Nursing, 29*(3), 221–228. doi:10.1177/0898010110393353.

Anselmo, J. (2013). Relaxation. In B. Dossey & L. Keegan (Eds.), *Holistic nursing: A handbook for practice* (6th ed., pp. 327–361). Sudbury, MA: Jones and Bartlett.

Balbuena, L., Baetz, M., & Bowen, R. (2013). Religious attendance, spirituality, and major depression in Canada: A 14-year follow-up study. *Canadian Journal of Psychiatry, 58*(4), 225–232.

Barrere, C. (2013). Teaching future holistic nurses: Integrating holism into an undergraduate nursing curriculum. In B. Dossey & L. Keegan (Eds.), *Holistic nursing: A handbook for practice* (6th ed., pp. 815–824). Sudbury, MA: Jones and Bartlett.

Bibby, R. (2011). *Beyond the gods and back: Religion's demise and rise and why it matters*. Lethbridge, AB: Project Canada Books.

Binda, J. (2011). *The renaissance of native spirituality: The journey of the spiritual seeker and traditional healing practices*. Bloomington, IN: iUniverse Books.

Borgatti, J. C. (2008). Tap your way to fast relief. *American Nurse Today, 3*(1), 32–33.

Canadian Association of Naturopathic Doctors. (2011). *Education & regulation*. Retrieved from http://www.cand.ca/index.php?40.

Canadian Association of Schools of Nursing & Canadian Federation of Mental Health Nurses. (2017). *Entry-to-practice mental health and addiction competencies for undergraduate nursing education in Canada*. Ottawa: Canadian Association of Schools of Nursing.

Canadian Chiropractic Association. (2011). *Chiropractic and you*. Retrieved from https://www.chiropractic.ca/.

Canadian Federation of Aromatherapists. (2011). *About us*. Retrieved from http://cfacanada.com/about/.

Canadian Holistic Nurses Association. (2011). *Specialization program in holistic nursing*. Retrieved from http://www.chna.ca/.

Cao, H., Pan, X., Li, H., et al. (2009). Acupuncture for treatment of insomnia: A systematic review of randomized controlled trials. *Journal of Alternative and Complementary Medicine, 15*, 1171–1186. doi:10.1089/acm.2009.0041.

Doidge, N. (2007). *The brain that changes itself: Stories of personal triumph from the frontiers of brain science*. New York: Viking.

Engebretson, J., & Wardell, D. W. (2007). Energy-based modalities. *Nursing Clinics of North America, 42*, 243–259. doi:10.1016/j.cnur.2007.02.004.

Esmail, N. (2007). Complementary and alternative medicine in Canada: Trends in use and public attitudes, 1997–2006. *Fraser Institute Public Policy Sources, 87*, 19–22.

Ford, A. H., Flicker, L., Thomas, J., et al. (2008). Vitamins B_{12}, B_6, and folic acid for onset of depressive symptoms in older men: Results from a 2-year placebo-controlled trial. *The Journal of Clinical Psychiatry, 69*(8), 1203–1209.

Fortney, L., & Bonus, K. (2012). Recommending meditation. In D. Rakel (Ed.), *Integrative medicine* (3rd ed., pp. 873–881). Toronto: Saunders.

Gurgevich, S. (2012). Self-hypnosis techniques. In D. Rakel (Ed.), *Integrative medicine* (3rd ed., pp. 836–842). Toronto: Saunders.

Health Canada. (2012a). *Drugs and health products: About natural health products: How can I use natural health products safely?* Retrieved from http://www.hc-sc.gc.ca/dhp-mps/prodnatur/about-apropos/cons-eng.php.

Health Canada. (2012b). *Drugs and health products: Natural health products*. Retrieved from http://www.hc-sc.gc.ca/dhp-mps/prodnatur/index-eng.php.

Health Canada. (2012c). *Natural health product tracking survey—2010 final report*. Ottawa: Author.

Health Canada. (2012d). *The regulation of natural health products (NHPs) in Canada: Myths and facts*. Ottawa: Author.

Hoffer, A. (1999). *Orthomolecular treatment for schizophrenia: Megavitamin supplements and nutritional strategies for healing and recovery*. Lincolnwood, IL: Keats.

Hofmann, S., Sawyer, A., Witt, A., et al. (2010). The effect of mindfulness-based therapy on anxiety and depression: A meta-analytic review. *Journal of Consulting and Clinical Psychology, 78*(2), 169–183. doi:10.1037/a0018555.

Jackson, C., & Keegan, L. (2013). Touch. In B. M. Dossey & L. Keegan (Eds.), *Holistic nursing: A handbook for practice* (6th ed., pp. 347–366). Sudbury, MA: Jones & Bartlett.

Jackson, C., & Latini, C. (2013). Touch and hand-mediated therapies. In B. M. Dossey & L. Keegan (Eds.), *Holistic nursing: A handbook for practice* (6th ed., pp. 417–437). Sudbury, MA: Jones & Bartlett.

Kalish, N. (2012). Evidence-based spiritual care: A literature review. *Current Opinions & Support in Palliative Care, 6*(2), 242–246.

Khorsan, R., Coulter, I. D., Crawford, C., et al. (2011). Systematic review of integrative health care research: Randomized control trials, clinical controlled trials, and meta-analysis. *Evidence-based Complementary and Alternative Medicine*, 1–10. doi:10.1155/2011/636134.

Kitko, J. (2007). Rhythmic breathing as a nursing intervention. *Holistic Nursing Practice, 21*, 85–88. doi:10.1097/01.HNP.0000262023.27572.65.

Koenig, H. (2011). *Spirituality & health research*. West Conshohocken, PA: Templeton.

Lake, J. (2009). *Integrative mental health care: A therapist's handbook*. New York: W. W. Norton.

Levine, P. (2010). *An unspoken voice: How the body releases trauma and restores goodness.* Berkeley, CA: North Atlantic Books.

Lichtenberg, P., Vass, A., Ptaya, H., et al. (2009). Shiatsu as an adjuvant therapy for schizophrenia: An open-label pilot study. *Alternative Therapies in Health and Medicine, 15*(5), 44–46.

Lloyd, L., & Dunn, L. (2007). Mind–body–spirit medicine: Interventions and resources. *JAAPA: Official Journal of the American Academy of Physician Assistants, 20*(10), 31–35.

Mariano, C. (2013). Holistic nursing: Scope and standards of practice. In B. Dossey & L. Keegan (Eds.), *Holistic nursing: A handbook for practice* (6th ed., pp. 59–84). Sudbury, MA: Jones & Bartlett.

Meade, C., Lukas, S., McDonald, L., et al. (2010). A randomized trial of transcutaneous electric acupoint stimulation as adjunctive treatment for opioid detoxification. *Journal of Substance Abuse Treatment, 38*, 12–21. doi:10.1016/j.jsat.2009.05.010.

Morris, D. (2006). Pilot study using reflexology. *Beginnings (American Holistic Nurses' Association), 26*(5), 28–29.

National Center for Complementary and Alternative Medicine. (2011a). *Ayurvedic medicine: An introduction.* Retrieved from http://nccam.nih.gov/health/ayurveda/introduction.htm.

National Center for Complementary and Alternative Medicine. (2011b). *Highlighted research results—acupuncture.* Retrieved from http://nccam.nih.gov/health/357/research.

National Center for Complementary and Alternative Medicine. (2011c). *Homeopathy: An introduction.* Retrieved from http://nccam.nih.gov/health/homeopathy/.

National Center for Complementary and Alternative Medicine. (2011d). *Mental health.* Retrieved from http://nccam.nih.gov/health/mentalhealth.htm.

National Center for Complementary and Alternative Medicine. (2011e). *Naturopathy.* Retrieved from http://nccam.nih.gov/health/naturopathy/.

National Center for Complementary and Alternative Medicine. (2011f). *NCCAM facts-at-a-glance and mission.* Retrieved from http://nccam.nih.gov/about/ataglance/.

National Center for Complementary and Alternative Medicine. (2011g). *Reiki information.* Retrieved from http://nccam.nih.gov/health/reiki/.

National Center for Complementary and Alternative Medicine. (2011h). *Spinal manipulation.* Retrieved from http://nccam.nih.gov/health/chiropractic/.

Native Mental Health Association of Canada. (2008). *Charting the future of Native mental health in Canada: Ten-year strategic plan 2008–2018.* Chilliwack, BC: Author.

Pinto, S., March, P., & Pravikoff, D. (2008). *Evidence-based care sheet: Spiritual needs of hospitalized patients.* Glendale, CA: Cinahl Information Systems.

Rakel, D., & Jonas, W. (2012). Creating optimal healing environments. In D. Rakel (Ed.), *Integrative medicine* (3rd ed., pp. 12–19). Philadelphia: Saunders.

Ramsay, C. (2009). *Unnatural regulation: Complementary and alternative medicine policy in Canada.* Retrieved from https://www.fraserinstitute.org/studies/unnatural-regulation-complementary-and-alternative-medicine-policy-canada.

Registered Psychiatric Nurses Association of Saskatchewan. (2011). *Position statement: The role of the RPN in relation to complementary and alternative healing.* Retrieved from http://www.rpnas.com/?s=position+statement.

Sarris, J. J., Moylan, S. S., Camfield, D. A., et al. (2012). Complementary medicine, exercise, meditation, diet, and lifestyle modification for anxiety disorders: A review of current evidence. *Evidence-based Complementary and Alternative Medicine*, 1–20. doi:10.1155/2012/809653.

Schaub, B., & Burt, M. (2013). Imagery. In B. M. Dossey & L. Keegan (Eds.), *Holistic nursing: A handbook for practice* (6th ed., pp. 363–396). Sudbury, MA: Jones & Bartlett.

Schneider, C., & Lovett, E. (2007). Depression. In D. Rakel (Ed.), *Integrative medicine* (2nd ed., pp. 73–83). Toronto: Saunders.

Scott Barss, K. (2012). T.R.U.S.T.: An affirming model for inclusive spiritual care. *Journal of Holistic Nursing, 30*(1), 24–34. doi:10.1177/0898010111418118.

Sedlmeier, P., Eberth, J., Schwartz, M., et al. (2012). The psychological effects of meditation: A meta-analysis. *Psychological Bulletin, 138*(6), 1139–1171. doi:10.1037/a0028168.

Shields, D. A., & Wilson, D. R. (2016). Energy healing. In B. M. Dossey & L. Keegan (Eds.), *Holistic nursing: A handbook for practice* (7th ed., pp. 345–363). Burlington: MA: Jones & Bartlett.

Slater, V. (2013). Energy healing. In B. M. Dossey & L. Keegan (Eds.), *Holistic nursing: A handbook for practice* (6th ed., pp. 752–774). Sudbury, MA: Jones & Bartlett.

Smith, M. C., & Kyle, L. (2008). Holistic foundations of aromatherapy for nursing. *Holistic Nursing Practice, 22*, 3–9. doi:10.1097/01.HNP.0000306322.03590.e9.

Ulbricht, C. (2011). *Davis's pocket guide to herbs and supplements.* Philadelphia: Natural Standard Research Collaboration/F. A. Davis.

vanderVaart, S., Gijsen, V., de Wildt, S., et al. (2009). A systematic review of the therapeutic effects of Reiki. *Journal of Alternative and Complementary Medicine, 15*(11), 1157–1169. doi:10.1089/acm.2009.0036.

Willison, K. D. (2008). Advancing integrative medicine through interprofessional education. *Health Sociology Review, 17*(4), 342–352. doi:10.5172/hesr.451.17.4.342.

World Health Organization. (2000). *General guidelines for methodologies on research and evaluation of traditional medicine.* Geneva, Switzerland: Author.

Young, C., & Koopsen, C. (2011). *Spirituality, health, and healing: An integrative approach* (2nd ed.). Toronto: Jones & Bartlett.

Zahourek, R. (2002). *Imagery in holistic health and healing.* Philadelphia: F. A. Davis Co.

Zhang, Z., Chen, H., Yip, K., et al. (2010). The effectiveness and safety of acupuncture therapy in depressive disorders: Systematic review and meta-analysis. *Journal of Affective Disorders, 124*, 9–21. doi:10.1016/j.jad.2009.07.005.

Standards of Practice, Code of Ethics, Beliefs, and Values

CANADIAN FEDERATION OF MENTAL HEALTH NURSES STANDARDS OF PRACTICE

Psychiatry/mental health is a specialized area of nursing practice, education, and research. The psychiatric mental health (PMH) nurse uses evidence-informed and experiential knowledge from nursing and related health sciences. This practice is grounded in the values as stated in the Canadian Standards for Psychiatric-Mental Health Nursing (Canadian Federation of Mental Health Nurses, 2014). Practice involves the promotion of mental health and the prevention, treatment, and management of mental disorders.

Standard I:

Provides Competent Professional Care Through the Development of a Therapeutic Relationship

Standard II:

Performs/Refines Client Assessments Through the Diagnostic and Monitoring Function

Standard III:

Administers and Monitors Therapeutic Interventions

Standard IV:

Effectively Manages Rapidly Changing Situations

Standard V:

Intervenes Through the Teaching–Coaching Function

Standard VI:

Monitors and Ensures the Quality of Health Care Practices

Standard VII:

Practices Within Organizational and Work-Role Structure

Beliefs/Values

Psychiatric-mental health nurses believe:
- The centrality of therapeutic nurse-client relationships, based on trust and mutual respect, to practice; 6 Canadian Standards of Psychiatric-Mental Health Nursing
- The alleviation of stigma and discrimination;
- The promotion of recovery and well-being for people of all ages living with mental health problems and illnesses;
- The conduct and utilization of research for improvement in care;
- Social action to promote political and social awareness to influence health and organizational policy;
- Working in collaborative relationships with the individual, family, community, different populations, and social agencies;
- A holistic approach that is essential to understanding the unique experience of the client;
- Equitable access to culturally competent care;
- Reflective ethical practice and a commitment to continuous learning;
- The protection of human rights in the context of civil commitment and relevant aspects of jurisprudence;
- Advocating for practice environments that facilitate and ensure safe and positive work relationships; and
- Fostering a legacy of moral and visionary psychiatric-mental health nursing leaders.

Source: Canadian Federation of Psychiatric Mental Health Nurses. (2014). Canadian standards for psychiatric-mental health nursing (4th ed.). Toronto, ON: Author.

REGISTERED PSYCHIATRIC NURSES OF CANADA

Standards of Psychiatric Nursing Practice

Psychiatric nursing, as a distinct profession, provides service to individuals whose care needs relate to mental, physical, and developmental health. Registered psychiatric nurses engage in various roles providing health services to individuals, families, groups, and communities. The practice of psychiatric nursing occurs within the domains of direct practice, education, administration, and research.

Standard 1: Therapeutic Interpersonal Relationships

Registered psychiatric nurses establish professional, interpersonal, and therapeutic relationships with individuals, groups, families, and communities.

Standard 2: Application and Integration of Theory-Based Knowledge

Registered psychiatric nurses apply and integrate theory-based knowledge relevant to professional practice derived from psychiatric nursing education and continued lifelong learning.

Standard 3: Professional Responsibility

Registered psychiatric nurses are accountable to the public for safe, competent, and ethical psychiatric nursing practice.

Standard 4: Professional Ethics

Registered psychiatric nurses understand, promote, and uphold the ethical values of the profession.

The Code of Ethics

Through the *Code of Ethics*, registered psychiatric nurses uphold the values of:
- Safe, competent, and ethical practice to ensure the protection of the public;
- Respect for the inherent worth, right of choice, and dignity of persons;
- Health, mental health, and well-being; and,
- Quality practice.

Source: Registered Psychiatric Nurses of Canada. (2010). *Code of ethics & standards of psychiatric nursing practice*. Edmonton: Author.

CANADIAN NURSES ASSOCIATION

The Canadian Nurses Association has established a code of ethics to serve as a foundation for ethical practice. It is built upon the specific values and ethical responsibilities expected of registered nurses practicing within Canada.

Values and Ethical Responsibilities

There are seven primary values that guide the practice of registered nurses. Listed below are the primary values are their corresponding ethical responsibilities.

1. Providing safe, compassionate, competence and ethical care.
   - Nurses have a responsibility to conduct themselves according to the ethical responsibilities outlined in this document and in practice standards in what they do and how they interact with persons receiving care as well as with families, communities, and other members of the health-care team.
   - Nurses engage in compassionate care through their speech and body language and through their efforts to understand and care about others' health-care needs.
   - Nurses build trustworthy relationships with persons as the foundation of meaningful communication, recognizing that building these relationships involves a conscious effort. Such relationships are critical to understanding people's needs and concerns.
   - Nurses question, intervene and report to address unsafe, non-compassionate, unethical or incompetent practice or conditions that interfere with their ability to provide safe, compassionate, competent and ethical care to those to whom they are providing care, and they support those who do the same.
   - Nurses admit mistakes and take all necessary actions to prevent or minimize harm arising from an adverse event. They learn from near misses and work with others to reduce the potential for future risks and preventable harms.
   - When resources are not available to provide appropriate or safe care, nurses collaborate with others to adjust priorities and minimize harm. Nurses keep persons, families and communities informed about potential and actual plans to delivery of care. They inform employers about potential threats to safety.
   - Nurses planning to take job action or practising in environments where job action occurs take steps to safeguard the health and safety of people during the course of the job action.
   - During a natural or human-made disaster, including a communicable disease outbreak, nurses have a duty to provide care using appropriate safety precautions.
   - Nurses support, use and engage in research and other activities that promote safe, competent, compassionate and ethical care, and they use guidelines for ethical research that are in keeping with nursing values.
   - Nurses work to prevent and minimize all forms of violence by anticipating and assessing the risk of violent situations and by collaborating with others to establish preventative measures. When violence cannot be anticipated or prevented, nurses take action to minimize risk to protect others and themselves.
2. Promoting health and well-being.
   - Nurses provide care directed first and foremost toward the health and well-being of the person, family or community in their care.
   - When a community health intervention interferes with the individuals rights of persons receiving care, nurses use and advocate for the use of the least restrictive measures possible for those in their care.

- Nurses collaborate with other health-care providers and other interested parties to maximize health benefits to persons with health-care needs and concerns, recognizing and respecting the knowledge, skills and perspectives of all.

3. Promoting and respecting informed decision-making.
   - Nurses, to the extent possible, provide persons with the information they need to make informed and autonomous decisions related to their health and well-being. They also work to ensure that health information is given to individuals, families, groups, populations and communities in their care in an open, accurate, understandable, and transparent manner.
   - Nurses respect the wishes of capable persons to decline to receive information about their health condition. 3
   - Nurses recognize that capable persons may place a different weight on individualism and may choose to defer to family, cultural expectations, or community values in decision-making.
   - Nurses ensure that nursing care is provided with the person's informed consent. Nurses recognize and support a capable person's right to refuse or withdraw consent for care or treatment at any time.
   - Nurses are sensitive to the inherent actual or potential power differentials between care providers and those receiving care. They do not misuse that power to influence decision-making.
   - Nurses advocate for persons in their care if they believe that the health of those persons is being compromised by factors beyond their control, including the decision-making of others.
   - When family members disagree with the decisions made by a person with health-care needs, nurses assist families in gaining an understanding of the person's decisions.
   - Nurses respect the informed decision-making of capable persons, including choice of lifestyles or treatment not conducive to good health.
   - When illness or other factors reduce a person's capacity for making choices, nurses assist or support that person's participation in making choices appropriate to their capability.
   - If a person receiving care is clearly incapable of consent, the nurse respects the law on capacity assessment and substitute decision-making in the nurse's jurisdiction.
   - Nurses, along with other health-care professionals and with substitute decision-makers, consider and respect the person receiving care and any previously known wishes or advance directives that apply in the situation.

4. Preserving dignity.
   - Nurses, in their professional capacity, relate to all persons with respect.
   - Nurses support persons in maintaining their dignity and integrity.
   - In health-care decision-making, in treatment and in care, nurses work with persons receiving care, including families, groups, populations and communities, to take into account their unique values, customs and spiritual beliefs, as well as their social and economic circumstances.

- Nurses intervene, and report when necessary, when others fail to respect the dignity of a person receiving care, recognizing that to be silent and passive is to condone the behaviour.
- Nurses respect the physical privacy of persons by providing care in a discreet manner and by minimizing intrusions as much as possible.
- When providing care, nurses utilize practice standards, best practice guidelines and policies concerning restraint usage.
- Nurses maintain appropriate professional boundaries and ensure their relationships are always for the benefit of the person. They recognize the potential vulnerability of persons and do not exploit their trust and dependency in a way that might compromise the therapeutic relationship. They do not abuse their relationship for personal or financial gain, and do not enter into personal relationships (romantic, sexual or other) with persons in their care.
- In all practice settings, nurses work to relieve pain and suffering, including appropriate and effective symptom and pain management, to allow persons to live and die with dignity.
- When a person receiving care is terminally ill or dying, nurses foster comfort, alleviate suffering, advocate for adequate relief of discomfort and pain and support a dignified and peaceful death. This includes providing a palliative approach to care for the people they interact with, across the lifespan and across the continuum of care and support for the family during and following the death, and care of the person's body after death.
- Nurses treat each other, colleagues, students and other health-care workers in a respectful manner, recognizing opportunities for sharing governance with those in formal leadership positions, staff and students. They work with others to preserve dignity and resolve differences in a constructive way.

5. Maintaining privacy and confidentiality.
   - Nurses respect the right of persons to have control over the collection, use, access and disclosure of their personal information.
   - When nurses are conversing with persons receiving care, they take reasonable measures to prevent confidential information in the conversation from being overheard.
   - Nurses collect, use and disclose health information on a need-to-know basis with the highest degree of anonymity required in the circumstances and in accordance with privacy laws.
   - When nurses are required to disclose information for a particular purpose, they disclose only the amount of information necessary for that purpose and inform only those necessary. They attempt to do so in ways that minimize any potential harm to the persons, family, or community.
   - When nurses engage in any form of communication, including verbal or electronic, involving a discussion of clinical cases, they ensure that their discussion of persons

is respectful and does not identify those persons unless necessary and appropriate.

- Nurses advocate for persons to receive access to their own health-care records through a timely and affordable process when such access is requested.
- Nurses respect policies that protect and preserve persons' privacy, including security safeguards in information technology.
- Nurses do not abuse their access to information by accessing health-care records, including a family member's or any other person's, for purposes inconsistent with their professional obligations.
- Nurses do not use phot or other technology to intrude into the privacy of a person receiving care.
- Nurses intervene if others inappropriately access sod disclose personal or health information of persons receiving care.

6. Promoting justice.
   - When providing care, nurses do not discriminate on the basis of a person's race, ethnicity, culture, political and spiritual beliefs, social or marital status, gender identity, sexual orientation, age, health status, place of origin, lifestyle, mental or physical ability or socioeconomic status or any other attribute.
   - Nurses refrain from judging, labelling, stigmatizing and humiliating behaviours toward persons receiving care, toward other health-care professionals or students and toward each other.
   - Nurses do not engage in any form of lying, punishment or torture or any form of unusual treatment or action that is inhumane or degrading. They refuse to be complicit in such behaviours. They intervene, and they report such behaviours.
   - Nurses make fair decisions about the allocation of resources under their control based on the needs of persons, groups or communities to whom they are providing care. They advocate for fair treatment and for fair distribution of resources.
   - Nurses support a climate of trust that sponsors openness, encourages the act of questioning the status quo and supports those who speak out in good faith to address concerns (e.g., whistle-blowing).

7. Being accountable.
   - Nurses, as members of a self-regulating profession, practise according to the values and responsibilities in the Code of Ethics for Registered Nurses and in keeping with the professional standards, laws and regulations supporting ethical practice.
   - Nurses are honest and practise with integrity in all of their professional interactions.
   - Nurses practise within the limits of their competence. When aspects of care are beyond their level of competence, they seek additional information or knowledge, report to their supervisor or a competent practitioner and/or request a different work assignment. In the meantime, nurses remain with the person receiving care until another nurse is available.
   - Nurses maintain their fitness to practise. If they are aware that they do not have the necessary physical, mental or emotional capacity to practise safely and competently, they withdraw from the provision of care after consulting with their employer. If they are self-employed, arranging that someone else attend to their clients' health-care needs. Nurses then take the necessary steps to regain their fitness to practise.
   - Nurses are attentive to signs that a colleague is unable, for whatever reason, to perform their duties. In such a case, nurses will take the necessary steps to protect the safety of persons receiving care.
   - Nurses clearly and accurately represent themselves with respect to their name, title and role.
   - If nursing care is requested that is in conflict with the nurse's moral beliefs and values but in keeping with professional practice, the nurse provides safe, compassionate, competent and ethical care until alternative care arrangements are in place to meet the person's needs or desires. If nurses can anticipate a conflict with their conscience, they have an obligation to notify their employers or, if the nurse is self-employed, persons receiving care, in advance so that alternative arrangements can be made.
   - Nurses identify and address conflicts of interest. They disclose actual or potential conflicts of interest that arise in their professional roles and relationships and resolve them in the interest of persons receiving care.
   - Nurses share their knowledge and provide feedback, mentorship and guidance for the professional development of nursing students, novice nurses and other health-care team members.

Source: Canadian Nurses Association. (2008). Code of ethics for registered nurses (2008 centennial edition). Ottawa: Canadian Nurses Association.

NANDA-International Nursing Diagnoses 2018–2020

There are 13 domains, 47 classes, and 244 diagnoses in the current NANDA taxonomy. The following identifies all of the domains, the classes within the domains, and the diagnoses within the specified domains and classes.

Domain 1: Health Promotion

Class 1: Health Awareness
  Decreased Diversional Activity Engagement
  Readiness for Enhanced Health Literacy
  Sedentary Lifestyle
Class 2: Health Management
  Frail Elderly Syndrome
  Risk for Frail Elderly Syndrome
  Deficient Community Health
  Risk-Prone Health Behaviour
  Ineffective Health Maintenance
  Ineffective Health Management
  Readiness for Enhanced Health Management
  Ineffective Family Health Management
  Ineffective Protection

Domain 2: Nutrition

Class 1: Ingestion
  Imbalanced Nutrition: Less Than Body Requirements
  Readiness for Enhanced Nutrition
  Insufficient Breast Milk Production
  Ineffective Breastfeeding
  Interrupted Breastfeeding
  Readiness for Enhanced Breastfeeding
  Ineffective Adolescent Eating Dynamics
  Ineffective Child Eating Dynamics
  Ineffective Infant Feeding Dynamics
  Ineffective Infant Feeding Pattern (00107)
  Obesity (00232)
  Overweight (00233)
  Risk for Overweight (00234)
  Impaired Swallowing (00103)

Class 2: Digestion
  This class does not currently contain any diagnoses.
Class 3: Absorption
  This class does not currently contain any diagnoses.
Class 4: Metabolism
  Risk for Unstable Blood Glucose Level
  Neonatal Hyperbilirubinemia
  Risk for Neonatal Hyperbilirubinemia
  Risk for Impaired Liver Function
  Risk for Metabolic Imbalance Syndrome
Class 5: Hydration
  Risk for Electrolyte Imbalance (00195)
  Risk for Imbalanced Fluid Volume
  Deficient Fluid Volume
  Risk for Deficient Fluid Volume
  Excess Fluid Volume (00026)

Domain 3: Elimination and Exchange

Class 1: Urinary Function
  Impaired Urinary Elimination
  Functional Urinary Incontinence
  Overflow Urinary Incontinence
  Reflex Urinary Incontinence
  Stress Urinary Incontinence
  Urge Urinary Incontinence
  Risk for Urge Urinary Incontinence
  Urinary Retention
Class 2: Gastrointestinal Function
  Constipation
  Risk for Constipation
  Perceived Constipation
  Chronic Functional Constipation
  Risk for Chronic Functional Constipation
  Diarrhea
  Dysfunctional Gastrointestinal Motility
  Risk for Dysfunctional Gastrointestinal Motility
  Bowel Incontinence

Class 3: Integumentary Function
    This class does not currently contain any diagnosis.
Class 4: Respiratory Function
    Impaired Gas Exchange

Domain 4: Activity/Rest

Class 1: Sleep/Rest
    Insomnia
    Sleep Deprivation
    Readiness for Enhanced Sleep
    Disturbed Sleep Pattern
Class 2: Activity/Exercise
    Risk for Disuse Syndrome
    Impaired Bed Mobility
    Impaired Physical Mobility
    Impaired Wheelchair Mobility
    Impaired Sitting
    Impaired Standing
    Impaired Transfer Ability
    Impaired Walking
Class 3: Energy Balance
    Imbalanced Energy Field
    Fatigue
    Wandering
Class 4: Cardiovascular/Pulmonary Responses
    Activity Intolerance
    Risk for Activity Intolerance
    Ineffective Breathing Pattern
    Decreased Cardiac Output
    Risk for Decreased Cardiac Output
    Impaired Spontaneous Ventilation
    Risk for Unstable Blood Pressure
    Risk for Decreased Cardiac Tissue Perfusion
    Risk for Ineffective Cerebral Tissue Perfusion
    Ineffective Peripheral Tissue Perfusion
    Risk for Ineffective Peripheral Tissue Perfusion
    Dysfunctional Ventilatory Weaning Response
Class 5: Self-Care
    Impaired Home Maintenance
    Bathing Self-Care Deficit
    Dressing Self-Care Deficit
    Feeding Self-Care Deficit
    Toileting Self-Care Deficit
    Readiness for Enhanced Self-Care
    Self-Neglect

Domain 5: Perception/Cognition

Class 1: Attention
    Unilateral Neglect
Class 2: Orientation
    This class does not currently contain any diagnoses.
Class 3: Sensation/Perception
    This class does not currently contain any diagnoses.
Class 4: Cognition
    Acute Confusion
    Risk for Acute Confusion
    Chronic Confusion

    Labile Emotional Control
    Ineffective Impulse Control
    Deficient Knowledge
    Readiness for Enhanced Knowledge
    Impaired Memory
Class 5: Communication
    Readiness for Enhanced Communication
    Impaired Verbal Communication

Domain 6: Self-Perception

Class 1: Self-Concept
    Hopelessness
    Readiness for Enhanced Hope
    Risk for Compromised Human Dignity
    Disturbed Personal Identity
    Risk for Disturbed Personal Identity
    Readiness for Enhanced Self-Concept
Class 2: Self-Esteem
    Chronic Low Self-Esteem
    Risk for Chronic Low Self-Esteem
    Situational Low Self-Esteem
    Risk for Situational Low Self-Esteem
Class 3: Body Image
    Disturbed Body Image

Domain 7: Role Relationship

Class 1: Caregiving Roles
    Caregiver Role Strain
    Risk for Caregiver Role Strain
    Impaired Parenting
    Risk for Impaired Parenting
    Readiness for Enhanced Parenting
Class 2: Family Relationships
    Risk for Impaired Attachment
    Dysfunctional Family Processes
    Interrupted Family Processes
    Readiness for Enhanced Family Processes
Class 3: Role Performance
    Ineffective Relationship
    Risk for Ineffective Relationship
    Readiness for Enhanced Relationship
    Parental Role Conflict
    Ineffective Role Performance
    Impaired Social Interaction

Domain 8: Sexuality

Class 1: Sexual Identity
    This class does not currently contain any
      diagnoses.
Class 2: Sexual Function
    Sexual Dysfunction
    Ineffective Sexuality Pattern
Class 3: Reproduction
    Ineffective Childbearing Process
    Risk for Ineffective Childbearing Process
    Readiness for Enhanced Childbearing Process
    Risk for Disturbed Maternal–Fetal Dyad

Domain 9: Coping/Stress Tolerance

Class 1: Post-Trauma Responses
  Risk for Complicated Immigration Transition
  Post-Trauma Syndrome
  Risk for Post-Trauma Syndrome
  Rape-Trauma Syndrome
  Relocation Stress Syndrome
  Risk for Relocation Stress Syndrome
Class 2: Coping Responses
  Ineffective Activity Planning
  Risk for Ineffective Activity Planning
  Anxiety
  Defensive Coping
  Ineffective Coping
  Readiness for Enhanced Coping
  Ineffective Community Coping
  Readiness for Enhanced Community Coping
  Compromised Family Coping
  Disabled Family Coping
  Readiness for Enhanced Family Coping
  Death Anxiety
  Ineffective Denial
  Fear
  Grieving
  Complicated Grieving
  Risk for Complicated Grieving
  Impaired Mood Regulation
  Powerlessness
  Risk for Powerlessness
  Readiness for Enhanced Power
  Impaired Resilience
  Risk for Impaired Resilience
  Readiness for Enhanced Resilience
  Chronic Sorrow
  Stress Overload
Class 3: Neurobehavioural Stress
  Acute Subacute Withdrawal Syndrome
  Risk for Acute Subacute Withdrawal Syndrome
  Autonomic Dysreflexia
  Risk for Autonomic Dysreflexia
  Decreased Intracranial Adaptive Capacity
  Neonatal Abstinence Syndrome
  Disorganized Infant Behaviour
  Risk for Disorganized Infant Behaviour
  Readiness for Enhanced Organized Infant Behaviour

Domain 10: Life Principles

Class 1: Values
  This class does not currently contain any diagnoses.
Class 2: Beliefs
  Readiness for Enhanced Spiritual Well-Being
Class 3: Value/Belief/Action Congruence
  Readiness for Enhanced Decision-Making
  Decisional Conflict
  Impaired Emancipated Decision-Making
  Risk for Impaired Emancipated Decision-Making

  Readiness for Enhanced Emancipated Decision-Making
  Moral Distress
  Impaired Religiosity
  Risk for Impaired Religiosity
  Readiness for Enhanced Religiosity
  Spiritual Distress
  Risk for Spiritual Distress

Domain 11: Safety/Protection

Class 1: Infection
  Risk for Infection
  Risk for Surgical Site Infection
Class 2: Physical Injury
  Ineffective Airway Clearance
  Risk for Aspiration
  Risk for Bleeding
  Impaired Dentition
  Risk for Dry Eye
  Risk for Dry Mouth
  Risk for Falls
  Risk for Corneal Injury
  Risk for Injury
  Risk for Urinary Tract Injury
  Risk for Perioperative Positioning Injury
  Risk for Thermal Injury
  Impaired Oral Mucous Membrane Integrity
  Risk for Impaired Oral Mucous Membrane Integrity
  Risk for Peripheral Neurovascular Dysfunction
  Risk for Physical Trauma
  Risk for Vascular Trauma
  Risk for Pressure Ulcer
  Risk for Shock
  Impaired Skin Integrity
  Risk for Impaired Skin Integrity
  Risk for Sudden Infant Death Syndrome
  Risk for Suffocation
  Delayed Surgical Recovery
  Risk for Delayed Surgical Recovery
  Impaired Tissue Integrity
  Risk for Impaired Tissue Integrity
  Risk for Venous Thromboembolism
Class 3: Violence
  Risk for Female Genital Mutilation
  Risk for Other-Directed Violence
  Risk for Self-Directed Violence
  Self-Mutilation
  Risk for Self-Mutilation
  Risk for Suicide
Class 4: Environmental Hazards
  Contamination
  Risk for Contamination
  Risk of Occupational Injury
  Risk for Poisoning
Class 5: Defensive Processes
  Risk for Adverse Reaction to Iodinated Contrast Media
  Risk for Allergy Reaction
  Latex Allergy Reaction

Risk for Latex Allergy Reaction

Class 6: Thermoregulation
Hyperthermia
Hypothermia
Risk for Hypothermia
Risk for Perioperative Hypothermia
Ineffective Thermoregulation
Risk for Ineffective Thermoregulation

Domain 12: Comfort

Class 1: Physical Comfort
Impaired Comfort
Readiness for Enhanced Comfort
Nausea
Acute Pain
Chronic Pain

Chronic Pain Syndrome
Labour Pain

Class 2: Environmental Comfort
Impaired Comfort
Readiness for Enhanced Comfort

Class 3: Social Comfort
Impaired Comfort
Readiness for Enhanced Comfort
Risk for Loneliness
Social Isolation

Domain 13: Growth/Development

Class 1: Growth
This class does not currently contain any diagnoses.

Class 2: Development
Risk for Delayed Development

Source: NANDA International, Inc. *Nursing Diagnoses: Definitions and Classification 2018–2020*. © 2017 NANDA International, ISBN 978-1-62623-929-6. Used by arrangement with the Thieme Group, Stuttgart/New York.

A

abandonment The relinquishment of responsibilities.

abnormal motor behaviour Alterations in behaviour, including bizarre and agitated behaviours. Grossly disorganized behaviours may include mutism, stupor, or catatonic excitement.

abuse The stage of addiction when the problems resulting from misuse of a substance or behaviour become much more regular and disabling.

acculturation The process by which members of one cultural group adopt the behaviours of another cultural group, generally due to close, prolonged contact with the other group.

active listening Awareness of the patient's verbal and nonverbal communications and the monitoring of personal verbal and nonverbal communications.

acupuncture A method of traditional Chinese medicine that involves the placement of needles into the skin at meridian points to modulate the flow of energy and stimulate physical changes such as in brain activity, blood chemistry, endocrine functions, blood pressure, heart rate, and immune system response.

acute dystonia Acute sustained contraction of muscles, usually of the head and neck.

acute phase The earliest of three phases of mania, during which the person experiences poor judgement, excessive and constant motor activity, probable dehydration, and difficulty evaluating reality. The overall outcome of the acute phase is injury prevention.

acute stress disorder A short-term reaction to a highly traumatic event. Occurs within 1 month of event and resolves within 4 weeks.

addiction The persistent, compulsive dependence on or use of a substance or behaviour despite its negative consequences and the increasing frequency of those consequences.

admission criteria Factors that justify the hospitalization of an individual. Admission criteria must include evidence of one or more of the following: (1) imminent danger of harming self, (2) imminent danger of harming others, and (3) inability to care for basic needs, placing individual at imminent risk of harming self.

adult support program There are three types of adult support programs: (1) social care, (2) adult health or medical treatment programs, and (3) maintenance care. In each type, older adults are cared for during the day and stay in a home environment at night.

advance directives Documents that express patients' treatment choices.

advanced-practice nursing (APN) Includes the roles of nurse practitioner and clinical nurse specialist. Clinical nurse specialists work as consultants, educators, and clinicians in inpatient and outpatient psychiatry throughout Canada. Nurse practitioners work as consultants or collaborative team members who can diagnose, prescribe and manage medications, and provide psychotherapy.

adventitious crisis A state of imbalance that results from events not part of everyday life, such as a natural disaster, a national disaster, or the results of crime.

affect The outward representation of a person's internal state of being, manifested in facial expression, tone of voice, and body language.

affective symptoms Symptoms involving emotions and their expression.

ageism A bias against older adults based solely on age.

aggravated sexual assault A legal term used when, during a sexual assault, the life of the survivor is endangered or the assault results in injury.

aggression An emotion that results in a verbal or physical attack. Aggression is not always inappropriate.

agnosia Loss of sensory ability to recognize objects.

agonist An agent that interacts with a specific receptor and enhances the normal response for that receptor.

agoraphobia Fear of being in an open, crowded, or public place, such as a field, tunnel, bridge, congested street, or busy department store, where escape is perceived as difficult or help as not available in the case of a sudden incapacitation.

agraphia Inability to read or write.

akathisia Psychomotor restlessness evident as pacing or fidgeting, sometimes pronounced and very distressing.

Alcoholics Anonymous (AA) A 12-step program (the prototype for all that were subsequently developed for various types of addiction) that offers the behavioural, cognitive, and dynamic structure needed by those in recovery from alcohol addiction.

alcohol poisoning A state of toxicity that results when an individual has consumed large amounts of alcohol either quickly or over time.

alcohol withdrawal A physical reaction to the cessation or reduction of alcohol (ethanol) intake that develops within a few hours of the last intake.

alcohol withdrawal delirium An altered level of consciousness, presenting with seizures, following acute alcohol withdrawal. Alcohol withdrawal delirium is a medical emergency and can result in death even if treated.

alternate personality (alter) Also called *subpersonality*. An additional personality within a single individual that has its own pattern of perceiving, relating to, and thinking about the self and the environment.

Alzheimer's disease (AD) A form of degenerative dementia.

anergia Lack of energy or passivity.

anger A strong feeling of displeasure or hostility.

anger control assistance Facilitation of the expression of anger in an adaptive, nonviolent manner

anhedonia The loss of ability to experience joy or pleasure in living.

anorexia nervosa An eating disorder characterized by a refusal to maintain a minimally normal weight for height and by an intense fear of gaining weight.

anosognosia An inability to recognize illness in oneself, which is caused by the illness itself.

antagonist An agent that interacts with a specific receptor site and blocks or depresses the normal response for that receptor.

antianxiety (anxiolytic) drugs Drugs that enhance $GABA_A$ receptors or increase 5-HT, norepinephrine, or both.

anticholinergic-induced delirium A potentially life-threatening medical emergency secondary to use of anticholinergic drugs and characterized by dry mucous membranes; reduced or absent peristalsis; mydriasis; nonreactive pupils; hot, dry, red skin; hyperpyrexia without diaphoresis; tachycardia; agitation; unstable vital signs; worsening of psychotic symptoms; delirium; urinary retention; seizure; and repetitive motor movements.

anticholinesterase drugs Drugs that interfere with the action of acetylcholinesterase with the result of elevated levels of the neurotransmitter acetylcholine.

anticipatory grief A patient's or loved one's experience of grief ahead of time, after a life-limiting diagnosis or when threatened with loss of ability to function independently, loss of identity, or changes in role definition.

anticonvulsant drugs A group of drugs (e.g., carbamazepine, valproic acid) used especially in treating people with mania that has been refractory to lithium therapy. These drugs are also useful in treating people who need rapid de-escalation and do not respond to other treatment approaches.

anxiety A feeling of apprehension, uneasiness, uncertainty, or dread resulting from a real or perceived threat.

aphasia Loss of language ability.

apraxia Loss of purposeful movement in the absence of motor or sensory impairment.

aromatherapy The use of essential oils for enhancing physical and mental well-being and healing.

assault Reasonable belief that a person means to cause one harm.

assent Expressed agreement to participate in health care or research.

assertive community treatment (ACT) An intensive type of case management developed in response to the community-living needs of people with serious, persistent psychiatric symptoms.

assimilation The process by which different cultural groups come to share a culture; generally, when a minority group adapts to the dominant culture and loses its uniqueness.

associative looseness Disorganized thinking, manifested as jumbled and illogical speech and impaired reasoning (also known as *looseness of association*).

asylums Retreats from society designed with the hope that, with early intervention and several months of rest, people with mental illness could be cured.

attention-deficit/hyperactivity disorder (ADHD) A disorder that causes an inappropriate degree of inattention, impulsiveness, and hyperactivity, all of which interfere with functioning or development.

737

automatic thoughts Rapid, unthinking, often irrational responses based on schemata. These responses are particularly intense and frequent in psychiatric disorders such as depression and anxiety. Also called *cognitive distortions*.

autonomy The rights of others to make their own decisions

B

barriers to treatment Factors that impede access to psychiatric care, including stigma, geographic challenges, financial limitations, policy issues, and system shortcomings.

battery Harmful or offensive touching.

Beck's cognitive triad Three thoughts that perpetuate depression: (1) a negative, self-deprecating view of self; (2) a pessimistic view of the world; and (3) the belief that negative reinforcement (or no validation for the self) will continue in the future.

behavioural family therapy A collection of psychological techniques for modifying maladaptive behaviours.

behavioural therapy A treatment method that is concerned with patterns of behaviour rather than inner motivations. Behavioural therapy is effective in treating people with phobias, alcoholism, schizophrenia, and many other conditions.

beneficence The duty to act to benefit or promote the good of others.

Benson's relaxation technique A method, influenced by Eastern practices, for switching from the fight-or-flight response to a state of relaxation; achieved by adopting a calm and passive attitude and focusing on a pleasant mental image in a calm and peaceful environment.

bereavement The period of grieving following a death.

bibliotherapy The use of literature for children or adolescents to help the individual express feelings in a supportive environment, gain insight into feelings and behaviour, and learn new ways to cope with difficult situations.

binge eating disorder An eating disorder characterized by repeated episodes of binge eating, after which patients experience significant distress but, in most cases, do not use compensatory behaviours.

bioethics Deontological principles that are irreducible and must be balanced in clinical situations.

biofeedback A form of behavioural therapy, especially effective in stress management, that uses sensitive instrumentation to provide immediate and exact information about physiological responses.

biopsychiatry A theoretical approach to understanding mental health disorders as biological malfunctions of the nervous system.

biopsychosocial model A model that takes a holistic view of the client, including the person's biology, social environment and skills, and psychological characteristics.

bipolar I disorder A chronic, recurrent illness marked by shifts in mood, energy, and ability to function and in which at least one episode of mania alternates with major depression. Psychosis may accompany the manic episode.

bipolar II disorder A chronic, recurrent illness marked by shifts in mood, energy, and ability to function and in which hypomanic episodes alternate with major depression. Psychosis is not present. Hypomania tends to be euphoric and often increases functioning; depression in this disorder tends to put people at particular risk for suicide.

bisexual A term to describe people who are attracted to both men and women when describing their sexual orientation.

blame Attachment of personal responsibility for the assault onto the victim.

blood alcohol level (BAL) A measure (by urinalysis or Breathalyzer) of the level of alcohol in the blood.

boundaries Distinctions made between individuals in the family. Boundaries may be clear, enmeshed, rigid, or inconsistent.

boundary impairment An impaired ability to sense where one's self ends and others' selves begin.

bulimia nervosa An eating disorder characterized by repeated episodes of binge eating followed by compensatory behaviours, such as self-induced vomiting; misuse of laxatives, diuretics, or other medications; fasting; or excessive exercise.

bullying A repetitive behaviour that sustains an imbalance of power.

C

callousness A lack of concern about the feelings of others; the absence of remorse or guilt except when facing punishment; and a disregard for meeting school, family, and other obligations.

Canadian Federation of Mental Health Nurses An organization of registered nurses across Canada who specialize in psychiatric mental health nursing. Under the umbrella of the Canadian Nurses Association and with consumer input, this organization set the standards of practice for psychiatric mental health nursing for registered nurses.

Cannabis sativa Marijuana (*Cannabis sativa*) is a member of the hemp family of plants with one major distinction: it contains delta 9-tetrahydrocannabinol (THC). This is the psychoactive ingredient found in the resin secreted from the flowering tops and leaves of the female cannabis plant

caregiver burden The physical, psychological, emotional, social, and financial stresses that individuals experience as a result of providing care.

case management Care coordination activities the nurse does with or for the patient; includes referrals, assistance with paperwork applications, connection to resources, and overall navigation of the health care system.

catastrophic reactions Over-reactions to a seemingly normal, nonthreatening situation, commonly experienced in Alzheimer's disease.

chiropractic medicine A system of medicine based on the relationship between the body's structure (mainly the spine) and function and its relationship to the preservation and restoration of health, using manipulative therapy as a treatment tool.

circadian rhythms The fluctuation of various physiological and behavioural parameters over a 24-hour cycle.

circumstantiality The inclusion of unnecessary and often tedious details in one's conversation.

cisgender A term that refers to one's gender identity being aligned with the gender assigned at birth.

clang associations The stringing together of words because of their rhyming sounds, without regard to their meaning.

classical conditioning Bringing about involuntary behaviour or reflexes through conditioned responses to stimuli.

clear boundaries Boundaries that are well understood by all members of the family and that give family members a sense of both "I-ness" and "we-ness."

clinical epidemiology A broad field that addresses what happens after people with illnesses are seen by clinical care providers.

clinical pathway A guideline that is used to describe and implement clinical standards. It helps to provide quality and efficient patient care.

clinical supervision A mentoring relationship characterized by evaluation and feedback and a gradual increase in autonomy and responsibility.

closed-ended questions Questions that elicit a "yes" or "no" response. They are useful for getting information efficiently, as in an assessment, but do little to encourage the sharing of feelings.

cluster suicide A term that describes deaths by suicide that follow a highly publicized suicide of a public figure, an idol, or a peer in the community

cognitive behavioural therapy (CBT) A commonly employed, effective, and well-researched therapeutic tool based on both cognitive psychology and behavioural theory that is used to treat a variety of psychiatric disorders (e.g., depression, anxiety, phobias, pain problems).

cognitive distortions Rapid, unthinking, often irrational responses based on schemata. Prevalent in many forms of mental illness. Also called *automatic thoughts*.

cognitive reframing The changing of an individual's perceptions of stress through the reassessment of a situation and the replacing of irrational beliefs ("I can't pass this course") with more positive self-statements ("If I choose to study for this course, I will increase my chances of success").

cognitive symptoms Difficulty with attention, memory, information processing, cognitive flexibility, and executive functions (e.g., decision making, judgement, planning, problem solving).

collaboration Formal links between mental health and addiction service personnel who work together to develop and implement a recovery plan.

colonization The process whereby a people are overcome by a more powerful group and the views, philosophies, values, and beliefs of the powerful group are imposed on the original inhabitants of the land.

command hallucinations "Voices" that direct the person to take an action.

community treatment orders (CTOs) Mandatory treatment provided in a less restrictive community setting.

comorbid condition Having more than one mental disorder at a time.

competency The capacity to understand the consequences of one's decisions.

complicated grief Grief that is prolonged, maladaptive, and dysfunctional, experienced after the loss of a loved one.

compulsions Ritualistic behaviours or thoughts an individual feels compelled to perform in an attempt to reduce anxiety.

compulsive behaviour Behaviour that does not have a biological element but only psychological and social elements. Some examples are exercising, gaming, gambling, Internet use, pornography viewing, shopping, smartphone use, studying, and work.

concrete thinking An impaired ability to think abstractly. The person interprets statements literally.

concurrent disorder The complex combination of a diagnosis of mental illness and a substance abuse disorder or addiction.

conditioning The pairing of a behaviour with a condition that reinforces or diminishes the behaviour's occurrence.

conduct disorder A disorder characterized by a persistent pattern of behaviour in which the rights of others are violated and age-appropriate societal norms or rules are disregarded.

confabulation The creation of stories or answers in place of actual memories to maintain self-esteem.

confidentiality A person's right to privacy of information.

conflict Open disagreement among members. Positive conflict resolution within a group is key to successful outcomes.

confusional arousal disorders Recurrent episodes of incomplete waking from sleep with or without terror or movement, usually occurring during the first third of the major sleep episode and contributing to impaired nighttime and daytime safety or functioning.

conscious One of Freud's levels of awareness. It contains all of the material a person is aware of at any one time, including perceptions, memories, thoughts, fantasies, and feelings.

consent A person's capacity to understand information and voluntarily to act on this information.

consequentialist theory The belief that every person in society has the right to be happy and that we have an obligation to make sure happiness results from our actions.

consultation A process that involves informal links between mental health and addiction service personnel along with additional human services as may be needed for the client.

contemplation The process through which patients become aware that they are stuck in a situation and must decide whether they wish to change or remain where they are.

contentious objection An individual refuses to perform a legal or professional responsibility because of moral or other personal beliefs.

continuation phase Lasts for 4 to 9 months. Although the overall outcome of this phase is relapse prevention, many other outcomes must be accomplished to achieve relapse prevention.

contract An agreement, either stated or written, that contains the place, time, date, and duration of the meetings between nurse and patient.

controlled style of coping A contained response to an event that may be ambiguous in appearance and reactions and exhibited by a lack of affective response or even calm or subdued behaviours.

conventional health care A system of medicine based largely on highly controlled, evidence-informed scientific research. Also known as *biomedical*, *allopathic*, or *mainstream medicine*.

conversion disorder Also called *functional neurological disorder*. An illness in the absence of a neurological diagnosis that presents with neurological symptoms such as deficits in voluntary motor or sensory functions, including paralysis, blindness, movement disorder, gait disorder, numbness, paresthesia (tingling or burning sensations), loss of vision or hearing, or episodes resembling epilepsy.

coping Navigating through challenges using skills, either learned or natural, to meet goals.

coping methods The thinking, behavioural, and emotional processes individuals use to support functioning in the face of stressors.

coping skills Healthier ways of looking at and dealing with illness (e.g., assertiveness training, cognitive reframing, problem-solving skills, social supports).

coping styles Personal attributes people develop to help manage stress.

correctional nursing Nursing practice organized by the location of the work or the legal status of the patient, rather than by the role or functions being performed. The role involves all aspects of nursing practice.

counter-transference The health care worker's unconscious personal response to the patient.

crisis An acute state of psychological imbalance resulting in poor coping with evidence of distress and functional impairment.

crisis intervention A process focused on resolution of the immediate problem through personal, social, and environmental resources.

crisis situation A situation that puts stress on a family that includes a violent member.

critical incident stress debriefing (CISD) A group-level crisis intervention carried out very soon after a traumatic event.

cultural competence The ability of nurses to apply knowledge and skill appropriately in cross-cultural situations and to adapt care delivery to meet the patient's cultural needs and preferences.

cultural concepts of distress Sets of signs and symptoms that are common in a limited number of cultures but virtually nonexistent in most other cultural groups.

cultural filters Filters through which each of us interprets ourselves, others, and the world.

cultural humility A process of self-reflection and humbly recognizing oneself as a learner about the experience of another, with the responsibility to grow and awareness that therapeutic relationships are reciprocal and formed, over time, with mutual respect.

cultural safety An awareness of power relations between health care professionals and clients; it is of particular importance in light of Indigenous peoples' experiences of colonization.

cultural violence When an individual is harmed as a result of practices that are part of her or his culture, religion, or tradition.

culture The shared beliefs, values, and practices of a group that shape members' thinking and behaviour in patterned ways. Culture can also be viewed as a blueprint for guiding actions that affect care, health, and well-being.

custodial care Assistance in performing the basic daily necessities of life, such as dressing, eating, using a toilet, walking, and so on.

cyclothymia Hypomanic episodes that alternate with minor depressive episodes of at least 2 years' duration. Individuals with cyclothymia tend to have irritable hypomanic episodes.

cyclothymic disorder Symptoms of hypomania alternate with symptoms of mild to moderate depression for at least 2 years in adults and 1 year in children.

D

death by suicide The act of taking one's own life. Also called *suicide*.

decompensation Deterioration of mental health.

de-escalation techniques Methods and tools, including advanced communication skills, used to defuse any incident of acting out, anger, aggression, or violence.

defence mechanisms Innate, unconscious means of preventing conscious awareness of threatening feelings or of denying or distorting reality to ward off anxiety.

deinstitutionalization The shift from caring for people with mental illness in institutions to caring for them in communities.

delirium A neurocognitive disturbance characterized by inattention, disorganized thinking, altered consciousness, and fluctuations in mental status.

delusions Alterations in *thought content* (what a person thinks about). Delusions are false fixed beliefs that cannot be corrected by reasoning.

dementia Global deterioration of cognitive functioning (e.g., memory, judgement, ability to think abstractly, orientation). Often progressive and irreversible, depending on the underlying cause.

deontology Duty-based ethics with the central concepts of reason and duty.

depersonalization A nonspecific feeling that a person has lost his or her identity, that the self is different or unreal, or that the person is an observer of his or her own body or mental processes. An aspect of depersonalization/derealization disorder.

depressive disorder due to another medical condition May be caused by disorders that affect the body's systems or from long-term illnesses that cause ongoing pain.

derealization An aspect of depersonalization/derealization disorder that results in individuals experiencing a recurring feeling that their surroundings are unreal or distant—an external or outside feeling of disconnect.

***Diagnostic and Statistical Manual of Mental Disorders*, fifth edition (*DSM-5*)** The official guideline for diagnosing psychiatric disorders.

dialectical behaviour therapy (DBT) Evidence-informed therapy used to treat chronically suicidal people with borderline personality disorder.

diathesis–stress model A general theory that explains psychopathology using a systems approach. This theory helps us understand how personality disorders emerge from the multifaceted factors of biology and environment.

diathesis–stress model of depression A theory that depression results from a dynamic interplay of biology and the environment.

disasters Events that threaten the well-being of citizens.

disenfranchised grief Grief that can promote a sense of isolation and occurs when losses are not always openly acknowledged, supported, or recognized as significant, such as a loss through a suicide, the loss of a friend, the loss of a pet, or the grief of someone thought incapable of grieving (e.g., a child, a person with dementia).

disorganized thinking The loosening of associations, manifested as jumbled and illogical speech and impaired reasoning.

disruptive mood dysregulation disorder Characterized by severe and recurrent temper outbursts that are inconsistent with developmental level.

dissent Expressed refusal to participate in health care or research.

dissociative amnesia An inability to recall important autobiographical information, often of a traumatic or stressful nature, that is too pervasive to be explained by ordinary forgetfulness.

dissociative disorders A group of illnesses in which mind–body connections are unconsciously altered.

dissociative fugue A subtype of *dissociative amnesia*, characterized by sudden, unexpected travel away from the customary location and an inability to recall one's identity and information about some or all of the past.

dissociative identity disorder (DID) An illness in which a person experiences two or more distinct personality states that alternately and recurrently take control of the person's behaviour.

distress A negative, draining energy that results in anxiety, depression, confusion, helplessness, hopelessness, and fatigue.

Dorothea Dix A passionate social reformer, she advocated for improved treatment and public care of people with mental illness and was influential in lobbying for the first public mental hospital in the United States and for reform in institutions in Britain and Canada.

double-bind messages Communication that contains two contradictory messages given by the same person at the same time, to which the receiver is expected to respond, putting the receiver in "a bind," or an impossible conflict. Constant double-bind situations result in feelings of helplessness, fear, and anxiety in the recipient of such messages.

double messages Conflicting messages (also known as *mixed messages*).

duty to protect Responsibility of the nurse when the nurse determines—or, pursuant to professional standards, should have determined—that the patient presents a serious danger to another.

duty to warn Responsibility to notify a potential victim of a threat to his or her well-being or to notify authorities of such a threat.

dyssomnias Sleep disturbances associated with the initiation and maintenance of sleep or with excessive sleepiness.

dysthymic disorder (DD) A chronic depressive syndrome that is usually present for most of the day, more days than not, for at least 2 years.

E

echolalia The pathological repeating of another's words, often seen in catatonia.

echopraxia The mimicking of the movements of another.

ecological model An analytical tool that identifies personal (victim or perpetrator) characteristics, family members, the immediate social context (often referred to as *community factors*), and the characteristics of the larger society to help understand the multilevel, multifaceted nature of violence.

ego One of three psychological processes that make up the Freudian system of personality (id, ego, superego). The ego is one's sense of self and provides such functions as problem solving, mobilization of defence mechanisms, reality testing, and the capability of functioning independently. The ego is said to be the mediator between one's primitive drives (the id) and internalized parental and social prohibitions (the superego).

electroconvulsive therapy (ECT) A procedure in which electric currents are passed through the brain, intentionally triggering a brief seizure.

electronic health care Health care services provided from a distance through the Internet.

elopement Absence from the unit without leave.

emotional dysregulation A term that describes poorly modulated mood characterized by mood swings.

emotional lability Moods that alternate rapidly from one emotional extreme to another.

emotional violence When someone says or does something to make a person feel belittled or worthless.

empathy The ability of one person to imagine him- or herself inside another's world and see things from the other person's perspective and to communicate this understanding to the other person.

enculturation The learning, usually passed from parents, about which behaviours, beliefs, values, and actions are "right" and which are "wrong."

engagement The connection between the self and another. It is through this connection that nurses can develop a meaningful understanding of another person's experience, perspective, and vulnerability.

enmeshed boundaries A blending together of the roles, thoughts, and feelings of the individual family members so that clear distinctions fail to emerge. Also called *diffuse boundaries*.

epidemiology The quantitative study of the distribution of mental disorders in human populations.

ethics An expression of the values and beliefs that guide practice.

ethnicity The sharing of common traits, customs, and race. Ethnic groups have a common heritage, history, and world view.

ethnocentrism A perception that one's own values, beliefs, and behaviours are superior.

euphoric mood When associated with mania, unstable mood during which the patient may describe an intense feeling of well-being. The overly joyous mood may seem out of proportion to the situation, and cheerfulness may be inappropriate for the circumstances, considering that the person is full of energy but has had little or no sleep.

eustress A positive, beneficial energy that motivates and results in feelings of happiness, hopefulness, and purposeful movement.

euthanasia A deliberate act undertaken by a person with the intention of ending the life of another person in order to relieve that person's suffering and where that act is the cause of death.

evidence-informed decision making Promoted by the Canadian Nurses Association in nursing practice as a model for decision making that incorporates the best available research evidence, with professional clinical judgement, client preference, and collaboration with other key health stakeholders.

evidence-informed practice Care based on the collection, interpretation, and integration of valid, important, and applicable patient-reported, clinician-observed, and research-derived evidence.

excessive sleepiness (ES) At least 1 month of prolonged sleep episodes or daytime sleep episodes that occur almost daily and cause significant distress and social and vocational impairment.

expressed style of coping An outwardly expressed behavioural response to an event (e.g., crying, withdrawing, smoking, abusing alcohol and drugs, talking about the traumatic event).

extinction The absence of reinforcement through the withholding of a reward that has become habitual.

extrapyramidal side effects (EPS) Adverse effects, including akathisia, acute dystonias, pseudoparkinsonism, and tardive dyskinesia, caused by blockage of D_2 dopamine receptor sites in the motor areas.

F

false imprisonment Detention of a voluntarily admitted patient, with no agency or legal policies to support detaining the patient.

family systems theory A theory of family therapy that downplays problem resolution, focusing instead on the long-term ability of family members to make autonomous choices. Its goals are to decrease emotional reactivity and encourage differentiation among individual family members.

family triangle A basic building block of interpersonal relationships; a third person is brought into a dyad to lower tensions once they build. All triangles contain a close side, a distant side, and a side in which conflict or tension exists between two people.

fear A reaction to a specific danger.

feedback Communication of one person's impressions of and reactions to another person's actions or verbalizations.

feeding disorder An inability or difficulty in eating or drinking sufficient quantities to maintain optimal nutritional status.

fight-or-flight response The body's way of preparing for a situation perceived as a threat to survival; this response results in increased blood pressure, heart rate, and cardiac output.

financial abuse The withholding of financial support or the illegal or improper exploitation of funds or other resources for one's personal gain.

first-generation antipsychotic drugs Also referred to as typical, traditional, or conventional antipsychotics developed in the 1950s to treat psychosis.

flashbacks Dissociative experiences during which the event is relived and the person behaves as though he or she is experiencing the event in the present.

flexibility Allowance for the changes inherent in normal growth and development.

flight of ideas A nearly continuous flow of accelerated speech, with abrupt changes from topic to topic that are usually based on understandable associations or plays on words.

forensic nursing The application of nursing science to public or legal proceedings. The practice combines the forensic and biopsychosocial aspects of health care in the scientific investigation of trauma or death of victims and perpetrators of abuse, violence, criminal activity, and traumatic accidents.

forensic psychiatric mental health nurse A nurse who integrates nursing philosophy and theory with knowledge of and skill in mental health care and legal proceedings in the investigation or treatment of the trauma of victims and perpetrators of criminal activity.

Four Gifts of Resolving Relationships A predictable sequence of communications about four processes that can be shared with a person who is dying (forgiveness, love, gratitude, farewell).

frotteurism Rubbing or touching a nonconsenting person.

G

gay A term that refers to a man being attracted to another man. Also called *homosexual*.

gender A person's identity and social classifications, often based on masculine or feminine qualities and traits.

gender dysphoria Feelings of unease about one's maleness or femaleness.

gender identity A person's sense of maleness or femaleness. Gender identity is not inborn but is usually established by the age of 3 years.

general adaptation syndrome (GAS) A three-stage theory of stress proposed by Hans Selye: (1) the *alarm* stage, the initial, brief, and adaptive response (fight or flight) to the stressor; (2) the *resistance* stage, during which sustained and optimal resistance to the stressor occurs; (3) the *exhaustion* stage (occurring only when attempts to resist the stressor prove futile)—resources are depleted, and the stress may become chronic, producing a wide array of psychological and physiological responses and even death.

generalized anxiety disorder (GAD) An anxiety reaction characterized by persistent and exaggerated apprehension and tension.

genogram A tool for efficiently providing a clinical summary of information and relationships across generations of a family.

genuineness Self-awareness of one's feelings as they arise within the nurse–patient relationship and the ability to communicate them when appropriate.

grandiosity A state in which people with mania may exaggerate their achievements or importance, say that they know famous people, or believe that they have great powers. Grandiosity is also apparent in behaviour. Boasts of exceptional powers and status can take delusional proportions. Also called *inflated self-regard*.

grief All of an individual's reactions to loss (e.g., depressed mood, insomnia, anxiety, poor appetite, shock, denial, guilt); sorrow experienced in anticipation of, during, and after a loss.

grounding techniques Promote awareness of in-the-moment physical reality and help to counter dissociative episodes.

group Two or more people who come together for the purpose of pursuing common goals, interests, or both.

group content All that is said in the group.

group norms Expectations for behaviour in the group that develop over time and provide structure for members (e.g., starting on time, not interrupting).

group process The dynamics of interaction among the members (e.g., who talks to whom, facial expressions, body language).

group psychotherapy A specialized treatment intervention in which a trained leader (or co-leaders) establishes a group for the purpose of treating people with psychiatric disorders.

group themes Members' expressed ideas or feelings that recur and have a common thread. The leader can clarify a theme to help members recognize it more fully.

group work A method whereby individuals with a common purpose come together and benefit by giving and receiving feedback within the context of group life.

guardianship An involuntary trust relationship in which one party, the guardian, acts on behalf of an individual, the ward.

guided imagery A process whereby a person is led to envision images that are both calming and health enhancing; can be used in conjunction with Benson's relaxation technique.

H

hallucinations The perception of a sensory experience for which no external stimulus exists (e.g., hearing a voice when no one is speaking).

hallucinogen A distinct psychoactive agent in that it does not primarily produce euphoria but rather disrupts the central and peripheral nervous systems, producing a disconnect between the physical world and the user's perception of the physical world.

harm reduction A range of programs, policies, and interventions designed to reduce or minimize the adverse consequences, such as overdose, infections, and spread of communicable diseases, associated with drug use.

healing touch A therapeutic modality related to therapeutic touch that combines several energy therapies and is based on the belief that the body is a complex energy system that can be influenced by another, through that person's intention for healing and well-being.

health teaching Includes identifying the health education needs of the patient and teaching basic principles of physical and mental health, such as giving information about coping, interpersonal relationships, social skills, mental health disorders, the treatments for such illnesses and their effects on daily living, relapse prevention, problem-solving skills, stress management, crisis intervention, and self-care activities.

heterosexual A term that means to be sexually attracted to the opposite sex.

holistic approach An approach to care that addresses both the psychological and the physiological needs of the patient.

holistic nurse A nurse who recognizes and integrates body–mind–emotion–spirit–environment principles and modalities in daily life and clinical practice.

homeopathy A system of treatment of disease that uses small doses (dilutions) of specially prepared plant extracts, herbs, minerals, and other materials to stimulate the body's defence mechanisms and healing processes.

homosexual A term that means to be sexually attracted to the same sex.

hospice palliative care Whole-person health care aimed at relieving suffering and improving quality of life rather than at a cure; grounded in the belief that each of us has the right to die pain-free and with dignity.

hypermetamorphosis A compulsion to touch everything in sight.

hyperorality The need to taste and chew, resulting in putting everything in one's mouth.

hypersomnia Excessive daytime sleep.

hypersomnia disorder Excessive sleepiness that occurs three or more times per week for 3 or more months despite a main sleep lasting 7 hours or longer.

hypnotic An effect, produced by drugs, of blunting the degree to which a person feels alert and focused, often resulting in drowsiness.

hypomania State in which people have voracious appetites for social engagement, spending, activity, and even indiscriminate sex. During hypomania, constant activity and a reduced need for sleep prevent proper rest.

I

id One of three psychological processes that make up the Freudian system of personality (id, ego, and superego). The id is the source of all primitive drives and instincts.

ideal body weight A weight that is believed to be maximally healthful for a person, based chiefly on height but modified by factors such as gender, age, build, and degree of muscular development.

ideas of reference The giving of personal significance to trivial events; the perception that events relate to one when they do not.

illness anxiety disorder An illness that results in the misinterpretation of physical sensations as evidence of a serious illness.

illusions Misperceptions or misinterpretations of a real experience.

implied consent Nonwritten consent.

impulse-control training Assisting the person to mediate impulsive behaviour through application of problem-solving strategies to social and interpersonal situations.

impulsivity Manifests in acting quickly in response to emotions without considering the consequences.

incidence The number of new cases of mental disorders in a healthy population within a given period of time.

Indigenous peoples A collective term used in this text to identify original peoples and their descendants living in Canada.

informed consent A patient's approval of recommended treatment with the knowledge of the potential positive and adverse effects of treatment; based on a person's right to self-determination and the ethical principle of *autonomy*.

inhalants Include volatile gases, substances that exist in a gaseous form at body temperature, refrigerants, solvents, general anaesthetics, and propellants.

insight-oriented family therapy A combination of behavioural therapy and education of families in better understanding their power struggles, defence mechanisms, and other negative behaviours.

insomnia disorder A state of constant hyperarousal, involving biological, psychological, and social factors, that disrupts sleep and impairs daytime functioning for 3 or more nights per week for 3 or more months.

institutionalized Dependent on the services and structure of institutions and therefore unable to function independently outside such institutions.

integrated use Refers to when a substance is used to enhance an already pleasurable and ongoing experience (e.g., a social occasion)

integration The provision of addiction and mental health services in a single treatment setting to meet the often multiple and high needs of the client.

integrative health care An interdisciplinary, nonhierarchical blending of both conventional health care and traditional, complementary, or alternative health care, with the intent to synergistically blend the best of all evidence-informed healing practices to provide relationship-based, holistic care.

intentional torts Voluntary acts intended to bring about a physical or mental consequence.

interdisciplinary A team approach that integrates separate discipline approaches. A common understanding of the patient issues is developed, and team members move beyond the silo of their discipline to work toward the best possible patient outcome.

intergenerational issues Various patterns of behaviour (e.g., involving geographical distance between members, suicide, divorce, addiction, affairs, grief, triangles, historical colonization, loss) that affect successive generations.

internalized homophobia A concept that refers to a set of negative beliefs and attitudes toward homosexuality and one's own homosexuality.

interpersonal psychotherapy An effective short-term therapy that is predicated on the notion that disturbances in interpersonal relationships can play a role in initiating or maintaining clinical depression. The goal of interpersonal psychotherapy is to reduce or eliminate psychiatric symptoms (particularly depression) by improving interpersonal functioning and satisfaction with social relationships.

interpersonal violence Includes child abuse, intimate partner violence, and older adult abuse and can involve all nine types of violence: physical, sexual, psychological, emotional, spiritual, cultural, verbal abuse, financial abuse, and neglect.

intersex A set of medical conditions that features a congenital anomaly of the reproductive system or genitals.

intrapsychic conflict A mental struggle, often unconscious, between the id, ego, and superego; it is no longer widely thought to be valid, and such therapy requires a lengthy period of treatment, making it prohibitively expensive for most.

intrusive thoughts Thoughts about a sexual assault that break into the survivor's conscious mind during the day and during sleep. May include flashbacks (re-experiencing of the traumatic event) or dreams with violent content.

J

journalling The keeping of an informal diary of daily events and activities; journalling can reveal surprising information on sources of daily stress.

justice The duty to distribute resources or care equally, regardless of personal attributes.

L

la belle indifférence Lack of emotional concern about the symptoms.

learned helplessness Martin Seligman's theory of depression in which individuals perceive a lack of control over a situation.

lesbian A term that refers to a woman being attracted to another woman. Also called *homosexual*.

lethality The degree of suicidal risk.

light therapy A treatment used in seasonal affective disorder (SAD) consisting of 30 to 45 minutes of exposure daily to a 10 000-lux light source.

limbic system Complex set of brain structures, including the hypothalamus, the amygdala, and the hippocampus, that plays a crucial role in emotional status and psychological function.

limit setting Establishing the parameters of desirable and acceptable personal behaviour.

lithium carbonate Mood stabilizer drug used in patients with bipolar disorder.

locus of control (LOC) An inherent factor in our experience and expression of mood.

M

maintenance/adaption Focuses on supporting and consolidating the gains made during the action stage and continued focus on avoiding lapse or more significant relapse.

maintenance phase A stage of change during which the patient focuses on actively working to maintain changes made and prevent relapse. Also, the final phase of bipolar disorder, the focus of which is prevention of relapse and limitation of the severity and duration of future episodes.

major depressive disorder (MDD) A history of one or more major depressive episodes without a history of manic or hypomanic episodes.

major neurocognitive disorders Commonly referred to as *dementia*, which is progressive and irreversible.

malpractice An act or omission of an act that breaches the duty of due care and results in or is responsible for a person's injuries.

mania An exaggerated euphoria or irritability.

manic episode Individuals experiencing a *manic episode* feel euphoric and energized, don't sleep or eat, and are in perpetual motion. They often take significant risks and engage in hazardous activities.

maturational crisis A critical period of increased vulnerability and heightened potential—a turning point.

medically assisted death Providing another with the knowledge or means to intentionally end his or her own life through medicine (e.g., a physician prescribes medication to a patient with advanced terminal illness, who uses the drugs to end his or her life).

medication reconciliation The process of developing the most accurate list possible of all medication a patient is taking.

medicine wheel An ancient symbol that can be interpreted in many ways—the four directions, the four grandfathers, the four components of human nature (physical, mental, spiritual, and emotional)—and that represents the interrelatedness of all aspects of the person, a holistic world view of health and illness based on deep personal connections to the natural world and the tribe.

meditation A discipline for training the mind to develop greater calm and then using that calm to bring penetrative insight into one's experience.

melatonin A naturally occurring hormone; although it is a popular over-the-counter nutraceutical, there are few data to support its use in the management of insomnia.

mental health A state of well-being in which the individual is able to realize his or her potential, cope with the normal stresses of life, work productively and fruitfully, and make a contribution to the community. Psychiatry's definition is continually evolving since it is shaped by the prevailing culture, societal values, and political climate.

mental health emergency A state of overwhelming anxiety that can lead to serious personality disorganization, depression, confusion, and behavioural disturbances.

mental health first aid (MHFA) The help provided to a person who is developing a mental health problem or experiencing a mental health crisis.

mental illness Alterations in cognition, mood, or behaviour that are coupled with significant distress and impaired functioning.

mental status examination (MSE) Analogous to the physical examination in general medicine. The purpose is to evaluate an individual's current cognitive, affective (emotional), and behavioural functioning.

metabolites The products that result from the body's breaking down a drug.

mild anxiety The level of anxiety that occurs in the normal experience of everyday living and that allows an individual to perceive reality in sharp focus. A person experiencing a mild level of anxiety sees, hears, and grasps more information, and problem solving becomes more effective.

mild neurocognitive disorders Result from changes in the brain that produce less pronounced deficits than do major neurocognitive disorders.

milieu therapy The use of a living, learning, or working environment, including people, setting, structure, and emotional climate, to treat psychiatric patients. Milieu therapy uses naturally occurring events in the environment as rich learning opportunities for patients.

mindfulness A centuries-old form of meditation that is based on the premise that we are not aware of ourselves moment to moment but operate on a sort of mental autopilot. Being mindful requires observing and monitoring the content of our consciousness and recognizing that thoughts are just thoughts and that negative interpretations can become positive.

misuse The stage of addiction when people begin to experience problems associated with their use of alcohol, other drugs, or other behaviours.

moderate anxiety A level of anxiety that interferes with what a person sees, hears, and grasps—the perceptual field narrows, and some details are excluded from observation.

monoamine oxidase inhibitors (MAOIs) Group of antidepressant drugs that prevent the destruction of monoamines by inhibiting the action of monoamine oxidase.

mood disorders A group of diagnoses related to disturbances in mood.

mood stabilizer Drug used to treat mood disorders by balancing brain neurotransmitters.

moral agent A person who has the power and capacity to do what is good and right.

moral distress A response to one's values and commitments being compromised.

moral residue Feelings that are carried forward from situations that resulted in moral distress or uncertainty.

moral resilience The ability and willingness to speak and take the most fitting action in the presence of moral and ethical dilemmas.

moral treatment Social and psychological approaches to treatment that included retreats from society, calm environments, and several months of rest.

moral uncertainty An uneasy feeling that results from a person's being unable to make an ethical decision.

motivational interviewing An approach to both assessment and treatment whereby nurses and other practitioners work with patients to facilitate movement through fluctuations between the stages of change.

mourning Things people do to cope with their grief, including shared, social expressions of grief, such as attending funerals and participating in bereavement groups.

multiculturalism The presence of diverse racial and ethnic minorities who identify themselves as different and wish to remain so; a set of ideals celebrating the cultural diversity of Canada adopted at the federal, provincial, and municipal levels.

multidisciplinary A team approach that consists of individuals from distinct disciplines approaching the patient from their own perspectives.

mutual aid Community-based (face-to-face or online) support that usually involves peer-to-peer support groups where people recovering from problematic substance use meet to share their challenges and successes in an effort to assist one another to achieve and maintain sobriety (e.g., Alcoholics Anonymous, Narcotics Anonymous). Mutual aid is also used by people to gain understanding and coping skills in the face of living with someone with problematic substance use (e.g., AlAnon or Alateen family groups).

mutual storytelling A psychodramatic technique developed to help young children express themselves verbally.

N

natural health products (NHPs) Substances such as vitamins and minerals, herbal medicines, homeopathic preparations, energy drinks, probiotics, and many alternative and traditional medicines.

naturopathy A system guided by a philosophy emphasizing the healing power of nature and restoring the body's natural ability to maintain and restore health using a variety of traditional and modern therapies.

negative reinforcement The removal of an unpleasant consequence of a behaviour; it is not the same as *punishment*. This concept is related to *positive reinforcement*.

negative symptoms The absence of something that should be present but is not (e.g., apathy, lack of motivation, anhedonia, poor thought processes).

neglect Failure to provide basic needs for a dependant. Includes physical neglect (failure to provide for basic needs or to protect from harm), emotional neglect (failure to attend to basic emotional needs and nurturing), educational neglect (failure to provide a child with experiences, including formal education necessary for intellectual growth and development), and medical neglect (failure to provide basic medical, dental, or psychiatric care).

negligence Carelessness.

neologisms Made-up words (or idiosyncratic uses of existing words) that have meaning for the person but a different or nonexistent meaning to others. This eccentric use of words represents disorganized thinking and interferes with communication.

neurocognitive disorders Result from changes in the brain and are marked by disturbances in orientation, memory, intellect, judgement, and affect.

neurodevelopmental disorders Disorders characterized by developmental deficits in the young (i.e., preschool-aged) child that produce impairments in social skills, intelligence, academic and occupational functioning, and communication skills.

neuroleptic malignant syndrome (NMS) A potentially fatal reaction to antipsychotic medications. Symptoms include muscular rigidity, hyperpyrexia, and sometimes oculogyric crises.

neurons Specialized nerve cells that process and transmit information through electrical and chemical signals.

neurotransmitters Chemicals that transmit signals from one neuron to the next across synapses.

nonmaleficence The duty to minimize harm and do no wrong to the patient.

nonsuicidal self-injury Characterized by self-harming behaviour with no intent to die.

nontherapeutic communication techniques Any method of communication that detracts from the therapeutic relationship.

nonverbal behaviours Behaviours such as body language, the crossing of arms or tapping of the foot or fingers on a surface, tone of voice, and other expressions other than the content of speech.

nonverbal communication Interpersonal communication conveyed through such nonverbal behaviours as body language, eye contact, facial expressions, tone of voice, or gestures.

normal anxiety A healthy reaction necessary for survival, providing the energy needed to carry out everyday tasks and strive toward goals.

nuclear family Parents and the children under their care.

Nursing Interventions Classification (NIC) A tool used to standardize, define, and measure nursing care.

Nursing Outcomes Classification (NOC) A reference that provides a comprehensive list of standardized outcomes, definitions, and measures to describe client outcomes influenced by nursing practice.

O

obsessions Thoughts, impulses, or images that persist and recur and cannot be dismissed from the mind. Obsessions often seem senseless to the individual who experiences them (*ego-dystonic*), and their presence causes severe anxiety.

open-ended questions Questions that encourage lengthy responses and information about experiences, perceptions, or responses to a situation and cannot be answered by a simple "yes" or "no" response.

operant conditioning A type of behaviour modification in which voluntary behaviours are increased or decreased through reinforcement or punishment.

opioid A drug that acts on endorphin receptors with a secondary effect on dopamine.

oppositional defiant disorder A recurrent pattern of negativistic, disobedient, hostile, defiant behaviour toward authority figures without going so far as to seriously violate the basic rights of others.

orientation phase The phase during which the nurse conducts the initial interview; can last for a few meetings or extend over a longer period.

outcome criteria The hoped-for outcomes that reflect the maximal level of patient health that can realistically be achieved through nursing interventions.

P

palliative care An interdisciplinary and collaborative approach to care for the treatment of pain and suffering of chronically and terminally ill patients.

panic The most extreme level of anxiety, marked by an inability to process the meaning of activity in the environment, noticeably disturbed behaviour, and, sometimes, a lost sense of reality.

panic attack The sudden onset of extreme apprehension or fear, usually associated with feelings of impending doom. The feelings of terror present during a panic attack are so severe that normal function is suspended, the perceptual field is severely limited, and misinterpretation of reality may occur.

panic disorder (PD) An anxiety disorder characterized by recurring severe panic attacks. It may also effect significant behavioural changes lasting at least a month and ongoing worry about having other attacks.

paranoia Any intense and strongly defended irrational suspicion.

perpetrators Those who initiate violence. Perpetrators often consider their own needs to be more important than anyone else's and look to others to meet their needs.

perseveration The repetition of phrases or behaviour.

persistent depressive disorder Diagnosed when feelings of depression occur for most of the day, for the majority of days.

persona Latin word meaning *mask* and the origin of the word *personality*. May refer to the person as other people see him or her.

personality The combination of qualities or characteristics that makes a person a distinct individual. Personality determines the quality of experiences among people and serves as a guide for one-to-one interaction and in social groups.

personality disorders Disorders that cause significant challenges in self-identity or self-direction and problems with empathy or intimacy within relationships.

personality trait A stable characteristic of a person, such as neuroticism, extraversion, openness to experience, agreeableness, and conscientiousness.

personality type A way to describe a cluster of traits.

pharmacodynamics Biochemical and physiological effects of drugs on the body, which include the mechanisms of drug action and its effect.

pharmacogenetics An approach to treatment that takes into consideration individual genetic differences when determining which and how much medication to prescribe.

pharmacokinetics The study of the action of drugs within the body; used to determine the blood level of a drug and to guide the dosage schedule.

phases of crisis Four distinct phases of physical and psychological experiences in response to a crisis as identified by Caplan.

Philippe Pinel Eighteenth-century reformer who, along with William Tuke, introduced the moral treatment era of psychiatry, which attempted to focus on providing peaceful, nurturing environments for people with mental illness.

physical dependency A physiological state of cellular adaptation that arises when the central and peripheral nervous systems become habituated to a psychoactive agent such that the person physically needs the drug to function or to avoid the physical pain of withdrawal.

physical stressors Negative changes to our environment (e.g., trauma, excessive cold or heat) or physical beings (e.g., infection, hemorrhage, hunger, pain).

physical violence The infliction of physical pain or bodily harm (e.g., slapping, punching, hitting, choking, pushing, restraining, biting, throwing, burning).

pica The persistent eating of non-nutritive substances without an aversion to eating food. Infants and toddlers may eat paint, plaster, string, or cloth.

play therapy Usually, a one-to-one session the therapist has with a child in a playroom. The therapist offers a choice of play materials to the child to aid self-expression, assess developmental and emotional status, determine diagnosis, and institute therapeutic interventions.

polysomnography (PSG) The most common sleep test; used to diagnose and evaluate people with sleep disorders related to breathing, nocturnal seizure disorders, and various parasomnias or with unusual sleep patterns that interrupt functioning.

positive reinforcement The presentation of a reward immediately following a behaviour, making the behaviour more likely to occur in the future.

positive symptoms The presence of something that is not normally present (e.g., hallucinations, delusions, bizarre behaviour, paranoia).

post-traumatic stress disorder (PTSD) An acute emotional response to a traumatic event or situation involving severe environmental stress.

postvention Interventions with the family and friends of a person who has died by suicide. Postvention aims to both reduce the traumatic aftereffects and explore effective means of addressing survivor problems using primary and secondary interventions.

preconscious One of Freud's levels of awareness. Just below the surface of awareness, it contains material that can be retrieved rather easily through conscious effort.

precontemplation The first stage of the Transtheoretical Model of Change (TTM), it recognizes that an individual will be resistant to change and typically has no intention of altering behaviour in the near future.

premenstrual dysphoric disorder A cluster of symptoms that occur in the last week before the onset of a woman's menstrual period.

preorientation phase The phase of the therapeutic relationship during which the nurse prepares for the orientation phase—for instance, by familiarizing himself or herself with the patient's background or engaging in self-reflection.

preparation Also known as the determination stage, it involves some commitment from the patient that changing his or her drug-using behaviour is being considered along with the anticipation of what this future action may look like.

prevalence The total number of cases, new and existing, in a given population during a specific period of time, regardless of when the subjects became ill.

primary care In terms of mental health care, care that promotes mental health and reduces mental illness to decrease the incidence of crisis.

primary dementia An irreversible, progressive dementia that is not secondary to any other disorder.

primary intervention In relation to suicide, activities that provide support, information, and education to prevent suicide.

primary prevention In regard to abuse, measures taken to prevent the occurrence of abuse.

principle of least restrictive intervention This principle requires that more restrictive interventions be used only after less restrictive interventions to manage the behaviour have been attempted.

progressive muscle relaxation (PMR) A stress relaxation technique performed by tensing groups of muscles (beginning with feet and ending with face) as tightly as possible for 8 seconds and suddenly releasing them.

pseudodementia A disorder that mimics dementia.

pseudoparkinsonism A medication-induced, temporary constellation of symptoms associated with Parkinson's disease: tremor, reduced accessory movements, impaired gait, and stiffening of muscles.

psychiatric consultation liaison nurse (PCLN) A nurse who functions as a consultant to other nurses in managing psychological concerns and symptoms of psychiatric disorders and who works directly with patients as a clinician to help them deal more effectively with physical and emotional problems.

psychodynamic therapy A therapy focused on the present that uses many of the tools of psychoanalysis, such as free association, dream analysis, transference, and counter-transference, but in which the therapist has increased involvement and interacts with the patient more freely.

psychoeducation An approach to care that emphasizes helping a person gain knowledge necessary to manage the illness.

psychoeducational family therapy Therapy that provides families with the information they need about mental illness and the coping skills that will help them deal with their loved one's psychiatric disorder.

psychoeducational groups Groups that aim to increase knowledge or skills about a specific subject and allow members to communicate emotional concerns.

psychological dependency When a drug becomes so important to an individual's thoughts and actions that the person believes she or he cannot manage without the substance.

psychological stressors Changes that are cognitive- or emotion-based (e.g., divorce, loss of a job, unmanageable debt, the death of a loved one, retirement, fear of a terrorist attack); psychological stressors also include changes we might consider positive (e.g., marriage, the arrival of a new baby, unexpected success).

psychological violence When someone uses threats and causes fear in an individual to gain control.

psychomotor agitation The need to fidget (e.g., constant pacing and wringing hands).

psychomotor retardation The slowing of physical movements and, often, of thoughts.

psychoneuroimmunology An area of study focused on the relationship between the mind, the nervous system, and the immune system.

psychosis Altered cognition, altered perception, or an impaired ability to determine what is or is not real (an ability known as reality testing).

psychosocial assessment An evaluation of the person's social functioning and the systems in which the person operates.

punishment An unpleasant consequence of a behaviour.

Q

queer A term often used as an umbrella term for individuals who do not identify as heterosexual.

R

rage An uncontrollable, violent state of anger that prevents a person from thinking clearly or logically, impeding psychosocial or cognitive behavioural interventions.

rape-trauma syndrome A variant of post-traumatic stress disorder that consists of an acute phase and a long-term reorganization process that occurs after an actual or attempted sexual assault.

rapid cycling Four or more mood episodes in a 12-month period. The term is used to indicate more severe symptoms, such as poorer global functioning, high recurrence risk, and resistance to conventional somatic treatments.

rapport A relationship characterized by trust, support, and understanding.

reality testing The ability to determine accurately whether or not an experience is based in reality.

receptors Protein molecules, embedded in a cell, to which one or more specific kinds of signalling molecules may attach.

recovery The ability of a patient to work, live, and participate in the community after an illness.

recovery model A patient-centred approach that stresses hope, living a full and productive life, and eventual recovery. Patients partner with health care providers and aim to extend their improvement beyond stability.

reflexology A form of manipulative therapy based on the understanding that zones and points of the body relate to one another. Focuses primarily on the feet to improve circulation and promote optimum function elsewhere in the body.

refugee A person who is seeking asylum in a new country due to threat of trauma or actual trauma and violation of human rights.

Registered Psychiatric Nurses of Canada An organization representing the four Western provincial associations for registered psychiatric nurses.

rehabilitation A program focused on managing patients' deficits and helping patients learn to live with their illnesses.

Reiki An energy-based therapy in which the practitioner's energy is connected to a universal source and is transferred to a recipient for physical or spiritual healing.

reinforcement An outcome that causes a behaviour to occur more frequently.

relapse prevention The process that occurs after formal treatment.

relational ethics A developing ethical theory with the core elements of mutual respect, engagement, embodied knowledge, interdependent environment, and uncertainty.

resilience A characteristic of mental health that aids people to recognize stressors and negative emotions, deal with them, and learn from the experience.

respect for autonomy Respecting the rights of others to make their own decisions (e.g., acknowledging the patient's right to refuse medication promotes autonomy).

reticular activating system (RAS) Part of the brain that helps to control sleep, motivation, and breathing.

reuptake Reabsorption of a neurotransmitter by a neuron following impulse transmission across a synapse.

right to privacy The assurance that only people with a right to know will have access to privileged information.

right to refuse treatment A person's ability to understand and appreciate his or her condition and determine if he or she will accept treatment.

rigid boundaries Boundaries in which the rules and roles are consistently adhered to no matter what. Rigid boundaries prevent family members from trying out new roles or, in some cases, from taking on more mature functions as time goes on. Also called *disengaged boundaries.*

rumination disorder The repeated regurgitation and rechewing of food without apparent nausea, retching, or gastrointestinal problems.

S

SAD PERSONS scale A simple and practical guide for triaging potentially suicidal patients.

safety plan A plan for a rapid escape when abuse recurs.

seclusion protocol An outline of the proper reporting procedure, through the appropriate channels, to be used when seclusion is used as a treatment.

secondary care In terms of mental health, care that includes intervention during an acute crisis to prevent prolonged anxiety from diminishing personal effectiveness and personality organization.

secondary dementia A form of dementia that occurs as a result of some other pathological process (e.g., metabolic, nutritional, or neurological).

secondary gains Benefits derived from the symptoms alone.

secondary intervention In relation to suicide, a treatment of the actual suicidal crisis. It is practised in clinics, hospitals, and jails and on telephone hotlines.

secondary prevention In regard to abuse, early intervention in abusive situations to minimize their disabling or long-term effects.

secondary victimization The sexual assault survivor's experiencing further stress or trauma when seeking help.

second-generation antipsychotic drugs Drugs used to treat psychosis that target both the positive and possibly the negative symptoms of schizophrenia and may produce fewer extrapyramidal side effects.

selective inattention An impairment in the ability to see or hear everything in the environment.

selective serotonin reuptake inhibitors (SSRIs) Medications that increase both serotonin and norepinephrine.

self-care activities Personal responsibility for activities of daily living (ADL).

self-help groups Groups (often run by the members themselves) that are structured for the purpose of providing members with the opportunity to maintain or enhance personal and social functioning through cooperation and shared understanding of life's challenges. Also called *support groups.*

serotonin syndrome A potentially life-threatening reaction caused by concurrently taking two medications that increase the level of serotonin.

serotonin–norepinephrine reuptake inhibitor (SNRI) A drug used to treat generalized anxiety disorder (GAD), social anxiety disorder (SAD), and panic disorder (PD).

severe anxiety A level of anxiety that seriously impairs the person's ability to notice his or her environment, even when it is pointed out by another. A person with severe anxiety may instead focus on one particular detail or many scattered details.

sexual assault Any sexual activity for which consent is not obtained or freely given. Also called *sexual violence.*

sexual assault nurse examiners (SANEs) Nurses who are specially trained in the care and assessment (including of psychological and emotional trauma) of adult and pediatric victims of sexual assault (*SANE-A* and *SANE-P,* respectively).

sexual orientation A person's sexual identity in relation to the gender to which they are attracted. Sexual orientation is biological; people are born heterosexual, homosexual, or bisexual.

sexual violence When a person is forced to unwillingly take part in sexual activity. Sexual violence against adults may be referred to as *rape,* or in legal terms as *sexual assault.*

sexuality The ways in which people experience and express themselves as sexual beings.

situational crisis Acute imbalance that arises from events that are extraordinary, external rather than internal, and unanticipated.

sleep architecture The structural organization of non–rapid eye movement (NREM) and rapid eye movement (REM) sleep.

sleep continuity The distribution of sleep and wakefulness across the sleep period.

sleep deprivation The discrepancy between hours of sleep obtained and hours of sleep required for optimal functioning.

sleep efficiency Ratio of sleep duration to time spent in bed.

sleep fragmentation Disruption of sleep stages as indicated by excessive amounts of stage 1 sleep, multiple brief arousals, and frequent shifts in sleep staging.

sleep hygiene Conditions and practices that promote continuous and effective sleep.

sleep latency The time it takes to go to sleep.

sleep restriction Limiting the total sleep time to create a temporary, mild state of sleep deprivation and strengthen the sleep homeostatic drive.

social determinants of health Elements of one's lifestyle that affect health, including economic status, genetics, job security, employment opportunities, access to safe and affordable housing, child care availability, food security, and inclusion and exclusion from society.

social phobia Also called *social anxiety disorder (SAD)*. Severe anxiety or fear provoked by exposure to a social or performance situation (e.g., fear of being scrutinized, saying something that sounds foolish in public, not being able to answer questions in a classroom, eating in public, performing on stage).

social relationship A relationship that is initiated primarily for the purpose of friendship, socialization, enjoyment, or accomplishment of a task. Mutual needs are met during social interaction (e.g., participants share ideas, feelings, and experiences).

social skills training The teaching of a wide variety of social and activities of daily living (ADL) skills.

sociocultural context The equal consideration of issues of gender, race, ethnicity, class, sexual orientation, and religion.

somatic symptom disorders Thoughts, feelings, and behaviours caused by excessive worry about physical signs and symptoms.

somatic therapies Also known as *sensorimotor psychotherapy*. These therapies combine talk therapy with body-centred interventions and movement to address dissociative symptoms.

somatization Emotional or psychological distress expressed as physical pain.

specific phobias High levels of anxiety or fear in response to specific objects or situations (e.g., an animal, dirt), activities (e.g., meeting strangers, leaving the familiar setting of a home), or physical situations (e.g., heights, open or closed spaces).

spiritual (religious) violence When someone uses an individual's spiritual beliefs to manipulate, dominate, or control that person.

splitting A primary defence or coping style used by people with borderline personality disorder. Splitting makes the person unable to incorporate positive and negative aspects of people (self or others) into a whole image.

standards of nursing practice Authoritative statements that promote, guide, direct, and regulate professional nursing practice.

stereotyped behaviours Repeated motor behaviours that do not presently serve a logical purpose.

stereotyping A generalized conscious or unconscious conceptualization of a group of people that does not allow for individual differences with the group.

stigma Negative attitudes or behaviours toward a person or group based on a belief that they possess negative traits.

stigmatized persons with medical conditions Patients assumed by health care workers to be bad, disgusting, or even just unusual; often include those who have mental illnesses, those who are HIV positive, and those who have undergone transgender surgeries or treatments.

stimulus control A strategy of adherence to five basic principles that decrease negative associations with the bed and bedroom and strengthen the stimulus for sleep.

stressors Psychological or physical stimuli that are incompatible with current functioning and require adaptation.

subpersonality Also called *alternate personality (alter)*. An additional personality within a single individual that has its own pattern of perceiving, relating to, and thinking about the self and the environment.

substance-induced anxiety disorder The onset of symptoms of anxiety, panic attacks, obsessions, or compulsions that develop with the use of a substance or within a month of discontinuing use of the substance.

substance/medication-induced depressive disorder A depressive disorder, such as major depressive disorder, that is a result of prolonged use of or withdrawal from drugs and alcohol.

suicidal behaviour Actions that cause self-harm (also referred to as self-injury) initiated with a clear intent to cause bodily harm or death by suicide.

suicidal ideation Also known as *suicidal thoughts*. These thoughts can range from a fleeting idea about one's own death (or about not being here) that does not include the act of killing oneself to a detailed plan, including the final act of killing oneself.

suicide The act of taking one's own life. Also called *death by suicide*.

sundowning Also known as *sundown syndrome*. Symptoms become more pronounced in the evening. This symptom-exacerbation pattern may occur in people who have either delirium or dementia.

superego One of three psychological processes that make up the Freudian system of personality (id, ego, superego). The superego consists of the conscience and the ego ideal. The superego represents the ideal rather than the real and seeks perfection rather than pleasure or reason.

support groups Groups (usually facilitated by a professional) that are structured for the purpose of providing members with the opportunity to maintain or enhance personal and social functioning through cooperation and shared understanding of life's challenges. Also called *self-help groups*.

supported-employment model A model of care that includes rapid job placement, on-the-job support, and provision of a job coach who is linked to the mental health team.

supportive psychotherapy An approach that stresses empathic understanding, a nonjudgemental attitude, and the development of a therapeutic alliance.

survivor A person who has endured abuse and recovered. This term recognizes the recovery and healing process that follows victimization.

survivors of suicide Family and friends of a person who has died by suicide.

synapse Structure that permits a neuron (or nerve cell) to pass an electrical or chemical signal to another cell.

T

tangentiality A departure from the main topic to talk about less important information; going off on tangents in a way that takes the conversation off topic.

tardive dyskinesia (TD or TDK) A persistent extrapyramidal side effect that usually appears after prolonged treatment and persists even after the medication has been discontinued. TD consists of involuntary tonic muscular contractions that typically involve the tongue, fingers, toes, neck, trunk, or pelvis.

temperament The style of behaviour habitually used to adapt to the demands and expectations of the environment. This style is present in the infant, is modified by maturation, and develops in the context of the social environment.

termination phase The final, integral phase of the nurse–patient relationship, during which the patient and nurse summarize the achievement of goals and discuss the continued implementation by the patient of strategies learned.

tertiary care In terms of mental health care, provision of support for those who have experienced a severe crisis and are now recovering from a disabling mental state.

tertiary intervention In relation to suicide, interventions with the family and friends of a person who has died by suicide. Tertiary interventions aim to both reduce the traumatic aftereffects and explore effective means of addressing survivor problems using primary and secondary interventions.

tertiary prevention In regard to abuse, the facilitating of the healing and rehabilitative process through counselling of individuals and families, provision of support for groups of survivors, and provision of assistance to survivors of violence to achieve their optimal level of safety, health, and well-being.

therapeutic communication skills and strategies Communication that reflects the use of skills such as warmth, respect, and empathy and strategies such as using silence, recognizing strengths, and making observations.

therapeutic encounter A brief, informal meeting between nurse and patient that is useful and important for the patient.

therapeutic factors Aspects of the group experience that facilitate therapeutic change.

therapeutic games Specific games played with children that elicit children's fears and fantasies and help with assessment and treatment.

therapeutic index The ratio of the lethal dose to the effective dose; a measure of overall drug safety regarding the possibility of overdose or toxicity.

therapeutic relationship A relationship in which the nurse maximizes his or her communication skills, understanding of human behaviours, and personal strengths to enhance the patient's growth.

therapeutic touch A healing modality based on the premise that healing is promoted by balancing the body's energies through hand movements and direct energy (but no physical touch) to the energy field of the body.

therapeutic use of self One's individual, genuine ways of being with another person based on one's personal values and beliefs of humanity and enhanced by the application of microcommunication skills to guide the process of developing, maintaining, and terminating a therapeutic relationship.

tidal model A model that focuses on the interpersonal relationships as the context for recovery.

tolerance A physiological experience that occurs when a person's reaction to a substance decreases with repeated administrations of the same dose.

tort law Law developed from obligations to another.

traditional, complementary, and alternative medicine (TCAM) A system of medicine that recognizes that many of the philosophical underpinnings for different approaches are derived from both non-Western cultural traditions and newer concepts from quantum physics and studies in the nature of energy and reality, which have not historically been a part of conventional health care delivery.

transcranial magnetic stimulation (TMS) A noninvasive treatment modality that uses magnetic resonance imaging (MRI)-strength magnetic pulses to stimulate focal areas of the cerebral cortex.

transference The patient's experience of feelings toward the nurse or therapist that were originally held toward significant others in his or her life.

transgender An incongruence between a person's gender identity and the gender assigned at birth.

Transtheoretical Model of Change A behaviour change model that is the basis for developing effective interventions to promote health behaviour change in addictions services.

trauma Experiencing or witnessing events that threaten an individual's very survival (physical or psychological).

trauma-informed care Care focused on patients' past experiences of violence or trauma and the role this violence or trauma currently plays in their lives.

trauma-informed practice An approach that recognizes the impacts of previous traumatic events on current health and mental health situations.

tricyclic antidepressants (TCAs) Drugs that block the reuptake of norepinephrine for the secondary amines and both norepinephrine and serotonin for the tertiary amines.

two-spirit A term used by some Indigenous people to describe their gender, sexual, or spiritual identity; it refers to a person who embodies both a male and a female spirit.

typology of interpersonal violence Four modes in which the abuse of power may be inflicted: physical abuse, sexual abuse, psychological or emotional abuse, and deprivation or neglect. (Economic abuse is another mode in which violence can be inflicted.)

U

unconscious One of Freud's levels of awareness. The unconscious includes all repressed memories, passions, and unacceptable urges lying deep below the surface. The unconscious exerts a powerful yet unseen effect on the conscious thoughts and feelings of the individual.

unintentional torts Unintentional acts that produce injury or harm to another person.

utilitarianism Bringing about the greatest good and the least harm for the greatest number of people.

V

vagus nerve stimulation (VNS) Electrical stimulation of the vagus nerve to increase the level of neurotransmitters and improve mood.

values Abstract standards that represent an ideal, either positive or negative.

vegetative signs of depression Alterations in those activities necessary to support physical life and growth (e.g., change in bowel movements and eating habits, sleep disturbances, disinterest in sex).

verbal abuse When someone uses language, whether spoken or written, to cause harm to an individual.

verbal communication All the words a person speaks.

vicarious trauma A term used to describe the disruptions in thinking and perspectives of those who are exposed to the stories of people who are traumatized; it is of concern for nurses and others working with sexual assault victims.

violence Any action that has the intent to harm. It can be directed at self, others, or objects.

virtue ethics An ethical theory that espouses that good people will make good decisions.

virtues Attitudes, dispositions, or character traits that enable us to be and to act in ways that develop ethical potential and ensure ethical outcomes.

vocational rehabilitation A program providing vocational training, financial support for attaining employment, or supported-employment services.

vulnerable person An adult or child who, as a result of illness, physical condition, or experiences, is at greater risk than the general population for being harmed.

W

Weir Report A report released in 1932 by the Canadian Medical Association and the Canadian Nurses Association. It concluded that drastic changes to nursing education programs were needed, including the standardization of curriculum, work hours, and instructor training, and that the care of people with mental illnesses needed to be integrated into all generalist programs.

Western tradition A world view based on the scientific biomedical model and aligned with values of autonomy, individualization, and independence.

William Tuke Eighteenth-century reformer who, along with Philippe Pinel, introduced the moral treatment era of psychiatry, which attempted to focus on providing peaceful, nurturing environments for people with mental illness.

withdrawal The experiences and physiological changes that occur when blood and tissue concentrations of a drug decrease in individuals who have maintained heavy and prolonged use of a substance.

word salad A jumble of words that is meaningless to the listener—and perhaps to the speaker as well—because of an extreme level of disorganization.

working phase The phase of the nurse–patient relationship during which the nurse and patient identify and explore areas that are causing problems in the patient's life.

world view A major paradigm that is used to explain the world and its mysteries, including beliefs about health, illness, and the hereafter. The major world views used to explain health and illness phenomena are attributed to the paradigms of magic and religion, empirical science, and holistic health.

INDEX

Page numbers followed by "*f*" indicate figures, "*t*" indicate tables, and "*b*" indicate boxes.

A

AA. *see* Alcoholics Anonymous
Abandonment, 111
ABCD-ER mnemonic tool, for abuse screening, 541, 543*b*
Abilify. *see* Aripiprazole
Abnormal Involuntary Movement Scale (AIMS), 192, 323, 326*f*–327*f*
Abnormal motor behaviour, with schizophrenia, 302
Aboriginal peoples
  alcoholism prevalence statistics in, 394
  federal government funding mental health care for, 27
Abstraction, 86*b*–87*b*
Abuse
  as adventitious crisis, 480
  case study and nursing care plan in, 554*b*–556*b*
  comorbidity of, 537, 537*b*
  define, 531
  epidemiology of, 535–536
  myth *vs.* fact in, 545*t*
  nursing process application in, 539–556
    assessment in, 539–546, 541*b*
    diagnosis in, 546, 546*t*
    evaluation in, 552–553
    implementation in, 547–552
    outcomes identification in, 546, 547*t*
    planning in, 546–547
  power and control in, 538, 539*f*
  prevention of, 550
  reporting, 547
  screening tools in, 541, 542*f*
Abuse Assessment Screen, 541, 542*f*
Acamprosate (Campral), 417
Accepting, as therapeutic communication technique, 160*t*–161*t*
Access to care
  as key strategy area for Canadian mental health care, 8, 9*b*
  of older adults, 618–619
Accidents
  concurrent with substance abuse disorders, 395
  due to sleep deprivation, 458
Accountability, of health care workers, 138
Acculturation, 123
Acetylcholine, 175, 176*t*
  in anger and aggression, 515
  depression and, 250
  first-generation antipsychotic drugs and, 192
  reduction of, 177*b*, 177*f*
  tricyclic drugs and, 187
Acetylcholinesterase, 175
Acrophobia, 207*t*
Actigraphy, 462
Action phase, of Transtheoretical Model of Change, 412
Action potential, 175
Active listening, as therapeutic communication technique, 157–158
Active negativism, 311
Acupuncture, 715–716, 718
Acute care
  for anorexia nervosa, 346
  for bulimia nervosa, 351
Acute confusion
  with dementia, 367
  NOC outcomes related to, 369*t*
Acute dystonia, from conventional antipsychotics, 323, 324*t*–325*t*
Acute intoxication, assessment of, 398–400, 399*b*
Acute phase
  of bipolar disorders
    implementation for, 286, 287*t*
    outcomes identification in, 284
    planning in, 285
  of depression, 257
  of rape-trauma syndrome, 562–563, 564*b*
  of schizophrenia, 306, 314, 316*t*
    interventions, 317
    setting, 316–317

Acute stress disorder, description of, 214, 214*b*
AD. *see* Alzheimer's disease
Adapting, resilience and, 5
Adaptive uses, of defences, 205*t*–206*t*
Addiction
  comprehensive conceptualization of, 391–392, 392*f*
  definition of, 394
  development, process of, 392–394, 393*f*
    excessive use, 393
    experimentation, 393
    integrated use, 393
    no contact, 392
  helping patients change and, 411–415
  psychological changes due to, 411
  self-assessment and self-awareness due to, 411
  services, funding of, 27–28
Addiction supportive housing (ASH), 423
Adenosine, 461
ADHD. *see* Attention deficit-hyperactivity disorder
Adherence
  to medication, 41
  as treatment issues, in serious mental illness, 638*b*
Admission assessment, by psychiatric nurse, 40
Admission criteria, for hospitalization, 33
Adolescent-onset conduct disorder, 604
Adolescents, 587–613
  anxiety disorders in, 606–607
    assessment guidelines for, 608*b*
    generalized anxiety disorder (GAD), 607
    Nursing Outcomes Classification (NOC) for, 608*t*
    separation anxiety disorder, 598*b*, 606–607
  assessment of, 83, 83*b*
  bipolar and related disorders in, 608–609
  bipolar disorders in, 278, 278*t*
  characteristics of mentally healthy, 592*b*
  depression in, 248
    assessment of, 254
    impact on, 588*b*
  depressive disorders in, 608–609
  disorders of, 587–613
    brain development and biochemicals in, 590
    comorbidity of, 589
    cultural factors, 591
    drug treatment of, 598*b*
    environmental factors, 591
    epidemiology of, 588–589
    genetic factors in, 590
    resilience factors, 591
    temperament in, 590
  disruptive, impulse control, and conduct disorders in, 603–604
    adolescent-onset conduct disorder, 604
    bullying, 604
    childhood-onset conduct disorder, 604
    conduct disorders, 598*b*, 603–604, 605*b*
    nursing process application to, 604–606, 605*b*, 605*t*
    oppositional defiant disorder, 603, 605*b*
    techniques for managing, 607*b*
  feeding and eating disorders, 609
  gender dysphoria in, 580*b*
  hostility toward lesbian, gay, bisexual and transgender, and queer, 592*b*
  mood disorders in, 608–609
  neurodevelopmental disorders in, 598–601
    attention deficit-hyperactivity disorder (ADHD), 598*b*, 599–600, 601*b*, 603*b*
    autism spectrum disorders, 599
    communication disorders, 599
    intellectual disabilities, 599
    motor disorders, 600–601
    Nursing Outcomes Classification (NOC) for, 602*t*
    nursing process application to, 601–603, 601*b*, 602*t*
    specific learning disorder (SLD), 600
    stereotypic movement disorder, 600
    Tourette's disorder, 600
  post-traumatic stress disorder (PTSD) in, 598*b*, 609
  psychiatric mental health nursing, 591–598

Adolescents *(Continued)*
    assessment data in, 592–594, 593*b*
    behavioural therapy, 594–595
    bibliotherapy, 597
    cognitive behavioural therapy, 595
    cultural factors in, 594
    data collection in, 591–592
    developmental assessment in, 593
    family therapy, 594
    group therapy, 594
    mental status examination in, 593
    milieu management, 595–596, 595*b*
    mind-body therapies, 596
    multimodal music therapy, 596
    mutual storytelling, 596–597, 597*b*
    play therapy, 596–597
    principle of least restrictive intervention, 594
    psychopharmacology, 598
    quiet room, 596
    risk assessment in, 593–594
    seclusion and restraint in, 595–596
    therapeutic drawing, 597
    therapeutic games, 597, 597*b*
    time out, 596
  risk factors for mental illness in, 589, 590*b*
  use of antidepressant drugs by, 266
  yoga for, 596*b*
Adrenal cortex, stress response and, 66
Adrenal glands, role of, in mental function, 173
α_1-adrenergic receptors, 192
α_2-adrenergic receptors, 188–189
Adult support programs, 630
Adults, gender dysphoria in, 580*b*
Advance directives, 106
  in Canadian hospice palliative care treatment model, 658
  nursing responsibilities with, 106
Advanced-practice interventions
  for anorexia nervosa, 347–348
  for bulimia nervosa, 351–352
  in sexual assault, 570–571
  in violence and abuse, 550–552
Advanced-practice nurses, 691
Advanced-practice nursing (APN), 22–23
Advanced-practice psychiatric mental health nurses, as members of psychiatric mental health treatment teams, 38*b*
Advanced-practice psychiatric mental health nurses interventions, 13*t*
Adverse effects, of lithium carbonate, 190, 191*t*
Advice, giving, 161–163, 162*t*
Affect
  assessment of, during mental status examination, 86*b*–87*b*
  depression assessment of, 253
Affection, for managing disruptive behaviours, in children and adolescents, 607*b*
Affective blunting, in schizophrenia, 311*t*
Affective symptoms, of schizophrenia, 307, 312
Age, considerations for, during assessments, 83–84
Ageism
  and drug testing, 620
  older adult, 619
  and public policy, 619–620
Aggravated sexual assault, definition of, 561
Aggression, 512–529
  considerations for, 520
  de-escalation techniques for, 519, 519*b*
  defining, 513, 531
  nursing process application to, 517–527, 518*b*, 519*t*, 521*b*–523*b*, 525*b*–526*b*
  safety and, 35
  signs and symptoms, nursing diagnoses, and outcomes for, 519*t*
  stages and assessment of, 518*b*, 519–520
  words describing different types of, 512
Aggressive behaviour
  goals with personality disorders, 448*t*
  with personality disorders, 447–450, 448*t*, 450*b*, 451*t*

Aging. *see also* Older adults
 as challenge to psychiatric mental health nurses, 12
 facts and myths about, 615*b*
 major theories of, 615, 615*b*
 mental health issues related to, 616–620
  anxiety disorders, 617
  depression in, 616–617
  late-life mental illness in, 616–618
  substance use disorders, 617–618
  suicide risk, 616–617
 normal, major neurocognitive disorder *vs.*, 371*t*
 of population, 614
Agitation
 with delirium, 367
 with dementia, 378
Agnosia, 374
Agonist, 184
 buspirone as, 186
Agoraphobia, 206, 206*b*, 207*t*
Agranulocytosis, from conventional antipsychotics, 324*t*–325*t*
Agreement, element of LEAP approach, 302
Aguilera, Donna, 479
Akathisia
 from conventional antipsychotics, 323, 324*t*–325*t*
 suicide and, 503
Al-Anon, 420–421, 424*b*–426*b*
Al-Ateen, 420–421
Alcohol abuse
 CAGE-AID screening tool, 617*b*
 Michigan Alcoholism Screening Test-Geriatric Version (MAST-G), 618*b*
 as most prevalent substance abuse disorder, 395
 by older adults, 617–618, 617*b*–618*b*
Alcohol dependence
 with depression, case study on, 424*b*–426*b*
 screening of immigrants for, 12–13
Alcohol intoxication, effects in nontolerant individuals, 401–403, 403*t*
Alcohol poisoning
 prevalence statistics in Canada, 394
 signs and symptoms of, 401
Alcohol use
 in LGBTQ, 584
 in violence and abuse, 545–546
Alcohol withdrawal
 alcohol withdrawal delirium, 403–404
 benzodiazepines for, 185
 pharmacological interventions during, 416–417
 signs and symptoms of, 401, 401*t*–402*t*
Alcoholics Anonymous (AA), 419–420, 422*b*, 617–618
Alcoholism
 Michigan Alcoholism Screening Test-Geriatric Version (MAST-G), 618*b*
 by older adults, 617–618, 617*b*–618*b*
 prevalence statistics in Canada, 394
Alcohol-related neurodevelopmental disorder (ARND), 395
Allies, 578
Allopathic medicine, 714–715
All-or-nothing thinking, 56*t*
 in cognitive distortions, 347*b*
Alogia, in schizophrenia, 311*t*
Alprazolam (Xanax), 185, 185*f*, 230*b*–231*b*, 521*b*
Alternate personality (alter), 216
Altruism, 685*b*
 as defence mechanism, 205*t*–206*t*
Alzheimer Society of Canada, 378
Alzheimer's disease (AD), 370–371, 371*t*
 brain injury and, 374
 in Canada, 373
 as challenge for psychiatric mental health nurses, 12
 drugs for, 195
 environmental factors in, 374
 epidemiology of, 373
 genetic factors in, 373–374
 genetics in, 373–374
 as most common cause of dementia, 370–373
 positron emission tomography scan of brain with, 180–183, 182*f*
 progression of, 371–373
 stages of, 371–372, 372*t*
 symptoms of, 374

Amino acids, 176*t*
Amitriptyline hydrochloride (Elavil), 230*b*–231*b*, 261*b*–262*b*, 263
Amphetamines, 194, 461
 description and medical uses for, 407–408
Amygdala, emotions and psychological function and, 177–178
β-amyloid, 180–183
Anergia
 in schizophrenia, 311*t*
 with seasonal affective disorder, 245
Anger, 512–529, 531
 during bereavement, 667*t*
 clinical picture of, 512–514, 513*b*
 comorbidity, 514
 considerations for, 520
 as counter-transference, 141*t*
 de-escalation techniques for, 519, 519*b*
 depression and, 253
 escalates, safety when, 143, 145*t*
 etiology of, 514–516
 feelings that precipitate, 512–513, 513*b*
 nursing process application to, 517–527, 518*b*, 519*t*, 521*b*–523*b*, 525*b*–526*b*
 stages and assessment of, 518*b*, 519–520
Anger control assistance, interventions for, 450*b*
Anhedonia
 depression and, 253
 in schizophrenia, 311*t*
Animal-assisted therapy, 720*b*
Animistic charms, 18
Anorexia nervosa, 343–348
 acute care in, 346
 advanced-practice interventions for, 347–348
 assessment of, 343–345, 345*b*
 case study and nursing care plan for, 353*b*–356*b*
 characteristics of, 339*b*
 clinical picture of, 338–340
 cognitive distortions in, 347*b*
 comorbidity of, 341–342
 criteria for hospital admission of, 344*b*
 culture and, 6
 depression co-occurring with, 259*t*
 diagnosis of, 345
 epidemiology of, 340–341
 etiology of, 342–343
 evaluation of, 348
 general assessment for, 345
 health teaching and health promotion for, 346
 implementation in, 346–348
 medical complications of, 344*b*
 milieu management of, 347
 NOC outcomes related to, 346*t*
 outcomes identification of, 345
 pharmacological interventions for, 346
 planning of, 345–346
 psychosocial interventions for, 346, 346*b*
 psychotherapy for, 347–348
 self-assessment of, 345
 signs and symptoms of, 344*t*
 state of treatment for, 348*t*
 thoughts and behaviours associated with, 344*b*
 vignette in, 347*b*–348*b*
Anosognosia, 312–313, 634, 637
Antagonism, *vs.* compliance, 445, 446*t*
Antagonist, 184
 buspirone as, 186
Anthony, Dr. William, on recovery model for depression, 256
Antiandrogens, in gender dysphoria, 579–580
Antianxiety (anxiolytic) drugs, 183
 for anxiety disorders, 230*b*–232*b*, 232–233
 for bipolar disorders, 290
 gamma-aminobutyric acid as, 183, 185
Anticholinergic-induced delirium, from antipsychotics, 323–325, 324*t*–325*t*
Anticholinesterase drugs, for Alzheimer's disease, 195
Anticipatory grief
 dementia and, 376
 signs of, 663, 663*b*
Anticonvulsants
 for anxiety disorders, 230*b*–231*b*, 233
 for bipolar disorders, 289–290, 291*b*
 for chronic aggression, 522*b*

Antidepressant drugs, 258–266
 for anxiety disorders, 186, 187*f*, 230*b*–231*b*, 232
 for bulimia nervosa, 351
 monoamine oxidase inhibitors, 261*b*–262*b*, 263–265, 265*f*
 monoamine oxidase inhibitors (MAOIs) as, 189, 189*f*
 selective serotonin reuptake inhibitors (SSRIs) as, 186, 188, 259–262, 261*b*–263*b*
 serotonin and norepinephrine disinhibitors (SNDIs) as, 188–189
 serotonin-norepinephrine reuptake inhibitors (SNRIs) as, 186, 188, 261*b*–262*b*, 262
 for sleep disorders, 471*b*
 suicide risk and, 190
 tricyclic antidepressants, 187–188, 188*f*, 261*b*–262*b*, 263, 264*b*
 use by children and adolescents, 266
 use by older adults, 266
 use by pregnant women, 265
Antihistamines
 for anxiety disorders, 230*b*–231*b*, 233
 for sleep disorders, 471*b*
Antimanic agents, 325
Antipsychotics
 for chronic aggression, 522*b*
 first-generation, 192, 192*f*
 for schizophrenia, 321
  adjuncts to, 325
  atypical, 321–322, 322*t*
  conventional, 322–323, 322*t*, 324*t*–325*t*
  issues in, 321
  potentially dangerous responses to, 323–325
  when to change, 325
 second-generation, 192–194, 193*f*
  aripiprazole (Abilify), 194
  clozapine (Clozaril) as, 193–194
  olanzapine (Zyprexa) as, 194
  paliperidone (Invega) as, 194
  quetiapine, 194
  risperidone (Risperdal) as, 194
  ziprasidone (Zeldox) as, 194
Antiseizure drugs, for bipolar disorder, 191
Antisocial personality disorder (ASPD)
 characteristics and behaviours associated with, 434, 441–442
 nursing and therapy guidelines for, 442, 449*t*
 treatment of, 442
Anxiety, 202–209
 clinical picture on, 204
 defences against, 203–204, 205*t*–206*t*
 defined by Sullivan, 51
  application of, by Peplau, 51–52
 definition of, 202
 depression assessment of, 253
 drugs for, 185–186
  antidepressants as, 186
  selective serotonin reuptake inhibitors (SSRIs), for, 186
 due to nonpsychiatric medical conditions, 209, 209*t*
 in eating and feeding disorder, 341–342
 fear *vs.*, 202
 flowchart illustrating, 204*f*
 Hamilton Rating Scale for, 218, 219*t*
 levels of, 202–203, 203*t*
  case study and nursing care plan for, 235*b*–236*b*
 mild, 202, 203*t*, 225, 225*t*
 moderate, 202, 203*t*, 225, 225*t*
 NANDA-I classifications of, 483
 normal, 202
 operationally defined, 70*f*
 panic, 203, 203*t*, 225–226, 226*t*
 reduction techniques in crisis situation, 485
 related to hospitalization, 524
 schizophrenia and, 303
 self-control, in anorexia nervosa, 346*t*
 with serious medical illness, 649–650, 649*b*
 severe, 202–203, 203*t*, 225–226, 226*t*
 in sexual assault, 565
 in Sigmund Freud's Psychoanalytic Theory, 47
 in violence, 544
Anxiety disorders, 200–243
 applying nursing process to, 218–241
  assessment of, 218–222, 219*b*, 219*t*, 220*f*, 222*t*
  evaluation for, 234
  implementation for, 225–234, 225*t*–226*t*

Anxiety disorders (Continued)
  nursing diagnosis of, 222, 223t
  outcomes of, 222–224
  planning for, 224–225
  behavioural therapy for, 233–234
  case study and nursing care plan for, 235b–236b
  in children and adolescents, 606–607
    assessment guidelines for, 608b
    generalized anxiety disorder (GAD), 607
    Nursing Outcomes Classification (NOC) for, 608t
    separation anxiety disorder, 598b, 606–607
  cognitive therapy for, 234
  comorbidity of, 209
  counselling for, 227
  culture-bound syndromes, 218
  drug treatment for, 230b–231b
  epidemiology of, 209
  etiology of, 216–218
    biological factors in, 216
    environmental factors in, 217
    psychological factors in, 216–217
    sociocultural factors in, 217–218, 218b
  health teaching and health promotion for,
      227–229
  integrative therapy for, 233, 233b
  milieu therapy for, 229
  pharmacological interventions for, 232–233
    antianxiety drugs, 230b–232b, 232–233
    antidepressants, 230b–231b, 232
  psychosocial interventions for, 226–227, 229b
  selective serotonin reuptake inhibitors for, 230b–231b,
      232
  selective serotonin-norepinephrine reuptake inhibitors
      for, 230b–231b
  self-care promotion for, 229–232
    elimination, 229
    nutrition and fluid intake, 229
    personal hygiene and grooming, 229
    sleep, 232
  suicide risk in, 497
  types of
    acute stress disorder, 214, 214b
    agoraphobia, 206, 206b
    generalized anxiety disorder, 207–208, 208b, 208t
    obsessive-compulsive disorders, 211–212, 211b,
        213b
    panic attack, 204–206, 204b
    panic disorder, 204–206, 204b
    phobias, 206–207, 206b, 207t
    post-traumatic stress disorder, 214
    substance-induced anxiety disorder, 209
Apathy, in dementia, 376t
Aphasia, 374
Apiphobia, 207t
APN. see Advanced-practice nursing
Apolipoprotein E (APOE), 374
Appearance, assessment of, during mental status
    examination, 86b–87b
Appetite
  changes with depression, 254
  serotonin regulating, 250
Approachability, in abuse screening, 543b
Approval, giving, 159–161, 162t
Apraxia, 374
Aripiprazole (Abilify), 194
  for bipolar disorders, 291b
  for schizophrenia, 321, 322t
ARND. see Alcohol-related neurodevelopmental
    disorder
Aromatherapy, 723–724
  for dementia, 384, 384b
Art therapists, as members of psychiatric mental health
    treatment teams, 38b
Asenapine (Saphris), 194
ASH. see Addiction supportive housing
ASPD. see Antisocial personality disorder
Assault, 109–110, 109t
  define, 531
  violence and, 513
Assent, in child health care decision making, 589, 591
Assertive communication, 164
Assertive community treatment, 34, 35b
  for serious mental illness, 640
Assertiveness, confrontational assertions, 520–521,
    522b

Assessment
  of adolescents, 83, 83b
  age considerations in, 83–84
  of anorexia nervosa, 343–345, 345b
  of bulimia nervosa, 349, 350b
  of children, 83
  cultural and social, 88–89
  language barriers and, 84
  of older adults, 84
  in psychiatric mental health, purpose of, 84–89
  psychosocial, 87, 88b
  rating scales for, 89, 89t
  religious, 87–88
  of schizophrenia, 307–314, 308f
  spiritual, 87–88
  Standards of Practice and, 82–89
  validation of, 89
Assimilation, 123
Assisted death, 500–501
Association of Registered Nurses of Newfoundland and
    Labrador, 23
Associative looseness, 309
  counselling and communication techniques for,
      318–319
Astraphobia, 207t
Asylums, 17–18
  Canadian, early, 18–19
  introduction of nurses to, 19, 19f
Ataque de nervios, 126b, 127
Atenolol (Tenormin), 230b–231b
Atlantic Canada, history of psychiatric nursing licensing
    in, 20–21
Atomoxetine (Strattera), 195
Atonia
  muscle during REM sleep, 460
  rapid eye movement behaviour disorder and,
      464
Attending behaviour, for patient's growth, 148
Attention, 86b–87b
  norepinephrine modulating, 250
Attention deficit-hyperactivity disorder (ADHD)
  assessment guidelines in, 601b
  as comorbid condition, 589
  description of, 599–600
  drugs for, 194–195, 598b, 603b
  prevalence statistics of, in Canada, 10t
Attitude
  in abuse screening, 543b
  behaviours in personality and, 445, 446t
Atypical antipsychotics
  for anorexia nervosa, 346
  aripiprazole (Abilify), 291b
  for bipolar disorders, 290, 291b
  olanzapine (Zyprexa), 291b
  quetiapine fumarate (Seroquel), 291b
  risperidone (Risperdal), 291b
  for schizophrenia, 321–322, 322t
  ziprasidone (Zeldox), 291b
Atypical features, with major depressive disorder, 245
Atypicals, 192–193
Audiovisual hallucinations, with substance abuse or
    behavioural addictions, 416
Auditory functions, area of brain responsible for, 178f
Auditory hallucinations, 310, 310t
  coping with, 319b
  with major depressive disorder, 245
Aura, 725
Authorization of treatment, 104
Autism spectrum disorders, 598b, 599
Autocratic leader, 687
Automatic obedience, 311
Automatic thoughts, 55–56
Autonomic dysfunction, from conventional
    antipsychotics, 324t–325t
Autonomic nervous system, regulation of, 173,
    174f
Autonomic physiological responses, as nonverbal
    behaviour, 156t
Autonomy
  defined, 99–100
  principle of, 104–105
  respect for, 97
Autoreceptors, 175
Aversion therapy, as behavioural therapy, 54
Avoidance training, 54

Avoidant personality disorder
  characteristics and behaviours associated with, 434,
      443–445, 444b
  nursing and therapy guidelines for, 444, 449t
  treatment of, 444
Avoidant/restrictive food intake disorder, 339–340
Avolition, in schizophrenia, 311t
Awareness, levels of, in Sigmund Freud's Psychoanalytic
    Theory, 46, 46f
Ayurvedic medicine, 718

B
Baby boomers, 615
Bachelor of science degrees in nursing (BScN), 21
Bad medicine, hit by, 126b
Baghdad, early asylums in, 17–18
BALs. see Blood alcohol levels
Bandura, Albert, 61t
Bariatric surgery, for binge eating disorder, 353,
    353b
Barriers
  to accurate pain assessment, in older adults, 620
  to treatment, as future issue in psychiatric mental
      health care, 41–42
Barry, Pat, 22
Basal ganglia, 179, 179f
Bath salts, description and medical uses for, 408
Bathing, in guidelines for self-care for individuals with
    cognitive impairment, 381b
Battery
  in cycle of violence, 535
  liability issues with, 109–110, 109t
  signs of, 532–533
Battlefords and District Co-operative Ltd. v. Gibbs,
    101
BDNF. see Brain-derived neurotrophic factor
Beauport asylum, 18
Beck, Aaron T., 55, 55f
Beck's cognitive triad, 251
Beers, Clifford W., 8
Behavioural contract, for managing disruptive
    behaviours, in children and adolescents,
    607b
Behavioural crises, management of, 41
Behavioural family therapy, 703, 704t
Behavioural health home care, 630
Behavioural theories, 52–55
  of anxiety disorders, 217
  behaviourism theory as, 53
  classical conditioning theory as, 53, 53f
  implications of, in nursing practice, 54–55
  operant conditioning theory as, 53, 53f
Behavioural therapy, 53–55
  for anxiety disorders, 233–234
  aversion therapy as, 54
  biofeedback as, 54
  for children and adolescents, 594–595
  modelling, 53–54
  operant conditioning, 54, 54t
  systematic desensitization as, 54
Behaviourism Theory, 53
Behaviours
  assessment of, during mental status examination,
      86b–87b
  attitudes in personality and, 445, 446t
  bipolar disorders and, 281
  with delirium, 367
  with dementia, 376t, 378
    medications for, 384
  nonverbal, 155, 156t
  norepinephrine modulating, 250
Beliefs
  in abuse screening, 543b
  in therapeutic relationships, 140–142
Belongingness, need for, 58
Beneficence, 98, 105–106
Benner, Patricia, 52t
Benson, Herbert, 73
Benson's relaxation technique, 73, 74b
Benzodiazepines, 185, 185f
  for alcohol withdrawal symptoms, 417b
  for anxiety disorders, 230b–231b
  for chronic aggression, 522b
  for schizophrenia, 325
  for sleep disorders, 471b

Bereavement, 665
  communication and, 668b
  depression with, 247
  guidelines for dealing with, 670b
  phenomena experienced during, 667t
Best action principle, 98
Best practice
  establishing, 102–103
  standards of practice, 102–103
Beta blockers
  for anxiety disorders, 230b–231b, 233
  for chronic aggression, 522b
Bettelheim, Bruno, 60
Bias, cultural, 164
Bibliotherapy, 597
Binet, Alfred, 48–49
Binet Intelligence Test, 48–49
Binge eating disorder, 352–358
  bariatric surgery for, 353, 353b
  characteristics of, 339b
  clinical picture of, 338–340
  comorbidity of, 341–342
  epidemiology of, 340–341
  etiology of, 342–343
  state of treatment for, 348t
Biochemical factors, with depression, 250, 250f
Bioelectromagnetic-based therapies, 726
Bioethics, 97–98
Biofeedback, 719
  as behavioural therapy, 54
  as relaxation technique, 75
Biofield energy, 725
Biologic endowment, as key social determinant of
    health, 14
Biological factors
  in aggression and violence, 514–515
  with depression, 249–251
  in nonsuicidal self-injury, 508
  with substance use disorders, 396–397, 396f
  in suicide, 498–500
Biological interventions, during psychiatric mental
    health nursing process, 92
Biological model, 60
  implications of, for nursing practice, 60
Biological theories, 60
  advent of psychopharmacology and, 60
  Biological model and, 60
Biological therapy, as basic-level psychiatric mental
    health nursing intervention, 13t
Biologically based integrative therapies, 721–724
  aromatherapy as, 723–724
  diet and nutrition as, 721–723
  herbal therapy as, 723
  megavitamin therapy as, 723
Biologically based mental illness, 633
Biopsychiatry
  as biological approach to nervous system
    malfunctions, 172
  and psychotropic drugs, 172
Biopsychosocial assessment, 36–37
Biopsychosocial care manager, 37–38
Biopsychosocial model, 36
Bipolar disorders, 275–298
  acute phase of
    implementation for, 286, 287t
    outcomes identification in, 284
    planning in, 285
  antiseizure drugs for, 191
  behavioural symptoms of, 281
  biological factors of, 279–280
  carbamazepine for, 191
  in children and adolescents, 608–609
  clinical picture on, 277–278
    bipolar I disorder, 277, 277b
    bipolar II disorder, 277–278
    cyclothymic disorder, 278
  cognitive symptoms of, 283
  comorbidity of, 279
  continuation phase of
    implementation for, 286
    outcomes identification in, 284
    planning in, 285
  continuum symptoms of, 276f
  cultural considerations for, 280b
  drug treatment for, 190–191

Bipolar disorders (Continued)
  electroconvulsive therapy for, 290
  environmental factors of, 280
  epidemiology of, 278–279, 278t
  etiology of, 279–280
  euphoric mood associated with, 281
  flight of ideas and, 282–283
  genetics and, 279
  health teaching and health promotion for, 292,
    292b
  hypomania in
    behaviour symptoms of, 281
    with bipolar II disorder, 277–278
    transition to mania, 281
  lamotrigine for, 191
  lithium carbonate, 190–191, 191t
  maintenance phase of
    implementation for, 286
    outcomes identification in, 285
    planning in, 286
  milieu management for, 290–292
  Mood Disorder Questionnaire for, 281, 282f
  nursing process application to, 281–297
    assessment in, 281–284, 282f, 284f
    case study and nursing care plan for, 294b–
      296b
    evaluation for, 293
    implementation for, 286–293
    nursing diagnosis of, 284, 285t
    outcomes identification in, 284–285
    planning in, 285–286
  pharmacological interventions for, 286, 291b
    antianxiety drugs, 290
    anticonvulsant drugs, 289–290, 291b
    atypical antipsychotics, 290
    lithium carbonate, 286–289, 288t, 289b, 291b
    omega-3 fatty acids, 291b
  prevalence statistics of, in Canada, 10t
  psychological factors of, 280
  psychotherapy for, 292–293
  suicide risk in, 497
  support groups for, 292
  thought and speech symptoms of, 282–283
  valproate for, 191
Bipolar I disorder, 277
  comorbidity of, 279
  diagnostic criteria for, 277b
Bipolar II disorder, 277–278
  comorbidity of, 279
Bisexual, 577–578
  hostility toward, 592b
Bladder function, in guidelines for self-care for
    individuals with cognitive impairment, 381b
Blame
  during family therapy, 700b
  in sexual assault, 569
Bleuler, Eugen, coined the term schizophrenia,
    302
Blood alcohol levels (BALs)
  limits in Canada, 458–459
  testing of, 398
Blurred boundaries, 139–140, 139t
Blurred vision, from conventional antipsychotics,
    324t–325t
Body language
  during clinical interview, 166
  as nonverbal behaviour, 156t
Borderline personality disorder
  case study and nursing care plan on, 453b–454b
  characteristics and behaviours associated with, 434,
    438–441, 441b
  nursing and therapy guidelines for, 440, 449t
  pathological personality traits seen in, 438–440,
    439f
  treatment of, 440–441
Boredom, as counter-transference, 141t
Boundaries
  blurred, 139–140, 139t
  establishing, 139
  in family therapies, 699, 699b
  relationship, 139–140
  self-check on, 140, 142f
Boundary impairment, 310
Bowel function, in guidelines for self-care for individuals
    with cognitive impairment, 381b

Brain
  activities of, 172–175
  biopsychiatry and, 172
  cellular composition of, 175–177, 175f
  control of biological drives and behaviour in, 173–174
  development and biochemicals, in child and
      adolescent disorders, 590
  functions of, 172–184, 173b
  homeostasis in, maintenance of, 173
  lobes and associated functions of, 178–179, 179f
  organization of, 177–179
    brainstem in, 177–178, 178f
    cerebellum, 178, 178f–179f
    cerebrum, 178–179, 179f
  structure of, 172–184
  visualization of, 179–183, 180t, 181f
Brain imaging, 375
Brain injury
  delirium, major neurocognitive disorders, depression,
      comparison of, 364t
  traumatic, in Alzheimer's disease, 374
Brain-derived neurotrophic factor (BDNF), monoamines
    and, 190
Brainstem, 177–178, 178f–179f
Breach of duty, 110–111
Breathing exercises, 74, 74b
Breathing-related disorders, affecting sleep, 464
Brexpiprazole, for schizophrenia, 321
Brief psychotic disorder, 303b
BScN. see Bachelor of science degrees in nursing
Bulimia nervosa, 348–349
  acute care for, 351
  advanced-practice interventions for, 351–352
  assessment of, 349, 350b
  case study and nursing care plan for, 356b–357b
  characteristics of, 339b
  clinical picture of, 338–340
  comorbidity of, 341–342
  counselling for, 351
  diagnosis of, 350
  epidemiology of, 340–341
  etiology of, 342–343
  evaluation of, 352
  general assessment of, 349
  health teaching and health promotion for, 351
  implementation in, 351–352
  medical complications of, 349b
  milieu management for, 351
  NOC outcomes related to, 351t
  outcomes identification of, 350
  pharmacological interventions for, 351
  planning for, 350–351
  psychotherapy for, 351–352
  self-assessment of, 349
  signs and symptoms of, 350t
  state of treatment for, 348t
  thoughts and behaviours associated with, 349b
  vignette in, 349b–350b, 352b
Bullycide, 497
Bullying
  in children and adolescents, 604
  culture in schools, 516, 516b
  suicide and, 497
Buprenorphine (Suboxone), 417
Bupropion (Wellbutrin), 261b–262b
  for bulimia nervosa, 351
  for depression, 189
Burden on family, in dementia, 376t
Buspirone (BuSpar), 186, 186f
  as alternative to addictive benzodiazepines, 233
Buspirone hydrochloride (Bustab), 230b–231b

C
Caffeine
  addiction to, 408–409
  associated with insomnia, 462
  physical complications related to abuse of, 395t
  reduction or cessation of intake of, as stress buster,
    70b
CAGE-AID Screening Tool, for substance abuse, 617b
Cairo, Egypt, early asylums in, 17–18
Calgary Family Assessment Model (CFAM), 698–699,
    705f
Calgary Family Intervention Model (CFIM), 698–699
Callousness, 441

CAM. *see* Confusion Assessment Method
Canada
　correctional nursing in, 679–680
　cultural landscape of, 120, 121*t*
　demographic shifts in, 102
　forensic mental health system in, 678
　residential schools among indigenous people in, 619*b*
Canada Health Act, 27–28, 97
Canadian Association for Suicide Prevention, 504*b*
Canadian Association of Schools of Nursing (CASN), 22
Canadian Community Health Survey Mental Health,
　　mental health and substance abuse statistics by,
　　41–42
Canadian Council of Psychiatric Nurses (CCPN), 21
Canadian Federation of Mental Health Nurses
　　(CFMHN), 22
　standards of practice, 11–12, 22, 97*b*
Canadian Gerontological Nursing Association, 624
Canadian Holistic Nurses Association (CHNA), 717
Canadian Hospice Palliative Care Association (CHPCA),
　658
Canadian Index of Wellbeing (CIW), 70–71
Canadian Medical Association, 20
Canadian Mental Health Association (CMHA), 8
　housing and support established by, 29
Canadian National Association of Trained Nurses, 20
Canadian Network for Mood and Anxiety Treatments
　　(CANMAT), 290
Canadian Nurses Association (CNA), 20
　on addiction in the workplace, 426
　certification by, 22
　code of ethics, 97–98, 97*b*
　confidentiality and, 106–107
　history of, 20
　standards of practice set by, 11–12
Canadian Tobacco, Alcohol and Drugs Survey (CTADS),
　394
Cancer
　anxiety caused by, 212*t*
　pain, visual analogue scale for, 623*f*
CANMAT. *see* Canadian Network for Mood and Anxiety
　　Treatments
Cannabis sativa, 409
Cannon, Walter, 66
Carbamazepine (Tegretol), 191, 230*b*–231*b*
　for bipolar disorders, 290, 291*b*
Cardiovascular diseases
　anxiety caused by, 212*t*
　in dementia, 374
　depression co-occurring with, 248*t*
　that may mimic psychiatric illness, 85*b*
Care theory, ethics of, 50
Caregiver
　families as, 698
　role strain, in dementia, 376
　service, for dementia, 379*t*–380*t*
Caregiver burden
　for older adults, 618
　serious mental illness and, 637
Caring, during end-of-life (EOL) care, 659
Cariprazine, for schizophrenia, 321
Case management, 39
　as basic-level nursing intervention, 29
CASN. *see* Canadian Association of Schools of Nursing
Catastrophic reaction, aggression and, 525–526
Catastrophizing, 56*t*
　in cognitive distortions, 347*b*
Catatonia, 311, 328
　associated with another medical condition, 303*b*
Catatonic features, with major depressive disorder, 245
Catharsis, 685*b*
Cathartic method, 46
Cause in fact, 111
CBT. *see* Cognitive behavioural therapy
CCPN. *see* Canadian Council of Psychiatric Nurses
Cellular composition, of brain, 175–177, 175*f*
Cellular reuptake, 175
Central nervous system (CNS)
　alcohol affecting, 395
　depressants, 248*t*, 400–404, 400*t*
　gamma-aminobutyric acid (GABA) and, 185
　stimulants, intoxication, overdose and withdrawal,
　　406–407, 407*t*
Cerebellum, 178, 178*f*–179*f*
Cerebral hypoxia, 368

Cerebrum, 178–179, 179*f*
CFAM. *see* Calgary Family Assessment Model
CFIM. *see* Calgary Family Intervention Model
CFMHN. *see* Canadian Federation of Mental Health
　Nurses
Chakras, 718, 725
Chamomile extract, 723, 724*t*
*Changing Directions, Changing Lives: The Mental Health
　Strategy for Canada*, 29
Child abuse, 530–559
　as adventitious crisis, 480
　in Canada, 535
　characteristics of abusive parents, 538*b*
　Duluth "Abuse of Children" wheel, 540*f*
　Duluth "Nurturing Children" wheel in, 553*f*
　epidemiology of, 535
　factors to assess in home visits in, 545, 546*b*
　interventions for, 549*b*
　neglect and, 535
　nursing process application in, 539–556
　　assessment in, 539–546, 541*b*
　　diagnosis in, 546, 546*t*
　　evaluation in, 552–553
　　implementation in, 547–552
　　outcomes identification in, 546, 547*t*
　　planning in, 546–547
　reporting suspected, 108–109, 108*b*
　risk factors for mental illness in, 589, 590*b*
　sexual, 533
　vulnerability in, 538, 540*f*
Childhood-onset conduct disorder, 604
Children
　anxiety disorders in, 606–607
　　assessment guidelines for, 608*b*
　　generalized anxiety disorder (GAD), 607
　　Nursing Outcomes Classification (NOC) for, 608*t*
　　separation anxiety disorder, 606–607
　assessment of, 83
　bipolar disorders in, 278, 608–609
　characteristics of mentally healthy, 592*b*
　depression in
　　assessment of, 254
　　stress leading to, 248
　depressive disorders in, 608–609
　disorders of, 587–613
　　brain development and biochemicals in, 590
　　comorbidity in, 589
　　cultural factors, 591
　　drug treatment of, 598*b*
　　environmental factors, 591
　　epidemiology of, 588–589
　　genetic factors in, 590
　　resilience factors, 591
　　temperament in, 590
　disruptive, impulse control, and conduct disorders in,
　　603–604
　　adolescent-onset conduct disorder, 604
　　bullying, 604
　　childhood-onset conduct disorder, 604
　　conduct disorders, 603–604, 605*b*
　　nursing process application to, 604–606, 605*b*, 605*t*
　　oppositional defiant disorder, 603, 605*b*
　　techniques for managing, 607*b*
　Duluth "Nurturing Children" wheel in, 553*f*
　feeding and eating disorders, 609
　mood disorders in, 608–609
　neurodevelopmental disorders in, 598–601
　　attention deficit-hyperactivity disorder (ADHD),
　　　599–600, 601*b*, 603*b*
　　autism spectrum disorders, 599
　　communication disorders, 599
　　intellectual disabilities, 599
　　motor disorders, 600–601
　　Nursing Outcomes Classification (NOC) for, 602*t*
　　nursing process application to, 601–603, 601*b*, 602*t*
　　specific learning disorder (SLD), 600
　　stereotypic movement disorder, 600
　　Tourette's disorder, 600
　post-traumatic stress disorder (PTSD) in, 609
　psychiatric mental health nursing, 591–598, 592*b*
　　assessment data in, 592–594, 593*b*
　　behavioural therapy, 594–595
　　bibliotherapy, 597
　　cognitive behavioural therapy, 595
　　cultural factors in, 594

Children *(Continued)*
　　data collection in, 591–592
　　developmental assessment in, 593
　　family therapy, 594
　　group therapy, 594
　　mental status examination in, 593
　　milieu management, 595–596, 595*b*
　　mind-body therapies, 596
　　multimodal music therapy, 596
　　mutual storytelling, 596–597, 597*b*
　　play therapy, 596–597
　　principle of least restrictive intervention, 594
　　psychopharmacology, 598
　　quiet room, 596
　　risk assessment in, 593–594
　　seclusion and restraint in, 595–596
　　therapeutic drawing, 597
　　therapeutic games, 597, 597*b*
　　time out, 596
　risk factors for mental illness in, 589, 590*b*
　use of antidepressant drugs by, 266
　vulnerable to abuse, 538, 540*f*
Chinese immigrants, in Canada, 616*b*
Chiropractic medicine, 724
Chlordiazepoxide hydrochloride (Librax), 230*b*–231*b*
Chlorpromazine (Largactil, Thorazine), 7, 60, 521*b*
　for anorexia nervosa, 346
　for schizophrenia, 322*t*
CHNA. *see* Canadian Holistic Nurses Association
Cholestatic jaundice, from conventional antipsychotics,
　324*t*–325*t*
Cholinergics, 176*t*
Cholinesterase inhibitors, for Alzheimer's disease, 195,
　381–382
CHPCA. *see* Canadian Hospice Palliative Care
　Association
Chronic fatigue syndrome, 466
Chronic sorrow, 665, 666*b*, 666*t*
Chronological age, 615
Circadian process, 460
Circadian rhythm sleep disorder, 464
Circadian rhythms, 174
　circadian rhythm sleep disorder, 464
Circumstantiality, in communication, 309
Cirrhosis, concurrent with substance abuse disorders,
　395
CISD. *see* Critical incident stress debriefing
Cisgender, 578–579
Citalopram (Celexa), 188, 230*b*–231*b*, 261*b*–262*b*
Civil obligations, 109–111, 109*t*
CIW. *see* Canadian Index of Wellbeing
Clang associations, 283
　in communication, 310
Clarification, for managing disruptive behaviours, in
　children and adolescents, 607*b*
Clarifying techniques, as therapeutic communication
　technique, 158–159, 160*t*–161*t*
Classical conditioning theory, 53
　vs. operant conditioning, 53*f*
Classical psychoanalysis, 48
　counter-transference in, 48
　transference in, 48
Claustrophobia, 207*t*
Clear boundaries, 699*b*
Cleverley, Kristin, 22
Clinical competence, of health care workers, 138
Clinical consultation, 687
Clinical epidemiology, 10
Clinical interview, 152–170
　attending behaviours during, 166–167
　clinical supervision during, 167
　helpful guidelines for, 166
　initiating, 165
　introductions during, 165
　pace of, 164
　preparation, 164–165
　process recordings during, 167, 168*t*
　setting of, 164
　tactics to avoid during, 165–166, 165*t*–166*t*
Clinical nurse specialist, province licensing regulations
　for, 22
Clinical Opiate Withdrawal Scale (COWS), 405–406,
　406*t*
Clinical pathway, discharge planning and, 34
Clinical supervision, 138

Clomipramine hydrochloride (Anafranil), 230b–231b, 261b–262b
Clonazepam (Rivotril), 185, 185f, 230b–231b
Clonidine (Catapres), 417
Closed group, 685b
Close-ended questions, 159
Clozapine (Clozaril), 193–194
  for schizophrenia, 321, 322t
Clozaril. see Clozapine
Cluster A personality disorders, 434
Cluster B personality disorders, 434
Cluster C personality disorders, 434
Cluster suicide, 500
CMHA. see Canadian Mental Health Association
CNA. see Canadian Nurses Association
Cocaine, 407
  physical complications related to abuse of, 395t
Code of ethics
  Canadian Nurses Association, 97–98, 97b
  Registered Psychiatric Nurses of Canada, 97–98, 99b
Code White responders, 520
Codeine, intoxication, overdose and withdrawal from, 405t
Cognition, 362
  assessment of, during mental status examination, 86b–87b
Cognitive behavioural therapy (CBT), 55–56, 57b, 689, 689t
  for anxiety disorders, 234
  for binge eating disorder, 353
  for bipolar disorders, 293
  for bulimia nervosa, 351
  for children and adolescents, 595
  for depression, 269
  for insomnia, 470–472
  internet-delivered, for obsessive-compulsive disorder, 213b
  for serious mental illness, 640
Cognitive deficits, aggression and, 525–526, 526b
Cognitive development, 48–49, 61t
Cognitive distortions, 55–56, 56t, 75
  in anorexia nervosa, 346, 347b
Cognitive disturbances, in delirium, 366
Cognitive enhancement therapy, for serious mental illness, 640
Cognitive function, 362–363
  bipolar disorders and, 283
Cognitive impairment
  case study and nursing care plan, 385b–387b
  self-care for individuals with, guidelines for, 381b
  with substance abuse or behavioural addictions, 415t
Cognitive reframing, 75, 75t
Cognitive symptoms, of schizophrenia, 307, 311–312
Cognitive theories, 55–58
  of anxiety disorders, 217
  Cognitive Behavioural Therapy and, 55–56, 57b
  of depression, 251
  Dialectic Behavioural Therapy as, 56–58
  implications of, in nursing practice, 58, 58b
  Rational Emotive Behaviour Therapy as, 55
Cognitive therapy, for anxiety disorders, 234
Cogwheel rigidity, from conventional antipsychotics, 324t–325t
Collaboration
  definition of, 423
  as key strategy area for Canadian mental health care, 8, 9b
  of primary health care and mental health care, 647, 648b
Collagen vascular diseases, that may mimic psychiatric illness, 85b
Colonization, 116
  defined, 122
Command hallucinations, 310–311
Communicable diseases, confidentiality and, 109
Communication, 152–170
  for associative looseness, 318–319
  for catatonia, 328
  for delusions, 318, 319b
  in dementia, 378, 380b
  depression and, 254
  disorders, in children and adolescents, 599
  for disorganization, 328
  dysfunctional, in family therapy, 699–700, 699b–700b
  factors affecting, 153–155

Communication (Continued)
  in group therapy, 689t
  for hallucinations, 318, 318b
  importance of effective, during end-of-life (EOL) care, 661–664, 662b
  nonverbal, 155
  for paranoia, 327
  process of, 153, 154f
  for schizophrenia, 317–319
  skills for nurses, 157–164
    assertive communication in, 164
    evaluation of, 164, 165f
    therapeutic communication strategies in, 157–163
  style, 163
  techniques
    of group leader, 688t
    with substance abuse patients, 413–415, 413t–415t
  therapeutic strategies, 157–163, 160t–161t
    accepting as, 160t–161t
    active listening as, 157–158, 160t–161t
    asking questions and eliciting patient responses as, 159
    clarifying techniques as, 158–159, 160t–161t
    exploring as, 159, 160t–161t
    listening with empathy as, 158
    paraphrasing as, 158
    reflecting as, 158–159, 160t–161t
    restating as, 158, 160t–161t
    silence as, 157, 160t–161t
    summarizing as, 160t–161t
  verbal, 155
Community mental health centres, 29–30, 30b
  deinstitutionalization and, 29
  interprofessional team model in, 30
  psychiatric mental health nurse in, 30
  recovery and, 29
Community mental health workers, as members of psychiatric mental health treatment teams, 38b
Community psychiatric mental health nursing, 36
Community supports, for Alzheimer's disease, 378–381, 379t–380t
Community treatment orders (CTOs), 105
Community violence, 122
Community-based programs, for older adults, 630
Comorbid condition, defined, 9
Comparison, encouraging, as therapeutic communication technique, 160t–161t
Compensation defence mechanism, 205t–206t
Competency, 104
  early defining of, in psychiatric mental health nurse, 23
  in older adult abuse, 547
  in relationship building, 136–137
Complaining member, 692–693, 693b
Complementary therapies, 714–728
Complete suicide, 496
Compliance, vs. antagonism, 445, 446t
Complicated grief, 665
Compulsions, 211, 213t
Compulsive behaviours, 392
Computed tomography (CT scans), description and psychiatric uses for, 180t
Concentration, 86b–87b
  difficulties with depression, 253
Concordance
  depression in identical twins and, 249
  in identical twin brain image research, 181f, 183
Concrete operational stage, of cognitive development, 48
Concrete thinking, in schizophrenia, 308–309, 311–312
Concreteness, 311–312
Concurrent disorders, 394–395, 636
  groups, 690
  programs, 28, 422–423, 422b
Conditioning
  classical, 53, 53f
  defined, 53
  operant, 53, 53f
Conduct disorders, in children and adolescents, 598b, 603–604, 605b
Confabulation, 374
Confidentiality
  in abuse screening, 543b
  adolescents and, 83
  after death, 109

Confidentiality (Continued)
  communicable diseases and, 109
  in nurse-patient relationship, 143–145
  rights regarding, 106–109
Conflict
  in groups, 685b
  nurse responses to, 144t–145t
Confrontational assertions, 520–521, 522b
Confusion Assessment Method (CAM), 365
Confusional arousal disorders, types of, 463–464
Connecting, during end-of-life (EOL) care, 659
Conscientious objection, 100
Conscious mental activity, brain function and, 174–175
Conscious mind, 46
Consensual validation, seeking, as therapeutic communication technique, 160t–161t
Consent
  in child health care decision making, 589, 591
  informed, 104
Consequentialist theory, 98
Consistency, in nurse-patient relationship, 147
Constipation
  from conventional antipsychotics, 324t–325t
  depression co-occurring with, 259t
Constraint, vs. impulsivity, 445, 446t
Consultation
  by advanced-practice psychiatric mental health nurses, 13t
  definition of, 422–423
Contemplation phase, of Transtheoretical Model of Change, 412
Content, of message, 156
Continuation phase
  of bipolar disorders
    implementation for, 286
    outcomes identification in, 284
    planning in, 285
  of depression, 257
Continuum of psychiatric mental health treatment, 28, 29f
Contract, for nurse-patient relationship, 143
Control
  in nurse-patient relationships, 147
  of perpetrators, 538
Controlled Drugs and Substances Act (CDSA), schedule IV drugs, 186
Controlled style, of coping, 564b, 565–566
Conventional antipsychotics
  for anorexia nervosa, 346
  for schizophrenia, 322–323, 322t, 324t–325t
Conventional health care, 714
Conversion defence mechanism, 205t–206t
Conversion disorder, 210, 211b
Coordination of care
  as basic-level psychiatric mental health nursing intervention, 13t
  in psychiatric mental health nursing, 92
Coping
  definition of, 478
  "ineffective" diagnosis in crisis situations, 483, 484t
  styles, assessment of, 71
Coping mechanisms
  four phases of crisis, 480
  in sexual assault, 565
  with stress and crisis, 478
  in violence, 544–545, 545t, 546b
Coping skills
  anger and aggression and
    healthy, overwhelmed, 524
    marginal, 524–525
  anxiety disorders and, 221
  factors compromising, 478
  as key social determinant of health, 14
  mental illness and, 648, 652–654, 652t, 654b
Copycat suicide, 500
Correctional nursing, 679–680, 680b–681b
Corrections and Conditional Release Act (1992), 680
Corticosteroids, stress response and, 68
Corticotropin, nerve cells of brain influenced by, 173
Corticotropin-releasing factor (CRF), depression and, 251
Corticotropin-releasing hormone (CRH), nerve cells of brain influenced by, 173

Cortisol
  depression and, 250
  nerve cells of brain influenced by, 173
Counselling
  for anorexia nervosa, 342
  for anxiety disorders, 227
  as basic-level nursing intervention, 28
  for bulimia nervosa, 351
  communication techniques with depression, 257,
    257*b*–258*b*
  for dementia, 378
  for managing disruptive behaviours, in children and
    adolescents, 607*b*
  for schizophrenia, 317–319
  for sexual assault, 569–570
  for sleep disorders, 469
  techniques in crisis situation, 485–486
  for violence and abuse, 548, 548*b*
Counsellors, as members of psychiatric mental health
    treatment teams, 38*b*
Counter-transference, 140, 141*t*, 312
  in classical psychoanalysis, 48
COWS. *see* Clinical Opiate Withdrawal Scale
Crack, 407
CRF. *see* Corticotropin-releasing factor
CRH. *see* Corticotropin-releasing hormone
Crime, Canada's National Crime Prevention Strategy,
    675, 676*b*
Criminal Code, 500–501, 678
  in reporting abuse, 547
  in sexual assault, 561
Criminal responsibility, 679
Criminalization
  decreased, crisis intervention team and, 31
  of mentally ill, 678
Crisis, 477–494
  Aguilera's paradigm on outcomes of, 478, 478*f*
  coping and coping methods, 478
  defining, 478
  "ineffective coping" diagnosis in, 483
  NANDA-I classifications of anxiety associated with,
    483
  phases of, 480
    phase 1, 480
    phase 2, 480
    phase 3, 480
    phase 4, 480
  resolution from the state of, 478, 478*f*
  situation, abuse and, 539
  theory, 478–480, 479*f*
  two necessary conditions (Roberts) for, 478
  types of, 479–480
    adventitious, 480
    maturational, 479–480
    situational, 480
Crisis intervention
  cultural considerations, 482*b*
  definition of, 478
  five elements of, 479
  foundation for, 481*b*
  guidelines for, 485, 486*t*
  nursing process application to
    assessment of, 478*f*, 480–483, 481*b*–483*b*
    case study and nursing care plan on, 489*b*–492*b*
    diagnosis of, 483, 483*b*, 483*t*
    evaluation of, 487, 487*b*
    implementation of, 485–486, 485*b*, 487*b*
    outcomes identification of, 484, 484*b*, 484*t*
    planning of, 485
  process of, 478
  Roberts's seven-stage model of, 479, 479*f*
  self-assessment in, 482–483
Crisis intervention team, 31–32, 31*b*
Crisis management, 41
  behavioural, 41
  medical, 41
Crisis theory, nursing process application to, 480
Critical incident stress debriefing (CISD), phases of, 486,
    487*b*
Crying, nurse responses to, 144*t*–145*t*
CTADS. *see* Canadian Tobacco, Alcohol and Drugs
    Survey
CTOs. *see* Community treatment orders
Cues, nonverbal, 155, 156*t*
Cultural awareness, 128

Cultural competence, 127–128
*Cultural Competency and Safety: A Guide for Health Care
    Administrators, Providers and Educators*, 127
Cultural concepts of distress, 126, 126*b*
Cultural considerations
  for bipolar disorders, 280*b*
  concept of weight, 343*b*
  crisis resolution, 478, 478*f*
  eye contact, 163
  on gender bias in diagnosing personality disorders,
    441*b*
  nonverbal communication, 163–164
  regarding sexual orientation and gender identity,
    578*b*
  regarding sleep in Canadian culture, 461*b*
  touch, 163–164
Cultural contexts, on end-of-life (EOL) care, 660
Cultural desire, 130
Cultural encounters, 128
Cultural factors
  of nonsuicidal self-injury, 508
  of suicide, 500, 501*b*
Cultural filters, 164
Cultural humility, 129–130
Cultural knowledge, 128
Cultural norms, 116
Cultural safety, 116
Cultural skill, 128–130
Cultural violence, 532*t*, 534
Culturally competent care, 127–130
Culturally sensitive assessment, 129, 129*b*
Culture
  assessment of, 88–89
  beliefs of, regarding mental illness, 6
  Chinese immigrants growing old in Canada, 616*b*
  defined, 116
  as key social determinant of health, 14
  as mediator of stress response, 69
  mental health and, 116
  nonverbal communication patterns and, 119,
    119*t*
  pharmacogenetics and, 184, 184*b*
  world view of, 116, 117*t*
Culture-bound syndromes, 6
  anxiety disorders and, 218
Custodial care, 18
Cutting, as self-harm, 501
Cycle of violence, 535, 536*f*
Cyclic stage, in cycle of violence, 535
Cyclothymic disorder, 278
  comorbidity of, 279
  epidemiology of, 279
Cytokines
  depression and, 68
  stress response and, 68

D
Damages, 111
Dance therapists, as members of psychiatric mental
    health treatment teams, 38*b*
Dantrolene, 323
Data collection
  definition of, 80
  primary source for, 82
Date rape, 562, 563*t*
Day treatment programs, 630
  for drug abuse, 422
  for schizophrenia, 317
DBT. *see* Dialectical behaviour therapy
Death
  Canadian hospice palliative care treatment model and,
    658
  confidentiality after, 109
  in eating disorders, 343–344
  guidelines when caring for the dying, 661*b*
  by suicide, 496
  Woodruff's Total Suffering Model, 661, 661*f*
Debriefing, 167
"Decade of the brain", 8
Decision making
  in crisis situations, 484*t*
  in dementia, 376*t*
Decompensation, 28
De-escalation techniques, 519, 519*b*

Defamation, of character, 109*t*
Defence mechanisms
  in Alzheimer's disease, 374
  in Sigmund Freud's Psychoanalytic Theory, 47
Defences
  adaptive and maladaptive uses of, 205*t*–206*t*
  against anxiety, 203–204, 205*t*–206*t*
Deficient fluid volume, in delirium, 367–368
Deinstitutionalization, 21, 675
  consequences of, 32
  lack of funding for, 29
  trend of, 29
Delirium, 363–365
  alcohol withdrawal, 403–404
  assessment of, 365–367, 367*b*
  clinical picture of, 363
  common causes of, 365*b*
  comorbidity and etiology of, 365
  diagnosis of, 367–368, 368*t*
  diagnostic criteria for, 364*b*
  epidemiology of, 365
  evaluation of, 370
  implementation in, 369–370, 369*b*
  major neurocognitive disorders, depression, and brain
    injury, comparison of, 364*t*
  outcomes identification in, 368, 369*t*
  planning for, 368
  vignette in, 367*b*
Delirium tremens (DTs), 403–404
Delusional disorder, 303*b*
Delusions
  coping with, 319*b*
  counselling and communication techniques for, 318
  with dementia, 378
  with major depressive disorder, 245
  people experiencing, 319*b*
  with schizophrenia, 302
  summary of, 309*t*
Dementia, 370
  from Alzheimer's disease, 370–371
  care at home, guidelines for, 382*b*
  as challenge for psychiatric mental health nurses, 12
  clinical picture of, 370–373
  communication, guidelines for, 378, 380*b*
  counselling and communication techniques for, 378
  cross-cultural differences in, 372*b*
  delirium, depression, and brain injury, comparison of,
    364*t*
  diagnostic criteria for, 370*b*
  epidemiology of, 373
  etiology of, 373–374
    biological factors in, 373–374
    environmental factors in, 374
  evaluation for, 384
  Functional Dementia Scale in, 377*f*
  health teaching and health promotion in, 378–381
  integrative therapy for, 384, 384*b*
  normal aging *vs.*, 371*t*
  nursing process, application of, 374–388
    assessment of, 374–375, 375*b*
    case study and nursing care plan in, 385*b*–387*b*
    diagnosis of, 375–376
    implementation in, 378–384, 379*b*
    outcomes identification in, 376, 376*t*, 377*b*
    planning for, 376–378
  palliative care for patients with, 669–670
  pharmacological interventions for, 381–384
  self-care for individuals with cognitive impairment,
    guidelines for, 381*b*
  services that may be available to people with,
    379*t*–380*t*
  types of, 371*t*
  vignette in, 373*b*
Democratic leader, 687
Demoralizing member, 693, 693*b*
Denial
  with Alzheimer's disease, 374
  as defence mechanism, 205*t*–206*t*
  with serious medical illness, 650–651, 650*b*
Deontology, defined, 97–98
Dependent personality disorder
  characteristics and behaviours associated with, 434,
    444, 444*b*
  nursing and therapy guidelines for, 444, 449*t*
  treatment of, 444

Depersonalization/derealization disorder, 215, 215b, 310, 568
  sexual assault and, 568
Depression
  advanced practice interventions for
    group therapy, 269
    psychotherapy, 269
  alcohol dependence with, case study on, 424b–426b
  antidepressant drugs for, 258–266
    by children and adolescents, 266
    choosing, 259
    monoamine oxidase inhibitors, 261b–262b, 263–265, 265b
    by older adults, 266
    by pregnant women, 265
    selective serotonin reuptake inhibitors (SSRIs), 259–262, 261b–263b
    serotonin-norepinephrine reuptake inhibitors (SNRIs), 261b–262b, 262
    tricyclic antidepressants, 261b–262b, 263, 264b
  assessment of, 251–256, 255b, 312
    age considerations in, 254
    areas to assess, 253–254
    in children and adolescents, 254
    guidelines in, 255b
    key findings in, 253
    in older adults, 254
    screening tools in, 251, 252f
    self-assessment in, 254–256
    suicidal ideation in, 251–253
  affecting basic sex and hunger drives, 173–174
  Beck's cognitive triad and, 251
  during bereavement, 667t
  case study and nursing care plan for, 269b–271b
  comorbidity of, 249
  cytokines and, 68
  delirium, major neurocognitive disorders, and brain injury, comparison of, 364t
  with dementia, 378
  diagnosis of, 256, 256t
  drug treatment for, 186–190, 187f
    potential receptor interactions of, 187f
  in eating and feeding disorder, 341–342
  epidemiology of, 248–249, 249f
    in children and adolescents, 248
    in older adults, 248–249
  etiology of, 249–251
    biochemical factors in, 250, 250f
    biological factors in, 249–251
    cognitive theory in, 251
    diathesis-stress model in, 251
    genetic factors in, 249–250
    hormones in, 250
    inflammation in, 251
    learned helplessness and, 251
    neurotransmitters and, 250
    psychological factors in, 251
    risk factors in, 249b
    stress factors in, 250
  evaluation for, 269
  Geriatric Depression Scale, 624, 626b
  vs. grief, 665–666
  impact on adolescents, 588b
  implementation for, 257–266
    acute phase, 257
    continuation phase, 257
    counselling and communication techniques in, 257, 257b–258b
    electroconvulsive therapy in, 266–267, 267f
    health teaching and health promotion, 257–258
    maintenance phase, 257
    milieu management in, 258
    pharmacological interventions in, 258–266, 260f
    promotion of self-care activities in, 258
    transcranial magnetic stimulation in, 267, 267f
    vagus nerve stimulation in, 267–268, 268f
    for vegetative signs, 259t
  integrative therapy for, 268b
    exercise, 268b
    light therapy, 268b
    St. John's wort, 268b
  in LGBTQ, 583–584
  monoamine theory of, 186, 187f, 190
  NOC outcomes related to, 256, 257t
  in older adults, 616–617

Depression (Continued)
  PET scan images, before and after medication, 250, 250f
  planning in, 256–257
  positron emission tomography scan of brain with, 180–183, 182f
  recovery model for, 256, 257t
  schizophrenia and, 303
  serious medical illness and, 649, 649b
  spirituality and religious beliefs influencing, 254
  subtypes and specifiers of, 245
    atypical features, 245
    catatonic features, 245
    melancholic features, 245
    postpartum onset, 245
    psychotic features, 245
    seasonal features, 245
  suicide risk in, 497
  symptoms of, 256t
    anger, 253
    anhedonia, 253
    communication difficulties, 254, 257, 257b
    grooming lapses, 254
    mood and feelings, 253, 256t
    physical behaviour, 253–254
    psychomotor agitation, 253
    psychomotor retardation, 253
    sleep issues, 254, 259t
    vegetative signs, 253–254, 256t, 259t
Depressive disorders, 244–274
  in children and adolescents, 608–609
  disruptive mood dysregulation disorder, 245–246
  due to another medical condition, 247, 248t
  major depressive disorder, 245
  persistent depressive disorder, 246–247
  premenstrual dysphoric disorder, 247
  substance/medication-induced depressive disorder, 247
Depressive episodes, treatment during bipolar, 286
Derealization, 310, 568
Desensitization, systematic, as behavioural therapy, 54
Desipramine hydrochloride (Norpramin), 230b–231b, 263
Desvenlafaxine (Pristiq), 188
Development, stages of
  Erikson's, 49t
  moral, 49–50
  psychosexual, 47, 47t
Developmental theories, 48–50
  cognitive development as, 48–49
  ethics of care theory and, 50
  implications of, for nursing practice, 50
  stages of moral development in, 49–50
  theory of psychosocial development and, 49, 49t
Dexamethasone, 250
Diagnostic and Statistics Manual of Mental Disorders, fifth edition (DSM-5), 5, 10, 119, 211–212
  in gender dysphoria, 579, 580b
  organizational structure of, 11
  for schizophrenia, 302
Dialectical behaviour therapy (DBT), 56–58, 691
  for binge eating disorder, 353
  engaging street-involved youth in, 62b
  for personality disorders, 452, 452f
  for violence, 551
Diarrhea, 415t
Diathesis, defining, 435
Diathesis-stress model, 7
  of depression, 251
  of personality disorders, 435
  of schizophrenia, 304
Diazepam (Valium), 185, 185f, 230b–231b, 521b
DID. see Dissociative identity disorder
Diet
  for integrative health care, 721–723
  restrictions in, with monoamine oxidase, 189
Differentiation, 701b, 703
Diffuse boundaries, 699b
Dignity, to the dying, 657
Diphenhydramine (Benadryl, Nytol), 471b
Disability Assessment Schedule 2.0, 11
Disapproval, giving, 159–161, 162t
Disaster response teams, 32

Disasters, 477–494
  as adventitious crisis, 480
  critical incident stress debriefing (CISD), 486, 487b
  five elements of intervention, 479
  resilience and, 5
Discharge planning, for anorexia nervosa, 342
Discrimination
  advocacy groups to fight Canadian mental health care, 8
  against mentally ill persons, 101
Disenfranchised grief, 665
Disengaged boundaries, 699b
Disorganization, 328
Disorganized thinking, with schizophrenia, 302
Disorientation
  with delirium, 366
  with dementia, 376, 376t
Disparities, reduction of, as key strategy for Canadian mental health care, 8, 9b
Displacement, 205t–206t
Disqualifying the positive, 56t
Disruptive, impulse control, and conduct disorders, in children and adolescents, 603–604
  adolescent-onset conduct disorder, 604
  bullying, 604
  childhood-onset conduct disorder, 604
  conduct disorders, 598b, 603–604, 605b
  nursing process application to, 604–606, 605b, 605t
  oppositional defiant disorder, 603, 605b
  techniques for managing, 607b
Disruptive mood dysregulation disorder, 245–246
Dissent, in child health care decision making, 589, 591
Dissociation, 86b–87b
  as defence mechanism, 205t–206t
Dissociative amnesia, 215–216
Dissociative disorders, 214–216
  assessment guidelines for, 221b
  comorbidity of, 216
  depersonalization/derealization disorder, 215, 215b
  dissociative amnesia, 215–216
  dissociative identity disorder, 216
  epidemiology of, 216
  nursing diagnoses for, 224t
  nursing interventions for, 228t
  sexual assault and, 568, 568b
Dissociative fugue, 215–216
Dissociative identity disorder (DID), 216
Distortions, cognitive, 55–56, 56t, 75
  in anorexia nervosa, 346, 347b
Distracting, during family therapy, 700b
Distress, 66
  cultural concepts of, 126, 126b
Disturbed thought processes, with delirium, 368
Diuretics, use of, 350b
Divalproex sodium (Epival), for bipolar disorders, 290, 291b
Diversion
  of drugs, 103–104
  signs with nurses, 426–427, 427b
Diversity
  increasing, as challenge for psychiatric mental health nurses, 12–13
  as key strategy area for Canadian mental health care, 8, 9b
Dix, Dorothea, 18–19, 18f
Documentation, 40–41
  in abuse screening, 543b
  of care, 107
  importance in seclusion protocol, 292
  legal considerations for, 93b
  as seventh step in nursing process, 92
  of suicide risk assessment, 502b
Donepezil (Aricept), 195
  for Alzheimer's disease, 382, 383f
Dopamine, 176t
  in anger and aggression, 515
  reduction of, 177b, 177f
  substance use disorders and, 396
  theory, of schizophrenia, 304
  use of, by neuronal circuitry, 184
  wakefulness and, 461
Dopamine system stabilizer, aripiprazole as, 194
Double messages, 156
Double-bind messages, 156

Doubt, voicing, as therapeutic communication technique, 160t–161t
Doxepin hydrochloride (Adapin, Sinequan), 230b–231b, 263
Dressing, in guidelines for self-care for individuals with cognitive impairment, 381b
Drug use
  in LGBTQ, 584
  in violence and abuse, 545–546
Drug-facilitated sexual assault, 562, 563t
Drugs
  effects that may mimic psychiatric illness, 85b
  mental health dysfunction and, 183
Dry eyes, from conventional antipsychotics, 324t–325t
Dry mouth, from conventional antipsychotics, 324t–325t
Dual Process Model, of coping with bereavement, 667–668
Duloxetine hydrochloride (Cymbalta), 188, 230b–231b
  for major depressive disorder, 261b–262b
Duluth "Abuse of Children" wheel, 540f
Duluth "Equality" wheel, 552f
Duluth "Nurturing Children" wheel, 553f
Duluth "Power and Control" wheel, 539f
Dutton, Dr. Donald, 535
Duty, 110
  breach of, 110–111
  to protect, 107
  vignette regarding, 110b
  to warn, 107
Dyssomnia, 457
Dysthymia, drug treatment for, 598b

E
Early-onset Alzheimer's disease, 373–374
Eastern Canada, history of psychiatric nursing licensing in, 20–21
Eating and feeding disorders, 338–361
  anorexia nervosa as, 343–348
    acute care in, 346
    advanced-practice interventions for, 347–348
    assessment of, 343–345, 345b
    case study and nursing care plan for, 353b–356b
    characteristics of, 339b
    clinical picture of, 338–340
    cognitive distortions in, 347b
    comorbidity of, 341–342
    criteria for hospital admission of, 344b
    diagnosis of, 345
    epidemiology of, 340–341
    etiology of, 342–343
    evaluation of, 348
    general assessment for, 345
    health teaching and health promotion for, 346
    implementation in, 346–348
    medical complications of, 344b
    milieu management of, 347
    NOC outcomes related to, 346t
    outcomes identification of, 345
    pharmacological interventions for, 346
    planning of, 345–346
    psychosocial interventions for, 346, 346b
    psychotherapy for, 347–348
    self-assessment of, 345
    signs and symptoms of, 344t
    thoughts and behaviours associated with, 344b
    vignette in, 347b–348b
  avoidant/restrictive food intake disorder as, 339–340
  binge eating disorder as, 352–358
    bariatric surgery for, 353, 353b
    characteristics of, 339b
    clinical picture of, 338–340
    comorbidity of, 341–342
    epidemiology of, 340–341
    etiology of, 342–343
  bulimia nervosa as, 348–349
    acute care for, 351
    advanced-practice interventions for, 351–352
    assessment of, 349, 350b
    case study and nursing care plan for, 356b–357b
    characteristics of, 339b
    clinical picture of, 338–340
    comorbidity of, 341–342
    counselling for, 351
    diagnosis of, 350
    epidemiology of, 340–341

Eating and feeding disorders (Continued)
    etiology of, 342–343
    evaluation of, 352
    general assessment of, 349
    health teaching and health promotion for, 351
    implementation in, 351–352
    medical complications of, 349b
    milieu management for, 351
    NOC outcomes related to, 351t
    outcomes identification of, 350
    pharmacological interventions for, 351
    planning for, 350–351
    psychotherapy for, 351–352
    self-assessment of, 349
    signs and symptoms of, 350t
    thoughts and behaviours associated with, 349b
    vignette in, 349b–350b, 352b
  in children and adolescents, 609
  coping with a family member who has, 348b
  NIC interventions for, 352, 352b
  not otherwise specified, 338–339
  pica as, 340
  prevalence statistics of, in Canada, 10t
  prevention of, 341b
  rumination disorder as, 340
  screening, 350b
  state of treatment for, 348t
Echolalia, in communication, 309
Echopraxia, 311
Economic abuse, 539f–540f
Education
  in abuse screening, 543b
  clinical levels of, in psychiatric mental health nursing, 12
  early university-based nursing curriculum and, 21–22
  as key social determinant of health, 14
  medication, 689, 690b, 690f
  shifts in control over nursing and, 20–21
  Weir Report and, 20
Ego, 46, 46f
Electrical conductivity, adverse effect of lithium on, 190, 191t
Electrical impulses, conducted by neurons, 175
Electroconvulsive therapy, 19
  for bipolar disorders, 290
  for depression, 266–267, 267f
Electroencephalograms (EEGs), measuring sleep, 459
Electrolyte imbalance
  with anorexia nervosa, 345
  with delirium, 367–368
Electronic documentation, guidelines for, 107–108
Electronic health care, affecting mental health care, 13
Elimination, anxiety disorders and, 229
Ellis, Albert, 55, 55f, 61t, 516
Ellis, Kathryn, 21
Elopement, safety and, 35
Embodied knowledge, as relational ethics principle, 99
EMDR therapy. see Eye movement desensitization and reprocessing (EMDR) therapy
Emergency care, mental health first aid (MHFA), 487b
Emotional dysregulation
  defining, 434
  emotional stability vs., 445, 446t
Emotional freedom technique, 725–726
Emotional lability, 438–439
Emotional reactions
  in coping, 564b
  in dementia, 376t
Emotional reasoning, 56t
  in cognitive distortions, 347b
Emotional stability, vs. emotional dysregulation, 445, 446t
Emotional trauma
  long-lasting, 562
  signs and symptoms of, 565–566, 565b
Emotional violence
  definition of, 532t, 533
  devastating consequences in children, 533
  in "Power and Control" wheel, 539f
Emotions
  control and regulation of, 514
  resilience and, 5

Empathy
  element of LEAP approach, 302
  listening with, 158
  for patients' growth, 148
  sympathy vs., 148
Employee assistance programs, for substance use disorders, 427
Employment, as key social determinant of health, 14
Employment Equity Act, 97
Empowering, during end-of-life (EOL) care, 659
Enculturation, 119–120
Endocrine disorders
  depression co-occurring with, 248t
  that may mimic psychiatric illness, 85b
Endocrine system, regulation of, 173, 174f
End-of-life care
  art, presence, and caring of nursing in, 659
  assessment for spiritual issues during, 659–660
  hospice palliative care nursing, 659
  importance of effective communication during, 661–664, 662b
  nursing care at, 659–664
Endorphins, stress response and, 66
Energy therapies, 725–726
  bioelectromagnetic-based, 726
  emotional freedom technique as, 725–726
  healing touch as, 725
  Reiki as, 725
  therapeutic touch as, 725
  thought field therapy as, 725–726
Engagement, as relational ethics principle, 99
Enmeshed boundaries, 699b
Environmental factors
  affecting communication, 154
  of nonsuicidal self-injury, 508
  in violence and abuse, 537–539
Environmental stressors, in schizophrenia, 305
Enzymes, that destroy neurotransmitter, 175
Epidemiology, defined, in mental health, 9
Epilepsy, 7
  in aggression and violence, 514–515
"Epp Report," Mental Health for Canadians: Striking a Balance, 3, 4f
EPSs. see Extrapyramidal side effects
Equality, in Canadian mental health care, 8
Erik Erikson's Ego Theory, 479
Erik Erikson's Maturational Crisis Theory, 479
Erikson, Erik, 49, 49t
Erotomanic delusion, 309t
Escitalopram oxalate (Cipralex), 188, 230b–231b, 261b–262b
Essential hypertension, anxiety caused by, 212t
Esteem, need for, 58–59
Estrogen, in gender dysphoria, 579–580
Ethical concepts, 97–100, 98f
Ethical dilemma, 99–100
Ethics, defined, 97
Ethnic groups, pharmacogenetics and, 184, 184b
Ethnicity, 116
Ethnocentrism
  cultural awareness and, 128
  defined, 120
Etiology, diagnostic titles and, 90
Etiquette, culture and, 120b
Euphoric mood, associated with mania, 281
Europe, early asylums in, 17–18
Eustress, 66
Euthanasia, 501
Evaluation
  definition of, 81
  in nursing process, 92
Evidence-informed decision making, 90–91, 91b
Evidence-informed practice, 12
Excessive questioning, 159, 162t
Excessive sleepiness (ES), due to sleep deprivation, 458
Excitotoxicity, 195
Exercises
  for depression, 268b
  physical, as relaxation technique, 75
  for relaxation, 72–73
  as stress buster, 70b
Existential resolution, 685b
Existentialism, 61t
Expert witnesses, forensic psychiatric mental health nurses as, 678

Exploring, as therapeutic communication technique, 159, 160t–161t
Expressed style, of coping, 564b, 565
Extinction, 53
Extrapyramidal side effects (EPSs), in conventional antipsychotics, 322
Extraversion, vs. introversion, 445, 446t
Eye cast, 156t
Eye contact
  during clinical interview, 166
  cultural beliefs and, 119t, 120
  cultural considerations to, 163
Eye movement desensitization and reprocessing (EMDR) therapy, for sexual assaults, 570

F
Facial expressions
  cultural beliefs and, 119t
  as nonverbal behaviour, 156t
Facilitative Skills Checklist, 165f
False imprisonment, 109–110, 109t
Falsely reassuring, 162t
Family, 697–698, 697b
  application of the nursing process, 704–711
    assessment, 704–708
    diagnosis, 708
    evaluation, 711
    implementation, 708–711, 709b
    interventions, 708b
    outcomes identification, 708
    planning, 708
  Canadian models of nursing care, 698–699
    Calgary Family Assessment Model (CFAM), 698–699, 705f
    Calgary Family Intervention Model (CFIM), 698–699
    McGill Model of Nursing, 698
  as caregivers, 698
  diversity, Canadian, 697
  emotional support from, 700
  functions, 698
  ideal form, 697
  identified patient, 700–701
  life cycle, 700
  and mental illness, 698
  socialization and, 700
  as system, 703–704
  triangles, 701–702, 702f
  working with, 700–702, 701b
Family assessment
  Calgary Family Assessment Model (CFAM), 698–699
  Calgary Family Intervention Model (CFIM), 698–699
  McGill Model of Nursing, 698
Family coping patterns, in violence, 544–545, 546b
Family education, therapeutic groups and, 689–690
Family interventions, 696–713
Family psychotherapy, in violence and abuse, 551, 553f
Family service, for dementia, 379t–380t
Family systems theory, 701b, 703
Family therapy, 699–702, 709–710
  boundaries, 699, 699b
  for children and adolescents, 594
  dysfunctional communication during, 699–700, 699b–700b
  psychoeducational, 710
  for schizophrenia, 329–330, 329b
  theory, 702–704
  traditional, 709–710
Family triangles, 701–702, 702f
Family violence, 122
  case study and nursing care plan in, 554b–556b
  coping responses in, 544, 545t
  diagnosis of, 546, 546t
  long-term effects of, 537b
  maintaining accurate records in, 542–544, 543b–544b
  myth vs. fact in, 545t
  nursing process application in, 539–556
    assessment in, 539–546, 541b
    diagnosis in, 546, 546t
    evaluation in, 552–553
    implementation in, 547–552
    outcomes identification in, 546, 547t
    planning in, 546–547
Family-centred care, 697
Family-focused therapy, for bipolar disorders, 293

Farewell, in death and dying situations, 663–664
FAS. see Fetal alcohol syndrome
FASD. see Fetal alcohol spectrum disorder
Fear
  anxiety vs., 202
  in delirium, 368
  of dependency, with serious medical conditions, 651, 651b
  phobias, 206–207, 206b, 207t
  systematic desensitization of, 54
Federal government, role of, in psychiatric mental health care funding, 27–28
Feedback, in communication process, 153, 154f
Feelings
  depression and, 253
  minimizing, 162t
Fentanyl, 405t
Fetal alcohol spectrum disorder (FASD), 395
Fetal alcohol syndrome (FAS), 395
Fiddler, Nettie, 20–21
Fidelity, principle of, 98
Fight-or-flight response, 66
  with anger and aggression, 515
Financial abuse, 532t, 534
First aid, psychological, 32
First Nations
  federal government role in funding mental health care for, 27–28
  as key strategy area for Canadian mental health care, 9b
  mental illness and, 619b
First Nations and Inuit Mental Wellness Advisory Committee (MWAC), 497
First Nations Health Authority (FNHA), 123, 123f
Fish oil, 724t
Flashbacks, 214
Flight of ideas, with bipolar disorders, 282–283
Flooding, for anxiety disorders, 234
Fluid intake issues, with substance abuse or behavioural addictions, 415t
Flunitrazepam (Rohypnol, "roofies"), 401
Fluoxetine hydrochloride (Prozac), 188
  for anorexia nervosa, 346
  for anxiety disorders, 230b–231b
  for bulimia nervosa, 351
  for depression, 261b–262b, 262
Flupentixol, for schizophrenia, 322t
Fluphenazine, for schizophrenia, 322t
Flurazepam (Dalmane, Som Pam), 185, 471b
Fluvoxamine maleate (Luvox), 188, 230b–231b, 261b–262b
FNHA. see First Nations Health Authority
Focusing, as therapeutic communication technique, 160t–161t
Follicle-stimulating hormone, 173
Follow-up care, in sexual assault, 570
Food and Drugs Act, 186
Forced treatment, advocacy groups to fight Canadian mental health care, 8
Forchuk, Cheryl, 22
Forensic correctional nurses, 676
Forensic geriatric or pediatric nurses, 676
Forensic nurse examiners, 676
Forensic nursing, 676–678
  education of, 676
  nurse coroner or death investigator, 677–678
  roles and functions of, 676–678
  sexual assault nurse examiner (SANE), 677
Forensic psychiatric mental health nurses, 678
  competencies associated with, 679b
  as expert witnesses, 678
  roles and functions of, 678–680
Forensic psychiatric nursing, 678–680
Forensics, 675–676
Foreseeability, of harm, 111
Forest bathing, 75
Forgetfulness. Forget-me-not pill, 563t
Forgiveness, in death and dying situations, 663
Formal contract, for nurse-patient relationship, 143
Formal operational stage, of cognitive development, 48–49
Fortune-telling error, 56t
Four Gifts of Resolving Relationships, 663–664, 664b
Frankl, Viktor, 61t

Free association, 46
Freud, Sigmund, 46, 500
  psychoanalytic theory by, 46–47
    defence mechanisms and anxiety, 47, 204, 205t–206t
    levels of awareness in, 46, 46f
    personality structure in, 46–47
    psychosexual stages of development in, 47, 47t
Frontotemporal dementia, 371t
Functional Dementia Scale, 377f
Functional magnetic resonance imaging (fMRI), description and psychiatric uses for, 180t
Functional neurological symptom disorder, 210
Funding, for psychiatric mental health care, 27–28, 27b

G
GABA. see Gamma-aminobutyric acid
Gabapentin (Neurontin), 191, 230b–231b, 291b
  for chronic aggression, 522b
GAD. see Generalized anxiety disorder
Galantamine (Reminyl), 195
  for Alzheimer's disease, 383f
Gambling, pathological, suicide risk in, 497
Gamma-aminobutyric acid (GABA), 176t
  in anger and aggression, 515
  antianxiety actions of, 183
  associated with substance abuse, 396
  types of receptors for, 185
Gamma-hydroxybutyrate (GHB), 563t
Gang involvement, 589
GAS. see General adaptation syndrome
Gastritis, concurrent with substance abuse disorders, 395
Gastrointestinal disorders, that may mimic psychiatric illness, 85b
Gay, 577–578
  hostility toward, 592b
Gender, 577–586
  bias in diagnosing personality disorders, 441b
  definition of, 578–579, 579b
  as key social determinant of health, 14
  nursing process application in, 580–582
    assessment, 580–581, 581b–582b, 582f
    diagnosis, 581
    evaluation, 584–585
    implementation, 582, 583b
    mental health issues, 582–585
    outcomes identification, 581, 582t
    planning, 582
Gender dysphoria, 579
  advanced interventions in, 579–580
  clinical picture of, 579
  criteria for, 580b
  epidemiology of, 579
  nursing care for, 579
Gender identity
  cultural considerations, 578b
  definition of, 578–579
Gender-affirming surgery, in gender dysphoria, 580
General adaptation syndrome (GAS), 66, 515, 648
Generalizations, making, 128
Generalized anxiety disorder (GAD)
  in children and adolescents, 607
  description of, 207–208, 208b, 208t
  prevalence statistics of, in Canada, 10t
  selective serotonin reuptake inhibitors for, 186
Generalizing, during family therapy, 700b
Genes, mapping of, neurological illness and, 8
Genetic endowment, as key social determinant of health, 14
Genetics
  anxiety disorders and, 216
  bipolar disorders and, 279
  in dementia, 373–374
  depression and, 249–250
  in eating and feeding disorders, 342
  Human Genome Project, 7–8, 13
  in identical twin brain image research, 181f, 183
  personality disorders and, 434
  substance use disorders and, 396
Genogram, 705–706, 706b, 707f
Genuineness
  element of LEAP approach, 302
  for patients' growth, 148
Geriatric Depression Scale, 254

Germ theory, 7
Gestures
  cultural beliefs and, 119t
  nonverbal communication through, 156t
  use of, for managing disruptive behaviours, in children and adolescents, 607b
GHB. see Gamma-hydroxybutyrate
Ghost sickness, 126b, 127
Gilligan, Carol, 50
Ginkgo biloba, 195, 723
Glossophobia, 207t
Glutamate, 176t, 461
  in anger and aggression, 515
  depression and, 250
Glycogen synthase kinase 3ß (GSK3ß), 190
Golden root, 724t
Graduate nursing programs, CFMHN recommendations for, 22
Grandeur delusion, 309t
Grandiosity, with mania, 283
Gratitude, in death and dying situations, 663
Grey matter, 178–179, 179f
Grey nuns, 18
Grief
  anticipatory grief, 663, 663b
  defined, 665, 665b
  guidelines for, 669t
  normal, 665
  nursing care for, 664–665
  psychoanalytic model of, 666–667
  with serious medical illness, 650, 650b
  theories of, 666–668
  types of, 665–666
Grieving, depression and, 247
Grooming
  anxiety disorders and, 229
  depression and, 254
  nonverbal communication through, 156t
Grounding techniques, for sexual assaults, 570
Group, 684
  cohesiveness, 685b
  development, phases of, 685–686
  observation, 688
  planning, 685
  psychoeducational, 689–691
  therapeutic factors in, 685, 685b
Group content, 685b
Group discussion, nurse-patient relationship and, 143
Group homes, in schizophrenia, 317
Group norms, 685b
Group process, 685b, 689t
Group psychotherapy, 691
  in violence and abuse, 551–552
Group themes, 685b
Group therapy, 40
  for children and adolescents, 594
  for depression, 269
  ethical issues in, 688–689
  modalities of, for older adults, 628t
  theoretical foundations for, 689t
Group work, 684, 685b
  terms describing, 685b
Growth, patients'
  attending behaviour, 148
  develop resources for, 149
  empathy for, 148
  factors that encourage and promote, 147–149
  genuineness for, 148
  positive regard for, 148–149
Guardianship, 106
Guided imagery, 74, 74b, 596, 719
Guilt
  during bereavement, 667t
  depression assessment of, 253
  with major depressive disorder, 245
Gustatory hallucination, 310t

H
Haldol. see Haloperidol
Hallucinations
  assessment of, during mental status examination, 86b–87b
  auditory, 310, 310t
  causes of, 310
  command, 310–311

Hallucinations (Continued)
  counselling and communication techniques for, 318, 318b
  with delirium, 367–368
  with dementia, 371, 378
  gustatory, 310t
  hypnagogic, 463
  illusions and, 310
  with major depressive disorder, 245
  olfactory, 310t
  with schizophrenia, 302
  with substance abuse or behavioural addictions, 415t
  summary of, 310, 310t
  tactile, 310t
  visual, 310t, 311
Hallucinogens, intoxication, overdose and withdrawal, 409–411, 410t
Haloperidol, 521b
  for schizophrenia, 322–323, 322t
Hamilton Anxiety Rating Scale, 218, 219t
Hamilton Depression Rating Scale, 251
Hamilton Psychiatric Hospital, 21–22
Harm Command Safety Protocol, 313, 315f
Harm reduction approaches, for drug abuse programs, 418–419
HAT. see Heroin assisted treatment
Head injury, in dementia, 374
HEADSSS psychosocial interview technique, 83b
Healing touch, 725
Healing Your Spirit: Surviving After the Suicide of a Loved One, 506–507
Health, culture and, 116
Health Canada
  approved drug treatment
    for anxiety, 230b–231b, 232
    for bipolar disorders, 290, 291b
  on natural health products, 195–196
Health care aides, as members of psychiatric mental health treatment teams, 38b
Health determinants, used in psychiatric mental health nursing, 14
Health indicators, 70
Health information acts, provincial and territorial, 83t
Health maintenance, pharmacological interventions during, 416
Health Professions Act (HPA), 102
Health promotion
  for anorexia nervosa, 346–347
  for bulimia nervosa, 351
  for dementia, 378–381
  interventions in psychiatric mental health nursing and, 92
  regarding sleep hygiene, 463b, 470
  for schizophrenia, 319–320
  in violence and abuse, 549–550
Health services, as key social determinant of health, 14
Health teaching
  for anorexia nervosa, 346–347
  as basic-level nursing intervention, 29
  as basic-level psychiatric mental health nursing intervention, 13t
  for bulimia nervosa, 351
  for dementia, 378–381
  interventions in psychiatric mental health nursing and, 92
  regarding sleep hygiene, 463b, 470
  for schizophrenia, 319–320
  in violence and abuse, 549–550
Healthy child development, as key social determinant of health, 14
Hearing
  area of brain responsible for, 178–179, 179f
  in communication, 153, 154f
  issues when assessing older adults, 84
Helplessness
  as counter-transference, 141t
  depression assessment of, 253, 256t
Hematophobia, 207t
Herbal teas, 723
Herbal therapy, 723
Heroin
  intoxication, overdose and withdrawal from, 405t
  physical complications related to abuse of, 395t
Heroin assisted treatment (HAT), 418–419
Heterogeneous group, 685b

Heterosexual, 577–578
Hierarchy, in families, 701b
Hincks, Clarence M., 8
Hippocampus, emotions and psychological function and, 177–178
Histamine, 176t
History
  of early Canadian asylums, 18–19
  of early psychiatric treatments, 19
  Rockwood Asylum Nursing School, 19, 19f
Histrionic personality disorder
  characteristics and behaviours associated with, 434, 442–443, 442b–443b
  nursing and therapy guidelines for, 442, 449t
  treatment of, 442–443
Holistic approach, 647
Holistic medicine, from indigenous peoples in Canada, 18
Holistic nurse, 717
Holistic world view, 117, 117t
Holmes, David, 22
Home care
  for dementia, 379t–380t
  guidelines for, 382b
Homeless, increase of individuals with mental illness in, deinstitutionalization and, 32
Homeopathy, 718–719
Homeostasis
  cycle of sleep and wakefulness and, 174
  maintenance of, brain and, 173
Homeostatic processes, for sleep drive, 460
Homicide
  in Canada, 675
  concurrent with substance abuse disorders, 395
  potential, in violence and abuse, 545
Homogeneous group, 685b
Homosexual, 577–578
Honesty, misuse of, as counter-transference, 141t
Honeymoon stage, in cycle of violence, 535
Hope
  bulimia nervosa and, 351t
  inspiration for anxiety disorders, 227b
  instillation, in therapeutic groups, 685b
Hopelessness, 122
  as counter-transference, 141t
  depression assessment of, 253, 256t
  with substance abuse or behavioural addictions, 415t
Hormones
  depression and, 250
  in gender transition, 579–580
  mental health dysfunction and, 183
  regulation of, 173, 174f
Hospice palliative care, 658–659, 658b
Hospital admission, of patients with eating disorders, 343–344, 344b
Hospital policies and procedures, 103
Hospitalizations, mental health-related, by youth and adults, 33b
Housing instability, serious mental illness and, 637
How a Nurse Helped Me, in LEAP approach, for schizophrenia, 301b, 302
HPA. see Health Professions Act
Human energy field, 725
Human Genome Project, 7–8, 13
Human immunodeficiency virus (HIV) infection, with dementia, 371t
Human rights abuses, of stigmatized persons with medical conditions, 651
Humanism, 61t
Humanistic Psychology Theory, 58–60
  hierarchy of needs, 58–59, 59b, 59f
Humanistic theories, 58–60
  Abraham Maslow's Humanistic Psychology Theory as, 58–60
Humour, 76
  for managing disruptive behaviours, in children and adolescents, 607b
Huntington's disease, with dementia, 371t
Hwa-Byung, 126–127, 126b
Hydromorphone (Dilaudid), intoxication, overdose and withdrawal from, 405t
Hydrophobia, 207t
Hydrotherapy, 19
5-hydroxyindoleacetic acid (5-HIAA), suicide and, 498–500

Hydroxyzine hydrochloride (Atarax), 230b–231b
Hydroxyzine pamoate (Vistaril), 230b–231b
Hygiene
    anxiety disorders and, 229
    with substance abuse or behavioural addictions, 415t
Hyperpyrexia, from conventional antipsychotics, 324t–325t
Hypersomnia disorders
    description and types of, 463
    with seasonal affective disorder, 245
Hypertension, sleep disorders and, 465
Hypnosis, 719
Hypnotics
    benzodiazepines used in Canada for, 185
    short-acting sedative, 186
Hypochondriasis, 210
Hypocretin, wakefulness and, 461
Hypomania
    behaviour symptoms of, 281
    with bipolar II disorder, 277–278
    transition to mania, 281
Hypotension, from conventional antipsychotics, 324t–325t
Hypothalamic-pituitary-thyroid-adrenal (HPTA) axis, associated with mood disorders, 280
Hypothalamus, 177–178
    emotions and psychological function and, 177–178
    role in mental function, 173
    stress response and, 66
Hypothyroidism
    associated with hypersomnia, 466
    depression and, 280
    mimicking depression, 84
Hypoxia, 368
Hysteria, 6, 46

I
IAFN. see International Association of Forensic Nurses
Id, 46, 46f
Ideal body weight, definition of, 346
Ideas of harming self or others, assessment of, during mental status examination, 86b–87b
Ideas of influence, in delusions, 309t
Ideas of reference, in delusions, 309t
Identical twins
    autism concordance rate for, 599
    brain image research on, 181f, 183
    depression concordance in, 249
Identification, as defence mechanism, 205t–206t
Identified patient, 700–701
Illness anxiety disorder, 210
Illusions
    assessment of, during mental status examination, 86b–87b
    with delirium, 367
Imaging, of brain, in anorexia nervosa, 342
Imipramine hydrochloride (Tofranil), 230b–231b
Immigrants
    health and alcohol-dependence screening of, 12–13
    mental health concerns of, 123, 124b
Immigration, culture and, 120, 121t
Immune stress response, 67–68
Impaired executive functioning, 312
Impaired impulse control, 311
Impaired information processing, 312
Impaired memory, 312
Impaired social interaction, with delirium, 368
Impaired verbal communication, in delirium, 368
Implementation
    definition of, 81
    within psychiatric mental health nursing process, 91–92
Implied consent, 104
Impossibility, principle of, 98
Impotence, from conventional antipsychotics, 324t–325t
Impulse control
    goals with personality disorders, 448t
    interventions for, 450b
Impulse self-control, in bulimia nervosa, 351t
Impulsivity
    constraint vs., 445, 446t
    manifestation of, 438–439
Incest, 561
Incidence, defined, in mental health epidemiology, 9

Income, as key social determinant of health, 14
Incontinence, in dementia, 376t
Indian Act, 121–122
Indigenous contexts, 120
Indigenous people
    culturally relevant and appropriate services for, 122–123, 123f
    defined, 120
    end-of-life care and, 660
    family structure of, 696–697
    impact of Canadian residential schools among, 619b
    mental health concerns of, 121–123
    residential school system, 696–697
Indigenous world view, 117, 117t
Individual psychotherapy, in violence and abuse, 550–551, 551b, 552f
Infections
    depression co-occurring with, 248t
    mental health dysfunction and, 183
    that may mimic psychiatric illness, 85b
Inflammation, depression and, 251
Inflammatory disorders, depression co-occurring with, 248t
Informal contract, for nurse-patient relationship, 143
Information
    giving, as therapeutic communication technique, 160t–161t
    imparting of, in groups, 685b
    Personal Information Protection and Electronic Documents Act, 82
    privacy of, right to, 106
Informed consent, 104
Inhalants, intoxication, overdose and withdrawal of, 404, 404t
Initial impressions, in nurse-patient relationship, 147
Inpatient psychiatric mental health programs, 32–34
    entry to, 32–33, 33b
    preparation for discharge to the community in, 34, 34b
Insight, 86b–87b
Insight-oriented family therapy, 703, 704t
Insomnia
    with delirium, 368
    with dementia, 378
    depression co-occurring with, 259t
    disorders
        description and types of, 462–463
        sleep hygiene and, 463, 463b
    drugs for, 185–186, 471b, 598b
    melatonin for, 463, 471b
    NANDA definition of, 469
    three factors contribute to, 462
Institutionalization, 29
Insulin shock treatment, 19
Insured services, defined, 27–28
Integration, definition of, 423
Integrative groups, 691
Integrative health care
    biologically based integrative therapies for, 721–724
        aromatherapy as, 723–724
        diet and nutrition as, 721–723
        herbal therapy as, 723
        megavitamin therapy as, 723
    in Canada, 715–716
    definition of, 714
    manipulative practices for, 724–725
        chiropractic medicine, 724
        massage therapy, 724–725
        reflexology, 725
    patients and, 716–717
    resources, 716b
    whole medical systems of, 717–719
        acupuncture, 715–716, 718
        Ayurvedic medicine, 718
        homeopathy and naturopathy, 718–719
        traditional Chinese medicine, 718
        traditional Indigenous medicine, 717–718
Integrative nursing care, 717
Integrative therapy, 714–728
    for anxiety disorders, 233, 233b
    as basic-level psychiatric mental health nursing intervention, 13t
    classification of, 717–726
    for dementia, 384, 384b

Integrative therapy (Continued)
    for depression, 268b
        exercise, 268b
        light therapy, 268b
        St. John's wort, 268b
        ma huang, 345b
        melatonin for insomnia, 471b
    during psychiatric mental health nursing process, 92
Intellectual disabilities, in children and adolescents, 599
Intellectualization, as defence mechanism, 205t–206t
Intelligence, fund of, 86b–87b
Intentional torts, 109–110, 109t
Interdependent environment, as relational ethics principle, 99
Interdisciplinary team, care plans and, 39
Intergenerational issues, with families, 701b, 705–706
Intergenerational trauma, 121–122
Interleukins, depression and, 68
International Association of Forensic Nurses (IAFN), 676
International Classification of Diseases-10-CA ICD-10-CA), 11
Interpersonal and social rhythm therapy, for bipolar disorders, 293
Interpersonal relations, Peplau's theory of, 51–52
Interpersonal Relations in Nursing, 51, 142
Interpersonal theories, 50–52
    implications of, for nursing practice, 52
    interpersonal psychotherapy in, 51
    Peplau's theory of Interpersonal Relations, 51–52
    by Sullivan, 51
    theory of object relations in, 50
Interpersonal therapy
    for binge eating disorder, 353
    in groups, 689t
Interpersonal violence, 530–559
    case study and nursing care plan in, 554b–556b
    clinical picture of, 531–535
    comorbidity of, 537, 537b
    define, 531f
    effective nursing intervention in, 531–532, 532b
    epidemiology of, 535–536
    etiology of, 537–539t
    myth vs. fact in, 545t
    nursing process application in, 539–556
        assessment in, 539–546, 541b
        diagnosis in, 546, 546t
        evaluation in, 552–553
        implementation in, 547–552
        outcomes identification in, 546, 547t
        planning in, 546–547
    typology of, 531, 531f
Interprofessional team model
    in community mental health centres, 30
    members of, 37, 38b
Intersex, 578–579
Interventions
    advanced-practice, 92
    basic-level, 92
    basic-level and advanced-practice psychiatric, 13t
    for detoxification or alcohol withdrawal treatment, 416–417, 417b
    for nicotine addiction, 417–418
    Nursing Interventions Classification (NIC), 12
    for opioid addiction, 417
    pharmacological, biological and integrative, 92
    substance abuse, for those resisting treatment, 416–427
    pharmacologic, 416–418
Interviewing techniques
    abuse and, 541–542, 542f, 543b
    HEADSSS psychosocial interview technique as, 83b
    motivational, in substance abuse cases, 413, 414b
    for older adults, 626b
Intimate partner abuse, 530–559
    in Canada, 535
    epidemiology of, 535–536
    interventions for, 549b
    nursing process application in, 539–556
        assessment in, 539–546, 541b
        diagnosis in, 546, 546t
        evaluation in, 552–553
        implementation in, 547–552
        outcomes identification in, 546, 547t
        planning in, 546–547
    safety planning interventions for, 541b

Intimate relationships, between patients, 34
Intoxication, assessment of acute, 398–400, 399b
Intrapsychic conflict, 48
Intravenous drugs, comorbid conditions in users, 395
Introjection, as defence mechanism, 205t–206t
Introversion, vs. extraversion, 445, 446t
Intrusive thoughts, of sexual assaults, 563
Inuit people
    federal government role in funding mental health care
        for, 27–28
    as key strategy area for Canadian mental health care,
        9b
Inventory of Voice Experiences, 313–314
Involuntary admission, 33
    criteria, 105
    vignette regarding, 104b
Isolation, with serious mental illness, 636

J
Jacobson, Edmund, 72–73
Jealousy delusion, 309t
Jet lag, 471b
Journaling, 76
Judgement, 86b–87b
    delaying, of health care workers, 138
Jumping to conclusions, 56t
Justice, 98
Justice view, of morality, 50

K
Kava kava, 195, 233b, 723, 724t
Keon, Wilbert, 29
Ketamine, 410, 410t, 563t
Kinesics, 166
Kirby, Michael, 29
Kleine-Levin Syndrome, 464
Knowledge, fund of, 86b–87b
Kohlberg, Lawrence, 49–50, 61t
Korsakoff's syndrome, 395
Kraepelin, Emil, coined the term schizophrenia, 302
Kübler-Ross, Dr. Elisabeth, 658
    Four Gifts of Resolving Relationships, 663–664

L
La belle indifférence, 210
Labelling, 56t
Laboratory data, during psychiatric mental health
    nursing assessments, 84
Laissez-faire leader, 687
Lamotrigine (Lamictal), 191
    for bipolar disorders, 290, 291b
    for schizophrenia, 325
Language, 86b–87b
    area of brain responsible for, 179, 179f
    barriers to, assessments and, 84
Laryngeal dystonia, from conventional antipsychotics,
    324t–325t
Late-onset Alzheimer's disease, 374
Latuda. see Lurasidone
Lavender, 724t
Leadership, 686–688
    clinical supervision for, 687
    as key strategy area for Canadian mental health care,
        8, 9b
    nurse as group leader, 688–693
    styles of, 687, 688t
        in therapeutic groups, 687
    as therapeutic communication technique, 160t–161t
LEAP approach, to schizophrenia, 301b, 302
Learned helplessness, depression and, 251
Learning theory, of anxiety disorders, 217
Least restrictive type, of mental health care, 105–106,
    106b
Leeching, 19
Leenars, Antoon, 497
Legal issues, documentation guidelines and importance,
    92, 93b
Legislation, mental health, 97, 100–102, 102b
Leininger, Madeleine, 116
Lesbian, 577–578
    hostility toward, 592b
Lethality, of suicide plan, 503
Letourneau, Nicole, 22
Level of consciousness, assessment of, during mental
    status examination, 86b–87b

Levels of awareness, in Sigmund Freud's Psychoanalytic
    Theory, 46, 46f
Levels of prevention, for substance use disorders,
    418–427
    primary, 418
    secondary, 418–421
        controlled drinking in, 419
        harm reduction in, 418–419
        heroin assisted treatment in, 418–419
        managed alcohol programs in, 419
        methadone treatment and methadone maintenance
            in, 418
        needle exchange programs in, 418
        relapse, 419–420, 420b, 420f
        self-help groups in, 420–421
        supervised injection sites in, 419
    tertiary, 421–427
        addiction supportive housing in, 423
        alternative living environment in, 423
        assessment and referral in, 421–422
        community-based (outpatient), 422
        day, 422
        nurses and addiction in the workplace, 426–427
        Onen'tó:kon Healing Lodge in, 423–424
        recovery homes in, 423
        short-term residential, 423
        withdrawal management services in, 422
Lewy bodies, dementia with, 371t
LGBT (lesbian, gay, bisexual, and transgender),
    578
LGBTQ (lesbian, gay, bisexual, transgender, and queer),
    578
LGBTTIQQ2SA (lesbian, gay, bisexual, transsexual,
    transgender, intersex, queer, questioning,
    two-spirited, and allies), 578
Liability issues, from failure to protect safety of patients,
    109
Libel, 109t
Libido, serotonin regulating, 250
Licensed Natural Health Products Database,
    195–196
Licensed practical nurses, as members of psychiatric
    mental health treatment teams, 38b, 39
Licensure
    province regulations regarding APN, 22
    for psychiatric nurse, history of, 20
Life After Service Studies, 496
Life changes, depression and, 250
Light therapy, for depression, 268b
Limbic system
    benzodiazepines and, 185
    roles and neurotransmitters associated with,
        177–178
Limit setting
    for managing disruptive behaviours, in children and
        adolescents, 607b
    with manipulative behaviour, 448–450, 448b
Lindemann, Erich, 478–479
Linehan, Marsha, 56–58
Listening
    active, 157–158
    element of LEAP approach, 302
    in nurse-patient relationship, 147
Lithium carbonate, 190–191, 191t
    for bipolar disorders, 286–289, 288t, 289b, 291b
    for chronic aggression, 522b
    contraindications to, 289
    indications for bipolar disorders, 288
    maintenance therapy for, 289
    therapeutic and toxic levels of, 288–289, 288t
Little Albert, 53
Liver
    disorders concurrent with substance abuse disorders,
        395
    drug metabolism and, 184
Lobotomies, 19
LOC. see Locus of control
Locus of control (LOC), 515–516
Loneliness, with serious mental illness, 636
Lone-parent families, 699
Long-term reorganization phase, of rape-trauma
    syndrome, 563
Loose ego boundaries, 310
Looseness of association, with schizophrenia,
    174–175

Lorazepam (Ativan), 185, 230b–231b, 521b
Loss
    helping people cope with, 668
    with serious medical illness, 650–651, 650b
Loss-oriented stressors, 668
Love
    in death and dying situations, 663
    need for, 58
Loxapac. see Loxapine
Loxapine, 521b
    for schizophrenia, 322t
LSD. see Lysergic acid diethylamide
Lurasidone (Latuda), 194
    for schizophrenia, 321
Luteinizing hormone, 173
Lysergic acid diethylamide (LSD), 183, 410, 410t

M
Ma huang, 345b
Magnetic resonance imaging (MRI), description and
    psychiatric uses for, 180t
Magnification, 56t
Mahler, Margaret, 50
Maintenance of wakefulness test (MWT), 462
Maintenance phase
    of bipolar disorders
        implementation for, 286
        outcomes identification in, 285
        planning in, 286
    of depression, 257
    of schizophrenia, 306, 314, 317
    of Transtheoretical Model of Change, 412–413
Major depressive disorder (MDD), 245
    case study on, 245b
    diagnostic criteria for, 246b
    drug treatment for, 598b
    epidemiology of, 248
    medical conditions and substances or medications
        associated with, 248t
    prevalence statistics of, in Canada, 10t
    subtypes and specifiers of, 245
        atypical features, 245
        catatonic features, 245
        melancholic features, 245
        postpartum onset, 245
        psychotic features, 245
        seasonal features, 245
Major neurocognitive disorder. see Dementia
Maladaptive uses, of defences, 205t–206t
Malpractice, 109t, 110
Managed alcohol programs (MAPs), 419
Mania
    with bipolar disorder, 277, 277b
    case study and nursing care plan for, 294b–296b
    euphoric mood associated with, 281
    spectrum of symptoms of, 281
Maniac episodes
    with bipolar disorder, 277
    treatment during bipolar, 286, 287t
Manipulative behaviour
    during family therapy, 700b
    with personality disorders, 446, 448–450, 448b, 448t,
        451t
Manipulative practices, 724–725
    chiropractic medicine, 724
    massage therapy, 724–725
    reflexology, 725
MAO. see Monoamine oxidase
MAOIs. see Monoamine oxidase inhibitors
MAPs. see Managed alcohol programs
Marijuana
    description and medical uses for, 409
    physical complications related to abuse of, 395t
Maslow, Abraham, Humanistic Psychology Theory by,
    58–60
Mass disasters, five elements of intervention, 479
Massage, 724–725
    as stress buster, 70b
Master biological clock, 460
MAST-G. see Michigan Alcoholism Screening
    Test-Geriatric Version
McGill Model of Nursing, 698
MDD. see Major depressive disorder
MDQ. see Mood Disorder Questionnaire
Media, in communication process, 153, 154f

Medical conditions
  anxiety caused by, 212t
  application of nursing process, 651–655
    assessment, 651–653, 652b, 652t
    diagnosis, 653
    evaluation, 654
    implementation, 653–654
    outcomes identification, 653
    planning, 653
  depression co-occurring with, 248t, 250
  human rights abuses of stigmatized persons with, 651
  psychiatric consultation liaison nurse (PCLN), 654
  psychological factors affecting, 647–649
  psychological responses to serious, 649–651
  psychosis associated with, 303b
  psychosocial assessment, 651–652, 652b
    coping skills, 652, 652t
    quality of life assessment, 651–652
    social and spiritual support, 652
  that may mimic psychiatric illness, 85b
Medical crises, management of, 41
Medical physicians, as members of psychiatric mental health treatment teams, 38b
Medical records
  as evidence, 108
  organizational use of, 108
Medically assisted death, 500–501
Medicare Act, 27–28
Medication adherence, 639b
Medication prescriptive authority, of advanced-practice psychiatric mental health nurses, 13t
Medication-induced dementia, 371t
Medication-induced psychotic disorder, 303b
Medications
  for anxiety disorders, 232–233
    antianxiety drugs, 230b–232b, 232–233
    antidepressants, 230b–231b, 232
  for behavioural symptoms, 384
  delirium from, 367
  for depression, 258–266, 260f, 261b–262b
  depression co-occurring with, 248t
  education group protocol, 689, 690b, 690f
Medicine wheel, 117–118, 118f
Meditation, 73–74, 719–720
Medulla oblongata, 178f
Megavitamin therapy, 723
Melancholic features, with major depressive disorder, 245
Melatonin, 724t
  for insomnia, 463, 471b
Memantine (Ebixa, Namenda), 195
  for Alzheimer's disease, 382, 383f
Memory
  assessment of, during mental status examination, 86b–87b
  brain and, 175
  impairment, in dementia, 376t
Memory deficits
  normal aging vs. major neurocognitive disorder, 371t
  with substance abuse or behavioural addictions, 415t
Menstrual periods, premenstrual dysphoric disorder, 247
Mental Disorder Continuum, 3–4, 4f
Mental disorders, classification of, 10–11
Mental filter, 56t
Mental function, disturbances of, 183–184, 183f
Mental health, 2–16, 3b
  contributing factors to, 5–7, 5f
  culture in, 116–120
  four possible outcomes of, 4–5, 4f
  Mental Health for Canadians: Striking a Balance, defining three major challenges, 8, 9b
  positive, attributes of, 3, 4f
  recovery of, 6, 6b
  two conceptualizations of, 3–5
  WHO definition of, 3
Mental Health and Well-Being of Recent Immigrants in Canada, 12–13
Mental health care
  barriers and facilitators to, in multicultural context, 125–127
    communication barriers as, 125–126, 126b
    discrimination as, 125
    misdiagnosis as, 126–127
    stigma as, 125
  continuum of, 28
    evolving venues of practice in, 28, 28b

Mental health care (Continued)
    least restrictive type of, 105–106, 106b
    primary health care and, 647, 648b
Mental Health Care Law: Ten Basic Principles, 101, 102b
Mental Health Commission of Canada (MHCC)
    Changing Directions, Changing Lives: The Mental Health Strategy for Canada, 8, 587
    defining strategies for mental health, 8, 9b
    on mental health issues related to aging, 616
    on mental illness, recovery from, 635
Mental health concerns
    of immigrants, 123, 124b
    of Indigenous people, 121–123
    of refugees, 124–125
Mental health emergency, defining in phase four of crisis coping, 480
Mental health first aid (MHFA), 484
Mental Health for Canadians: Striking a Balance, "Epp Report", 3, 4f
    three major challenges/goals identified by, 8, 9b
Mental health nursing practice, psychiatric, ethical responsibilities and legal obligations for, 96–114
Mental illness, 2–16, 3b
    definition of, 3
    early care for, 17–19
    families and, 698
    historical beliefs regarding, 17–18
    vs. physical illness, 7
    psychiatric definitions of, 3
    stigma of, 42
Mental status examination, 85, 86b–87b
    of children and adolescents, 593
Meperidine (Demerol), addiction effects of, 405t
Mephedrone, 408
Mescaline (peyote), 410, 410t
Mesnick, Janice, 479
Mesocortical pathways, 177–178
Mesolimbic pathways, 177–178
Messages
    in communication process, 153, 154f
    double, 156
    double-bind, 156, 701b
Metabolic disorders, that may mimic psychiatric illness, 85b
Metabolites, 184
Methadone (Metadol), 405t, 417
Methadone maintenance (MM), 418
Methadone treatment (MT), 418
Methamphetamine, description and medical uses for, 407–408, 408t
Methylenedioxypyrovalerone, 408
Methylphenidate (Biphentin, Concerta, Ritalin), 194, 601–603
Métis
    federal government role in funding mental health care for, 27–28
    as key strategy area for Canadian mental health care, 9b
Meyer, Adolph, 51
MHCC. see Mental Health Commission of Canada
MHFA. see Mental health first aid
Michigan Alcoholism Screening Test-Geriatric Version (MAST-G), 618b
Midbrain, 178f
Middle Eastern Islamic societies, historical beliefs regarding, 17–18
Mild Alzheimer's disease, 372t
Mild anxiety, 202, 203t
    interventions for, 225, 225t
Mild neurocognitive disorder, 363, 370–374, 370b
Milieu
    for children and adolescents, 595–596, 595b
    defined, 60
    management, 40
        for anorexia nervosa, 347
        for bipolar disorders, 290–292
        for bulimia nervosa, 351
        for catatonia, 328
        for depression, 258
        for disorganization, 328
        in older adults, 627–629
        for paranoia, 327
        for schizophrenia, 317
        as suicide precautions, 505, 505t
    therapeutic factors in, 595b

Milieu therapy, 60
    for anxiety disorders, 229
    as basic-level psychiatric mental health nursing intervention, 13t
    implications of, for nursing practice, 60
    as part of psychiatric mental health nursing process, 92
Mind-body therapies, 71
    for children and adolescents, 596
Mind-body-spirit approaches, to integrative health care, 719–721
    biofeedback, 719
    guided imagery, 719
    hypnosis, 719
    meditation, 719–720
    rhythmic breathing, 720
    spirituality, 720–721
    therapeutic suggestion, 719
    T.R.U.S.T. model, 720–721, 721f, 722b
Mindfulness, 76
    for schizophrenia, 320b
Mindfulness-based therapy, 719–720
Mind-reading, 56t
Minimization, 56t
Mino-Pimatisiwin, 701b
Mirtazapine (Remeron), 188–189, 261b–262b
Misperceptions, with delirium, 367
Mistaken beliefs, in dementia, 376t
Mixed messages, 156
MM. see Methadone maintenance
Mnemonic tool ABCD-ER, 541, 543b
Mobile crisis outreach, 487b
Mobile mental health units, 28
MoCA. see Montreal Cognitive Assessment
Moclobemide (Aurorix, Manerix), 261b–262b
Modecate. see Fluphenazine
Model of care, for mental illness, 635, 635b
Modelling
    for anxiety disorders, 233–234
    as behavioural therapy, 53–54
    for managing disruptive behaviours, in children and adolescents, 607b
Moderate Alzheimer's disease, 372t
Moderate anxiety, 202, 203t
    interventions for, 225, 225t
Monoamine oxidase (MAO)
    definition of, 189
    as destructive enzyme, 175
Monoamine oxidase inhibitors (MAOIs), 189, 189f
    actions and effects of, 261b–262b
    adverse reactions and toxic effects of, 265, 265t
    for anxiety disorders, 230b–231b, 232
    definition of, 189
    for depression, 261b–262b, 263–265, 265b
    drugs that can interact with, 263, 264b
    foods that can interact with, 263, 264t
Monoamine theory, of depression, 186, 190
Monoamines, 176t
    definitions, 189
    normal release, reuptake, and degradation of, 186, 187f
Monophobia, 207t
Monopolizing member, 692, 692b
Montreal Cognitive Assessment (MoCA), in delirium, 366
Mood
    assessment of, during mental status examination, 86b–87b
    bipolar disorders and, 281
    in delirium, 367
    depression assessment of, 253
Mood Disorder Questionnaire (MDQ), 281, 282f
Mood disorders, 245
    in children and adolescents, 608–609
    in eating and feeding disorder, 341–342
    Mood Disorder Questionnaire for, 281, 282f
    prevalence statistics of, in Canada, 10t
Mood stabilizers, 190, 325
    for bipolar disorders, 286–290
Moral agent, 99–100
Moral development, stages of, 49–50, 61t
    conventional level of, 50
    postconventional level of, 50
    preconventional level of, 50
Moral distress, 100, 101b
Moral residue, 100

Moral resilience, 100, 100*b*
Moral treatment, 18
Moral uncertainty, 100
Morphine, intoxication, overdose and withdrawal from, 405*t*
Motivation theory, implications of, for nursing practice, 60
Motivational interviewing, 639*b*
    in substance abuse cases, 413, 414*b*
    supplementing goal setting for families using, 155*b*
Motor disorders, in children and adolescents, 600–601
Motor functions, area of brain responsible for, 179, 179*f*
Mount, Balfour, 658
Mourning, 665
    four tasks of, 668
    goals of, 667
MT. *see* Methadone treatment
Multiculturalism, 120
Multiculturalism Act, 120
Multiculturalism policy, 121*t*
Multidisciplinary teams, care plans and, 39
Multimodal music therapy, 596
Multiple sleep latency test, 462
Muscarinic receptors, 187, 192
Muscle atonia, rapid eye movement behaviour disorder, 464
Music, as stress buster, 70*b*
Music therapists, as members of psychiatric mental health treatment teams, 38*b*
Must statements, 56*t*
Mutual aid, 419–420
Mutual avoidance, defined, 147
Mutual storytelling, 596–597, 597*b*
MWT. *see* Maintenance of wakefulness test
Mysophobia, 207*t*

N

NA. *see* Narcotics Anonymous
Naltrexone (ReVia)
    for detoxification or alcohol withdrawal treatment, 417
    for opioid addiction, 417
NANDA-I. *see* North American Nursing Diagnosis Association International
Narcissistic personality disorder
    characteristics and behaviours associated with, 434, 443, 443*b*
    nursing and therapy guidelines for, 443, 449*t*
    treatment of, 443
Narcolepsy, 463
Narcotics Anonymous (NA), 420
National Aboriginal Youth Suicide Prevention Strategy (NAYSPS), 497
National Center for Complementary and Alternative Medicine (NCCAM), 716
National Crime Prevention Strategy (NCPS), 675, 676*b*
National Eating Disorder Information Centre (NEDIC), 351
National Inuit Suicide Prevention Strategy, 500
National Native Alcohol and Drug Abuse Program (NNADAP), 122
National Network for Mental Health, 691*b*
National Sleep Foundation, recommended hours of sleep per night, 458
Natural disasters, critical incident stress debriefing (CISD), 486, 487*b*
Natural health products (NHPs), 195
    in Canada, 715
Natural Health Products Directorate (NHPD), 715
Natural Health Products Regulations (NHPR), 715
Nature *vs.* nurture, 7
Naturopathy, 718–719
Navane. *see* Thiothixene
Navigation, resilience and, 5
NAYSPS. *see* National Aboriginal Youth Suicide Prevention Strategy
NCCAM. *see* National Center for Complementary and Alternative Medicine
NCPS. *see* National Crime Prevention Strategy
NDRIs. *see* Norepinephrine-dopamine reuptake inhibitors
NEDIC. *see* National Eating Disorder Information Centre

Needle exchange programs, 418
Needs
    for belongingness, 58
    for esteem, 58–59
    hierarchy of, 58–59, 59*b*, 59*f*
    for love, 58
    physiological, 58
    safety, 58
Negative reinforcement, 53
Negative symptoms, of schizophrenia, 302, 307, 311, 311*t*
Negativism, 311
Neglect, 532*t*, 534–535
    as risk factor for mental illness, 589
Negligence, 110
    as liability issue, 109*t*
    by peers, 103
Negotiation, resilience and, 5
Neologisms, in communication, 309
Neoplastic disorders, depression co-occurring with, 248*t*
Nervous system, 173, 174*f*
Neuman, Betty, 52*t*
Neurasthenia, 126–127, 126*b*
Neurochemical factors, in aggression and violence, 515
Neurochemical hypotheses, of schizophrenia, 304
Neurocognitive disorders, 362–389
    case study and nursing care plan in, 385*b*–387*b*
    delirium as, 363–365
        assessment of, 365–367, 367*b*
        clinical picture of, 363
        common causes of, 365*b*
        comorbidity and etiology of, 365
        diagnosis of, 367–368, 368*t*
        diagnostic criteria for, 364*b*
        epidemiology of, 365
        evaluation of, 370
        implementation in, 369–370, 369*b*
        major neurocognitive disorders, depression, and brain injury, comparison of, 364*t*
        outcomes identification in, 368, 369*t*
        planning for, 368
        vignette in, 367*b*
    dementia as, 370
    major, 363, 370–374, 370*b*
    mild, 363, 370–374, 370*b*
    types of, 371*t*
Neurodevelopmental disorders
    in children and adolescents, 598–601
        attention deficit-hyperactivity disorder (ADHD), 598*b*, 599–600, 601*b*, 603*b*
        autism spectrum disorders, 599
        communication disorders, 599
        intellectual disabilities, 599
        motor disorders, 600–601
        Nursing Outcomes Classification (NOC) for, 602*t*
        specific learning disorder (SLD), 600
        stereotypic movement disorder, 600
        Tourette's disorder, 600
    nursing process application to, 601–603, 601*b*, 602*t*
Neuroimaging techniques, 279–280
    refinement of, 8
Neuroleptic malignant syndrome (NMS), from conventional antipsychotics, 323, 324*t*–325*t*
Neurological disorders
    anger, aggression and violence, 514–515
    depression co-occurring with, 248*t*
    that may mimic psychiatric illness, 85*b*
Neuromodulators, receptors and mental disorders associated with, 176*t*
Neurons, 175
    activity of, 175*f*
    as psychotropic drug targets, 185
Neuropathic pain, antidepressant drugs for, 188
Neuropeptides, 175–177
Neurotensin, 176*t*
Neurotransmitters
    associated with bipolar disorder, 279
    associated with depression, 250
    circadian rhythms and, 174
    destruction of, 175
    excess transmission of, 183*f*
    of limbic system, 177–178
    normal transmission of, 183*f*
    as psychotropic drug targets, 185
    reduction of, in the synapse, 177*b*, 177*f*
    release of, 175

Neurotransmitters (*Continued*)
    stress response and, 66–67
    substance use disorders and, 396
Neurotrophic factors, 177
NHPD. *see* Natural Health Products Directorate
NHPR. *see* Natural Health Products Regulations
NHPs. *see* Natural health products
NIC. *see* Nursing Interventions Classification
Nicotine
    dependence, in schizophrenia, 303
    description and medical uses for, 409
    pharmacological treatment of, 417–418
    physical complications related to abuse of, 395*t*
Nightingale, Florence, 21–22
Nightmare disorder, 463–464
Nightmares, muscle atonia preventing acting out of, 460
Nitrazepam (Mogadon), 185, 471*b*
N-methyl-D-aspartate (NMDA) receptor antagonist, for Alzheimer's disease, 382–384
NMS. *see* Neuroleptic malignant syndrome
NNADAP. *see* National Native Alcohol and Drug Abuse Program
NOC. *see* Nursing Outcomes Classification
Nonadherence, as treatment issues, in serious mental illness, 637
Nonbenzodiazepines, for anxiety disorders, 230*b*–231*b*
Nonmaleficence, 97, 105–106
Non-rapid eye movement (NREM) sleep
    description and EEG illustration of, 459
    patterns and efficiency of, 461
Nonspecific bruising, in abuse, 533
Nonsteroidal anti-inflammatory drugs (NSAIDs), for Alzheimer's disease, 382
Nonsuicidal self-injury, 495–511
    assessment of, 508
    biological factors, 508
    clinical picture of, 508
    comorbidity of, 508
    cultural factors, 508
    diagnosis of, 508
    environmental factors, 508
    epidemiology of, 507
    evaluation of, 509
    interventions for, 509
    outcomes criteria of, 508
    plan of care for, 508–509
    risk factors for, 508
    societal factors, 508
Nontherapeutic communication techniques, 159, 162*t*
    asking "why" questions as, 162*t*, 163
    excessive questioning as, 159, 162*t*
    giving advice as, 161–163, 162*t*
    giving approval or disapproval as, 159–161, 162*t*
Nontherapeutic relationships, 147
Nonverbal clues, suicide and, 502–503
Nonverbal communication, 155
    cultural considerations for, 163–164
    interaction with verbal communication, 156–157, 156*b*
    patterns, culture and, 119, 119*t*
Noradrenaline, 176*t*
Norepinephrine, 176*t*
    circadian rhythms and, 174
    depression and, 250
    reduction of, 177*b*, 177*f*
    selective serotonin reuptake inhibitors (SSRIs), 186, 188
    substance use disorders and, 397
    wakefulness and, 461
Norepinephrine reuptake inhibitors (NRIs), for depression, 261*b*–262*b*
Norepinephrine-dopamine reuptake inhibitors (NDRIs), for depression, 261*b*–262*b*
Normal anxiety, 202
North American Nursing Diagnosis Association International (NANDA-I), 12
    crisis-related anxiety issues, 483
    Nursing Diagnoses: Definitions and Classification 2012-2014, 12
    sleep disorders, 469
Nortriptyline hydrochloride (Aventyl, Norventyl), 187, 230*b*–231*b*, 261*b*–262*b*
NRIs. *see* Norepinephrine reuptake inhibitors
NSAIDs. *see* Nonsteroidal anti-inflammatory drugs

Nuclear family, 700
  emotional system, 702
Nurse
  addiction in the workplace and, 426–427, 427b
  as group leader, 688–693
Nurse coroner or death investigator, 677–678
Nurse practitioners, province licensing regulations for, 22
Nurse therapist, 691
Nurse-patient relationship, 136–140
  boundaries of, 139–140
  confidentiality in, 143–145
  counter-transference in, 140, 141t
  establishing rapport in, 143
  factors that enhance, 147
  factors that hinder, 147
  formal or informal contract in, 143
  goals and functions of, 137
  parameters of, 143
  Peplau's model of, 142–147
    orientation phase of, 143–146
    preorientation phase of, 143, 144t–145t
    termination phase of, 146–147
    working phase of, 146
  Registered Psychiatric Nurses of Canada (RPNC) on, 91–92
  social vs. therapeutic, 137–138
  transference in, 139–140
Nursing
  care for those who grieve, 664–665
  end-of-life (EOL) care, 659
  self-care and, 664, 664b
  shifts in control over, 20–21
Nursing care, 39–41, 40b
  crisis management and, 41
  documentation and, 40–41
  establishing a therapeutic relationship in, 39–40
  medical administration in, 41
    adherence to, 41
    for pain management, 41
  mental and physical health assessment in, 40
  milieu management and, 40
  structured group activities and, 40
Nursing diagnosis
  definition of, 81
  North American Nursing Diagnosis Association International (NANDA-I), 12
    Nursing Diagnoses: Definitions and Classification 2012-2014, 12
  within psychiatric mental health nursing process, 89–90
  structural components of, 90
Nursing help boxes
  on anxiety disorders, 201b
  on bipolar disorders, 276b
  on co-worker abuse reporting, 391b
  on critical incident stress debriefing, 488b
  on dementia, 363b
  on eating and feeding disorders, 339b
  on major depressive disorder, 245b
  on personality disorders, 433b
  on worrying and insomnia, 458b
Nursing Interventions Classification (NIC), 12
  for aggressive, manipulative and impulsive behaviours, 448–450, 448b, 450b
  for anxiety disorders, 226, 227b
  for delirium, 369–370, 369b
  for eating disorders, 352, 352b
  within psychiatric mental health nursing process, 91
  for sexual assault, 569
  for sexuality, 582, 583b
Nursing Outcomes Classification (NOC), 12, 90, 517
  for aggressive, manipulative and impulsive behaviours, 448t
  for anorexia nervosa, 345, 346t
  for anxiety disorders, 222–223, 224t
  for bipolar disorders, 284
  for bulimia nervosa, 351t
  for crisis-related anxiety issues, 484, 484t
  for delirium, 368, 369t
  for depression, 256, 257t
  related to neurocognitive disorders, 377b
  for sexual assault, 568
  for sexuality, 581, 582t
  for sleep disorders, 469, 470t

Nursing practice, relevant theories and therapies for, 45–64
Nursing process, standards of care for psychiatric mental health nursing and, 80–95, 81f, 82b
  advanced-practice interventions in, 92
  assessment and, 82–89
  basic-level interventions, 92
  documentation of, 92
  evaluation in, 92
  implementation, 91–92
  nursing diagnosis in, 89–90
  outcomes identification in, 90, 90t
  planning for, 90–91, 91b
Nursing shortage, in mental hospitals, 20–21
Nutrition
  anxiety disorders and, 229
  in guidelines for self-care for individuals with cognitive impairment, 381b
  for integrative health care, 721–723
Nutritional disorders, that may mimic psychiatric illness, 85b
Nutritional status, in anorexia nervosa, 346t
Nyctophobia, 207t

O
Obesity
  in Canada, 343
  sleep disorders and, 465
Object, defined, 50
Object relations, theory of, 50
Observation, making, as therapeutic communication technique, 160t–161t
Obsessions, 211, 213t
Obsessive-compulsive disorder (OCD)
  with anorexia nervosa, 342
  characteristics and behaviours associated with, 434, 445, 445b
  comorbidity of, 212
  description of, 211–212, 211b, 213b
  drug treatment for, 598b
  epidemiology of, 212
  medications for, 230b–231b
  nursing and therapy guidelines for, 445, 449t
  positron emission tomography scan of brain with, 180–183, 181f
  prevalence statistics of, in Canada, 10t
  selective serotonin reuptake inhibitors for, 186
  treatment of, 445
  Yale-Brown Obsessive Compulsive Scale (YBOCS) for, 218
Obstructive sleep apnea hypopnea syndrome, description and types of, 464
Occupational therapists, as members of psychiatric mental health treatment teams, 38b
OCD. see Obsessive-compulsive disorder
Oculogyric crisis, from conventional antipsychotics, 324t–325t
Olanzapine (Zyprexa), 194, 521b
  for anorexia nervosa, 346
  for bipolar disorders, 291b
  for schizophrenia, 321, 322t
Older adult abuse, 530–559
  competency in, 547
  epidemiology of, 536
  factors to assess in home visits in, 545, 546b
  interventions for, 549b
  neglect and, 535
  nursing process application in, 539–556
    assessment, 539–546, 541b
    diagnosis, 546, 546t
    evaluation, 552–553
    implementation, 547–552
    outcomes identification, 546, 547t
    planning, 546–547
  vulnerability in, 538–539
Older adults
  access to care in, 618–619
  ageism, 619
  aging of the population, 614
  assessment of, 84
  care giver burden and, 618
  care settings in, 629–630
    behavioural health home care, 630
    community-based programs, 630
    day treatment programs, 630

Older adults (Continued)
    long-term care facilities, 629
    partial hospitalization, 629–630
    respite care, 630
  depression in, 616–617
    assessment of, 254, 624, 626b
      Geriatric Depression Scale, 624, 626b
    and suicide risk, 616–617, 624
  factors to assess in home visits in, 545, 546b
  facts and myths regarding, 615b
  group therapy modalities for, 628t
  late-life mental illness in, 616–618
  milieu management, 627–629
  nursing care of, 624–630
    assessment strategies for, 624–626, 625f, 626b
    health teaching and health promotion, 627, 628b
    intervention strategies, 626–629
    interview and, 626b
    pharmacological interventions, 627
    promotion of self-care activities in, 627
    psychosocial interventions in, 626–627, 627b, 628t
    standards of care, six categories of, 624
  pain in, 620–624, 620f–621f, 622b, 623f
    pharmacological pain management in, 623b
  psychosocial needs of, 614–632, 616b
  serious mental illness in, 634, 634b
  sleep hypnogram vs. young adults, 460, 460f
  suicide rate among, 616–617
  trauma in, 618, 619b
  vulnerable to abuse, 538–539
Olfactory hallucination, 310t
Omega-3 fatty acids, 724t
  for bipolar disorders, 291b
Onen'tó:kon Healing Lodge, 423–424
Open group, 685b
Open-ended questions, 159
Opening Minds campaign, to address mental illness stigma, 125
Operant conditioning, 594
  as behavioural therapy, 54, 54t
Operant conditioning theory, 53
  vs. classical conditioning, 53f
Operation, defined, 48
Operational Stress Injury Social Support (OSISS) programs, 27–28
Opioids
  addiction to, 404–406, 405b
    case example, 391b
  intoxication, overdose and withdrawal, 405t
  pharmacological treatment of, 417
  physical complications related to abuse of, 395t
  withdrawal, 405–406, 406t
Opisthotonos, from conventional antipsychotics, 324t–325t
Opium (paregoric), intoxication, overdose and withdrawal from, 405t
Oppositional defiant disorder, in children and adolescents, 603, 605b
Orap. see Pimozide
Orem, Dorothea, 52t
Orientation, to reality, 86b–87b
Orientation phase
  of Peplau's model of nurse-patient relationship, 143–146
  in therapeutic group, 686
Orthomolecular therapy, 723
OSISS programs. see Operational Stress Injury Social Support (OSISS) programs
Out of the Shadows at Last, 29, 42, 588–589
Outcome criteria, 90, 90t
Outcome identification, definition of, 81
Outcomes, seven domains of, 12
Overeating, with seasonal affective disorder, 245
Overgeneralization, 56t
  in cognitive distortions, 347b
Overidentification, as counter-transference, 140, 141t
Overinvolvement, as counter-transference, 141t
Oxazepam (Serax), 185, 230b–231b
Oxcarbazepine (Trileptal), 191

P
Pacing, 147
Pain
  barriers to accurate pain assessment, in older adults, 620

Pain (Continued)
in older adults, 620–624
Pain Assessment in Advanced Dementia (PAINAD)
scale, 620, 621f, 622b
pharmacological pain management in older adults,
623b
visual analogue scale, for cancer pain, 623f
Wong-Baker FACES Pain Rating Scale, 620, 620f
Pain Assessment in Advanced Dementia (PAINAD) scale,
620, 621f, 622b
Pain management
medication administration for, 41
in older adults, 623b
PAINAD scale. see Pain Assessment in Advanced
Dementia (PAINAD) scale
Paliperidone (Invega), 194
for schizophrenia, 322t
Palliative care, 658
cultural contexts of, 660, 660b
guidelines when caring for the dying, 661b
patient-centred, 657–658
for patients with dementia, 669–670
symptom management, 660–661
Pancreatitis, concurrent with substance abuse disorders,
395
Panic, 203, 203t
interventions for, 225–226, 226t
and school phobia, drug treatment for, 598b
Panic attack, description of, 204–206, 204b
Panic disorder, 204–206, 204b
generic care plan for, 207t
Panic Disorder Severity Scale (PDSS) for, 218
prevalence statistics of, in Canada, 10t
selective serotonin reuptake inhibitors for, 186
Panic Disorder Severity Scale (PDSS), 218
Paranoia, 325–327
communication guidelines for, 327
milieu needs for, 327
in schizophrenia, 330b–332b
self-care needs for, 327
Paranoid personality disorder
characteristics and behaviours associated with,
434–436, 436b
nursing and therapy guidelines for, 436, 449t
treatment of, 436
Paraphrasing, as therapeutic communication technique,
158
Parasympathetic nervous system, regulation of, 173, 174f
Parents, characteristics of abusive, 538b
Parkinson's disease, with dementia, 371t
Paroxetine (Paxil), 188, 230b–231b, 261b–262b
Partial hospitalization
in older adults, 629–630
programs, 32, 32b
criteria for referral to, 32
in schizophrenia, 316
Participant observer, 52
Partnership
element of LEAP approach, 302
and family support, for serious mental illness, 640
Passive negativism, 311
Paternalism, 104
Patient and family teaching
on bipolar disorder, 292b
coping with a major medical illness, 654b
coping with auditory hallucinations or delusions, 319b
guidelines for care at home, 382b
guidelines for self-care for individuals with cognitive
impairment, 381b
on lithium therapy, 289b
regarding selective serotonin reuptake inhibitors, 263b
regarding tricyclic antidepressants, 263, 264b
in schizophrenia, 320b
Patient Health Questionnaire-9 (PHQ-9), 251, 252f
Patient Health Questionnaire-15 (PHQ), 219, 220f
Patient safety, as liability issue, 109, 109t
Patients
intimate relationships between, 34
tracking whereabouts and activities of, 34
Patient's rights, under law, 104–109
Pauly, Bernie, 22
Pavlov, Ivan, 53
PCLN. see Psychiatric consultation liaison nurse
PCP. see Phenylcyclohexyl piperidine
PDSS. see Panic Disorder Severity Scale

Peer supervision, 687
Penitentiary system, increase of individuals with mental
illness in, deinstitutionalization and, 32
Peplau, Hildegard, 21–22, 51, 51f, 142
theory of interpersonal relations by, 51–52
Peplau's model of nurse-patient relationship, 142–147
orientation phase of, 143–146
preorientation phase of, 143, 144t–145t
termination phase of, 146–147
working phase of, 146
Peptic ulcer, anxiety caused by, 212t
Peptides, receptors and mental disorders associated with,
176t
Perceived Stress Scale, 71, 73f
Perception, 55
assessment of, during mental status examination,
86b–87b
encouraging description of, as therapeutic
communication technique, 160t–161t
as mediator of stress response, 69
Perceptual disturbances
assessment of, during mental status examination,
86b–87b
in delirium, 366
Peripheral nerves, 173, 174f
Perpetrators
sexual assault, 562, 570–571
of violence, 538, 538b, 539f
Perpetuating factors, of insomnia, 462
Perphenazine, for schizophrenia, 322t
Persecution, in delusions, 309t
Perseveration, 374
Persistent depressive disorder, 246–247
Persona, as origin of term "personality", 432
Personal appearance, as nonverbal behaviour, 156t
Personal factors, affecting communication, 153–154
Personal health practices, as key social determinant of
health, 14
*Personal Information Protection and Electronic Documents
Act*, 82
Personal question, nurse responses to, 144t–145t
Personal space
cultural beliefs and, 119t
in nurse-patient relationships, 139
Personality
defined by Sullivan, 51
defining, 432–433
five dimensions of, 445, 446t
from Latin word persona, 432
as mediator of stress response, 69
structure of, in Sigmund Freud's Psychoanalytic
Theory, 46–47
Personality disorders, 432–456
advanced-practice interventions for, 452
aggressive behaviour with, 447–450, 448t, 450b, 451t
case management of, 451–452
clinical picture of, 433–434
cluster A
paranoid personality disorder, 434–436, 436b
schizoid personality disorder, 434, 436–437, 437b
schizotypal personality disorder (STPD), 434, 437,
437b
cluster B
antisocial personality disorder (ASPD), 434,
441–442
borderline personality disorder, 434, 438–441, 441b
histrionic personality disorder, 434, 442–443,
442b–443b
narcissistic personality disorder, 434, 443, 443b
cluster C
avoidant personality disorder, 434, 443–445, 444b
dependent personality disorder, 434, 444, 444b
obsessive-compulsive personality disorder, 434, 445,
445b
comorbidity of, 434
dialectical behaviour therapy treatment for, 452, 452f
in eating and feeding disorder, 342
epidemiology of, 434
etiology of, 434–435
biological factors in, 434–435
environmental factors in, 435
genetics in, 434
neurobiology and neurochemistry in, 435
psychological factors in, 435
system factors in, 435

Personality disorders (Continued)
impulsive behaviour with, 447–450, 448t, 450b, 451t
manipulative behaviour with, 447, 448b, 448t, 450,
451t
nursing process application to
assessment of, 445–446, 447b, 453t
case study and nursing care plan on, 453b–454b
diagnosis of, 446, 447t
evaluation of, 453
implementation of, 448–452, 448b, 450b, 454t
outcomes identification of, 447, 448t
patient history in, 446
planning of, 447–448
self-assessment in, 446
pharmacological interventions of, 450–451
psychotherapy for, 452
safety and teamwork for, 450, 451t
suicide risk in, 497
Personality trait, defining, 432–433
Personality type, defining, 432–433
Personalization, 56t
in cognitive distortions, 347b
Pets, as stress buster, 70b
Pharmacists, as members of psychiatric mental health
treatment teams, 38b
Pharmacodynamics, 184
ethnic variation in, 127
Pharmacogenetics, 184
Pharmacokinetics, 184
Pharmacological interventions
for Alzheimer's disease, 381–384, 383f
for anorexia nervosa, 346
as basic-level psychiatric mental health nursing
intervention, 13t
for bulimia nervosa, 351
for older adults, 627
during psychiatric mental health nursing process, 92
for schizophrenia, 321–325
Phases of crisis, 480
phase 1, 480
phase 2, 480
phase 3, 480
phase 4, 480
Phenelzine sulphate (Nardil), 230b–231b, 261b–262b
Phenylcyclohexyl piperidine (PCP), 410, 410t
Phobias, 206–207, 206b
common types of, 207t
social, 207
specific, 206–207
Photosensitivity, from conventional antipsychotics,
324t–325t
PHQ. see Patient Health Questionnaire-15
PHQ-9. see Patient Health Questionnaire-9
Physical activities, for anxiety disorders, 227b
Physical behaviours
in delirium, 367
depression and, 253–254
Physical characteristics, as nonverbal behaviour, 156t
Physical dependency, 391–392
Physical distance, for managing disruptive behaviours, in
children and adolescents, 607b
Physical environments, as key social determinant of
health, 14
Physical exercise, 75
Physical illness
vs. mental illness, 7
psychological factors affecting, 647
schizophrenia and, 303
Physical needs
in delirium, 366–367
in dementia, 376t
Physical restraint, for managing disruptive behaviours, in
children and adolescents, 607b
Physical trauma
mental health dysfunction and, 183
signs and symptoms of, 566
Physical violence
common presenting problems in, 533b
definition of, 532–533, 532t, 533b
Physiological needs, 58
Piaget, Jean, 48–49, 61t
Pibloktoq, 6
Pica, 340
Pimozide, for schizophrenia, 322t
Pinel, Philippe, 18

Pituitary glands, role of, in mental function, 173
Placating, during family therapy, 700*b*
Placebo effect, 717
Planned ignoring, for managing disruptive behaviours, in children and adolescents, 607*b*
Planning
    definition of, 81
    within psychiatric mental health nursing process, 90–91, 91*b*
    for terms of termination, in nurse-patient relationship, 146
Play therapy, 596–597
Pollard, Cheryl L., 22
Polypharmacy, aging and, 615
Polysomnography (PSG), 462
Pons, 178*f*
Positive regard, for patients' growth, 148–149
Positive reinforcement, 53
Positive symptoms, of schizophrenia, 307
Positron emission tomography (PET) scan
    for depression, before and after medication, 250, 250*f*
    description and psychiatric uses for, 180*t*
        in Alzheimer's disease, 180–183, 182*f*
        in depression, 180–183, 182*f*
        in obsessive-compulsive disorder, 180–183, 181*f*
        in schizophrenia, 180, 181*f*
Postpartum onset, with major depressive disorder, 245
Postsynaptic neuron, 175
Post-traumatic stress disorder (PTSD)
    with adventitious crisis, 480
    case study and nursing care plan for, 239*b*–240*b*
    in children and adolescents, 598*b*
    description of, 214
    flashbacks and, 214
    prevalence statistics of, in Canada, 10*t*
    selective serotonin reuptake inhibitors for, 186
Postural hypotension, from conventional antipsychotics, 324*t*–325*t*
Posture, nonverbal communication through, 156*t*, 166
Postvention, for survivors of suicide, 506–507, 507*b*
Potlatch, 18
Poverty
    of content of speech, in schizophrenia, 311*t*
    serious mental illness and, 637
    of speech, in schizophrenia, 311*t*
Power, of perpetrators, 538
"Power and Control" wheel, 539*f*
Prayer, 69
Precipitating factors, of insomnia, 462
Preconscious mind, 46
Precontemplation phase, of Transtheoretical Model of Change, 411–412
Predisposing factors, of insomnia, 462
Prednisone, mental health dysfunction and, 183
Pregnancy, violence and, 538
Prejudice, cultural, 164
Premenstrual dysphoric disorder, 247
Prenatal stressors, in schizophrenia, 305
Preoperational stage, of cognitive development, 48
Preorientation phase, of Peplau's model of nurse-patient relationship, 143, 144*t*–145*t*
Preparation phase, of Transtheoretical Model of Change, 412
Prepsychotic phase, of schizophrenia, 307
Prescription medications, for suicide, 503
Present, giving, nurse responses to, 144*t*–145*t*
Presenting reality, as therapeutic communication technique, 160*t*–161*t*
Presynaptic neuron, 175
Prevalence, defined, in mental health epidemiology, 9
Prevention, as key strategy area for Canadian mental health care, 8, 9*b*
Primary alveolar hypoventilation, 464
Primary care, for crisis intervention, 485–486
Primary central sleep apnea, 464
Primary prevention, of abuse, 550
Principle of least restrictive intervention, 594
Prion, 371*t*
Prison, in Canada, 674
Privacy
    adolescents and, 83
    electronic documentation and, 108
    Personal Information Protection and Electronic Documents Act, 82
    right to, 106–107

Problem, in nursing diagnoses, 90
Process, of message, 156
Process of Cultural Competence in the Delivery of Healthcare Services, Campinha-Bacote model, 128
Process recordings, 51, 167, 168*t*
Profile, of sexual perpetrators, 562
Progressive muscle relaxation, 72–73
Projection, as defence mechanism, 205*t*–206*t*
Promotion, as key strategy area for Canadian mental health care, 8, 9*b*
Propranolol (Inderal), 230*b*–231*b*
Protective factors, for suicide, 499*b*
Protein kinase A (PKA), suicide and, 500
Provincial governments
    health professions acts in, 103*t*
    mental health acts in, 101–102, 102*t*
Proxemics, 166
Proximate cause, 111
Pseudodementia, 374–375
Pseudoparkinsonism, in conventional antipsychotics, 323, 324*t*–325*t*
Psilocybin (mushrooms), 410, 410*t*
Psychiatric consultation liaison nurse (PCLN), 654
Psychiatric mental health advanced-practice nurses, as members of psychiatric mental health treatment teams, 38*b*
Psychiatric mental health care
    funding for, 27–28
    future issues in, 41–42
        barriers to treatment as, 41–42
        meeting changing demands as, 42
    roles and responsibilities in, 36–41
        biopsychosocial assessment as, 36–37
        biopsychosocial care manager as, 37–38
        community psychiatric mental health nursing as, 36
        interprofessional team member as, 37, 38*b*
        nursing care as, 39–41
        relevant to educational preparation, 37*t*
        treatment goals and interventions as, 37
        treatment team as, 38–39
    settings of, 28–36
        assertive community treatment as, 34, 35*b*
        characteristics, treatment outcomes, and interventions by, 36*t*
        community mental health centres as, 29–30, 30*b*
        crisis intervention team as, 31–32, 31*b*
        disaster response teams as, 32
        ensuring safety in, 34–36
        inpatient psychiatric mental health programs as, 32–34
        partial hospitalization programs as, 32, 32*b*
Psychiatric mental health nurse, roles and responsibilities of, 36–41
    biopsychosocial assessment as, 36–37
    biopsychosocial care manager as, 37–38
    community psychiatric mental health nursing as, 36
    in community setting, 30
    interprofessional team member as, 37, 38*b*
    nursing care as, 39–41
    relevant to educational preparation, 37*t*
    treatment goals and interventions as, 37
    treatment team as, 38–39
Psychiatric mental health nursing, 11–14
    assessment in, 84–89
    of children and adolescents, 591–598
        assessment data in, 592–594, 593*b*
        behavioural therapy, 594–595
        bibliotherapy, 597
        cognitive behavioural therapy, 595
        cultural factors in, 594
        data collection in, 591–592
        developmental assessment in, 593
        family therapy, 594
        group therapy, 594
        mental status examination in, 593
        milieu management, 595–596, 595*b*
        mind-body therapies, 596
        multimodal music therapy, 596
        mutual storytelling, 596–597, 597*b*
        play therapy, 596–597
        principle of least restrictive intervention, 594
        psychopharmacology, 598
        quiet room, 596
        risk assessment in, 593–594
        seclusion and restraint in, 595–596

Psychiatric mental health nursing (*Continued*)
        therapeutic drawing, 597
        therapeutic games, 597, 597*b*
        time out, 596
    clinical practice of, levels of, 12
    cultural competence in, 127
    cultural considerations for, 115–133
    defined, 11–12
    future challenges and roles in, 12–14
    future of, 23
    historical overview of, 17–24
    levels of psychiatric mental health clinical nursing practice and, 12
    national organizations for, 22
    nursing diagnosis in, 89–90
    shifts in control over, 20–21, 20*b*
    twelve key social determinants of health used in, 14
Psychiatric mental health programs, for inpatients, 32–34
    entry to, 32–33, 33*b*
    preparation for discharge to the community in, 34, 34*b*
Psychiatric mental health treatment, continuum of, 29*f*
Psychiatrists, as members of psychiatric mental health treatment teams, 38*b*
Psychiatry, early treatments in, 19
Psychic secretion, 53
Psychoactive substance use and treatment, 390–431
    addiction and
        compulsive behaviour *vs.*, 391–392
        development, process of, 392–394
    comorbidity and, 394–395
        medical, 395, 395*t*
        psychiatric, 394–395
    concurrent disorders and, 394–395
    definitions associated with
        addiction definition, 394
        tolerance, 394
        withdrawal stage, 394
    epidemiology of, 394
    etiology of, 396–398
        biological factors in, 396–397, 396*f*
        psychological factors in, 397
        sociocultural factors in, 397–398
    initial and active, 416
    nursing process application to, 398–427
        assessment of, 398–411, 399*b*–400*b*
        case study and nursing care plan on, 421*b*, 424*b*–426*b*
        diagnosis of, 415, 415*t*
        evaluation of, 427, 428*f*
        helping patients change in, 411–415
        implementation of, 416
        interventions of, 416–427
        outcomes identification of, 415–416
        planning of, 416, 424*b*–426*b*
Psychoanalysis, classical, 48
    counter-transference in, 48
    transference in, 48
Psychoanalytic theories, 46–48
    classical psychoanalysis, 48
        counter-transference in, 48
        transference in, 48
    implications of, for nursing practice, 48
    psychodynamic therapy and, 48
    Sigmund Freud's, 46–47
        defence mechanisms and anxiety in, 47
        as foundation for group therapy, 689*t*
        levels of awareness in, 46, 46*f*
        personality structure in, 46–47
        psychosexual stages of development in, 47, 47*t*
Psychobiological intervention, as basic-level nursing intervention, 28
Psychodrama groups, 691
Psychodynamic theories, of anxiety disorders, 216–217
Psychodynamic therapy, 48
    in groups, 689*t*
Psychoeducation, adherence to treatment and, 638*b*
Psychoeducational family therapy, 710
Psychoeducational groups, 689–691
Psychological dependency, 391–392
Psychological effects, of sexual assault, 562
Psychological factors
    anger and, 515–516
    with depression, 251
    with substance use disorders, 397

Psychological first aid, 32
Psychological stressors, in schizophrenia, 305
Psychological violence, 532t, 534
Psychologists, as members of psychiatric mental health treatment teams, 38b
Psychomotor agitation, 311
  depression and, 253
Psychomotor retardation, 311
  depression and, 253
Psychoneuroimmunology, 68
  mind-body therapies and, 71
Psychopharmacology
  advent of, 60
  for children and adolescents, 598
Psychosexual stages of development in, 47, 47t
Psychosis, 301
  associated with another medical condition, 303b
  drugs for, 192–194
  family psychoeducation interventions for, 329b
  prevalence statistics of, in Canada, 10t
Psychosocial assessment, 87, 88b
Psychosocial factors, of suicide, 500
Psychosocial interventions
  for anorexia nervosa, 346, 346b
  in older adults, 626–627, 627b, 628t
Psychostimulants
  for chronic aggression, 522b
  depression co-occurring with, 248t
Psychotherapy
  by advanced-practice psychiatric mental health nurses, 13t
  for anorexia nervosa, 347–348
  for bipolar disorders, 292–293
  for bulimia nervosa, 351–352
  for depression, 269
  for serious mental illness, 640–641, 641b
Psychotic disorders
  aggression and violence and, 525
  other than schizophrenia, 303b
Psychotic features, with major depressive disorder, 245
Psychotic symptoms, drug treatment for, 598b
Psychotropic drugs, 171–198, 172b, 184b
  adverse effects of, serious mental illness and, 638
  for Alzheimer's disease, 195
  for anxiety and insomnia, 185–186
  for attention-deficit/hyperactivity disorder, 194–195
  biopsychiatry and, 172
  for bipolar disorders, 190–191
  for depression, 186–190, 187f
  nonadherence to, 185
  for psychosis, 192–194
  use of, 184–196
PTSD. see Post-traumatic stress disorder
Punishment, 53
Pyrophobia, 207t

Q
Qi, 718
Quality of life, psychosocial assessment of, 651–652
Quality palliative care, 658–659
Queer, 577–578
  hostility toward, 592b
Questions, avoidance of, in Alzheimer's disease, 374
Quetiapine, 194
  for schizophrenia, 321, 322t
Quetiapine fumarate (Seroquel), for bipolar disorders, 291b
Quiet room, 596

R
Race, mental health and, 116
Rage, defining, 513
Rape. see also Sexual assault
  date, 562, 563t
  myth vs. fact in, 567t
  sexual violence and, 561
Rape-trauma syndrome, 562–563
  acute phase of, 562–563, 564b
  diagnosis of, 567–568
  interventions for, 569, 569b
  long-term reorganization phase of, 563
Rapid cycling, with bipolar disorder, 278
Rapid eye movement (REM), sleep
  description and EEG illustration of, 459
  patterns and efficiency of, 461

Rapid eye movement behaviour disorder (RBD), 464
Rapport, in nurse-patient relationship, 143
RAS. see Reticular activating system
Rating scales, for assessment, 89, 89t
Rational Emotive Behaviour Therapy (REBT), 55
Rationalization, as defence mechanism, 205t–206t
RBD. see Rapid eye movement behaviour disorder
Reaction formation, as defence mechanism, 205t–206t
Readiness for enhanced sleep, NANDA definition of, 469
Reality testing, in schizophrenia, 308
Reattribution treatment, for anxiety disorders, 227, 229b
REBT. see Rational Emotive Behaviour Therapy
Receiver, in communication process, 153, 154f
Recent Life Changes Questionnaire, 71
Receptor desensitization, 190
Receptors, 175, 176t
  as psychotropic drug targets, 185
Recognition
  in abuse screening, 543b
  as therapeutic communication technique, 160t–161t
Recovery
  as critical aspect ot improving well-being, 29
  importance with bipolar disorder, 292
  as key strategy area for Canadian mental health care, 8, 9b
Recovery model, for depression, 256, 257t
Recreational therapists, as members of psychiatric mental health treatment teams, 38b
Redirection, for managing disruptive behaviours, in children and adolescents, 607b
Refeeding syndrome, 345–346
Reflecting, as therapeutic communication technique, 158–159, 160t–161t
Reflexes, role of medulla oblongata in, 178f
Reflexology, 725
Refugees
  defined, 124
  mental health concerns of, 124–125
Registered nurses, as members of psychiatric mental health treatment teams, 38b, 39
Registered Nurses' Association of Ontario (RNAO), 128
  document on cultural diversity, 128
  history of psychiatric nursing licensing and, 20–21
Registered practical nurses, as members of psychiatric mental health treatment teams, 38b, 39
Registered Psychiatric Nurse Regulators of Canada (RPNRC), 21
Registered psychiatric nurses, as members of psychiatric mental health treatment teams, 38b
Registered Psychiatric Nurses Act, 21
Registered Psychiatric Nurses of Canada (RPNC)
  baccalaureate and graduate programs for, 22
  code of ethics, 22, 97–98, 99b
  on nurse-patient relationships, 91–92
  standards of practice, 11–12, 22, 97–98, 99b
Regression, as defence mechanism, 205t–206t
Rehabilitation, concept of, for serious mental illness, 635
Reiki, 725
Reincarnation, 117
Reinforcement, 53
Reis Typology, 422, 422b
Rejection, giving, nurse responses to, 144t–145t
Relapse, prevention strategies, 419–420, 420b, 420f
Relational ethics, 97, 99
Relationship factors, affecting communication, 154–155
Relaxation techniques
  for anxiety disorders, 227b
  Benson's, 71–76, 74b
  biofeedback as, 75
  breathing exercises and, 74, 74b
  cognitive reframing as, 75, 75t
  exercises, 72–73
  guided imagery as, 74, 74b
  humour as, 76
  journaling as, 76
  mediation as, 73–74
  mindfulness as, 76
  physical exercise as, 75
  progressive muscle relaxation as, 72–73
  for stress, 71–76
Religion, 87
  anxiety disorders and, 221
  assessment of, 87–88
  medical conditions and, 652

Religious beliefs
  depression and, 254
  as mediator of stress response, 69
Religious world view, 117t
Reminiscence therapy, 628t
Remotivation therapy, 628t
Repetitiveness, in dementia, 376t
Repression, as defence mechanism, 205t–206t
Rescue, as counter-transference, 141t
Research, evidence-informed practice and, 12
Research highlight boxes
  adolescents' experiences of internet-delivered cognitive behavioural therapy for obsessive-compulsive disorder, 213b
  animal-assisted therapy, 720b
  on borderline personality disorder, 447b
  on crisis interventions in rural vs. urban settings, 488b
  depression impact on adolescents, 588b
  DSM-5 classifications of, 462
  factors that contribute to under-recognition of delirium, 366b
  family interventions, 710b
  family psychoeducation interventions for psychosis and schizophrenia, 329b
  on fear of cancer recurrence, 648b
  First Nations communities and palliative care, 660b
  group intervention for vulnerable children, 692b
  in intimate partner violence, 541b
  on mental health first aid (MHFA), 485b
  mental health of immigrants, 124b
  Miyo-mahcihoyān, 137b
  moral distress, 101b
  nursing students' knowledge, attitude, and cultural competence, 583b
  population health burden of depression, 255b
  post-traumatic stress disorder (PTSD) for sexual assault, 571b
  prevention of eating disorders, 341b
  recovery communities for people with serious mental illness, 635b
  screening eating disorders, 350b
  self-harm and suicidal behaviour, 499b
  on sleep education for nursing students, 459b
  smoking cessation via mobile texting, 409b
  supplementing goal setting for families using motivational interviewing, 155b
  survivors' satisfaction with nurse-led sexual assault and domestic violence care, 677b
  in violence, 515b
  on youth with bipolar disorder seeking health information online, 283b
Residential crisis centres, in schizophrenia, 316
Residential schools, trauma and, in indigenous people in canada, 619b
Resilience
  of children and adolescents, 591
  definition of, 5–6
  goals with personality disorders, 448t
  Resilience Factor Test, 6b
Resources, helping patients develop, 149
Respect
  in abuse screening, 543b
  for autonomy, as principle of bioethics, 97
  as relational ethics principle, 99
Respiratory disorders, that may mimic psychiatric illness, 85b
Respiratory retraining, 74
Response prevention, for anxiety disorders, 234
Restating, as therapeutic communication technique, 158, 160t–161t
Restitution, for managing disruptive behaviours, in children and adolescents, 607b
Restless leg syndrome (RLS), 464, 465b
Restlessness, with delirium, 367
Restoration-oriented stressors, 668
Restraint
  abuse, 532
  for children and adolescents, 595–596
  contraindications to, 106b
  least restrictive, 105
  liability issues with, 109–110
  with violence, 523–524, 523b
Restrictive food intake disorder, 339–340

Restructuring, for managing disruptive behaviours, in children and adolescents, 607b
Reticular activating system (RAS), 177
Reuptake, cellular, 175, 177b
Rexulti. see Brexpiprazole
Rhodiola, 724t
Rhythmic breathing, 720
Rights
    as key strategy area for Canadian mental health care, 8, 9b
    to privacy, 106–107
    to refuse treatment, 104–105, 105b
    regarding confidentiality, 106–109
Rigid boundaries, 699b
Risk
    in home, 376t
    for injury, with delirium, 368
    outside the home, 376t
    for self-mutilation, 508
Risk factors, with depression, 249b
Risperdal. see Risperidone
Risperidone (Risperdal), 194
    for bipolar disorders, 291b
    for schizophrenia, 321, 322t
    for violent behaviour, 521b
Rivastigmine (Exelon), 195
    for Alzheimer's disease, 382, 383f
RLS. see Restless leg syndrome
RNAO. see Registered Nurses' Association of Ontario
Road rage, 512
Rockwood Asylum Nursing School, 19, 19f
Rogers, Carl, 61t
Rohypnol, 563t
Role performance, in crisis situations, 484t
Role-playing, for managing disruptive behaviours, in children and adolescents, 607b
"Roofies", 563t
Roy, Sister Callista, 52t
RPNC. see Registered Psychiatric Nurses of Canada
RPNRC. see Registered Psychiatric Nurse Regulators of Canada
Rumination disorder, 340
Running amok, 6
Russell, E. Kathleen, 21
Ryan-Nicholls, Kimberley, 22

S
SAD. see Seasonal affective disorder; Social anxiety disorder
SAD PERSONS scale, 503, 503t
Safe environment, in guidelines for care at home, 382b
Safety
    Accreditation Canada, patient safety practices required by, 34
    considerations during planning, 90
    in delirium, 367
    needs, 58
    plan, in violence and abuse, 548
    in psychiatric mental health care settings, 34–36
        goals for, 35b
    of staff, violence and, 520
    of traditional, complementary, and alternative medicine, 716–717, 717b
SAMe, 724t
SANE. see Sexual assault nurse examiner
SARI. see Serotonin antagonist and reuptake inhibitor
SARTs. see Sexual assault response teams
Saunders, Dame Cicely, 658
Scapegoating, 701b
Schizoaffective disorder, 303b
Schizoid personality disorder
    characteristics and behaviours associated with, 434, 436–437, 437b
    nursing and therapy guidelines for, 436, 449t
    treatment of, 436–437
Schizophrenia
    advanced-practice interventions for, 328–330, 329b
        family therapy in, 329–330, 329b
    assessment of, 307–314
        affective symptoms, 312
        cognitive symptoms, 307, 311–312
        general, 307–312, 308f
        guidelines for, 314b
        interventions for overcoming obstacles to, 313t
        negative symptoms, 307, 311, 311t

Schizophrenia (Continued)
        positive symptoms, 307–311
        during prepsychotic phase, 307
        self-assessment, 312–314, 313f, 315f
    case study and nursing care plan in, 330b–332b
    catatonia in, 328
    clinical picture of, 302
        abnormal motor behaviour, 302
        delusions, 302
        disorganized thinking, 302
        hallucinations, 302
        negative symptoms, 302
    comorbidity of, 303
    counselling and communication techniques in, 317–319, 318b–319b
    course of, 305–306
    delusions, summary of, 308, 309t
    diagnosis of, 314, 316t
    epidemiology of, 302
    etiology of, 303–307
        brain structure abnormalities, 304
        environmental stressors, 305
        genetic factors, 304
        neurobiological factors, 304
        prenatal stressors, 305
        psychological stressors, 305
    evaluation of, 330
    hallucinations, summary of, 310, 310t
    health teaching and health promotion in, 319–320, 320b
    implementation of, 315–330
    interventions of, 317
    LEAP approach in, 301b, 302
    maintenance of, 317
    milieu management of, 317
    nursing process, application of, 307–333
    outcomes identification in, 314, 316t
    paranoia in, 325–327
    pharmacological interventions for, 321–325
        additional medication administration issues, 321
        adjuncts to, 325
        atypical antipsychotics, 321–322, 322t
        conventional antipsychotics, 322–323, 324t–325t, 326f–327f
        potentially dangerous responses to, 323–325
    phases of, 306–307
    planning for, 314–315
    positron emission tomography scan of brain with, 180, 181f
    prevalence statistics of, in Canada, 10t
    prognosis of, 306
    psychotic disorders other than, 302, 303b
    reality testing in, 308
    settings in, 316–317
    stabilization of, 317
    stigma of, 305b
    suicide risk in, 497
    word salad with, 174–175
Schizophrenia spectrum and other psychotic disorders, 300–337, 303b
    LEAP approach in, 301b, 302
Schizophreniform disorder, 303b
Schizotypal personality disorder (STPD)
    characteristics and behaviours associated with, 434, 437, 437b
    nursing and therapy guidelines for, 437, 449t
    treatment of, 437
Scientific world view, 117t
Seasonal affective disorder (SAD)
    depressive features of, 245
    light therapy for, 245, 268b
Seasonal features, with major depressive disorder, 245
Seclusion
    for children and adolescents, 595–596
    contraindications to, 106b
    history of, 105–106
    liability issues with, 109–110
    protocol, careful documentation of bipolar, 292
    with violence, 523–524, 523b
Secondary care, for crisis intervention, 486
Secondary gains, 217, 221
Secondary prevention, of abuse, 550
Secondary traumatic stress, 482–483
Secondary victimization, 561
Secret, keeping, nurse responses to, 144t–145t

Security operations, defined by Sullivan, 51
Sedation, benzodiazepines causing, 185
Seeing, in communication, 153
Selective inattention, 202
Selective serotonin reuptake inhibitors (SSRIs), 186, 188
    actions and side effects of, 261b–262b
    for anorexia nervosa, 346
    for anxiety disorders, 230b–231b, 232
    for binge eating disorder, 353
    for bulimia nervosa, 351
    for chronic aggression, 522b
    for depression, 259–262, 261b–262b
    disorders treated by, 186
    patient and family teaching regarding, 263b
    serotonin syndrome, 262, 262b
Selective serotonin-norepinephrine reuptake inhibitors (SSNRIs), for anxiety disorders, 230b–231b
Self-actualization, 59
    characteristics of persons who have, 59b
Self-assessment
    in abuse, 544, 544t
    in nonsuicidal self-injury, 508
    in sexual assault, 566–567
    in suicide, 503
Self-awareness, in therapeutic relationships, 140–142
Self-care
    guidelines for, when caring for the dying, 664, 664b
    promotion of
        for anxiety patients, 229–232
        elimination, 229
        nutrition and fluid intake, 229
        in older adults, 627
        personal hygiene and grooming, 229
        sleep, 232
Self-care activities
    for anorexia nervosa, 346–347
    promotion of
        as basic-level nursing intervention, 28
        in psychiatric mental health nursing, 92
        in violence and abuse, 549
    in sexual assault, 570
Self-care deficits
    with delirium, 368
    depression co-occurring with, 259t
    with substance abuse or behavioural addictions, 415t
Self-care needs
    for catatonia, 328
    for disorganization, 328
    for paranoia, 327
Self-check, on boundaries, 140, 142f
Self-determination, right to, 104
Self-esteem
    in anorexia nervosa, 346t
    enhancement, for anxiety disorders, 227b
Self-harm, 497, 497t
    in LGBTQ, 584, 584b
    risk factors associated with, 497
    suicidal behaviour and, research highlight on, 499b
Self-help groups, 69, 690–691, 691b, 710, 711b
Self-injurious behaviours, in eating and feeding disorder, 341
Self-injury, nonsuicidal, 495–511
    assessment of, 508
    biological factors, 508
    clinical picture of, 508
    comorbidity of, 508
    cultural factors, 508
    diagnosis of, 508
    environmental factors, 508
    epidemiology of, 507
    evaluation of, 509
    interventions for, 509
    outcomes criteria of, 508
    plan of care for, 508–509
    risk factors for, 508
    societal factors, 508
Self-mutilation, 508
    with borderline personality disorder (BPD), case study and nursing care plan, 453b–454b
Selye, Hans, 66
    on general adaptation syndrome, 648
Selye's general adaptation syndrome, 515
Sender, in communication process, 153, 154f
Sensorimotor stage, of cognitive development, 48

Sensory functions, area of brain responsible for, 179, 179*f*
Separation, 122
Separation anxiety disorder, in children and adolescents, 598*b*, 606–607
Serious mental illness
    across the lifespan, 634
        in older adults, 634, 634*b*
        in younger adults, 634, 634*b*
    adherence, treatment issues, 638*b*
    anosognosia, 634, 637
    chronic or recurrent, 634
    comorbid conditions and, 636
    current issues on, 643
        criminal offences and incarceration, 643
        involuntary treatment, 643
    definition of, in Canada, 633
    depression and suicide, 636
    development of, 635
    economic challenges, 637
    establishing a meaningful life and, 635
    evidence-informed treatment approaches with, 640–641
        assertive community treatment, 640
        cognitive behavioural therapy, 640
        cognitive enhancement therapy, 640, 640*b*
        family support and partnership, 640
        social skills training, 640
        supportive psychotherapy, 640–641, 641*b*
        vocational rehabilitation and related services, 641
    exercise for, 641
    impairments associated with, 634
    isolation and loneliness, 636
    nonadherence, treatment issues, 637
    nursing care of patients with, 641–643, 642*b*, 642*t*
    rehabilitation *vs.* recovery for, 635
    resources for, 639
        comprehensive community treatment, 639
        consumer-run programs, 641
        exercise, 641
        substance abuse treatment, 639, 640*b*
        wellness and recovery action plans, 641
    social problems with, 636–637
    stigma of, 636
    substance abuse, 636
    victimization, 636–637
Seroquel. *see* Quetiapine
Serotonin, 176*t*
    in anger and aggression, 515
    circadian rhythms and, 174
    depression and, 186, 250
    in eating disorders, 342
    reduction of, 177*b*, 177*f*
    for sleep promotion, 461
    stress response and, 66–67
    substance use disorders and, 397
Serotonin and norepinephrine disinhibitors (SNDIs), 188–189
    for depression, 261*b*–262*b*
Serotonin antagonist and reuptake inhibitor (SARI), 189–190
Serotonin modulator and stimulator, 188
Serotonin syndrome, 195, 262, 262*b*
Serotonin-norepinephrine reuptake inhibitors (SNRIs), 186, 188
    for depression, 261*b*–262*b*, 262
Sertraline hydrochloride (Zoloft), 188, 230*b*–231*b*, 261*b*–262*b*
Severe Alzheimer's disease, 372*t*
Severe anxiety, 202–203, 203*t*
    case study and nursing care plan for, 235*b*–236*b*
    interventions for, 225–226, 226*t*
Sex offenders, defining, 561
Sexual abuse, as risk factor for mental illness, 589
Sexual advances, nurse responses to, 144*t*–145*t*
Sexual assault, 560–575
    clinical picture of, 562–563
    date rape and, 562, 563*t*
    definition of, 560–561
    epidemiology of, 561–562
    myth *vs.* fact in, 567*t*
    nursing process application to, 564–573
        assessment, 564–567, 565*b*–567*b*
        case study and nursing care plan for, 571*b*–573*b*
        diagnosis, 567–568, 568*b*

Sexual assault *(Continued)*
        evaluation, 571
        implementation, 569–571, 569*b*
        outcomes identification, 568
        planning, 568–569
        trauma-informed approach, 564, 564*b*
    secondary victimization in, 561
    sexual assault nurse examiner (SANE) and, 565–566
Sexual assault nurse examiner (SANE), 565–566, 570–571, 677
    adults, 677
    pediatric, 677
Sexual assault response teams (SARTs), 677
Sexual exploitation, 561
Sexual functioning, 581, 582*t*
Sexual history, algorithm for taking, 581, 582*b*, 582*f*
Sexual identity, 581, 582*t*
Sexual interest, depression and, 254
Sexual orientation
    considering culture in, 578*b*
    definition of, 577–578
Sexual reassignment surgery, in gender dysphoria, 580
Sexual violence, 560–561
    in Canada, 535
    definition of, 532*t*, 533
Sexuality, 577–586
    definition of, 577–578, 578*b*
    North American Nursing Diagnosis Association International (NANDA-I) classification of, 581
    nursing process application in, 580–582
        assessment, 580–581, 581*b*–582*b*, 582*f*
        diagnosis, 581
        evaluation, 584–585
        implementation, 582, 583*b*
        mental health issues, 582–585
        outcomes identification, 581, 582*t*
        planning, 582
Shaken baby syndrome, 533
Shea, Shawn, 156
Shelters, for abused person, 548
Shiatsu massage, 724–725
Shift-work disorder, 471*b*
Short-Acting Sedative-Hypnotic Sleep Drugs, 186
Should statements, 56*t*
Signals, use of, for managing disruptive behaviours, in children and adolescents, 607*b*
Signs and symptoms
    of anxiety disorders, 223*t*
    of bipolar disorders, 285*t*
    of depression, 256*t*
    within nursing diagnoses, 90
Silence
    nurse responses to, 144*t*–145*t*
    as therapeutic communication technique, 157, 160*t*–161*t*
Silent member, 693, 693*b*
Similarities test, 308–309
SISs. *see* Supervised injection sites
SKA2 gene expression, suicide and, 500
Skinner, B. F., 53
Slander, 109*t*
SLD. *see* Specific learning disorder
Sleep, 458. *see also* Sleep-wake disorders
    anxiety disorders and, 232
    in Canadian culture, 461*b*
    circadian process or drive, 460
    dyssomnia, 457
    efficiency, 461
    functions of, 461
    general health and, 466, 466*b*
    in guidelines for self-care for individuals with cognitive impairment, 381*b*
    hypnogram illustrating young *vs.* older adult, 460, 460*f*
    loss, consequences of, 458–459
    normal cycle and stages of, 459–460
    patterns and efficiency, 461, 466–469
    readiness for enhanced, 469
    regulation of, 460–461
    serotonin regulating, 250
    as stress buster, 70*b*
    studies, 468
    requirements, 461
Sleep and wakefulness, cycle of, 174

Sleep architecture, hypnogram illustrating young adult *vs.* older adult, 460, 460*f*
Sleep continuity, definition of, 460
Sleep deprivation
    consequences of
        accidents, 458, 463
        economic burden, 459
        excessive sleepiness, 458, 462
        hypersomnia, 458, 463
        medical disorders associated with, 465
        psychiatric disorders associated with, 465
    definition of, 458
    in delirium, 368
    NANDA definition of, 469
Sleep diary, 467*f*, 470
Sleep disturbances, 470*t*
Sleep efficiency, 461
Sleep fragmentation, definition of, 460
Sleep hygiene
    health teaching and health promotion regarding, 463*b*, 470
    importance for bipolar patients, 292
Sleep latency, 459–460
Sleep paralysis, 464
Sleep restriction, to strengthen homeostatic drive, 470
Sleep terrors, 463
Sleep-wake cycle, with substance abuse or behavioural addictions, 415*t*
Sleep-wake disorders, 457–475
    advanced-practice intervention of, 472, 472*b*
    anxiety and, 472
    Canadian Sleep Society research on, 457–458
    clinical picture of, 462–464
    cognitive behavioural therapy for, 470–472
    comorbidity of, 465–466
    epidemiology of, 465
    functioning and safety for, 468
    identifying, 468, 468*b*
    medications to treat, 469, 470*t*
    mental illness and, 465–466, 466*b*
    nonpharmacological methods for, 470
    nursing process application to, 466–472
        assessment, 466–468
        diagnosis, 469
        evaluation, 472
        implementation, 469–472
        outcomes identification, 469
        planning, 469
    pharmacological interventions for, 470
    self-assessment of, 469
    types of
        breathing-related disorders, 464
        circadian rhythm sleep disorder, 464
        confusional arousal disorders, 463–464
        hypersomnia disorders, 463
        insomnia disorders, 462–463
        Kleine-Levin Syndrome, 464
        narcolepsy, 463
        nightmare disorder, 463–464
        obstructive sleep apnea hypopnea syndrome, 464
        primary alveolar hypoventilation, 464
        primary central sleep apnea, 464
        rapid eye movement behaviour disorder, 464
        restless legs syndrome, 464, 465*b*
        sleep paralysis, 464
        sleep terrors, 463
        sleepwalking, 463
        substance-induced sleep, 466
Sleepwalking, 463
Smoking
    cessation
        bupropion for, 189
        research via mobile texting, 409*b*
        in LGBTQ, 584
        in schizophrenia, 303
SNDIs. *see* Serotonin and norepinephrine disinhibitors
SNRIs. *see* Serotonin-norepinephrine reuptake inhibitors
Social anxiety disorder (SAD)
    description of, 207, 207*t*
    selective serotonin reuptake inhibitors for, 186
Social assessment, 88–89
Social determinants of health, 116
    in psychiatric mental health nursing, 14
Social environments, as key social determinant of health, 14

Social interaction
    impaired, with delirium, 368
    skills, goals with personality disorders, 448t
Social learning theory, 61t
Social phobia
    anxiety symptoms with, 207, 207b, 207t
    drug treatment for, 598b
Social relationships, 137
Social skills
    brain functioning and, 175
    training, for serious mental illness, 640
Social status, as key social determinant of health, 14
Social support
    as mediator of stress response, 69
    medical conditions and, 652
    networks, as key social determinant of health, 14
Social workers, as members of psychiatric mental health
    treatment teams, 38b
Societal factors
    of nonsuicidal self-injury, 508
    of suicide, 500–501
Sociocultural context, of family, 704–705
Sociocultural factors, with substance use disorders,
    397–398
Sociological factors, aggression and, 516, 516b
Somatic delusion, 309t
Somatic reaction, in coping, 564b
Somatic symptom disorders, 209–211
    assessment guidelines for, 220b
    case study and nursing care plan for, 237b–238b
    clinical picture on, 210
    comorbidity of, 211, 212t
    conversion disorder, 210, 211b
    epidemiology of, 211
    illness anxiety disorder, 210
    interventions for, 228t
    nursing diagnoses for, 223t
    somatic symptom disorder, 210
Somatic therapy
    for dissociative disorders, 234
    for sexual assaults, 570
Somatization, 126, 209
Somatostatin, 176t
Somnambulism, 463
Soporific drugs, benzodiazepines as, 185
Spatial processing, 86b–87b
Specific learning disorder (SLD), in children and
    adolescents, 600
Specific phobias, anxiety and, 206–207
Speech
    area of brain responsible for, 179, 179f
    assessment of, during mental status examination,
        86b–87b
    patterns, bipolar disorders and, 282–283
Spinning, 19
Spiritual carers, as members of psychiatric mental health
    treatment teams, 38b
Spiritual issues, assessment for, during end-of-life (EOL)
    care, 659–660
Spiritual support, medical conditions and, 652
Spiritual violence, 532t, 534
Spirituality, 87
    anxiety disorders and, 221
    assessment of, 87–88
    depression and, 254
    as integrative health care, 720–721
    as mediator of stress response, 69
Splitting
    characteristics and behaviours associated with, 440
    as defence mechanism, 205t–206t
SSNRIs. see Selective serotonin-norepinephrine reuptake
    inhibitors
SSRIs. see Selective serotonin reuptake inhibitors
St. John's wort, 723, 724t
    for depression, 268b
    interactions of, with conventional medications, 195
Stabilization phase, of schizophrenia, 306, 314, 317
Standards of care, 103
    guidelines for ensuring adherence to, 103–104
    nursing process and, for psychiatric mental health
        nursing, 80–95, 82b
        assessment, 82–89
        documentation, 92
        evaluation, 92
        implementation, 91–92

Standards of care (Continued)
        nursing diagnosis, 89–90
        outcomes identification, 90, 90t
        planning, 90–91, 91b
Standards of practice, 102–103
Standards of Psychiatric Nursing Practice, Registered
    Psychiatric Nurses of Canada, 97–98, 99b
Starson v. Swayze, 104–105, 105b
Stereotyped behaviours, 311
Stereotypic movement disorder, in children and
    adolescents, 600
Stereotyping
    culture and, 119
    making generalizations vs., 128
    of older adults, 84
Stevens-Johnson syndrome, 191
Stigma
    advocacy groups to fight Canadian mental health care,
        8
    human rights abuses of stigmatized persons with
        medical conditions, 651
    of schizophrenia, 305b
    of serious mental illness, 636
Stigmatized persons with medical conditions, 651
Stimulus
    in communication process, 153, 154f
    control, in CBT sleep-improvement techniques,
        470–471
STPD. see Schizotypal personality disorder
Strategic model of family therapy, 703, 703b
Stress
    acute, reactions to, 68t
    anxiety flowchart and, 204f
    coping mechanisms during crisis and, 484t
    depression and, 250
    diathesis-stress model and, 7, 435
    effective busters of, 70b
    effects of, 66–68
    management groups, 690
    measurement of, 70–71, 71f, 72t
    mental health and, 648
    operationally defined, 70f
    prolonged, reactions to, 68t
    recovery, 68b
    reduction of, benefits of, 71
    relaxation techniques for, 71–76
        Benson's, 71–76, 74b
        biofeedback as, 75
        breathing exercises and, 74, 74b
        cognitive reframing as, 75, 75t
        exercises, 72–73
        guided imagery as, 74, 74b
        humour as, 76
        journaling as, 76
        mediation as, 73–74
        mindfulness as, 76
        physical exercise as, 75
        progressive muscle relaxation as, 72–73
        for stress, 71–76
    responses to, 66–68
        early theories in, 66, 67f
        immune, 67–68
        mediators of, 68–69
        neurotransmitters and, 66–67
        nursing management of, 70–76
        positive and negative, 73
        understanding of, 65–78
    substance use disorders and, 397
Stressors, 68–69
    defined, 66
    physical, 68–69
    psychological, 68–69
    in schizophrenia, 305
Structural model of family therapy, 703
Structured group activities, 40
Subgroup, 685b
Subject, changing, 162t
Sublimation, as defence mechanism, 205t–206t
Subpersonality, 216
Substance abuse
    depression co-occurring with, 248t
    in LGBTQ, 584
    in peers, 103–104
    substance-induced anxiety disorder, 209
Substance P, 176t

Substance use, 122
    serious medical illness and, 650
Substance use disorders
    in eating and feeding disorder, 342
    etiology of, 396–398
        biological factors in, 396–397, 396f
        psychological factors in, 397
        sociocultural factors in, 397–398
    motivational interviewing for, 413, 414b
    nursing process application to, 398–427
        assessment, 398–411, 399b–400b
        case study and nursing care plan, 421b, 424b–426b
        diagnosis, 415, 415t
        evaluation, 427, 428f
        helping patients change, 411–415
        implementation, 416
        interventions, 416–427
        outcomes identification, 415–416
        planning, 416, 424b–426b
    in older adults, 617–618
    prevalence statistics of, in Canada, 10t
    psychological changes due to, 411
    schizophrenia and, 303
    self-assessment and self-awareness due to, 411
    suicide risk in, 497
Substance-induced anxiety disorder, 209
Substance-induced dementia, 371t
Substance-induced psychotic disorder, 303b
Substance-induced sleep disorder, 466
Substance/medication-induced depressive disorder, 247
Subsyndromal depression, 248–249
Suicidal behaviour, 496, 501
    self-harm and, research highlight on, 499b
Suicidal ideation
    among Inuit in Canada, 248b
    with anger, helplessness and hopelessness, 253
    assessment in depressed patients, 251–253
    definition of, 497
    verbal and nonverbal clues of, 502–503
Suicidal patients, long and short-term goals for, 90t
Suicide, 495–511
    assessment of, 502–503, 502b
        guidelines for, 504b
        tools for, 503, 503t
        in young child, 594
    biological factors, 498–500
    in Canada, 674
    cultural beliefs regarding, 6, 500, 501b
    in eating and feeding disorder, 341
    epidemiology of, 496–498
    etiology of, 498–501
    in Indigenous peoples, 122
    interventions for
        case management for, 506
        counselling for, 505
        health teaching and health promotion for, 506
        implementation of, 503–507
        milieu management for, 505
        pharmacological, 506
        primary, 504–505, 504b
        secondary, 505
        tertiary, 505
    in LGBTQ, 584
    nurse responses to, 144t–145t
    nursing process application to, 501–507
        assessment, 502–503
        evaluation, 507
        implementation, 503–507
    potential, in violence and abuse, 545
    precautions, 505, 505t, 506b
    prevalence statistics of, in Canada, 10t
    protective factors, 499b
    psychosocial factors, 500
    racial and ethnic statistics of, 496–497
    risk
        antidepressant drugs and, 190
        in older adults, 616–617, 624
    risk factors for, 497–498, 497t, 498f, 499b–500b
    in schizophrenia, 303
    self-assessment of, 503
    societal factors, 500–501
    warning signs of, 500b
Suicide Risk Assessment Guide: A Resource for Health Care
    Organizations, 502
Sullivan, Harry Stack, 51, 217

Summarizing, in therapeutic communication, 160t–161t
Sundance, 18
Sundowning, 366
Superego, 46–47, 46f
Supervised injection sites (SISs), 419
Supervision, of health care workers, 138
Supervisory liability, 109t
Support groups, 690–691, 691b
  for bipolar disorders, 292
Support system
  in abuse, 545
  available, in sexual assault, 565
Supported play, 83
Supported-employment model, for serious mental illness, 641
Supporting data, within nursing diagnoses, 90
Supportive psychotherapy, for serious mental illness, 640–641, 641b
Supportive therapies, 48
Suppression, as defence mechanism, 205t–206t
Survivor
  of abuse, 538
  of sexual assaults, 561, 570
  of suicide, 495–496
Susto, 126b, 127
Sweat lodge, 18
Sympathy, empathy *vs.*, 148
Synapse, 175
  reduction of neurotransmitters in, 177b, 177f
Systematic desensitization
  for anxiety disorders, 234
  as behavioural therapy, 54
Systemic medications, depression co-occurring with, 248t

T
Tachycardia, from conventional antipsychotics, 324t–325t
Tacrine (Cognex), for Alzheimer's disease, 382
Tactile hallucination, 310t
Talk therapy, Freud's use of, 46
Tangentiality, in communication, 309
Tarasoff v. Regents of University of California, 107
Tardive dyskinesia, from conventional antipsychotics, 323, 324t–325t
TCAM. *see* Traditional, complementary, and alternative medicine
TCAs. *see* Tricyclic antidepressants
Technology
  community care and, 28
  expanding, mental health and, 13–14
Tegretol. *see* Carbamazepine
Telemedicine, 13–14
Telepsychiatry, 13–14
Temazepam (Restoril), 185, 471b
Temperament
  in child and adolescent disorders, 590
  defining, 435
Tension headache, anxiety caused by, 212t
Tension-building stage, in cycle of violence, 535
Terminal illness
  assessment for spiritual issues, 659–660
  caring for patients with, 657, 658b, 661b
  Kübler-Ross, Dr. Elisabeth, 658
Termination phase
  of Peplau's model of nurse-patient relationship, 146–147
  of therapeutic group, 686
Territorial governments
  health professions acts in, 103t
  mental health acts in, 101–102, 102t
Terrorism, 480
Tertiary care, for crisis intervention, 486
Tertiary prevention, of abuse, 550
Testosterone, in gender dysphoria, 579–580
Theories
  behavioural, 52–55
    Behaviourism theory as, 53
    Classical Conditioning Theory as, 53, 53f
    implications of, in nursing practice, 54–55
    Operant Conditioning Theory as, 53, 53f
  biological, 60
    advent of psychopharmacology and, 60
    Biological Model and, 60

Theories *(Continued)*
  cognitive, 55–58
    Cognitive Behavioural Therapy and, 55–56, 57b
    Dialectic Behavioural Therapy as, 56–58
    implications of, in nursing practice, 58, 58b
    Rational Emotive Behaviour Therapy and, 55
  comparison of, 57t
  developmental, 48–50
    cognitive development as, 48–49
    ethics of care theory and, 50
    implications of, for nursing practice, 50
    stages of moral development in, 49–50
    theory of psychosocial development and, 49, 49t
  humanistic, 58–60
    Abraham Maslow's Humanistic Psychology Theory as, 58–60
  interpersonal, 50–52
    implications of, for nursing practice, 52
    interpersonal psychotherapy in, 51
    Peplau's theory of Interpersonal Relations, 51–52
    by Sullivan, 51
    theory of object relations in, 50
  psychoanalytic, 46–48
    classical psychoanalysis, 48
    implications of, for nursing practice, 48
    psychodynamic therapy and, 48
    Sigmund Freud's, 46–47
  selected nursing theorists in, 52t, 61t
Therapeutic communication
  basic *vs.*, 152
  strategies, 157–163, 160t–161t
    accepting as, 160t–161t
    active listening as, 157–158, 160t–161t
    asking questions and eliciting patient responses as, 159
    clarifying techniques as, 158–159, 160t–161t
    exploring as, 159, 160t–161t
    listening with empathy as, 158
    paraphrasing as, 158
    reflecting as, 158–159, 160t–161t
    restating as, 158, 160t–161t
    silence as, 157, 160t–161t
    summarizing as, 160t–161t
Therapeutic drawing, 597
Therapeutic encounter, 138
Therapeutic factors, in groups, 685, 685b
Therapeutic games, 597, 597b
Therapeutic groups, 684–695
  member roles, 686, 687t
  support and self-help groups, 690–691
  terms central to, 685b
Therapeutic index, 191, 191t
Therapeutic nurse-patient relationships, Registered Psychiatric Nurses of Canada (RPNC) on, 91–92
Therapeutic relationships, 39–40, 135–151, 136b
  beliefs in, 140–142
  blurred boundaries in, 139–140, 139t
  establishing boundaries in, 139
  Peplau's model of, 142–147
    orientation phase of, 143–146
    preorientation phase of, 143, 144t–145t
    termination phase of, 146–147
    working phase of, 146
  phases of, 147f
  self-awareness in, 140–142
  social *vs.*, 137–138
  values in, 140–142
Therapeutic suggestion, 719
Therapeutic touch, 725
Therapeutic use of self, 136
Thiothixene, for schizophrenia, 322t
Thought broadcasting, in delusions, 309t
Thought field therapy, 725–726
Thought insertion, in delusions, 309t
Thought processes
  area of brain responsible for, 178–179, 179f
  bipolar disorders and, 282–283
  depression assessment of, 253
  disturbed, with delirium, 368
Thought stopping, for anxiety disorders, 234
Thought withdrawal, in delusions, 309t
Thoughts
  assessment of, during mental status examination, 86b–87b
  automatic, 55–56

Tidal model, 52
Time out, 596
"To Everything There Is a Season": Mental Health-Related Hospitalizations by Youth and Adults, 33b
Token economy, 54
Tolerance, definition of substance, 394
Topiramate (Topamax), 191, 417
  for bipolar disorders, 291b
Tort law, 109–111
Touch
  in communication process, 153, 154f
  control, for managing disruptive behaviours, in children and adolescents, 607b
  cultural beliefs and, 119t
  cultural considerations to, 163–164
Tourette's disorder, in children and adolescents, 600
Toxicity, of lithium carbonate, 288–289, 288t
Traditional, complementary, and alternative medicine (TCAM), 714–715, 715t
  biologically based integrative therapies for, 721–724
    aromatherapy as, 723–724
    diet and nutrition as, 721–723
    herbal therapy as, 723
    megavitamin therapy as, 723
  in Canada, 715–716
  definition of, 714
  jurisdiction over, 715–716
  manipulative practices for, 724–725
    chiropractic medicine, 724
    massage therapy, 724–725
    reflexology, 725
  patients and, 716–717
  research on, 716b
  resources, 716b
  safety of, 716–717, 717b
  whole medical systems of, 717–719
    acupuncture, 715–716, 718
    Ayurvedic medicine, 718
    homeopathy and naturopathy, 718–719
    traditional Chinese medicine, 718
    traditional Indigenous medicine, 717–718
Traditional Chinese medicine, 718
Traditional Indigenous medicine, 717–718
Traditional medicine, definition of, 714–715
Traditional practice knowledge, 103
Transcranial magnetic stimulation, for depression, 267, 267f
Transference, 139–140
  in classical psychoanalysis, 48
Transgender, 578–579
  hostility toward, 592b
Translators
  for overcoming communication barriers, 125
  professional health care, 84
Transmitters, 176t
Transtheoretical Model of Change, stages of, 411–413, 412f
  action, 412
  contemplation, 412
  evaluation/termination, 413
  maintenance/adaption, 412–413
  precontemplation, 411–412
  preparation, 412
Tranylcypromine sulphate (Parnate), 230b–231b, 261b–262b
Trauma
  as adventitious crisis, 480
  impact of Canadian residential schools among indigenous people in Canada, 619b
  on older adults, 618
  physical, mental health dysfunction and, 183
  resilience and, 5
  as risk factor for mental illness, 589
Trauma-informed approach, to sexual assault, 564, 564b
Trauma-informed care, 517
Trauma-informed practice, 116
Traumatic brain injury, 371t
  in dementia, 374
Travelbee, Joyce, 52t
Trazodone (Oleptro, Trazodone, Trazorel), 471b
  for depression, 189–190
TRD. *see* Treatment-resistant depression
Treatment, Nursing Interventions Classification (NIC), 12
Treatment plans, clinical pathway and, 34

Treatment team, 38–39, 39b
  collaboration of, 107–108
Treatment-resistant depression (TRD), 267
Triangulation, 701, 701b, 702f
Triazolam (Halcion), 185, 471b
Tri-Council Policy Statement: Ethical Conduct for Research Involving Humans, 100
Tricyclic antidepressants (TCAs), 187–188, 188f
  actions of, 261b–262b, 263
  adverse reactions and toxic effects of, 263
  for anxiety disorders, 230b–231b
  for bulimia nervosa, 351
  for depression, 261b–262b, 263
  patient and family teaching regarding, 263, 264b
Triskaidekaphobia, 207t
T.R.U.S.T. Model for Inclusive Spiritual Care, 720–721, 721f, 722b
Tryptophan, 342
Tuberculosis, with long term alcohol abuse, 395
Tuke, William, 18
Two-spirit, 578–579
Typology of interpersonal violence, 531, 531f
Tyramine, 189, 263, 264t

U
UBC. see University of British Columbia
Uncertainty, as relational ethics principle, 99
Unconscious mind, 46
Unconventionality, 445, 446t
Undoing, as defence mechanism, 205t–206t
Unemployment, with serious mental illness, 637
Unintentional torts, 110–111
Universality, 685b
University of Alberta, 21–22
University of British Columbia (UBC), 21
University of Saskatchewan, 21–22
University of Toronto, 21
University of Western Ontario, 21–22
University-based nursing curriculum, 21–22
Unpleasant Voices Scale, 313, 313f
Urban tree canopy, 68b
Urinary retention, from conventional antipsychotics, 324t–325t
Useful activities, in guidelines for care at home, 382b
Utilitarianism, 98
Utility, principle of, 98

V
Vagus nerve stimulation, for depression, 267–268, 268f
Valerian root, 723, 724t
Valproic acid (Depakote, Depakene), 191, 230b–231b
  for bipolar disorders, 290, 291b
  for schizophrenia, 325
Value judgements
  making, 162t
  suspending, for patient's growth, 148–149
Values, in therapeutic relationships, 140–142
Valuing, during end-of-life (EOL) care, 659
Vanier Institute of the Family, 698
Vascular dementia, 371t
Vegetative signs, of depression, 253–254, 256t, 259t
Venlafaxine hydrochloride (Effexor), 188, 230b–231b, 261b–262b
Ventral tegmental pathway, 177–178
Verbal abuse, 532t, 534
Verbal clues, suicide and, 502–503
Verbal communication, 155
  interaction with nonverbal communication, 156–157, 156b

Verbal tracking, during clinical interview, 166–167
Vicarious liability, 109t
Vicarious trauma, 482–483, 566–567
Victimization
  in inmates with a mental illness, 675
  with serious mental illness, 636–637
  in sexual assault, 563t
  perpetrators and, 562
Vignette, 346–347
Violence, 512–529, 532–535, 675
  coping responses in, 544, 545t
  cycle of, 535, 536f
  de-escalation techniques for, 519, 519b
  defining, 513, 531
  drugs treatments for emergency management of, 521b
  ecological model of, 537, 537f
  epidemiology of, 514
  milieu characteristics conducive to, 514, 514b
  nursing process application in, 517–527, 518b, 519t, 521b–523b, 525b–526b, 539–556
    assessment in, 539–546, 541b
    diagnosis in, 546, 546t
    evaluation in, 552–553
    implementation in, 547–552
    outcomes identification in, 546, 547t
    planning in, 546–547
  restraints or seclusion use with, 523–524, 523b
  as risk factor for mental illness, 589
  safety and, 35
  stages and assessment of, 518b, 519–520
  types of, 532–535, 532t
Virtue ethics, 98–99
Virtues, defined, 98–99
Vision, area of brain responsible for, 178–179, 179f
Visitors, safety and, 34
Visual hallucinations, 310t, 311
Visual processing, 86b–87b
Vital signs, in bulimia nervosa, 351t
Vocal quality, during clinical interview, 166
Vocational rehabilitation, for serious mental illness, 641
Voice-related behaviours, as nonverbal behaviour, 156t
Voices, in hallucinations, 310
Vomiting
  with anorexia nervosa, 347
  with bulimia nervosa, 339, 349, 349b, 351
  with substance abuse or behavioural addictions, 415t
Vortioxetine (Trintellix), 188
Vraylar. see Cariprazine
Vulnerability
  coping with crisis and, 480
  ethical dilemma and, 100
  as relational ethics principle, 99
Vulnerable population, as target of abuse
  children, 538, 540f
  older adult, 538–539
  women, 538

W
Wakefulness, neurotransmitters responsible for, 461
Wandering
  with dementia, 378
  in guidelines for care at home, 382b
War, as adventitious crisis, 480
Watson, John B., 53
Waxy flexibility, 311
Weight gain behaviour, in anorexia nervosa, 346t
Weight maintenance behaviour, in bulimia nervosa, 351t
Weir Report, 20
Wernicke's encephalopathy, 395

Western Canada, history of psychiatric nursing licensing in, 21
Western tradition, 117, 117t
White matter, 178–179, 179f
Whole medical systems, of integrative health care, 717–719
  acupuncture, 715–716, 718
  Ayurvedic medicine, 718
  homeopathy and naturopathy, 718–719
  traditional Chinese medicine, 718
  traditional Indigenous medicine, 717–718
"Why" questions, asking, 162t, 163
Wieman, Corniela, 129–130
Wind illness, 126c
Withdrawal stage
  definition of addiction, 394
  management services, 422
  pharmacological interventions during, 416
Women
  sexual assault of, 536
  vulnerability of, in abuse, 538
Wong-Baker FACES Pain Rating Scale, 620, 620f
Woodruff's Total Suffering Model, 661f
Word salad, 310
  with schizophrenia, 174–175
Working conditions, as key social determinant of health, 14
Working phase
  of Peplau's model of nurse-patient relationship, 146
  of therapeutic groups, 686
Workplace
  addiction in nurses, 426–427, 427b
  violence, 512
World Health Organization (WHO)
  defining traditional medicine, 714–715
  Disability Assessment Schedule 2.0, 11
  in ecological model of violence, 537, 537f
  in interpersonal violence, 531
  Mental Health Care Law: Ten Basic Principles, 101, 102b
World view, 116, 117t
  indigenous, 117, 118t
  non-indigenous, 118t

Y
Yale-Brown Obsessive Compulsive Scale (YBOCS), 218
YBOCS. see Yale-Brown Obsessive Compulsive Scale
Yin and yang, 718
Yoga, 719
  for adolescents, 596b
Young
  serious mental illness in, 634, 634b
  sleep hypnogram vs. older adults, 460, 460f

Z
Z-drugs, 186
Zeitgebers, 460
Zeldox. see Ziprasidone
Ziprasidone (Zeldox), 194
  for bipolar disorders, 291b
  for schizophrenia, 321, 322t
Zoophobia, 207t
Zopiclone (Imovane, Rhovane), 186, 471b
Zuclopenthixol, 521b
  for schizophrenia, 322t
Zung Self-Rating Depression Scale, 251
Zyprexa. see Olanzapine